Postgraduate Orthopaedics

Viva Guide to the FRCS (Tr & Orth) Examination

Second edition

Postgraduate Orthopaedics

Viva Guide to the FRCS (Tr & Orth) Examination

Second edition

Edited by

Paul A. Banaszkiewicz FRCS (Glas) FRCS (Ed) FRCS (Eng) FRCS (Tr & Orth) MClinEd FAcadMEd FHEA

Consultant Orthopaedic Surgeon, Queen Elizabeth Hospital and North East NHS Surgical Centre (NENSC), Gateshead, UK
Visiting Professor
Northumbria University, Newcastle-upon-Tyne, UK

Deiary F. Kader FRCS (Glas) FRCS (Ed) FRCS (Tr & Orth) MFSEM (UK)

Consultant Orthopaedic Surgeon, Academic Unit South West London Elective Orthopaedic Centre
Visiting Professor in Sport and Exercise Science, Northumbria University, Newcastle-upon-Tyne, UK

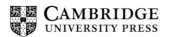
CAMBRIDGE
UNIVERSITY PRESS

CAMBRIDGE
UNIVERSITY PRESS

University Printing House, Cambridge CB2 8BS, United Kingdom

One Liberty Plaza, 20th Floor, New York, NY 10006, USA

477 Williamstown Road, Port Melbourne, VIC 3207, Australia

314–321, 3rd Floor, Plot 3, Splendor Forum, Jasola District Centre, New Delhi – 110025, India

79 Anson Road, #06–04/06, Singapore 079906

Cambridge University Press is part of the University of Cambridge.

It furthers the University's mission by disseminating knowledge in the pursuit of
education, learning, and research at the highest international levels of excellence.

www.cambridge.org
Information on this title: www.cambridge.org/9781108722155
DOI: 10.1017/9781108686624

© Cambridge University Press 2012, 2020

First published 2012

Second edition 2020

Printed in Singapore by Markono Print Media Pte Ltd

A catalogue record for this publication is available from the British Library.

ISBN 978-1-108-72215-5 Paperback

Contents

Section 1 – The FRCS (Tr & Orth) Oral Examination

Section 2 – Adult Elective Orthopaedics and Spine

Section 3 – Trauma

Section 4 – Children's Orthopaedics/ Hand and Upper Limb

Section 5 – Applied Basic Sciences

Section 6 – Drawings for the FRCS (Tr & Orth)

Contributors

Fazal Ali FRCS (Tr & Orth)
Chesterfield Royal Hospital, Chesterfield, UK

Mohammed Al-Maiyah MBChB FICMS FRCS Msc Orthop FRCS (Tr & Orth)
James Cook University Hospital, Middlesbrough, UK

Sattar Alshryda MBChB MRCP (UK) MRCS SICOT EBOT FRCS (Tr & Orth) MSc PhD
Royal Manchester Children's Hospital, Manchester, UK

Firas Arnaout MD MSc MRCS FEBOT FRCS (Tr & Orth)
Bristol University Hospitals, Bristol, UK

Paul A. Banaszkiewicz FRCS (Glas) FRCS (Ed) FRCS (Eng) FRCS (Tr & Orth) MClinEd FAcadMEd FHEA
Queen Elizabeth Hospital, Gateshead and Northumbria University, Newcastle, UK

Tomas B. Beckingsale MSc FRCS (Tr & Orth)
Freeman Hospital, Newcastle-upon-Tyne, UK

Rajarshi Bhattacharya MBBS MRCSEd MRCS (Glas) MSc FRCS (Tr & Orth)
Imperial College Healthcare NHS Trust and North West London Major Trauma Centre, London, UK

David J. Bryson MBChB MRCS FRCS (Tr & Orth)
Queen's Medical Centre, Nottingham, UK

Clare Carpenter BSc (Hons) MRCS Pg Dip Sports Med FRCS (Tr & Orth) MD
University Hospital of Wales and the Noah's Ark Children's Hospital for Wales, Cardiff, UK

Nick Caplan BSc (Hons) PhD PgCert FHEA
Northumbria University, Newcastle, UK

Kim Weng Chan FRCS (Tr & Orth)
Woodend Hospital, Aberdeen, UK

Jeevan Chandrasenan FRCS (Tr & Orth) BMBS BMed Sci
Chesterfield Royal Hospital, Chesterfield, UK

Jonathan A. Clamp MB ChB (Hons) MRCS (Eng) FRCS (Tr & Orth)
Royal Derby Hospital, Derby, UK

John Dabis MBBS MRCS FRCS (Tr & Orth)
Basingstoke and North Hampshire Foundation Trust, Basingstoke, UK

John Davies MBChB, MSc (Eng), FRCS (Tr & Orth)
Hull University Teaching Hospitals NHS Trust, Hull, UK

Aravind Desai MBBS MS (Orth) MRCS MSc MCh (Orth) FRCS (Tr & Orth)
North Lincolnshire NHS Foundation Trust, Scunthorpe, UK

Will Eardley MSc PgCertMedEd, DipSEM (UK&I) MD FRCSEd (Tr & Orth)
South Tees Hospitals NHS Trust, UK

Simon Freilich MBBS (Dist) BSc (Hons) FRCP (UK) AICSM
Luton and Dunstable University Hospital, Luton, UK

Kanishka Milton Ghosh MD FRCS (Tr & Orth)
Great North Trauma and Emergency Centre, Royal Victoria Hospital, Newcastle-upon-Tyne, UK

Mohamed Hafez FRCS (Tr & Orth)
Sheffield's Children's Hospital, Sheffield, UK

John W. K. Harrison MSc FRCS (Ed) FRCS (T &Orth) MFSEM (UK)
Queen Elizabeth Hospital and NENSC, Gateshead, UK

Stan Jones MBChB MSc BioEng FRCS (Tr & Orth)
Al Ahli Hospital, Qatar

Deiary F. Kader FRCS (Glas) FRCS (Ed) FRCS (Tr & Orth) MFSEM (UK)
Academic Unit South West London Elective Orthopaedic Centre, London, UK

Rajesh Kakwani MBBS MRCS MS (Orth) FRCS (Tr & Orth)
Northumbria Healthcare NHS Trust, Newcastle upon Tyne, UK

Prasad Karpe MRCS (Ed) MS (Orth) FRCS (Tr & Orth)
University Hospital of North Tees, Stockton-on-Tees, UK

Sarah Kleinka MBChB FRCS (Tr & Orth) MD
Sunderland Royal Hospital, Newcastle upon Tyne, UK

Gunasekaran Kumar FRCS (Tr & Orth)
Royal Liverpool University Hospital, Liverpool, UK

David Limb BSc FRCS Ed (Orth)
Chapel Allerton Orthopaedic Centre, Leeds Teaching Hospitals Trust, Leeds, UK

Catherine McCauley MBChB MRCGP DRCOG PGCmedE
Grassendale Medical Practice, Liverpool, UK

Iain McNamara MA (Cantab) BM BCh (Oxon) MRCP FRCS (Tr & Orth) MD
Norfolk and Norwich University Hospital & Honorary Professor University of East Anglia, Norwich, UK

N. Jane Madeley FRCS (Tr & Orth)
Glasgow Royal Infirmary, Glasgow, UK

William Marlow FRCS (Tr & Orth)
Royal Manchester Children's Hospital, Manchester, UK

Lyndon Mason MB BCh MRCS (Eng) FRCS (Tr & Orth)
Aintree University Hospital, Liverpool, UK

Paul Middleton FRCS (Tr & Orth)
Borders General Hospital, Melrose, UK

Munier Hossain MSc (Orth Eng) MSc (EBHC) FRCS (Glas) FPG Cert FHEA
Royal Manchester Children's Hospital, Manchester, UK

Matthew Nixon MBChB MRCS PGCAPHE MD FRCS (Tr & Orth)
Royal Manchester Children's Hospital, Manchester, UK

Jeya Palan BSc (Hons) MBBS FRCS (Tr & Orth)
Nottingham City Hospitals, Nottingham University Hospitals NHS Trust, UK

Bodil Robertson MBChB FRCA
Queen Elizabeth Hospital and NENSC, Gateshead, UK

Matthew Jones MBChB (Hons) MRCS FRCS (Tr & Orth) Dip Hand Surg
University Hospital of Coventry and Warwick, Coventry, UK

Terence Savaridas MBChB MRCSEd FRCS (Tr & Orth) MD
Forth Valley NHS Trust, Stirling, UK

Majeed Shakokani MBBS, MRCS, FRCS (Tr & Orth)
Norfolk and Norwich University Hospital NHS Foundation Trust, Norwich, UK

Khaled Sarraf BSc (Hons) MBBS FRCS (Tr & Orth) MFSTEd
Imperial College Healthcare NHS Trust, London, UK

Kiran Singisetti FRCS (Tr & Orth)
Queen Elizabeth Hospital and NENSC, Gateshead, UK

Tom Symes MBChB MSc FRCS (Tr & Orth)
Hull and East Yorkshire Hospitals NHS Trust, UK

Roger Walton MBChB (Hons) FRCS (Tr & Orth)
Alder Hey Children's Hospital, Liverpool, UK

Christopher Watkins MBChB, MRCS
Royal Victoria Hospital (RVI), Newcastle upon Tyne Hospitals NHS Foundation, UK

James Widnall MBChB FRCS (Tr & Orth)
Aintree University Hospital, Liverpool, UK

Patrick Williams MBBS MRCS PGCertClinEd
James Cook University Hospital, Middlesbrough, UK

Preface

With the first-edition viva book we were keen to write a viva book to complement our main orthopaedic textbook.

We had a reasonable surplus of material available that we had been unable to fit into the second-edition book. We were keen to go into a more detailed, structured answer to use in the viva situation rather than just going ahead with revision bullet points. We were attempting (but perhaps not realizing at the time) to provide examples of higher-order thinking and judgement for candidates to use in their exam preparation.

We had already published two books previously and so were experienced in the 'know how' of 'how to get a book done'. Like any new book it was certainly more difficult writing from scratch, but there was no great master plan of what we wanted to achieve.

We approached a number of post FRCS (Tr & Orth) registrars who did an excellent job of taking on the task of writing the allocated book chapters. As such, the viva book came together with the minimum of fuss.

The main orthopaedic book had been the first of its kind combining all parts of the FRCS (Tr & Orth) syllabus together in one volume. The viva book was a very different challenge in that there were lots of similar viva-type books already out on the market.

When released, the complexity within some model answers in the viva book took a while to be fully appreciated by our audience. In due course there was a realization that perhaps two or three chapters didn't quite hit our own expected high standards. The book was published very close to similar competing titles that ended up muddying the waters. The book became something of a slow burner, but over time increased in popularity.

The exam format keeps changing, and as time went on the viva book started to age. A decision was needed as to whether to update the book or just let it go out of date. It wasn't a difficult decision as we wanted to improve the quality of the viva book. During the intervening years the standard of FRCS (Tr & Orth) exam books had significantly improved and we wanted to keep up with the newer titles emerging. We also realized that the vast majority of the book was well written and could be improved even further to do the book its full justice.

The two main areas that we concentrated on were basic science and trauma. Basic science is by and large by far the most difficult subject for candidates to revise and we wanted to significantly raise the bar in this section. Trauma was becoming more subspecialized with the MTC, but candidates still needed a good working knowledge of the material. Diagrams needed to be more professionally drawn.

Although the whole exam is based on the Tr & Orth curriculum, the mechanics of the viva exam are very different to that of the MCQs and clinicals. The viva exam allows for a more formal assessment of communication skills. If you are a gifted, silver-tongued candidate with inherit tactical nous in answering viva questions that's great, but most candidates need some guidance.

A standardized method of approach to answering a viva question needs to be learnt and thoroughly practised to avoid mishaps.

We hope the book realizes its aim of moving the material up a level and that it will guide you better in your exam preparation. Again, like all books of the Postgraduate Orthopaedics book series we make no claim to the originality of the material. We are distilling orthopaedic knowledge from the wider orthopaedic community specifically for exam-related subjects. We have attempted to acknowledge our sources wherever possible and our sincere apologies if we have inadvertently missed anyone out.

We thank Cambridge University Press for all their patience and advice with the project, again remembering that the grass is still not greener elsewhere.

Overall, we are generally happy with the end result. We could have continued writing material for another year and still not be finished, as the Tr & Orth curriculum is vast. Some of the chapters are very specialized and candidates may struggle to find similar information on the internet, but this material somehow still gets asked by the ICB. If the basic science or general adult pathology answer to the question is unGoogleable but we have managed to provide for a model answer, then we have mostly succeeded in what we wanted to achieve.

This book was much more difficult to write than the first edition and didn't come together all that easily. We were surprised by this and went through a few Peroni tests to get there! Will we write a third-edition viva book? Never say never, but probably not!

Paul Banaszkiewicz

Acknowledgements

Special thanks to all the authors involved with the Postgraduate Orthopaedics book series over the years. Without your input no books would be possible.

Special thanks to Nicholas Dunton at Cambridge University Press for his help, guidance and strong support over the years, a constant springboard of advice throughout the evolution of the Postgraduate Orthopaedics book series. Also special thanks to Simon Freilich for providing the answers to un-Googleable nerve conduction study questions for the second edition.

Thanks to Steve Atkinson and Clive Kelly for implant photography and putting up with the hassles of multiple repeated requests for photos to get that final book implant photo just right.

A very special thanks to Harry Heyes and the team for their help in drawing medical illustrations at short notice (Graphics Section, Clinical Photography & Medical Illustration, Manchester University NHS Foundation Trust (Oxford Road site), Saint Mary's Towers).

Thanks to Lois Lincoln, senior operating department practitioner at QEH, keen marathon runner and triathlon trainer for the surgical approaches pictures and Penny Day for additional help with photography.

Lastly, a special thank you to Jo McStea, who helps coordinate the Postgraduate Orthopaedics book and lecture programme. This involves a huge amount of behind-the-scenes organization skills and problem solving such that that we couldn't manage without her input.

Abbreviations

1,2-ISCRA	1,2-intercompartmental supraretinacular artery
A&E	Accident and Emergency
AAOS	American Academy of Orthopaedic Surgeons
ABC	airway, breathing, circulation
ABG	arterial blood gas
ABI	ankle–brachial index
ABPB	axillary brachial plexus block
ABPI	Ankle–Brachial Pressure Index
AC	acromioclavicular
ACDF	anterior cervical decompression and fusion
ACI	autologous chondrocyte implantation
ACJ	acromioclavicular joint
ACL	anterior cruciate ligament
ACR	American College of Rheumatology
AD	autosomal dominant
ADL	activities of daily living
AER	apical ectodermal ridge
AFO	ankle–foot orthosis
AGE	advanced glycation end product
AIDS	acquired immunodeficiency syndrome
AIIS	anterior inferior iliac spine
AIN	anterior interosseous nerve
AIS	Abbreviated Injury Scale
AIS	adolescent idiopathic scoliosis
AJCC	American Joint Committee on Cancer
AKA	above-knee amputation
ALIF	anterior lumbar interbody fusion
ALL	anterior longitudinal ligament
ALVAL	aseptic lymphocyte-dominated vasculitis-associated lesions
AM	anteromedial
AMTS	abbreviated mental test score
ANOVA	analysis of variance
AOFAS	American Orthopaedic Foot and Ankle Society
AORI	Anderson Orthopaedic Research Institute
AP	anteroposterior
APB	abductor pollicis brevis
APL	abductor pollicis longus
APT	all polyethylene tibial
AR	autosomal recessive
ARCO	Association Research Circulation Osseous
ARDS	acute respiratory distress syndrome
ARMD	adverse reactions to metal debris
AS	ankylosing spondylitis
ASIA	American Spinal Injury Association
ASIS	anterior superior iliac spine
ATFL	anterior talofibular ligament
ATL	atypical lipoma
ATLS°	Advanced Trauma Life Support°
ATP	adenosine triphosphate
AVN	avascular necrosis
BASS	British Association of Spine Surgeons
BDGF	bone-derived growth factor
bFGF	basic fibroblast growth factor
BHN	bone homeostasis, healing and non-union
BHS	British Hip Society
BKA	below-knee amputation
BMD	bone mineral density
BMES	bone marrow oedema syndrome
BMI	body mass index
BMP	bone morphogenetic protein
BMU	basic multicellular unit
BOA	British Orthopaedic Association

BOAST	British Orthopaedic Association Standards for Trauma
BP	blood pressure
BPBG	bone–patella–bone graft
BPBT	bone–patella–bone–tendon
BPI	brachial plexus injury
BPN	bisphosphonate
BPTB	bone–patella–tendon–bone
BR	brachioradialis
BSSH	British Society for Surgery of the Hand
BW	body weight
CAVE	cavus, adductus, varus, equinus
CC	costoclavicular
CCK	constrained condylar knee
CCS	central cord syndrome
CDH	congenital dislocation of the hip
CDR	cervical disc replacement
CEA	carcinoembryonic antigen
CECI	cauda equina syndrome incomplete
CES	cauda equina syndrome
CESR	cauda equine syndrome retention
CFL	calcaneofibular ligament
CFU	colony-forming units
CLPE	cross-lined polyethylene
CMAP	compound muscle action potential
CMC	carpometacarpal
CMN	cephalomedullary nail
CMT	Charcot–Marie–Tooth
CNB	central neuraxial block
CNS	central nervous system
CNS	Congress of Neurological Surgeons
CoC	ceramic on ceramic
CoP	ceramic on polyethylene
COPD	chronic obstructive pulmonary disease
CP	cerebral palsy
CPSP	central post-stroke pain
CR	cruciate retaining
CROW	Charcot restraint orthotic walker
CRP	C-reactive protein
CRPS	complex regional pain syndrome
CS	cannulated screw
CSF	cerebrospinal fluid
CSM	cervical spondylotic myelopathy

CT	computed tomography
CTEV	congenital talipes equinovarus
CTGF	connective tissue growth factor
CTS	carpal tunnel syndrome
CVA	cerebrovascular accident
CVT	congenital vertical talus
DAIR	debridement, antibiotics and implant retention
DASH	Disabilities of the Arm, Shoulder and Hand
DB	Denis Browne
DCO	damage control orthopaedics
DCP	dynamic compression plate
DCS	dynamic condylar screw
DDH	developmental dysplasia of the hip
DEXA	dual energy x-ray absorptiometry
DGH	district general hospital
DHS	dynamic hip screw
DIP	distal interphalangeal
DIPJ	distal interphalangeal joint
DISH	diffuse idiopathic skeletal hyperostosis
DMAA	distal metatarsal articular angle
DMARDs	disease modifying anti-rheumatoid drugs
DRUJ	distal radioulnar joint
DVT	deep vein thrombosis
ECA	extensor compartment artery
ECM	extracellular matrix
ECRB	extensor carpi radialis brevis
ECRL	extensor carpi radialis longus
ECU	extensor carpi ulnaris
EDB	extensor digitorum brevis
EDC	extensor digitorum communis
EDL	extensor digitorum longus
EDM	extensor digiti minimi
EF	external fixation
EGF	epidermal growth factor
EHL	extensor hallucis longus
EIP	extensor indicis proprius
EJS	effective joint space
EMA	epiphyseal–metaphyseal angle
EMG	electromyography
EMIs	extended matching items
EPB	extensor pollicis brevis
EPI	epicondylitis
EPL	extensor pollicis longus

EPS	extracellular polymeric substance	HA	hyaluronic acid
ER	external rotation	HA	hydroxyapatite
ERAS	enhanced recovery after surgery	HCLPE	highly cross-linked polyethylene
		HIV	human immunodeficiency virus
ERCB	extensor carpi radialis brevis	HO	heterotopic ossification
ERCL	extensor carpi radialis longus	HSMN	hereditary sensorimotor neuropathies
ESR	erythrocyte sedimentation rate	HTO	high tibial osteotomy
ETO	extended trochanteric osteotomy	HU	Hounsfield units
		HVA	hallux valgus angle
EUA	examination under anaesthesia	HVI	hallux valgus interphalangeus
EULAR	European League Against Rheumatism	IASP	International Association of the Study of Pain
EWS	early warning score	ICB	Intercollegiate Board
FAOS	foot and ankle outcome score	ICSRA	intercompartmental supraretinacular artery
FBC	full blood count	IGF	insulin-like growth factor
FCL	fibular collateral ligament	II	image intensifier
FCR	flexor carpi radialis	IL	interleukin
FCU	flexor carpi ulnaris	IM	intramedullary
FDB	flexor digitorum brevis	IMA	intermetatarsal angle
FDG	fluorodeoxyglucose	INR	International Normalized Ratio
FDL	flexor digitorum longus	IP	interphalangeal
FDP	flexor digitorum profundus	IPJ	interphalangeal joint
FDQ	flexor digiti quinti	ISB	interscalene block
FDS	flexor digitorum superficialis	ITB	iliotibial band
FFP	fresh frozen plasma	ITOH	idiopathic transient osteoporosis of the hip
FGF	fibroblast growth factor		
FGF23	fibroblast growth factor 23	ITU	Intensive Care Unit
FGFR3	fibroblast growth factor receptor gene 3	IV	intravenous
		IVC	inferior vena cava
FHL	flexor hallucis longus	IVDU	intravenous drug user
FMDA	femoral metaphyseal–diaphyseal angle	JBJS	*Journal of Bone and Joint Surgery*
FNB	femoral nerve block	JCIE	Joint Committee on Intercollegiate Examinations
FPL	flexor pollicis longus		
FPPS	farnesyl pyrophosphate synthase	JLCA	joint line convergence angle
		JRF	joint reaction force
FTR	femoral tibial ratio	KAFO	knee–ankle–foot orthosis
GA	general anaesthetic	LA	local anaesthetic
GAGs	glycosaminoglycans	LAST	local anaesthetic systemic toxicity
GCS	Glasgow Coma Score		
GCT	giant cell tumour	LAT	lateral
GHL	glenohumeral ligaments	LBP	low back pain
GI	gastrointestinal	LC	lateral compression
GIRFT	get it right first time	LCDCP	low-contact dynamic compression plates
GMC	General Medical Council		
GRAFO	ground reaction ankle foot orthosis	LCL	lateral collateral ligament
		LCP	low compression plates
GRF	ground reaction forces	LCPD	Legg Calves Perthes disease
GT	greater trochanter		

LDFA	lateral distal femoral angle	NF	neurofibromatosis
LFA	low-friction arthroplasty	NF-1	neurofibromatosis type 1
LFTs	liver function tests	NF-2	neurofibromatosis type 2
LHB	long head of biceps	NGAL	neutrophil gelatinase-associated lipocalin
LLD	limb length discrepancy		
LMWH	low molecular weight heparin	NICE	National Institute for Health and Clinical Excellence
LP	lumbar puncture		
LRTI	ligament reconstruction tendon interposition	NIDDM	non-insulin-dependent diabetes mellitus
LUCL	lateral ulnar collateral ligament	NJR	National Joint Registry
MA	metatarsus adductus	NMJ	neuromuscular junction
MAD	mechanical axis deviation	NOGG	National Osteoporosis Guideline Group
MCFA	medial circumflex femoral artery		
MCL	medial collateral ligament	NPV	negative predictive value
MCP	metacarpophalangeal	NSAIDs	non-steroidal anti-inflammatory drugs
MCQs	multiple choice questions		
MCSF	macrophage-colony stimulating factor	OA	osteoarthritis
		OATS	osteochondral autograft transfer system
MDA	metaphyseal–diaphyseal angle		
MDP	methylene diphosphonate	OCD	osteochondritis dissecans
MDT	multidisciplinary team	OCL	osteochondral lesions
MED	multiple epiphyseal dysplasia	ODEP	Orthopaedic Data Evaluation Panel
MFC	medial femoral condyle		
MHRA	Medicines and Healthcare products Regulatory Agency	OHS	Oxford hip score
		OI	osteogenesis imperfecta
MIPO	minimally invasive plate osteosynthesis	OKS	Oxford knee score
		OLT	osteochondral lesion of the talus
MMP	metalloproteinase	ON	osteonecrosis
MoM	metal on metal	OPG	osteoprotegerin
MoP	metal on polyethylene	OPLL	ossification of the posterior longitudinal ligament
MPC	2-methacryloyloxyethyl phosphorylcholine		
		ORIF	open reduction internal fixation
MPFL	medial patellofemoral ligament	OSCAR	Orthosonics System for Cemented Arthroplasty Revision
MPTA	medial proximal tibial angle		
MR	magnetic resonance	OSCE	objective structured clinical examination
MRC	Medical Research Council		
MRI	magnetic resonance imaging	PA	posterior anterior
MS	multiple sclerosis	PACS	picture archive and communication system
MSC	mesenchymal stem cell		
MSCC	malignant spinal cord compression	PAO	periacetabular osteotomy
		PCA	patient-controlled analgesia
MSK	musculoskeletal	PCL	posterior cruciate ligament
MSTS	Musculoskeletal Tumor Society	PCT	procalcitonin
MSU	monosodium urate	PD	proximodistal
MTC	Major Trauma Centre	PDFA	posterior distal femoral angle
MTP	metatarsophalangeal	PDGF	platelet-derived growth factor
MTPJ	metatarsophalangeal joint	PDNP	peripheral diabetic neuropathic pain
MUA	manipulation under anaesthetic		
NAI	non-accidental injury	PE	polyethylene
NCS	nerve conduction studies	PE	pulmonary embolism

PET	positron emission tomography
PF	patellofemoral
PFJ	patellofemoral joint
PFO	proximal femoral osteotomy
PFR	proximal femoral replacement
PG	proteoglycan
PGE2	prostaglandin E2
PHN	postherpetic neuralgia
PI	pelvic incidence
PIN	posterior interosseous nerve
PIP	proximal interphalangeal
PIPJ	proximal interphalangeal joint
PIS	pinning-in-situ
PJI	periprosthetic joint infection
PL	posterolateral
PLC	posterior ligamentous complex
PLIF	posterior interbody lumbar fusion
PLRI	posterolateral rotatory instability
PMMA	polymethylmethacrylate
PMN	polymorphonuclear neutrophil
PPF	periprosthetic fracture
PPP	preperitoneal pelvic packing
PPTA	posterior proximal tibial angle
PPV	positive predictive value
PQ	pronator quadratus
PR	per rectum
PROM	patient-reported outcome measure
PROSTALAC	prosthesis of antibiotic-loaded acrylic cement
PRP	platelet-rich plasma
PS	posterior stabilized
PSA	posterior sloping angle
PSA	prostate-specific antigen
PSF	posterior spinal fusion
PSIS	posterior superior iliac spine
PT	pronator teres
PTFL	posterior talofibular ligament
PTH	parathyroid hormone
QAP	questions, answers and prompting
RA	rheumatoid arthritis
RANK	receptor activator of nuclear factor κβ
RANKL	receptor activator of nuclear factor kB ligand
RC	radial collateral
RCT	randomized controlled trial

RDS	respiratory distress syndrome
RF	rheumatoid factor
RHK	rotating-hinge knee
RLN	recurrent laryngeal nerve
ROM	range of movement
ROTEM	rotational thromboelastometry
RR	relative risk
RTA	road traffic accident
SACH	solid ankle cushioned heel
SAR	structures at risk
SBA	single best answer
SCA	sickle cell anaemia
SCB	supraclavicular block
SCD	sickle cell disease
SCFE	slipped capital femoral epiphysis
SCH	supracondylar fracture of the humerus
SCI	spinal cord injury
SCM	sternocleidomastoid
SD	standard deviation
SER	supination external rotation
SERMs	selective oestrogen receptor modulators
SI	sacroiliac
SIRS	systemic inflammatory response syndrome
SLAC	scapholunate advanced collapsed
SLAP	superior labrum from anterior to posterior
SLE	systemic lupus erythematosus
SLR	straight leg raise
SMA	second moment area
SMAC	Standing Medical Advisory Committee
SNAC	scaphoid non-union advanced collapsed
SNAP	sensory nerve action potential
SNB	sciatic nerve block
SOL	space occupying lesion
SPECT	single photon emission computed tomography
SPN	superficial peroneal nerve
SR	sarcoplasmic reticulum
SRN	superficial radial nerve
SRS	Scoliosis Research Society
ST3	surgical trainee year 3
STACIS	Surgical Timing in Acute Spinal Cord Injury Study

STAR	Scandinavian total ankle replacement	TSF	thread shape factor
STC	Specialist Training Committee	TT	tibial tubercle
STIR	short-tau inversion recovery	TTO	tibial tubercle osteotomy
STT	scaphotrapeziotrapezoid	TT–TG	tibial tuberosity–trochlea groove
SUFE	slipped upper femoral epiphysis	U&E	urea and electrolytes
TA	tibialis anterior	UA	uric acid
TB	tuberculosis	UCL	ulnar collateral ligament
TCA	tricyclic antidepressant	UCS	Unified Classification System
TEG	thromboelastography	UHMWPE	ultra-high-molecular-weight polyethylene
TENS	transcutaneous electrical nerve stimulation	UKR	unicompartmental knee replacement
TER	total elbow replacement	UMN	upper motor neuron
TFA	tibiofemoral angle	URTI	upper respiratory tract infection
TFCC	triangular fibrocartilage complex		
TFL	tensor fascia lata	US	ultrasound
TGF	transforming growth factor	UTI	urinary tract infection
TGF-β	transforming growth factor-beta	UTS	ultimate tensile strength
THA	total hip arthroplasty	UV	ultraviolet
THR	total hip replacement	VACTERL	vertebral, anorectal, cardiac, tracheal, oesophageal, renal and limb
TIMPs	tissue inhibitory metalloproteinases		
TIVA	total intravenous anaesthesia	VAS	visual analogue scale
TKA	total knee arthroplasty	VEGF	vascular endothelial growth factor
TKR	total knee replacement		
TLICS	Thoracolumbar Injury Classification and Severity	VFG	vascularized fibular graft
TLIF	transforaminal lumbar interbody fusion	VTE	venous thromboembolism
		WBC	white blood cell
TLSO	thoracolumbar spinal orthosis	WCC	white blood cell count
TM	trabecular metal	WDL	well-differentiated lipoma
TMT	tarsometatarsal	WHO	World Health Organization
TNF	tumour necrosis factor	WOMAC	Western Ontario and McMaster Universities Arthritis Index
TRAP	tartrate resistance acid phosphatase	ZPA	zone of polarizing activity

Interactive website

The website to accompany the book:
www.postgraduateorthopaedics.com

This website accompanies the textbook series: Postgraduate Orthopaedics. It includes:

- Postgraduate Orthopaedics: The Candidate's Guide to the FRCS (Tr & Orth) Examination, third edition
- Postgraduate Orthopaedics: Viva Guide for the FRCS (Tr & Orth) Examination, second edition
- Postgraduate Paediatric Orthopaedics

The aim is to provide additional information and resources in order to maximize the learning potential of each book.

Additional areas of the website provide supplementary orthopaedic material, updates and web links. *Meet the editorial team* provides a profile of authors who were involved in writing the books. There is also a list of Postgraduate Orthopaedics courses available for candidates to fine-tune their examination skills. Details of the next diet of exams are also provided.

There is a link to additional orthopaedic websites that are particularly exam-focused.

It is very important our readership gives us feedback. Please email us if you have found any errors in the text that we can correct. In addition, please let us know if we haven't included an area of orthopaedics that you feel we should cover. Likewise, any constructive suggestions for improvement would be most welcome.

Chapter

General guidance

David Limb

Introduction

The structured oral (viva) examinations are the second component of Section 2 of the Intercollegiate examinations, usually occurring over a two-day period after the clinical section, but for any individual candidate the four vivas will occur on the same day. It is perhaps worth putting the vivas into context: between them the vivas contribute 48 of the 96 marking episodes in Section 2. The clinicals (intermediate and short cases) together make up the other 48 episodes, but in general it is more common for a poor mark in the vivas to be compensated for by a good mark in the clinicals than vice versa. Employing the training principles of a heptathlete, effort may be better spent on the weaker disciplines than becoming better at one's strengths.

This chapter will review the overall marking structure for the exam and outline the contribution of the structured clinical orals to the overall result. The process will then be explained in detail so that you, the candidate, can understand why the exam has evolved into its current form (incidentally, one of the most reliable high-stakes professional examinations in the world). By understanding this process you will be in the best position to prepare yourself for assessment against the examination standards. These standards are not set to ensure examination income for colleges, or to impose a limit on the supply of qualified professionals. The standards are set to reassure the regulator (GMC), employers and, most importantly, patients that those being awarded a certificate of completion of training today are of the same high standard as those awarded it last year and the year before. The FRCS (Tr & Orth) is one component of that assessment and if everyone presenting for the examination shows themselves to meet that standard, then every candidate will pass!

Overall structure of Section 2

To reach Section 2 of the Intercollegiate examination candidates must first pass Section 1. Section 1 is a computer-based test using 'single best answer', which over the past few years has evolved to focus principally on higher-order thinking. The large majority of factual, knowledge-based questions have been removed from the question bank. Therefore, to arrive at Section 2 you have already shown that you have a knowledge base and can apply that knowledge to solve problems posed in clinically relevant scenarios. Section 2 moves us higher up the ladder of higher-order thinking: it enables professional behaviours to be observed while the application of knowledge to real clinical problems in a time-pressured environment gives insight into how candidates might behave in independent clinical practice. Decisions have to be made on information elicited by the candidate and these have to be in the patients' best interests.

There are two components to Section 2: the clinical examinations (usually taking place in a hospital facility on a Sunday) and the structured oral examinations on the following two days, in an examination hall, often the ballroom of a hotel. The clinical examination will involve two 15-minute intermediate cases, one upper limb/cervical spine and one lower limb/thoracolumbar spine, and two 15-minute short case examinations with the same upper/lower limb split and each with three cases for 5 minutes each.

This chapter focuses on the structured oral examinations and each candidate will undertake four such vivas, each 30 minutes in length. Together these broadly cover the curriculum and are themed thus:

- Trauma (including spine)
- Basic science
- Adult and pathology (including spine)
- Children and hands (including upper limb)

Note there are qualifications against some viva titles – this is to ensure that wide syllabus coverage is possible, and this is facilitated by each candidate being preceded at the viva table by a topic sheet indicating the specific questions they have been asked to that point. Thus, if supracondylar fracture is a topic in the trauma viva it will not reappear in the children's viva. If spine has been omitted from trauma and children's vivas it is very likely to be asked in the adult and pathology viva.

Each viva is now quite rigidly structured – a 30-minute viva with two examiners will consist of 15 minutes with each examiner. Each examiner will ask on three topics for 5 minutes each (with a bell sounding to indicate each 5-minute interval). Each viva therefore involves six topics and each of these is marked independently by the two examiners, giving a total of 12 marking episodes for each of the four vivas. The practicalities of sitting the viva will be described later.

Marking scheme

In Section 2 of the FRCS (Tr & Orth) an examiner has only five choices of mark to award for each marking episode. A mark of 6 is a pass mark; 7 is a good pass and 8 a very good pass; 5 is a fail and 4 a bad fail. As noted above, the vivas carry a total of 48 marking episodes and that is matched by 48 marking episodes in the clinical section: 24 in the intermediate cases and 24 in the short cases. Altogether, therefore, there are 96 marking episodes and a score of 6 in every episode reaches the pass mark for the exam, which is therefore 576.

In the past a mark of 4 in any part of the clinical examination meant an automatic fail, no matter what marks were achieved in the vivas. This skewed examiner behaviour and now no such 'killer' mark exists. It is possible to compensate for a 4 in one marking episode by achieving an 8 in another episode, or indeed by two 7s in two separate marking episodes. The disaster of course would be to pass 95 episodes with marks of 6 and therefore fail the exam because of a single score of 5. There is no discussion around the marks at the end: no vouching for candidates by examiners who know them is possible. Examiners award a mark at the end of each marking episode independently of their co-examiner and enter it in their tablet computer. The sum of 96 episodes determines the total mark and if this is 576 or above the candidate has passed. If it is 575 or below the candidate has failed.

The mark awarded is not simply a grading based on the examiners' whim. There is a marking scheme which ascribes descriptors to levels of quality in response and this determines the mark that should be awarded. Although it is still up to the examiner to assess your performance and allocate the appropriate mark, the quality of response needed to achieve a 6, 7 or 8 is agreed at the examiner standard-setting meeting, which will be described later. Examiners are not allowed to confer before awarding their marks (except to clarify matters of fact, such as might occur if the co-examiner mishears something but is not allowed to interrupt), and they should mark according to the standards agreed at the standard setting discussion. Therefore, marks do not vary significantly – although it is acceptable for the examiners to give different marks, only a difference of one mark is accepted and examiners are not allowed to change their mark after allocating it. A discrepancy of two marks triggers an investigation, but fortunately this is rare.

Practicalities

For examiners the day is split into three or four sessions with three to six vivas in each session. Candidates are examined in groups, which may therefore have vivas either side of a coffee break. Each group of candidates receives a briefing from the Chairman of the Board immediately before their block of vivas begins.

The examiners use the same batch of standardized questions for each session. Resist the temptation to find ways of discovering what others in your group have been asked – this could give you an unfair advantage and is unprofessional. The GMC would take a dim view of any attempt to gain such an advantage in the examination process and a GMC referral is not helpful in gaining access to a consultant post.

You will be led into the examination hall and accompanied to your table by a member of intercollegiate staff who will identify your table and indicate your candidate number to the examiners. The examiners will stand, greet you and check your candidate number. They will not know whether you are a trainee or out of training. They will not know if this is your first attempt or if you are a returning candidate. Your heart will be racing and your mouth dry, but the examiners will be aware of this. It is their job to find out how well you can perform, not to humiliate you, so expect a polite introduction, a check of your candidate number, an orientation to which viva you are about to sit and an outline of how the next 30 minutes will be spent ('three questions of 5 minutes from myself with a bell between, followed by three more from my colleague'). The actual questioning doesn't start until the first bell sounds, ensuring that all candidates receive the same time, particularly when the hall is long, and some candidates have further to walk to their examiners than others. Commonly the topic is introduced by asking you to look at an image or diagram on a tablet computer screen and describe what you see, which leads into the questioning.

There will follow 30 minutes that seem to rush by, punctuated by bells at 5-minute intervals. When a bell sounds the examiner moves on to the next question – you will not be interrupted if you are part-way through a sentence in response to the previous question, but the examiner will simply stop the line of inquiry related to the previous question and introduce the next question. After six questions, three with each examiner, the final bell will be met with a polite but swift termination of the viva and you will be invited to leave the hall with the other candidates. Outside the Intercollegiate staff will organize you in preparation for your next viva, or allow you to leave if you have come to the end.

Examiner behaviour

Examiners are human beings and will naturally be different. However, they are trained to get the best from you and to minimize the chances that your performance in one component of the exam will affect it in another. There is a significant amount to consider in an examiner's training course, and examiners then attend an exam as 'examiners in training', so what follows is a very brief outline of how that training should impact on you.

Apart from being polite and courteous, examiners can steer you through a viva question and give you opportunities to elicit responses that show that you have reached a certain level in the marking scheme. In doing so you should find that most of the examiners' responses are emotionally flat, encouraging you to impart more or steering you away from areas that do not gain marks. They should not give you the impression that you are performing very well ('*Excellent! Well done!*') or very badly, as this may influence your performance in subsequent questions and vivas. They should not harass you and co-examiners are trained to intervene appropriately if

unacceptable examiner behaviour is witnessed. Of course, personalities will come through and you may hear beforehand of examiners who are reputed to be fierce – it may interest you to know that the marking behaviour of examiners is very strictly observed and analysed and bears no relation to candidates' perceptions.

Each viva will involve two examiners, each asking three questions. The examiner who is not asking questions is still actively participating and will be marking you. This examiner may also take some notes – do not be concerned if you see this happening. Of course, notes may be made for feedback purposes or to indicate why a low mark has been given. They can also be made simply to document areas discussed, identify any clarification the co-examiner might want from the examiner before marking or even to indicate why an '8' was awarded. Notes can also be for more mundane reasons, such as completing a topic sheet (which is passed ahead of the candidate so that examiners know what the candidate has been asked about previously – including a note of the short and intermediate cases). When optical marking sheets were used a candidate even apparently complained that he saw the examiner award him two 4s and a 5 before the viva was over, when in fact the examiner had been filling in his unique three-digit examiner number on the mark sheet.

The general pattern of a viva will be that the examiner asks you a series of questions. Eventually you will be asked a question that you cannot answer, or you can only partly answer. The examiner may rephrase the question or ask it in a different way. You may or may not be able to answer it, but the examiner then moves on to a related path of questions. This pattern is the same for all vivas, whether the candidate ends up with a 4 or an 8. If the examiner is having to rephrase the basic 'competence questions' that gain you a 6, then you may not pass. If you have quickly responded to the competence questions early on you may soon be in to the questions determining whether you should get a 7 or an 8 and in many cases candidates at this level are asked more questions that they cannot answer. The basic message is do not try to second-guess what mark you have achieved by the way you have been asked questions and answered them. Just treat every bell as a new start and try not to be influenced by whatever experience you perceived in the previous question.

Who are the examiners?

Examiners are not selected for their sadistic tendencies or cold hearts. They are consultants who have been in practice for at least 5 years and in that time have demonstrated an interest in, and continuing involvement in, training and education. They have put themselves forwards with the support of their medical director and usually have ongoing roles in regional and national training committees, teaching roles and the supervision of trainees. They must also demonstrate that they have remained active in research and that they can make the time to fulfil the role (which includes unpaid weekends away from home).

Applications are considered by the Intercollegiate Board and successful applicants are invited to attend an examiners training course. Successful completion of this allows them to attend an examination as an 'examiner in training', where they will observe and learn, and discuss marking (without influencing it) until eventually they can examine with an experienced examiner. Only after completion of the training exam does the examiner's term begin, but that is not where the oversight ends.

In every diet of the examination there will be a small team of 'examiner assessors'. They report back to the Intercollegiate Board on all aspects of the examination, from facilities and case mix to catering arrangements and environment. These assessors are also trained (usually after finishing the maximum 10-year term as an examiner) to assess and feedback on examiner performance. As a candidate you may have an assessor sitting out of your eyeline, slightly behind you, during vivas or clinicals. The assessors are actually assessing the examiners. Usually each examiner is assessed four times during one examination – twice during clinicals and twice during vivas.

The assessors ensure the standard of examining remains high, but this is supplemented by detailed analysis of the marking behaviour of examiners afterwards, again being fed back to the examiners after the event. Each examiner gets to see how they marked candidates compared to their peers. Hawkish or Dovish tendencies can be observed and reflected upon. Rest assured that stories of the examiner who routinely fails all candidates simply could not be true – such an examiner would be a wide outlier and could not continue thus.

How are marks allocated?

The key to this question is the examiners' standard-setting meeting, which takes place the day before the clinical examinations. Examiners attend a day earlier than candidates and are organized into groups according to which vivas they are examining. Each group then receives the questions that are to be asked in the vivas, with a different block of questions for each session of the two viva days. The questions themselves are taken from the Section 2 question bank and the Section 2 question writing committee has a lead examiner for each section, who chooses the questions to be used in each viva ensuring a spread of questions covering the curriculum widely. Thus, at standard-setting the trauma examiners, for example, will receive tablet computers preloaded with all of the trauma questions to be used. The questions have been written with a structure that begins with an opening statement or question that orientates the candidate to the topic, moves on through questions that stimulate discussion that should show whether the candidate is competent in the topic, before opening up into advanced questions that enable high marks to be reached. An accompanying data sheet from the bank will include information on where in the question competence is identified, either from the question writers or from previous diets of the exam. As a group the examiners agree what level has to be achieved to reach a '6', what higher-order responses will take the candidate to a '7' or '8' and what unsatisfactory or dangerous responses might earn the candidate a '4'. Examiners can annotate the data sheet with the group decision and this can inform future diets. This also ensures that the standard of the 'day one consultant' can be identified and agreed and should be consistently applied.

This process means that candidates examined by different pairs of examiners have the same chance of achieving a pass mark, and candidates being asked different questions in a later session still have the same standard to achieve to obtain a pass. It is accepted that marking a discussion will inevitably introduce some variation, but the standard setting process minimizes this and, when it is applied to the 48 different sets of marks a candidate will be awarded across the vivas, ensures the same standard is required to pass the examination for all candidates.

What do the marks mean?

A closed marking system is used from 4 to 8 and this equates to the following.

- 4 – Bad fail.
- 5 – Fail.

- 6 – Pass.
- 7 – Good pass.
- 8 – Exceptional pass.

Examiners assess nine trainee characteristics during the standardized oral examination.

1. Personal qualities.
2. Communication skills.
3. Professionalism.
4. Surgical experience.
5. Organizational and logical, step-wise sequencing of thought processes, ability to focus on the answers quickly.
6. Clinical reasoning and decision making.
7. Ability to handle stress.
8. Ability to deal with grey areas in practice and complex issues.
9. Ability to justify an answer with evidence from the literature.

This has been simplified into three domains.

Overall professional capability/patient care

- Personal qualities, professionalism and ethics, surgical experience, ability to deal with grey areas.

Knowledge and judgement

- Knowledge, ability to justify, clinical reasoning.

Quality of response

- Communication skills, organisation and logical thought process. Assess questions, answers and prompting (QAP).

Detailed marking descriptors indicate the behaviours typical of each mark: this helps examiners identify the mark boundaries during the standard setting meeting before the vivas take place. These can be interpreted as follows:

4 – Unsafe and potentially dangerous. A very poor answer. Gross basic mistakes and poor knowledge. Should not be sitting the exam. The examiners have severe reservations about the candidate's performance and are essentially flagging this up. Too ignorant of the fundamentals of orthopaedic practice to pass. Candidate is scoring a 4 in the first instance. Did not get beyond the default questions, fails in all/most competencies. Poor basic knowledge/judgement/understanding to a level of concern.

5 – Some hesitancy and indecisiveness. The answer is really not good enough with too many deficiencies. Too many basic errors and not getting to the nub of the issue. Wandering off at tangents and not staying focused on the question. Misinterpreting the question. Repeats the same ATLS and/or radiograph talk with each oral viva question. Difficulty in prioritizing, large gaps in knowledge, poor deductive skills, patchy performance, struggled to apply knowledge and judgement. Confused or disorganized answer. Poor higher-order thinking.

6 – Satisfactory performance. Covered the basics well, safe and would be a sound consultant. No concerns. Performance OK, but certainly not anything special or outstanding. Good knowledge and judgement of common problems. Important points mentioned, no major errors and required only occasional minor prompting.

7 – Good performance. Would make a good consultant. Articulate and to the point. Able to identify some literature to support their answers, knows various guidelines and publications. Coped well with difficult topics/problems. Goes beyond the competency questions. Logical answers. Strong interpretation/judgement but wasn't able to quote specific literature effectively. Good supporting reasons for answers. No prompting needed for answers but prompting required to identify the literature.

8 – Potential gold medal or prize-winning performance. Smooth, articulate and polished. Able to succinctly discuss controversial orthopaedic issues in a sensible way. Excellent command of the literature. Switched on and makes the examiners feel very reassured. Looks and talks the part. Stretches the examiners, no prompting necessary. Confident, clear, logical and focused answers.

While it is impossible to reference this list while computing an answer, knowledge of the principles of 'what makes a good answer' can certainly help your preparation.

Answering questions

From the above it should be apparent that advice to 'steer the examiners to ask about something you know about' is a tactic that is doomed to failure. You will obtain marks as you pass through mark boundaries agreed at Standard Setting by the examiners. You will therefore be steered to these mark boundaries by the examiner's questions. If you attempt to move the examiner into a different line of questioning, you will be moving them into an area where no marks are available. Of course, the examiners will resist and steer you back to the line of discussion they had started, but in the process you will have wasted time.

The wise candidate will answer the question posed by the examiners. It is entirely appropriate to develop the answer by starting to talk about options, or justifying your answer by referring to literature or whatever – follow the examiner's cues. If the examiner is listening intently then continue. If the examiner seems to be wanting to interrupt then allow this, as they are probably saving you from wasting your time or you have said something ambiguous that they need you to clarify before they can move on.

If one considers some of the underpinning educational theory, it may help understand the marking structure and how you can best approach answering questions (and even preparing for the exam). Bloom's taxonomy describes levels of complexity in using learned material:

1. Knowledge/recall.
2. Comprehension or understanding.
3. Application.
4. Analysis.
5. Synthesis.
6. Evaluation.

Level 1, factual recall, has almost been removed from the Intercollegiate exam. You may still be asked a question that demands a factual answer at some point in a viva, and there may have been occasional level 1 questions (particularly basic sciences) in the SBA paper. In general terms, however, the exam will be checking that you understand the facts and that you can apply your factual knowledge to help you analyse a problem and synthesize a solution, then suggest how to evaluate the outcome. The vivas will be structured where possible to take you along this pathway.

Thus, a viva might start by describing a clinical scenario. From a set of described symptoms and signs, or by looking at a radiograph, your first question might be 'what do you think is going on here?' Even interpreting a radiograph, for instance classifying loosening of a hip prosthesis or identifying an AP3 pelvic fracture, shows that not only do you have knowledge and understand it, but that you can apply it.

The examiners will then move you on to adding further clinical detail, for example, which require you to analyse the impact of this new information and predict its impact on the scenario. It is easy to see how the viva becomes an excellent method for testing higher-order thinking, whereas the constraints of the written section mean that although it can test the curriculum very broadly, it is largely restricted to level 2 and 3 knowledge.

What the examiners are looking for, therefore, is not simply that you 'know stuff', but that you can use it. You can work with limited or incomplete information to make sensible choices. You can make safe decisions on how to initiate management and you will initiate the next steps to fill in the missing data that allow you to come to a conclusion that is effective. Finally, why do you do it like that? What are the alternatives? You should be prepared to justify your choices not just by saying 'because that's what my trainer does' but by showing that you have thought about the alternatives and have come to a reasoned choice. To score 7s and 8s an argument based on good-quality evidence quoted from the literature and justified by your own training and experience gets you there.

Preparation

It is easy to fall into the trap of believing that you need to spend months working in the library and working through textbooks in order to pass the examination. There is an awful lot to learn in a six-year training programme so that you can be safe to manage a general trauma take and screen referrals to a general orthopaedic service, managing the majority and identifying those that need more specialist care. However, demonstrating that you have level 1 knowledge far wider even than the examiners does not help if you can't apply the more mainstream elements of that knowledge base to solve clinical problems. Sure, the books will help a lot, especially with basic sciences and rare conditions that you may not have met, but for the most part your day job is the best preparation you can get. However, transferring this to the exam environment can feel hard.

Vivas are about discussing clinical scenarios – solving a problem based on information, building on that solution and using the options to identify the best way to a good outcome. It's therefore more about getting used to talking through that process rather than looking somewhere to find all the answers. There are a few ways to approach this.

Probably the best way is what the best candidates have unconsciously done through their training – discussing cases with peers and with trainers. Take every opportunity to ask questions about cases. Add in '*what if?*' questions whenever you get an answer. Talk through cases from presentation through management to outcome. Talk about the alternatives and why some people do one thing and others another. This is how you will decide on your own practice when you become a consultant and the examiners want to see how you make such decisions.

Talking over cases with trainers and peers can be morphed into 'viva practice' as the exam draws near. Instead of a wide-ranging discussion of all the possibilities, try to hone it down to specific circumstances and try to become concise. Focus on the sort of case in which decision making can be critical, such as rare cases that might turn up in clinic, and it is important that you recognize them. There are well-publicized lists of the sort of cases that have been asked, so nothing should be a surprise. It is no surprise that the most commonly asked questions in the children's viva, for example, relate to DDH, SUFE, clubfoot, septic arthritis of the hip and cerebral palsy. Courses are available that specifically offer viva practice, and many find these useful, if only to get them into the frame of mind to work and to give them some idea of what to expect. Remember, however, that examiners are not allowed to take part in 'crammer courses' to prepare individuals for the exam. Examiners can, however, help their own trainees to prepare as they will never be called on to examine their own trainees in the real exam. Most such crammer courses involve enthusiastic trainers and trainees who have relatively recently passed the exam. Most will not have had any examiner training, so the practice may not be a good mirror of the genuine event.

Finally, I would recommend that you try doing some preparation for vivas in the same way that gymnasts can train for complex routines even between training sessions – just think it through in your head. In gymnasts the engram – that cerebrally encoded complex pattern of muscle movement and contraction required to perform a particular skill –

can be reinforced by imagining it in real time. 'Thinking through' the routine can actually improve physical execution. The same could be said for viva practice – imagine you are asked a question; how will you answer it? Think through in real time what words you would use in your answer to avoid ambiguity. Think what the examiner might say in response and how you will react. You may find that the form of words that comes to your mind in the first instance is clumsy – could you say it better? For the more commonly asked viva topics prepare in advance the phrases you will use to indicate your personal preference for treatment and the evidence that backs this up. In this way a lot of useful viva preparation can actually be done while 'relaxing' or sitting on the journey to and from work each day.

On the day

Don't panic. Don't stay up late trying to pack in last-minute revision and miss out on sleep as a consequence. Think about your appearance – it is not a beauty contest, but the exam is one of the few occasions in your training where professionalism is formally assessed. How will you present yourself to patients in the future? You will not be marked down for your choice of shirt or blouse, but if you are scruffy and unkempt for such an important event the examiners will probably assume that you will present yourself in no better a light in the outpatient clinic, where you are supposed to be gaining the patient's trust and confidence.

Undoubtedly you will be nervous. The examiners expect this and will try to put you at ease. Remember that anxiety improves performance up to a point, so nerves can be helpful. Go in expecting a robust discussion on a number of topics with a series of questions culminating in you running out of answers. That is the pattern of all vivas and each viva will end with you in the realms of questions you aren't sure you are answering correctly. Each bell is therefore a new opportunity to score points and just forget about what has gone before.

Listen to the examiners and answer the questions they pose – do not volunteer an answer to a related question because you know the subject better. If you really are unsure about what has been asked, request clarification. However, do not deliberately try to slow things down as you will only restrict the opportunity for yourself to progress through the marking structure. If your mouth is dry take a sip of water – it is always provided. Expect to finish your sentence when the bell rings then be moved on to the next question. Do not try to pack in more detail on the last question as you will be receiving no marks after the bell and will eat into the opportunities to score on the next question.

Be human! The examiners want to see how you will work under some time pressure and when faced with real clinical problems. They want a discussion with a colleague, to be able to assess how you will behave when you start as a consultant, potentially in a very general post and with a trauma take that includes the full range of emergencies that can present anywhere at any time.

Summary

The viva section of the Intercollegiate examination is rather like a clinical examination without patients. It is used to see if you have the knowledge base needed to work as a day one consultant in the generality of orthopaedics and trauma. More importantly, however, it tests whether you can use that knowledge base to solve clinical problems, identify solutions and test that your proposed solutions have worked. It also gives some opportunity to test professional behaviours; after all, it is a discussion between colleagues. Analysis suggests that the FRCS (Tr & Orth) is one of the most reliable high-stakes professional examinations in the world. Go into it with the ambition that you will be back five or so years later as an examiner!

Candidate guidance

Firas Arnaout and John Davies

Introduction

The FRCS (Tr & Orth) structured oral viva is a daunting prospect because of its high-stakes nature and the uncertainty surrounding it. The aim of this chapter is to consolidate insights from successful former candidates as well as the perspective of a senior examiner to guide you through the difficult challenges and achieve exam success!

The structured, standardized oral exam

The FRCS (Tr & Orth) represents the standard of knowledge and aptitude required for clinical practice by a day one consultant in the generality of Trauma and Orthopaedics. Passing the exam is an important milestone which symbolizes the pinnacle of a stressful period of intensive study. It is also seen as an opportunity to demonstrate the learning and knowledge you have accumulated over many years of training!

Achievement of the FRCS (Tr & Orth) enables the erstwhile candidate to apply for his or her Certificate of Completion of Training and therefore a consultant post. In turn, it leads to largely unsupervised surgical practice.

The examiners expect a competent candidate to have a broad knowledge, possess sound basic principles and demonstrate the requisite key skills and attitudes in their judgement and professionalism. In effect, they are someone with whom they could entrust the treatment of a family member, or work with as a fellow colleague.

In contrast to examiners in other postgraduate objective structured clinical examinations (OSCEs), in the FRCS (Tr & Orth) oral viva examiners are not forced to recite verbatim a prescriptive text. As detailed in David Limb's account, they follow a predetermined mark scheme ensuring reproducibility and fairness. However, to make certain each candidate can achieve their highest possible score, by

the process of exploring the limits of their knowledge, this culminates in the experience of a particular viva station being unique to that individual. For instance, despite being asked the same initial starter question from an image as a prompt, the ensuing discussion depends upon whether a candidate correctly identifies the problem from the information, or picks up on hints if they start to veer off topic. Candidates who are well rehearsed at answering problems in clinical scenarios will score highly, compared to those who are unable to apply their knowledge to hypothetical dilemmas, which the examiners believe you should be able to manage competently as a day one consultant in practice.

Viva preparation

1. Aptitude and mind set

During the exam, your knowledge aptitude only becomes evident to the examiners when you demonstrate it talking around a subject in a competent fashion. Crucially, you must be prepared to do this for all of the important topics on the curriculum. For most candidates, this means a broad rather than narrow knowledge base will allow them to deliver an answer that displays higher-order thinking.

It is important to focus your preparation on the high-yield topics during viva practice, so that you stand the best chance of maximizing your score. For each viva station, you will often be tested on topics from the curriculum encountered in daily practice that are critical to manage correctly for patient safety. You should be able to generate a list of topics that are recurrently asked every year based on: those that you have already been quizzed on in deanery and departmental teaching; questions from good viva revision textbooks; as well as a list from any past candidate or consultant with FRCS (Tr & Orth) accreditation.

For instance, in the trauma viva, you must be conversant on all of the topics discussed in a departmental trauma meeting from the management of elbow Terrible Triad to the classification of acetabular fractures. The examiners will expect a comprehensive knowledge because turning up to be quizzed in the morning trauma meeting should have been part of your normal day job for the last five years. In the basic science viva, surgical approaches are often asked after being shown a photograph of an anatomical prosection. Being able to draw a brief line diagram and confidently talk about the important biomechanical principles involved is routinely expected for high-ranking topics such as articular cartilage or the stress–strain curve. To ensure your answer is fluent and that the diagram contains all of the essential features means repeated practice.

2. Speech and communication in the viva

It is important to realize before commencing preparation for the vivas that when it comes to answering questions, universally without exception at the start, every single candidate due to sit the exam has a poor technique. Much hard work is needed in rehearsing for the viva beforehand to stand a chance of success.

Preparation for the viva is an individual process, but it bears many similarities to how you might go about rehearsing to give a vast number of podium presentations scheduled at a scientific conference for the same day with the added feature that you will be doing it without the use of notes. Part of that preparation would involve several months memorizing every day the content of what you will say. It would also be imperative to prepare answers on areas that are likely to invite interested questions. If some of the audience appeared hostile or indifferent this would not affect your performance, because you know the material well and can talk about it confidently. Many candidates find the use of index or flash cards an invaluable memory aid during this process (Figure 2.1a,b). Alternatively, recording your speech onto a Dictaphone and playing this back can be a powerful revision tool, especially when commuting to work.

For many candidates, it is essential to work on your public speaking so that on the spot, you sound credible to a consultant to whom you have just been formally introduced. Even the late Alan Apley, of Apley's System of Orthopaedics and Fractures,[1] painstakingly memorised 'off-the-cuff' comments and repartee, so that he delivered a polished performance during a presentation. According to the JCIE marking descriptors, to achieve a level 7 or 8 answer you should be fluent and confident without prompting.

Before the start of the viva, while in the holding bay of the exam hall, the myriad candidates flicking through reams of notes in their bags is a testament to how desperate a situation the majority of people find themselves in! Unfortunately, it is extremely difficult under pressure to be able to read something, internalize it and then speak it aloud minutes later in a flawless performance. That is why it is so important to rehearse the answers. For some, this even extends to rehearsing the phrases or 'discourse markers' that occur during your conversation:

'I would want to discuss with a consultant who specialises in … but essentially, the treatment principles are …'

'My primary concern is that I'd want to establish this was in fact a closed, isolated injury. What is the state of the soft tissue envelope … Whilst a cast is an option there is a likelihood it will displace, and managing late displacement is a difficult situation.'

'I'm really sorry. I've made a mistake. I've started on completely the wrong track. Can I please start again?'

'Excuse me. I'm very sorry it's quite noisy. Can I please clarify what you've asked?'

Remember that constantly asking for clarification every time you are asked a question quickly becomes irksome, but you are allowed to do this once or twice because it gets noisy in the exam hall. Typically, there is a key point your answer needs to cover so that you initially demonstrate competence. Thereafter, once you've surpassed this and your answer takes off, you can achieve the attributes of a fluent and confident higher-level answer. Bear in mind that anything you say to the examiner often becomes the basis of their next question in a predictable sequence. For example, in the following scenario on paediatric septic hip the follow-on questions would be anticipated:

CANDIDATE: From the clinical picture of febrile, non-weight-bearing, raised CRP and white cell count, I would get an ultrasound to look for an effusion. The child meets Kocher's criteria …

EXAMINER: What are Kocher's criteria?

CANDIDATE: Kocher's paper published in 1999 is almost 20 years old. It was a retrospective multivariate analysis differentiating septic arthritis from an irritable hip in children.[2] It has been superseded by other studies but is still relevant to practice, apart from one criterion being an elevated ESR which in some hospitals is difficult to obtain out-

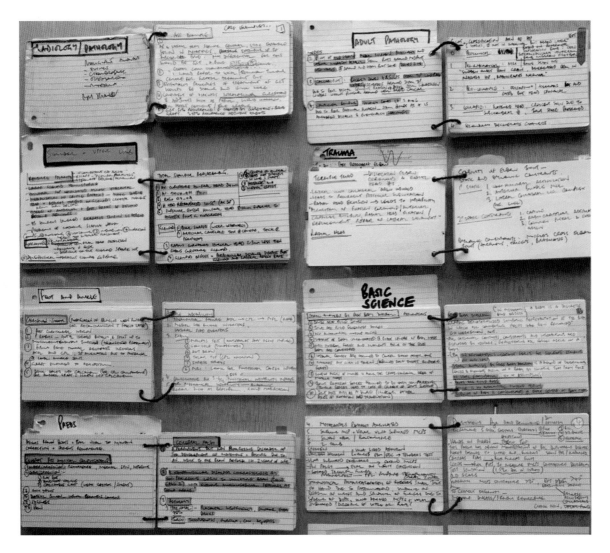

Figure 2.1a,b Revision cards.

of-hours nowadays. With 4 out of 4 criteria, there was a 99% probability predictive for septic arthritis.

EXAMINER: The scan shows an effusion.

CANDIDATE: I would take him to theatre to wash him out via an anterior approach.

EXAMINER: What is the anterior approach?

CANDIDATE: Supine, sandbag, bikini incision. Interval between sartorius and TFL, gluteus medius and rectus femoris. The internervous plane is superior gluteal and femoral nerves. It isn't necessary to go up proximally over the iliac crest or split the apophysis. The structure at risk is the lateral cutaneous nerve. I would want to visualize the articular cartilage of the femoral head to confirm I'm in the joint. To do this, some people excise a small square of capsule by a cruciform incision . . .

If you struggle answering questions aloud, rehearsing the commonly asked topics in your study group pays dividends. As you become more familiar with the viva process you can then predict the ensuing questions the examiner moves on to for each topic.

3. Study group practice

The merits of a study group cannot be overstated. It is a major leap from reading material to articulating

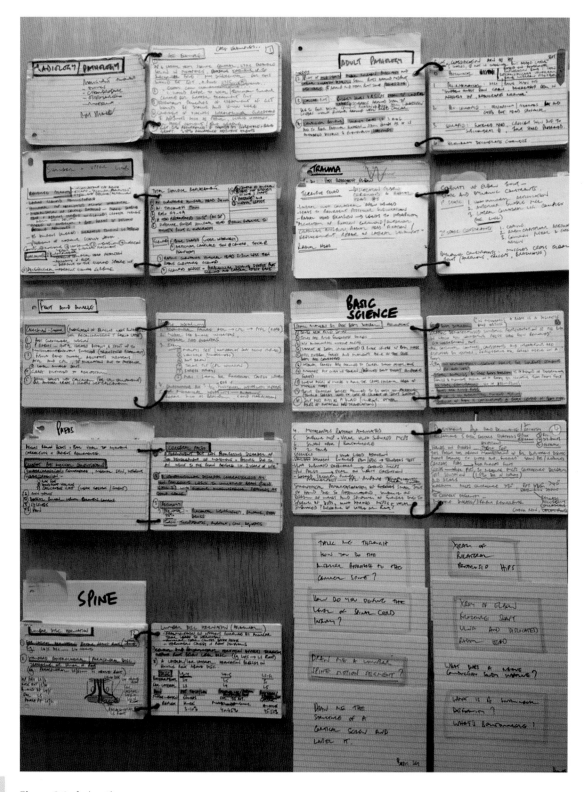

Figure 2.1a,b (cont.)

a viva answer. Meeting regularly to discuss your answers will improve the quality of what you say, as well as highlighting areas where your deficiencies lie. Often each member of the group has a particular subspecialist interest that they want to pursue as a long-term career. In this way you are able to complement each other and fill outstanding gaps in knowledge. By far this represents the most efficient use of your time in the final months; and will yield the greatest improvement.

It is important that in your viva study group you pool resources and help each other. Remember that every deanery has a set of consultants who are fully expecting you to approach them for viva practice. Typically, they will be FRCS examiners already, or have a role in the deanery mock exam or viva courses. Often they have a FRCS viva PowerPoint presentation on their laptop. To make it the most efficient use of time, you should attend these as a group. These sessions are absolutely invaluable because they often recreate what you will be asked. You have the opportunity to see how other people answer questions that you will be asked in the real thing. For instance, if you come across an exceptional answer which you think is close to perfect, it is self-evident you should make a note, write it out later and practise it, so that it becomes committed to memory. Should you be asked the same question in the viva, you can recite a brilliant answer and almost certainly score 7–8. First impressions make a significant contribution in a time-pressured environment. If you are in the fortunate position of being able to do this on the first question, you have a high chance of passing that station because the other examiner will also be silently impressed with the level of knowledge you demonstrate on the starting question.

Skyping and FaceTime can be useful if there are difficulties arranging a regular meeting due to on call commitments or long distances that have to be travelled. However, there is no substitute to the actual experience of being quizzed face-to-face with a consultant or post-FRCS trainee acting as an examiner critiquing your answer. There are many subtle nuances and non-verbal communication skills you will acquire; and any irritating mannerisms which you weren't consciously aware of doing will be highlighted to you.

4. Assigned educational supervisor practice

It is important in the run-up to the exam that you let all the trainers know in your unit that you have the Part 2 coming up, and you need help! There are many reasons for this, not least the fact if you have any non-essential clinical commitments these can be temporarily dropped. For instance, if any spare time arises in your timetable, they know you have to focus on viva and clinical revision. Now is the time to be forthright and tell them where your deficiencies lie. If you have not done a paediatric placement, and need to go to elective paediatric clinic, they need to be told! There is absolutely no way you can pass the exam without attending these clinics. Similarly, if your placement in hand surgery was lacking, you need to make amends for this.

Your educational supervisor and the other consultants you work with can play a vital role in the last few months. Every time you do a fracture clinic, or for that matter any other clinic, ask them to go through an FRCS case or 'watch you examine a patient with pathology'.

The number of vivas that have a plain radiograph as the starting point is ridiculously commonplace. How to deal with a peri-prosthetic fracture in a patient with loosening, for instance, or a complex primary hip in a patient with protrusio or ankylosing spondylitis, are everyday topics that you see in clinic, and likewise will be almost certain to get in the viva. These will be prefaced by 'Have a look at this iPad, and tell me what you think' in the viva. In effect, this is the same as being sat in the clinic in between patients, with your trainer saying 'Have a look at this X-ray on PACS and tell me what you think.'

5. FRCS viva courses

It is not essential to have done a course to do well in the viva. However, an FRCS viva or clinical revision course can be a saving grace if you know that your technique is lacking and you have deficiencies. For example, to cover the entire basic science syllabus for the viva is a substantial amount of work and going on a good course that covers basic science will save you considerable time, as it recaps the numerous weighty topics such as: stress–strain, free body diagrams, viscoelastic material properties, types of lever, nerve action potential and numerous others that sequester hours of revision. If you go with members of your group, you can spend the evenings practising in your hotel room, which again is quality revision time.

It is true that there is some variability in the quality of the teaching on courses. As a rule, you are bound to gain some helpful information and knowledge, and there will likely be negative and positives aspects for each course that you go on. If you strongly believe your time and money were wasted, then you are entitled to let the organizers know. It would be worth bearing in mind, however, that almost all courses are run by practising consultants who have to make time to organize them for little or no recompense; and if they stopped doing it altogether most candidates would be the worse off. Also, most reputable courses will have a current or previous FRCS examiner in the faculty, although this may not be openly advertised, who will provide valuable insights.

General approach and what to do when things go wrong

The format for oral viva questions is detailed in David Limb's account. Vivas are structured so that the examiners have preset questions, with which they start an exchange and then quiz the candidate as things progress beyond initial competence to the discussion stages involving higher-order thinking. Oral exam questions are prepared so as to be crystal clear and explicit, with default competence questions if candidates are unable to discuss the more challenging topic areas in the syllabus.

At some point, most candidates require help from the examiner. Now and again, most people will experience some prompting if they stray off topic. The examiner's answer sheet contains a list of prompts to guide the candidate back to the subject. It is the responsibility of the examiners to ensure that the requisite points are covered, and the answer sheets contain more information than all but the highest-flying candidates will be expected to cover.

Occasionally you may experience the unpleasant sensation of becoming completely unstuck. This is often because you have inadvertently missed the point of the original question from the outset. This is why it is so important to listen extremely carefully to every word the examiner says, as this will contain all of the clues you need to arrive at the correct answer. While sometimes it appears examiners may ask something in an innocuous fashion, it is absolutely imperative that you have listened to every single word and think carefully before launching into an answer. It is also important to have some means to compensate for a bad score by being strong elsewhere in a particular viva subject.

Likewise, examiners expect that if a candidate knows a topic well, unprompted they will start confidently reciting vast amounts of knowledge to score

highly. This can be done if you have practised your answers well and rehearsed what the likely questions are. This form of prolific data dump is often rewarded with the examiner sitting back in their chair, and then interrupting only to change to start a new topic after 5 minutes. In this situation it can sometimes be observed the examiner will subtly nod as you deliver a well-prepared answer, which indicates they agree with what you are saying. Examiners are highly trained so that they are not supposed to reveal any conscious encouragement, but during the course of a long day they can sometimes fail to maintain a deadpan face all the time.

Formulating answers to oral questions

Before you answer the question, take a few seconds to mentally construct a checklist of the main points you want to make and then start calmly with your answer. This avoids blurting out the first thing that comes into your head and gives the examiners the impression you are giving a logical, considered response.

If you are confident on a topic keep talking, keep to the question that was asked, and go for it! Avoid going off on a tangent as you don't score points for this. If you can direct the answer onto a topic you know well this can be a rewarding position to be in. Once you have finished your answer stop, smile at the examiners and calmly wait for the next question. Avoid the temptation to fill the silence by adding superfluous information to the end of your answer, as this falsely gives an impression that you are waffling. This annoys the examiners because you don't appear to be giving a straightforward answer to a direct question. It can also bring you into an area you really didn't want to talk about. The examiners may cut you off mid-sentence, it can happen whether you are doing well or not so don't let this put you off. Just concentrate on the next question.

If the examiner asks you if you are sure about your answer this generally means you have answered incorrectly, so unless you are very self-assured, take the hint. If the examiner asks you to clarify an answer, they are usually checking to make sure they actually heard what they thought they heard, which again is usually the wrong answer!

It is better not to argue with the examiners if they point out your answer is wrong, even if deep down you are convinced it reflects the latest evidence or opinion. You may get the sense the examiner is unhappy because your answer does not match what is written on their sheet, so it is reasonable to explain your justification. Although to defuse some of the tension in this situation you can preface this with 'In my humble opinion', or 'there is some controversy in this area, and I'm aware of this evidence'. Remember, part of what you are being tested on in the viva is your professionalism and attitude. Being a consultant involves skills in navigating through controversial areas. Offer your considered reasoning of the issue without being patronizing.

Quoting the literature

Being able to discuss the evidence for a particular treatment or justifying how and why you do something is the hallmark of understanding in the exam and a clear sign that you are someone suitable for consultant practice. Likewise, being unprepared to the extent that you don't have any relevant papers which you can discuss in your knowledge base effectively means you are putting yourself at a serious disadvantage to the other candidates. It is extremely difficult to remember every important paper that exists in every topic. Realistically, if your time is limited then you will have to be selective about what things you look at and prepare answers for. This means that trawling through every JBJS in the last 12 months is not necessarily a good use of time. However, making an index card on a seminal paper is worthwhile because it means you can quote something when being asked for the evidence. You will not be expected to know the length and breadth of the orthopaedic literature. It is more important to have some appropriate papers to talk about, which either you will have come across from your study group, from a revision course lecture or from listening to your peers being quizzed.

One guide for the important hallmark papers is to look through any FRCS viva revision textbook, this one included, for the references for papers mentioned in the model answers in the endnotes of each chapter. If the same paper is recurrently signposted over many topics – such as the Lidwell[3] paper on the effect of ultraclean air theatres on deep infection in joint replacement, which is a reference for prosthetic joint infection in adult pathology as well as theatre sterility in basic science – this probably means you should be familiar with it. If you are pushed for time then one shortcut is to read the abstracts only, but be warned there is a risk to this! The danger is if you mention a paper the examiner may well ask you the details of that study, so preparing in this fashion is based on whether you feel you can carry it off in the exam under pressure. The National Joint Registry is something you are expected to be able to discuss. One perennial topic is the relative advantages and disadvantages of using registries to guide practice, whether these are regional or national. How survivorship favours more established prostheses or the effect of data collection and the measurement of endpoints are among some of the other discussion points you will come across in your study group.

Final advice

It rapidly becomes apparent to the examiners how well a candidate has prepared for the structured oral exam. Usually within the first two minutes most candidates will have demonstrated their knowledge and aptitude to indicate what their score should be. Unfortunately, in the unlucky situation that a candidate rapidly draws a blank from the start and cannot progress from the initial competence question this usually spells bad news. However, even if this does happen, all is not lost due to the marking system allowing a second chance by means of compensating for a poor score in another viva station. Grasping that second chance is dependent on being practised sufficiently so that you can perform under the inevitable pressure that you will feel in the next viva station, as well as having an adequate knowledge to raise your score. This is why if you put in the hard work and preparation early, then you will be able to withstand the setbacks which almost inevitably occur on the day, and come through the viva with a pass!

References

1. Blom A. (Ed.) *Apley and Solomon's System of Orthopaedics and Trauma*, 10th Edition. Boca Raton: CRC Press; 2017.

2. Kocher MS, Zurakowski D, Kasser JR. Differentiating between septic arthritis and transient synovitis of the hip in children: an evidence-based clinical prediction algorithm. *J Bone Joint Surg Am*. 1999;81(12):1662–1670.

3. Lidwell OM, Lowbury EJ, Whyte W *et al*. Effect of ultraclean air in operating rooms on deep sepsis in the joint after total hip or knee replacement: a randomized study. *Br Med J*. 1982;285:10–14.

Chapter

3

Hip

Jeya Palan and Paul A. Banaszkiewicz

Introduction

There has been a change in emphasis in the oral questions in the last 2 years to higher-order thinking and judgement. Exam revision should be less book reading and more being practical and adept at managing complex clinical conditions. Examiners would argue if you have been well trained in the basics it isn't too difficult to apply these basic principles to various clinical situations that you may be tested on in the oral exam. If you haven't managed periprosthetic joint infection (PJI) then it's going to be doubly difficult to answer the real-life practical questions that are related to managing a patient with this condition.

We have aimed the candidates' answers for a 7–8 score, so they are significantly more detailed than what would be required for a bare pass. Aiming for the minimum to pass will generally be unsuccessful and is not recommended.

Structured oral examination question 1

EXAMINER: These are the radiographs of a 65-year-old gentleman who had a primary left THA 14 years ago (Figure 3.1a and b). Over the last 2 weeks, he has had increasing pain in the left hip and he has contacted his GP who has referred him back to you on an urgent basis. Postoperatively, he was progressing well, and he has no history of any trauma. He is now unable to weight bear fully on the left leg and has night pain.

CANDIDATE: This is an AP pelvic radiograph showing a left cemented Exeter THA. I am concerned that there is an area of radiolucency around the tip of the greater trochanter. The acetabular component appears well fixed. My worry here is that this gentleman may have a periprosthetic joint infection. Every painful prosthetic joint is potentially infected.

EXAMINER: So how are you going to proceed with this patient?

CANDIDATE: I would want to take the patient to theatre and perform an aspiration of the hip to rule out infection.

EXAMINER: You are sure? Are you not jumping in a bit fast? Is there anything else you might want to find out beforehand?

CANDIDATE: I would want to take a full history from the patient. A number of patients who develop infection have early wound problems such as

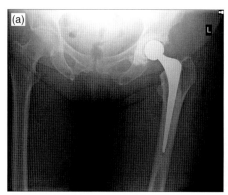
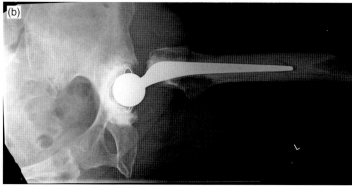

Figure 3.1a and 3.1b Anteroposterior (AP) pelvis and lateral radiographs demonstrating a left Exeter THA.

prolonged redness, induration, swelling or discharge. There may be a history of repeated courses of antibiotics. The wound may have become frankly infected requiring washout in theatre.

Onset of hip pain following a problem-free interval and an episode of sepsis is suggestive of haematogenous seeding of infective organisms from elsewhere. I would enquire if there was a history of bacteraemia from a UTI, chest infection or dental extraction.

Pain from an infected prosthesis is typically non-mechanical and unrelated to physical activity and not relieved by rest.

I would also like to explore more fully host risk factors for infection such as diabetes, rheumatoid arthritis, depression, obesity, hypothyroidism, immunosuppression (steroids, DMARDs), smoking and poor dentition. Lifestyle factors such as heavy alcohol intake and smoking.

Having taken a full history, I would perform a comprehensive clinical examination, looking at the scar for any evidence of infection such as erythema, warmth, a sinus, etc. What is the hip ROM and is there pain associated with ROM? I would also like to examine the abdomen, knee and lumbar spine to exclude other potential sources of haematogenous infection/cause for the hip pain. I would then request an FBC, CRP and ESR to look for evidence of raised inflammatory markers.

EXAMINER: How helpful are these?

CANDIDATE: They have relatively low sensitivity and low specificity as markers of prosthetic joint infection. Berbari et al. (level 2) published a systematic review in the JBJS American edition in 2010 on the use of inflammatory markers for diagnosis of prosthetic joint infection.[1] They concluded that IL-6 is a much more sensitive test for infection. Unfortunately, IL-6 assays are not readily available in most NHS hospitals and certainly not in my trust at present.

EXAMINER: What about diabetes as a risk factor for PJI?

CANDIDATE: The association between diabetes and PJI may be mediated by impaired leukocyte function and microvascular complications which may impair wound healing.

In addition, factors associated with diabetes, such as hyperglycaemia, hyperlipidaemia, hypertension and increased oxidative stress, upregulate cellular and inflammatory reactions and play a part in atherothrombosis that may cause impaired wound healing. Hyperglycaemia has also been shown to increase biofilm formation.

EXAMINER: The paper actually reported that IL-6 was more accurate than CRP or ESR rather than sensitive. The wound was oozy postoperatively but settled down. A large part of picking up periprosthetic infection is obtaining a good history and examination along with a high index of clinical suspicion.[2]

How useful is a hip aspiration in diagnosing infection?

CANDIDATE: Spangehl et al. (level 1) demonstrated a sensitivity of 0.86, a specificity of 0.94, a positive predictive value of 0.67 and a negative predictive value of 0.98 with initial image-guided aspiration in 180 patients undergoing revision hip arthroplasties.[3] They reported that aspiration alone is not sufficient for the diagnosis because of the risk of false positive and false negative results. They suggested that aspiration was not necessary in low-probability cases with a normal ESR and CRP. Aspiration would be indicated if pretest probability for infection was high (acute onset of pain, systemic illness, sinus formation), particularly if the CRP/ESR was normal, or in all cases where the CRP or ESR was high. A normal CRP and ESR does not always exclude a PJI, however.

EXAMINER: How would you perform a hip aspiration?

CANDIDATE: I would perform this in theatre under II control. I would fully prepare and drape the skin. I would incise the skin with a small nick to minimize the risk of skin contamination and also perform two separate aspirations to reduce the risk of false positives. If both are positive with the same organism this would be suggestive of infection.

EXAMINER: What about if one aspirate only is positive?

CANDIDATE: If only one aspirate is positive then it is a tricky situation. It is a soft positive result and I think it would be reasonable to repeat hip aspiration 2 weeks later.

EXAMINER: Joint aspiration did not grow any organisms after 48 h of culture. Is there anything else you may wish to consider in terms of establishing a diagnosis of a periprosthetic joint infection?

CANDIDATE: 48 h for bacterial culture may not be long enough to identify certain bacteria. For example, low-virulence organisms such as *Propionibacterium acnes* may take up to 2 weeks to culture successfully. I would speak to the microbiology lab and make sure they are performing extended cultures on the material sent.

EXAMINER: Isn't that normal for most labs to do?

CANDIDATE: My own local hospital policy is to perform extended culture for 5 days on any suspected PJI, but I am not sure if this has been universally agreed on. I would speak to the microbiology lab regardless to make sure I was notified promptly if extended culture grew any organism as this may significantly change my management plans. Synovial fluid culture has a sensitivity of 52% and specificity of 95%. Sensitivity at 52% is poor.

The differential white cell count from synovial fluid analysis is useful in diagnosing a PJI. For hips, a WCC > 4200/μl and/or a granulocyte percentage > 80% has a sensitivity of 85% and a specificity of 90%. I realize there are some difficulties getting the microbiology department to perform regular counts. Pus swabs are not regarded as useful anymore.

The Gram stain itself has a very low sensitivity (< 25%). Use of antibiotics prior to the aspiration of the hip joint can lead to reduced sensitivity of the synovial fluid analysis. Ideally, any antibiotics the patient is still on should be discontinued for up to 2 weeks in order to improve the pick-up rate of any synovial fluid culture.

There are modern biomarkers such as α-defensin (Synovasure, Zimmer Biomet), neutrophil elastase 2 (ELA2), bactericidal/permeability increasing protein, neutrophil gelatinase-associated lipocalin (NGAL) and lactoferrin which have recently shown promise in diagnosing PJI, but there are still no reliable data to prove their sensitivity and specificity to date.[4] One potential advantage of such biomarkers is the fact that they are not reliant on the bacteria and, therefore, pre-administered antibiotics should not affect their sensitivity. Synovial tissue biopsy can also be taken which can improve the sensitivity of microbiological culture and samples should also be sent for histology. A minimum of three tissue samples should be taken and ideally more than six samples.

Neutrophil granulocytes are indicators of bacterial infections (in acute infections). Leucocyte esterase has been shown as being as sensitive and specific as Synovasure and much more cost effective.

EXAMINER: What is α-defensin?

CANDIDATE: α-defensin is an antimicrobial peptide secreted by neutrophils to fight infection.

EXAMINER: Are there any other tests you might want to perform that could diagnose infection before going ahead with surgery?

CANDIDATE: The use of nuclear imaging (technetium-99 triple-phase bone scan, gallium imaging, labelled-leukocyte scans or FDG-PET imaging) for the detection of periprosthetic joint infection is worth considering but controversial. The AAOS clinical practice guidelines summary from 2010 reported a weak recommendation for their use.[5,6]

EXAMINER: How do you classify periprosthetic hip infection?

COMMENT: It may be enough just to mention the uncertainties with nuclear imaging or you may have to quantify your answer more fully. It is a judgement decision, but don't persist with your answer if the examiners want to move on. Technetium-99 bone scans are sensitive but not specific. Some investigators have found that a negative scan rules out infection, others report that a scan can occasionally be negative with infection if there is inadequate blood supply to the bone. A technetium-99m bone scan identifies areas of increased bone activity through preferential uptake of the diphosphonate by metabolically active bone. Increased uptake occurs with loosening, infection, heterotopic bone formation, Paget's disease, stress fractures, modulus mismatch of a large uncemented stem, neoplasm, reflex sympathetic dystrophy and other metabolic conditions. In the uncomplicated THA, uptake around the lesser trochanter and shaft is usually insignificant by 6 months, but in 10% of cases, uptake may persist at the greater trochanter, prosthesis tip and acetabulum for more than 2 years. The pattern of uptake has not been found to consistently reflect the presence or absence of infection. Gallium imaging likewise has a poor sensitivity and accuracy. The use of leukocyte scans is generally preferred, having a higher sensitivity (88–92%) and specificity (73–100%), but their usefulness for the diagnosis of infection

19

Table 3.1 MSIS Workgroup standard definition for PJI.

Musculoskeletal Infection Society (MSIS) diagnostic criteria		
Major criteria	**or**	**Minor criteria**
A sinus tract communicating with the prosthesis		Elevated ESR and CRP (ESR [30 mm/h; CRP [10 mg/l])
A pathogen is isolated by culture from two separate tissue or fluid samples obtained from the affected prosthetic joint		Elevated synovial fluid WBC count (3000 cells/l)
		Elevated synovial fluid neutrophil percentage (65%)
		Isolation of a microorganism in one periprosthetic tissue or fluid culture
		5 neutrophils per high-powered field in 5 high-power fields observed from histologic analysis of periprosthetic tissue at ×400 magnification

continues to be debated. FDG-PET is expensive and limited to a few institutions, and although very sensitive does not allow differentiation between an inflamed aseptically loosened prosthesis and an infected one.

CANDIDATE: Tsukayama *et al.* proposed a four-stage system consisting of early postoperative, late chronic, and acute hematogenous infections, and positive intraoperative cultures of specimens obtained during revision of a presumed aseptically loose THA.[7,8]

Early postoperative infection presents less than 1 month after surgery with a febrile patient and a red swollen discharging wound. With late postoperative infection, the patient is well, the wound has healed well, there is a worsening of hip pain and a never pain-free interval. Acute haematogenous infection can occur several years after surgery with a history of bacteraemia (UTI or other source of infection) and severe hip pain in a previously well-functioning hip. Positive intraoperative culture (at least three samples from different locations taken with clean instruments) occurs when a preoperative presumptive diagnosis of aseptic loosening was made.

McPherson *et al.* have also developed a staging system for periprosthetic hip infections that included three categories: infection type (acute versus chronic), the overall medical and immune health status of the patient, and the local extremity (wound) grade.[9]

EXAMINER: How do you diagnose PJI?

CANDIDATE: I would use the criteria of the musculoskeletal infection society. PJI can be diagnosed when one out of two major and four out of six minor criteria exist (Table 3.1).

Major criteria are (1) a sinus tract communicating with the prosthesis and (2) two positive periprosthetic cultures with phenotypically identical organisms.

A pathogen is isolated by culture from at least two separate tissue or fluid samples obtained from the affected prosthetic joint.

The six minor criteria are (1) elevated ESR and CRP, (2) elevated synovial leukocyte count, (3) elevated synovial neutrophil percentage (PMN%), (4) presence of purulence in the affected joint, (5) single positive culture, (6) positive histological analysis of periprosthetic tissue.

PJI may be present if fewer than four of these criteria are met.

COMMENT: The MSIS criteria were modified in 2013. Essentially three from five minor criteria (Table 3.1).

EXAMINER: How will you manage this patient assuming that your diagnosis of an acute PJI is now made?

CANDIDATE: As the diagnosis of a PJI has been made within 2 weeks and assuming that there are positive microbiological results with a known organism and sensitivities to antimicrobial therapy, there remains the option of undertaking a DAIR-type procedure. DAIR stands for Debridement, Antibiotics and Implant Retention, in which the prosthesis is retained with exchange of any mobile components such as a liner and head exchange while keeping the acetabular socket and stem in place. A DAIR should only be undertaken if the PJI is acute and ideally within 3 weeks of the PJI starting, although some units such as Oxford will undertake a DAIR at up to 6 weeks or so. The optimum management of a PJI involves a multidisciplinary team approach with MSK radiologists, bone infection microbiologists, histopathologists, plastic surgeons and experienced revision arthroplasty surgeons with a specialist interest in managing PJIs. The success rate of DAIR procedures is around 90–95%.[10] The Oxford group have recently published a case control study comparing DAIR versus a two-stage revision and showed a 98% 5-year survivorship rate with DAIR and better outcome with DAIR.[11]

EXAMINER: This patient had a delay in diagnosing the PJI and was only seen 2 months after the onset of their clinical presentation. How would you manage the patient now?

CANDIDATE: The patient is now outside the window of opportunity to undertake a DAIR. If there was a microbiological result with a known organism and sensitivities, then a single-stage revision could be undertaken, especially if the patient had multiple comorbidities and the surgical stress of having a two-stage procedure might compromise the patient. In this case, it is critical that all cement is removed as well as all the components and a thorough debridement with complete excision of infected soft tissues is undertaken.

EXAMINER: What are the prerequisites for a one-stage procedure?

CANDIDATE: Prerequisites include a known organism sensitive to antibiotics, no pus present, elderly patients or patients with multiple medical problems. It is also indicated in healthy individuals devoid of re-infection risk who have adequate bone and soft tissue for reconstruction and a low-virulence pathogen.

EXAMINER: What are the reported success rates for a single-stage revision?

CANDIDATE: Buchholz et al., who pioneered one-stage revisions at the Endo-Klinic in Hamburg, reported a success rate of 77% in 583 revisions, but only after extensive bone and soft-tissue resection, which compromised long-term function.[12] These results were published in 1981 and can be viewed as somewhat historic now. Raut et al. from Wrightington reported a success rate of 86% in 57 cases at average follow-up of 7 years despite many discharging sinuses.[13,14] Hanssen and Rand summarized the results of single-stage exchange and found a cumulative success rate of 83% when antibiotic-loaded cement was used, but only 60% when it was not.[15] A recent RCT has been started to compare a single- versus two-stage revision.[16] In 11 studies

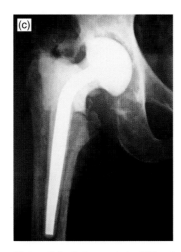

Figure 3.1c Anteroposterior (AP) radiograph of first-stage PROSTALAC spacer.

with 1225 patients with a hip PJI receiving exclusively one-stage revision, the rate of re-infection at 2 years was 8.6% (95% CI 4.5–13.9). After two-stage revision exclusively in 28 studies with 1188 patients, the rate of re-infection at 2 years was 10.2% (95% CI 7.7–12.9). The authors conclude that on the basis of a systematic review of published data, there is no difference in the re-infection rate between one-stage and two-stage revision THA for PJI.

EXAMINER: What are the advantages to performing a two-stage procedure?

CANDIDATE: It is particularly important to perform a two-stage revision with more severe infections or virulent organisms, as the success rate of a single-stage procedure is much less in these situations.

EXAMINER: That's not what I asked.

CANDIDATE: It is more versatile for reconstruction allowing the use of either cemented or cementless components and bone allograft in patients with severe bone loss. It allows clinical assessment of the response to antibiotics prior to re-implantation.

EXAMINER: What are the disadvantages of a two-stage procedure?

CANDIDATE: It can be difficult to nurse patients between stages and the second-stage surgery can be difficult due to soft-tissue scarring, limb shortening, disuse atrophy, loss of bone density and distortion of anatomy.

EXAMINER: Have a look at this radiograph below (see Figure 3.1c). What is going on with the right hip?

CANDIDATE: This is a cement spacer in a patient who has had a first-stage revision for infection and an articulating cement spacer such as a PROSTALAC spacer has been used. The potential complications of using such a spacer are that it can dislocate or fracture and it costs more money to perform a two-stage procedure. An alternative would be to use a nail or multiple wires with cement coating around the wires to act as a temporary spacer. There is also the option of loosely cementing a THA in place (using a polished tapered stem and cementing a liner for the socket) ((The "Kiwi" Prostalac)) which has the advantage of allowing the patient to mobilize full weight bearing postoperatively and, if necessary, the THA spacer could be left in more permanently if the patient's medical condition precludes further surgery or the patient decided against second-stage revision.

EXAMINER: So, you perform the first-stage revision, how long will you keep the patient on antibiotics?

CANDIDATE: The duration of antibiotic treatment and timing between stages remains controversial. Current practice suggests delaying the second stage for at least 6 weeks pending good clinical progress with antibiotics and wound healing. A number of surgeons re-implant at 3 months, treating the patient with 6 weeks antibiotics and then a further 6 weeks without antibiotics, regularly monitoring the CRP/ESR for any signs of elevation and checking clinical progress for any signs of reoccurrence of infection such as sinus discharge or increasing hip pain. Antimicrobial therapy will be guided by the microbiology advice given and this is why the management of PJI is best undertaken as part of an MDT review. In general, however, 2 weeks of targeted intravenous antibiotics followed by a further 4 weeks or so of oral antibiotics is the norm.

EXAMINER: Five of my last six THAs have become infected. What should I do?

CANDIDATE: Stop operating and investigate. I would undertake a root-cause analysis to identify the source or cause of these infections.

EXAMINER: Go on.

CANDIDATE: I would want to know if the same organism had been identified in the five cases, particularly if the organism was *Staphylococcus aureus* as this may suggest a nasal carrier in theatre. Nasal swab cultures would need to be taken of relevant theatre staff and appropriate treatment started.

We would want to investigate for a breakdown in theatre sterility. I would involve microbiology and investigate the laminar flow system to see if it was correctly working.

There may be issues with the preparation of the instruments set such as packaging integrity and expiry date. A sterilization indicator should be present, and the packaging must be dry.

There may be a breakdown in the precautions that must be taken by the scrub practitioner during the procedure, such as the sterile field not being constantly observed and too much movement around the sterile field, including the opening and closing of doors and a wide space not being observed between scrubbed staff.

Taylor *et al.* showed that sets opened outside the confines of the laminar hood have significantly higher colony-forming unit (CFU) counts during and after surgery.[17] Very few centres follow Sir John Charnley's technique of opening the instrument sets under the canopy at each stage of the operation.

Madhavan's paper from Bristol in the *Annals of the Royal College of Surgeons England* specifically looked at breakdown in theatre discipline during total joint replacement.[18] They noted that slackness had crept into the theatre protocol, such as corridor from changing room to theatre and theatre personnel attire.

EXAMINER: Screening has shown that you, the surgeon, were found to be a *Staphylococcus aureus* nasal carrier. You have been treated with decolonization and are now clear. Would you mention this to your patients when you are listing them for joint arthroplasty?

CANDIDATE: Yes.

EXAMINER: Are you sure?

CANDIDATE: Yes, patients should be informed that I was a nasal carrier at the time of listing for surgery.

EXAMINER: Are you absolutely sure?

CANDIDATE: Yes, patients need to be told to make sure they are happy.

COMMENT: Wrong answer. It is not expected that a surgeon informs patients when he/she is listing them for surgery that they were previous nasal carriers but have been successfully treated and are now clear.

EXAMINER: Do you know any papers that have looked at theatre sterility?

CANDIDATE: The classic paper on theatre sterility was published by Lidwell *et al.* in 1982.[19] This was an MRC randomized study which showed a decrease in infection rates following joint replacements carried out in ultraclean theatres.

The deep infection rate was 3.4% in conventional theatres, 1.7% with ultraclean air and body exhaust and 0.2% when this was combined with prophylactic antibiotics.

EXAMINER: That's fine. Let's move on.

Reading list

Focus on *BJJ* 2012:

One stage exchange arthroplasty: the devil is in the detail

D. Kendoff; T. Gehrke

ENDO-Klinik Hamburg

Structured oral examination question 2

EXAMINER: This is an AP radiograph of a 52-year-old female who presents to your clinic with non-specific right hip pain. She had a right metal-on-metal hip resurfacing procedure performed 3 years ago (Figure 3.2a).

CANDIDATE: The AP radiograph demonstrates a higher abduction angle (lateral opening) than normal. The current recommendations are for an acetabular abduction angle of 40°. Several studies have demonstrated the importance of optimal cup positioning with regard to wear, metal ion levels and the revision rate. High cup angle has been consistently reported to lead to greater wear and higher serum metal ion levels. The head size appears small; the current recommendations are that unless a minimum 46-mm head size can be used the procedure should not be performed because of the risks of ALVAL and pseudotumours. There is no

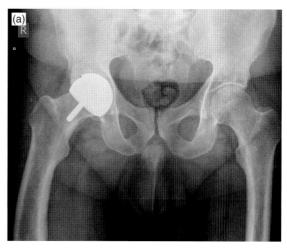

Figure 3.2a Anteroposterior (AP) radiograph right MoM hip resurfacing implant.

radiolucency about the metaphyseal stem, no obvious narrowing of the neck and no divot sign.

EXAMINER: What do you mean by a divot sign?[20]

CANDIDATE: A divot sign is a depression in the neck contour just below the junction with the femoral component often associated with a reactive exostosis. It is believed to be caused by repetitive bone to component abutment due to impingement.

EXAMINER: What is a pseudotumour and what is the difference between ALVAL and pseudotumour?

CANDIDATE: ALVAL (aseptic lymphocyte-dominated vasculitis-associated lesion) is a histological diagnosis caused by metal particulate debris. Patients present with localized hip pain and a localized osteolytic reaction. A more severe inflammatory reaction is termed a pseudotumour. This is diagnosed on an MRI scan. The umbrella term 'adverse reactions to metal debris' (ARMD) is now preferred to cover a wide spectrum of destructive involvement including metallosis, pseudotumours and ALVAL.

COMMENT: Pseudotumour, aseptic lymphocytic vasculitis-associated lesions (ALVAL) and metallosis are terms often used interchangeably to describe the same process. In June 2008, the NJR first introduced the term ARMD for surgeons to select as an indication for revision surgery, given ARMD is

23

Table 3.2 MHRA management recommendations for patients with metal-on-metal hip replacements.

	Hip resurfacing (no stem): - Female - Male (femoral head diameter ≤ 48 mm) - All DePuy ASR hip resurfacing devices **Stemmed total hip replacement (THR):** - Femoral head diameter > 36 mm	**Hip resurfacing (no stem):** - Male (femoral head diameter > 48 mm) **Stemmed total hip replacement (THR):** - Femoral head diameter < 36 mm		
Device implanted				
Patient and device group	Symptomatic and asymptomatic	**Symptomatic**	**Asymptomatic** • All stemmed THR • Resurfacing devices without 10A ODEP rating	Resurfacing devices with 10A ODEP rating
Frequency of follow-up after primary operation date	Annually while the device remains implanted	Annually while the device remains implanted	Annually for the first 5 years, 2-yearly to 10 years and 3-yearly thereafter	First year, once at 7 years and 3-yearly thereafter
Questionnaire	Oxford Hip Score assessment	Oxford Hip Score assessment	Oxford Hip Score assessment	Oxford Hip Score assessment
Imaging	• MARS MRI or ultrasound recommended if negative change in Oxford Hip Score is observed and/or elevated/rising blood metal levels	• MARS MRI or ultrasound in all cases	• Plain radiographs • MARS MRI or ultrasound recommended if negative change in Oxford Hip Score is observed and/or elevated/rising blood metal levels	• Plain radiographs • MARS MRI or ultrasound recommended if negative change in Oxford Hip Score is observed and/or elevated/rising blood metal levels
Blood metal level test	All patients	All patients	All patients	All patients
Consider need for revision	If imaging is abnormal and/or blood metal levels rising, and/or hip-related clinical function/Oxford Hip Score deteriorating	If imaging is abnormal and/or blood metal levels rising, and/or hip-related clinical function/Oxford Hip Score deteriorating	If imaging is abnormal and/or blood metal levels rising, and/or hip-related clinical function/Oxford Hip Score deteriorating	If imaging is abnormal and/or blood metal levels rising, and/or hip-related clinical function/Oxford Hip Score deteriorating

Whole blood should be used to test for cobalt and chromium metal levels.

considered the most inclusive term for these abnormal reactions.

CANDIDATE: Several studies have described an association between pseudotumours and increased wear of retrieved components. Influencing factors include implant size and implant design (clearance and cover [arc angle]). In addition, acetabular component positioning and femoral head–neck offset influence the risk of impingement and edge loading usually associated with high wear rates.

Despite this, Campbell *et al.* reported that in 32 THA revised due to pseudotumour several patients demonstrated minimum wear features, suggesting a hypersensitivity cause.[21]

Therefore, the origin of pseudotumours is probably multifactorial caused either by excessive wear, metal hypersensitivity, a combination of the two, or an as yet unknown cause. Pseudotumour-like reactions have also been reported in non-metal-on-metal bearings. In these cases, the histological findings showed accumulations of macrophages and giant cells again suggesting an excessive wear origin.

EXAMINER: What are the risk factors for pseudotumours?

CANDIDATE: Significant risk factors for the development of pseudotumour include female sex, age less than 40 years, small component size, hip dysplasia and specific implant designs (ASR).

EXAMINER: How are you going to investigate this patient?

CANDIDATE: A careful history and examination of the patient is required. It is crucial to determine if the pain is arising from intrinsic (indicating hip pathology) or extrinsic sources (referred pain).

Extrinsic sources would include referred pain from the spine or pelvis, peripheral vascular disease, stress fracture, tendinitis or bursitis about the hip.

Intrinsic causes include aseptic loosening, avascular necrosis, infection. (Long pause.)

EXAMINER: What are the latest Medicines and Healthcare Products Regulatory Agency (MHRA) recommendations (2017) (Prompt)? (Table 3.2.)

CANDIDATE: In essence, the latest MHRA guidelines with input from the BHS and BOA risk stratifies patients into high-risk and low-risk groups based on patient factors, device implanted and whether they are symptomatic. Having an ASR hip is automatically high-risk and therefore patients should have annual surveillance together with cobalt and chromium levels, MARS MRI and OHS. On the other hand, a Birmingham hip resurfacing, which is an ODEP 10A device, in patients who are asymptomatic, should be followed-up in the first year, at 7 years and then every 3 years after that. Stemmed large MoM devices are higher risk than resurfacing hips and therefore the follow-up guidance is different, and these patients require closer review.

EXAMINER: Anything else?

CANDIDATE: I am not sure.

EXAMINER: ALVAL may occur in both asymptomatic and symptomatic patients and early detection should give a better revision outcome if this is necessary. Essentially all MoM/resurfacing hips require some sort of clinical follow-up for life and should not be discharged even if well functioning.

COMMENT: Additional clinic slots are required for follow-up of MoM hip patients and this can be a significant burden on resources. Interferes with new/follow-up ratios.

EXAMINER: This is the MRI scan obtained. What does it show? (Figure 3.2b and 3.2c.)

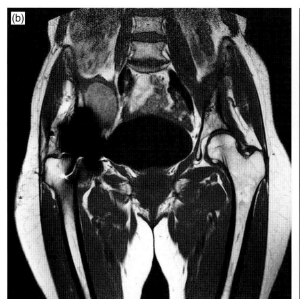

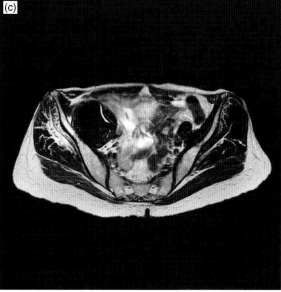

Figure 3.2b and c T1 coronal and transverse MRI of right MoM hip resurfacing implant demonstrating ALVAL mass.

25

CANDIDATE: The MRI is a T2-weighted image coronal view, which demonstrates an intra-pelvic mass.

EXAMINER: This was a pseudotumour. In fact, the mass could be felt clinically when examining the abdomen.

What are you going to do?

CANDIDATE: This patient requires urgent revision surgery to the hip.

EXAMINER: She is very scared of surgery and would prefer to avoid it.

CANDIDATE: I would stress the importance of early revision surgery as the longer the MoM resurfacing implant is left in place the more extensive the soft-tissue destruction will likely be.

EXAMINER: What are the principles of surgery for pseudotumours?

CANDIDATE: The pseudotumour needs to be managed with aggressive debridement of all involved soft tissue. It is important to do a thorough debridement of the abnormal tissue similar to the treatment of infection. The surgery should be performed by an experienced hip surgeon.

Although she is still relatively young I would use a metal and PE bearing surface. I would want to use first- or second-generation highly cross-linked PE. A ceramic bearing surface has the potential for catastrophic fracture. We are already revising for a rare complication and we don't want anything to go wrong again. However, I would use an uncemented implant. I would keep the option of using a dual mobility acetabular cup as the soft tissues may be so poorly compromised that the hip is unstable. Another possibility is to use a constrained cup if the hip is unstable with significant abductor muscle destruction, but I would prefer to avoid using this implant if possible as components will loosen early in this situation.

It would be sensible to get a second opinion from an experienced hip surgeon as per British Hip Society guidelines to confirm and support the appropriateness of my management plan. In my region, all revision arthroplasty cases are discussed as part of a revision clinical network involving several hospitals within a geographical region. I would certainly ensure that this case is discussed with other colleagues within the revision network meeting.

EXAMINER: What is the evidence that highly cross-linked PE improves clinical outcomes?

CANDIDATE: There was a double-blinded study from New Zealand (level 1 evidence) recently published in the American JBJS edition comparing HXLPE to conventional PE. HXLPE liners had significantly reduced wear present and were associated with a greater implant survival rate at 10 years compared to conventional UHMWPE liners.[22]

EXAMINER: Why did surgeons bother with MoM hip resurfacing procedures? The old Charnley cemented hip replacement with trochanteric osteotomy worked equally as well with excellent long-term results reported from the surgeons at Wrightington.

CANDIDATE: The perceived advantages of MoM hip resurfacings included better restoration of hip biomechanics, improved proprioceptive feedback, improved wear characteristics with no PE-induced osteolysis, increased levels of postsurgical activity, greater range of movement, reduced risk of dislocation, improved femoral bone stock mass because the neck and most of the head are retained and ease of conversion to a THA if the implant should fail.

EXAMINER: What are the contraindications for resurfacing?

CANDIDATE: These include severe osteoporosis, insufficient bone stock in the femoral head, large cysts at the femoral neck or head, a narrow femoral neck, notching of the femoral neck, extensive ON and severe obesity (BMI > 35 kg/m^2).

Other contraindications include a history of chronic renal disease, metal hypersensitivity, those with anatomical abnormalities in the acetabulum or proximal femur and certainly caution in women of childbearing age.

EXAMINER: Is resurfacing contraindicated in women of childbearing age?

CANDIDATE: No, although most surgeons would now avoid a resurfacing procedure in a female regardless of whether they were of childbearing age.

EXAMINER: Is there a role for resurfacing at all?

CANDIDATE: Data from the latest NJR annual report showed that less than 1% of all hip replacements were resurfacings. There may be a role for this implant to be used in young male individuals who are likely to trash their hip.

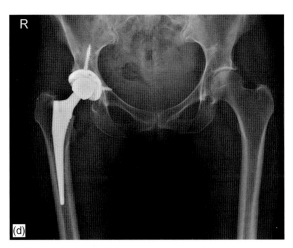

Figure 3.2d Anteroposterior (AP) radiograph of revised hip demonstrating uncemented THA with screw fixation acetabulum.

EXAMINER: What do you mean by trashing your hip?

CANDIDATE: A patient who has to do very heavy manual work as part of his job or who just wants to play football or rugby regardless.

COMMENT: Candidates should mention that:
- Nowadays very few resurfacing hips are performed (< 1% NJR data 14th report 2017).
- Although they are not contraindicated they would generally only be indicated in a very small, select number of individuals.
- Surgery should ideally be performed by a specialized hip resurfacing surgeon.[23]
- Cases should ideally be discussed with hip colleagues and a consensus view reached as to whether to proceed with resurfacing.

Candidates should be able to discuss:
- The poorly performing implants (ASR) and subgroups of patients at risk for ARMD (female sex, age < 40 years, small component size, malpositioning of the acetabular component, hip dysplasia, known nickel allergy).
- Complications of MoM hips.
- A follow-up clinic protocol.

Large MoM jumbo hip replacements are now contraindicated as a primary procedure due to metal wear and corrosion at the trunnion.

EXAMINER: These are her postoperative radiographs (Figure 3.2d). We kept her non-weight bearing for 6 weeks as there was quite an extensive anterior wall defect in the acetabulum, but she has done very well. The hip pain has settled, and the abdominal mass resolved. We were very lucky as the extensive soft-tissue destruction that sometimes can be seen with this condition was absent[24].

EXAMINER: What are the outcomes of hip resurfacing compared to conventional THA?

CANDIDATE: Several recent studies report identical Harris hip scores but a greater percentage of patients with resurfacing involved in high-demand activities. There is a higher revision rate in hip resurfacing compared to conventional THA.[25]

EXAMINER: What factors are associated with higher revision rates for hip resurfacing procedures?

CANDIDATE: These would include ON (relative contraindication), hip dysplasia (technically difficult, more suitable reconstructive options available), female sex, inflammatory arthritis (relative contraindication), increased age (deteriorating bone quality), a small femoral implant and specific implant designs (ASR).

COMMENT: Causes of revision primary hip resurfacing procedure include fracture (39%), loosening/lysis 29%, infection 9%, ARMD (6%), pain (5%), dislocation (3%), other (8%). Australian Joint Registry 1999–2008.

COMMENT: MoM hips are still a hot topic, but viva themes would be more about how to manage ARMD, when to revise and clinic follow-up protocol. Resurfacing is rarely performed these days (< 1%), so the safest option is not to mention this as a possible arthroplasty option unless specifically brought into the discussion by the examiners.

Structured oral examination question 3

EXAMINER: This is an AP radiograph of a 78-year-old man presenting with increasing right hip pain. He had a THA performed 17 years ago (Figure 3.3a).

CANDIDATE: The AP radiograph demonstrates severe osteolysis of both femoral and acetabular components. There are radiolucent lines at the bone cement interface located circumferentially around all three Dee and Charnley zones in the acetabulum. The femoral component has separated from the femoral cement with lucencies in all seven Gruen zones.

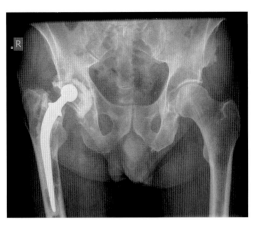

Figure 3.3a Anteroposterior (AP) radiograph of loose cemented right THA.

I am unfamiliar with the type of implant used for the femur. On the radiograph shown i can not determine if a cement plug has been used or not.

COMMENT: Score 6 candidates should ideally be able to recognize a Charnley and Exeter stem. Score 7 candidates should recognize a Stanmore prosthesis (banana-shaped). Score 8 candidates should be able to weave in somewhere in the discussion that when revising a Stanmore prosthesis, it is particularly important due to its banana shape to clear the shoulder of the prosthesis removing any cement or bone overhanging the proximal aspect of the greater trochanter. Otherwise stem removal will be obstructed and/or difficult or a greater trochanter fracture will occur.

EXAMINER: What are the different generations of cementing techniques?

CANDIDATE: First-generation cementing techniques involved hand-mixing of cement and finger packing of bone cement in the doughy phase into an unplugged, unwashed femoral canal. Clinical results with first-generation cementing have been variable and in general have produced some disappointing results due to the inability to produce a consistent cement mantle.

Second-generation technique involved plugging the medullary canal, cleaning the canal with pulsed lavage and inserting cement in a retrograde manner using a cement gun. This reduced the incidence of gross voids and filling defects in the mantle.

EXAMINER: Are you sure pulsed lavage was used?

CANDIDATE: Yes.

COMMENT: Take the hint that your answer may be wrong. Second-generation technique involves essentially using a gun and bone plug (restrictor) and nothing else. The bone is thoroughly cleaned before cement insertion but not pulsed lavage.

EXAMINER: What else?

CANDIDATE: Third-generation techniques involved porosity reduction via vacuum mixing or centrifugation and cement pressurization.

Fourth-generation cementing techniques include stem centralization both proximally and distally to ensure an adequate and symmetrical cement mantle. This is important as uneven and excessively thin cement mantles are associated with early failure and revision.

COMMENT: Distal centralizers are often included as a third generation technique. Some books list only 3 generations of cementing techniques omitting the fourth.

EXAMINER: How is cementing technique graded?

CANDIDATE: The quality of the cement mantle has been described by Harris and Barrack using a scale of A to D.[26]

Complete filling of the medullary cavity by cement, a so-called 'white-out' at the cement–bone interface, is graded 'A'. Slight radiolucency of the cement–bone interface was defined as 'B'. Radiolucency involving 50–99% of the cement–bone interface or a defective or incomplete cement mantle was graded 'C'. Grade 'C2' was given to a defect where the tip of the stem abuts the cortex with no intervening cement. Radiolucency at the cement–bone interface of 100% in any projection, or a failure to fill the canal with cement such that the tip of the stem was not covered, was classified 'D'.

EXAMINER: What are you going to do?

CANDIDATE: I would want to take a full history from the patient. I would enquire about pain.

I would also want to exclude the possibility of infection (septic loosening) and would ask about problems with the hip postoperatively such as wound infection requiring washout or a prolonged course of antibiotics. A history of fever, chills or a sinus tract suggests infection. Night pain, rest pain or constant pain would also suggest infection.

With aseptic loosening typically, the pain is aggravated by weight bearing. Pain is significant with the first few steps of walking (start-up pain) which improves slightly with further walking, only to worsen again with further walking. The pain is always improved with rest and rarely constant.

With aseptic loosening of a THA examination may reveal shortening of the affected limb, an antalgic gait and a Trendelenberg positive test is usually present. Pain at the extremes of movement suggest loosening.

It is important to exclude other causes of local extrinsic hip pain such as trochanteric bursitis, tendinitis or impingement. Extrinsic remote sources of hip pain should also be excluded, particularly the lumbar spine, especially if the pain has neurogenic features such as radiation below the knee, numbness, paraesthesia or dysesthesias. Pulses and skin temperature should be checked to rule out a vascular cause for pain.

EXAMINER: Assume there is no infection in the hip and referred causes of pain have been ruled out. What are you going to do?

CANDIDATE: I would assess the patient. Find out how bad the pain is and whether the hip should be revised or whether symptoms are manageable, and the patient can be reviewed regularly at the orthopaedic follow-up clinic. Based on the current radiographic appearances I would have some concerns with the natural progression of the condition and the possibility of catastrophic periprosthetic fracture occurring.

EXAMINER: The patient can only walk about 200 yards before severe pain.

CANDIDATE: I would offer him revision hip surgery provided comorbidity issues have been optimized and the risks of surgery had been discussed and understood. Both components would need to be revised.

EXAMINER: What are the complications that you would need to mention to the patient when consenting for surgery?

CANDIDATE: I would mention
- Infection.
- Dislocation. Usually component malpositioning or laxity of soft tissues around the hip.

Table 3.3 AAOS classification system for femoral defects.

I Segmental defect
- proximal (partial or complete)
- intercalary
- greater trochanter

II Cavitary defect
- cancellous
- cortical
- ectasia (dilatation)

III Combined segmental and cavity defect

IV Malalignment
- rotational
- angular

V Femoral stenosis

VI Femoral discontinuity

- Fracture/perforation femoral shaft.
- Nerve palsy (peroneal, sciatic, femoral) 2–7%.
- Vascular injury (femoral, iliac, obturator).
- Leg-length discrepancy.
- Heterotopic ossification.
- Death (cardiac/pulmonary).
- DVT/PE.

In addition, the patient has significant bone loss on both the femoral and acetabular side, so I would plan to use donor femoral head allograft to attempt to restore bone stock. An ETO is helpful if there is a large amount of cement to remove distally but will increase operating time and blood loss. An osteotomy site can also go on to either malunion or non-union. I would prefer to avoid its use in this particular case.

I would warn him that he might need a period of partial weight bearing if there were concerns with initial implant stability due to excessive osteolysis and bone loss.

EXAMINER: You mentioned about the bone loss. How do you plan for this?

CANDIDATE: Bone loss can be classified on the femoral side by using either the AAOS (Table 3.3) or the Paprosky classification system (Table 3.4).

The Paprosky classification evaluates the femoral diaphysis for its ability to support an uncemented, fully porous coated prosthesis. It is less detailed than the AAOS classification but is more useful in decision making if an uncemented revision is to be performed.

Table 3.4 Paprosky classification system for femoral defects.

I Minimal metaphyseal cancellous bone loss with normal intact diaphysis

Type I defects are seen after removal of uncemented component without biological ingrowth on surface. Usually seen with Austin Moore type prosthesis or resurfacing procedures. The diaphysis and metaphysis are intact and there is partial loss of the calcar and anteroposterior (AP) bone stock

II Extensive metaphyseal cancellous bone loss with normal intact diaphysis

Often seen after removal of cemented prosthesis. Calcar deficiency and major AP bone loss

IIIA Metaphysis severely damaged with > 4 cm diaphyseal bone for distal fixation

• Grossly loose femoral component

• First-generation cementing techniques

IIIB Metaphysis severely damaged with < 4 cm diaphyseal bone for distal fixation

Type IIIB defects extend slightly further than Type IIIA; however, reliable fixation can be achieved just past the isthmus of the femur

• Cemented with cement restrictor

• Uncemented with substantial distal osteolysis

IV Extensive metaphyseal and diaphyseal bone loss/isthmus non-supportive

Extensive defect with severe metaphyseal and diaphyseal bone loss and a widened canal that cannot provide adequate fixation for a long stem

Acetabular bone loss

Acetabular defect classification systems are used to predict the extent of intraoperative bone loss and guide reconstructive options.

Several classification systems exist; the three most commonly used are the American Academy of Orthopaedic Surgeons (AAOS) system (Table 3.5), the Gross and associates system (Table 3.6) and the Paprosky classification system (Table 3.7).

Gross and associates classification system (Table 3.6)

This classification is based on the nature of the bone graft needed for reconstruction determined on standard preoperative AP and lateral radiographs. A bone defect is considered uncontained if morselized bone graft cannot be used to fill the defect.

Paprosky acetabular bone loss classification

This classification is based on information that can be obtained from AP radiographs. Four radiographic criteria are assessed:

1. **Superior migration of the hip centre**
   • Indicates damage to anterior and posterior columns
   • Supero-medial indicates greater damage to anterior column

Table 3.5 AAOS classification system for acetabular defects.

Type I Segmental defects

Peripheral – superior/anterior/posterior

Central – medial wall absent

Type II Cavitary defects

Peripheral – superior/anterior/posterior

Central – medial wall intact

Type III Combined segmental and cavitary bone loss

Type IV Pelvic discontinuity

Separation of anterior and posterior columns

Type V Arthrodesis

Table 3.6 Gross and associates classification system.

Type	Description
I	No substantial loss of bone stock
II	Contained loss of bone stock (columns and/or rim intact)
III	Uncontained loss of bone stock (< 50% acetabulum)
IV	Uncontained loss of bone stock (> 50% acetabulum)
V	Contained loss of bone stock with pelvic discontinuity

Table 3.7 Paprosky classification of acetabular bone defects.

Type	Radiographic finding	Intraoperative finding	Trial stability
I Minimum bone loss	No cup migration No substantial bone loss	Intact rim and no distortion. No major osteolysis. Bone loss minimal Small focal areas contained bone loss Columns intact	Full
II Anterior and posterior columns intact and supportive Migration less than 2 cm supcromedially or laterally Minimal ischial lysis Minimal tardrop lysis			
IIA Cavitary defect medial to a thinned superior rim	Superior (or superomedial) migration of < 2 cm Up and in	Superomedial bone loss but intact superior rim (contained cavity)	Full
IIB Superior acetabular rim is missing	Superior (or superolateral) migration of < 2 cm Up and out	Uncontained superior rim defect < 1/3	Full
IIC	Straight medial wall defect Cup medial to Kohler line Teardrop may be obliterated Protrusio	Uncontained medial wall defect Rim intact and rim columns supportive	Full
III Columns non-supportive			
IIIA	Superolateral cup migration > 3 cm Up and out Moderate ischial lysis Partial teardrop destruction Kohler line intact	Unsupportive dome Columns intact Host–bone contact of 40–60%	Partial
IIIB	Superomedial migration > 3 cm Up and in Severe ischial destruction Teardrop loss Migration medial to Kohler line	Risk of pelvic discontinuity Bone contact of < 40% Rim defect of > 50%	None

- Supero-lateral indicates greater damage to posterior column

2. **Ischial osteolysis**
   - Bone loss inferior posterior column and posterior column

3. **Teardrop osteolysis**
   - Inferior anterior column and medial wall

4. **Position of the implant relative to Kohler's line**
   - Deficiency of anterior column and/or medial wall deficiency

A trial component with full inherent stability does not change position when the surgeon pushes its rim or performs a trial reduction. A trial component with partial inherent stability does not change position with removal of the inserter, but does not withstand the force of pushing on the rim or performance of a trial reduction. A trial component with no inherent stability changes position with the simple act of removing the inserter.

The Paprosky classification (Table 3.7) is often used clinically in preference to the AAOS classification as it not only predicts bone loss encountered intraoperatively, but also assists in determining reconstructive options.

EXAMINER: How would you plan for surgery?

CANDIDATE:
- I would counsel the patient regarding the natural history of the condition and recommend revision is undertaken on an urgent basis as the situation is likely to deteriorate and may lead to catastrophic periprostatic fracture.

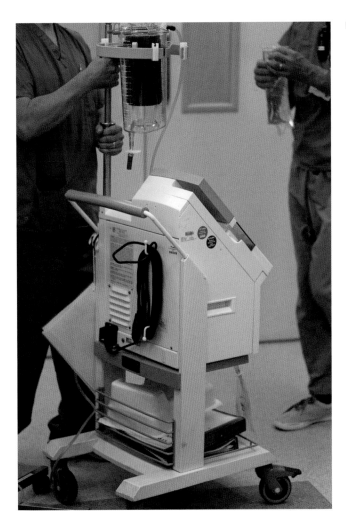

Figure 3.3b Cell saver.

- I would get an anaesthetic review to make sure the patient was fit enough for surgery, the risks acceptable and also so they could order any special tests such as echocardiogram or pulmonary function tests if required.
- I would cross-match for 4 units and make sure the cell saver(Figure 3.3b) was available.
- I will give tranexamic acid at the time of induction.

EXAMINER: What dose of tranexamic acid?

CANDIDATE: 1 g IV and if needed a further dose of 1 g IV at closure.

- I would order one femoral head frozen allograft and have freeze-dried allograft available if required.
- I would liaise with my anaesthetic colleagues in case an HDU bed was needed postoperatively.

- I would obtain the original operative notes to check what surgical approach was used and which implants were inserted.
- I would make sure the company rep is available at the time of surgery.
- I would ask the theatre coordinator to make sure there was an appropriate skill mix and experience in theatre on the scrub side to deal with complicated revision hip cases.
- I would ideally make sure the case wasn't performed at the weekend when fewer staff are generally available or last case on a Friday with the possibility of a long theatre overrun.[27]
- I would need to make sure the implant removal kit would include curved and straight osteotomies for the cemented cup and femur, ultrasonic tools, high-speed burrs, rongeurs, cement splitters, reverse hooks, drills and Dall miles cabling system.

- I would need a flexible light source for visualizing the medullary canal of the femur.
- I would prefer to use uncemented components if possible if previously cement was used for fixation. The femoral bone surface after cement removal is often sclerotic, hard and resistant to cement interdigitation. I would also hesitate to use cement as long-term results in revision cases can be poor.
- I would plan to use a long-stem uncemented modular tapered fluted revision femoral implant, aiming for a good scratch fit distally. If this could not be achieved, I would use a long-stem uncemented implant with a distal interlocking screw option.

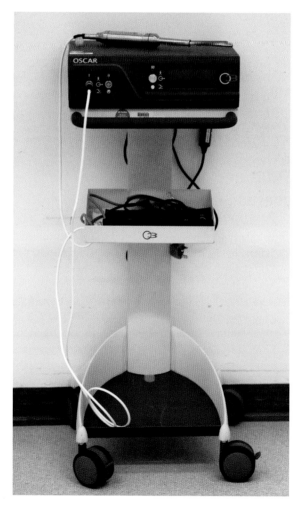

Figure 3.3c OSCAR system.

- I would use a multihole TM revision acetabular shell and a metal on polyethylene bearing surface. I would attempt to use at least a 32-mm head but preferably a 36-mm head, as this will significantly reduce the risk of postoperative dislocation.
- I would prefer to use a posterior approach, incorporating the old incision into this if possible.
- If the risk of dislocation was deemed very high I would consider using an anterolateral approach or more preferably a posterior approach but with the use of a dual-motion acetabular cup.

COMMENT: 'I would' is what YOU would do. It is probably the most appropriate turn of phrase to use for the exam.

CANDIDATE: I would clear soft tissue and overhanging cement away from the proximal femur to expose the proximal edge of the bone–cement interface.

Flexible osteotomes and a small burr can then be used to further disrupt the cement/implant interface.

An ETO would simplify implant and cement removal, but as mentioned, in this particular situation I would prefer to avoid it.

I would use cement splitters to remove cement along with ultrasonic tools. Cement is split radially and longitudinally and then removed.

OSCAR (Figure 3.3c) (or a similar ultrasonic cement removal system) is useful for getting through a distal cement plug. A combination of sharp cement splitters, cement osteotomes (straight and curved), a Midas Rex high-speed burr, ultrasonic tools and patience is the key to removing the cement mantle. I would be careful about losing cement down the femoral canal and the use of mastoids down the canal can be helpful. I would avoid levering the cement out as this risks an iatrogenic fracture, especially around the greater trochanteric region.

EXAMINER: What about the acetabular component, if it's cemented?

CANDIDATE: The safest way is to disrupt the PE cup from the cement using curved gouges. This prevents inadvertent damage to the bone of the acetabulum bed. After removal of the cup the cement is removed piecemeal. Sometimes a threaded acetabular extractor can be used, threading into a drilled hole until its metal plate is flush with the rim of the acetabular component. The extractor is then toggled to disrupt the

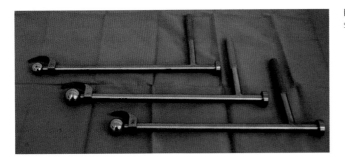

Figure 3.3d Explant (Innomed) acetabular cup removal system.

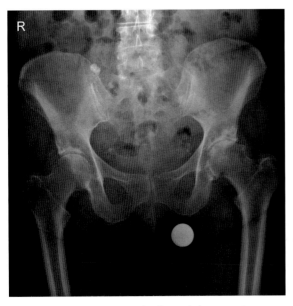

Figure 3.4 Anteroposterior (AP) radiograph demonstrating severe osteoarthritis left hip.

fixation interface and allow removal of the component. High-speed burrs are sometimes needed to debulk cement within acetabular anchoring holes.

EXAMINER: And if the socket is uncemented?

CANDIDATE: The order of removal is component liner removal then screw removal (if there are supplementary screws) and finally metal shell removal. If the liner is polyethylene, then drilling into the centre of the liner followed by inserting a screw into the liner hole will usually lift off the liner.

If the liner is ceramic, then the principle is first to disengage the smooth taper lock by a sharp tap into the liner. This is followed by the use of a suction cup with its attached three scallops that contact the peripheral rim of the metal acetabular

to remove the liner. Different implants will have their own extraction devices, so it is critical to know all about the implant one is revising and to ensure that the relevant and appropriate kit is available. That is why it is important to have a good system in place whereby old medical records can be easily retrieved to look over well in advance of surgery.

Removing any supplementary screws can be challenging and I would always have the Timex broken screw set available as well as a burr in case the screw heads are gone. Finally, to remove the metal-backed shell, the essential tool required here is the Explant (Figure 3.3d). This has been revolutionary in making the removal of an uncemented acetabular shell easier.

Structured oral examination question 4

EXAMINER: These are the radiographs of a 78-year-old lady who has been referred to the orthopaedic clinic by her GP because of increasing pain in her right hip. Would you care to comment on the radiographs? (Figure 3.4)

CANDIDATE: This is an AP radiograph, demonstrating lower lumbar vertebrae, both hips and proximal femur. The most obvious features in the right hip are loss of joint space, osteophytes, sclerosis and bone cysts. The radiographic features are highly suggestive of osteoarthritis (OA) of the hip.

EXAMINER: How is osteoarthritis classified?

CANDIDATE: OA is classified into primary OA when an obvious cause can be identified, and secondary OA caused by such conditions as osteonecrosis (ON), DDH, posttraumatic, Paget's disease, slipped capital femoral epiphysis, protrusio acetabuli, and Perthes disease.

EXAMINER: What are the percentages of each type of OA?

CANDIDATE: Various studies have suggested that almost 90% of cases of OA are secondary.

EXAMINER: How are you going to manage this patient?

CANDIDATE: I would take a full history and examination from the patient. Specifically, I would want to know the location of pain and exclude referred pain from the spine. Hip pain is classically located in the buttock or groin radiating to the knee. Pain radiating below the knee to the foot is strongly suggestive of radicular-type pain from the spine. I would inquire whether the patient had difficulty putting shoes and socks on, tying shoe laces, bending to pick up an object from the floor, getting in and out of a car, [Examiner interrupts]

EXAMINER: The patient struggles to walk a quarter of a mile. She has typical symptoms of advanced OA. What are you going to do?

CANDIDATE: Assuming that all conservative options had been tried and have been unsuccessful I would offer her THA.

EXAMINER: What type of hip arthroplasty would YOU perform?

CANDIDATE: I would use a cemented Exeter THA.

EXAMINER: Why this particular implant?

CANDIDATE: The Exeter THA has excellent peer-reviewed long-term data. It is an implant that I am very comfortable using, I have been trained to use this implant by my consultants, the instrumentation is straightforward and simple to use, the neck cut is not critical, and the introducer allows for even pressure when inserting the implant.

This hip system provides me with the ability to deal with anatomical variants and to recreate offset and leg length and gives me a choice of bearing surfaces and head sizes.

It allows good initial fixation and excellent long-term survival.

It is an ODEP (Orthopaedic Data Evaluation Panel) 13A* rated stem.

EXAMINER: What do you mean by anatomical variants?

CANDIDATE: The shape of the femur.

EXAMINER: The shape of the femur is a more important consideration when using an uncemented implant and is less applicable for a cemented implant.

CANDIDATE: The Exeter stem has different offset sizes, which improves hip abductor function and stability. In recent years smaller offsets and shorter-length 'CDH' stems have been introduced to deal with smaller femoral geometry. In smaller femurs oversizing of a femoral component may result in an incomplete or insufficient cement mantle of less than the recommended 2 mm uniform thickness. This may lead to early failure.

EXAMINER: What is the problem with using smaller stems?

CANDIDATE: I am not sure.

EXAMINER: If you use a smaller stem there are concerns with stem breakage and implant failure.

COMMENT: The viva could have gone on to discuss stem geometry affecting cement stresses (avoidance of sharp edges, broad lateral curve), factors predisposing to stem breakage, bending and torsional rigidity of stems, etc.

EXAMINER: What do we mean by a Dorr grading of the femur?

CANDIDATE: There are three types of femoral shape based on metaphyseal–diaphyseal anatomy. Dorr type A femurs have wide metaphyses and narrow diaphyses, type B have a smooth metaphyseal–diaphyseal transition and type C do not have much difference in the sizes of these two regions.

EXAMINER: So how does this apply to uncemented implants?

CANDIDATE: We tend to avoid using uncemented implants in patients with Dorr C femurs.

COMMENT: Candidates should try to avoid mentioning any loose terms they don't fully understand as it can lead on to difficult questions.

EXAMINER: What are the survival figures like for the Exeter implant?

COMMENT: Know some papers to quote for your chosen implant.

CANDIDATE:
1. Lewthwaite *et al.* CORR 2008[28]
Results of Exeter THA in younger patients < 50 years at 10–17 years FU

- Survivorship of the femoral stem from all causes was 99%
- No stem was revised for aseptic loosening

2. Petheram *et al. Bone Joint J* 2016[29]
Results of Exeter THA at 20–25 years.
FU study of 382 cemented Exeter THA (350 patients) at a mean age of 66.3 years (17–94).

- With an endpoint of revision for aseptic loosening or lysis, survivorship of the stem at 22.8 years was 99.0%

EXAMINER: What are the design principals of the Exeter Stem?

CANDIDATE: The Exeter implant is a loaded taper model and becomes lodged as a wedge in the cement mantle during axial loading, reducing peak stresses in the proximal and distal cement mantle. The stem is allowed to subside initially until radial compressive forces are created in the adjacent cement and transferred to the bone as hoop stresses.

EXAMINER: What approach would you use to the hip?

CANDIDATE: I am happy to use either the Hardinge or posterior approach to the hip.

EXAMINER: Make up your mind. Which one are YOU going to do?

CANDIDATE: For the majority of cases I would prefer to use the posterior approach to the hip. In rare instances, I would use a Hardinge anterolateral approach if the risk of dislocation was considered to be high such as neurological or muscular weakness around the hip (Paget's/CVA), early dementia or substance abuse.

The posterior approach is considered easier to perform and is generally a quicker procedure, limiting operative complications such as blood loss and anaesthetic issues.

The abductor muscles are not disturbed significantly so there is generally no gait abnormality, but the acetabulum is more difficult to see and can make prosthesis positioning difficult, possibly causing an increased dislocation rate due to component malpositioning. The sciatic nerve is at slightly more risk of being injured as well.

EXAMINER:[30] There is about double the risk of sciatic nerve injury using the posterior approach.

COMMENT: Most surgeons would say that there is no significant difference in time between the two approaches; the posterior approach can take just as long as the anterolateral approach. The posterior approach is marginally technically easier than the anterolateral approach, but this also depends on surgeon training, experience with using either approach and personal preference. I would argue about the acetabulum being less easy to visualize posteriorly as most surgeons believe the posterior approach provides better acetabular visualization, especially for revision cases. The pelvis tends to tilt more and so the degree of cup anteversion is usually underestimated, leading to an increased risk of dislocation. Where I think the posterior approach does make a difference is a reduced incidence of Trendelenberg gait postoperatively and improved Harris hip scores compared to the anterolateral approach. While results have been a bit contradictory the risk of posterior dislocation is slightly higher posteriorly even with a careful repair of the soft tissues. Larger head sizes are being used now so this is becoming less of an issue.

EXAMINER: Talk me through the posterior approach to the hip.

CANDIDATE: Assuming full informed consent has been obtained, all relevant case notes and radiographs have been obtained, the leg has been marked, WHO checklist performed and she has been suitably anaesthetized. In the anaesthetic room I would position the patient laterally, affected leg uppermost, with hip supports. I would then prepare and drape the patient and make an incision centred over the greater trochanter, approximately 15 cm in length.

I would cut through the skin, subcutaneous tissue, and open up the fascia lata, splitting the gluteus maximus along the line of muscle fibres, and then release the short external rotators from the greater trochanter. Finally, I would perform a capsulectomy and then dislocate the hip.

I would protect the sciatic nerve, being aware of its position and avoid dissecting too close to it.

I would place a large retractor over the anterior edge of the acetabulum at 2–3 o'clock. I would perform a releasing incision into the inferior capsule. I would then place a Charnley spike into the posterior wall of the acetabulum and an additional Hohmann retractor inferiorly. This should give me a 360° view of the whole face of the acetabulum as recommended by BOA guidelines.

EXAMINER: What are the pathological processes involved in the development of osteoarthritis of the hip?

CANDIDATE: Disruption of the integrity of the collagen network occurs early in OA allowing hyperhydration. The increased water content of cartilage causes softening, decreases Young's modulus of elasticity and reduces its ability to bear load.

Initial changes in OA involve damage to the tangential zone immediately below the articular surface, with disorganization of the collagen network, loss of proteoglycans and swelling. This leads to a hypertrophic repair response with increased synthesis and accumulation of proteoglycan. However, the repair process fails with loss of surface integrity, and fibrillation parallel to the surface. In regions of severe damage, there is a loss of cellularity and sporadic formation of cell clusters or clones.

Normal cartilage metabolism is a highly regulated balance between synthesis and degradation of the various matrix components. With OA the equilibrium between anabolism and catabolism is weighted in favour of degradation.

Cartilage catabolism results in release of breakdown products into synovial fluid, which then initiates an inflammatory response by synoviocytes.

These breakdown products include: chondroitin sulphate, keratan sulphate, PG fragments, type II collagen peptides and chondrocyte membranes.

Activated synovial macrophages then recruit PMNs, establishing a synovitis. They also release cytokines, proteinases and oxygen free radicals (superoxide and nitric oxide) into the adjacent synovial fluid. These mediators act on chondrocytes and synoviocytes, modifying synthesis of PGs, collagen, and hyaluronan as well as promoting the release of catabolic mediators.

Cartilage changes in OA are characterized by increases in:

- Water content.
- Chondrocyte activity and proliferation.
- Stiffness of articular cartilage.
- Interleukin-1.
- Metalloproteinase levels.
- Cathepsins B and D levels.

And by decreases in:

- Quality of collagen.
- Proteoglycan quality and size.

Histology classically demonstrates:

- Loss of superficial chondrocytes.
- Replication and breakdown of the tidemark.
- Fibrillation.
- Cartilage destruction with eburnation (polished, shiny smooth with an appearance like ivory) of subchondral bone.

EXAMINER: Is OA simply an ageing process of cartilage?

CANDIDATE: Several differences between ageing cartilage and OA cartilage have been described suggesting a separate disease entity. For example, OA and normal ageing cartilage differ in the amount of water content and the ratio of chondroitin sulphate to keratin sulphate constituents.

EXAMINER: [Interrupting] That's fine that's OK.[31] What molecules are responsible for degrading the cartilage matrix?

CANDIDATE: The primary enzymes responsible for the degradation of cartilage are the matrix metalloproteinases (MMPs). These enzymes are secreted by both synovial cells and chondrocytes and are categorized into three general categories: (a) collagenases; (b) stromelysins; and (c) gelatinases.

Under normal conditions, MMP synthesis and activation are tightly regulated at several levels. They are secreted as inactive proenzymes that require enzymatic cleavage in order to become activated. Once activated, MMPs become susceptible to the plasma-derived MMP inhibitor, alpha-2-macroglobulin, and to tissue inhibitors of MMPs (TIMPs) that are also secreted by synovial cells and chondrocytes.

In OA, synthesis of MMPs is greatly enhanced and the available inhibitors are overwhelmed, resulting in net degradation. Interestingly, stromelysin can serve as an activator for its own proenzyme, as well as for procollagenase and prostromelysin, thus creating a positive feedback loop of proMMP activation in cartilage.

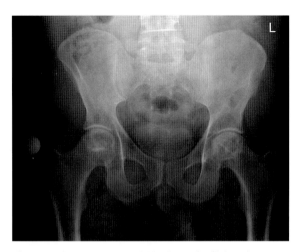

Figure 3.5a Anteroposterior (AP) radiograph of bilateral osteonecrosis.

EXAMINER: What factors are responsible for inducing metalloprotease synthesis?

CANDIDATE: IL-1 is a potent pro-inflammatory cytokine that, in vitro, is capable of inducing chondrocytes and synovial cells to synthesize MMP. In addition, IL-1 suppresses the synthesis of type II collagen and proteoglycans and inhibits transforming growth factor-β-stimulated chondrocyte proliferation. Therefore, in OA, IL-1 actively promotes cartilage degradation and may also suppress attempts at repair.

Structured oral examination question 5

Osteonecrosis (ON)

EXAMINER: This is the anteroposterior (AP) radiograph of a 48-year-old man who presents to your clinic with several weeks history of progressively worsening bilateral hip pain. What do you think of the radiograph? (Figure 3.5a)

CANDIDATE 1: This is an anteroposterior (AP) view of the pelvis. The most obvious abnormality is patchy diffuse sclerosis with increased density in the superolateral aspect of the right femoral head (Ficat 2).

The left femoral head has a possibly minimal osteoporosis and/or blurring and poor definition of the bony trabeculae (Ficat 1).

The radiograph is suspicious of bilateral osteonecrosis. I would like to obtain a frog-leg lateral radiograph of both hips. I would look for the crescent sign, indicating subchondral fracture, a feature of osteonecrosis that is more obvious on a frog-leg lateral than AP projection. This is because the anterior and posterior margins of the acetabulum on the AP projection are superimposed over the superior portion of the femoral head, the usual location of the sign. When osteonecrosis is bilateral, it usually occurs in each hip at different times, and the staging of disease in each hip is often different. [Candidate score 7–8]

CANDIDATE 2: This is an AP pelvic radiograph showing both hips. There is nothing very obvious staring at me. There are no features of osteoarthritis such as joint space narrowing, osteophytes or sclerosis.[32] [Candidate score 4]

EXAMINER: What do you mean by osteonecrosis?

CANDIDATE: Osteonecrosis occurs due to interruption of the blood supply to the femoral head leading to ischaemia and cellular death.

COMMENT: The term osteonecrosis is preferred to commonly used AVN because it best describes the histopathological processes involved and does not imply a specific aetiology.

EXAMINER: What is the aetiology of osteonecrosis?

CANDIDATE: A number of conditions are associated with osteonecrosis. The most common cause is trauma secondary to fracture and/or dislocation of the femoral head. Other conditions include:

- Corticosteroid use.
- Alcohol abuse.
- Smoking.
- Coagulopathies.
- Sickle cell anaemia.
- Caisson disease.
- Hypercholesterolaemia.
- Organ transplantation.
- Systemic lupus erythematosus.
- Gaucher disease.
- Hypertriglyceridaemia.
- Intramedullary haemorrhages.
- Chronic pancreatitis.

AS IT GRIPS 3Cs (mnemonic)

Alcohol

Steroids

Idiopathic

Trauma

Gout, Gauchers

Rheumatoid/radiation

Infection/increased lipids/inflammatory arthritis

Pancreatitis/pregnancy

SLE/sickle cell/smoking

CRF/chemotherapy/Cassion's disease

In approximately 10–20% of cases no cause can be identified.

EXAMINER: What is the pathophysiology of osteonecrosis?

CANDIDATE: Aetiologic factors in osteonecrosis are usually related to underlying pathologic conditions that alter blood flow, leading to cellular necrosis and ultimately to collapse of the femoral head. This damage can occur in one of five vascular areas around the femoral head: arterial extraosseous, arterial intraosseous, venous intraosseous, venous extraosseous and extravascular extraosseous.

1. *Extraosseous arterial factors* are the most important. The femoral head is at increased risk because the blood supply is an end-organ system with poor collateral development. Blood supply can be interrupted by trauma, vasculitis (Raynaud disease), or vasospasm (decompression sickness).

2. *Intraosseous arterial factors* may block the microcirculation of the femoral head through circulating microemboli. These can occur in sickle cell disease (SCD), fat embolization or air embolization from dysbaric phenomena.

3. *Intraosseous venous factors* affect the femoral head by reducing venous blood flow and causing stasis. These factors may accompany conditions such as Caisson disease, SCD or enlargement of intramedullary fat cells.

4. *Intraosseous extravascular factors* affect the hip by increasing the pressure, resulting in a femoral head compartment syndrome. For example: fat cell hypertrophy after steroid administration or abnormal cells, such as Gaucher and inflammatory cells, can encroach on intraosseous

capillaries, reducing intramedullary circulation and contributing to compartment syndrome.

5. *Extraosseus extravascular (capsular) factors* involve the tamponade of the lateral epiphyseal vessels located within the synovial membrane, through increased intracapsular pressure. This occurs after trauma, infection and arthritis, causing hip effusion that may affect the blood supply to the epiphysis.

EXAMINER: Specifically, how do steroids cause osteonecrosis?[33]

CANDIDATE: The mechanism postulated for steroid-induced ON is still unclear.

Johnson proposed that fat cell hypertrophy within the bone marrow increases femoral head pressure resulting in sinusoidal vascular collapse and necrosis of the femoral head.[34] The exact mechanism of fat cell hypertrophy remains obscure, but a disorder in fat metabolism is implicated.

Jaffe *et al.* believe patients undergoing steroid treatment are in a hyperlipidaemic state, which can increase the fat content within the femoral head and raise intracortical pressure producing sinusoidal collapse and finally necrosis.[35]

Other investigators have proposed that this hyperlipidaemic state leads to fat embolism occluding the femoral head microvasculature, which initiates the pathophysiologic process.[36]

A recent study in rabbits suggests that the use of steroids can also damage endothelial and smooth muscle cells within the vasculature. This may result in interruption of the venous drainage from the femoral head, leading to blood stasis, an increase in intraosseous pressure, and osteonecrosis.[37]

Other studies suggest primary osteocyte cell death without any other features. This is seen with steroid use, in transplant patients and those who consume significant amounts of alcohol.

EXAMINER: How common is steroids as a cause of osteonecrosis?

CANDIDATE: High-dose corticosteroids are the most common cause of non-traumatic osteonecrosis accounting for 10–30% of cases. However, only 10% of patients exposed to corticosteroids may develop osteonecrosis. Dosage is typically steroids > 2 g of prednisone, or its equivalent, within a 2–3-month period.

The period from the start of corticosteroid treatment to the diagnosis of osteonecrosis ranges from 1 to 16 months (mean 5.3 months), and the majority of patients are diagnosed within 1 year.

EXAMINER: You mentioned the crescent line, what is its significance?

CANDIDATE: Therapeutic interventions are less likely to halt progression of the disease once this sign appears.

EXAMINER: How does osteonecrosis of the hip present?

CANDIDATE: Although osteonecrosis can be clinically silent, typically a patient complains of pain, usually localized to the groin area but occasionally to the ipsilateral buttock and knee. It is usually a deep intermittent, throbbing pain, with an insidious onset that eventually occurs at rest and may be present or even worsen at night. Physical examination reveals pain with both active and passive range of motion, especially with passive internal rotation. Range of motion is important as this helps determine the extent of the disease. In general, more limited flexion and abduction indicates more extensive articular damage, whereas limited rotation alone may indicate less destruction. A careful examination of the contralateral hip should always be undertaken, as osteonecrosis is bilateral in 40–80% of cases.

EXAMINER: How is osteonecrosis classified?

CANDIDATE: Several classification systems for osteonecrosis exist. Ficat and Arlet is the most commonly known and consists of four stages.[38] Hungerford and Lennox later added a fifth stage (Stage 0) when MRI became available.[39]

Stage 0 (preclinical). Suspected disease in the contralateral hip when the index joint has definitive findings. No clinical symptoms. MRI non-diagnostic.

Stage I (preradiological). Normal findings on radiographs and positive findings on MRI or bone scan. The MRI shows a double-line sign, consistent with a necrotic process.

Stage II (pre-collapse). Osteopaenia, demineralization, sclerosis or cysts. A late finding is the crescent sign, a linear subcortical lucency, situated immediately beneath the subcortical bone, representing a fracture line and impending femoral head collapse.

Stage III (collapse). The femoral head is flattened and collapsed with the presence of

Table 3.8 Staging system of Steinberg et al.

Stage	Radiographic feature
0	Normal X-ray findings; normal bone scan and MRI. Diagnosed on histology
I	Normal X-ray findings; abnormal bone scan and/or MR findings IA: Mild (< 15% of femoral head affected) IB: Moderate (15–30% of femoral head affected) IC: Severe (> 30% of femoral head affected)
II	Cystic and sclerotic changes in the femoral head IIA: Mild (< 15% of femoral head affected) IIB: Moderate (15–30% of femoral head affected) IIC: Severe (> 30% of femoral head affected)
III	Subchondral collapse (crescent sign) without flattening IIIA: Mild (< 15% of femoral head affected) IIIB: Moderate (15–30% of femoral head affected) IIIC: Severe (> 30% of femoral head affected)
IV	Flattening of femoral head IVA: Mild (< 15% of surface and < 2 mm depression) IVB: Moderate (15–30% of surface or 2–4 mm depression) IVC: Severe (30% of surface)
V	Joint narrowing and/or acetabular changes (this stage can be graded according to severity)
VI	Advanced degenerative changes

sequestration manifested by a break in the articular margin without acetabular involvement.

Stage IV (progressive degenerate disease). Severe collapse and destruction of the femoral head, acetabular osteophytes. Osteoarthritis superimposed on a deformed femoral head.

EXAMINER: Any other classification systems?

CANDIDATE: Steinberg (Table 3.8) expanded the staging system into seven stages and quantified the amount of involvement of the femoral head into mild (< 15%), moderate (15–30%) and severe (> 30%), based on radiographs.[40] It is considered more useful than Ficat because it grades the severity and extent of the involvement, both of which are thought to affect prognosis.

EXAMINER: Any others?

CANDIDATE: Other classification systems include the ARCO (Association Research Circulation Osseous) classification, University of Pennsylvania system and the Mitchell MRI classification.

EXAMINER: What is the Kerboull necrotic angle and its importance?

CANDIDATE: The Kerboull necrotic angle is used to calculate the size of the necrotic segment. It is the sum of the angle of the necrotic segment as measured on both the anteroposterior and frog-lateral radiographs. Patients with a Kerboull angle > 200° more commonly have poor results with certain bone-preserving procedures.

EXAMINER: How are you going to manage this patient?

CANDIDATE: I would perform bilateral core decompression. The osteonecrosis is still at an early stage where it may be successful (Ficat stages I and II osteonecrosis). The procedure has no role in the management of Ficat stages III or IV disease. Results have been satisfactory when core decompression is combined with either non-vascularized or vascularized fibula grafts in patients with Ficat stage II lesions.

EXAMINER: What are the pre-requisites for performing a free vascularized fibular graft (VFG)?

CANDIDATE: VFG for AVN is a major operative procedure with a long rehabilitation time and therefore patient selection to minimize the potential for an unsuccessful operation is critical.

McKee from Toronto suggests the operation should be limited to patients [scoring 7–8]:[41]

1. With 2 mm or less of femoral head collapse as measured on plain radiographs.
2. Who are 45 years of age or younger (and have a reasonable life expectancy).
3. Have had withdrawal of an identified aetiologic agent.
4. Have no contractures about the hip.
5. Have a supple joint.

These are obviously general guidelines that may be adjusted somewhat depending on the individual patient.

EXAMINER: What are the advantages of performing a free VFG?

CANDIDATE: The advantages of vascularized fibular grafting include:
- Being able to perform a core decompression of the femoral head.

- The ability to perform curettage and removal of the osteonecrotic focus.
- Impaction of autogenous cancelleous graft to fill the defect created by removal of the osteonecrotic bone.
- The structural support of the subchondral surface provided by the fibular graft.
- The addition of vascularized bone and blood supply to the area of osteonecrosis enhances the revascularization process.

EXAMINER: What complications can occur with a free vascularized fibular graft?

CANDIDATE: Gaskill *et al.* from a tertiary centre in North Carolina performing a large volume of VFG reported a 16.9% complications rate, 4.3% of complications require reoperation or chronic pain management.[42,43]

Donor site morbidity:
- Great-toe flexion contracture (4.3%). Majority asymptomatic, noticeable only on clinical examination with the ankle fully dorsiflexed. Occasionally requires z-lengthening of the FHL tendon at the level of the medial malleolus. Flexion contracture of the second and third toes may coexist in a small number of patients.
- Persistent weakness in the operated extremity (0.6%) either long toe flexors or peroneal group.
- Mild persistent pain and tenderness at the ankle or distal osteotomy site (4.1%) usually after prolonged standing or moderate activity such as jogging.
- Sensory deficits (1.7%). The sensory deficit was not always consistent with peripheral nerve or dermatomal distributions.
- Superficial infection.

Graft site complication

- Symptomatic lateral pin migration (2.4%). A Kirschner wire was used routinely to secure the fibular graft in its final position after placement in the femoral head.
- Symptomatic heterotopic ossification (1.4%).
- Femoral fracture (0.7%). All occurred in the intertrochanteric and subtrochanteric region after a fall.
- Superficial infection (4%).
- Deep infection (4%).
- Haematoma (1%).

- Trochanteric bursitis (1%).

EXAMINER: What are the other techniques that can be used to manage osteonecrosis of the hip?

CANDIDATE: The trapdoor procedure is performed with an arthrotomy to dislocate the hip anteriorly, followed by curettage of the necrotic segment of the head and packing of the defect with iliac crest bone graft through a cartilage window in the femoral head. This can be used for Ficat stage III and early Ficat stage IV and reasonable results have been reported.

EXAMINER: You have to be more specific than that; what do you mean by reasonable results?[44]

CANDIDATE: Michael Mont reported on a series of 30 hips Ficat stage III/IV at 5 years with 73% having good to excellent results.[45]

EXAMINER: Any other options?

CANDIDATE: Osteotomy has been used to treat Ficat stage III and IV disease, but results have been variable because it is difficult to rotate the necrotic segment out from the weight bearing area, especially when the lesion is large. Sugioka et al. reported good to excellent results at 3–16 years of follow-up in 78% of 229 hips treated with the transtrochanteric anterior rotational osteotomy.[46] Their results with this technically demanding procedure have not been reproduced by others.

A success rate of approximately 30% at 5 years is common, with the best results reported in patients whose lesions do not result from trauma and who have less than 30% of the head involved.

EXAMINER: Any new technique that has emerged in the last 2 or 3 years?

CANDIDATE: Stem cells have been used to manage ON.

EXAMINER: Go on – do you know about the technique or results?

CANDIDATE: Two techniques are being promoted. One is a three-stage procedure and the other is a single-stage procedure. The first method is by stem cell culture in the lab to multiply the number of cells several million fold. These cultured stem cells are reinjected into a previous core decompression site.

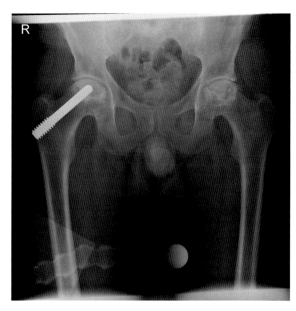

Figure 3.5b Anteroposterior (AP) radiograph of pelvis with tantulum rod inserted into the right hip.

In the second method, bone marrow obtained from the pelvis is centrifuged in the operating room to yield a bone marrow concentrate rich in stem cells. The patient is supine on a traction table with a C-arm image intensifier. Percutaneous core decompression drilling with a Kirschner wire (diameter 2.7 mm) is performed to perforate the interface between the necrotic lesion and healthy bone. Following this, concentrated autologous bone marrow aspirate is slowly transplanted into the necrotic area under fluoroscopic control. This is still an experimental procedure, but early results seem promising for early disease.

EXAMINER: The patient had surgery on both hips. These are his postoperative radiographs (Figure 3.5b).

CANDIDATE: The AP radiograph demonstrates a metal core rod in the right hip.

EXAMINER: What do we call this?

CANDIDATE: The patient has had a tantalum rod inserted into the femoral head. The implant achieves decompression, supports the subchondral plate of the necrotic areas and probably induces bone regeneration.

EXAMINER: Anything else?

CANDIDATE: The use of a trabecular metal 'AVN rod' has a number of attractive theoretical advantages, including no donor site morbidity, improved rehabilitation, structural support of the femoral head and the potential for 'osseointegration' of the biologically friendly material.

EXAMINER: The patient had core decompression performed on the left hip and a core decompression with tantulum rod inserted in the right hip. He initially got good pain relief from the procedures for about a year or so, but he returns to the orthopaedic clinic complaining both hips are now painful. The left side is worse than the right. What do you think of the radiographs?

CANDIDATE: The AP radiograph suggests osteonecrosis has progressed.

EXAMINER: What will you do?

CANDIDATE: I would offer him bilateral hip arthroplasty, the left one being more symptomatic first.

EXAMINER: What type of hip replacement would you use?

CANDIDATE: In view of his relatively young age I would perform an uncemented THA with a ceramic on HCLPE bearing surface.

EXAMINER: What are the results like at 10 years for this bearing surface? What will you tell the patient about how long his hip will last?

CANDIDATE: Sorry, I am not sure, I think it is around 95%.

COMMENT: The latest NJR report (15th, 2018) has shown a *5.33% (3.77% to 7.50%) RR* at 14 years for males aged *under 55* with an *uncemented THA CoP* surface.

EXAMINER: Are there any other bearing surface options available?

CANDIDATE: A ceramic-on-ceramic (CoC) bearing surface.

EXAMINER: What are the advantages of using a ceramic bearing surface?

CANDIDATE: The advantages of using a ceramic bearing surface include superior lubrication, friction and wear properties compared with other bearing surfaces in clinical use. Specifically, it is an extremely hard material very resistant to wear, and has a low coefficient of friction, excellent abrasive resistance and excellent wettability properties for improved lubrication. It is presumed that the lower wear rates lead to a lower rate of aseptic loosening and the need for revision surgery.

Disadvantages include potential for catastrophic fracture, squeaking, and cost.

EXAMINER: What is the incidence of squeaking?

CANDIDATE: The reported incidence of squeaking with alumina ceramic bearings varies widely from 0.45% in a series of 2716 ceramic implants to 7.0% in a series of 159 ceramic implants. Most reported series note that squeaking is rare and without clinical significance; however, on rare occasions, major squeaking has led to revision surgery.[47]

EXAMINER: What are the results like for ceramic-on-ceramic hips?

CANDIDATE: UK NJR data report a 6.43% (5.17–7.98%) revision rate at 14 years for males aged *under 55* with an *uncemented THA CoC* surface.

COMMENT: Latest data from the 15th NJR report have shown a steady decline since 2011 in CoC THA use due to the concerns with squeaking, catastrophic failure and high cost.

The use of a CoP bearing surface is steadily increasing and if used with a second-generation HCLPE becomes a highly attractive option in a young patient. Better NJR survival figures in males under 55 at 14 years are reported for CoP compared to CoC.

Definitely avoid mentioning MoM resurfacing as an option in a viva scenario unless specifically brought up in the discussion by the examiners.[48]

Ceramic on X3 poly is becoming the preferred bearing option for young patients with most hip arthroplasty surgeons moving away now from ceramic-on-ceramic use.

EXAMINER: Will there be any special issues removing the tantulum rod and performing THA?

CANDIDATE: I would contact the manufacturers of the implant as there is a special implant removal kit. Otherwise not using the removal kit makes the surgery more difficult. I would use a Gigli and reciprocating saw to section the head, implant removal corer to take out the tantulum rod and then perform a conventional uncemented THA.

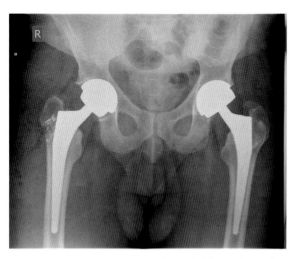

Figure 3.5c Anteroposterior (AP) radiograph left MoM hip and right ceramic large jumbo hip arthroplasty.

EXAMINER: Are there any worries with tantalum material?

CANDIDATE: Studies suggest a trend towards an inferior outcome in patients following conversion of tantalum rod to THA.[49] There is also concern of residual tantalum metal within the joint space found in the majority of conversions. Although there is no catastrophic wear seen in studies there is the potential for accelerated joint damage in the medium to long term.

EXAMINER: These are his radiographs (Figure 3.5c). He had a large jumbo MoM performed on the left side and a large ceramic jumbo head THA performed on the right side. Do you have any worries?

CANDIDATE: Following the BHS meeting in Manchester 2012 a statement was released advising that stemmed large-diameter MoM total hip replacements using bearing of 36 mm or above should no longer be performed.

A higher than anticipated early failure rate for large jumbo head MoM hips had been reported. Concern was expressed regarding the trunnion at the 'Morse' taper where the large diameter metal head attaches to the stem with damage occurring from either wear or corrosion or both resulting in either loosening of the acetabular component, loosening of the femoral component or a metal reaction with necrosis and soft tissue damage. Excluding the ASR implant these devices have a reported revision rate of 22.14% at 13 years (14th NJR data).

EXAMINER: What about follow up?

CANDIDATE: This should be as per recent MHRA and BHS guidelines for MoM bearing surfaces, yearly for the first 5 years and continuing on for life. Pain in this group of patients should be taken seriously and investigated appropriately with cobalt chromium levels, a MARS MRI scan of the hip and OHS. This patient should be considered at high risk for implant failure as he has a stemmed implant with a femoral head ≥ 36mm.

I would review this patient at least yearly as ARMD may occur in symptomatic and asymptomatic patients and earlier detection should give a better revision outcome if needed.

Although each patient needs to be assessed individually I would have a low threshold for obtaining blood level ion measurements and MARS MRI even for asymptomatic patients if I had concern about ARMD.

EXAMINER: What would you look for in the MARS MRI of the hip?

CANDIDATE: I would look for any soft-tissue local reaction or masses (pseudotumour), abductor muscle detachment, the presence and extent of any osteolysis and any periprosthetic fluid collections. A fluid collection by itself around the joint in an asymptomatic patient, unless very large can be safely observed with interval scanning.

MARS MRI scan is more important in the decision-making process to revise a MoM hip replacement than elevated cobalt/chromium levels.

I would have significant concerns in any patients with surrounding muscle/bone damage visualized on MARS MRI. Solid lesions seen on MARS MRI are more worrying than cystic. Synovial thickness has a high sensitivity and specificity for ALVAL.

EXAMINER: Is there a role for US of the hip?

CANDIDATE: Ultrasonography is a good screening tool, is cheap and has no radiation hazard. However, the detection of small or deep lesions is difficult and the use of ultrasound is highly dependent on the operator's experience.

EXAMINER: What about the other ceramic hip?

And while a large femoral head may potentially cause elevated trunnion stresses, trunnion corrosion is likely to be multifactorial with taper design, contact area, preparation of the taper, impact force, head–neck junction alloy composition also playing a part.

Structured oral examination question 6

EXAMINER: This is an anteroposterior (AP) radiograph of a 73-year-old male who had a cemented THA performed 14 years ago (Figure 3.6).

CANDIDATE: The AP radiograph demonstrates a cemented THA. I am unfamiliar with the implant, but both the cup and femoral stem have been cemented and most likely a 28-mm head size has been used. The cup does not appear excessively worn or loose. There are no significant lucencies in any of the DeLee and Charnley acetabular zones. However, there is a continuous radiolucency at the femoral cement–bone interface in all seven Gruen zones suggestive of gross femoral stem loosening.

EXAMINER: What are Gruen zones?

CANDIDATE: This is a widely used system in which the femoral component interface is considered in seven zones. These allow the location of cement fractures and of lucent lines either at the cement–bone or the cement–prosthesis interface. It is the progressive changes that are seen in serial radiographs that are important in diagnosing osteolysis and femoral stem loosening.

EXAMINER: What mode of cemented femoral stem failure has occurred?

CANDIDATE: This is Gruen mode 1b failure. Pistoning subsidence of stem and cement within bone.

EXAMINER: Briefly, what are the other modes of failure?

CANDIDATE: There is mode 1, a pistoning subsidence of stem within cement mantle; mode 2, medial midstem pivot; mode 3, calcar pivot and bending cantilever fatigue (distal pivot).

EXAMINER: OK, what will you see radiographically with each mode of failure?

CANDIDATE: There is one mode of failure like a car windscreen wiper, but I am not sure which one,

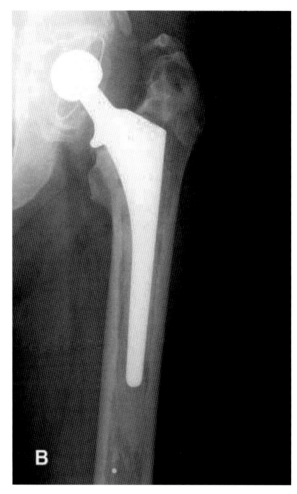

Figure 3.6 Anteroposterior (AP) radiograph of a loose cemented left THA.

CANDIDATE: There are some worries again regarding the trunnion where the large ceramic head attaches to the stem, which may be the source of excessive wear or corrosion leading again to early failure, although the evidence isn't as strong.

EXAMINER: Why choose a Delta ceramic head over a cobalt chrome head?

CANDIDATE: It was originally thought that this would result in a lower revision rate with decreased clinically relevant wear rates. The use of a large ceramic head provides an advantageous head–neck ratio that theoretically reduces the risk of impingement and subluxation and provides for an increased ROM.

I think it may be medial stem pivot mode 2, no sorry I think it is mode 4.

COMMENT: Far better for the candidate to say they aren't sure and leave it at that rather than guessing and getting all mixed up.

EXAMINER: What do we mean by the term wear?

CANDIDATE: Wear is defined as a progressive loss of bearing surface from a material as a result of chemical (corrosive) or mechanical action. Types of mechanical wear include adhesive, abrasive and fatigue.

EXAMINER: What do you mean by abrasive and adhesive wear?

CANDIDATE: Abrasive wear occurs when two surfaces with microscopic irregularities or asperities slide past one another while in intimate contact. The interaction generates particles mainly from the softer material.

Adhesive wear occurs when two opposing materials bond under contact load. Actual transfer of material from one surface to the other may occur, forming transfer films. When motion resumes between the two surfaces, particles may be broken free from one or both surfaces. These new particles then further contribute to wear from third-body abrasive wear.

The wear of UHMWPE in THA is mainly adhesive and abrasive.

EXAMINER: What is fretting wear?

CANDIDATE: Fretting occurs with small cyclic motions of one surface relative to another.

EXAMINER: What are the wear sources in joint replacement surgery?

CANDIDATE: Wear sources include the primary articulation surface, secondary articulation surfaces, cement/prosthesis micromotion, cement/bone or prosthesis/bone micromotion and third-body wear.

EXAMINER: What are the modes of wear in joint replacement surgery?

CANDIDATE: There are four modes of wear.

1. Mode 1 is the generation of wear debris that occurs with motion between the two bearing surfaces as intended by the designers.

2. Mode 2 refers to a primary bearing surface rubbing against a secondary surface in a manner not intended by the designers (for example, a femoral head articulating with an acetabular shell following wear-through of the polyethylene).

3. Mode 3 refers to two primary bearing surfaces with interposed third-body particles (such as bone, cement, metal and so on).

4. Mode 4 refers to two non-bearing surfaces rubbing together (such as back-sided wear of an acetabular liner, fretting of the Morse taper, stem–cement fretting).

While several modes of wear often occur simultaneously, mode 1 accounts for the majority of wear in well-functioning hip or knee replacements.

EXAMINER: What do we mean by effective joint space?

CANDIDATE: Schmalzreid et al. coined the term 'effective joint space' to refer to all periprosthetic regions to which joint fluid, and hence wear debris, can gain access.[50] In the acetabulum, wear debris can reach the interface through unfilled screw holes or via non-ingrown areas of the shell. On the femoral side, use of circumferential porous coating has reduced the incidence of diaphyseal osteolysis by blocking access of wear particles.

Table 3.9 Implant-specific factors affecting joint wear.

Implant design choices
- Modularity versus monoblock
- UHMWPE component thickness
- Bearing couple conformity
- Fixation (cemented versus ingrowth)
- Implant constraint
- Implant impingement

Material
- Metallic alloy (Co–Cr–Mo alloy versus titanium alloy)
- Ceramic (alumina, zirconia, oxidized zirconium alloy)
- UHMWPE (highly cross-linked versus conventional)

Bearing couple
- Metal-on-UHMWPE
- Ceramic-on-UHMWPE
- Metal-on-metal
- Ceramic-on-ceramic

Quality control
- Lot-to-lot variability
- Shelf-life and packaging of UHMWPE components
- Sterilization process (radiation versus ethylene oxide)

Table 3.10 Surgical factors affecting joint wear.

- Surgical approach
- Component position
- Restoration of appropriate mechanical and rotational axes
- Initial stability and method of component fixation
- Soft-tissue balance (laxity versus overconstraint)
- Subluxation or dislocation
- Third-body wear
- Surgeon experience

Table 3.11 Patient-specific factors affecting joint wear.

- Activity level (activities of daily living, pivot-shift activities). Patients with active lifestyles often return to recreational activities that markedly increase joint-loading conditions (e.g. running, jumping, pivoting, stair climbing)
- Body mass index and body weight. Increased body weight can be associated with increased magnitude of force and altered kinematics, although the detrimental effects of excessive weight can be counterbalanced by decreased activity levels and loading cycles that accompany a sedentary lifestyle
- Gait mechanics (level and stairs)
- Limb alignment
- Implant time in situ
- Preoperative diagnosis post-traumatic arthritis and AVN have been associated with higher prosthesis failure rates as usually arthroplasty is performed in younger, more active patients
- Comorbidities. ACL and meniscal injuries predispose to osteoarthritis in a young age group
- Special cultural demands (e.g. kneeling in Middle Eastern and Asian populations). Deep flexion for kneeling, load implants beyond current design characteristics (TKA)
- Revision versus primary surgery

EXAMINER: What is osteolysis?

CANDIDATE: Osteolysis is a biological phenomenon that can result in the loosening of the implant principally caused by the UHMWPE wear particles. Metal or ceramic wear particles that are produced at the articulating surfaces of a hip prosthesis are also implicated but to a much lesser degree. Osteolysis is influenced by the size and morphology of the UHMWPE particles. Macrophages actively phagocytose (engulf) wear debris at the bone–implant interface. These cells release various enzymes and osteolytic mediators such as interleukin, tumour necrosis factor (TNF-α) and prostaglandin. These cytokines cause inflammation and trigger bone dissolution or resorption around the implanted region.

EXAMINER: What factors influence osteolysis (wear)?

CANDIDATE: Osteolysis (wear) is a multifactorial process dependent on surgical factors, implant design, patient factors and material composition.

Implant-specific factors that affect wear performance of THA (and TKA) include (see Table 3.9):[51,52]

Surgical factors (e.g. component position, soft-tissue balancing) that affect joint loads and kinematics influence wear performance of THA (and TKA) (see Table 3.10).

Patient-specific factors that affect wear performance of THA (and TKA) include (see Table 3.11).

EXAMINER: What do you know about osteoblastic regulators?

CANDIDATE: Three osteoblastic regulators (RANK, RANKL and OPG) are involved in bone resorption. This is linked to TNF-α, a cytokine responsible for encouraging osteolysis through the facilitation and augmentation of osteoclast differentiation and activation of pre-existing osteoclasts.

Gold medal candidates

Periprosthetic osteolysis is the loss of bone surrounding an artificial implant. The formation of a periprosthetic interfacial membrane between the bone and the implant is implicated in bone resorption. The interfacial membrane is composed primarily of two cell types, the macrophage and the fibroblast.

Aseptic osteolysis is thought to occur through a mechanism involving expression of bone resorptive cytokines such as interleukin-1β (IL-1β), interleukin-6 (IL-6), tumour necrosis factor-α (TNF-α), platelet-derived growth factor (PDGF), and receptor activator of nuclear factor-κ B ligand (RANKL).

RANKL is a potent bone resorptive cytokine present on the membranes of bone marrow stromal cells, osteoblasts in bone, as well as on T cells, and as a soluble molecule secreted into the bone microenvironment by these cells. Receptor activator of nuclear factor-κ B (RANK), a RANKL receptor, is expressed on the cell surface of preosteoclasts.

Macrophages express RANK and, when exposed to RANKL in the presence of macrophage colony-stimulating factor (M-CSF), have been shown to differentiate into mature osteoclasts capable of bone resorption. Osteoprotegerin (OPG) acts as a decoy receptor for RANKL by binding to RANKL and preventing the functional interaction of RANKL with RANK, thereby blocking the osteoclast formation and the bone resorptive effects of RANKL. Osteoclast activation is thus blocked.

EXAMINER: What factors affect PE cup wear in THA?

CANDIDATE: Implant factors associated with an increased wear rate include non-cross-linked PE, longer shelf-life for liners γ-irradiated in air, thickness of PE.

Patient factors include younger age due to higher activity levels, obesity due to increased joint loading.

Surgeon factors include position of the cup relative to Kohler's line, increase in cup abduction angle.

EXAMINER: What is the current thinking about UHMWPE?

CANDIDATE: Three approaches are currently being investigated in an attempt to modify highly cross-linked UHMWPE so that the increased wear resistance provided by cross-linking can be maintained without the reduced fracture resistance that accompanies cross-linking:[53]

1. Stabilization of free radicals through the impregnation of irradiated ultra-high molecular weight polyethylene with vitamin E. Vitamin E protects polyethylene against oxidation, which renders the melting step that normally follows cross-linking with radiation unnecessary. Vitamin E also quenches free radicals.

2. A second approach involves sequentially irradiating and annealing polyethylene. Irradiation is conducted in three steps with interspersed annealing processes that together improve oxidative stability compared with that resulting from a single large dose of irradiation followed by annealing.

3. The third approach involves the photo-induced graft polymerization of

2-methacryloyloxyethyl phosphorylcholine (MPC) onto cross-linked polyethylene (CLPE). The concept is to create a hydrophilic layer with better wettability than a conventional polyethylene surface, thus increasing the chance for lubrication.

Structured oral examination question 7

EXAMINER: This is a radiograph of a 68-year-old woman who has been referred up to the orthopaedic clinic by the physiotherapist-led musculoskeletal clinic with an 18-month history of left hip pain and difficulty walking (Figure 3.7).

CANDIDATE: This is an anteroposterior (AP) radiograph of the pelvis demonstrating a coarsened trabecular pattern of the left hip, a thickened left cortex compared to the opposite hip, and increased density of the left hip compared to the right side. Both iliopectineal (Brim sign) and ilioischatic lines are thickened. There is sclerosis involving the left pelvis (ileum, ischium and pubic rami), left femora and lower lumbar spine. The radiograph is highly suspicious of Paget's disease.

Differential diagnosis would include other causes of increased and disorganized bone turnover such as sclerotic bony metastasis (prostatic carcinoma), renal osteodystrophy, fibrous dysplasia, multiple myeloma, lymphoma, osteopetrosis and hyperparathyroidism.

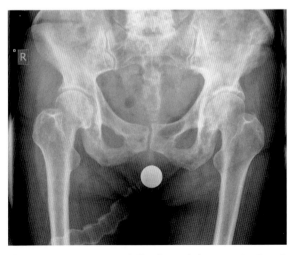

Figure 3.7 Anteroposterior (AP) radiograph demonstrating Paget's disease of the left hemipelvis.

EXAMINER: What is Paget's disease?

CANDIDATE: Paget's disease is a metabolic bone disorder of unknown aetiology characterized by a disorganized increase in osteoclastic bone resorption and compensatory osteoblastic new bone formation. There is accelerated but chaotic bone remodelling in which the bone is biomechanically weak and prone to deformity and fracture.

The disease can be divided into three major phases, lytic, mixed lytic/sclerotic and sclerotic, each of which is associated with distinctive clinical, radiological and pathological features.

EXAMINER: What causes Paget's disease? What is the pathophysiology of Paget's disease?

CANDIDATE: The primary abnormality of Paget's disease is an intense focal resorption of normal bone by abnormal osteoclasts. These osteoclasts are abnormal in size, activity and quantity. The abnormal osteoclasts make large resorption cavities in the bone matrix. In response to the osteoclast resorption, osteoblasts are recruited, resulting in bone formation. The osteoblast activity is rapid such that the newly formed bone is not organized and remains irregular and woven in nature, less-resistant and more elastic than typical lamellar bone; prone to deformity and fracture.

EXAMINER: What are the other radiographic features of Paget's disease?

CANDIDATE: Radiographic features of Paget's include:
- Advanced disease in the long bones is characterized by coarsened trabecula, bony sclerosis, bony enlargement, and deformity. A 'candle flame' or 'blade of grass' sign represents a wedge- or V-shaped pattern of advancing lysis in the diaphysis of long bones. The femur develops a lateral curvature while the tibia develops an anterior curvature that may result in fracture. Fine cracks may appear (stress fractures) which resemble Looser zones but occur on the convex bone surface.
- Lateral radiographs of the lumbar spine demonstrate a 'picture-frame' vertebral body that is secondary to severe osteoporosis centrally and a thickened, sclerotic cortex.
- The skull is involved in 29–65% of cases. Inner and outer table involvement leads to diploic widening. Osteoporosis circumscripta is a well-defined lysis, most commonly involving the frontal bone producing well-defined geographic lytic lesions in the skull. It is seen in the early or lytic phase when osteoclastic resorption overwhelms bone production. At a later stage a 'cotton wool appearance' represents mixed lytic and blastic pattern of thickened calvarium.
- Protrusio deformity of the pelvis is a common occurrence with advanced Paget's disease.

EXAMINER: What are the current theories regarding the aetiology of Paget's disease?

CANDIDATE: The aetiology of Paget's disease is still unknown. Proposed theories include viral, genetic and environmental causes. Paramyxoviruses such as measles virus, respiratory syncytial virus and canine distemper virus have been implicated. Electron microscopy has shown virus-like structures that resemble the paramyxovirus in osteoclast nuclei and cytoplasm of cells affected by Paget's disease. However, more recent studies have been unable to confirm the presence of specific viral antibodies in patients with Paget's disease. Environmental factors implicated include high levels of arsenic and an uncertain association with cats and dogs. Genetically, 5–40% of patients have first-degree relatives with the disease.

EXAMINER: That's fine. I am, however, a bit sceptical about the cats and dogs theory. Moving on – what are the complications of Paget's disease?

CANDIDATE: Complications of Paget's disease include:
- Compression fractures of the vertebral body (commonest complication of spinal Paget's).
- Pagetic spinal stenosis, defined as compression of the spinal cord, cauda equina or spinal nerves by expanded Pagetic bony tissue of the spine. Most common in the lumbar region and typically single level, causing cord or nerve root compression.
- An enlarged and deformed skull can lead to increased intra-cranial pressure, hydrocephalus or cranial nerve deficits such as facial palsy (narrowing of neural foramina), hearing loss or blindness (pressure on optic nerve).
- High cardiac output secondary to increased bone vascularity (rare).

- Insufficiency fractures.
- Osteosarcoma, chondrosarcoma, malignant fibrous histiocytoma and giant cell tumours all have been reported with Paget's disease.

EXAMINER: What are the indications for THA in Paget's disease?

CANDIDATE: The indications are similar to non-Pagetoid disease. It is important to make sure that the pain is arising from the joint surface and not the bone. Bone pain with active Paget's is suggested by an increased alkaline phosphatase value. It is also important to exclude insufficiency fractures, neurological compression in the spine or Paget's sarcoma as a cause of pain.

EXAMINER: How do you assess disease activity?

CANDIDATE: Patients with active Paget's disease have raised alkaline phosphatase (AlkPhos) and urine hydroxyproline values. The higher the level the more active the disease is. Patients with very high AlkPhos levels are thought to be at higher risk of bleeding and heterotrophic ossification formation.

EXAMINER: If the Paget's disease is active what will you do?

CANDIDATE: I would refer him to one of my rheumatoid colleagues for a Pamidronate (Aredia) injection. This is a bisphosphonate, which is a potent inhibitor of osteoclastic activity and hence bone resorption. This reduces bone vascularity and bleeding and possibly the incidence of heterotopic ossification. The other option is the use of bisphosphonates or calcitonin to reduce bone-related pain, reduce postoperative bone resorption and decrease bleeding should surgery be required.

EXAMINER: What are the technical issues of performing THA in Paget's disease?

CANDIDATE: There is a tendency for excessive bleeding at surgery due to increased vascularity. Blood should ideally be cross-matched or at the least available from a group and saved within 10 minutes. Bone can be very hard and sclerotic making it difficult to ream and broach. Burrs may be needed to enter the bone prior to reaming and/or broaching. Varus deformity of the proximal end of the femur predisposes to varus placement of the femoral component.

Protrusio, as we have mentioned, is a common finding and I would consider using bone graft medially to compensate. Some surgeons use lateral offset liners and antiprotrusio cages, although this complicates surgery.

As Paget's bone is brittle there is a higher risk of both intraoperative and postoperative fracture.

There is some controversy as to whether there is an increased risk of heterotopic ossification occurring from the abnormalities of osteogenic differentiation in Paget patients. Some surgeons routinely give prophylaxis to reduce the risk of HO [Score 6].

EXAMINER: There is a bit more than that when planning THA.

CANDIDATE: As bone pain is common in Paget's disease and does not necessarily improve with THA a diagnostic local anaesthetic injection to rule out concurrent bone pathology may be indicated. It is also important to exclude referred pain from spinal stenosis or radiculopathy and other causes of musculoskeletal pain.

Good-quality, full-length radiographs to assess the degree of deformity and the extent of bone involvement. Radiographs should be scrutinized for the presence of a stress fracture that could account for hip pain. The fractures may be in the region of the femoral neck, intertrochanteric area or femoral shaft. They usually present as incomplete or fissure fractures on the tension side of the bone. Unrelenting hip pain and radiographic bone destruction suggests sarcomatous change.

Consider using cell salvage, hypotensive anaesthesia and predonation of autologous blood if intraoperative blood loss is anticipated to be high with active disease. Concurrent osteotomy may be needed if component alignment is difficult.

Marked protrusio can make hip dislocation very difficult.

EXAMINER: You mentioned osteotomy, how often do you perform osteotomy when you perform THA for Paget's disease?

CANDIDATE: In the majority of patients with Paget's THA can be performed without need for osteotomy. However, if deformity is severe, precluding implantation with a standard stem, then planning for reduction osteotomy to correct the deformity and/or the use of modular stems must be done preoperatively.

EXAMINER: What type of hip replacement would you use?

CANDIDATE: Although there has been a trend in recent years to use uncemented components in Paget's disease, in this patient I would use a cemented THA. She is 68 and has Paget's disease and I think it is a reasonable option in this situation. If the patient is younger, then the choice becomes more controversial. Although previous studies have recommended the use of cement in the last 20 years there has been a trend to use uncemented components. The worry that the altered morphology of pagetoid bone adversely influences ingrowth into cementless implants has not been borne out in practice. In addition, previous concerns for the problem with osseointegration are mostly unfounded. The biology of bone ingrowth for initial fixation of uncemented components depends, in part, on the ability of bone to proceed through the early phase of fracture healing. Patients with Paget's disease are not known to have compromised ability for fracture healing and these patients progress through the biological process of fracture healing at normal speed.

Parvizi et al. reported on 21 cementless THA implanted against pagetoid bone; all were stable and demonstrated radiographic evidence of ingrowth at 7-year follow-up.[54] Lusty et al. from Sydney, Australia reported medium-term results of 23 uncemented THA at 6.7 years follow up.[55] There were three revisions, one stem for aseptic loosening and two stems after periprosthetic fracture.

Some surgeons prefer cementless components especially when bone is very sclerotic, or a concurrent osteotomy is done. Extremely sclerotic bleeding bone will make interdigitation of cement difficult and cement extravasation into the fracture gaps may occur after osteotomy. If using a cementless cup the use of adjuvant acetabular screws is recommended.

EXAMINER: Any special complications that can occur postoperatively?

CANDIDATE: There is a reported greater incidence of heterotopic ossification.

EXAMINER: Anything else?

CANDIDATE: Dislocation.

EXAMINER: No, I am not aware of an increased risk of dislocation.

COMMENT: Several studies have documented osteolysis following THA in patients with Paget's disease.[56] This is thought to be related to the increased metabolic turnover of the pathologic bone. Other authors have reported that osteolysis is not a problem following THA in Paget's disease.[57]

Other complications include periprosthetic fracture around total hip implants; and the continuation of bone pain following arthroplasty, microfractures, and malignant transformation to osteosarcoma.

Gold medal candidates

EXAMINER: What causes have been identified for the increased number and activity of Pagetic osteoclasts?

CANDIDATE: Causes identified include:
1. Osteoclastic precursors are hypersensitive to calcitriol (1,25(OH) 2D3).
2. Osteoclasts are hyper-responsive to RANK ligand (RANKL), the osteoclast stimulatory factor that mediates the effects of most osteotropic factors on osteoclast formation.
3. Marrow stromal cells from Pagetic lesions have increased RANKL expression.
4. Osteoclast precursor recruitment is increased by interleukin (IL)-6, which is increased in the blood of patients with active Paget's disease and is over-expressed in pagetic osteoclasts.
5. The antiapoptotic oncogene Bcl-2 in Pagetic bone is over-expressed.
6. Expression of the proto-oncogene c-fos, which increases osteoclastic activity, is increased.
7. Numerous osteoblasts are recruited to active resorption sites and produce large amounts of new bone matrix. As a result, bone turnover is high and bone mass is normal or increased, not reduced.

Structured oral examination question 8

DDH is one of the most common hip viva questions that regularly gets asked in the oral viva examination.

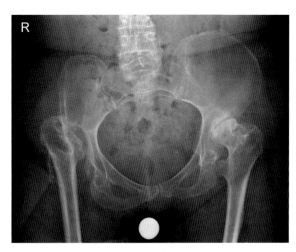

Figure 3.8 Anteroposterior (AP) radiograph of the pelvis of severe bilateral DDH.

We think this is because it is a fairly common hip condition with a lot to talk about. The story can go in many different directions.

EXAMINER: These are the anteroposterior (AP) radiographs of a 66-year-old woman with bilateral hip pain (Figure 3.8). Would you like to pass comment on them?

CANDIDATE 1: The AP radiograph demonstrates a severely dysplastic hip on the right side with secondary OA changes. On the left side again, there is dysplasia but to a lesser degree with again secondary OA changes present. [Score 5]

CANDIDATE 2: This is an AP radiograph of the hips and pelvis of a 66-year-old woman taken on the 16/5/11, which demonstrates severe bilateral dysplasia.[58] There is a high dislocation on the right side, Crowe IV or Hartofilakidis III hip. There is no contact between the true and false acetabulum. The femoral head appears poorly developed, probably absent, with the femoral neck articulating against the iliac crest. The view of the proximal portion of the femoral canal on the right side suggests a very narrow medullary canal. On the left side there is a Crowe III hip or Hartofilakidis II hip. There is a low dislocation and secondary osteoarthritis.[59] [Score 6–7]

  COMMENT[60]: The left side is a Hartofilakidis I hip as the femoral head is still contained within the original acetabulum. With a low dislocation the femoral head is in contact, at least in part, with the true acetabulum and in this situation, this is

the most severe deformity. In high dislocation, the femoral head and acetabulum make no contact and the head has migrated superiorly and posteriorly. Often in this situation the true acetabulum is reasonably well-preserved, although underdeveloped and osteoporotic.

EXAMINER: What do you mean by dysplasia?

CANDIDATE: Dysplasia is lack of coverage of the femoral head, whether it is subluxed or dislocated.

EXAMINER: How do you classify dysplasia?

CANDIDATE: Crowe classified dysplasia radiographically into four categories based on the proximal migration of the femoral head. The migration is calculated on an AP radiograph by measuring the vertical distance between the inter-teardrop line and the junction between the femoral head and medial edge of the neck.

  Crowe I is less than 50% subluxation, Crowe II hips have between 50% and 75% subluxation.

EXAMINER: [Interrupting] That's fine. That's OK. Any other classification systems that you know?

CANDIDATE: [Sharp intake of breath, shaking of head and then silence.] No.

EXAMINER: Have you heard of the Hartofilakidis classification?

CANDIDATE: I have, but I can't remember the specifics.

EXAMINER: The Hartofilakidis classification system, which divides DDH in adults into three types: dysplasia, low dislocation and high dislocation. Many surgeons prefer this system, as it is more practical and simpler to use.

  What are the anatomical issues associated with DDH?

CANDIDATE: The anatomical differences are divided into acetabular, femur and soft-tissue issues. The acetabulum is shallow and anteverted; the femur has a small deformed head and short anteverted valgus neck.

EXAMINER: That's not all the differences. There are some you have missed. Do you know any more?

CANDIDATE: Muscles around the hip are usually shortened and, er, er . . .

EXAMINER: The greater trochanter is small and posteriorly displaced, the femoral canal narrow, the acetabulum is usually small with poor bone quality, hip capsule elongated and redundant, psoas tendon hypertrophied, and abductors orientated transversely as a result of the superior migration of the femoral head. The femoral and sciatic nerves may be shortened and therefore more vulnerable to injury during arthroplasty surgery.

What is the role of a CT scan in planning an operation for DDH?[61]

CANDIDATE 1: CT scans can be used to determine the available acetabular coverage and to estimate the degree of femoral anteversion.

CANDIDATE 2: CT scans are useful in assessing available bone stock, and the morphology, dimensions and orientation of both the acetabulum and femur.

Any leg length discrepancy can be precisely evaluated and allow for design of custom femoral implants.

Various measurements include: femoral neck shaft angle, anteversion of the femoral neck, medial head offset, position of the isthmus and height.

The AP size of the acetabulum as measured by CT is often different from the supero-inferior size evaluated on plain radiographs.

Proximal femoral anteversion is calculated by measuring the angle between the posterior bicondylar axis and the mediolateral dimensions of the medullary canal 20 mm above the lesser trochanter.

EXAMINER: These measurements are useful to know but how are they actually going to help you to plan surgery?

CANDIDATE: In the acetabulum following the abnormal anatomy too closely might lead to anterior instability if the cup is overanteverted. It is important to recognize that a substantial amount of acetabular anteversion and deformity can be present with a relatively normal-looking AP pelvic radiograph.

In addition, femoral anteversion may be difficult to recognize. Even in normal-looking AP radiographs a significant amount of anteversion may be present. Attempting to implant an uncemented stem in a deformed anteverted femur may result in a proximal femoral fracture.

EXAMINER: What are the technical difficulties in performing a THA in a DDH patient?

CANDIDATE: Crowe type II and III hips have a marked superolateral rim deficiency and anterior

wall defect. Bulk autografting of the superolateral acetabulum with bone from the femoral head can be used to increase the cover and stability of the acetabular component. The graft and its bed need careful preparation, stable fixation and precise positioning. Graft resorption can occur, leading to cup migration and loosening.

Although it is technically difficult for anatomic placement of the acetabular component the forces on the THA are significantly reduced. Linde et al. found a 42% rate of loosening of cemented Charnley components after a mean of 9 years if the component was positioned outside the true acetabulum compared to 13% if placed inside.[62,63]

EXAMINER: Any other options to deal with deficient superior coverage of the cup?

CANDIDATE: A small, uncemented cup can be placed in a high hip centre location. In this position the cup is completely covered with host bone and avoids the need for grafting. Disadvantages include decreased polyethylene thickness associated with a small acetabular component, difficulties with correction of leg length inequality and altered hip biomechanics. Hip instability is increased due to the use of a small femoral head component along with the risk of femoral–pelvic impingement either in flexion or extension.

EXAMINER: What do we mean by cotyloplasty?

CANDIDATE: Cotyloplasty involves a deliberate fracture of the medial wall of the acetabulum in order to place the acetabular component within the available iliac bone. The acetabulum is advanced medially by the creation of a controlled comminuted fracture of the medial acetabular wall. Mixed results have been reported, but there is a worry that future revisions may be difficult because issues with restoration of bone stock have not been addressed.[64]

EXAMINER: How do you preoperatively plan for DDH surgery?

CANDIDATE: On the acetabulum side the position of the true acetabulum should be identified, and a decision made whether to restore the acetabulum to its true position or not. The degree of anteversion of the acetabulum should be defined as well as the adequacy of bone stock for satisfactory cup fixation and coverage.

Preoperative planning would also include an estimation of the acetabular component size, the

53

preferred method of fixation (cement/uncemented) and need for bone graft.

On the femoral side the size of the femoral canal and the need for special or custom implants should be assessed.

The need for femoral shortening should be made preoperatively. The method and amount of femoral shortening need to be worked out beforehand.

Preoperative planning should also include the surgical approach to be used, solutions to deal with the hypoplastic acetabulum and femur, management of LLD and restoration of abductor function.

EXAMINER: What is the effect of anteversion of the femoral stem on THA?[65]

CANDIDATE: When there is more than 40° of anteversion, a corrective rotational osteotomy or a modular implant in which the version of the femoral neck can be varied may be necessary.

EXAMINER: That's not really the question I asked.

CANDIDATE: A large amount of femoral anteversion increases the risk of dislocation.

EXAMINER: That's correct, but not the whole story. You have already partly answered the question earlier on.

CANDIDATE: I am sorry, I don't understand.[66]

COMMENT: Attempting to implant an uncemented stem in a deformed femur may result in a proximal femoral fracture. In this situation you may want to use either a cemented or modular stem that allows control of anteversion. Also, excessive anteversion of the femoral component can lead to internal rotational contracture of the hip.

EXAMINER: How do you correct length inequality in DDH?

CANDIDATE: With Crowe type III and IV hips, if the cup is placed in the anatomic position femoral shortening is required. Without femoral shortening it is very difficult to reduce the prosthetic head into the acetabular component because of soft-tissue contractures.

If one attempts to fully correct a significant leg length discrepancy a sciatic nerve palsy may occur. If permanent this can be a disabling complication from surgery and which patients are less willing to

accept these days. The exact amount of lengthening that results in sciatic nerve palsy is not known. Acute limb lengthening of more than 2–4 cm during arthroplasty is associated with an increased risk of neural injury. Therefore, as a general rule the hip should be lengthened the minimum amount required to re-establish reasonable function and hip stability. Any lengthening more than 4 cm becomes very risky for a sciatic nerve injury and is generally not advised.

Shortening is performed either by sequential resecting of the proximal femur or by performing a shortening subtrochanteric osteotomy.

Sequential proximal resection results in a small, straight femoral tube with a small metaphyseal flare which is usually unsuitable for an uncemented femoral implant. Typically, a small cemented DDH stem needs to be used with a straight proximal medial geometry and without a metaphyseal flare.

Advantages of a subtrochanteric shortening osteotomy include preservation of the metaphyseal femoral region (which provides most of the rotational stability of the implant) and allowing concomitant correction of angular and anteversion deformities. It is technically difficult and there is a risk of non-union.

EXAMINER: How do you reduce the risk of non-union?

CANDIDATE: Different subtrochanteric osteotomy geometries can be used. These include transverse, oblique, stepcut and double Chevron osteotomies. A transverse osteotomy is simplest and the resected bone can be used as an onlay graft.

Avoiding the use of a cemented stem prevents the risk of the cement interfering with healing of the osteotomy site. A press fit achieves distal fixation of the prosthesis. Strut allograft and circlage cables may also be needed for support.

EXAMINER: What are the principles of revision hip surgery with DDH?

CANDIDATE: Two major concerns are deficient acetabular bone stock and the position of the acetabular cup, particularly if the centre of the hip has not been restored during the primary procedure.

Several surgeons have advocated the use of a high hip centre in order to take advantage of the remaining bone stock and to avoid the use of a structured graft.

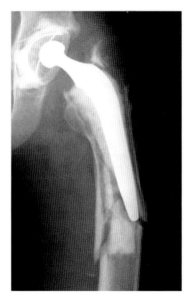

Figure 3.9a Vancouver B3 periprosthetic fracture left THA.

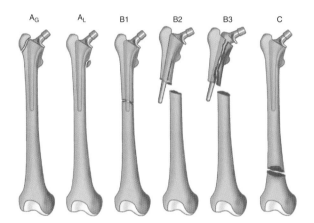

Figure 3.9b Vancouver classification of PPF around the hip.

However, a high hip centre does not correct leg length discrepancy, does not provide good bone stock for revision hip surgery and is associated with early acetabular loosening and a higher rate of dislocation because of ischial impingement.

The pattern of bone loss associated with DDH is a reduced AP diameter combined with poor superior support. This loss is further increased by surgical bone loss at the time of the index operation, migration of the cup and osteolysis.

Bone graft would need to be ordered along with special equipment such as universal screwdrivers, screw extractors, high-speed burrs and metal cutters.

Structured oral examination question 9

Periprosthetic fracture (PPF) around the hip

EXAMINER: This is a 70-year-old man who was admitted to the orthopaedic ward last night after a fall. He is generally fit and healthy although is on Warfarin for a mitral value replacement. These are his radiographs that were presented at the trauma meeting in the morning (Figure 3.9a). What do you see?

CANDIDATE: This is an AP radiograph showing a left Vancouver B2 periprosthetic fracture around a Charnley cemented total hip replacement.

EXAMINER: What makes you state that this is a Vancouver B2 periprosthetic fracture?

CANDIDATE: A B2 fracture is around the distal stem or tip with significant communtion and a loose stem with adequate bone stock.

EXAMINER: Any difficulties with the Vancouver classification (Figure 3.9b)?

CANDIDATE: There are some difficulties differentiating between type B1 and type B2 on plain radiographs. What you think is a well-fixed stem may in fact be loose. If you haven't thought through a plan B to deal with the possibility of a loose stem, then this will significantly increase the complexities and difficulties of managing the case intraoperatively.

EXAMINER: Are you aware of any more recent classification system?

CANDIDATE: The Vancouver group have recently published their Unified Classification System (UCS) for periprosthetic fractures around a hip or knee arthroplasty in 2014.[67] Fractures are categorized A to F.

Type A fractures involve the apophysis, e.g. greater trochanter fracture around a THA.

Type B fractures involve the 'bed' of the implant, e.g. femoral shaft fracture around a stem, and are still graded B1, B2 and B3 as per the original Vancouver classification system.

Type C fractures are 'clear' from the implant, e.g. distal to the stem but within the same bone.

Type D is a PF in a bone between two joint replacements, e.g. femoral shaft fracture between a hip and knee replacement.

Type E is a fracture in which two bones support one joint replacement, e.g. an acetabular and femoral fracture around a THA.

Type F fractures involve a joint surface that has not been replaced or resurfaced, e.g. acetabular fracture around a hip hemiarthroplasty.

EXAMINER: What advantages does this classification system have over the Vancouver classification system?

CANDIDATE: The Vancouver classification system was based on the key principles of management of periprosthetic fractures. It has demonstrated good inter- and intra-observer reliability and has become widely accepted.

However, there was felt to be a need to expand the Vancouver classification system to include three other types of fracture that may occur in combination or in isolation, and to deal with the pelvis as a whole (not just the acetabulum).

EXAMINER: This is actually a B3 fracture as there is poor bone stock around the stem, which is loose. This patient is a 70-year-old male who had a left THA 20 years ago and had a fall sustaining this PPF. He has had a previous mitral valve replacement and is on warfarin. He is a diet-controlled type 2 diabetic. He is otherwise quite fit, well, is fully active and independent and still drives a car. What will be your management plan?

CANDIDATE: This is a difficult and complex case. The review article by Schwarzkopf provides a good treatment algorithm for dealing with periprosthetic fractures[68] (Figure 3.9c). Firstly, I would like to get details of the original operation and implants if at all possible, although in this case, it may prove impossible given the length of time since the original hip replacement. I would also seek advice from other senior colleagues who were experienced hip surgeons or discuss this case in a regional revision hip network.

I would need to consider the following: whether to just deal with the femoral stem or also deal with the acetabular component. I would additionally need to take into account the patient's ability to cope physiologically with a complex and prolonged procedure. This patient is still very active and healthy with few comorbidities, and this will influence my surgical plan. His Warfarin will need to be stopped but he must be covered with an alternative anticoagulant because of his MVR.

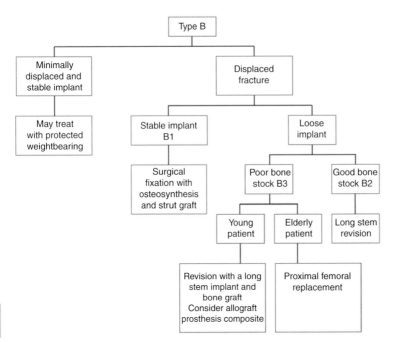

Figure 3.9c Treatment algorithm B3 PF.

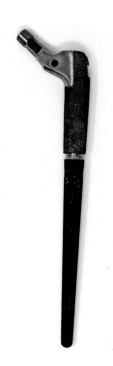

Figure 3.9d ARCOS uncemented revision femoral stem. Grit-blasted, anatomic bow.

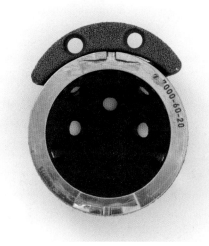

Figure 3.9e TM revision shell with augment.

I would use a posterior approach as this is an extensile approach and provides excellent acetabular and femoral exposure. I can also extend the incision distally if I needed to, along the length of the femur. Assuming the patient is fit enough, I would plan to also revise the socket as the radiographs show acetabular component loosening. This is a B3 fracture, which necessitates revision of the femoral stem, and I would bypass the fracture using a long-stem, titanium, modular fluted revision hip such as the ZMR or ARCOS system (which I am familiar with) (Figure 3.9d) in order to get distal fixation and provide rotational and axial stability. I would ensure that I had templated preoperatively the different stem options available. Using such a stem helps deal with the issues of poor proximal bone quality, bone loss and stress shielding. I would also use cerclage cables or wires distally and around the diaphysis of the femur to help maintain control of the femoral tube and prevent fracture propagation distally. The modular stem allows for greater flexibility in controlling for leg length, offset and version. I would also consider doing an ORIF for the fracture with or without an allograft to help maintain the integrity and stability of the femoral tube.

For the acetabular component, I would use an uncemented socket (such as a trabecular metal (TM) backed socket) with supplementary screws, but have augments available in case there are significant acetabular bone defects present (Figure 3.9e). A preoperative CT scan of the hip would be useful in helping identify significant acetabular bone defects, although from what I can determine on the radiograph shown to me, there doesn't appear to be significant bone loss or any protrusio. My bearing surfaces of choice would be a ceramic head (36 mm ideally) with a highly crosslinked lipped polyethylene liner to help minimize the risk of a posterior dislocation.

EXAMINER: Why not just fix the fracture with a long femoral plate and leave the stem in situ?

CANDIDATE: The evidence suggests that reoperation rates are higher when B3 fractures only have an ORIF performed and are not revised. The systematic review in the BJJ 2017 by Khan *et al.*[69] from Nottingham showed almost 30% reoperation rate compared to around 15% for revision ± ORIF.

EXAMINER: Are there any other surgical options available?

CANDIDATE: A distally locked, uncemented, hydroxyapatite-coated long femoral stem prosthesis such as the Cannulok hip could be used. The paper by El-Bakoury in 2017[70] looking at B2 and B3 fractures in 28 patients aged 75 and over showed a 95% fracture union rate and 100% survivorship of the revised hip at a mean 4 years follow-up. The Exeter group have reported on their experience using impaction bone grafting, supported by a plate to contain the graft, with a long cemented femoral stem for situations with extensive femoral bone loss including B2 and 3 periprosthetic fractures.[71]

EXAMINER: Are there any other options available that you might need to consider if the patient was very frail and the bone quality very poor?

CANDIDATE: Another potential option would be to do a proximal femoral replacement (PFR). The study from Parvizi's group[72] looking at 21 patients with a B3 PPF showed a good outcome using a PFR. They advised using a constrained liner in such patients if the hip was unstable intraoperatively (as is often the case because the abductor mechanism is often disrupted in such patients and the risk of dislocation is high). They also advised trying to maintain as much of the proximal femoral bone as possible even if the bone quality is very poor to help maintain bone stock and reapproximate the proximal bone onto the PFR.

EXAMINER: You perform the operation revising the femoral and acetabular components using an uncemented acetabular socket, a long uncemented femoral fluted titanium stem and a ceramic-on-polyethylene bearing couple. All went well during the operation. Postoperatively, on Day 1, he appeared quite comfortable and had no neurovascular complications. On Day 2, you see him and he has developed a foot drop on the left (operated) side. What will you do?

CANDIDATE: This patient has developed a foot drop secondary to some form of sciatic nerve injury. He was well immediately postoperatively, and this implies that the sciatic nerve must have been intact and working then. It is therefore unlikely that the nerve was injured iatrogenically intraoperatively. I would firstly establish exactly when the patient started to get neurological symptoms and signs. I would look at the incision site. Is there excessive bruising or swelling? Are the distal pulses intact? I would review the operation notes and anaesthetic notes. What type of anaesthesia was used (spinal/epidural, etc.) although,

again, there was no foot drop initially postoperatively.

EXAMINER: The patient has noticed that the thigh has swollen significantly and there is quite a lot of bruising and the soft tissues feel tense.

CANDIDATE: I note that the patient was on warfarin. Has this been restarted? I would get an urgent INR and clotting screen. My concern is that the patient has an evolving large haematoma, and this could be causing a sciatic nerve neuropraxia leading to a foot drop 48 hours after surgery. The difficulty is balancing the need to protect his mitral valve replacement and minimize the risk of getting a haematoma that is now causing a foot drop. I would also seek urgent advice from the cardiologists and haematologists as to whether we can stop the warfarin and put the patient on an alternative anticoagulant such as IV heparin or LMWH. I would prepare to take this patient to theatre and evacuate the haematoma urgently. An MRI might be helpful preoperatively to identify the location of any significant haematoma. An urgent CT angiogram may also help identify any significant bleeding vessels which may be amenable to embolisation.

Structured oral examination question 10

EXAMINER: What does the radiograph show (Figure 3.10)?

CANDIDATE: This is an AP radiograph of a cemented Exeter THA. The acetabular cup and stem are well fixed with an adequate cement mantle thickness which is greater than 2 mm.

EXAMINER: Anything else?

CANDIDATE: The stem is in slight varus, but the cup is well aligned with no suggestion of excessive anteversion or retroversion or being too closed or open.

EXAMINER: Anything else?

CANDIDATE: His femoral artery has a large amount of calcification present in its wall.

EXAMINER: Anything else?

CANDIDATE: Not sure.

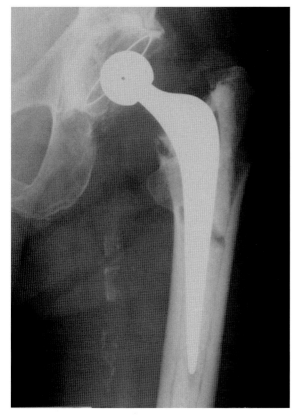

Figure 3.10 Anteroposterior (AP) radiograph cemented Exeter hip with broken cement mantle.

EXAMINER: Look here; what do you think this lucency is?

CANDIDATE: This is a cement fracture.

EXAMINER: What are the reasons for a broken cement fracture?

CANDIDATE: Cement mantle fractures are worrying as they are associated with early loosening and the need for revision surgery.

The early development of stem–cement interface debonding (separation) and subsequent cement fracture are thought to be the initiating events of aseptic loosening.

Studies suggest that the initiating events that result in cement failure are due to stresses.

COMMENT: Listen to the question the examiner asks you. Trying to waffle through a question isn't going to score you any marks.

Studies suggest that the initiating events that result in cement failure are due to stresses experienced at the cement mantle that exceed the fatigue endurance limit of both the stem–cement interface and the cement material itself.

It is important to reduce cement stresses so as to minimize the risk of cement debonding and fracture.

EXAMINER: So how can high cement stresses be avoided?

CANDIDATE: By the creation of an optimally thick, symmetric, and homogeneous cement mantle.

EXAMINER: So how do we achieve this?

CANDIDATE: Stresses experienced in the cement mantle have been shown to be highest at the stem tip and secondarily at the proximal–medial cement mantle.

Stem malalignment produces non-uniform cement mantle thickness in key areas.

Defects or voids in the cement mantle reduce bulk cement thickness and have a substantial effect on cement stresses.

Variations in implant geometry (e.g. diameter and contour) and material have also been shown to affect stresses experienced in the cement mantle.

EXAMINER: Can you be more specific?[73]

CANDIDATE: A varus femoral stem is associated with higher incidence of aseptic loosening. This results in thin or non-existent cement mantle in the proximal medial and distal lateral zones.

Large voids up to 5 mm in diameter are detrimental. Location of voids is important. Small voids in areas of the cement mantle known to experience high strains may result in premature fixation failure.

A proximal–medial cement mantle greater than 10 mm or less than 2 mm in thickness is associated with a significant increase in cement fracture, radiolucent lines at the prosthesis–cement and progressive component loosening when compared to proximal–medial cement mantles that measure 2–5 mm in thickness.[74]

An asymmetrical distal cement mantle significantly increases the risk of implant failure.

Inadequate centralization of the stem or malrotation will result in excessively thinned areas of distal cement, increased cement strains and prosthesis bone contact.

COMMENT: Best results for femoral components allow for 2–5 mm proximal medial thickness of cement mantle, less than 2 mm of proximal medial thickness of cancellous bone, a stem that fills more than half the distal part of the meduallary canal and a stem in neutral orientation.

Worst results for femoral components occur with a cement mantle thickness >10 mm or in a femur with more than 2 mm proximal medial cancellous bone, those that filled half or less of the medullary canal and those in varus orientation.

In general, too thin a layer of cement will occur if there is lack of removal of proximal medial cancellous bone whilst too much removal of proximal medial cancellous bone results in poor cement interdigitation and fixation with bone, as the bone surface is mostly cortical.

EXAMINER: What is the optimal cement mantle thickness?

CANDIDATE: The femoral stems of hips that have a 2–5 mm thick cement mantle in the proximal medial region have a better outcome than stems implanted with a thicker (>10 mm) or thinner (<2 mm) cement mantle.

EXAMINER: What about the cement, how can this be improved?

CANDIDATE: Improvements in the inherent properties of the cement (increased strength, reduced brittleness, improved interface adherence) to increase strain resistance and thus retard early debonding and microfractures will aid in the quality and long-term success of the cement.

EXAMINER: What measures can be taken intra-operatively to improve the quality of the cement mantle?

CANDIDATE :
1. Canal preparation
Use of correctly sized broaches that allow a mantle of adequate thickness, pulsatile lavage, and brushing and drying of the prepared canal before and during insertion (clean dry bone).
Packing of the femoral canal with adrenaline soaked swabs, hypotensive analgesia to reduce bleeding, suction catheter and avoidance of blood/cement occlusions.
2. Cement preparation
Centrifugation or vacuum mixing to minimize pore formation and timing of cement injection to achieve optimal viscosity during insertion improves the cement mantle quality.

Occlusion of the canal using a distal plug, retrograde filling of the canal and cement gun pressurization of the cement column with a tight proximal seal are essential in achieving an interdigitating, uniform, and homogeneous cement mantle.

EXAMINER: Have you heard of boneloc bone cement?

CANDIDATE: This is a bone cement that was withdrawn quite soon after introduction because of unacceptable revision rates with its use.

Mean fracture toughness and mean tensile strengths were significantly lower than other conventional bone cements.

EXAMINER: What is the function of a centralizer?

CANDIDATE:
- Femoral stem centralizers were originally designed for double tapered, straight stems.
- A stem centralizer guides the femoral prosthesis to a neutral position within the cement and guarantees an even cement layer between the bone and prosthesis.
- Use of a centralizer improves the quality of the distal cement mantle as well as improves stem position (central within mantle).
- Means the stem is "Non-end bearing", the void below the stem allows a degree of stem subsidence without directly bearing onto the cement thus preventing cement cracking and deterioration.
- This subsidence also seals off the stem-cement interface to prevent any fluid flow that may lead to loosening (effective joint space).
- Stem subsidence into an air filled centralizer leads to low shear stresses, high compressive stresses and almost no tensile stress

EXAMINER: What is the ideal cement mantle thickness?

CANDIDATE: I would aim for a cement mantle thickness greater than 2 mm as any less than this increases the risk of cement mantle fracture.

EXAMINER: Have you heard of the French paradox?

CANDIDATE: No, I am sorry I haven't.

COMMENT: The ideal cement mantle thickness is still uncertain. Two philosophies about cement mantle thickness exist. In the UK and USA, the first technique aims to produce a complete cement

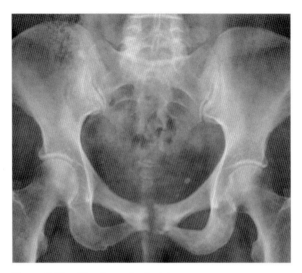

Figure 3.11a AP radiograph of pelvis.

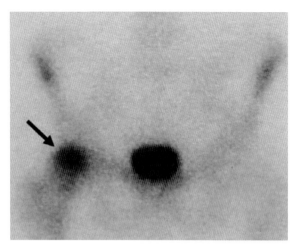

Figure 3.11b Nuclear bone scan.

mantle of at least 2 mm in thickness and without 'windows'. It is believed that 'windows' may allow debris to reach the interface and that thin cement mantles will be highly stressed and may fracture.

The second technique used in France is the use of a thinner cement mantle in which the possibility of windows is accepted. This has been called the French paradox in which implantation of a canal filling femoral component in a line to line manner is associated with a thin cement mantle[75]. The reason for good results is thought to be the fact that a thin cement mantle in conjunction with a canal filling stem was supported mainly by cortical bone and subjected to low stresses.

This is Score 8 material not expected for the average Score 6 pass candidate.

The discussion could move on to any number of topics related to cement use in arthroplasty surgery depending on how the viva is progressing.

- Barracks grading of cement.[76,77]
- Generations of cementing technique.
- Categories of loosening of cemented stems (Harris).
- Exeter vs. Charnley stem design.

Structured oral examination question 11

EXAMINER: A 52-year-old man has been referred to the orthopaedic clinic with a 6-week history of (right)[78] hip pain. The pain was unrelated to trauma and was a severe, deep aching groin pain worse at night. The patient has a limp with pain on weight bearing and a positive Trendelenburg sign.

These are his radiographs (Figure 3.11a). What do you see?

CANDIDATE: The anteroposterior (AP) pelvis radiograph shows no significant abnormality. At most there is a suggestion that the right femoral head may be more opaque than the left.[79]

OR The anteroposterior (AP) pelvis radiograph reveals diffuse osteopenia of the right femoral neck and head. There is no joint space narrowing, scalloping or fracture noted. The left hip appears normal.

Do we have a lateral radiograph of the right hip?

EXAMINER: That's all we have got. What further investigations would be appropriate?

CANDIDATE: I would start by taking a full history and examining the patient.[80]

EXAMINER: That's all been done. He has severe hip pain keeping him off work.

CANDIDATE: I would like to perform blood tests (FBC, UE, bone profile, LFT, clotting, ESR, CRP, PSA and serum electrophoresis).

My first choice investigation would be an MRI of the hips and pelvis.

Other investigations may involve a nuclear bone scan which would provide information about other possible skeletal abnormalities.

A CT scan is another option that would provide more information about the bone architecture.

EXAMINER: This is his bone scan (Figure 3.11b). What does it show?

CANDIDATE: The bone scan shows heterogeneous intense uptake of isotope in the femoral head (mainly anterosuperior) and neck region.

EXAMINER: These are his MRI hip images (Figure 3.11c). What do you see?

CANDIDATE: This is a coronal MR image of both hips short-tau inversion recovery (STIR sequence) characterized by a heterogeneous bone marrow oedema pattern in the right femoral head and neck regions. In the superior aspect of the head in the subchondral area, there are areas of low signal surrounded by rims of high signal.

MRI images of the hips demonstrate decreased marrow signal on T1 images of the right hip with striking T2 hyperintensity in the same area. No masses are noted.

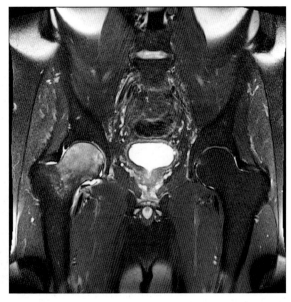

Figure 3.11c The likely diagnosis is bone marrow oedema syndrome (BMES) or idiopathic transient osteoporosis of the hip (ITOH). The main differentiating feature from osteonecrosis is the lack of focal lesions typically seen in osteonecrosis.

EXAMINER: What is the differential diagnosis?

CANDIDATE: The differential diagnosis is due to other conditions that cause bone marrow oedema on MRI that include infection (septic arthritis), osteonecrosis, osteochondromatosis and reflex sympathetic dystrophy. Other conditions that should be considered are: malignancy (primary and secondary), stress fracture of the femoral neck, osteoarthritis and inflammatory arthritis. Benign tumours including osteoid osteoma, osteoblastoma, chondroblastoma and malignant lesions such as leukaemia, osteosarcoma, Ewing's sarcoma and chondrosarcoma have been reported to be associated with bone marrow oedema.

In this case the history and imaging would suggest either ITOH or osteonecrosis. The radiographs are unremarkable (sometimes may show osteopenia). The reduced range of movement on examination can be seen with either osteonecrosis or BMES. In BMES one would usually find diffuse oedema but no focal defects or subchondral changes on T2 MRI. One would see low-signal intensity on T1-weighted images, high-intensity signal on T2-weighted images and short-tau inversion recovery (STIR) images. These changes reflect increased intracellular and extracellular fluid of the bone marrow resulting from the inflammatory process. The bone scan in BMES is sensitive for early disease typically showing homogeneous increased uptake in the head and neck and sometimes the trochanteric region.

In ON the isotope uptake is more localized and on MRI there are corresponding focal lesions in the same area (double line sign and subchondral changes), typically seen in the anterosuperior femoral head.

EXAMINER: What other joints are commonly affected?

CANDIDATE: Regional migratory osteoporosis can affect several joints. The hip is the most frequently affected joint (75%), followed by the knee, ankle, foot and tibial shaft. Rare cases affecting the upper extremities and the spine have also been reported.

EXAMINER: What are the features of this condition?

CANDIDATE: The syndrome is characterized by acute disabling pain in the hip and functional disability without a history of previous trauma. It is a rare condition.

Men are more commonly affected than women (3:1).

Two distinct groups are seen:
- BMES rarely presents in women other than in the third trimester of pregnancy.
- Middle-aged men.

Most cases are unilateral. Up to 40% of patients may show involvement of other joints.

The aetiology is largely unknown. The ESR may be raised. There is thought to be a relationship with clotting abnormalities and impaired venous return with marrow oedema and increased intramedullary pressure. There is controversy as to whether BMES may represent a very early reversible stage of osteonecrosis.

EXAMINER: What is the natural history of this condition?

CANDIDATE: The disease is usually self-limiting and will resolve over a period of 6–12 months, restoration of bone density and normal MRI are seen by 6–12 months. Turner *et al.* reported five patients in which the condition evolved into ON with head collapse; however, these patients may have actually had ON at the time of initial presentation.[81] Patients should be followed-up with an MRI at around 2 months, with the focus on reducing oedema.

EXAMINER: What are the treatment options?

CANDIDATE: Treatment is usually symptomatic consisting of analgesia, protected weight-bearing, rest and physiotherapy to help maintain strength and mobility of the hip.

Various studies have reported that bisphosphonates improve the symptoms. Other options are prostacycline infusion and there is limited evidence for hyperbaric oxygen.

Some may consider operative treatment in the form of core decompression for intractable pain which may allow for a faster recovery than in the conservatively treated group of patients.

Key points

- Around 10,000–20,000 new cases of osteonecrosis (ON) are reported each year in the United States. Bone marrow oedema syndrome (BMES) is a relatively rare disease.
- ON and BMES similarly present in young and middle-aged patients with hip or groin pain.
- Magnetic resonance imaging (MRI) is the most sensitive and specific diagnostic tool for both ON and BMES.
- ON progresses to end-stage arthritis in as many as 80–90% of patients. BMES has an excellent prognosis, typically resolving within 2–9 months.
- BMES should be treated non-operatively with protected weight-bearing and analgesics.

References

1. Berbari E, Mabry T, Tsaras G *et al.* Inflammatory blood laboratory levels as markers of prosthetic joint infection: a systematic review and meta-analysis. *J Bone Joint Surg Am.* 2010;92(11):2102–2109.

2. This is teaching a candidate not examining them, and is no longer allowed by the ICB.

3. Spangehl MJ, Masri BA, O'Connell JX, *et al.* Prospective analysis of preoperative and intraoperative investigations for the diagnosis of infection at the sites of two hundred and two revision total hip arthroplasties. *J Bone Joint Surg Am.* 1999;81:672–682.

4. Wyatt MC, Beswick AD, Kunutsor SK, Wilson MJ, Whitehouse MR, Blom AW. The alpha-defensin immunoassay and leukocyte esterase colorimetric strip test for the diagnosis of periprosthetic infection: a systematic review and meta-analysis. *JBJS.* 2016;98(12):992–1000.

5. It may be enough just to mention the uncertainties with nuclear imaging or you may have to quantify your answer a bit more fully. It is a judgement decision, but don't persist with your answer if the examiners want to move on.

   Technetium-99 bone scans are sensitive but not specific. Some investigators have found that a negative scan rules out infection, while others have reported that a scan can occasionally be negative in the presence of infection if there is inadequate blood supply to the bone. A technetium-99m bone scan identifies areas of increased bone activity through preferential uptake of the diphosphonate by metabolically active bone. Increased uptake occurs with loosening, infection, heterotopic bone formation, Paget's disease, stress fractures, modulus mismatch of a large uncemented stem, neoplasm, reflex sympathetic dystrophy and other metabolic conditions. In the uncomplicated THA, uptake around the lesser trichinae and shaft is usually insignificant by 6 months, but in 10% of cases, uptake may persist at the greater trochanter, prosthesis tip and acetabulum for more than 2 years. The pattern of uptake has not been found to consistently reflect the presence or absence of infection. Gallium imaging likewise has a poor sensitivity and accuracy. The use of leukocyte scans is generally preferred, having a higher sensitivity (88–92%) and specificity (73–100%), but their usefulness for the diagnosis of infection continues to be debated. FDG-PET is expensive and limited to a few institutions, and although very sensitive does not allow differentiation between an inflamed aseptically loosened prosthesis and an infected one.

6. This is sometimes referred to as Gustilo's classification.

7. Tsukayama DT, Estrada R, Gustilo RB. Infection after total hip arthroplasty. A study of one hundred and six infections. *J Bone Joint Surg Am*. 1996;78:512–523.

8. This is sometimes referred to as Gustilo's classification.

9. McPherson EJ, Woodson C, Holtom P, Roidis N, Shufelt C, Patzakis M. Periprosthetic total hip infection. Outcomes using a staging system. *Clin Orthop Relat Res*. 2002;403:8–15.

10. Lötscher PO, Clauss M, Sendi P, Kessler B, Graber P, Zimmerli W. Debridement and implant retention in the management of hip periprosthetic joint infection: outcomes following guided and rapid treatment at a single centre. *Bone Joint J*. 2017;99(3):330.

11. Grammatopoulos G, Bolduc ME, Atkins BL et al. Functional outcome of debridement, antibiotics and implant retention in periprosthetic joint infection involving the hip. *Bone Joint J*. 2017;99(5):614–622.

12. Buchholz HW, Elson RA, Engelbrecht E et al. Management of deep infection of total hip replacement. *J Bone Joint Surg [Br]*. 1981;63B:342–353.

13. Raut VV, Siney PD, Wroblewski BM. One-stage revision of infected total hip replacements with discharging sinuses. *J Bone Joint Surg [Br]*. 1994;76B:721–724.

14. With due respect, although Raut is the first author, I think 'Wroblewski from Wrightington has shown' is easier to remember. There is enough to learn already without making things difficult for yourself!

15. Hanssen AD, Rand JA. Evaluation and treatment of infection at the site of a total hip or knee arthroplasty. *J Bone Joint Surg [Am]*. 1998;80A:910–922.

16. Strange S, Whitehouse MR, Beswick AD et al. One-stage or two-stage revision surgery for prosthetic hip joint infection – the INFORM trial: a study protocol for a randomised controlled trial. *Trials*. 2016;17(1):90.

17. Taylor GJS, Bannister GC. Infection and interposition between ultraclean air source and wound. *J Bone Joint Surg Br*. 1993;75:503–504.

18. Madhavan P, Blom A, Karagkevrakis B, Pradeep M, Huma H, Newman JH. Deterioration of theatre discipline during total joint replacement – have theatre protocols been abandoned? *Ann R Coll Surg Engl*. 1999;81:262–265.

19. Lidwell OM, Lowbury EJ, Whyte W et al. Effect of ultraclean air in operating rooms on deep sepsis in the joint after total hip or knee replacement: a randomised study. *BMJ*. 1982;285:10–14.

20. Occasionally if an examiner doesn't know what a candidate is discussing they will enquire further. Equally the examiner may let it pass so as not to reveal their own knowledge gap. Skilful wily candidates may be able to bait and tempt the examiner into asking for clarification so as to then appear very studious and knowledgeable. Be careful, however, as there is a very real danger you may irritate the examiners by coming across as a 'know-all'.

21. Campbell P, Ebramzadeh E, Nelson S, Takamura K, De Smet K, Amstutz HC. Histological features of pseudotumor-like tissues from metal-on-metal hips. *Clin Orthop Relat Res*. 2010;468:2321–2327.

22. Devane PA, Horne JG, Ashmore A, Mutimer J, Kim W, Stanley J. Highly cross-linked polyethylene reduces wear and revision rates in total hip arthroplasty: a 10-year double-blinded randomized controlled trial. *JBJS*. 2017;99(20):1703–1714.

23. Ideally, they should have published their resurfacing results in peer-reviewed journals and perform enough cases to justify continuing on with this procedure (GIRFT – getting it right first time).

24. This is an old-style viva as this type of going on background case discussion is no longer allowed.

25. Huo MH, Stockton KG, Mont MA, Parvizi J. What's new in total hip arthroplasty. *J Bone Joint Surg Am*. 2010;92 (18):2959–2972.

26. Barrack RL, Mulroy RD Jr, Harris WH. Improved cementing techniques and femoral component loosening in young patients with hip arthroplasty: a 12-year radiographic review. *J Bone Joint Surg Br*. 1992;74:385–389.

27. Real-life working in the NHS understanding inherent practical difficulties rather than reading facts from a book. Examiners score candidates higher if they manage to include the 'NHS working environment' into their answer.

28. Lewthwaite SC, Squires B, Gie GA, Timperley AJ, Ling RS. The Exeter™ universal hip in patients 50 years or younger at 10–17 years' follow-up. *Clin Orthop Rel Res*. 2008;466(2):324–331.

29. Petheram TG, Whitehouse SL, Kazi HA, et al. The Exeter Universal cemented femoral stem at 20 to 25 years: a report of 382 hips. *Bone Joint J*. 2016;98B:1441–1449.

30. Examiners should not teach candidates in the exam. Their role is to score candidates on their knowledge. They should not use up candidates' precious scoring opportunities by talking too much!

31. Know the biochemical differences between ageing and osteoarthritis in cartilage as your examiners may want candidates to continue answering the question. If all else fails, with ageing the cartilage 'dries out'.

32. If you initially miss a subtle AVN spot diagnosis it is difficult to recover the viva past a bare 6 pass, especially if the candidates before and after you spot it without prompting.

33. Take your pick. On the day steroids, but you may be asked about alcohol, smoking, Caisson disease, sickle cell anaemia and transplant recipients, etc. A few buzzwords may be sufficient to bluff your way through, although it is more likely the examiner will want a more detailed explanation.

34. Johnson LC. Histiogenesis of avascular necrosis. Presented at the Conference on Aseptic Necrosis of the Femoral Head, St Louis, 1964.

35. Jaffe WL, Epstein M, Heyman N, Mankin HJ. The effect of cortisone on femoral and humeral heads in rabbits. An experimental study. *Clin Orthop Relat Res.* 1972;82:221–228.

36. Jones JP Jr. Fat embolism, intravascular coagulation, and osteonecrosis. *Clin Orthop Relat Res.* 1993;292:294–308.

37. Nishimura T, Matsumoto T, Nishino M, Tomita K. Histopathologic study of veins in steroid treated rabbits. *Clin Orthop Relat Res.* 1997;334:37–42.

38. Ficat RP. Idiopathic bone necrosis of the femoral head. Early diagnosis and treatment. *J Bone Joint Surg (Br).* 1985;67(1):3–9.

39. Hungerford DS, Lennox DW. The importance of increased intraosseous pressure in the development of osteonecrosis of the femoral head: implications for treatment. *Orthop Clin North Am.* 1985;16(4):635–654.

40. Steinberg ME, Hayken GD, Steinberg DR. A quantitative system for staging avascular necrosis. *J Bone Joint Surg (Br).* 1995;77:34–41. (Level 2/3 evidence.)

41. McKee MD, Waddell JP, Kudo PA, Schemitsch EH, Richards RR. Osteonecrosis of the femoral head in men following short-course corticosteroid therapy: a report of 15 cases. *Canadian Med Assoc J.* 2001;164:205–206.

42. Gaskill TR, Urbaniak JR, Aldridge JM 3rd. Free vascularized fibular transfer for femoral head osteonecrosis: donor and graft site morbidity. *J Bone Joint Surg Am.* 2009;91(8):1861–1867.

43. Standard protocol is that Gaskill should be mentioned as the first author when quoting papers. Rules sometimes need to be bent and as Urbaniak is a recognized world expert in VFG the examiners may be more familiar with his research and therefore mentioning him as the lead author may be tactically more astute. There were 215 complications (a 16.9% rate) at the time of follow-up, at an average of 8.3 years, after the 1270 procedures. Quote papers and results but be sensible about it.

44. Sometimes you will get away with this type of general statement regarding results; other times the examiners will press you.

45. Mont MA, Einhorn TA, Sponseller PD, Hungerford DS. The trapdoor procedure using autogenous cortical and cancellous bone grafts for osteonecrosis of the femoral head. *J Bone Joint Surg Br.* 1998;80:56–62.

46. Sugioka Y, Hotokebuchi T, Tsutsui H. Transtrochanteric anterior rotational osteotomy for idiopathic and steroid-induced necrosis of the femoral head: indications and long-term results. *Clin Orthop.* 1992;277:111–120.

47. Jarrett CA, Ranawat A, Bruzzone M, Yossef B, Rodriguez J, Ranawat C. The squeaking hip: a phenomenon of ceramic-on-ceramic total hip arthroplasty. *J Bone Joint Surg Am.* 2009;91:1344–1349.

48. Less risk of viva meltdown.

49. Lewis P, Olsen O, Mckee M, Waddell J, Schemitsch E. Total Hip Arthroplasty Following Failure of Core Decompression and Tantalum Rod Insertion for Femoral Head Avascular Necrosis. 11th Congress Effort E poster content, 2–5 June 2010, Madrid, Spain.

50. Schmalzreid TP, Jasty M, Harris WH. Periprosthetic bone loss in total hip arthroplasty: polyethylene wear debris and the concept of the effective joint space. *J Bone Joint Surg [Am].* 1992;74A:849–863.

51. Tsao AK, Jones LC, Lewallen DC. What patient and surgical factors contribute to implant wear and osteolysis in total joint arthroplasty? *J Am Acad Orthop Surg.* 2008;16:S7–13.

52. For ease of learning and memorizing we have provided the information in table form. Be aware of the need to carefully apply this knowledge into an appropriate usable answer in the exam. If the radiograph demonstrates a malaligned THA (cup open or stem in varus, etc.) tell this to the examiners as a probable cause of accelerated wear and then follow up with other surgeon-related factors. Be proactive and mention this sooner rather than later on, especially if the topic is travelling down the wear rather than revision route. If the patient is young mention patient-related factors associated with wear such as activity or diagnosis (osteonecrosis).

53. Ramage SC, Urban NH, Jiranek WA, Maiti A, Beckman MJ. Expression of RANKL in osteolytic membranes: association with fibroblastic cell markers. *J Bone Joint Surg Am.* 2007;89(4):841–848.

54. Parvizi J, Schall DM, Lewallen DG, Sim FH. Outcome of uncemented hip arthroplasty components in patients with Paget's disease. *Clin Orthop Relat Res.* 2002;403:127–134.

55. Lusty PJ, Walter WL, Walter WK, Zicat B. Cementless hip arthroplasty in Paget's disease at medium-term follow-up (average of 6.7 years). *J Arthroplasty.* 2007;22(5):692–696.

56. Alexakis PG, Brown BA, Howl WM. Porous hip replacement in Paget's disease: an 8–2/3-year follow-up. *Clin Orthop Relat Res.* 1998;350:138–142.

57. Ludkowski P, Wilson-MacDonald J. Total arthroplasty in Paget's disease of the hip: a clinical review and review of the literature. *Clin Orthop Relat Res.* 1990;255:160–167.

58. It is not unreasonable to mention the patient's age and when the radiograph was taken to the examiners with the first radiograph shown in the viva exam. Just like the trauma viva and the 'I would initially manage the patient with the ATLS protocol', if you keep repeating the catchphrase it will severely annoy the examiners. Once is reasonable to let the examiners know it is part of your standard practice. Any is more irritating and wastes time.

59. The score is 6–7, as the candidate didn't classify the left side correctly. If the candidate had correctly identified a Hartofilakidis I hip it would be more towards the 7–8 mark.

The candidate would have correctly used two classification systems to grade the severity of the DDH. He/she has already pre-empted questions on DDH classification.

60. Examiners aren't allowed to teach. See first edition viva book.

61. This is probably one of the pre-agreed oral viva questions that the examiners need to ask. The examiners have a set standard answer with various bullet points provided so as to be able to mark candidates accordingly.

62. Linde F, Jensen J, Pilgaard S. Charnley arthroplasty in osteoarthritis secondary to congenital dislocation or subluxation of the hip. *Clin Orthop.* 1988;227:164–171.

63. The candidate's answer isn't particularly well structured.

64. Candidates can either volunteer this extra information or perhaps wait for the examiners to ask it!

65. Technically, the candidate hasn't really answered the question.

66. The candidate is not quite appreciating what the examiner wants and has just gone a bit blank in the stress of the moment.

67. Duncan C. The Unified Classification System (UCS): improving our understanding of periprosthetic fractures. *Bone Joint J.* 2014;96B:713–716.

68. Schwarzkopf R, Oni JK, Marwin SE. Total hip arthroplasty periprosthetic femoral fractures: a review of classification and current treatment. *Bull Hosp Jt Dis.* 2013;71(1):68–78.

69. Khan T, Grindlay D, Ollivere BJ, Scammell BE, Manktelow AR, Pearson RG. A systematic review of Vancouver B2 and B3 periprosthetic femoral fractures. *Bone Joint J.* 2017;4(Suppl B):17–25.

70. El-Bakoury A, Hosny H, Williams M, Keenan J, Yarlagadda R. Management of Vancouver B2 and B3 periprosthetic proximal femoral fractures by distal locking femoral stem (Cannulok) in patients 75 years and older. *J Arthroplasty.* 2017;32(2):541–545.

71. Tsiridis E, Amin MS, Charity J, Narvani AA, Timperley J, Gie GA. Impaction allografting revision for B3

periprosthetic femoral fractures using a Mennen plate to contain the graft: a technical report. *Acta Orthop Belg.* 2007;73:332–338.

72. Klein GR, Parvizi J, Rapuri V, *et al.* Proximal femoral replacement for the treatment of periprosthetic fractures. *J Bone Joint Surg Am.* 2005;87(8):1777–1781.

73. Dennis DA, Lynch CB. Optimizing the femoral component cement mantle in total hip arthroplasty. *Orthopedics.* 2005;28(8):S867–871.

74. Ebramzadeh E, Sarmiento A, McKellop HA, *et al.* The cement mantle in total hip arthroplasty: analysis of long-term radiographic results. *J Bone Joint Surg Am.* 1994;76:77–87.

75. El Masri F, *et al.* Is the so-called 'French paradox'a reality? *Bone Joint J.* 2010;92(3):342–348.

76. Barrack RL, Mulroy R, Harris WH. Improved cementing techniques and femoral component loosening in young patients with hip arthroplasty. A 12-year radiographic review. *Bone Joint J.* 1992;74(3):385–389.

77. Banaszkiewicz PA. Improved cementing techniques and femoral component loosening in young patients with hip arthroplasty: a 12-year radiographic review. In PA Banaszkiewicz, DF Kader (Eds.), *Classic Papers in Orthopaedics.* London: Springer; 2014:31–34.

78. The examiners may not specify a particular side, which will make the radiograph slightly more difficult to interpret.

79. Although the radiograph doesn't show anything significant, try to avoid the terms 'there is no obvious abnormality of bone' or 'there may be perhaps slightly more opacity in the right femoral head'. Be definite in your answer.

80. You have to play safe and default to this standard reply for your first couple of viva questions, but it can start to irritate the examiners by your fifth viva question.

81. Turner DA, Templeton AC, Selzer PM, Rosenberg AG, Petasnick JP. Femoral capital osteonecrosis: MR finding of diffuse marrow abnormalities without focal lesions. *Radiology.* 1989;171(1):135–140.

Knee

John Dabis and Deiary F. Kader

Structured oral examination question 1

TKA in valgus knee

EXAMINER: This is a radiograph of a 72-year-old lady complaining of pain and gradual deformity of her left knee (Figure 4.1a and 4.1b). She has been referred to your clinic to be considered for total knee arthroplasty. What can you see?

CANDIDATE: This is a weight bearing AP radiograph of a 72-year-old female demonstrating severe osteoarthrosis of the left knee with moderate valgus deformity. The cardinal features of osteoarthritis are demonstrated here, which include loss of joint space, subchondral sclerosis, osteophyte formation and subchondral cysts.

EXAMINER: How will you manage this patient?

CANDIDATE: Firstly, I would establish what are the symptoms the patient is suffering from. I would focus on pain, loss of function and severity of symptoms. I would like to know the exact location of the pain, alleviating and relieving factors, and where the pain is radiating to. How the pain is affecting activities of daily living such as cutting toenails, putting shoes and socks on, how easy it is to go up and down stairs are all questions I would ask. Treatment to date is also important; has the patient had any physiotherapy/rehabilitation, trialled any analgesics? Previous surgical procedures need to be established. Assessment of the effect of osteoarthritis on the patient's function, quality of life, occupation, mood, relationships and leisure activities is also important. Clinical examination findings such as assessment of the soft tissue envelope is also important. Severity of the deformity in the coronal plane will need to be established. A fixed flexion deformity should also be noted. The competency of the knee collateral ligaments and degree of deformity correction should be assessed in order to plan the type of implants.

EXAMINER: OK, after the history and examination, what are you actually going to do?

CANDIDATE: The management should commence with non-surgical options and generally should be exhausted before surgical options are explored. As per the NICE guidelines, strengthening, low-impact aerobic exercise and neuromuscular education should all be recommended. Acetaminophen and NSAIDS and Tramadol should be the first analgesics offered. Interventions to lose weight, as there is moderate evidence that this will influence osteoarthritis of the knee. Obese patients generally have an increased risk of infection and tend to have an earlier onset of symptoms [1]. Other non-pharmacological treatments include education, social support, physical therapy, exercise and orthotics devices. Acupuncture and herbal remedies have limited evidence; however, they are still popular methods of treatment.

EXAMINER: What conditions are associated with this pattern of joint disease?

CANDIDATE: The valgus deformity of the knee with arthritis is commonly seen in women and in inflammatory joint conditions such as rheumatoid arthritis. It can also occur in primary osteoarthritis, overcorrection of high tibial osteotomy (HTO), post-traumatic arthritis following lateral meniscectomy and osteonecrosis of the lateral femoral condyle.

EXAMINER: What are your technical goals of treatment?

CANDIDATE: My aims are the following:

- Restoring neutral mechanical axis of 0° (±3°).
- Balancing the flexion/extension gap.
- Ensuring the joint line perpendicular to the mechanical axis.
- Preserving the joint line height.

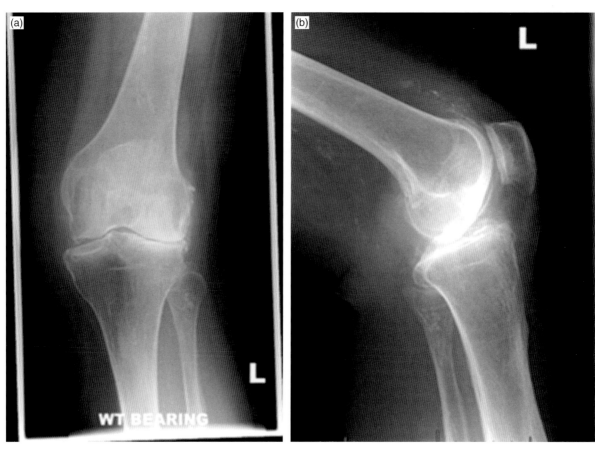

Figure 4.1a,b Anteroposterior (AP) and lateral radiographs of left knee.

- Balancing ligaments (2–3 mm symmetrical opening).
- Restoring normal joint alignment and Q angle.

EXAMINER: How would you restore the mechanical alignment?

CANDIDATE: The bony cuts of the femur and tibia should both be made perpendicular to the mechanical axis of the limb. The mechanical axis is a line bisecting the centre of the hip, knee and ankle. This is to ensure equal loading and even contact pressure of both medial and lateral compartments. The natural tibia has 3° of natural varus to the mechanical axis; however, we do cut perpendicular to the anatomical/mechanical axis. Deformity within the tibia needs to be taken into consideration and the cut should be made perpendicular to the mechanical axis and not the anatomical axis. Long leg mechanical axis views can be helpful for preoperative planning. The mechanical and anatomical axes of the femur are different, and it is this difference which creates the distal femoral valgus angle. This is usually 5–7°. The femoral component must be externally rotated by 3° with respect to the femoral neutral axis to create a rectangular flexion gap with the tibia. As the tibia was cut perpendicular to the mechanical axis, hence in 3° of valgus relative to the native plateau, the femoral component rotation will create a rectangular flexion gap.

EXAMINER: Tell me more about the intraoperative considerations.

CANDIDATE: In valgus knees the lateral femoral condyle is often deficient. This is important to remember because if you perform posterior femoral condylar referencing for femoral component rotation the resultant position of the femoral component will be internally rotated with reference to the transepicondylar axis. In this situation, the AP axis (Whiteside line) can be used to prevent malrotation in the form of internal rotation. The medial structures are stretched while lateral and posterior structures are contracted. The vastus lateralis acts as a subluxing or dislocating force to patella. In severe valgus deformity (7–10°) a distal femoral cut of 5 or 6° can improve patella tracking and avoid the need for lateral retinacular release. Patients with severe valgus deformity may require a lateral retinacular release to achieve normal patella tracking. Excessive PCL release usually requires cruciate-sacrificing implants in order to balance the knee. With correction of significant valgus deformity, one has to be cautious of the common peroneal nerve palsy in the postoperative period. It may be wise to identify the nerve to ensure no increased tension or damage occurs.

EXAMINER: OK, so what will be your choice of implant?

CANDIDATE: I would use a cemented implant. From the latest report of our National Joint Registry, over 84% of the primary TKA procedures performed are cemented, with less than 5% being uncemented and the remaining being a hybrid fixation. The advantages are that the cemented knee is less prone to aseptic loosening. There is, however, growing evidence for the use of uncemented knees [2]. There is an association with higher failure rates of cemented TKR in younger, heavier men. There are theoretical advantages of mobile bearing devices over fixed bearing devices, such as reduction in shear stresses and subsequent wear as the tibial insert will be able to rotate on a smooth tibial platform. However, I would use a fixed bearing insert; the Knee Arthroplasty Trial Group, after a large multicentre RCT, concluded that there is no advantage with the mobile bearing designs [3–5]. There are advantages and disadvantages of both cruciate-retaining and posterior stabilized knee replacements; however, I use a posterior stabilized knee, i.e. a cruciate-sacrificing knee replacement. There are many advantages, such as this implant design will facilitate deformity correction and provide anterior posterior stability with the CAM-post mechanism. I find it is technically easier to balance a PCL-sacrificing TKR and the results are more consistent. It can also be used in patients with previous patellectomy.

EXAMINER: How would you manage gap imbalance?

CANDIDATE: Ligament balancing is essential for proper knee stability and range of movement. When both the flexion and extension gaps are tight, options would be to reduce the polyethylene thickness or resect proximal tibia as this will equally alter both the flexion and extension gaps. If the extension and flexion gap are both equally loose, a larger polyethylene insert can be used. A tight flexion gap with a normal extension gap would require downsizing of the femoral component or shifting of the femoral component anteriorly [6,7]. With normal knee flexion, a flexion contracture would indicate a tight extension gap and may be an indication of an overstuffed extension spacer. Options of management would be to remove posterior osteophytes initially and release some posterior capsule. If the knee is still tight in extension the next step would be to resect some distal femur. Again, a normal flexion gap but a loose extension gap would indicate excessive distal femoral resection and distal femoral augmentation would be required. Flexion instability results when the flexion gap is larger than the extension gap and is often a result of undersized implants, incompetent PCL or excessive tibial slope. When the extension gap is normal the femoral component can be shifted posteriorly or one can augment the posterior condyles. It is imperative to ensure there is no anterior femoral cortex notching as a result of this shift.

References

1. Perry KI, MacDonald SJ. The obese patient: a problem of larger consequence. *Bone Joint J.* 2016;98(1 Supple A):3–5.

2. Arnold JB, Walters JL, Solomon LB, Thewlis D. Does the method of component fixation influence clinical outcomes after total knee replacement? A systematic literature review. *J Arthroplasty.* 2013;28(5):740–746.

3. Campbell MK, Fiddian N, Fitzpatrick R, *et al.* The Knee Arthroplasty Trial (KAT): design features, baseline characteristics and two-year functional outcomes after alternative approaches to knee replacement. *J Bone Joint Surg Am.* 2009;91(1):134–141.

4. Fransen BL, van Duijvenbode DC, Hoozemans MJ, Burger BJ. No differences between fixed-and mobile-bearing total knee arthroplasty. *Knee Surg Sports Traumatol Arthrosc.* 2017;25(6):1757–1777.

5. Van der Voort P, Pijls BG, Nouta KA, Valstar ER, Jacobs WC, Nelissen RG. A systematic review and meta-regression of mobile-bearing versus fixed-bearing total knee replacement in 41 studies. *Bone Joint J.* 2013 Sep 1;95(9):1209–1216.

6. Bercik MJ, Joshi A, Parvizi J. Posterior cruciate-retaining versus posterior-stabilized total knee arthroplasty: a meta-analysis. *J Arthroplasty.* 2013;28(3):439–444.

7. Huang T, Long Y, George D, Wang W. Meta-analysis of gap balancing versus measured resection techniques in total knee arthroplasty. *Bone Joint J.* 2017;99(2):151–158.

Structured oral examination question 2

Basic science: anatomy

EXAMINER: This young gentleman sustained a varus type injury to the knee and there is a suspected posterolateral (PLC) injury. Can you describe the lateral structures of the knee by layers (Figure 4.2)?

CANDIDATE: The lateral side of the knee comprises three main layers. Layer one, i.e. the most superficial layer, consists of the iliotibial tract and biceps femoris. The patella retinaculum is the primary constituent of the second layer. The common peroneal nerve lies between layers one and two. Layer three is split into superficial and deep layers. The lateral collateral ligament (LCL), fabellofibular ligament and anterolateral ligament (ALL) lie superficially. Within the deep layer are the arcuate ligament, coronary ligament, popliteus tendon and popliteofibular ligament. The lateral genicular artery lies between the deep and superficial layers.

EXAMINER: How about the medial side of the knee?

CANDIDATE: The medial side of the knee, similarly to the lateral side of the knee, is split into three layers. Layer one, most superficial, contains the sartorius and patella retinaculum. Layer two contains the semimembranosus, superficial MCL and the MPFL. The deepest layer consists of the deep MCL, capsule and the coronary ligament. Gracilis, semitendonosis and the saphenous nerve run between layers one and two.

EXAMINER: So, what is the function of the PLC and how commonly is it injured?

CANDIDATE: The role of the PLC is to resist external tibial rotation, varus and posterior tibial translation. The integrity of varus and external rotation stability ultimately depends on the integrity of the fibular collateral ligament (FCL), popliteus, the popliteofibular ligament and the lateral capsule. The PLC is rarely injured in isolation and is often

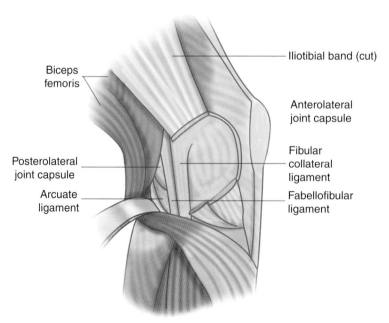

Figure 4.2 Diagram representing lateral side of the knee.

Biceps femoris

Iliotibial band (cut)

Anterolateral joint capsule

Posterolateral joint capsule

Fibular collateral ligament

Arcuate ligament

Fabellofibular ligament

associated with multiligament knee injuries; the PCL is injured less often than the ACL.

EXAMINER: Are you aware of any clinical tests to detect a PLC injury?

CANDIDATE: Hyperextension of the limb on passive extension testing can indicate a PLC injury. Initial gait examination may reveal a varus thrust. Lateral compartment gapping is assessed and compared with the contralateral side. If there is more gapping of the lateral compartment in flexion, then injury to the secondary stabilizers such as popliteus should be suspected. The dial test essentially measures external rotation of the tibia relative to the femur. I place the patient prone, and flex both knees to 30°. If there is more than 10° external rotation compared with the normal side, a PLC injury is diagnosed. I then flex both knees to 90° and repeat this manoeuvre. An increase in external rotation would suggest a combined PCL and PLC injury. I also use the reverse pivot shift test. I place the patient supine with the knee flexed to 90°. A valgus load is applied through the knee joint as well as an external rotation moment around the tibia. The knee is then brought out into extension. If the posteriorly subluxed tibia reduces at 40° of extension, this is interpreted as a positive result. The tibia reduces as a result of the ITB changing from a knee flexor to a knee extender.

EXAMINER: What investigations would you perform?

CANDIDATE: A routine radiograph work up should be performed including anteroposterior (AP), lateral and axial views. Mechanical axis long leg views should also be performed to assess the lower limb alignment. If there is any malalignment, an osteotomy should be performed prior to or at the time of reconstruction. These should be done to exclude fractures. Varus and PCL stress radiographs are reliable to assist in PCL and PLC injuries respectively.[1] Lateral compartment varus gapping of 2.7–4 mm is consistent with isolated FCL injuries, whereas more than 4 mm indicates a severe-grade PLC injury. Kneeling stress radiographs are best to assess PCL injuries and an opening of 4–12 mm would indicate an isolated PCL injury. Arthroscopy and MRI also have a role to assess for associated chondral, ligamentous and meniscal pathology. Double varus injuries can lead to a varus thrust as the LCL is injured. A triple varus can also lead to hyperextension and recurvatum, indicating a PLC injury.

EXAMINER: What are the options of management?

CANDIDATE: PLC injuries are usually part of a multi-ligament injury spectrum. It is rare to sustain an isolated PLC injury; however, if this were expected, the majority can be managed non-operatively.[2] If part of a multi-ligament injury, the PLC should be addressed. Patients with ACL ruptures should be assessed for PLC injuries and, depending on the grading of injury, should have a reconstruction to assess this deficiency. Grade 3 injuries are a different entity and there is good evidence to suggest poor functional outcomes and degenerative changes if non-operative measures are pursued. Options of operative approaches for grade 3 PLC injuries include acute repairs, which generally are reserved for bone or soft tissue avulsion injuries such as fibular head avulsions. This is normally done within 2–3 weeks and offers the advantage of fixing avulsed bony fragments and other structures anatomically. The ACL and PCL will need to be reconstructed acutely. Delayed reconstruction involves reconstruction of all structures including the PCL, ACL and PLC. Earlier evidence by Levy and Stannard *et al.* have both demonstrated higher failure rates with repair compared to delayed reconstruction.[3,4] However, more recent evidence by Westermann *et al.* has suggested good outcomes can be achieved with both repair and reconstruction of PLC injuries treated concurrently with ACL reconstruction at 6-year follow-up.[5] Anatomical reconstruction using tendon allograft and all three static stabilizers has been shown biomechanically to restore native knee biomechanics with improved outcomes. The common peroneal nerve needs to be identified and protected. I would use a modified Larson's technique for a grade I associated PLC injury, an Arciero for grade II and a LaPrade PLC reconstruction for a grade III injury.

References

1. LaPrade RF, Heikes C, Bakker AJ, Jakobsen RB. The reproducibility and repeatability of varus stress radiographs in the assessment of isolated fibular collateral ligament and grade-III posterolateral knee injuries: an in vitro biomechanical study. *J Bone Joint Surg Am*. 2008;90(10):2069–2076.

2. Krukhaug Y, Mølster A, Rodt A, Strand T. Lateral ligament injuries of the knee. *Knee Surg Sports Traumatol Arthrosc*. 1998;6(1):21–25.

3. Levy BA, Dajani KA, Morgan JA, Shah JP, Dahm DL, Stuart MJ. Repair versus reconstruction of the fibular collateral ligament and posterolateral corner in the multiligament-injured knee. *Am J Sports Med*. 2010;38 (4):804–809.

4. Geeslin AG, LaPrade RF. Outcomes of treatment of acute grade-III isolated and combined posterolateral knee injuries: a prospective case series and surgical technique. *J Bone Joint Surg Am*. 2011;93(18):1672–1683.

5. Westermann RW, Spindler KP, Huston LJ, Wolf BR. Posterolateral corner repair versus reconstruction: 6-year outcomes from a prospective multicenter cohort. *Orthop J Sports Med*. 2017;5(7_suppl6).

Structured oral examination question 3

Meniscus

EXAMINER: Tell me about the anatomy and function of the meniscus.

CANDIDATE: The menisci are crescentic cartilaginous structures interposed between the tibia and femoral condyles. They are triangular in cross-section. The peripheral borders are attached to the joint capsule. The medial meniscus is nearly semicircular with a wider posterior than anterior horn. This is attached anterior to the ACL insertion while the mid aspect is firmly attached to the deep MCL. The lateral meniscus is circular with a larger surface than the medial meniscus. The posterior horns of both menisci attach to the posterior intercondylar eminence. The attachment of the lateral meniscus to the capsule is interrupted by the popliteus tendon. Due to the loose attachment to the capsule, the lateral meniscus has twice the excursion to that of the medial meniscus. The anterior horns of both menisci are connected by intermeniscal ligaments. Histologically, the menisci have an extracellular matrix composed mainly of water (70%) and primarily type 1 collagen fibres (60%), proteoglycans, elastin and glycoproteins. The main cellular component is the fibrochondrocytes that synthesize and maintain extracellular matrix. The blood supply to the meniscus comes from the lateral, middle and medial geniculate vessels with 20–30% of the peripheral portion being vascular. The main functions of the menisci are load transmission with estimated 50% in extension and 85% in flexion, joint conformity and articular congruity, distribution of synovial fluid aiding nutrition and joint lubrication. The menisci also have proprioceptive function, act as shock absorbers and prevent soft tissue impingement during joint motion.

EXAMINER: What are the vascular zones of meniscus?

CANDIDATE: The menisci are relatively avascular structures with peripheral blood supply from the premeniscal capillary plexus formed by branches from lateral and medial geniculate vessels. Studies have shown that the degree of peripheral vascular penetration is 10–30% of medial meniscal width and 10–25% of lateral meniscal width. This gives rise to the three zones of meniscal vasculature from peripheral to central, namely red–red, red–white and white–white. Therefore, peripheral tears are suitable for repair while central tears may not be suitable due to lack of healing capacity.

EXAMINER: These are the images which belong to a young professional footballer (Figures 4.3b and 4.3c). What can you see?

CANDIDATE: The first is a sagittal T1 MRI image and the second is a T2-weighted image. The coronal image does not show any medial meniscal tissue indicating a peripheral detachment. There is a 'double PCL sign' on the sagittal image suggestive of bucket handle tear of the medial meniscus.

EXAMINER: How would you manage this patient?

CANDIDATE: I would start by taking a detailed history and clinical examination ... [EXAMINER interrupts].

EXAMINER: How would you treat this patient? [EXAMINER getting impatient]

CANDIDATE: I would offer this patient EUA, arthroscopy, repair or excision of bucket handle tear.

EXAMINER: Good. What factors affect the prognosis following meniscal repair?

CANDIDATE: Firstly, the patient's age dictates what I would do for the bucket handle tear. As he is a young professional footballer I would do my best to preserve the meniscus. Older patients have less cellularity and

(a)

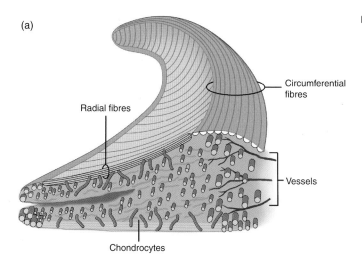

Figure 4.3a Cross-sectional anatomy of the meniscus.

Circumferential fibres

Radial fibres

Vessels

Chondrocytes

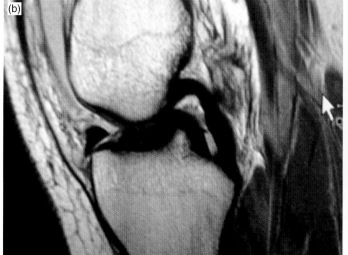

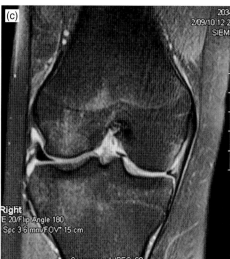

Figure 4.3b and 4.3c T2-weighted sagittal and coronal MRI scan images of the knee.

decreased healing response. Re-tears are common in patients above the age of 30. Location of the tear and the tear pattern are also important factors. The chronicity of the tear will also dictate what I do. I am also much more inclined to preserve the lateral meniscus than the medial meniscus. Other factors include location and pattern, and associated pathology, i.e. ligamentous malalignment and pre-existing arthritis.

EXAMINER: Are you aware of any meniscal repair techniques?

CANDIDATE: The four main meniscal repair methods are open repair, inside out, outside in and all inside. The 'outside in' method is versatile and safe but is reserved for anterior horn tears. [EXAMINER interrupts again]

EXAMINER: Let's move on . . .

References

Arnoczky SP, Warren RF. Microvasculature of the human meniscus. *Am J Sports Med.* 1982;10:90–95.

Structured oral examination question 4

Infected total knee arthroplasty (TKA)

EXAMINER: This gentleman had a TKA performed 3 months ago. Ten days after surgery he developed a large blister that was drained on the ward. Two weeks later he developed a draining abscess at the proximal aspect of the wound. He was taken to theatre and the abscess was washed out. The skin was debrided and closed primarily. Have you got any concerns?

CANDIDATE: This patient has a periprosthetic joint infection (PJI) until proven otherwise. He clearly developed an acute infection following the surgery. An acute infection is defined by the American Academy of Orthopaedic Surgeons and the International Consensus on PJI as infection within 3 weeks of the procedure, or in the case of late haematogenous infection, within 3 weeks of development of symptoms. Any infection developing after this time is considered as late. This is irrespective of bone stock and stability of the components.

EXAMINER: These are the most recent radiographs and there are no other postoperative radiographs available (Figures 4.4a and 4.4b). What would you like to do for this patient?

CANDIDATE: I would start by taking a detailed history of the perioperative events, general health as well as current problem. I would like to know the date of index operation, if there was prolonged discharge from the wound, redness or persistent swelling in the immediate postoperative period. A pain-free interval after the operation followed by sudden deterioration may be suggestive of haematogenous spread precipitated by bacteraemia from UTI, URTI or dental procedure.

EXAMINER: Are you aware of any staging systems with the use of periprosthetic joint infection?

CANDIDATE: McPherson advocated the concept of staging, which consists of timing of infection, i.e. early, acute haematogenous or late. The systemic medical and immune status of the patient is used. Systemic compromising factors include excessive alcohol, diabetes, smoking, liver, renal and lung failure. Immune status assessment includes CD4 count and neutrophil counts. Local compromising factors are also recorded and include whether active infection is present, synovial cutaneous fistula presence and a subcutaneous abscess of more than 8 cm^2. Each category has different grades according to what they score.[1]

EXAMINER: So how would you diagnose a periprosthetic joint infection?

CANDIDATE: I would always start with the history and clinical examination of the patient. I would focus on the events around the procedures this gentleman has had. Even without signs of infection, a painful TKR can manifest as a low-grade infection. I am aware of the AAOS clinical guideline practice summary for diagnosis of periprosthetic joint infection of the knee. The working group strongly recommend:

- Testing ESR and CRP.
- Joint aspiration.
- The use of intraoperative frozen sections.
- Obtaining multiple intraoperative cultures, against initiating antibiotic treatment until after cultures and against the use of intraoperative Gram stain.
- Nuclear imaging was weakly recommended as an option in patients in whom diagnosis of periprosthetic joint infection has not been established and who are not scheduled for reoperation.[2]

I refer to the diagnostic criteria set out by the workgroup of the MSK infection society. The major criteria include either a sinus tract communicating with the prosthesis or if a pathogen is isolated by culture from at least two separate tissue or fluid samples obtained from the affected prosthetic joint, or four of the following six minor criteria: (a) elevated CRP and ESR, (b) elevated synovial leucocyte count, (c) elevated synovial neutrophil percentage, (d) presence of purulence in the affected joint, (e) isolation of a microorganism in one culture of periprosthetic joint fluid or tissue and (f) > 5 neutrophils per high power field observed at ×400 magnification.[3] The isolation of the infecting organism and the corresponding antibiotic profile are essential.

EXAMINER: Anything else?

CANDIDATE: Analysis of the joint fluid which should include a leucocyte esterase assessment . . .

EXAMINER: Anything more recent in the literature?

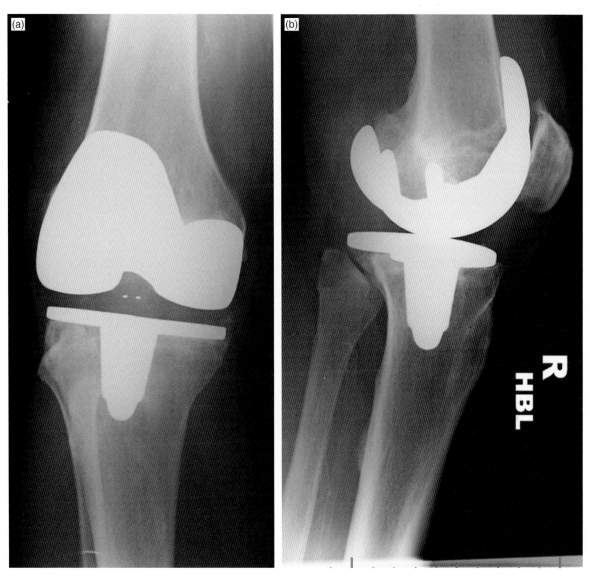

Figure 4.4a and 4.4b Anteroposterior (AP) and lateral radiographs of left TKA.

CANDIDATE: The alpha-defensin test, which is an immunoassay, has recently been shown to have a sensitivity and specificity of 100% in the diagnosis of PJI. Advantages include the specimen could also be assessed when blood was in the synovial fluid.[4]

EXAMINER: So how are you going to manage this case?

CANDIDATE: It is unfortunate, but I think this gentleman cannot be treated as an acute infection. He has missed the window of opportunity of debridement, antibiotic treatment and implant retention. He has already undergone a soft-tissue debridement and I am worried about the soft tissue envelope. It may require a plastic surgeon to review the wound. I would offer this patient a revision knee arthroplasty.

EXAMINER: And how would you do this?

CANDIDATE: It can be done over a one-stage or two-stage procedure. One stage has many advantages including low treatment costs and shorter hospital stays. The infecting organism and its sensitivity should be established preoperatively.

There are, however, contraindications to this, including infection with a highly virulent organism, sepsis with substantial systemic manifestations and culture-negative PJI where appropriate antibiotic treatment cannot be determined.

EXAMINER: So . . . ?

CANDIDATE: I would plan for a two-stage exchange procedure where I would remove all the material, including the cement, and perform an aggressive debridement of the soft tissues and bone. I would insert an antibiotic-loaded dynamic cement spacer. This should preserve the joint space, reduce soft-tissue contractures, and provide better ROM and knee function scores while eluting high doses of IV antibiotics.[5] Debridement is the most essential part of the procedure with meticulous handling of soft tissues to remove all septic membranes.

References

1. McPherson EJ, Woodson C, Holtom P, Roidis N, Shufelt C, Patzakis M. Periprosthetic total hip infection: outcomes using a staging system. *Clin Orthop Relat Res.* 2002;403:8–15.

2. Della Valle C, Parvizi J, Bauer TW, *et al.* Diagnosis of periprosthetic joint infections of the hip and knee. *J Am Acad Orthop Surg.* 2010;18(12):760–770.

3. Parvizi J, Zmistowski B, Berbari EF, *et al.* New definition for periprosthetic joint infection: from the Workgroup of the Musculoskeletal Infection Society. *Clin Orthop Relat Res.* 2011;469(11):2992.

4. Deirmengian C, Kardos K, Kilmartin P, *et al.* The alpha-defensin test for periprosthetic joint infection outperforms the leukocyte esterase test strip. *Clin Orthop Relat Res.* 2015;473(1):198–203.

5. Ding H, Yao J, Chang W, Liu F. Comparison of the efficiency of static versus articular spacers in two-stage revision surgery for the treatment of infection following total knee arthroplasty: a meta-analysis. *J Orthop Surg Res.* 2017;12(1):151.

Structured oral examination question 5

Unicondylar knee arthroplasty (UKA) vs high tibial osteotomy (HTO)

EXAMINER: This is a radiograph of a 42-year-old man who works as a bricklayer (Figure 4.5). He complains of pain over the medial aspect of the knee and has failed non-surgical management. He has come to your clinic for a consultation. What can you see?

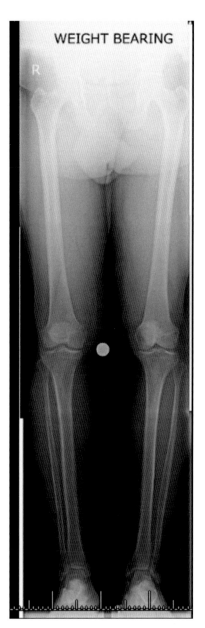

Figure 4.5 Standing anteroposterior (AP) lower limb alignment views.

CANDIDATE: These are long leg x-rays demonstrating moderate medial tibiofemoral compartment osteoarthritis. The lateral compartment appears normal. Crude assessment of the tibiofemoral angle appears to show a varus deformity of less than 10°. I cannot comment on the patellofemoral joint, hence I would like to see a lateral and a skyline view. There is no joint subluxation, long bone deformity or adjacent joint disease. The soft tissues appear to have normal body habitus. I would like to take a targeted history and examine the patient. The examination should be focused on eliciting localized tenderness in the medial compartment, range of motion, if the varus deformity is correctable and the stability of the knee.

EXAMINER: The patient is fit and well, states that the pain is affecting his job and he would like to consider surgical option 5. What would you offer him?

CANDIDATE: The options of surgical management include a valgizing osteotomy such as a high tibial osteotomy (HTO), medial unicondylar knee arthroplasty or total knee replacement. As this patient has a high-demand physical job and is young, I would offer him an osteotomy.

EXAMINER: What are the prerequisites of an HTO? And what are your indications?

CANDIDATE: The ideal candidate for HTO is a patient with physiological age of < 65 years, fixed varus deformity < 15° or valgus deformity < 12°, fixed flexion deformity of < 15° and a flexion arc of more than 90°. Patients with pain primarily on the medial aspect of the knee and less than 4 mm of space on the medial compartment on weight-bearing views with mechanical overload and varus deformity are prime candidates for a valgizing osteotomy. Young patients undergoing medial meniscal transplantation and articular cartilage restoration procedures may require an unloading osteotomy. Preoperative varus must exist and even patients with as little as 4° of varus can benefit from an HTO.

EXAMINER: Are you aware of any contraindication for HTO?

CANDIDATE: I would avoid an HTO in a patient with marked decreased range of movement, i.e. flexion of less than 90° if possible. The main contraindications are inflammatory arthropathy such as rheumatoid arthritis and psoriatic arthropathy, incompetent medial collateral ligament or ACL, large varus thrust with coronal subluxation of > 1 cm, although there are times one can adjust the tibial slope to compensate for ligament deficiency. Obesity is also a relative contraindication because valgus knee is poorly tolerated due to medial thigh contact. However, ensuring stable fixation can improve the success in obese patients. A small lateral plate to fix the hinge in addition to

the medial plate in a medial opening wedge HTO has been described. Any patient who smokes really should stop as this can cause a non-union. Consideration of a closing osteotomy or cancellous grafting are options.

EXAMINER: The patient tells you that he has heard about closing wedge osteotomy arthroscopies and partial knee replacements and is keen to consider the alternative options. How do you proceed?

CANDIDATE: I would explain that UKA is an option; however, I would not recommend UKA for this particular patient because of his young age and the high physical demand of his job could result in accelerated wear of a UKA. In the absence of an acute fixed flexion deformity and locked knee I would not offer him an arthroscopy. There have been numerous randomized controlled trials failing to show benefit when comparing arthroscopic debridement and partial meniscal resections against other controlled interventions. Thorlund et al. published a systematic review and meta-analysis of the benefits and harms of arthroscopy to the degenerative knee [1]. The evidence does not support this option in this situation. There is also a recent randomized controlled trial, by Barton et al., demonstrating that an arthroscopy in the year prior to a TKA were linked with significantly reduced Oxford Knee scores; also this cohort had a higher revision rate over a four-year period [2].

EXAMINER: So which patients would you offer UKA?

CANDIDATE: The indications and prerequisites for HTO and UKA are more or less the same between the ages of 55 and 65 years of age. However, women prefer the UKA because they do not tolerate the angular deformity created by an HTO very well. In addition, patients who have low physical demands may benefit from a UKA. A frank discussion regarding the pros and cons of each procedure needs to occur between the patient and surgeon. A meta-analysis by Fu et al. demonstrated with careful patient selection that both HTO and UKA demonstrate effective and reliable results [3].

EXAMINER: Are there any contraindications to performing a UKA?

CANDIDATE: Accepted contraindications include inflammatory arthritis, large fixed flexion deformities, ligamentous laxity and prior meniscectomy in the contralateral compartment. Previously old age, high activity level [4], obesity and pattern of OA were seen as contraindications. However, recent evidence has shown this is not the case [3]. There is good evidence to offer octogenarians a UKA with good outcome data [5]. Increasing BMI has also been found not to be associated with an increased failure rate [6].

EXAMINER: What are the advantages of a UKA?

CANDIDATE: By retaining the cruciate ligaments and remaining healthy joint surfaces, UKA restores the normal ligament driven kinematics of the native knee [7]. The procedure generally requires a smaller incision, avoiding the need to evert the patella. There is a shorter hospital stay and lower rates of infection, morbidity and mortality. Patients undergoing UKA are half as likely to have a major complication such as a myocardial infarction or stroke within the first 30 days after surgery. There is also evidence to suggest better PROMs and increased range of movement in patients undergoing UKA. It is technically not too challenging to revise a UKA to a TKA.

EXAMINER: So how about the outcomes? Are they comparable? And what does the NJR state?

CANDIDATE: There is a lot of evidence published from the designer group with regards to the outcomes of UKR. Lisowski et al. published a 10–15-year outcome prospective study. These are results from a non-designer group. Only medial UKAs were included. PROMs including the OKS, VAS and WOMAC scores were recorded. There was a mean follow-up of 11.7 years and results demonstrated excellent long-term functional and radiological outcomes with a 90% 15-year survival rate [8]. The 10-year revision rate published in the 13th annual report of the National Joint Registry was 12.38%. It has been suggested by Baker et al. that high-volume centres and surgeons specializing in UKA have superior results compared to their low-volume counterparts. The low-volume surgeon and low-volume centres will have skewed the NJR revision rate [9].

EXAMINER: Right let's get back to our patient, how about the results of TKA following HTO? Are they worse?

CANDIDATE: There is evidence to suggest the outcomes of TKA following HTO, especially an opening wedge osteotomy, are as good as TKA without

a HTO [10]. However, there is added difficulty with performing the procedure such as additional removal of hardware if a one-staged procedure is decided upon. [11]. There is no evidence demonstrating any differences in the outcomes between opening and closing wedge osteotomies [4].

EXAMINER: Let's say this patient has decided to go ahead with a HTO. How would you go about this? What would be your preference?

CANDIDATE: I always obtain full-length weight-bearing mechanical axis hip–knee–ankle radiographs. The mechanical and anatomical axes should be drawn. Native tibiofemoral varus alignment, medial joint space degeneration and lateral capsuloligamentous laxity need to be assessed. This can be compared with the contralateral side. The Coventry group suggest overcorrection to 8° of anatomical valgus. The difference between the preoperative anatomic axis and the planned anatomic axis should be calculated. The angle of correction can also be calculated using the Miniaci method. Firstly, the true mechanical axis is drawn from the centre of the femoral head to the centre of the tibiotalar joint, Line A. A second line is dropped from the centre of the femoral head to pass through the knee at the intended Mikulicz point (in a varus knee, aiming for 55% – width from medial tibial plateau), Line B. Now we need to create a hinge point, Point H. Two lines creating an angle are drawn connecting the caudal points of Line A and B.

EXAMINER: You mentioned difficulty with conversion of HTO to TKA. Tell me more about this.

CANDIDATE: Problems which can be encountered include patella baja which can make eversion of the patella and access very difficult, also tracking of the patella will be more challenging. There will be more distorted landmarks for proper tibial component orientation. The incision may well not be ideal for my joint replacement. I may need to consider staging the removal of metal-work and taking some deep samples to ensure infection is not present. Bone stock may be deficient laterally following a closing wedge osteotomy. The anterior tibial slope is also of importance and should be addressed. The tibial shaft offset can be medially deviated, which may require offset stems. Soft tissue balancing can be more challenging. More recent studies show that closing wedge osteotomy increases patellar height, whereas opening wedge osteotomy lowers patellar height, and this can have implications following TKA. Van Raaij *et al.* performed a systematic review and reported prolonged surgical time, extra operative procedures and less postoperative knee range of motion (ROM), but no increase in revision surgeries for patients receiving TKA after prior HTO compared to patients receiving primary TKA.

References

1. Thorlund JB, Juhl CB, Roos EM, Lohmander LS. Arthroscopic surgery for degenerative knee: systematic review and meta-analysis of benefits and harms. *Br J Sports Med.* 2015;49(19):1229–1235.

2. Barton SB, McLauchlan GJ, Canty SJ. The incidence and impact of arthroscopy in the year prior to total knee arthroplasty. *Knee.* 2017;24(2):396–401.

3. Fu D, Li G, Chen K, Zhao Y, Hua Y, Cai Z. Comparison of high tibial osteotomy and unicompartmental knee arthroplasty in the treatment of unicompartmental osteoarthritis: a meta-analysis. *J Arthroplasty.* 2013;28(5):759–765.

4. Preston S, Howard J, Naudie D, Somerville L, McAuley J. Total knee arthroplasty after high tibial osteotomy: no differences between medial and lateral osteotomy approaches. *Clin Orthop Relat Res.* 2014;472(1):105–110.

5. Tadros BJ, Dabis J, Twyman R. Short-term outcome of unicompartmental knee arthroplasty in the octogenarian population. *Knee Surg Sports Traumatol Arthrosc.* 2018;26(5):1571–1576.

6. Ali AM, Pandit H, Liddle AD, *et al.* Does activity affect the outcome of the Oxford unicompartmental knee replacement? *Knee.* 2016;23(2):327–330.

7. Pandit H, Jenkins C, Gill HS, *et al.* Unnecessary contraindications for mobile-bearing unicompartmental knee replacement. *J Bone Joint Surg Br.* 2011;93(5):622–628.

8. Lisowski LA, Meijer LI, Bekerom MP, Pilot P, Lisowski AE. Ten- to 15-year results of the Oxford Phase III mobile unicompartmental knee arthroplasty: a prospective study from a non-designer group. *Bone Joint J.* 2016; 98B(10 Supple B):41–47.

9. Baker P, Jameson S, Critchley R, Reed M, Gregg P, Deehan D. Center and surgeon volume influence the revision rate following unicondylar knee replacement: an analysis of 23,400 medial cemented unicondylar knee replacements. *J Bone Joint Surg Am.* 2013;95(8):702–709.

10. Meding JB, Wing JT, Ritter MA. Does high tibial osteotomy affect the success or survival of a total knee replacement? *Clin Orthop Relat Res.* 2011;469(7):1991–1994.

11. Niinimäki T, Eskelinen A, Ohtonen P, Puhto AP, Mann BS, Leppilahti J. Total knee arthroplasty after high tibial osteotomy: a registry-based case–control study of 1,036 knees. *Arch Orthop Trauma Surg.* 2014;134(1):73–77.

Structured oral examination question 6

Dislocated UKA PE spacer

EXAMINER: Have a look at these radiographs (Figure 4.6a and 4.6b). What can you see?

CANDIDATE: Weight-bearing AP and lateral radiographs of 54-year-old man showing a left medial UKA in situ. The components look well fixed and aligned. There are no obvious periprosthetic fractures. The lateral compartment and PFJ look relatively normal.

EXAMINER: What else can you see?

CANDIDATE: [A bit hesitant and moving closer to the computer screen. This is followed by a period of silence before the Examiner prompts]

EXAMINER: The patient tells you that he fell while coming down the stairs, sustaining injury to the left knee. He complains of global pain and swelling of the left knee and inability to flex it. What's going through your mind?

CANDIDATE: There is a faint radio-opaque line behind the femoral component and on the AP radiograph, a vertical lucency can be seen proximal to the medial tibial eminence. I would like to compare this with previous radiographs. The history and radiographs are suggestive of dislocation of the mobile-bearing spacer.

EXAMINER: How common is meniscal dislocation?

CANDIDATE: The meniscal dislocation rate for medial UKA is 1 in 200 and 10% in lateral UKA. Dislocation in medial UKA is usually anterior and rare in other directions.

There may be a history of trauma and it usually presents with severe onset of knee pain with difficulty weight-bearing.

Mobile-bearing knee implants are less tolerant of soft tissue imbalance. There is increased risk of bearing instability and dislocation with poor soft tissue balancing or unequal flexion and extension gaps.

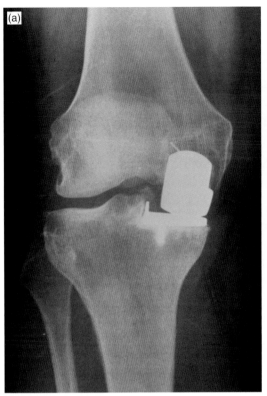
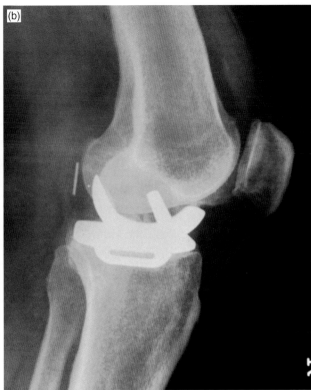

Figure 4.6a and 4.6b Anteroposterior (AP) and lateral radiographs UKA.

EXAMINER: Any other possible causes for dislocation?

CANDIDATE: Other causes could include intraoperative MCL damage, progressive stretching of the medial collateral ligament or bearing impingement on unresected osteophytes.

EXAMINER: Why is there an increased risk of dislocation in lateral UKA?

CANDIDATE: The increased dislocation rate in lateral UKA is mainly due to the fact that the medial collateral ligament is tight and lateral collateral ligament lax in flexion. Therefore, the medial compartment gets distracted about 2 mm on average in comparison with 7 mm on the lateral side.

EXAMINER: How are we going to manage this case?

CANDIDATE: The spacer could be exchanged for a larger one, but it may dislocate again with continued flexion/extension imbalance.

Definitive management would be revision to PS knee replacement.

Structured oral examination question 7

Posterior cruciate ligament and anterior cruciate ligament reconstruction

EXAMINER: These are images of a 26-year-old rugby player who has given a history of falling awkwardly. What can you see (Figures 4.7a–4.7d)?

CANDIDATE: These are plain radiographs and MRI of the right knee which show a displaced avulsion fracture of the posterior intercondylar tibial spine. This is where the PCL inserts, with the origin of the PCL being the lateral wall of the medial femoral condyle.

EXAMINER: How would you treat this patient?

CANDIDATE: I would offer this patient reattachment of the PCL avulsion through open procedure.

EXAMINER: What approach would you use?

CANDIDATE: The posterior approach.

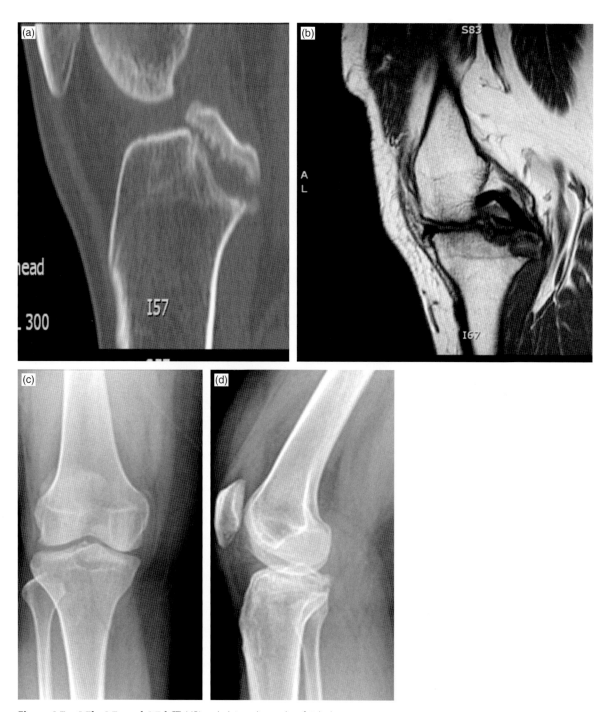

Figure 4.7a, 4.7b, 4.7c and 4.7d CT, MRI and plain radiographs of right knee.

EXAMINER: Tell me about the posterior approach to the knee.

CANDIDATE: The indications include removal of popliteal cysts and neoplasms, posterior synovectomy, open reduction and internal fixation of posterior tibial plateau shear fractures, fixation of bone avulsions associated with a posterior cruciate ligament (PCL) injury, repair of posterior

81

vascular injuries, and more recently, posterior inlay PCL reconstructions. The patient is usually positioned prone with tourniquet high up in the thigh. The S-shaped incision is centred over the popliteal fossa with the oblique section overlying the joint. The incision can be extended proximally along the tendon of semitendinosus and continued distally over the head of the lateral head of gastrocnemius. The medial sural cutaneous nerve is identified beneath the fascia. Just lateral to the nerve is the short saphenous vein. The deep fascia is incised in the midline. The medial sural cutaneous nerve is traced proximally where it pierces deep fascia from the tibial nerve trunk. At the apex of the fossa, the common peroneal nerve separates from the tibial nerve. The tibial nerve lies posterior to the popliteal vein, which in turn is superficial to the popliteal artery. Popliteal vessels are displaced laterally and this usually requires ligation of the middle geniculate and superior medial geniculate vessels. The medial head of the gastrocnemius is identified, traced proximally and can be detached from its origin then retracted towards the midline to expose the medial joint capsule. Similarly, the lateral head of the gastrocnemius can be detached to expose the posterolateral corner of the joint. The main structures at risk are the popliteal vessels, small saphenous vein and common peroneal nerve and tibial nerve.

EXAMINER: Can you tell me about the anatomy of the ACL?

CANDIDATE: The ACL is an intra-articular structure but extra-synovial with a blood supply from the middle genicular artery. It arises from the medial border of the lateral femoral condyle and inserts proximally into the tibial spines. It has an anteromedial (AM) and a posterolateral (PL) bundle. The AM bundle tightens in flexion and the PL bundle tightens in extension. This, however, is an oversimplification. It has been recently described as a ribbon-like structure. It primarily functions to prevent excessive anterior translation relative to the femur. It also primarily resists internal rotation of the tibia relative to the femur. It is a secondary stabilizer to varus and valgus stress. The main consistency is type 1 collagen; however, there is some type III collagen.

EXAMINER: When considering an ACL reconstruction, which graft would you use and why?

CANDIDATE: The two main options are autograft and allograft. The two most popular autografts are

hamstring and bone–patella–bone tendon grafts (BPBG) [1]. The advantages of using autografts are that they are biologically friendly and readily available, there are no additional costs and no risk of disease transmission. There are advantages of a BPBG over the hamstring graft, such as direct bone-to-bone healing within the femoral and tibial tunnels and avoiding loss of hamstring proprioception and strength, which can be detrimental to a high-level athlete. There is said to be less anterior knee pain with hamstring reconstructions. Smaller incisions and a higher maximum load to failure being almost twice that of the BPBG are other potential advantages.

However, hamstring grafts have slow healing properties because of tendon to bone incorporation, which can take 8–12 weeks. There are several studies comparing outcome of BPTB versus hamstring graft. Most studies show arthroscopic reconstruction with either graft results in similar functional outcome but increased morbidity in BPTB in the form of early OA and increased knee laxity [2–4].

EXAMINER: How about in revision ACL reconstruction? Does the type of graft affect the outcome?

CANDIDATE: Grassi et al. [5] published a meta-analysis looking into just this. Autografts had better outcomes than allografts in revision ACL reconstruction. There were lower rates of postoperative laxity and lower rates of re-operations and complications. Interestingly, if irradiated allografts are excluded, outcomes are similar between auto- and allografts.

EXAMINER: Now tell me about the optimum tunnel placement of your bony tunnels in an ACL reconstruction.

CANDIDATE: The principles of ACL reconstruction are placement of tunnels anatomically and isometrically, using biologically active grafts which are adequately tensioned to allow early rehabilitation. My aim is to stabilize the knee, restore normal kinematics and prevent early-onset degenerative arthrosis. The clockface method is a method for assessing femoral tunnel height; however, without proper alignment of the arthroscope it can be imprecise. In order to achieve 'graft isometry' the optimal position of the femoral tunnel was thought to be 11 or 1 o'clock depending on the side of surgery. This will place the femoral tunnel high and deep in the lateral femoral condyle. This would be ideal for isometric positioning. As someone who adopts anatomic tunnel placement, I believe isometry is not the most crucial factor. The ACL femoral attachment is oval in appearance and is defined by two bony ridges. These ridges, the lateral intercondylar ridge and the bifurcate ridge, will dictate where I place the femoral tunnel; however, this does require some extensive ACL remnant resection. The preserved remnant can actually enhance biological healing and provides mechanical support to the ACL reconstruction. The most common mistake is to place the femoral tunnel too 'shallow' on the so-called 'resident's ridge'. This restricts flexion of the knee and may result in elongation of the graft, causing incompetence and recurrent instability. Similarly, too 'deep' a tunnel placement results in excessive tightening of the graft when the knee is extended. It has been shown that an abnormally narrow intercondylar notch correlates directly with increased incidence of ACL tears. Careful assessment of the notch should be done prior to graft insertion to ensure no impingement on the lateral femoral condyle. The presence of impingement with correct placement of the tunnels necessitates notchplasty of the anterior portion of the lateral femoral condyle.

EXAMINER: How would you manage a child with an ACL injury who came to your clinic? Say she was 12 years old?

CANDIDATE: I would counsel the patient with regards to rehabilitation and activity modification. However, compliance with bracing and limitation of activity can be very difficult. My aim is to limit damage to the menisci and chondral surfaces. One should always consider the physis when planning reconstruction, as damage to the distal femoral physis can cause deformity. Reconstructions can be either extraphyseal or intraphyseal or even extra- or intra-articular. Extra-articular lateral-based procedures like a Macintosh or a Lemaire tenodesis are an option. Intra-articular reconstructions can be physeal-sparing. If transphyseal reconstruction is considered, then soft tissue grafts need to be used and bone plugs need to be avoided.

References

1. Xie X, Liu X, Chen Z, Yu Y, Peng S, Li Q. A meta-analysis of bone–patellar tendon–bone autograft versus four-strand hamstring tendon autograft for anterior cruciate ligament reconstruction. *Knee*. 2015;22(2):100–110.

2. Xie X, Xiao Z, Li Q, *et al.* Increased incidence of osteoarthritis of knee joint after ACL reconstruction with bone–patellar tendon–bone autografts than hamstring autografts: a meta-analysis of 1,443 patients at a minimum of 5 years. *Eur J Orthop Surg Traumatol*. 2015;25(1):149–159.

3. Howell SM, Taylor MA. Failure of reconstruction of the anterior cruciate ligament due to impingement by the intercondylar roof. *J Bone Joint Surg Am*. 1993;75 (7):1044–1055.

4. Webster KE, Feller JA, Hartnett N, Leigh WB, Richmond AK. Comparison of Patellar tendon and hamstring tendon anterior cruciate ligament reconstruction: a 15-year follow-up of a randomized controlled trial. *Am J Sports Med*. 2016;44(1):83–90.

5. Grassi A, Nitri M, Moulton SG, *et al.* Does the type of graft affect the outcome of revision anterior cruciate ligament reconstruction? A meta-analysis of 32 studies. *Bone Joint J*. 2017;99B(6):714–723.

Structured oral examination question 8

Revision knee replacement

EXAMINER: Have a look at these images and tell me what you can see (Figure 4.8a and 4.8b).

CANDIDATE: These are AP and lateral radiographs of a failed left total knee replacement. The implants appear to be loose with widespread osteolysis and bone loss on both the femoral and tibial sides. The tibial component is stemmed and has a medial augment, suggesting that this in itself is a revision implant. Bone stock on the tibial side is certainly an issue which needs to be addressed. There is calcification of soft tissues including the popliteal vessels. I would like to see immediate postoperative and most recent radiographs for comparison. The radiographs are suggestive of infection until proven otherwise.

EXAMINER: OK. After investigation you conclude this is aspetic loosening. The patient is keen to consider single-stage revision surgery. What are your concerns with regards to these radiographs?

CANDIDATE: The collateral ligaments are likely to be dysfunctional, especially the MCL as the tibial

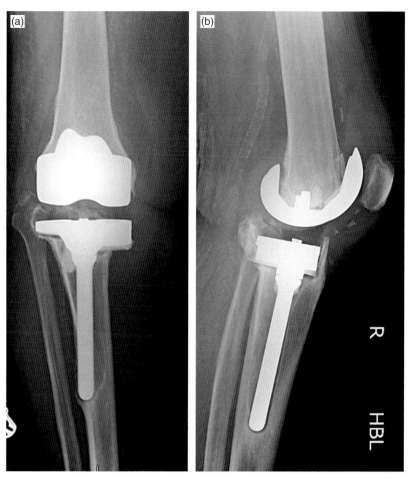

Figure 4.8a and 4.8b Anteroposterior and lateral radiographs revision TKA.

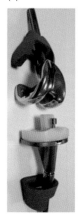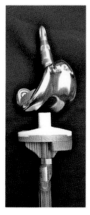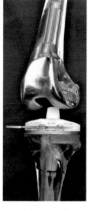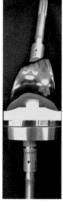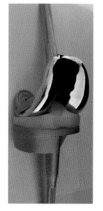

| NexGen (Zimmer) | Triathlon TS (Stryker) | Legion (Smith & Nephew) | Vanguard SSK (Biomet) | PFC Sigma TC3 (DePuy) |

Figure 4.8c Commonly used CCK systems.

component has subsided significantly and may be compromising the insertion of the MCL. Therefore, a constrained knee replacement may be required. The soft tissue envelope shadow on the radiograph appears contracted and calcified which may lead to wound complications. I would always take deep samples in all revisions to exclude infection as PJI can often be misdiagnosed.[1] The extensive bone loss will require a stemmed implant to promote load-sharing of the diaphysis. A fracture of the tibia may occur; however, the use of the stem will bypass this area. A metaphyseal sleeve will be needed to help with significant bone loss. I would be worried about the state of the extensor mechanism and if the patella tendon would remain attached after removal of the implants. The joint line needs to be restored and this may be a challenge.

EXAMINER: And what are your goals of surgery?

CANDIDATE: I would want to restore the joint line by achieving well-fixed implants and achieve a stable knee joint in a balanced fashion. I would also like to restore bone deficiencies and extract all the components with minimal bone loss while preserving the extensor mechanism.

EXAMINER: Are you aware of any classification system for bone loss around knee arthroplasty?

CANDIDATE: The most commonly used classification system is that of the Anderson Orthopaedic Research Institute (AORI), which classifies the femur (F) and tibia (T) separately as follows:

Type-1 – Intact metaphysical bone with minor defects which will not compromise the stability of a revision component.

Type-2 – Damaged metaphysical bone. Loss of cancellous bone in the metaphyseal segment which will need to be filled with cement, augments or a bone graft at revision in order to restore the joint line. Defects can occur in one femoral condyle or tibial plateau (2A) or in both condyles or plateau (2B).

Type-3 – Deficient metaphysical bone. Bone loss which comprises a major portion of either condyle or plateau. These defects are occasionally associated with detachment of the collateral or patellar ligaments and usually require long-stemmed revision implants with bone grafts or a custom-made hinged prosthesis.

EXAMINER: What are the factors you need to consider in the preoperative planning?

CANDIDATE: It is important to establish, prior to surgery, what components are present, their sizes, the level of constraint, and the surgical approaches previously used. Where vertical incisions have been used, I follow the most lateral incision. Transverse incisions can be crossed at right angles. Bone stock and soft tissue integrity should be considered as well as current deformity. The extraction of the implants and fixation methods all need to be planned prior to surgery.

EXAMINER: How would you optimize your exposure in a revision knee replacement?

CANDIDATE: I would utilize a longer skin incision to identify virgin territory. This will also allow the scar tissue to be mobilized from the underlying quadriceps, which we call debulking. A full synovectomy needs to be performed and there is a plane which needs exploiting between the muscle and synovium. A partial lateral release can help release the lateral gutter and aid the mobilization of the patella. If there are concerns about the patella tendon insertion, subluxing the patella may be a better option. I may need to use a rectus snip or quadriceps turn down or even a tibial tubercle osteotomy (TTO). A TTO provides excellent exposure and avoids an extensor lag which may be seen with a V-Y turndown as it avoids any violation of the quadriceps tendon. Patella baja can be corrected with TTO as well. The main problem is a non-union following fixation. There is a possibility of lengthening or shortening the quadriceps with techniques such as the V-Y turndown. The PCL should be sacrificed to aid balancing and assessment of the tibial plateau.

EXAMINER: You mentioned that a constrained implant may be required. What are the levels of constraints?

CANDIDATE: The constraint ladder within knee implant design includes:

PCL-retaining (cruciate-retaining or CR) rotating platform more constrained due to conformity.

↓

PCL-substituting (posterior stabilized or PS).

↓

Unlinked constrained non-hinged condylar implant (varus–valgus constrained) provides anteroposterior and varus–valgus stability (substitute for deficient collaterals), e.g. constrained condylar knee (LCCK, NexGen), TC3 (Figure 4.8c).

High central post which will substitute for a MCL deficiency and requires medullary stem support.

↓

Linked, constrained condylar implant (rotating-hinge knee or RHK). Rarely indicated. Used for global instability (total collateral disruption/recurvatum) and severe distal femoral bone loss, osteolysis/fracture.

↓

Fusion – may be required for chronically infected unstable knee with a poor soft tissue envelope.

EXAMINER: What is your intraoperative plan for revising a knee replacement with bone loss?

CANDIDATE: Removal of implants, i.e. extraction, is the first step. Bone preservation is critical and making sure fine or flexible osteotomes and a narrow reciprocating saw are available. My aim is to achieve stable fixation at the epiphysis, but often one has to use stemmed implants to achieve diaphyseal fixation as well as metaphysical sleeves to achieve press-fit metaphysical fixation, especially when there is a significant amount of bone loss. Once the tibial platform is established the flexion and extension gaps can be assessed. An intramedullary stem can guide the positioning of the femoral component. Gap balancing should be used to assess flexion and extension gaps. Distal femoral augments can be used to match the flexion gap.

EXAMINER: [Going back to the radiographs] What are the principles of management of bone loss in revision knee replacement in this patient?

CANDIDATE: The options of management of the extensive bone loss are:

1. The use of cement, either alone or combined with screws and mesh.
2. The use of bone grafting with structural or morsellized graft.
3. The use of modular augmentation of the components with wedges or blocks of metal. Recent studies show modular porous coated press fit metaphyseal sleeves may be used to fill AORI type 2 and 3 defects and provide for stable ingrowth.
4. The utilization of custom-made, tumour or hinge implants.

The method of reconstruction and the materials for revision surgery are largely dependent on the potential for future further revision and the life expectancy, functional demand and comorbidities of the patient. In this patient who is reasonably young, restoration of bone stock is preferable, because of the likelihood of further revision surgery.

References

1. Koh IJ, Cho WS, Choi NY, Parvizi J, Kim TK; Korea Knee Research Group. How accurate are orthopaedic surgeons in diagnosing periprosthetic joint infection after total knee arthroplasty? A multicenter study. *Knee.* 2015;22(3):180–185.

Structured oral examination question 9

Patellar instability

EXAMINER: A 17-year-old lady is referred to your patella clinic by her GP due to recurrent bilateral patella dislocations. How would you assess this patient?

CANDIDATE: I would start by taking a detailed history followed by clinical examination. In the history, I would enquire about age at first dislocation, frequency of dislocations, traumatic or atraumatic, any associated syndromes such as bone or connective tissue dysplasia and generalized joint laxity. I would also enquire about any mechanical symptoms, the presence and localization of pain.

I would start with a general hypermobility assessment using the Beighton score. Examination of the patella includes assessment of coronal and rotational alignment and patella height. We should also assess patella apprehension and patellofemoral crepitus. Quadriceps function and hamstring tightness should also be recorded.

EXAMINER: What are the risk factors for patella instability?

CANDIDATE: The risk factors for patellar instability are complex and multifactorial; however, they can be subcategorized in the following sections:

1. Bony factors (static).
   - Trochlear dysplasia.
   - Excessive lateral patella tilt.
   - Patella alta.
   - Femoral or tibial malrotation.

2. Malalignment.
   - Patellar malalignment is an abnormal rotational or translational deviation of the patella along any axis.

- External tibial torsion/foot pronation increased femoral anteversion and genu valgum especially in adolescence – miserable malalignment syndrome.
- Increased Q angle or abnormal tibial tuberosity–trochlea groove (TT–TG) distance.

3. Soft tissue (dynamic).
- Ligamentous laxity (medial patellofemoral ligament rupture/insufficiency).
- Muscle and soft tissue imbalance around the knee.
- Core muscle instability in the hip.

4. Abnormal gait.
- Walking with a valgus thrust.

5. Genetic factors such as connective tissue disorder syndromes and generalized hypermobility.

Two-thirds of patients are known to have multiple anatomical factors predisposing to recurrent patella dislocations.

EXAMINER: Tell me about the important stabilizers of the patella.

CANDIDATE: Patella stability results from a complex interplay of local, distant, static and dynamic factors. Dynamic muscular restraints, static soft-tissue restraints, bony morphology and lower limb alignment all stabilize the patellofemoral joint.

The distant static factors are femoral anteversion, knee rotation and external tibial torsion. The distant dynamic factors include the iliotibial band complex, hip abductors and foot rotation.

The primary local static restraint to the lateral patellar displacement is the medial patellofemoral ligament. It provides 50–60% of the total medial restraining force and resists lateral translation in early knee flexion (20–30°). MPFL sectioning can lead to substantial changes in patellar tracking.

The femoral attachment of the medial patellofemoral ligament (MPFL) has been the centre of much debate. Amis et al. concluded that the origin was the medial epicondyle [1]. Following on from his work, Schöttle et al., in a cadaveric study, identified a radiographic point for the origin, 1 mm anterior to the posterior cortex extension line, 2.5 mm distal to the posterior origin of the medial femoral condyle and proximal to the level of the posterior point of the Blumensaat line on a lateral radiograph with both posterior condyles projected in the same plane, which represented the mean femoral MPFL isometric centre [2]. Intraoperative fluoroscopy

can be used to accurately identify this position. However, it is now believed to be a point just anterior to the confluence of the Blumensaat line, a curving line of the posterior femoral cortex and posterior to the straight extension line from the posterior cortex in a true lateral radiograph. Hence it is named the confluence point.

During acute patellar dislocation there is a 90–95% incidence of damage to the MPFL. Femoral attachment is commonly affected. In the past 10 years, MPFL reconstruction has become a popular procedure for treatment of recurrent patellar dislocation.

Dejour et al. examined CT scans on 134 patients treated for patellar instability. They identified four common factors of unstable symptomatic knees: (1) trochlear dysplasia (85%), (2) quadriceps dysplasia (83%), (3) patella alta (24%), (4) tibial tuberosity–trochlear groove distance, pathological when greater than or equal to 20 mm (56%) [3].

EXAMINER: How would you investigate this patient?

CANDIDATE: I would perform the following investigations:

1. A true lateral radiograph is the most helpful view for assessment of patella height and trochlear depth.
2. Axial radiographs (Merchant's view) to assess patellar tilt angle (normal < 10°), congruence, lateral patellofemoral angle (normal 138°) and trochlear dysplasia.
3. Rotational profile CT scans assess femoral anteversion which normally is 5–15°, external tibial torsion, patellar tilt and index, TT–TG (tibial tuberosity–trochlear groove) distance. If the TT–TG is more than 19 mm this is pathological.
4. MRI for articular surface assessment (OCD), integrity of the MPFL, patella height, TTTG and trochlear dysplasia (Figure 4.9a).

When assessing the patella height, I use the Caton–Deschamps method. This is the ratio between the distance from the inferior border of the patella articular surface to the upper edge of the tibial plateau and the length of the patella articular surface. A ratio of more than 1.2 indicates patella alta. I use the lateral view with the knee in at least 30° of flexion.

EXAMINER: When would you offer a lateral release?

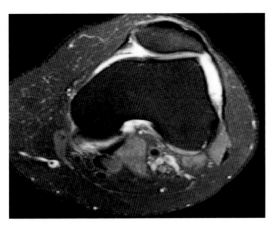

Figure 4.9a MRI scan, T2 axial view demonstrating lateral patella subluxation, knee effusion and shallow trochlea groove.

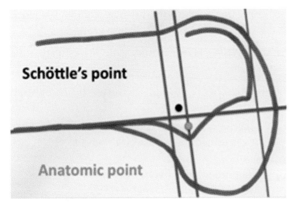

Figure 4.9b Schöttle's point.

CANDIDATE: I would only perform a lateral release if there were isolated lateral patellar tilt. I would not perform this procedure independently.

EXAMINER: What are the options of surgical treatment?

CANDIDATE: Generally, surgical procedures for chronic patellofemoral instability are often used in combination and include bony and soft-tissue procedures at the level of the joint, proximal or just distal to it. The realignment procedures are determined by direction of tibial tubercle (TT) transfer: medial transfer to treat malalignment, anteromedial transfer for malalignment and PFJ chondrosis, anterior when there is distal PFJ chondrosis.

Operative intervention for acute isolated first-time dislocation is only indicated if there is evidence of a large osteochondral defect. There are several reports of lower redislocation rates following surgical treatment of primary acute patella dislocations; however, there is no difference in the long term. Decision-making using patient-specific instability predictors can identify patients who would benefit from operative intervention. The parameters in the Patellar-Instability Severity Score (PIS-Score) include age, patellar tilt, patellar alta, TT–TG distance, trochlear dysplasia and positive anamnesis of contralateral patella dislocation. A score of more than 4 indicates a higher risk of redislocation.

MPFL reconstruction is a very successful procedure. An ideal candidate for this should have a history of recurrent dislocation and a physical examination demonstrating excessive lateral patella translation and a normal trochlea [4]. A Caton–Deschamps index up to 1.3 can be acceptable, except where there is a very short trochlea or significant knee hyperextension. The key bony procedures for patella instability are: trochleoplasty, tibial tuberosity osteotomy and femoral osteotomy (derotation or angular) [5].

References

1. Amis AA, Firer P, Mountney J, Senavongse W, Thomas NP. Anatomy and biomechanics of the medial patellofemoral ligament. *The Knee*. 2003;10(3):215–220.

2. Schöttle PB, Schmeling A, Rosenstiel N, Weiler A. Radiographic landmarks for femoral tunnel placement in medial patellofemoral ligament reconstruction. *Am J Sports Med*. 2007;35(5):801–804.

3. Dejour H, Walch G, Nove-Josserand L, Guier C. Factors of patellar instability: an anatomic radiographic study. *Knee Surg Sports Traumatol Arthrosc*. 1994;2(1):19–26.

4. Yeung M, Leblanc MC, Ayeni OR, *et al.* Indications for medial patellofemoral ligament reconstruction: a systematic review. *J Knee Surg*. 2016;29(7):543–554.

5. Steensen RN, Bentley JC, Trinh TQ, Backes JR, Wiltfong RE. The prevalence and combined prevalences of anatomic factors associated with recurrent patellar dislocation: a magnetic resonance imaging study. *Am J Sports Med*. 2015;43:921–927.

Structured oral examination question 10

Pain after TKA

EXAMINER: A 70-year-old gentleman has been referred to your clinic with ongoing pain in his knee following his primary uncomplicated TKA.

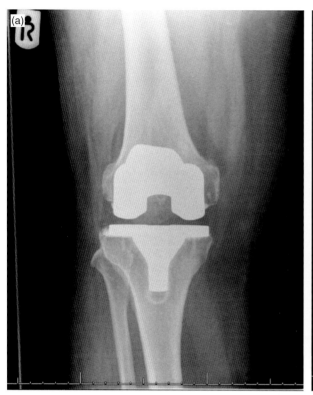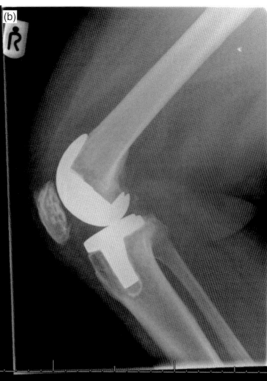

Figure 4.10a and 4.10b Anteroposterior and lateral radiographs right TKA.

He states the knee has never been quite right since his surgery three years ago. Please describe these radiographs (Figure 4.10a and 4.10b).

CANDIDATE: These radiographs demonstrate a cemented cruciate-sacrificing posterior stabilized implant. The patella has been resurfaced with a polyethylene button. There is no evidence of gross loosening of the implant neither are there any fractures. There is no evidence of tibial tray overhang or over-/under-sizing of the femoral component. The overall alignment is adequate.

EXAMINER: This patient is complaining of generalized knee pain. How would you proceed?

CANDIDATE: Firstly, I would take a history. I would like to know if there have been wound issues and if antibiotics have been prescribed previously. Were there any issues with wound healing? If infection has been excluded it is important to differentiate between extra- and intra-articular causes of pain. Lack of pain relief immediately after the TKA could suggest that the pain was not actually originating from the knee. It is also important to establish if the patient was initially pain-free, as pain developing after months or years is quite characteristic of component loosening or failure.

EXAMINER: OK, so this gentleman states his pain was no different following his TKA. What do you think of that?

CANDIDATE: Extra-articular causes of pain around the knee need to be excluded. Firstly, the hip should be assessed; pain may be radiating from the hip to the knee via the obturator nerve. Pain can radiate to the anterior or posterior aspects of the knee. Pathologies such as osteoarthritis, stress fractures, dysplasia and implant loosening after total hip replacement can all cause radiating pain to the knee. Posterior tibial tendon dysfunction causing planovalgus will lead to a valgus hindfoot alignment. This will subsequently cause changes in the ground reaction forces and increased lateral loading of the knee [1].

EXAMINER: So, you have suggested causes of pain above and below the knee. What else can cause the pain?

CANDIDATE: Vascular insufficiency with peripheral artery disease can cause leg pain in the elderly. Thrombosis is very common following TKR and should be excluded. An ankle–brachial pressure index is non-invasive and not costly. The history will also identify lumbar spinal stenosis which may require further imaging for assessment. Other neurological disorders such as chronic regional pain syndrome and cutaneous neuromas contribute to the incidence of knee pain following TKR. Posterolateral knee pain secondary to a posterolateral tibial tray overhang, a retained posterolateral osteophyte or cementophyte can cause biceps tendonitis and/or popliteus tendon impingement. Posteromedial pain can be caused by semimembranosus tendonitis. There are multiple periarticular bursae such as the infrapatellar, pes anserine and semimembranosus bursae which can cause pain and inflammation. Lateral pain with movement between 20 and 80° classically is a result of iliotibial band dysfunction.

EXAMINER: OK, but these causes are all outside the knee. What are the intrinsic pathologies which you should exclude?

CANDIDATE: Aseptic loosening is common and is frequently described as 'start-up pain'. A higher constrained implant, higher BMI, varus alignment and malrotation can contribute to implant loosening. Malalignment and wear are frequently responsible for late loosening.

EXAMINER: I agree. Aseptic/septic loosening needs to be excluded. What else?

CANDIDATE: Pain can be caused by instability as the soft tissues are overloaded. Early failure related to instability may be associated with trauma or more importantly surgical technique. Surgical considerations such as suboptimal alignment or positioning, improper balancing of flexion–extension gaps and medial collateral and posterior cruciate ligament rupture can cause persistent pain.

EXAMINER: Tell me how you would assess for malalignment of components?

CANDIDATE: I would organize a standard radiological series including a skyline view and a CT scan.

EXAMINER: What are the consequences of rotational malalignment?

CANDIDATE: Rotational alignment of the tibial and femoral component plays an important role in TKA. Once correct frontal alignment and proper soft tissue balancing has been achieved, the rotational placement of the components represents the 'third dimension' in knee TKA. Femoral component malposition has been implicated in patellofemoral maltracking following TKA, which is associated with anterior knee pain, subluxation, fracture, wear and aseptic loosening [1,2]. Internal rotation of the femoral component by resection of excessive amounts of posterior lateral femoral condyle or insufficient resection of the posterior medial femoral condyle moves the anterior femoral patellar groove portion of the femoral component medially, making it more difficult for a relatively laterally placed patella to be captured by the patellofemoral groove. In addition, internal rotation of the femoral component results in a tight flexion gap on the medial side of the knee.

EXAMINER: Do you know anything about how you determine rotational alignment of a TKA on CT?

CANDIDATE: Rotational component malalignment is difficult to access on standard AP and lateral radiographs. Patients with painful early TKA should be assessed for evaluation of malrotated components.

EXAMINER: Anything else?

CANDIDATE: [Silence]

COMMENT: Berger et al. have described methodology to quantitatively measure component rotational alignment using CT scanning [3].

Based on the published values, essentially the surgical transepicondylar axis (TEA) is on average 3° externally rotated in relation to the posterior condylar axis while the perpendicular axis to the trochlear anteroposterior axis is 4° externally rotated to the posterior condylar axis and finally the anatomical TEA is on average 5° externally rotated to the posterior condylar axis (Figure 4.10c). None of the above are entirely reliable, especially the TEA. Surgeons may have to use more than one reference point when placing the femoral and tibial components.

(c)

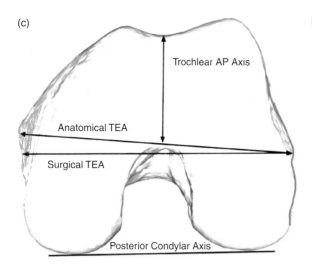

Figure 4.10c Femoral component rotational alignment.

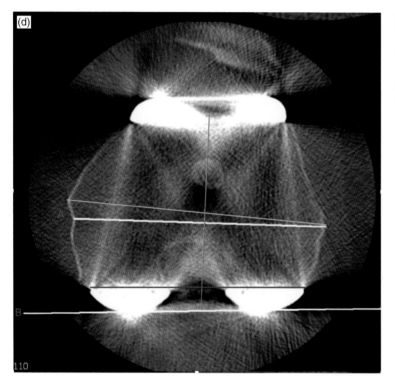

Figure 4.10d CT measurement of femoral implant rotation. The posterior condylar bone cut (red line) is 1–2° internally rotated in relation to the surgical TEA (white line A). However, the white line B represents the line of the posterior condyle of the femoral component. The yellow line represents the anatomical TEA and the orange line represents Whiteside's line.

The rotation of the tibial component (tibial posterior component axis) is measured in relation to the posterior tibial plateau axis, medial/middle third of the tibial tubercle, patellar tendon, PCL attachment, transverse axis of the tibia, midsulcus of the tibial spine and anteromedial margin of the tibial plateau.

Tibial component axis normal value = 18°.

References

1. Mandalia V, Eyres K, Schranz P, Toms AD. Evaluation of patients with a painful total knee replacement. *J Bone Joint Surg Br.* 2008;90(3):265–271.

2. Nicoll D, Rowley DI. Internal rotational error of the tibial component is a major cause of pain after total knee replacement. *J Bone Joint Surg Br.* 2010;92B: 1238–1244.

3. Berger RA, Crossett LS, Jacobs JJ, Rubash HE. Malrotation causing patellofemoral complications after total knee arthroplasty. Clin Orthop Rel Res. 1998;356:144–153.

Structured oral examination question 11

Osteotomies around the knee

EXAMINER: A 28-year-old gentleman who works as a postman attends your clinic, complaining of knee pain. He has had it for many years but is now unable to work. What do you think (Figure 4.11a)?

CANDIDATE: The weight-bearing AP radiograph demonstrates narrowing of the medial tibiofemoral joint space. There is a defect in the lateral aspect of the medial femoral condyle and it seems to be involving the subchondral bone.

EXAMINER: What are the pertinent features in the history and examination?

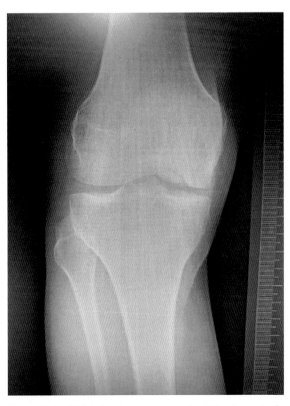

Figure 4.11a Weight-bearing anteroposterior (AP) radiograph of the right knee.

CANDIDATE: I would like to find out if this is traumatic or atraumatic, take a detailed pain history including site, severity and if he has mechanical symptoms. Clinically I would like to assess his overall alignment and see if he is tender over the medial femoral condyle (MFC). I would also like to get an MRI of the knee to elucidate the nature of this defect in the condyle. I would assume this patient has had osteochondritis dissecans in the past.

EXAMINER: OK, let's assume he has been through all conservative treatment and is keen to undergo surgery. Tell me about your management plan.

CANDIDATE: Firstly, I would like to assess his lower limb alignment. If I were to offer him a chondral procedure, I would certainly ensure his overall alignment is not in varus.

EXAMINER: What would you like to see?

CANDIDATE: I would like to see some long leg alignment views including the hip and ankle to perform some deformity analysis. I would also like to see a lateral and some further imaging of the joint surface would be helpful to plan further surgery.

EXAMINER: OK, so what information would you like?

CANDIDATE: Firstly, I would like to assess the deformity in the frontal plane, and according to Paley, should include the mechanical axis of the lower limb, overall malalignment, lateral distal femoral angle (LDFA), medial proximal tibial angle (MPTA) and the joint line convergence angle (JLCA). The tibial width is given a percentage of 100% starting medially (0%) and ending laterally (100%). Where the mechanical axis crosses the tibial plateau, this is named the Mikulicz point (and is a percentage value). I would also assess the sagittal alignment for the anatomical posterior proximal tibia angle (aPPTA), which reflects the tibial slope, and the anatomical posterior distal femur angle (aPDFA), which represents the flexion/extension positioning of the distal femur.

EXAMINER: Tell me, what are the key biomechanical parameters and normal values for frontal alignment?

CANDIDATE: The LDFA is normally 87° (85–90°) and the MPTA is normally 87° (85–90°). The JLCA is 0–2° [1] (Table 4.1).

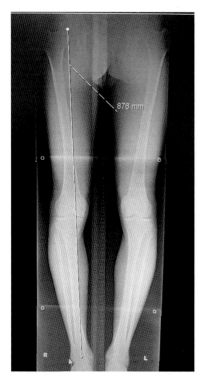

Figure 4.11b Standing anteroposterior (AP) long leg radiographs.

EXAMINER: So, what do you think of this patient's full-leg standing radiographs (Figure 4.11b)?

CANDIDATE: He looks to be in varus. The weight-bearing line is passing well into the medial compartment.

EXAMINER: So, the MRI demonstrates the OCD in the MFC, the meniscus is preserved and there is some chondral thinning of the medial tibial plateau. What would you offer him?

CANDIDATE: Firstly, I would offer him a valgizing osteotomy. Once his alignment is corrected, I will be able to safely perform some form of chondral surgery, if needed.

EXAMINER: OK . . . Please explain the rationale.

CANDIDATE: Well, as this patient is in varus, I would like to offload them and perform a valgizing osteotomy in the form of a high tibial osteotomy or distal femoral osteotomy. It depends where the deformity lies.

EXAMINER: Explain?

CANDIDATE: I perform an osteotomy in the bone where the deformity lies. As we can see from the

Table 4.1 Limb alignment analysis.

Angle	
mLPFA	86°
mLDFA	89°
mMPTA	80°
mLDFA	86°
JLCA	0°

limb alignment analysis (Table 4.1), the MPTA is 80°, which is abnormal. If we performed a femoral osteotomy, we would be introducing joint line obliquity to the knee and ultimately uneven joint loading. As the MPTA is 80°, normal being 87°, the deformity lies in the proximal tibia. The distal femur is normal and the proximal tibia is in varus.

EXAMINER: What kind of osteotomy would you offer him?

CANDIDATE: We can perform opening and closing wedge osteomies to both the medial and lateral sides of the femur and tibia. Given the proximal tibia is in varus, and this is where the deformity lies, we will need to increase the MPTA to the normal 87°. The two options are a medial opening wedge HTO or a lateral closing wedge HTO. The most efficient way to do this would be a medial opening wedge HTO.

EXAMINER: Why?

CANDIDATE: The opening wedge HTO has gained popularity because it does not require a fibular osteotomy, common peroneal nerve dissection, disruption of proximal tibiofibular joint, and bone stock loss (Bonasia *et al.*, 2014). If we were to perform a lateral closing wedge, this would create two bone surfaces which would be in direct contact and promote healing. Opening a wedge and potentially leaving a gap could reduce the time to union; this, however, has not been proven in the literature [3], therefore I may consider filling the gap, with either synthetic or allograft.

EXAMINER: So, if you've decided on a medial opening wedge HTO, how would you go about it and tell me the considerations intraoperatively?

CANDIDATE: I would prepare the patient supine on a radiolucent table under tourniquet with intravenous antibiotics at induction. An image

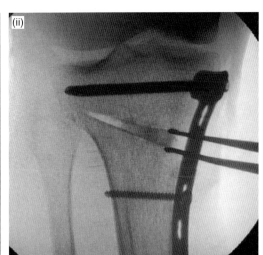

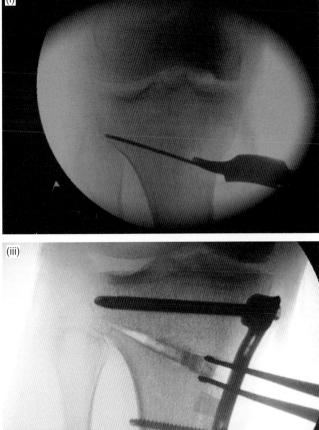

Figure 4.11c Intraoperative images of opening wedge HTO.
(i)   Positioning of the first guide wire, note the position of the hinge point.
(ii) Application of the Tomofix plate following opening of the wedge.
(iii) Image demonstrating maintenance of the gap opening following gap filling and application of the plate.

intensifier would be available to me approaching from the lateral side. I would approach the proximal tibia via a direct anteromedial oblique approach. I would identify the pes and release the hamstrings. I would release the MCL distal fibres subperiosteally in one layer with diathermy until I can see the posterior border of the tibia. After careful dissection posteriorly, I would use a curved brown-handled osteotome to clear the posterior structures off the tibia and place a radiolucent Homann in position to protect the neurovascular bundle. I would mark out my biplane osteotomy to increase the stability of the construct. A precision saw is safe and should be used with the radiolucent retractor. To ensure the trajectory of the saw cut is in the plane of the joint, I place 2 K-wires parallel with the joint under fluoroscopy. The callipers are then used to measure the exact distance for the opening wedge as per the preoperative plan to 0.1 mm (see Figure 4.11c).

EXAMINER: What would be your postoperative rehabilitation programme?

CANDIDATE: Rest, ice, a cryotherapy cuff would be advantageous, routine observations including neurovascular monitoring. Using a plate like the Tomofix system allows full weight bearing immediately. I would like to see an X-ray at the six weeks mark to ensure there has been no less of correction.

References

1. Paley D, Herzenberg JE, Tetsworth K, McKie J, Bhave A. Deformity planning for frontal and sagittal plane corrective osteotomies. *Orthop Clin North Am*. 1994;25(3):425–465.

2. Bonasia DE, Dettoni F, Sito G, *et al*. Medial opening wedge high tibial osteotomy for medial compartment overload/arthritis in the varus knee: prosthetic factors. *Am J Sports Med*. 2014;42(3): 690–698.

3. Staubli AE, Jacob HAC. Evolution of open-wedge high-tibial osteotomy: experience with a special angular stable device for internal fixation without interposition material. *Int Orthop*. 2010;34(2): 167–172.

Foot and ankle

N. Jane Madeley and Stan Jones

Structured oral examination question 1

Lateral ligament instability of the ankle

EXAMINER: Tell me what this diagram (Figure 5.1) represents and name the structures labelled 2, 3 and 5.

CANDIDATE: This diagram is a representation of the lateral aspect of the ankle showing the bony and ligamentous structures. Structure 2 is the anterior talofibular ligament, structure 3 is the calcaneofibular ligament and structure 5 is the posterior distal tibiofibular ligament.

EXAMINER: What structures are injured in a lateral ligament injury?

CANDIDATE: The mechanism is usually a rotational injury with sequential failure of the ligaments from front to back, hence the anterior talofibular ligament or ATFL is most commonly injured followed by the calcaneofibular ligament or CFL and the posterior talofibular ligament is the least frequently injured.

EXAMINER: How would you go about diagnosing a lateral ligament injury to the ankle?

CANDIDATE: In the acute setting I would expect the patient to give a history of an episode of a twisting incident resulting in significant pain and swelling. There may be a history of recurrent sprains and instability. Acutely the lateral side of the ankle anterior and inferior to the distal end of the fibula would be swollen and tender but discomfort may make it difficult to elicit definite signs of instability.

In a patient with a chronic history the clinical signs of instability would be a positive anterior drawer test or talar tilt test.

EXAMINER: Tell me more about those two tests.

CANDIDATE: The patient is examined sitting with their legs over the edge of the couch or sitting in a chair to relax the gastrocnemius soleus complex.

For the anterior drawer test the distal tibia is stabilized in one hand. The other hand is used to grasp the heel then draw the foot anteriorly in relation to the talus. Pain or excess anterior translation or a sulcus sign developing at the anterolateral corner of the ankle are signs of an ATFL injury. The other ankle must be examined for comparison. The talar tilt test involves inversion of the ankle while placing a finger on the anterolateral corner of the joint. The lack of a firm endpoint or tilt in excess of the normal side suggests instability and the CFL is considered to be injured if this test is positive.

EXAMINER: What other clinical findings may be positive in a patient with recurrent ankle sprains?

CANDIDATE: Ankle sprains are more common in patients with a cavus foot or hypermobility.

EXAMINER: If you suspect a lateral ligament injury how will you proceed in managing this patient?

CANDIDATE: The first step in management would be rehabilitation with physiotherapy, concentrating on peroneal strengthening and proprioceptive training. If the dynamic stabilizers of the ankle are well-conditioned the majority of patients recover well from a ligament injury. Bracing may be of benefit.

EXAMINER: What percentage of patients recover?

CANDIDATE: The vast majority.

EXAMINER: [That's a bit vague] Do you know a figure?

CANDIDATE: Sorry.

COMMENT: Around 20% of patients develop symptoms of chronic ankle instability such as recurrent

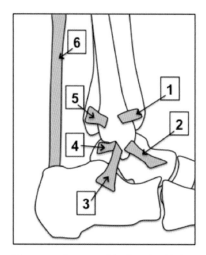

Figure 5.1 Diagram of the lateral ankle ligaments.

sprains, weakness and instability. Candidates should know this and may lose a mark.

EXAMINER: How do you determine severe injuries?

CANDIDATE: Severe extensive bruising, severe pain on moving the foot, inability to bear weight are features of a severe injury. The options for acute grade III injuries include cast immobilization or functional management. Cast immobilization involves 3 weeks in a below-knee walking cast followed by 12 weeks proprioceptive rehabilitation. Functional management involves early mobilization with external support and a protocol of rest, ice, compression and elevation. This is followed by a rehabilitation programme that comprises ROM exercises, muscle strengthening, proprioception (wobble boards) and activity-specific training.

EXAMINER: What if the patient continues to have significant symptoms despite adequate rehabilitation?

CANDIDATE: A patient that fails to recover would require investigation. I would begin with simple weight-bearing radiographs of the ankle. Other investigations include stress X-rays of the ankle and/or ultrasonography to assess the degree of ligamentous injury and if the patient is still having significant pain and swelling an MRI scan to look for additional pathology.

EXAMINER: What other conditions would you be looking for?

CANDIDATE: My differential diagnosis for an ankle sprain that does not improve would be peroneal tendon pathology such as a split tear or subluxing tendons, intra-articular pathology such as an osteochondral defect of the talus or loose body, or non-union of an anterior calcaneal process fracture.

EXAMINER: Do you know any scoring systems for chronic lateral instability?

CANDIDATE: No, sorry.

COMMENT: Karlsson score, American orthopaedic foot and ankle score (AOFAS) and the foot and ankle outcome score (FAOS).

EXAMINER: What are the surgical options for management of an isolated lateral ankle ligament complex injury in a young patient who has failed to respond to non-operative treatments?

CANDIDATE: The options fall into three broad categories. (1) Anatomic repair, (2) non-anatomic reconstruction, (3) anatomic tenodesis reconstruction.

EXAMINER: What is an anatomic repair?

CANDIDATE: Anatomic repair involves the use of endogenous ligamentous tissue to restore the ligament. This is considered in cases when adequate tissue is present.

The Broström and the 'modified Broström' are the most widely used procedures for anatomic repair of the lateral ligament complex.

The complication rate is lower (fewer wounds, less risk of injury to the superficial peroneal nerve and decreased incidence of degenerative joint disease) compared to non-anatomical reconstructions with minimal effect on subtalar movement and a quicker rehab.

Failures have been attributed to a variety of factors, including generalized ligamentous laxity, poor tissue quality, previous surgical repair, long-standing instability, and cavo-varus deformity.

EXAMINER: What do you mean by a non-anatomic reconstruction (check-rein procedure)?

CANDIDATE: Non-anatomic reconstruction does not replicate the normal course and anatomy of the ATFL and CFL.

Examples of non-anatomic reconstructive procedures include the Chrisman–Snook procedure, the Watson-Jones procedure and the Evans reconstruction, all utilizing the neighbouring peroneus brevis tendon to restrict motion without repair of the injured ligaments.

EXAMINER: What do we mean by anatomical reconstruction?

CANDIDATE: These procedures utilize autogenous tendon grafts such as semitendinosus, gracilis or plantaris that are rerouted in such a way as to replicate the anatomic positions of the ATFL and CFL origin and insertion sites.

EXAMINER: Are intra-articular lesions common in this group?

CANDIDATE: Various studies have found chondral injuries in a significant proportion of patients with chronic ankle instability. In one study associated intra-articular pathology amenable to arthroscopic treatment was identified in 83% of patients undergoing Brostrom repair [1]. Arthroscopic abrasion, curettage, drilling or microfracture can be used for the OCLs.

EXAMINER: A patient asks how successful a ligament repair will be, what will you tell them?

CANDIDATE: I would expect a successful result in approximately 80% of patients.

EXAMINER: What are the reported results of using a free hamstring graft?

CANDIDATE: The reports are good but there are some reports of weakness of knee flexion beyond 70°, particularly when both gracilis and semitendinosus tendons are harvested.

COMMENT: This ligament reconstruction can be performed through short incisions, effectively making it a minimally invasive technique. The harvested graft (semitendinosus or gracilis) is secured in a tunnel in the calcaneum using interference or biotendinosis screws then passed through a tunnel in the fibula and finally secured under tension into a further tunnel in the talus. This leaves the stabilizing evertor muscles intact together while reconstructing the ATFL and CFL and so may also be considered to be an anatomic repair.

The selected fixation device should be secure enough to maintain appropriate graft tension intraoperatively to support healing and potentially allow for early joint motion

EXAMINER: Thank you.

Structured oral examination question 2

Ankle arthritis

EXAMINER: Describe the findings on this X-ray (Figure 5.2).

CANDIDATE: This is an AP weight-bearing radiograph of a left ankle showing narrowing of the joint space and some subchondral sclerosis. There is also evidence of a previous fibula fracture superior to the syndesmosis and varus angulation of the ankle. These findings are consistent with post-traumatic arthritis.

EXAMINER: What are the most common causes of arthritis of the ankle?

CANDIDATE: The most common cause of ankle arthritis is post-traumatic arthritis. Other causes include inflammatory, neuropathic and septic arthritis. Primary osteoarthritis is thought to be relatively uncommon.

COMMENT: In a recent epidemiological survey, the onset of ankle osteoarthritis was attributable to a previous rotational fracture (37.0% of cases), recurrent sprains (14.6%), a single sprain (13.7%), pilon fracture (9.0%), tibial shaft fracture (8.5%) and osteochondral lesion of the talus (OLT) (4.7%) [2].

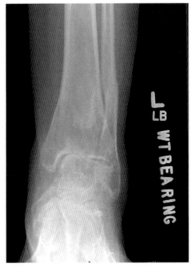

Figure 5.2 X-ray showing ankle arthritis.

EXAMINER: How is this patient likely to present?

CANDIDATE: The patient is likely to complain of pain, restriction of movement, deformity and difficulty in undertaking activities of daily living (ADLs).

EXAMINER: Are you aware of any classification systems for arthritis of the ankle?

CANDIDATE: No, I am not aware of any classification systems specific to the ankle.

COMMENT: The Kellgren and Lawrence Radiographic Criteria can be used [3].

EXAMINER: The X-ray you have been shown belongs to a 42-year-old manual worker who had an ankle fracture 7 years ago that was managed non-operatively. Describe your management strategy for this patient.

CANDIDATE: I would first want to take a full history and examine him, then obtain a lateral standing radiograph.

EXAMINER: Tell me about the management options available for ankle arthritis.

CANDIDATE: I would start with conservative measures and the options include NSAIDs, activity modification, footwear modification with a cushioned sole and rocker bottom shoe, an ankle brace or AFO, intra-articular steroid injection or visco-supplementation and physiotherapy.
PRP injections have been used in patients with osteoarthritis.
One study reported a strong positive effect on pain and function after four PRP injections at weekly intervals [4].

EXAMINER: What surgical options are available?

CANDIDATE: There are two types of surgical option available, those aimed to 'buy time' or provide temporary relief and definitive treatments. The temporizing measures are debridement of the joint which can be performed arthroscopically or open depending on the extent of disease and should be aimed at treating identifiable causes of symptoms such as removing loose bodies, trimming anterior osteophytes which may give impingement symptoms, or debriding loose areas of articular cartilage and areas of synovitis. The other option is distraction arthroplasty [5].
The definitive surgical options are ankle fusion or ankle replacement.

EXAMINER: What about arthroscopic debridement and osteophyte resection?

CANDIDATE: This may be helpful in patients with mild arthritis with a large osteophyte restricting motion or causing painful impingement at the extremes of motion. Rest pain is unlikely to be relieved. This operation is unlikely to be successful with this particular patient.

EXAMINER: What about distraction arthroplasty?

CANDIDATE: Distraction arthroplasty can be used on several joints including the hip, knee and ankle to preserve the joint space and decrease the weight-bearing load by using an external fixator to distract the respective joint. This is usually combined with an attempt at articular cartilage repair such as subchondral drilling or microfracture. Results of motion distraction are better than fixed distraction. Continuous joint movement is essential for cartilage regeneration and reduces overloading protecting fibrocartilage regeneration. Distraction arthroplasty is best suited for post-traumatic ankle osteoarthritis.

EXAMINER: Would you offer him distraction arthroplasty?

CANDIDATE: My concerns about offering him distraction arthroplasty are that he is a young patient with a physical occupation. The distraction device needs to be kept in place for at least 3 months, which is a significant treatment commitment. Ankle function declines following joint distraction such that at 5 years around 50% of patients will either have gone on to ankle arthrodesis or replacement. Due to the relatively small number of studies with only level 4 evidence and no long-term follow-up I would rather offer him ankle arthrodesis [6].

EXAMINER: Isn't fusion an outdated treatment now that ankle replacements are available?

CANDIDATE: No, total ankle replacements are not suitable for every patient and ankle fusion is still considered the 'gold standard', especially so for younger patients with severe post-traumatic ankle arthritis.

EXAMINER: So which patients should be considered for ankle replacement surgery?

CANDIDATE: Ankle replacement surgery could be considered in low-demand patients over the age of 60 years who have inflammatory arthritis or osteoarthritis. Bilateral disease or arthritis affecting adjacent joints is a relative indication. Contraindications include younger, more-active patients, significant ankle instability, particularly deltoid ligament insufficiency, significant deformity, especially varus or valgus of more than 10°, peripheral vascular disease, a poor soft-tissue envelope, marked osteoporosis or avascular necrosis of the tibial plafond or talar dome.

EXAMINER: Do you know anything about the types of ankle replacement available?

CANDIDATE: The earlier designs involved a two-component design such as the Agility total ankle replacement, which required fusion of the distal tibiofibular joint. Most modern designs are three-component uncemented mobile bearing prostheses.

EXAMINER: A patient wants to know how long an ankle replacement will last. What will you tell them?

CANDIDATE: The 10-year survival is about 85%, but there are fewer data available compared to knee and hip replacements [7–10].

EXAMINER: The 42-year-old patient we began by discussing wants an ankle replacement. What would you tell him?

CANDIDATE: He is a young patient in a manual job. He wouldn't be a candidate for total ankle replacement and I would explain to him that if his symptoms have not been controlled by non-operative measures then he requires definitive surgical treatment and an ankle fusion would be a better option for him.

EXAMINER: He still wants a replacement, as he is keen to get back to hill walking and sports and doesn't want a stiff ankle. What will you tell him now?

CANDIDATE: He would be at risk of early failure with an ankle replacement due to his age and level of activity. Postoperative complications of total ankle replacement include infection, loosening, progressive intracomponent instability or deformity, subsidence and polyethylene failure.

A fusion would provide a stable, pain-free ankle that would allow him to return to the majority of activities that he wishes to do. I would explain that many patients return to sports after ankle fusion. I would also explain that an ankle fusion would

only sacrifice the residual movement that he has at his ankle joint and that his subtalar, midfoot and forefoot movements would still be present.

EXAMINER: What position should his ankle be fused in?

CANDIDATE: The ankle should be fused in 5° of hind-foot valgus, 10° of external rotation and the foot should be plantigrade.

EXAMINER: What complications will you warn him about?

CANDIDATE: Infection, wound healing problems, neurovascular injury, DVT/PE, delayed union, malunion, non-union, hardware failure and the risk of exacerbating or developing arthritis in other joints (subtalar joint).

EXAMINER: Anything new on the horizon?

CANDIDATE: Ankle osteochondral allograft reconstruction involves replacing all or a large part of the arthritic ankle joint with a cadaveric bulk osteochondral allograft. Although in theory this procedure is a potentially desirable option for a young patient with advanced ankle arthritis, reported results suggest a high failure rate.

EXAMINER: Thank you.

Structured oral examination question 3

The rheumatoid foot

EXAMINER: Please have a look at this radiographic print and tell me what you see. (See Figure 5.3.)

CANDIDATE: This is an AP radiograph of a forefoot. There is a hallux valgus deformity with subluxation of the second metatarsophalangeal joint and destructive change of all the metatarsophalangeal joints. There may be deformities of the lesser toes and I would like to see a lateral view to clarify this.

EXAMINER: A lateral view would be very helpful. What do you think is the underlying diagnosis?

CANDIDATE: The changes suggest that this is an inflammatory polyarthropathy such as rheumatoid arthritis.

EXAMINER: Could it be anything else?

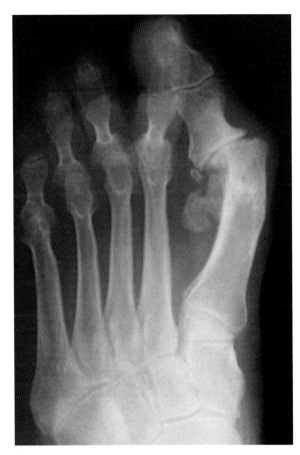

Figure 5.3 AP radiograph of rheumatoid forefoot.

CANDIDATE: The appearances could be secondary to a neuropathic process.

EXAMINER: What might be the commonest neuropathic process that could cause these appearances?

CANDIDATE: A peripheral neuropathy such as that associated with diabetes mellitus would be the commonest.

EXAMINER: How would you confirm your diagnosis?

CANDIDATE: A detailed history would be most informative. Specifically, I would enquire about pain, swelling and sensory alteration.

EXAMINER: OK. This lady gives a clear history of progressive, painful, bilateral small joint swelling and post-immobility stiffness. She has great difficulty finding comfortable shoes and describes the feeling of walking on pebbles. She is not aware of

any diabetes or sensory loss. What are your thoughts at this stage?

CANDIDATE: This appears to be an inflammatory arthropathy.

COMMENT: Candidates may be asked about the revised diagnostic criteria of the American College of Rheumatology (ACR)/European League against Rheumatism (EULAR).

This requires confirmed synovitis of one or more joints, with absence of alternative explanation for the synovitis, and achieving a score of 6 or greater out of 10 from domains including:
- Numbers and location of the involved joint(s).
- Serological abnormality.
- Elevated acute-phase response.
- Symptom duration.

These criteria replaced the previous set from 1987, which were felt to lack sensitivity in early disease. The advent of increasingly effective treatment paradigms, incorporating the use of conventional and biologic DMARDs, has made it possible to prevent destructive disease in patients who are identified early in the course of disease rather than after progression to irreversible radiographic changes.

EXAMINER: Yes. Her feet are making her life pretty miserable and she would like you, as an orthopaedic surgeon, to do something to make them better. Your examination finds marked active synovitis and plantar tenderness under the metatarsal heads as well as a minimally correctable hallux valgus. There is some hammering of the lesser toes with a cock-up deformity of the second toe. Sensation and perfusion appear good. What are you going to do?

CANDIDATE: First, I would want to know if she is known to a rheumatology service and has had any attempt at non-operative intervention.

EXAMINER: She has never seen a rheumatologist and has never sought help for her feet other than from you via her GP.

CANDIDATE: I would advise her that operations are helpful but that she should be formally assessed by a rheumatologist to confirm the diagnosis and achieve disease control using DMARDs. I would also advise review by the local podiatry and/or orthotics service as simple footwear modification may be all that is necessary to control her symptoms.

COMMENT: The key buzz phrase to mention (if appropriate) is that patients with rheumatoid arthritis require a (contemporary) multidisciplinary approach to their management. This may also include involvement of vascular surgeons, occupational therapists and physiotherapists.

EXAMINER: I think that is appropriate advice at this stage. However, she returns to you a year later. Her synovitis is controlled by biological agents, but she has not found insoles and modified shoes helpful. How would you manage her at this point?

CANDIDATE: I would suggest surgery in the form of forefoot reconstruction. This consists of excision of the lesser metatarsal heads, correction of lesser toe deformities and excision or fusion of the first metatarsophalangeal joint.

EXAMINER: Why?

CANDIDATE: This is a proven intervention with good results.

EXAMINER: How good?

CANDIDATE: More than 80% of patients report significant improvement.

EXAMINER: Would you fuse or excise the first metatarsophalangeal joint?

CANDIDATE: I would be guided by her age and functional demand in combination with the quality of the soft-tissue envelope of her foot. I would prefer to fuse the joint as I believe this aids maintenance of gait but, in a low-demand patient, excision is associated with reduced complications and more rapid rehabilitation [11].

EXAMINER: How would you secure the arthrodesis?

CANDIDATE: I would use an oblique compression screw augmented by a dorsal locking plate as biomechanical and clinical studies have shown this to be the most reliable method.

EXAMINER: Would you always excise the lesser metatarsal heads in a patient of this age who now appears to have their disease under control?

CANDIDATE: No. It would be appropriate to perform shortening osteotomies such as Weil osteotomies to preserve the metatarsal heads if they are not badly diseased.

EXAMINER: Surely that just prolongs the procedure and increases the risk of complication?

CANDIDATE: Yes, but it is very difficult to salvage a rheumatoid foot without metatarsal heads if the disease progresses in subsequent years.

EXAMINER: Tell me about the principles of surgery in rheumatoid arthritis.

CANDIDATE: Surgery is indicated when symptoms and/or deformity are uncontrolled or getting worse. The overall objective is to produce a stable, plantigrade foot. Arthrodesis is the favoured procedure, but the risk of complications as a result of osteopenia, reduced vascularity and immunosuppression are to be borne in mind.

EXAMINER: What steps can a surgeon take to minimize the risk of complications?

CANDIDATE: A drug history is vital, as patients may well be on medications such as antiplatelet therapy, steroids or immune-modifying drugs which may have to be stopped or modified perioperatively.

Biological agents should be stopped in the run up to surgery and not resumed until there is good evidence of postoperative healing. It should go without saying that meticulous handling of soft tissues is necessary. Incisions must be planned with care, both to maintain adequate skin bridges and to ensure satisfactory wound closure if significant deformities are being corrected.

EXAMINER: How long would you stop biological agents for?

CANDIDATE: Two weeks pre- and postoperatively [12,13].

EXAMINER: What about other disease-modifying anti-rheumatic drugs? Which other ones would you stop?

CANDIDATE: Studies have shown that there is generally no need to stop drugs such as methotrexate or leflunomide.

COMMENT: Perioperative management of RA medications [14]:
- Steroids: low dose (≤ 7.5 mg/day) or any dose if for < 3 weeks should be given as usual daily dose.
- Methotrexate: continue, as does not impair wound healing or increase perioperative infection risk.
- Other DMARDs: hold postoperatively until bowel and renal function are restored.
- TNF antagonists: stop one dose cycle preoperatively and restart when wound healed.

EXAMINER: I would like to backtrack a bit. Would you alter your management if she also had signs and symptoms of hindfoot arthritis?

CANDIDATE: Generally, I would plan to address the most symptomatic area first. However, a less symptomatic and fixed hindfoot deformity should be corrected before proceeding to the forefoot. Flexible hindfoot deformity could be left until more symptomatic.

EXAMINER: Which hindfoot joints are most commonly affected in rheumatoid arthritis?

CANDIDATE: The talo-navicular joint is most commonly affected, followed by the subtalar and calcaneocuboid joints.

EXAMINER: Can you outline the arguments for and against isolated talo-navicular fusion in RA?

CANDIDATE: Isolated talo-navicular fusion is a lesser procedure than triple fusion for both patient and surgeon and effectively eliminates hindfoot motion. Historically, a non-union rate of up to 37% has been reported, although more recent studies suggest the non-union rate using contemporary fixation is much less. A triple arthrodesis is more reliable and allows greater deformity correction.

EXAMINER: Thank you.

Structured oral examination question 4

Cavus foot

EXAMINER: These are photographs of the left foot of a 20-year old man (Figure 5.4). Describe them.

CANDIDATE: These clinical photographs show the anterior, medial and posterior views of a left foot with a cavus deformity. The hindfoot is in varus and there is a high medial arch. There doesn't appear to be any significant clawing or abnormality of the toes. There is some shortening of the medial column of the foot and I can't see any obvious callosities beneath the metatarsal heads.

EXAMINER: What is the likely underlying cause?

CANDIDATE: The causes of a cavus foot may be broken down into congenital or acquired. The common causes of congenital deformities are idiopathic, a sequelae of clubfoot or due to arthrogryposis. The acquired deformities may be

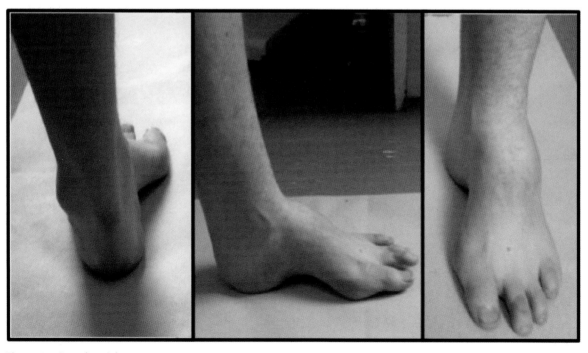

Figure 5.4 Cavus foot deformity.

due to trauma (compartment syndrome, crush injury) or neuromuscular conditions.

The neuromuscular causes may be grouped into central nervous system disease such as cerebral palsy or Friedrich's ataxia, spinal cord lesions such as spina bifida or spinal dysraphism, peripheral nervous system lesions such as an HSMN or muscular causes such as muscular dystrophy.

COMMENT: A cavus foot develops a high arch as the result of imbalance in the musculature of the foot. In the cavovarus foot the heel is in varus and the forefoot in equinus with pronation of the first and sometimes second ray.

It is important to distinguish between a cavovarus foot and a calcaneocavus foot. In the calcaneocavus foot the calf muscles are weak and the heel is in calcaneus and often valgus.

EXAMINER: HSMN?

CANDIDATE: Hereditary sensorimotor neuropathies. These are a group of inherited neurological conditions. Charcot–Marie–Tooth is the most common of these conditions.

EXAMINER: Can you go into more detail? How do these conditions lead to a cavus foot deformity?

CANDIDATE: The hereditary sensorimotor neuropathies are a group of related conditions that may lead to cavus foot deformity due to muscle imbalance. The conditions are diagnosed by the pattern of deformity and a positive family history. The most commonly recognized is Charcot–Marie–Tooth (CMT) disease, which affects approximately 1 in 2500 people. These patients commonly have weakness of the intrinsic muscles, tibialis anterior and peroneus brevis. Type I with an autosomal-dominant inheritance pattern tends to present in the second decade and patients have peroneal muscle weakness, abnormal (slow) nerve conduction studies, absent reflexes and hand involvement.

Type II presents in the third or fourth decade. Reflexes and nerve conduction are normal; however, the foot deformity may be more pronounced. Genetic analysis is able to diagnose and group these conditions more accurately and at least 17 types of CMT have been described.

EXAMINER: What causes the deformity in CMT?

CANDIDATE: In CMT the tibialis anterior and peroneus brevis muscles are weak and the strength of the antagonistic muscles tibialis posterior and peroneus longus causes the deformity. In detail, the peroneus longus contracts stronger than the weak tibialis anterior causing plantar flexion of the first ray. The posterior tibialis contracts harder than the weak peroneus brevis causing forefoot adduction. In addition, the long extensors to the toes are recruited to assist ankle dorsiflexion, causing claw toe deformities.

EXAMINER: What symptoms is this patient likely to complain about?

CANDIDATE: Common complaints include pain to the forefoot under the metatarsal heads, lateral aspect of the foot, instability of the ankle with a history of frequent ankle sprains and deformity of the foot with problems fitting footwear or alteration of gait.

EXAMINER: What are the main findings you would look for in the examination of a cavus foot?

CANDIDATE: On general inspection I would be looking to see if the deformity was bilateral and whether there were stigmata of a generalized condition such as intrinsic muscle wasting involving the hands.

With the patient standing I would look to see if the heel was in varus, neutral or valgus alignment, assess the height of the longitudinal arch by inspection and also look for any toe deformities. While the patient was standing I would also look at the spine for any stigmata of an underlying abnormality, such as a hairy patch or scoliosis.

With the patient sitting I would inspect the soles of the feet for callosities or areas of ulceration and look for any clawing of the toes.

I would undertake a neurological examination of the lower limbs to assess sensation, deep tendon reflexes and power of the major muscle groups, particularly the tibialis anterior (ankle dorsiflexion), tibialis posterior (inversion), peroneal longus (resisted plantar flexion) and peroneus brevis (eversion).

I would also like to see the patient walk to see if they had a broad-based ataxic gait (Friedrich's ataxia) or drop-foot gait.

EXAMINER: What is shown in these diagrams (Figure 5.5)?

CANDIDATE: These diagrams show the Coleman block test.

EXAMINER: And what is that?

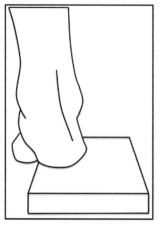 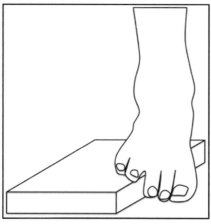

Figure 5.5 Coleman block test.

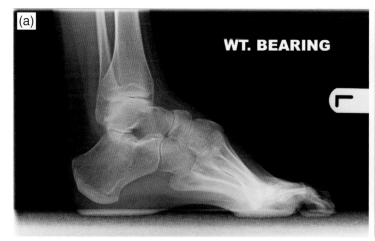 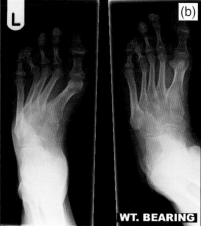

Figure 5.6a,b AP and lateral radiographs of a cavus foot.

CANDIDATE: The Coleman block test assesses flexibility of the hindfoot deformity by eliminating the deforming drive of the forefoot. In a cavus foot the first ray is plantar flexed so to place the foot on the ground the hindfoot has to move into varus. In the Coleman block test the foot is positioned so that the lateral border of the foot and the heel are placed on a block and the medial forefoot is allowed to hang off the edge of the block. If the heel assumes neutral to 5° valgus alignment when viewed from behind the hindfoot deformity is considered flexible and driven by the forefoot [15].

EXAMINER: What investigations would you use to evaluate this foot further?

CANDIDATE: In terms of evaluating the foot itself I would first obtain weight-bearing radiographs of the foot and ankle. An MRI scan of the spine is required if the patient has any signs or symptoms suggesting an underlying spinal cause.

EXAMINER: What information does the lateral X-ray provide?

CANDIDATE: The magnitude of the cavus deformity can be quantified using Meary's angle, the angle between the long axis of the talus and the first metatarsal shaft. Normally this lies between ±5°.

Hibb's angle is the angle between the long axis of the first metatarsal shaft and the long axis of the calcaneum. This angle is normally 150° but

105

decreases as the cavus worsens. The calcaneal pitch angle, the angle between the floor and the undersurface of the calcaneum, should be less than 30° but may be elevated in a cavus foot. The radiographs will also show any evidence of degenerative changes to the joints.

EXAMINER: What are the principles of managing this condition?

CANDIDATE: Firstly, it is important to identify and if necessary address the underlying cause of the cavus. The patient should be assessed for neuromuscular causes and referred for a neurological opinion if appropriate.

The patient's symptoms need to be understood as well as the likelihood of progression. Management can be non-operative with the use of orthotics to try and offload pressure areas, prevent rubbing of the toes and improve stability.

Surgical treatment needs to be tailored to the individual patient's underlying pathology, risk of progression, level of deformity and muscular imbalance. No single surgical procedure is appropriate for all patients, and frequently, multiple procedures are required. Correction of deformity without addressing muscular imbalance will not be successful.

Surgical procedures are broadly categorized into soft-tissue and bony procedures. Tendon transfers and osteotomies can provide correction of the deformity without the need for arthrodesis. Arthrodesis is usually required for severe arthritic joint disease or if complete muscle paralysis is present.

EXAMINER: Thank you.

Surgery

1. Soft-tissue releases

Plantar fascia release

In young children, surgical release of the plantar fascia and short toe flexors may be helpful. This is on the assumption that the deforming force of a contracted plantar fascia leads to a narrow arch base, plantar flexed first metatarsal and heel varus due to the windlass effect.

Gastrocnemius/Achilles lengthening

Occasionally required for contracture, but it is important to make sure a true equinus is present on standing lateral radiographs.

2. Tendon transfers

The most common tendon transfer in cavo varus foot is peroneus longus to brevis transfer to improve power of eversion. It helps stabilize the ankle.

3. Osteotomies

Patients with hindfoot involvement usually require a calcaneal osteotomy to correct the deformity. The osteotomy can include a closing wedge, a vertical displacement, or a combination (triplanar osteotomy).

4. Fusion

For a rigid painful foot in a young adult a triple arthrodesis can be used as a salvage stabilizing procedure that relieves pain but sacrifices joint motion.

Complications include development of ankle arthritis, pseudo-arthrosis, residue deformity, midfoot arthritis, overcorrection and AVN talus.

Structured oral examination question 5

Acquired adult flatfoot

EXAMINER: I would like you to look at this clinical photograph and tell me what you see (see Figure 5.7a).

CANDIDATE: This shows the posterior view of feet in a weight-bearing stance. There is marked heel valgus, loss of the medial longitudinal arch and too many toes are visible [16].

EXAMINER: What term is used to describe this situation?

CANDIDATE: Pes planus or flatfoot.

EXAMINER: Yes. In adults, what are the causes of this condition?

CANDIDATE: The commonest cause is tibialis posterior dysfunction.

Other causes include inflammatory arthritis, Charcot arthropathy, midfoot osteoarthritis and trauma (malunited calcaneum, missed Lisfranc injury, cuboid fracture).

EXAMINER: OK. How common is adult flatfoot?

CANDIDATE: It is commoner in females and the incidence increases with age.

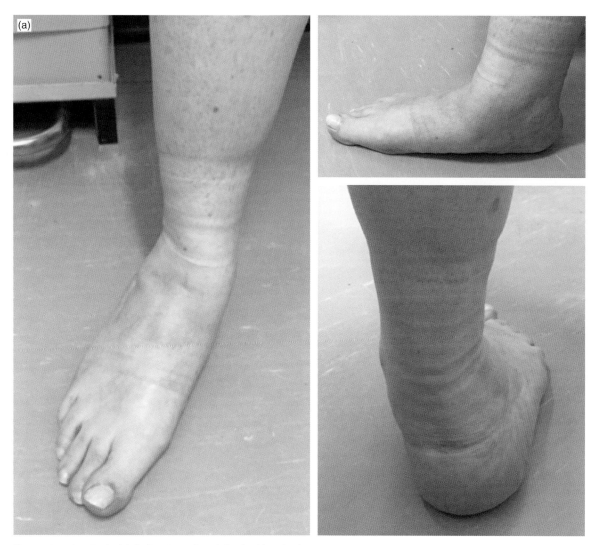

Figure 5.7a Acquired adult flatfoot. Loss of medial arch. Valgus heel, 'too many toes sign'.

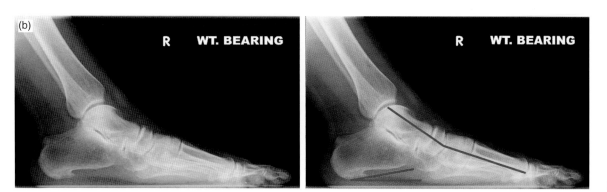

Figure 5.7b Midfoot sagittal radiographs. Meary's angle negative (> 10°). Reduced calcaneal pitch angle (10° approx., normal 20–30°).

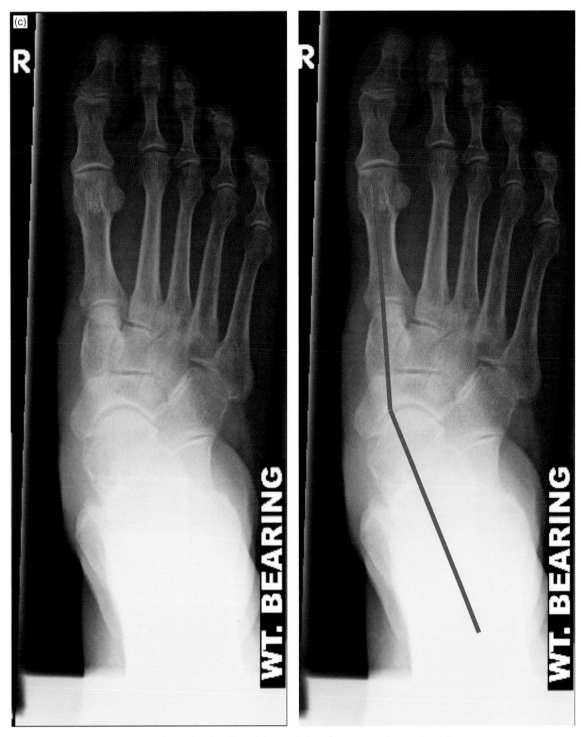

Figure 5.7c Anteroposterior (AP) radiographs of midfoot abduction. Talo to first metatarsal an angle > 10°.

EXAMINER: Okay. Let's stick with tibialis posterior dysfunction. Describe a typical patient.

CANDIDATE: The classic patient would be a female aged between 45 and 65 years with pain along the course of the tibialis posterior tendon exacerbated by activity. Standing on tip toe may be painful and difficult.

There is likely to be later development of increasing planovalgus deformity which may be associated with lateral impingement pain as the distal fibula contacts the calcaneum.

EXAMINER: What are the key examination points you would look for?

CANDIDATE: The most useful test is the ability to perform a single heel raise. I would also assess for hindfoot flexibility. These would guide classification and treatment.

EXAMINER: What are the origins and insertions of the tibialis posterior tendon?

CANDIDATE: It arises from the posterior tibia, interosseous membrane and the fibula in the proximal third of the leg and runs in the deep posterior compartment of the leg. The tendon then passes in a groove directly behind the medial malleolus, where it is tightly bound by the flexor retinaculum.

The main insertion is onto the navicular tuberosity but equally importantly it also fans out under the plantar aspect of the foot with extensive insertions to the second through fourth metatarsals, all three cuneiforms, the sustentaculum tali and the cuboid.

EXAMINER: How do you assess the strength of the tibialis posterior tendon?

CANDIDATE: The strength of the tendon is evaluated by asking the patient to attempt to invert the foot from a plantar flexed and everted position. This position isolates the posterior tibial tendon, neutralizing synergistic inversion from the anterior tibialis muscle.

EXAMINER: How does tibialis posterior dysfunction cause a flat foot?

CANDIDATE: The function of the posterior tibial tendon is threefold: it acts as an invertor of the subtalar joint, plantar-flexor of the ankle and an adductor of the forefoot. The combination of these actions serves to elevate the medial arch.

The inversion pull of tibialis posterior on the subtalar joint locks the transverse tarsal joint, providing a rigid lever arm with which to push off following the heel-raise phase of gait. With a diseased or poorly functioning tibialis posterior tendon, the unopposed action of the peroneus brevis pulls the forefoot into abduction and the subtalar joint into valgus. It is inactive during the swing phase. After heel contact the tibialis posterior contracts eccentrically to prevent excess hindfoot eversion.

The Achilles tendon is a powerful secondary inverter of the heel. It relies on the initial inversion power of the tibialis posterior to shift its mechanical axis more medially, thereby exerting a further inversion force.

As the function of the tibialis posterior fails, the Achilles tendon remains close to the subtalar axis, thereby reducing its function as both an inverter and a stabilizer of the subtalar joint. As the imbalance between lateral and medial soft tissues progresses, the hindfoot valgus and forefoot abduction increase. The static stabilizers on the medial side, in particular the spring ligament and the deltoid ligament, attenuate further.

EXAMINER: As you have mentioned classification of tibialis posterior dysfunction, could you tell me any more about this?

CANDIDATE: Yes. Johnson and Strom proposed a three-stage classification in 1989. Myerson later added a fourth stage [17].

In stage 1 disease, there is no deformity but pain from the tendon. A single heel raise is usually possible but painful. The tendon is inflamed, tender and swollen.

In stage 2 disease, there is a flexible planovalgus deformity and weakness of single heel raise. The tendon degenerates and lengthens with the foot changing shape going into valgus.

In stage 3 disease, the valgus hindfoot deformity has become fixed and reconstruction is not possible.

With stage 4, there is additional tilting of the talus in the ankle mortise leading to significant ankle arthritis secondary to valgus strain.

EXAMINER: OK. How would you investigate this patient?

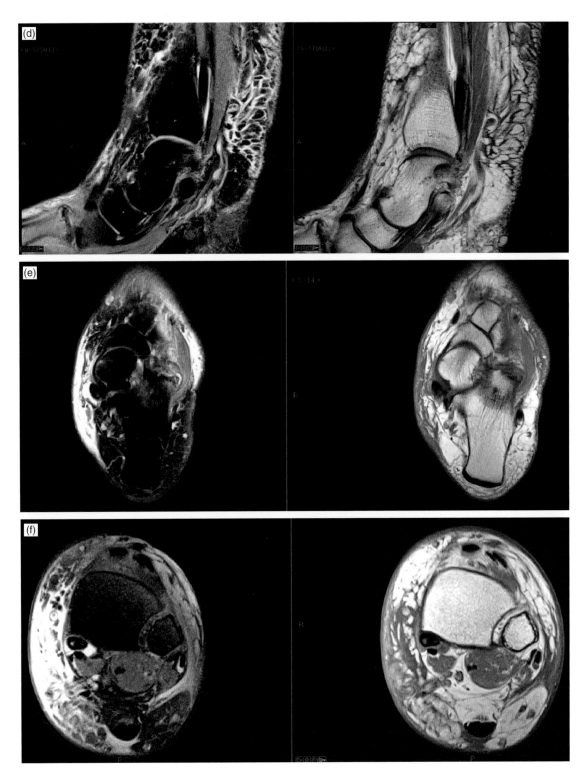

Figure 5.7d–f MRI tibialis posterior tendinopathy with fluid around tendon. Some increased signal within the tendon substance.

CANDIDATE: Weight-bearing AP and lateral radiographs of both the foot and ankle would help to assess structural change and exclude other causes of flatfoot. They could also show associated degenerate change. The arch index could also be measured.

EXAMINER: Would the arch index influence your management?

CANDIDATE: No. It is mainly used as a research tool.

EXAMINER: Is there a place for MRI?

CANDIDATE: MRI is not routinely needed for the diagnosis of flat feet. It is useful in detecting early changes within the tendon if there is any diagnostic doubt.

MRI is valuable if surgical management is being planned. It is also useful for assessing the medial structures such as the deltoid and spring ligaments and also the peroneal tendon [18].

Figure 5.7d–f. MRI tibialis posterior tendinopathy with fluid around tendon. Some increased signal within the tendon substance.

EXAMINER: Tell me what the treatment options are.

CANDIDATE: For stage 1, I would offer debridement of the tendon followed by 6–8 weeks of casting or splintage, then provision of a definitive arch support orthosis [19]. For stage 2 disease I would offer either a lateral column lengthening or a medializing calcaneal osteotomy in conjunction with a FDL transfer to augment or replace the tibialis posterior [20]. The Achilles tendon occasionally needs to be percutaneously released if it is tightened and is preventing full correction.

In stage 3 disease, triple arthrodesis is recommended [21].

For stage 4 disease, the treatment depends upon the flexibility of the ankle deformity. If it is flexible, a triple arthrodesis combined with ankle bracing or deltoid ligament reconstruction may be adequate, otherwise a triple arthrodesis combined or followed by ankle arthrodesis would be indicated.

EXAMINER: You seem very clear about surgical options. What about non-operative treatment?

CANDIDATE: I should have mentioned that. It is appropriate to offer analgesia and orthotic treatment to most patients initially. An orthotic providing medial arch support with a heel cup to control heel valgus would be appropriate. There are two aims of orthotic treatment. First, this may offer adequate symptom relief. Second, it may control progressive heel valgus and flattening of the medial arch.

COMMENT: It's not great viva tactics to jump straight in to discussing surgical options for a condition unless it is very clear that's what the examiners want to discuss.

EXAMINER: You spoke about an FDL transfer. Tell me about this procedure.

CANDIDATE: After obtaining informed consent I would make an incision in the line of the posterior tibial tendon, starting posterior to the medial malleolus. I would debride or resect the tendon according to the clinical appearances. The flexor digitorum longus sheath lies directly posterior to the tibialis posterior tendon and would be opened longitudinally as far distally as possible before the FDL tendon is divided. The free FDL tendon is then passed through a tunnel drilled in the navicular and sutured back to itself under tension.

EXAMINER: In what direction would you pass FDL through the navicular?

CANDIDATE: From plantar to dorsal.

EXAMINER: What is the aim of a medializing calcaneal osteotomy?

CANDIDATE: The calcaneal osteotomy directly reduces the heel valgus and brings the weight-bearing axis closer to the long axis of the leg. In addition, it displaces the Achilles tendon insertion medially to prevent it acting as an everter of the hindfoot.

EXAMINER: When obtaining consent, what would you advise about flexion of the toes after harvesting the flexor digitorum longus?

CANDIDATE: I would expect flexion of the lesser toes to be maintained by the flexor hallucis longus via the knot of Henry.

EXAMINER: Can you tell me a little more about the knot of Henry?

CANDIDATE: The flexor digitorum longus crosses the flexor hallucis longus at the knot of Henry. There are a number of fibrous interconnections between the two tendons that afford a degree of cooperation in movement. This means that flexion of the digits can continue after harvest of either FDL or FHL.

EXAMINER: What would you tell the patient about the success rate of the operation?

CANDIDATE: Chadwick *et al.* [22] reported that FDL transfer with medializing calcaneum osteotomy provided long-term pain relief and improved function in 85% of patients after a mean follow-up of 15.2 years. Substantial improvements were noted in the American Orthopaedic Foot & Ankle Society (AOFAS), visual analogue scale (VAS), and SF-36 scores.

COMMENT: This is scoring a 7. Appropriate up-to-date knowledge of the literature to justify a management decision.

EXAMINER: Is there a place for any additional procedures such as first ray fusions or lateral column lengthening?

CANDIDATE: One concern with stage 2 adult-acquired flatfoot deformity is that there is a large variability in disease severity within the classification group including hindfoot valgus, medial column stability, forefoot abduction and supination. The treatment remains controversial with numerous soft-tissue and bony procedures being described. How extensive a procedure is required remains unknown.

EXAMINER: What approach would you use for a triple arthrodesis to correct significant, fixed valgus heel deformity?

CANDIDATE: This is a potentially difficult situation. The joint preparation is straightforward if a lateral utility approach or similar is combined with a dorsal incision over the talonavicular joint. If a significant deformity is being addressed there can be difficulty in closing the lateral incision once the deformity is corrected. There are advocates of triple arthrodesis via a single medial approach, but this is difficult and not always possible.

EXAMINER: One final question. Any new developments?

CANDIDATE: PRP injections have recently been used in the early stages of posterior tendon dysfunction. We are awaiting randomized controlled data.

EXAMINER: Thank you.

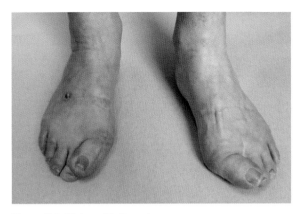

Figure 5.8 AP view of hallux valgus.

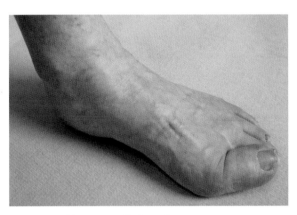

Figure 5.9 Oblique view of hallux valgus.

Structured oral examination question 6

Hallux valgus

EXAMINER: Please have a look at these clinical photographs and tell me what you see (see Figures 5.8 and 5.9).

CANDIDATE: These show a frontal view of a pair of feet and an oblique view of the left foot. There are bilateral hallux valgus deformities with the hallux over-riding the right second toe. I can only count three lesser toes for the left foot and there is a scar in the web space lateral to the hallux and a medial longitudinal scar over the metatarsophalangeal joint. The toenails appear friable and there is some excoriation around the lesser toes of the right foot.

EXAMINER: OK. This 65-year-old lady had her left second toe removed some years ago for a presentation similar to that which she now has on the right. Her left-sided symptoms have also recurred. How would you assess her further?

CANDIDATE: I would obtain a detailed history, looking to clarify the main source of her symptoms. Can I ask what symptoms she has?

EXAMINER: What do you think they are likely to be?

CANDIDATE: I would expect she has pain from her bunions and toes caused by rubbing on footwear and each other. I would also anticipate she has symptoms due to degenerative change involving the great toe MTP joint or metatarsalgia of the lesser rays.

EXAMINER: Let's say she has all these symptoms to varying degrees. Tell me about your further assessment.

CANDIDATE: I would complete the history, including questioning about relevant conditions such as diabetes, inflammatory arthritis, vascular disease and neuropathy, and proceed to examination.

I would assess her gait and the posture of the weighted foot as hallux valgus is often associated with a planus foot. I would palpate for areas of tenderness, paying particular attention to the hallux MTP joint and lesser metatarsal heads. I would assess the range of movement of the involved joints and look for gastrocnemius tightness. Finally, I would also undertake a grind test to assess pain from loading the MTP joint. Neurovascular status will also be assessed.

EXAMINER: You spoke about assessing the range of movement of the involved joints. Can you be more specific?

CANDIDATE: I would want to assess the range of plantar and dorsiflexion of the hallux MTP joint. It is also important to assess the movement at the first tarso-metatarsal joint as excessive mobility will influence the surgical choice.

EXAMINER: Okay, we might come back to that. Outline the value of plain radiographs in the management of hallux valgus.

CANDIDATE: I would obtain weight-bearing AP and lateral radiographs of the foot. These would allow me to objectively measure various angles,

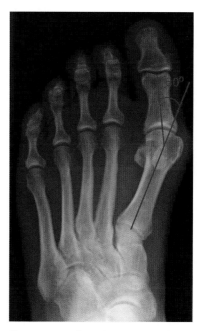

Figure 5.10 Hallux valgus angle (HVA). Angle between long axis of first metatarsal shaft and long axis of first proximal phalanx. Normal < 15°. Mild 15–20°. Moderate 20–40°. Severe > 40°.

assess uncovering of the sesamoids and look for evidence of arthritic change.

EXAMINER: Why weight-bearing?

CANDIDATE: Non-weight-bearing views tend to underestimate the severity of hallux valgus, and may give misleading information about alignment and relative metatarsal length.

EXAMINER: Keep going. What angles?

CANDIDATE: I would measure the intermetatarsal, hallux valgus and the distal metatarsal articular angles.

EXAMINER: What is the normal range of these angles and how would these influence your management? Can you demonstrate these angles on the radiographs (Figures 5.10–5.13)?

CANDIDATE: The intermetatarsal angle is normally less than 9°, the hallux valgus angle should be less than 15° and the distal metatarsal articular angle is normally a maximum of 15°. The degree of deformity helps determine the surgical options.

EXAMINER: What about these radiographs?

113

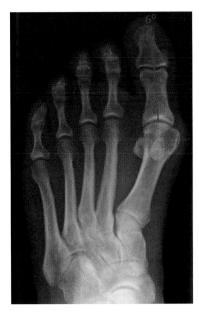

Figure 5.11 Hallux valgus interphalangeus angle (HVI). Angle between long axis of first distal phalanx and long axis of first proximal phalanx. Associated with congruent hallux valgus. Normal < 10°.

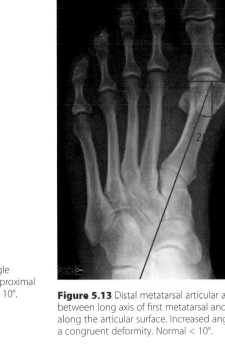

Figure 5.13 Distal metatarsal articular angle (DMAA). Angle between long axis of first metatarsal and perpendicular to a line along the articular surface. Increased angle associated with a congruent deformity. Normal < 10°.

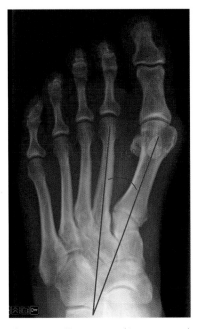

Figure 5.12 First to second intermetatarsal angle (IMA). Angle between long axis of first and second metatarsal shaft. Normal < 9°. Mild < 11°. Moderate 12–15°. Severe > 15°.

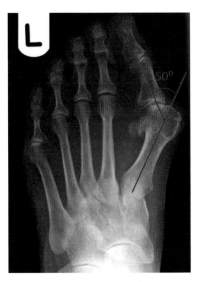

Figure 5.14 Hallux valgus angle (HVA) (pronation of toe). Normal < 15°.

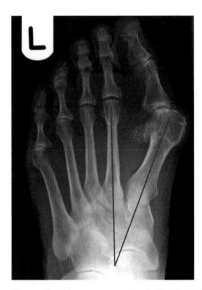

Figure 5.15 Intermetatarsal angle (IMA) 22°. Normal < 9°.

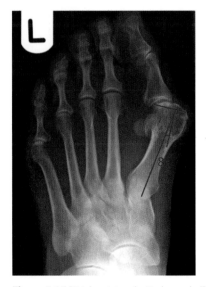

Figure 5.16 Distal metatarsal articular angle (DMAA). Normal < 10°.

CANDIDATE: These demonstrate severe hallux valgus with an HVA 50°, IMA 22° and DMAA 8° (Figures 5.14–5.16).

EXAMINER: If this lady had an intermetatarsal angle of 15° on the right with a hallux valgus angle of 35° and minimal passive correction of the hallux, what surgery would you plan?

CANDIDATE: If the first tarso-metatarsal joint is not lax, I would plan a scarf osteotomy combined with a lateral release and an Akin osteotomy of the proximal phalanx if necessary.

EXAMINER: Why would you choose a scarf osteotomy?

CANDIDATE: It is a very versatile procedure with stable fixation allowing early postoperative mobilization without a cast. It maintains the length of the metatarsal and facilitates translation, angulation and depression of the metatarsal head as necessary. It can also be used to shorten or lengthen the metatarsal [23].

EXAMINER: How would you secure the osteotomy?

CANDIDATE: With two headless compression screws.

EXAMINER: Why not use a simpler procedure such as a chevron or Mitchell osteotomy?

CANDIDATE: For the degree of deformity described, combined with the lack of passive correction of the hallux, I believe the correction that could be achieved with a distal osteotomy would be inadequate. A further disadvantage of a Mitchell osteotomy is that it produces shortening of the first metatarsal, which could lead to transfer metatarsalgia.

EXAMINER: Can you draw a scarf osteotomy?

CANDIDATE: No, sorry.

EXAMINER: For your proposed management, what complications would you discuss when seeking consent?

CANDIDATE: Firstly, I would advise that while early weight-bearing is possible with a scarf osteotomy, it takes up to a year for the foot to fully settle after such surgery, but that typically 85% of patients are pleased with the outcome. I would advise a 1% risk of deep infection and a slightly higher risk of superficial infection. Recurrence is possible with time, although the risk of this is greatest in adolescent cases. A minority of patients will have significant stiffness of the MTP joint afterwards and there can be sensory loss if the dorsomedial sensory nerve is injured. I would mention the possibility of hallux varus as a complication as this is difficult to

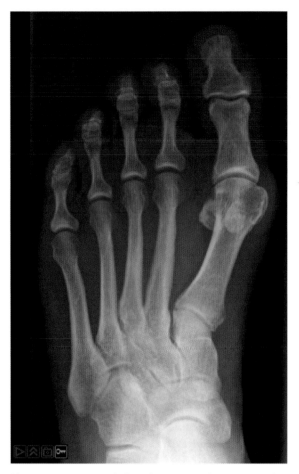

Figure 5.17 Congruent hallux valgus. Increased HVA, increased DMAA and congruent joint.

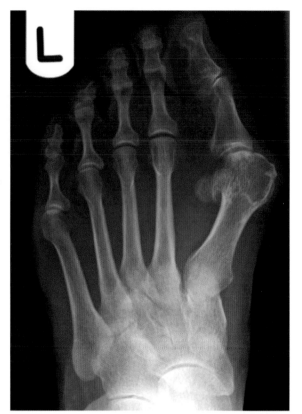

Figure 5.18 Incongruent hallux valgus. Increased HVA, normal DMAA and incongruent joint.

treat. I would also mention the possibility of intraoperative and postoperative metatarsal fracture.

EXAMINER: How would you treat hallux varus?

CANDIDATE: A subtle varus may improve as the patient returns to normal foot wear. While soft-tissue procedures such as abductor hallucis and medial capsular release or transfer or a slip of EHL are described for flexible deformity, arthrodesis of the first MTP joint arthrodesis is a reliable option in the presence of significant stiffness or arthrosis.

EXAMINER: So, you have successfully treated this lady's right foot and she is pleased with the result. Would you go ahead and do the same on the left?

CANDIDATE: No. The absence of the second toe predisposes to recurrence and I would propose arthrodesis of the hallux MTP joint.

EXAMINER: One final question. What do we mean by a congruent versus incongruent hallux valgus (see Figures 5.17 and 5.18)?

CANDIDATE: If there is no lateral subluxation then the joint is congruent.

COMMENT: A congruent first MTP joint is present when alignment of the articular joint surfaces of the metatarsal head and proximal phalanx base occurs in a slight valgus position. An incongruent joint exists when the toe is in a valgus orientation and the articular surfaces do not align properly or concentrically.

EXAMINER: Thank you.

Structured oral examination question 7

Hallux rigidus

EXAMINER: This 45-year-old male patient has presented with pain and stiffness of his right big toe. Describe the X-ray findings (see Figure 5.19).

CANDIDATE: This is a radiograph of a right foot showing loss of joint space, osteophyte formation and sclerosis of the first metatarso-phalangeal joint in keeping with osteoarthritis. There is also a mild hallux valgus deformity.

EXAMINER: So, what is this commonly called in orthopaedics?

CANDIDATE: Hallux rigidus.

EXAMINER: Tell me the range of movement of a healthy first MTP joint.

CANDIDATE: The joint should be able to dorsiflex between 70 and 90° and plantarflex between 24 and 40°.

EXAMINER: How would you manage this patient?

CANDIDATE: First of all, I would take a full history and examine the foot. I would also obtain a weight-bearing lateral and an oblique X-ray of the foot in addition to the AP view we have here.

EXAMINER: OK. If we concentrate on the clinical examination, what specific findings are you looking for to help with your management decision?

CANDIDATE: I would need to assess the integrity of the skin and the neurovascular status of the foot. I would then palpate for osteophytes and assess the range of movement of the first MTPJ and look to see whether the patient has pain limited to the extremes of movement or throughout the arc of motion. Often the first MTPJ is enlarged, erythematous and swollen. There may be medial-sided numbness present if the medial dorsal cutaneous nerve is compressed by an osteophyte. A grind test of the joint would be informative [24]. This test is usually done with the MTPJ in relative neutral dorsiflexion and can be a pointer to articular cartilage involvement [25]. I also need to evaluate the range of motion and look for any sign of degenerative change at the interphalangeal joint (IPJ).

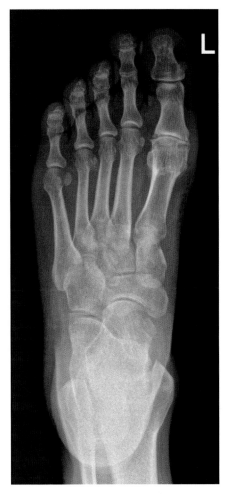

Figure 5.19 X-ray showing hallux rigidus.

EXAMINER: What is the importance of the IPJ?

CANDIDATE: Fusion of the first MTPJ may accelerate degeneration in the surrounding joints so if the IPJ is already symptomatic a motion-preserving procedure at the MTPJ may be more appropriate.

EXAMINER: Are you aware of any grading systems for this condition?

CANDIDATE: The most widely used is a radiographic grading by Hattrup and Johnson in which Grade 1 is a well-preserved joint space with mild to moderate osteophytes, Grade 2 has a reduced joint space with moderate osteophytes and Grade 3 is complete loss of joint space, marked osteophytes and there may be subchondral cysts within the metatarsal head [26].

EXAMINER: Right, so talk me through the management options for a patient with hallux rigidus.

CANDIDATE: In the first instance I would advise non-operative treatment. The options include activity modification, NSAIDS, footwear modification or an intra-articular steroid injection.

EXAMINER: And the operative options?

CANDIDATE: The operative options include cheilectomy with or without a dorsal closing wedge osteotomy of the phalanx (Moberg), fusion and arthroplasty. The choice depends on the grade of the arthritis, patient symptoms and expectations.

EXAMINER: So then, back to the operative options for treatment.

CANDIDATE: In Grade 1 or 2 disease, a cheilectomy, in which the osteophytes and the dorsal 25–30% of the articular surface are resected. No more than one-third of the dorsal metatarsal head articular surface should be excised otherwise there is the risk of dorsal subluxation or overload on the remaining articular surface.

Satisfaction rates of 90% have been reported, with improvement in dorsiflexion from 20 to 40°.

For Grade 2 or 3 disease in patients who are young and still highly active I would combine a cheilectomy with a Moberg dorsal closing wedge osteotomy of the proximal phalanx. This shifts the arc of movement further into the dorsiflexion range, reducing symptoms.

For patients with severe disease and no ligamentous instability total joint replacement is an option, but early loosening has been a problem. Good results have been reported with hemiarthroplasty of either the metatarsal head or the base of the proximal phalanx, but few large series exist and neither is commonly used in the United Kingdom [28,29].

Arthrodesis of the first MTPJ is still the mainstay of treatment for severe disease and joint preparation with dome-shaped reamers and a lag screw and dorsal plate construct is the most biomechanically sound fixation [30].

Keller's arthroplasty is an option in elderly, low-demand patients; however, cock-up deformities and transfer metatarsalgia may develop.

EXAMINER: So, back to arthrodesis. What is the optimal position for fusion?

CANDIDATE: Dorsiflexion of 25° across the MTPJ, valgus of 10–15° and neutral rotation to ensure an effective plane of motion of the IPJ.

EXAMINER: How will you consent a patient for arthrodesis of the first MTPJ?

CANDIDATE: I will explain that the aim of surgery is to relieve pain and optimize mobility. The risks and complications include wound healing problems, infection, damage to the medial cutaneous nerve, delayed union, malunion, non-union, metalwork irritation and accelerated degeneration in surrounding joints.

EXAMINER: If we return to the patient we started discussing. He is a 45-year-old male who is a keen walker. He has significant stiffness and pain on mobilization and dorsiflexion, but a grind test is negative. He has exhausted non-operative measures. What treatment will you offer him?

CANDIDATE: I would offer him a cheilectomy with a proximal phalanx osteotomy as this has the added benefit of improving range of movement over a cheilectomy on its own, although he will be made aware that the risks of this procedure are greater than a cheilectomy.

I would also discuss fusion with him and explain that this may become necessary if a cheilectomy failed to provide sufficient relief or he had later progression of disease.

EXAMINER: He is not keen on the joint being stiffened up and has read on the internet about joint replacements and is keen for this.

CANDIDATE: I would inform him that for his age group there would be a significant risk of loosening of the prosthesis resulting in failure, thus the need for revision surgery. A recent systematic review of the literature by Stevens *et al.* indicated that arthrodesis is superior for improving clinical outcome and reducing pain with fewer complications and revisions compared to total joint replacement.

They reported a 20.9% rate of prosthesis loosening causing instability and pain during gait and an 11% chance of revision surgery being required.

EXAMINER: He is still not convinced.

CANDIDATE: I would refer him to a colleague for a second opinion.
[Bell]

COMMENT: For the FRCS (Tr & Orth) exam joint replacement is very controversial.

References

1. Kibler WB. Arthroscopic findings in ankle ligament reconstruction. *Clin Sports Med*. 1996;15 (4):799–804.

2. Saltzman CL, Salamon ML, Blanchard GM, *et al*. Epidemiology of ankle arthritis: report of a consecutive series of 639 patients from a tertiary orthopaedic center. *Iowa Orthop J*. 2005;25:44–46.

3. Kellgren JH, Lawrence JS. Radiological assessment of osteoarthrosis. *Ann Rheum Dis*. 1957;16:494–501.

4. Repetto I, Biti B, Cerruti P, Trentini R, Felli L. Conservative treatment of ankle osteoarthritis: can platelet-rich plasma effectively postpone surgery? *J Foot Ankle Surg*. 2017;56(2):362–365.

5. van Valberg AA, van Roermund PM, Marijnissen AC, *et al*. Joint distraction in treatment of osteoarthritis: a two-year follow-up of the ankle. *Osteoarthritis Cartilage*. 1999;7:474–479.

6. Nguyen MP, Pedersen DR, Gao Y, Saltzman CL, Amendola A. Intermediate-term follow-up after ankle distraction for treatment of end-stage osteoarthritis. *J Bone Joint Surg Am*. 2015;97 (7):590–596.

7. Wood PLR, Prem H, Sutton C. Total ankle replacement: medium term results in 200 Scandinavian total ankle replacements. *J Bone Joint Surg Br*. 2008;90B (5):605–609.

8. Bonnin M, Gaudot F, Laurent J-R, *et al*. The Salto total ankle arthroplasty: survivorship and analysis of failures at 7 to 11 years. *Clin Orthop Relat Res*. 2011;469:225–236.

9. Mann JA, Mann RA, Horton E. STAR ankle: long-term results. *Foot Ankle Int*. 2011;32(5):473–484.

10. Labek G, Klaus H, Schlichtherle R, *et al*. Revision rates after total ankle arthroplasty in sample-based clinical studies and national registries. *Foot Ankle Int*. 2011;32 (8):740–745.

11. Rosenbaum D, Timta B, Schmiegel A, *et al*. First ray resection arthroplasty versus arthrodesis in the treatment of the rheumatoid foot. *Foot Ankle Int*. 2011;32(6):589–594.

12. Lee MA, Mason LW, Dodds AL. The perioperative use of disease-modifying and biologic therapies in patients with rheumatoid arthritis undergoing elective orthopedic surgery. *Orthopedics*. 2010;33 (4):257–262.

13. Howe CR, Gardner GC, Kadel NJ. Perioperative medication management for the patient with rheumatoid arthritis. *J Am Acad Orthop Surg*. 2006;14:544–551.

14. Scanzello CR, Figgie MP, Nestor BJ, Goodman SM. Perioperative management of medications used in the treatment of rheumatoid arthritis. *HSS J*. 2006;2 (2):141–147.

15. Coleman S, Chestnut W. A simple test for hindfoot flexibility in the cavovarus foot. *Clin Orthop Relat Res*. 1977;123:60–62.

16. A 'too many toes sign' will be present where more than one to two toes are seen along the lateral aspect of the affected foot.

17. Myerson MS, Corrigan J. Treatment of posterior tibial tendon dysfunction with flexor digitorum longus tendon transfer and calcaneal osteotomy. *Orthopedics*. 1996;19:383–388.

18. Abousayed MM, Alley MC, Shakked R, Rosenbaum AJ. Adult-acquired flatfoot deformity: etiology, diagnosis, and management. *JBJS Rev*. 2017;5(8):e7.

19. Teasdall RD, Johnson KA. Surgical treatment of stage I posterior tibial tendon dysfunction. *Foot Ankle Int*. 1994;15(12):646–648.

20. Myerson MS, Badekas A, Schon LC. Treatment of stage II posterior tibial tendon deficiency with flexor digitorum longus tendon transfer and calcaneal osteotomy. *Foot Ankle Int*. 2004;25 (7):445–450.

21. Kelly IP, Easley ME. Treatment of stage 3 adult acquired flatfoot. *Foot Ankle Clin*. 2001;6: 153–166.

22. Chadwick C, Whitehouse SL, Saxby TS. Long-term follow-up of flexor digitorum longus transfer and calcaneal osteotomy for stage II posterior tibial tendon dysfunction. *Bone Joint J*. 2015;97 (3):346–352.

23. Barouk LS, Toullec ET. Use of scarf osteotomy of the first metatarsal to correct hallux valgus deformity. *Tech Foot Ankle Surg*. 2003;2(1):27–34.

24. This is done by rotating and axially loading the hallux MTPJ with the toe in relative neutral dorsiflexion and can be a pointer to articular cartilage involvement.

25. Patients who experience grind test pain with the MTPJ in neutral or plantar flexion often have more extensive disease than realized.

26. Hattrup SJ, Johnson KA. Subjective results of hallux rigidus following treatment with cheilectomy. *Clin Orthop Relat Res*. 1988;226:182–191.

27. Moberg E. A simple operation for hallux rigidus. *Clin Orthop Relat Res*. 1979;142:55–56.

28. Taranow WS, Moutsatson MJ, Cooper JM. Contemporary approaches to Stage II and Stage III hallux rigidus: the role of metallic hemiarthroplasty of the proximal phalanx. *Foot Ankle Clin N Am.* 2005;10:713–728.

29. Carpenter B, Smith J, Motley T, *et al.* Surgical treatment of hallux rigidus using a metatarsal head resurfacing implant: mid-term follow-up. *J Foot Ankle Surg.* 2010;49:321–325.

30. Politi J, Hayes J, Njus G, *et al.* First metatarsal–phalangeal joint arthrodesis: a biomechanical assessment of stability. *Foot Ankle Int.* 2003;24(4): 332–337.

Spine

Prasad Karpe

Introduction

Spine questions can feature at any station for viva. They are frequently asked in adult pathology, but can pop up in basic science (structure of intervertebral disc), trauma (thoracolumbar fractures and their management) or paediatrics (adolescent scoliosis).

For many candidates learning spine for the exam is a daunting task. But with smart preparation, these questions are actually gifts. There is a set methodology to answer them. Also, spine is like maths – neurology and level of pathology should add up. Besides, indications for surgery are specific and usually encompass neurology or instability.

Each question is to be answered in 5 minutes. This is not a lot of time. This needs a lot of planning and practice. It is not only the knowledge you know, but also a smart and tactful way of getting it across in a timely manner.

By this time, you will be well aware of the marking process: minimum 6 pass for each question. But being humans, due to occasional anxiety or bad luck, there will be some setbacks (marking 5). So, plan for 7 or 8 at most stations. Try to stay calm and be positive. And no matter how bad the previous question was, forget it and recompose for the next question. Candidates who failed the exam are usually surprised as to how agonisingly close they were to passing and wished they had got the bad table out of their mind.

The usual format for a viva would be that a candidate would be shown a radiological picture (X-ray/CT/MRI) or a clinical picture and asked to describe it. This is followed by questions taking you to management. In other words, the sequence will be description of the picture or X-ray, followed by history, examination, investigations and treatment.

Describing an X-ray

Describe what X-ray it is first

PA and lateral standing X-ray of lumbar/thoracic/cervical/full spine showing . . .

Mention immature skeleton if you see a physis.

Lateral X-ray

1. Normal curves – cervical and lumbar lordosis, thoracic kyphosis.
2. Abnormal curves – exaggerated thoracic kyphosis, loss of lumbar/cervical lordosis, cervical kyphosis.
3. Disc height maintained or lost at any level. Fuzzy end plates could be a sign of discitis.
4. Facet arthritis.
5. Primary canal stenosis as evident by short pedicles.
6. Fracture – compression, burst, stable or unstable fracture.
7. Sagittal balance of full spine weight-bearing lateral – normal, positive or negative.
8. Listhesis – is it isthmic (if lysis of pedicles seen) or degenerative (facet arthropathy)?
   - Meyerding grading.
   - Pelvic tilt, sacral slope and pelvic incidence.

AP view

1. Cancer – winking owl sign – destruction of pedicle due to cancer.
2. Degenerative – facet arthritis or scoliosis (curve can be in either direction).
3. Idiopathic scoliosis – usually right convex in the thoracic spine (away from the heart).
4. Prolapsed disc – list away from nerve compression.
5. Evaluate pedicles always on AP view. Absent pedicle may be seen in metastases, aneurysmal bone cyst, osteoblastoma, trauma or congenital absence of pedicle.

Detecting the correct level

1. Highest point on the iliac crest usually points to L4/5 on the lateral view.
2. Count from C2 downwards if you have a full spine X-ray.
3. The twelfth rib can be helpful.

If confusion still exists between sacralization of L5 and lumbarization of S1, then it would be safe to comment on pathology based on the *last mobile level*. This is the level that has no bony connection to the pelvis, such as the large transverse process articulating with the ilium. This is usually the level where disc degeneration occurs.

History and examination

Unlike clinical cases, the advantage in a viva is that you won't be utilizing precious time in waiting for answers from a patient. By the time you have described the radiograph, you know what the clinical scenario is and so a focused history is not a difficult task.

Every clinical scenario has some important questions that need to be asked. Examples include:

- Sciatica – it is necessary to know the exact location of the leg pain (dermatome) as this will clinch the nerve root on the history alone.
- Night pain – cancer in elderly.
- Back pain worse than leg pain or significant back pain could mean instability.
- An immunocompromised patient such as IVDU or a diabetic gives a clue of infection.

Please read the spine clinical cases chapter in the Postgraduate Orthopaedics book for the relevant questions in history-taking and examination.

As for clinical examination, always divide into general and local/spine examination. So, points like EWS in sepsis or chest expansion in ankylosing spondylitis in the general examination will not be missed.

Specific points of importance in the clinical examination are:

1. PR and perianal sensations in cauda equina.
2. Reflexes is a must – this helps to decide if the lesion is in the brain or the cervical cord (brisk in all four limbs) or thoracic spine (brisk only in lower limbs). It differentiates upper motor neuron lesion from a lower motor neuron.
3. Pulsations in feet to differentiate vascular pathology.
4. Location of tenderness – lumbar facet, sacroiliac joint, hip (groin).

Relevant investigations and management are discussed in each scenario.

Contents

1. Infection.
2. Spine metastases.
3. Benign tumour.
4. Cervical spondylotic myelopathy.
5. Lumbar prolapse disc with cauda equina.
6. Spondylolisthesis.
7. Ankylosing spondylitis.
8. Idiopathic scoliosis.
9. Non-idiopathic scoliosis.
10. Cervical disc prolapse.

Structured oral examination question 1

Infection (discitis)

EXAMINER: You are on call and you are asked to see a 45-year-old diabetic patient on the medical wards with back pain. The medics are concerned as she has raised blood markers and they can't find any septic focus from their end.

CANDIDATE: Diabetic patients are immunocompromised and are prone for sepsis. I would like to take a detailed history, first wanting to know details of her back pain.

1. What is the onset, duration and progress of her back pain? Any trauma?
2. What's the exact location? Cervical/thoracic/lumbar.
3. Is she able to mobilize? (Non-ambulatory usually suggests sinister pathology or advanced disease or instability.)

EXAMINER: What next?

CANDIDATE: I need to know more from her history.

1. Fever.
2. Neurology including bowel and bladder involvement.
3. Other joints if painful? Other red flags?
4. More details of her diabetes, is it Type 1 or 2, how well has it been controlled, is she diet-controlled/oral medications or insulin?

5. Any other septic focus including chest, urine, abdomen? Any other significant past history including medications?

EXAMINER: She is a Type 2 diabetic now poorly controlled, on insulin. The medics have ruled out all other septic focus. Nothing else significant on history and she is bedridden. She is struggling to sit or stand. No history of trauma.

CANDIDATE: I will then do a general and spine examination. What's her EWS?

EXAMINER: This patient has no fever but a low temperature of 35 degrees. She also appears to be confused. What are you concerned about?

CANDIDATE: Sepsis is my major concern in this patient. Sepsis is SIRS with documented infection. I need to rule out an orthopaedic cause, primarily discitis, as this patient is complaining of back pain.

EXAMINER: (interrupting): What is SIRS?

CANDIDATE: SIRS is systemic inflammatory response syndrome and characterized by two or more of the following:
- Fever (> 38°C) or hypothermia (< 36°C).
- Tachycardia (> 90).
- Tachypnea (> 20).
- WBC >12 or < 4.
- Altered mental state.
- Blood glucose > 6.6 in absence of diabetes.

This patient already has two criteria needed for SIRS, namely altered mental state and hypothermia. My concerns are that she may progress to septic shock.

EXAMINER: She also has low blood pressure and tachycardia.

CANDIDATE: I need to rule out the spine or any other joint as a septic focus. I will do a detailed spine examination looking for specific *point tenderness* and progress to neurological examination.

EXAMINER: She has significant tenderness in her lower lumbar spine. No sensory–motor deficit in any of her limbs. PR normal. What next?

CANDIDATE: Point tenderness in the back is suggestive of discitis. What are her reflexes like?

EXAMINER: Does it matter?

CANDIDATE: Brisk reflexes could suggest upper motor neuron lesion. If only in lower limbs it will mean a lesion in the thoracic spine. If in all four limbs this suggests a lesion in the cervical spine or brain.

EXAMINER: Reflexes are normal.

CANDIDATE: I would then proceed to investigations. I will look at her bloods FBC, U/E, RFT, serum lactate. The trend is more important in WBS, ESR and CRP than actual values. Also, I will request for portable radiographs of her lumbar spine.

I will then follow the *Sepsis 6* pathway. This includes:
- High-flow oxygen.
- Blood cultures.
- IV antibiotics.
- IV fluids.
- Check haemoglobin and lactate levels.
- Measure urine output.

If feasible, I will ask for an MRI of her lumbar spine which is the primary diagnostic modality for spine infections.

EXAMINER: Please read this X-ray (Figure 6.1a,b).

CANDIDATE: These are AP and lateral views of the lumbar spine showing destruction of the vertebral end plates at L4/5 on the lateral view. There is no evidence of vertebral collapse. There is slight reduction on disc height at L5/S1.

EXAMINER: These are her MRI scans (Figure 6.1c–g).

CANDIDATE: This is an MRI scan showing a hypointense signal at L4/5 on sagittal T1 (Figure 6.1c) and hyperintense on sagittal T2 (Figure 6.1d). There is loss of end plate definition on both sides of the disc. There is hyperintense vertebral marrow signal of L4 and L5 on fat-saturated T2 WI or STIR (Figure 6.1e). These changes are classical of discitis. There is no evidence of canal compromise on axial cuts (Figure 6.1f and Figure 6.1g). Also, there is no evidence of any epidural, subdural or intradural abscess.

EXAMINER: Could this be metastases?

CANDIDATE: Although metastases can lead to hypointense T1 and hyperintense T2 vertebral lesions, the disc space is always spared in malignancy. Also, the posterior elements are commonly involved in metastases.

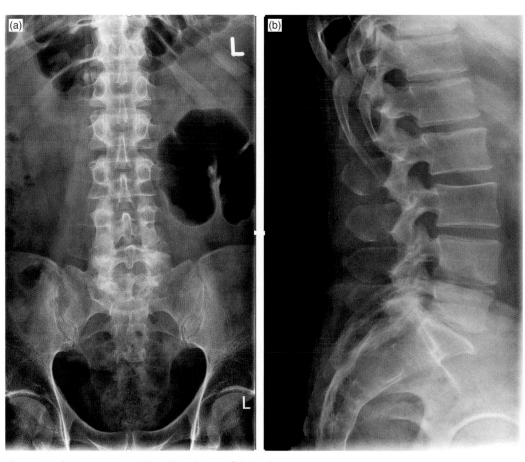

Figure 6.1a,b Anteroposterior(AP) and lateral views of the lumbar spine.

EXAMINER: What will you do next?

CANDIDATE: The management of this patient will need a multidisciplinary approach. Treatment at this point of time is essentially supportive with the *Sepsis 6* pathway. Her diabetes needs to be under strict control. I will start her on early empirical antibiotics after discussion with a microbiologist and infectious disease specialist until the causative organism is isolated. Parenteral antibiotics for 6–8 weeks in addition to a spinal brace for 6–12 weeks. At this point, she will need escalation of care and I will speak to HDU regarding the same.

Ideally, a biopsy would be ideal to decide the antibiotic. This can be done CT-guided depending on how stable the patient is. Also, a blood culture may provide a clue on the causative organism that should be done when the patient spikes a temperature.

I will keep a watch on her for worsening neurology and any further deterioration of her vital signs.

EXAMINER: What is the role of surgery?

CANDIDATE:
1. Epidural abscess – if significant neurology or worsening neurology.
2. Abscess with poor vitals to reduce the infective load, if fit for surgery. Interventional radiology may play a role.
3. Open biopsy in some cases to find exact organism and check drug sensitivity (e.g. *Mycobacterium tuberculosis*). Rarely done as CT-guided biopsy has replaced it.
4. Instability – healed infection with instability. Controversial as implant/surgery can lead to flare up of infection.

EXAMINER: What's the most common pathogen? What's the mode of spread?

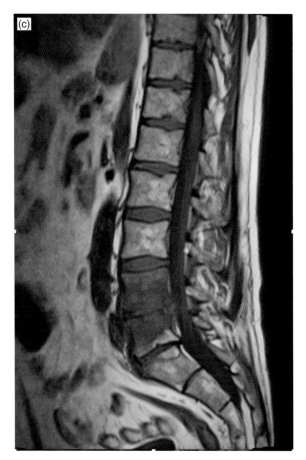

Figure 6.1c MRI lumbar spine (T1 sagittal).

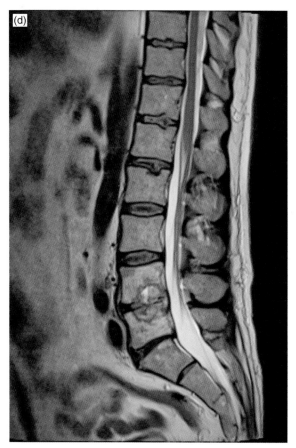

Figure 6.1d MRI lumbar spine (T2 sagittal).

CANDIDATE: Like most orthopaedic infections, *Staphylococcus* is the most common organism. *E. coli* is common within Gram-negative bacilli.

Bacteraemia (haematogenous – arterial) from an extra spinal primary source is the most common route of infection. This could be pulmonary, cardiac, urogenital, gut, cutaneous or mucous. Vascularized subchondral bone seeding occurs primarily with secondary involvement of the disc space and adjacent vertebrae. In children, however, the disc space infection is primary owing to vascular channels across the growth plate.

Other modes of spread are haematogenous – venous (Batsons plexus), lymphatic (more common in tuberculosis), direct (e.g. decubitus ulcer) or along cerebrospinal fluid pathways.

EXAMINER: How do you monitor response to therapy?

CANDIDATE: Symptomatic improvement like generalized feeling of well-being, reduction of back pain, increased mobility. Blood parameters like ESR, CRP and WBC. Also, serial MRI can be helpful.

EXAMINER: This MRI is done 5 weeks after therapy. Please comment.

CANDIDATE: The hypointense marrow signal seems to be improving on the T1 image (Figure 6.1h). So is the hyperintense T2 (Figure 6.1i) signal, suggesting that she is responding to the treatment.

EXAMINER: Thank you.

Learning points

1. Answer in a logical sequence of history, examination (general and local spine), investigations and management. Requesting blood cultures if a patient is pyrexic helps to isolate and identify a pathogen.

125

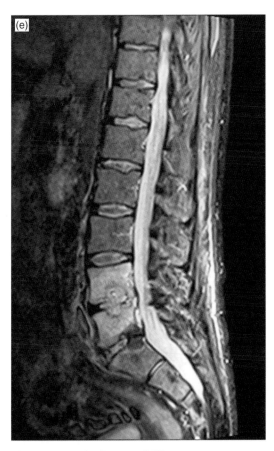

Figure 6.1e MRI lumbar spine (STIR) image.

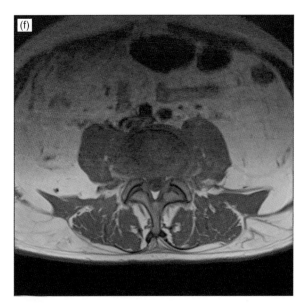

Figure 6.1f MRI lumbar spine axial cut.

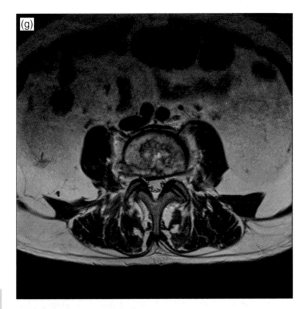

Figure 6.1g MRI lumbar spine axial cut.

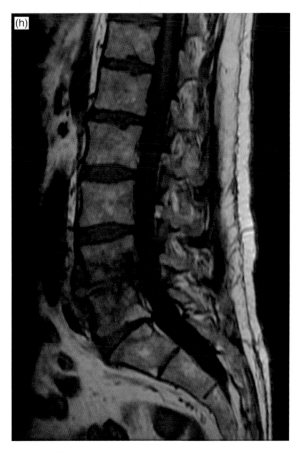

Figure 6.1h MRI lumbar spine.

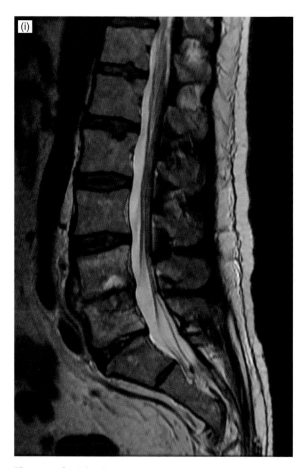

Figure 6.1i MRI lumbar spine.

2. An immunocompromised patient with either fever or joint/back pain = BONE/JOINT INFECTION.

3. Fever is variable and can be present in less than 50% of cases. Some patients may not have an inflammatory response and fever may be absent.

4. Indications of surgery in infective spine usually are:

    4.1. Neurology – worsening or advanced.

    4.2. Instability (read White and Punjabi definition for instability).

    4.3. Biopsy – if no improvement with antibiotics to find the causative organism, drug sensitivity or alternative pathology such as tumour.

    4.4. Abscess – if no improvement with antibiotics and worsening of systemic features or neurology due to compression of neural structures by the abscess.

5. The above scenario tests management of a septic patient as well as spinal infection.

6. Adult versus paediatric spinal infection differences: vascular channels across the growth plate in children leading to primary infection of the disc.

7. Similar infective scenarios could be vertebral osteomyelitis, epidural abscess, spinal cord abscess, septic facet joint arthritis or paraspinal abscess.

Structured oral examination question 2

Metastases

EXAMINER: You see a 68-year-old man in your clinic with progressive back pain that's worse at night and significant weight loss. How would you approach this patient?

CANDIDATE: His age, nocturnal pain and weight loss is suggestive of a sinister pathology such as infection or cancer. I will take a detailed history and examine . . . [being interrupted]

EXAMINER: What else do you want to know with history?

CANDIDATE:

1. Back pain.
    • Onset, duration, progress and its location (any point tenderness).
    • Aggravating or relieving factors, any trauma, radiation.
    • Severity and associated radiculopathy.

2. Neurology including bowel/bladder or gait involvement.

3. Other joints if painful? Other red flags?

4. For infections – any immunocompromised state such as being on steroids, diabetes or IVDU. Any other septic focus including chest, urine, abdomen?

5. Any other significant past history including medications, radiation or previous cancer?

6. Symptoms of other systems such as cough, abdominal pain and prostate symptoms to suggest any primary? Habits like smoking . . . [being interrupted]

EXAMINER: He is a chronic smoker with chronic cough and no other significant past medical history. He does complain of gait disturbances, though. His back pain is throughout thoracic and lumbar spine that is 8/10 on the VAS scale. There is no history of trauma. Nothing else is relevant on history.

CANDIDATE: I will proceed towards general and spine examination . . . [being interrupted]

EXAMINER: Nothing specific on general examination. Spine examination reveals tenderness along the entire thoracic and lumbar spine. He has no neurology in upper limbs but grade 3 power in lower limbs. PR is normal. Sensations are grossly normal.

CANDIDATE: What are the reflexes like?

EXAMINER: Brisk only in the lower limbs with upgoing plantar.

CANDIDATE: I am concerned about compression of cord in the thoracic spine, possible neoplastic aetiology with chronic smoking history and significant weight loss. I will get urgent blood investigations and radiological investigations.

Blood
- Infective – FBC, CRP, ESR.
- Metabolic – Ca, PO_4, Alk PO_4.
- Neoplastic – Se electrophoresis, Se PSA, CEA.

Radiological
- X-rays – full spine and chest in clinic.
- MRI full spine.

EXAMINER: These are his X-rays of lumbar spine (Figures 6.2a, 6.2b).

CANDIDATE: AP (Figure 6.2a) and lateral view (Figure 6.2b) of the lumbar spine. There is normal lordosis on the lateral view, but I can see compression of T11 vertebrae. I will need to see full-spine X-rays considering the fact that he has UMN signs in the lower limbs.

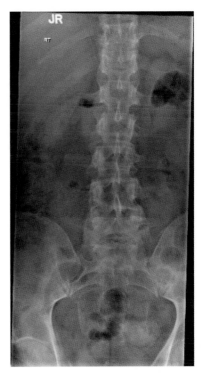

Figure 6.2a Anteroposterior (AP) radiograph of lumbar spine.

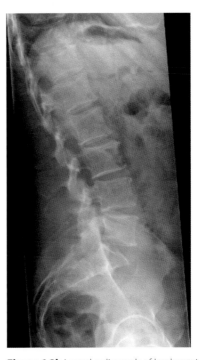

Figure 6.2b Lateral radiograph of lumbar spine.

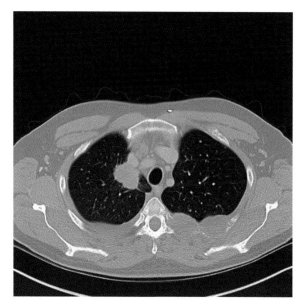

Figure 6.2c CT of chest.

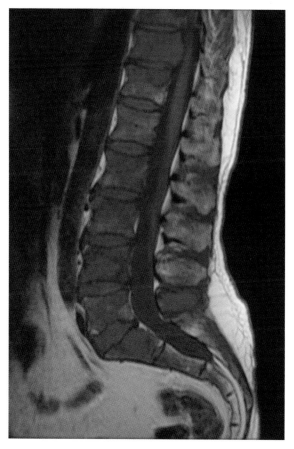

Figure 6.2d MRI lumbar spine, T1-weighted images.

EXAMINER: T11 is the only abnormality on X-rays. What next?

CANDIDATE: Disc height is fairly preserved (not infective). I am thinking more of metastases. Because this patient has neurology, I will get him admitted and get an urgent MRI within 24 hours. My aim will be to find out the primary as well. I will request urgent CT chest/abdomen/pelvis and bone scan to see for extra-spinal metastases/primary.

EXAMINER: This is his CT chest (Figure 6.2c).

CANDIDATE: There is a lesion in the right side of his chest, suggesting a primary in the lung. I will now manage this according to NICE guidelines for metastatic cord compression 2014 [1]. I will need an MRI and treatment plan within 24 hours.

EXAMINER: Please comment on the MRI scan (Figure 6.2d).

CANDIDATE: MRI T1-weighted images of lumbar spine (Figure 6.2d) showing loss of normal signal of the marrow with a replacement of hypointense signal with involvement of multiple vertebral bodies. The T2 (Figure 6.2e) shows variable signal from hypointense to hyperintense to normal bone marrow. The T11 vertebral body is the most involved with compression of the cord, which can explain the UMN signs in the lower limbs. However, I need to see axial cuts as well as full-spine MRI.

EXAMINER: Cervical MRI is normal. This is the thoracic MRI (Figure 6.2f and Figure 6.2g).

CANDIDATE: Thoracic MRI sagittal images (Figure 6.2f and Figure 6.2g) show multiple-level marrow infiltration with the cancer. T11 seems to be the major level of cord compression, but I would like to see the axial cuts as well.

EXAMINER: Yes, T11 is the major level of compression. What next?

CANDIDATE: As previously mentioned, this needs to be managed according to NICE guidelines for metastatic cord compression 2014. I will involve the local MSCC coordinator who will aid in decision-making, investigations, treatment and rehabilitation.

EXAMINER: Any further investigations?

129

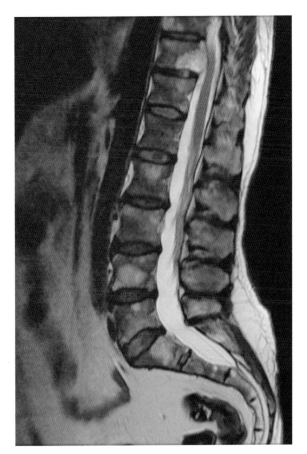

Figure 6.2e MRI lumbar spine, T2-weighted images.

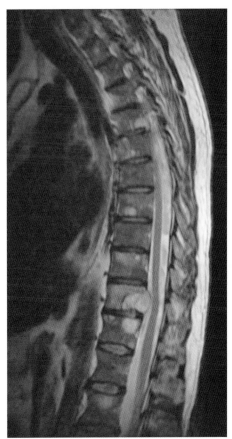

Figure 6.2f MRI lumbar spine.

CANDIDATE: I need to grade and stage this tumour.

Staging is to see the extent of spread of the tumour. This involves local and systemic staging. Local staging is MRI scan. Systemic staging is done by bone scan, CT of chest/abdomen/pelvis, PET scan or full-body MRI and is done to detect the primary and seek distant metastases.

Grading, on the other hand, is histology and is done by biopsy. Grading is the extent of differentiation of the tumour – low-grade undifferentiated or high-grade undifferentiated. Following the general principles applicable to all musculoskeletal tumours this biopsy should be done within the unit that will treat the tumour and samples should also be sent for culture. *Biopsy all infections and culture all tumours.*

Care must be taken in some metastases such as renal metastases that are very vascular and may need preoperative embolization prior to biopsy. Biopsy is needed if the primary is unknown.

EXAMINER: How would you decide about subsequent treatment?

CANDIDATE: The scoring system proposed by Tokuhashi [2] is useful in establishing indications for treatment and subsequent surgical goal. A poorer prognosis is correlated with a lower score. Six parameters are given a score from 0 to 2. A score of less than 5 indicates a life expectancy under 1 year and a palliative approach is suggested. A score of over 9 indicates a longer life expectancy and suggests resection/excision to be considered.

EXAMINER: His general condition is good otherwise and spine is the only metastases. What next?

CANDIDATE: Treatment options include:
- Surgical decompression and stabilization.
- Radiotherapy.
- Vertebroplasty/embolization.
- A combination of the above.

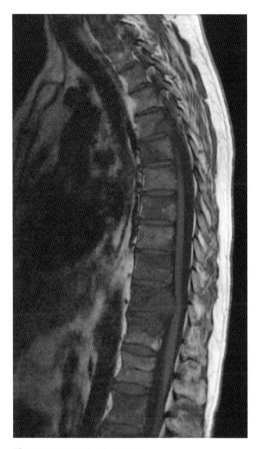

Figure 6.2g MRI lumbar spine.

Radiotherapy is mainly for palliative treatment and reduces bulk. Radiotherapy is more reserved for prostate, most breast and lymphoreticular tumours. Also, it can be given pre- and postoperatively. There should be an interval of 6 weeks between radiotherapy and surgery to avoid wound problems.

Vertebroplasty/kyphoplasty probably has no role in this case as the patient has neurology. Besides, it is done to stabilize the spine while minimizing soft-tissue trauma facilitating a faster postoperative recovery in patients with limited life expectancy.

Embolization will be decided depending on the vascularity of the metastases on angiography that is usually an issue in renal metastases.

Here, I am more inclined for surgical instrumented decompression ± fusion depending on his fitness for anaesthesia and major surgery. Decompression of compressed neural structures may lead to functional improvement even with

prolonged paraplegia. Simple laminectomy to 'decompress' the tumour is rarely indicated. This is because the presence of the tumour most frequently found in the vertebral body is likely to lead to mechanical instability and thus kyphosis. Instrumented stabilization is frequently undertaken.

Surgical resection of the tumour is aimed at improving survival. Resection may be undertaken anteriorly or posteriorly or both, and depending on the size and location of the lesion. In general terms, if a curative resection is hoped for, or survival is likely to extend beyond 6 months, intervertebral bony fusion should be undertaken to avoid instrumentation failure. If life expectancy is short and a palliative procedure is being considered, fusion may not be required, and posterior surgery is more commonly undertaken.

EXAMINER: How do metastases spread to the spine?

CANDIDATE: The spinal column is the most common site of osseous metastases of which thoracic spine is the most common. Spread can occur via:
- Direct extension – lung cancer extending into the chest wall into vertebral bodies and posterior elements.
- Haematogenous – Batson's plexus, which is a longitudinal plexus of valveless veins running parallel to the spinal column. Tumours in multiple sites can metastasize to the spinal column without liver or lung involvement, e.g. prostate cancer.
- Lymphatic.
- CSF pathways.

EXAMINER: Why do spine metastases in vertebral bodies show reduced signal on T1?

CANDIDATE: Vetebral bodies contain bone marrow that has fat. This fat shows as a bright signal on T1. In metastases, this fat is replaced by cancer cells, leading to a reduced signal.

EXAMINER: Thank you.

Learning points

1. In cancers, the first aim is to confirm the diagnosis, then extent of spread and finally management.
2. Ask relevant questions to examiners when taking a history or asking about the findings

of examination. This is just like an everyday clinic scenario.

3. Unless you ask for a relevant investigation, the examiner may not even show you the X-ray or MRI images.

4. Tokuhashi staging:
   - *General condition* (poor 0, moderate 1, good 2).
   - *Number of extra-spinal metastases* (three or more scores 0, one or two scores 1, zero scores 2).
   - *Number of spinal bony metastases* (three or more scores 0, two scores 1, one scores 2).
   - *Number of metastases to major internal organs* (not removable 0, removable 1, no mets 2).
   - *Tissue of origin* (lung/stomach 0, kidney/liver/uterus 1, other/breast/thyroid/prostate/rectum 2).
   - *Spinal cord palsy* (complete 0, incomplete 1, none 2).

Excisional surgery > 9.

Palliative treatment < 5.

5. Neurology generally points to surgery unless in a very unfit patient or a very radiosensitive tumour such as lymphoma/myeloma, where radiotherapy is recommended.

6. Myeloma – CRAB (HyperCalcaemia, Renal failure, Anaemia, Bone lesions).

7. Prognosis – median survival in patients with metastatic bone disease.
   a. thyroid: 48 months.
   b. prostate: 40 months.
   c. breast: 24 months.
   d. kidney: variable depending on medical condition but may be as short as 6 months.
   e. lung: 6 months.

8. Types of metastases:
   - Blastic – bone production exceeds bone destruction.
     - Prostate in adults.
     - Medulloblastoma, neuroblastoma, Ewing's in children.
   - Lytic – bone destruction exceeds bone production.

   - Renal, lung, breast and thyroid.

9. Differential diagnosis.
   - Blastic – haemangioma, Paget's disease, osteosarcoma, benign osteoporotic compression fractures, renal osteodystrophy.
   - Lytic – multiple myeloma, lymphoma, spondylodiscitis (destruction of disc space with abnormal signal on either side of disc space).

10. Factors to be considered in offering treatment.
    - Neurology.
    - Type of cancer – radio-resistant, -sensitive.
    - Systemic disease – limited or extensive.
    - Instability.

References

1. NICE. Metastatic spinal cord compression in adults. Quality Standard 56. February 2014.

2. Tokuhashi Y, Matsuzaki H, Toriyama S, Kawano H, Ohsaka S. Scoring system for the preoperative evaluation of metastatic spine tumor prognosis. *Spine*. 1990;15(11):1110–1113.

Structured oral examination question 3

Benign lesion

EXAMINER: You see a 35-year-old fit and healthy man complaining of insidious onset LBP, more severe at night. There is no history of trauma and no red flags on history.

CANDIDATE: Is the pain localized to one specific point in his back? Any neurology?

EXAMINER: Pain is localized to the right side of his back, for 6 months now. No neurology with no bowel or bladder symptoms. Nothing else is significant on history.

CANDIDATE: Night pain is a concern for me. If there is no other relevant history, I would like to go ahead with a general and spine examination.

EXAMINER: Nothing remarkable on general examination. Spine examination shows right-sided point

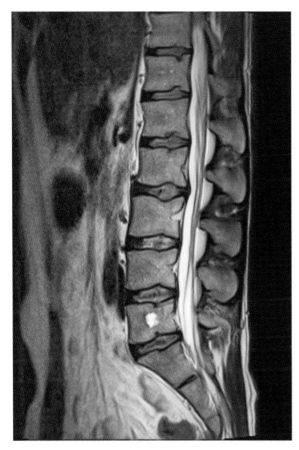

Figure 6.3a MRI lumbar spine T2 sagittal image.

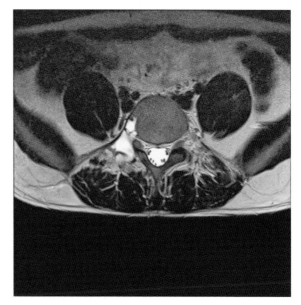

Figure 6.3b MRI lumbar spine, T2 axial image.

tenderness in the L45 region with normal neurology. Other joints and distal pulsations are normal.

CANDIDATE: I will then proceed for investigations.

Blood
- Infective – FBC, CRP, ESR.
- Metabolic – Ca, PO_4, Alk PO_4.
- Neoplastic – Se electrophoresis, Se PSA, CEA.

Radiological
- X-rays and MRI full spine.

EXAMINER: Why X-rays?

CANDIDATE: Night pain is a red flag. I need X-rays.

EXAMINER: X-ray of the full spine is normal. All blood investigations are within normal limits.

CANDIDATE: I will proceed for MRI.

EXAMINER: This is a midsagittal T2 image (Figure 6.3a). Please comment.

CANDIDATE: T2 sagittal image (Figure 6.3a) showing hyperintense signal in the L5 body. I want to see T1, axial and parasagittal images, please.

EXAMINER: Please comment, axials at L5.

CANDIDATE: Axial T2 and T1 and fat-suppressed images (Figures 6.3b–6.3d) showing cystic mass with fluid collections in right-side lamina, pedicle and extending into the body of L5. There is no evidence of thecal sac compression. I cannot appreciate infiltration of soft tissues.

EXAMINER: What are your differentials?

CANDIDATE: Aneurysmal bone cyst, infections, telangiectatic osteosarcoma or vascular metastases. Unlikely to be infective as bloods are normal. However, can't rule this out until a biopsy is done along with culture.

EXAMINER: What next?

CANDIDATE: I will like to refer this patient to regional oncology and the spinal team for their opinion. Also, I will get this MRI reported by a musculoskeletal radiologist.

EXAMINER: You are the regional team.

CANDIDATE: I will get a CT scan.

133

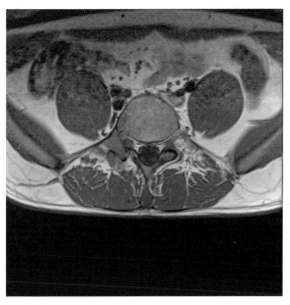

Figure 6.3c MRI lumbar spine, T1 axial image.

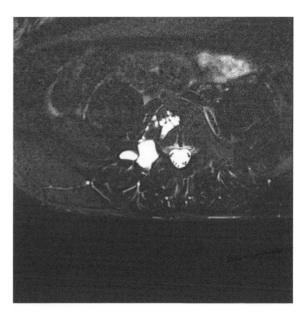

Figure 6.3d MRI lumbar spine, fat suppression axial image.

EXAMINER: Why?

CANDIDATE: Infection is less likely as bloods are normal and there is no fever. I am considering this either ABC, telangiectatic osteosarcoma or vascular metastases. I need to see whether this is an isolated lesion or if there are additional lesions like vascular metastases. So, CT chest/abdomen/pelvis and bone scan for additional lesions. I need to be wary of renal cell carcinoma that can have vascular metastases that can bleed torrentially during biopsy.

CT spine will also help me differentiate between ABC and telangiectatic osteosarcoma. ABC will have a narrow zone of transition and a lack of infiltration of surrounding soft tissues. CT angio is preferable to differentiate it from vascular metastases of renal cell carcinoma.

EXAMINER: CT confirms this is an isolated lesion. Please comment (Figure 6.3e).

CANDIDATE: Axial CT showing an expansile mass centred over the right-side pedicle, lamina, transverse process and extending into the body. The cortex appears thinned out. There is no soft-tissue infiltration and a small zone of transition. This needs biopsy to confirm it's an ABC and not telangiectatic osteosarcoma, preferably a CT-guided biopsy. Also, infection needs to be ruled out.

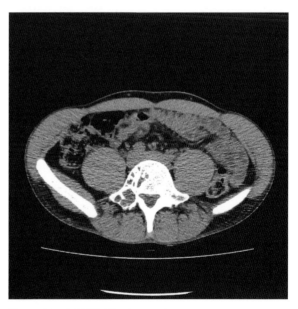

Figure 6.3e Axial CT of lumbar vertebra.

EXAMINER: Biopsy confirms your diagnosis of ABC. What next?

CANDIDATE: When doing a biopsy, I will make sure a specimen goes for culture and Gram staining. After confirming there is no growth, as this patient is symptomatic, I will probably offer resection or curettage. As this may lead to iatrogenic instability after resection, consent for instrumentation ± fusion. Also, the patient should be counselled for recurrence as 20% of cases can recur.

EXAMINER: Thank you.

Learning points

1. Final confirmation of benign, malignant or infection is only by biopsy (send specimen for microbiology as well).
2. Always mention local and systemic staging for tumours.
   - Local – X-rays, CT.
   - MRI (better for soft tissue, vascularity, micro metastases, intramedullary extension).
   - Systemic – bone scan, PET, CT chest/abdomen/pelvis.
3. Biopsy all infections and culture all tumours.
4. Know principles of biopsy.

Structured oral examination question 4

Cervical spondylotic myelopathy

EXAMINER: A 64-year-old man arrives in your clinic with neck pain. How would you approach this patient?

CANDIDATE: I will take a history first. Onset, duration and progress of the neck pain. Any radiculopathy?

EXAMINER: Axial neck pain that is not severe and since the past 6 months. No radiculopathy.

CANDIDATE: Does he have any gait disturbances? Any bowel or bladder disturbances? Does he have any weakness in any of his limbs? Any red flags?

EXAMINER: He does give a history of repeated falls. Mild clumsiness in his hands, but no bowel or bladder disturbances. No other red flags or any other significant history.

CANDIDATE : I am concerned about his repeated falls. Although there could be many causes for falls in this age group from vision problems to postural hypotension to heart disease, a patient

with neck pain and weakness of hand muscles, I am thinking of cervical spondylotic myelopathy.

EXAMINER: What next?

CANDIDATE: Proceed with examination. Start with gait and do a Romberg's test.

EXAMINER: He has a wide-based gait. How do you perform Romberg's and what is its significance?

CANDIDATE: Ask the patient to stand with feet close and check whether he sways with eyes open and closed.
  Romberg's test relies on the brain (cerebellum) receiving three sensory inputs. These are vision, vestibular apparatus in the inner ear and joint position (proprioception) carried by the dorsal columns of the spinal cord. If the visual pathway is removed by closing the eyes and the proprioceptive and vestibular pathways are intact, balance will be maintained. However, if proprioception is defective, two of the sensory inputs will be absent and the patient will sway and lose balance when his eyes are closed. If he stays with eyes open, then there is a problem with the brain (cerebellum).

EXAMINER: Romberg's test is positive with eyes open.

CANDIDATE: This means the joint position sense (or proprioception) carried by the dorsal columns of the spinal cord is not reaching the brain. I am thinking of cord compression, cauda equina compression or peripheral neuropathy. I need to complete the rest of the examination.

EXAMINER: Cervical movements are good range. Grade 3 power in hand muscles but rest all grade 5. Sensations are grossly normal except proprioception.

CANDIDATE: Reflexes in all four limbs? Hoffmans' and Babinski's? Any clonus?

EXAMINER: Reflexes brisk in all four limbs. Hoffmans' and Babinski's are positive. There is sustained clonus in the lower limbs. Rest all joints normal with good distal pulsations.

CANDIDATE: This suggests UMN lesion in all four limbs, so a lesion in brain or cervical cord. Less likely a lesion in the brain, as he does not have any

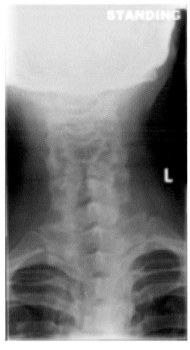

Figure 6.4a Anteroposterior (AP) radiograph lumbar spine.

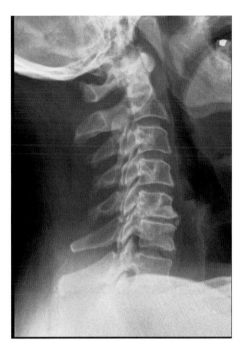

Figure 6.4b Lateral view of cervical spine.

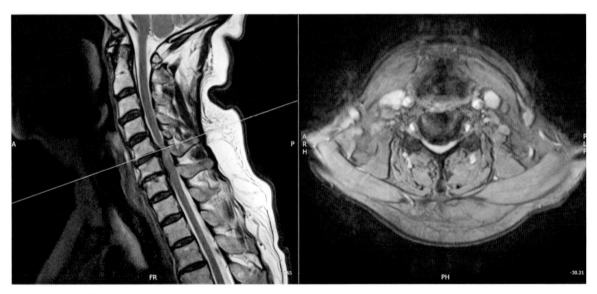

Figure 6.4c MRI (T2 sagittal and axial C5/6).

symptoms of the same, but I will need to check cranial nerves. Additional compression could be present in thoracic and lumbar spine.

EXAMINER: Brain is normal. What next?

CANDIDATE: X-rays of cervical spine and MRI scan of his full spine.

EXAMINER: Please comment on these X-rays (Figures 6.4a and 6.4b).

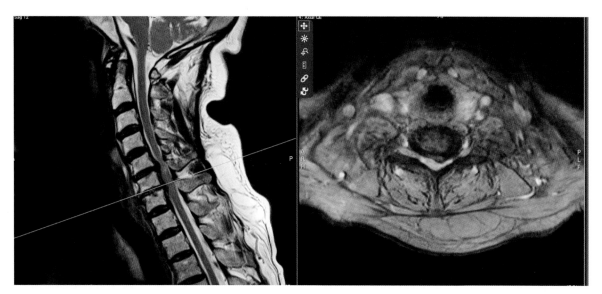

Figure 6.4d MRI (T2 sagittal and axial C6/7).

CANDIDATE: AP and lateral view of the cervical spine showing reduced disc height, osteophyte formation at C5/6 on the lateral view. Cervical lordosis is mildly lost.

EXAMINER: Please comment on the MRI (Figures 6.4c and 6.4d).

CANDIDATE: T2 MRI with axial cuts at C5/6, C6/7. There is significant compression at the disc level with cord compression. This MRI can explain all his symptoms. I need to make sure he has no compression elsewhere in his spine. A scout MRI would be preferred. Also, I need to see T1 axial and sagittal of the cervical spine.

EXAMINER: The rest of his spine is normal on MRI. T1 does not add much.

CANDIDATE: This is cervical spondylotic myelopathy confirmed on clinical examination and radiology. Treatment is essentially surgical as the disorder is typically progressive without surgery. I will refer him to a spinal surgeon for early surgical intervention for favourable outcome before permanent damage occurs within the spinal cord.

EXAMINER: What surgery do you know for this condition?

CANDIDATE: There are various options available.

- Anterior decompression with fusion (discectomy or corpectomy).
- Laminectomy with fusion.
- Laminectomy alone (limited role, leads to kyphosis).
- Laminoplasty with fusion.

As he has compression at the disc level and mainly anterior, I think he needs anterior cervical discectomy C5/6, C6/7 and fusion. This is done by the Smith Robinson approach.

EXAMINER: What about isolated laminectomy?

CANDIDATE: Laminectomy is rarely done due to risk of post-laminectomy kyphosis. This kyphosis can lead to further neck pain and the risk of recurrent myelopathy due to the cord getting compressed over the kyphosis.

Laminectomy with fusion can be done for compression mainly posteriorly or with involvement of more than three levels. But if pre-existing kyphosis is significant, then anterior or combined anterior–posterior surgery is recommended.

EXAMINER: How would you consent this patient?

CANDIDATE: After explaining the pathology, I will tell this patient that the main aim of the surgery is to prevent the progression of the disease process. However, many patients will notice improvement in neurology after cervical decompression and fusion surgery. I will explain all the complications of cervical spine surgery that include pain, neurology, non-union, metal problems, dysphagia, revision surgery.

EXAMINER: [Interrupting] What if patient has asymptomatic cord compression on the MRI?

CANDIDATE: Treatment then is controversial. Consideration should be given for surgery if cord changes are present. Alternatively, close follow-up is needed with patient counselling with warning about spinal cord injury with minor trauma (e.g. central cord syndrome).

EXAMINER: Thank you.

Learning points

1. Surgery is the mainstay for cervical spondylotic myelopathy unless the patient is unwilling or poor medically for surgery.

2. Tandem stenosis or combined cervical and lumbar stenosis can happen in 7–20% of patients. Always check for upper motor neuron signs in all four limbs to pick up cervical cord compression in patients referred for lumbar canal stenosis.

3. Smith Robinson's approach is frequently asked for exams.

4. The role of cervical disc replacement for myelopathy. This can be performed in

   selected cases with compression only anteriorly, no facet arthritis, no significant neck pain. –2.

5. Causes of myelopathy.
   - CSM (cervical spondylotic myelopathy).
   - OPLL (ossified posterior longitudinal ligament).
   - Infective – epidural abscess.
   - Trauma – fractures, bilateral facet subluxation.
   - Tumours.
   - Congenital stenosis – Pavlov ratio < 0.8 (ratio of width of canal to width of body).

References

1. Ikenaga M, Shikata J, Tanaka C. Long-term results over 10 years of anterior corpectomy and fusion for multilevel cervical myelopathy. *Spine*. 2006;31:1568–1574.

2. Gornet MF, Lanman TH, Burkus JK, et al. Cervical disc arthroplasty with the Prestige LP disc versus anterior cervical discectomy and fusion, at 2 levels: results of a prospective, multicenter randomized controlled clinical trial at 24 months. *J Neurosurg Spine*. 2017;17:1–15. doi:10.3171/2016.10. SPINE16264

Structured oral examination question 5

Lumbar disc prolapse with cauda equina

EXAMINER: You are on call and asked to see a 32-year-old lady with history of a fall from stairs and sustaining a fractured humerus. This fracture is closed and neurovascularly intact. There are no other injuries. How will you proceed?

CANDIDATE: I will first take a history. I will want to know mechanism of injury, any relevant past history.

EXAMINER: [Interrupting] She says she lost balance. She has had repeated falls over the past 1 month. She is otherwise fit and well. She has been to her GP for this balance problem, who has referred her to a neurologist.

CANDIDATE: This history is concerning. Loss of balance can be caused by many problems that affect the skeletal, visual, ear, nervous system, etc. I would like to know more from the history.

1. Does she have any hearing, visual problems?
2. Any headaches, medications, cranial nerve deficits?
3. Any weakness in any of the limbs, back pain, altered sensations, bowel or bladder disturbances?

EXAMINER: She has bilateral lower limb radiculopathy. She also has bladder disturbances with reduced desire to void, straining and altered urinary sensations.

CANDIDATE: I am now worried if she has cauda equina that was probably missed in the first place. This can also explain her gait disturbances.

EXAMINER: How does cauda equina lead to gait disturbances?

CANDIDATE: Cauda equina carries afferent inputs such as joint sense, position sense, touch, proprioception, etc. that provide signals to the brain to decide on balance and locomotion. Also, efferent pathways to the lower limbs for motor function exits via the cauda equina. With this pathway blocked, imbalance is inevitable.

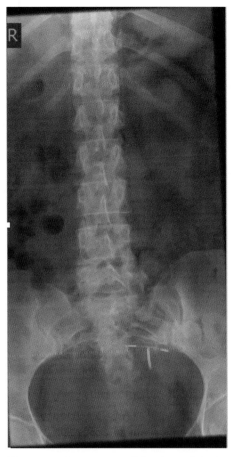

Figure 6.5a Anteroposterior (AP) radiograph lumbar spine.

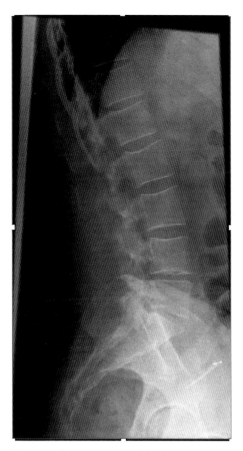

Figure 6.5b Lateral radiograph lumbar spine.

EXAMINER: What would you like to do now?

CANDIDATE: There are two issues here. First is the closed fracture humerus that has no neurovascular deficit and second is the more urgent suspected cauda equina. I will like to provide analgesia, keep the patient fasting, splint the fracture and do a detailed neurological examination.

This will include tone, power, reflexes, sensations in all four limbs, specifically check for plantars in lower limbs and Hoffman's in upper limbs. I will do a per rectal examination and check for perianal sensations, anal tone. I also will request a bladder scan. I will also check for bilateral SLR to see if positive, suggesting nerve root tension signs.

EXAMINER: Neurology is normal in the upper limbs. Reflexes are sluggish in the lower limbs, reduced sensations, equivocal plantars and motor deficit in L4–S1 dermatomes.

Perianal sensations are reduced, reduced anal tone. Bladder scan is not available. SLR bilaterally 30°.

Humerus fracture is undisplaced and can be managed in a plaster. It is now 4 pm and you are working in a DGH. What next?

CANDIDATE: This is cauda equina which is essentially a clinical diagnosis and needs an urgent MRI as well as lumbar spine X-rays.

EXAMINER: Please comment on these X rays (Figures 6.5a and 6.5b).

CANDIDATE: X-ray AP (Figure 6.5a) and lateral view (Figure 6.5b) of the lumbar spine. The lateral view shows reduced disc height at L4/5 and L5/S1. There is also facet arthritis at these levels. AP X-ray shows facet degeneration in the lower lumbar spine. I need urgent MRI for this patient.

EXAMINER: MRI busy but CT is available.

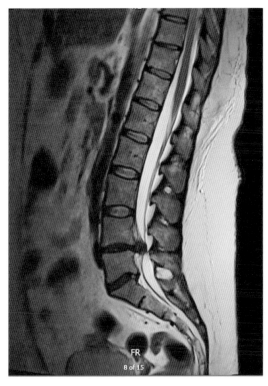

Figure 6.5c MRI sagittal T2 image.

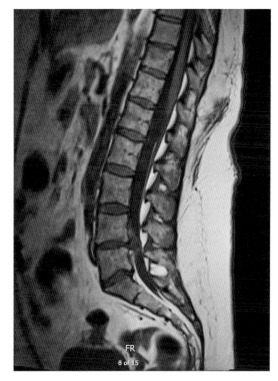

Figure 6.5d MRI sagittal T1 image.

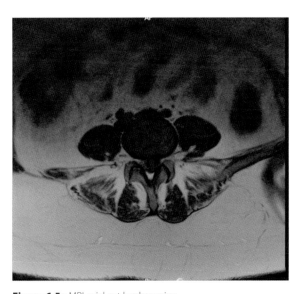

Figure 6.5e MRI axial cut lumbar spine.

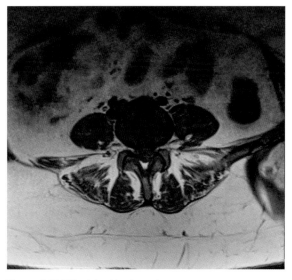

Figure 6.5f MRI axial cut lumbar spine.

CANDIDATE: MR imaging is the modality of choice for cauda equina as it has greater soft-tissue sensitivity and specificity as compared to a CT scan. Besides, CT may not be able to diagnose abscess or haematoma that can be a differential diagnosis. I will speak to the radiologist about the need for urgent MRI in this patient.

EXAMINER: Please comment on the MRI (Figures 6.5c–6.5f).

CANDIDATE: MRI T2 (Figure 6.5c) and T1 (Figure 6.5d) sagittal images show a large disc at L4/5 level. The axial cuts (Figures 6.5e and 6.5f) show significant compression of the cauda equina. Looking at her symptoms, she is CESI (cauda equina syndrome incomplete) and I will urgently refer her to a spinal surgeon for decompression.

EXAMINER: What do you mean by CESI?

CANDIDATE: Todd *et al.* [1] provided standards of care for cauda equina. They divided CES into:

1. CESS (cauda equina syndrome suspected) – bilateral radiculopathy.
   Management – Admission, operate or wait and watch.
2. CESI (cauda equina syndrome incomplete) – patient with urinary difficulties.
   Management – emergency surgery.
3. CESR (cauda equina syndrome retention) – painless retention of urine with overflow incontinence.
   Management – emergency surgery – early CESR (< 12 hours), uncertain CESI/CESR, residual sacral nerve function present.

   – Next acute list – prolonged CESR.

4. CESC (cauda equina syndrome complete) – loss of all cauda equina function (absent perianal sensations, patulous anus and paralyzed insensate bladder and bowel).
   Management – next acute list – prolonged CESR.

EXAMINER: You mentioned emergency surgery. Would you prefer this patient to be operated on at night if it is incomplete cauda equina syndrome?

CANDIDATE: The longer the duration of the compression, the worse the bladder outcome. So also the risk of progressing to CES retention and complete CES. Patients operated within 24 or 48 or over 48 h after CESI had normal bladder function in 89%, 79% and 44% of patients, respectively [2]. The British Association of Spine Surgeons (BASS) in their guidelines suggests decompressive surgery should be undertaken at the earliest opportunity, taking into consideration the duration of the pre-existing

symptoms and the potential for increased morbidity while operating in the small hours [3].

In other words, do not wait for symptoms and signs of CESR and CESC as the outcomes are poor despite surgical intervention. So, if safe, these cases should be operated upon as emergencies.

The principle of emergency decompressive surgery for all cauda equina is also gaining support [4,5].

EXAMINER: Take me through the surgery for this case.

CANDIDATE: The surgical approach could be unilateral or bilateral, fenestration or laminectomy. There are no data suggesting one is better over the other. But, in already compressed nerves, minimal handling with laminectomies tailored to the disc prolapse anatomy is recommended.

EXAMINER: Anything specific regarding consent for this patient for surgery?

CANDIDATE: Besides the routine risks of discectomy, I would counsel the patient that the main aim is to prevent progression of neurology, although recovery can be expected but can't be promised. The bladder, bowel, sexual dysfunction may not improve and may be permanent.

Also, there is a chance of actually worsening, not only due to iatrogenic damage of the compressed nerves (retracting for discectomy), but because the pathology is progressing by the time the patient has had the cauda equina decompressed (time to theatre, anaesthesia, etc.). In other words, documentation of the neurology just prior to anaesthesia would be wise from a medicolegal perspective as litigation is common in the event of persistent neurological deficit.

EXAMINER: Thank you.

Learning points

1. Clinical assessment has low sensitivity for CES.
2. There is no agreed definition for CES, but the five characteristics are bilateral sciatica, reduced perianal sensations, altered bladder function ultimately leading to painless urinary retention, loss of anal tone and sexual dysfunction.
3. Reflexes will narrow down the search for

pathology into upper motor neuron lesion (brain, spinal cord) or lower motor neurons (cauda equina, peripheral nerves). So also, Babinski and Hoffmann signs are prudent to be performed.

References

1. Todd NV, Dickson RA. Standards of care in cauda equina syndrome. *Br J Neurosurg*. 2016;30(5):518–522.

2. Srikandarajah N, Boissaud-Cooke MA, Clark S, Wilby MJ. Does early surgical decompression in cauda equina syndrome improve bladder outcome? *Spine*. 2015;40:580–583. doi:10.1097/BRS.

3. Germon T, Ahuja S, Casey AT, *et al*. British Association of Spine Surgeons standards of care for cauda equina syndrome. *Spine J*. 2015;15:S2–4.

4. Bydon M, Gokaslan ZL. Time to treatment of cauda equina syndrome: a time to re-evaluate our clinical decision. *World Neurosurg*. 2014;82:344–345.

5. Sonntag VKH. Why not decompress early? The cauda equina syndrome. *World Neurosurg*. 2014;82:70–71.

Structured oral examination question 6

Spondylolisthesis

EXAMINER: A 30-year-old female, otherwise fit and active, presents to your clinic with a 1-year history of back pain. These are her X-rays (Figures 6.6a and 6.6b), please comment.

CANDIDATE: AP (Figure 6.6a) and lateral X rays (Figure 6.6b) of the lumbar spine. The lateral view shows defect in the pars interarticularis. This is isthmic spondylolisthesis and I would say it is grade 1 according to Meyerding grading. There is also loss of disc height of the L5/S1 disc space suggesting disc degeneration. Lumbar lordosis is maintained.

The AP view does not show any deformity in the coronal plane. The 'Napoleon Hat' sign is positive (the hat is inverted with the crown representing L5 body and brim being the transverse process).

Ideally, I would like to do standing X-rays as the spine can behave differently when loading. Also, I want to see the entire sacrum with the hip joints to see the pelvic incidence, pelvic tilt and sacral slope. Additionally, flexion–extension lateral

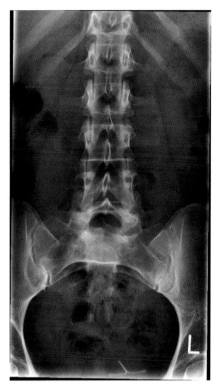

Figure 6.6a Anteroposterior (AP) radiograph lumbar spine.

views to look for > 4 mm translation suggesting instability.

EXAMINER: What types of spondylolisthesis do you know?

CANDIDATE: Spondylolisthesis is graded according to *Meyerding's grading system*, which is graded I–V depending on the degree of displacement of the cranial vertebral body.

Grade I is less than 25%.

Grade II is 25–50%.

Grade III is 50–75%.

Grade IV is 75–100%.

Grade V is spondyloptosis (> 100%).

Five different types of spondylolisthesis were described by *Wiltse–Newman*:

I. Dysplastic – congenital abnormalities of the sacrum or L5 allow the slip to occur.

II. Isthmic – here the defect is in the pars.

- IIA – pars fatigue fracture.
- IIB – pars elongation due to multiple healed fractures.
- IIC – pars acute fracture.

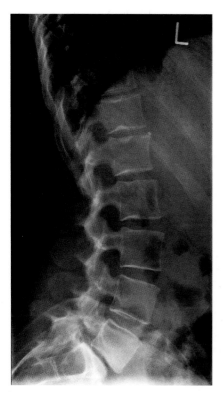

Figure 6.6b Lateral radiograph lumbar spine.

III. Degenerative – this is due to a degenerative change that produces intersegmental instability (due to changes in disc, joint capsules and facet joints).

IV. Traumatic – due to a fracture (but not of the pars, e.g. pedicle).

V. Pathological – caused by local bone disease (disease may not be localized).

EXAMINER: How would you proceed?

CANDIDATE: I would like to take a detailed history, do spine examination and request further investigations. History-wise:

1. Back pain – onset, duration, progress and its location (any point tenderness).

   - Aggravating or relieving factors, any trauma, radiation.
   - Severity.

2. Lower limb radiculopathy.

3. Neurology including bowel/bladder or gait involvement, any red flags.

4. Treatment she has had so far, expectations.

EXAMINER: What radiculopathy you expect in this case? How do you differentiate symptoms from degenerative listhesis?

CANDIDATE: Degenerative listhesis is more common at L4/5 as the more sagittal-oriented facets predispose to the pathology. Isthmic listhesis, on the other hand, happens due to repetitive hyperextension forces that are prevalent at L5/S1.

   This case being an isthmic spondylolisthesis at L5/S1, the patient may have either unilateral or bilateral L5 radiculopathy. This is unlike degenerative listhesis where the lower root is involved, so L5 radiculopathy for degenerative L4/5 listhesis.

EXAMINER: This lady has chronic back pain, L5 radiculopathy with no neurology. Her GP has exhausted all options including pain team, activity modifications and physiotherapy. Her back pain is worse than her legs and she says she will do whatever you feel is best for her.

CANDIDATE: I need to do an examination.

EXAMINER: [Interrupting] Anything specific you want to see on examinations?

CANDIDATE: Her gait, tenderness, step sign, range of movements, nerve root tension signs and neurology.

EXAMINER: No neurology, ROM restricted, hamstrings are tight, nothing else significant on examination. What next?

CANDIDATE: I will request an MRI scan of her lumbar spine.

EXAMINER: Why do you need an MRI? Is the diagnosis not evident on X-rays? She also has no neurology to warrant an MRI.

CANDIDATE: This lady has exhausted non-operative options and is now looking at surgery. MRI will provide more information that is needed to plan surgery. This includes the anatomy and extent of compression of the L5 nerve, status of the L4/5 disc (decide on level of fusion, facet hypertrophy, ligamentum flavum hypertrophy and also whether it is a unilateral or bilateral defect).

EXAMINER: Please comment on this MR image (Figures 6.6c and 6.6d).

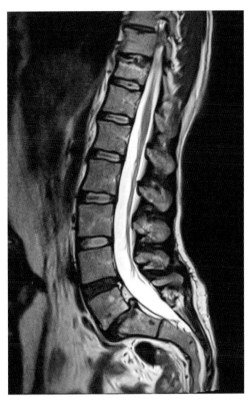

Figure 6.6c MRI T2 mid-sagittal image spine.

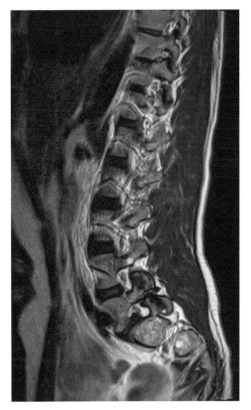

Figure 6.6d MRI para-sagittal image spine.

CANDIDATE: The T2 mid-sagittal image (Figure 6.6c) shows reduced disc height at L5/S1 with disc degeneration. There is also disc degeneration at the L4/5 level with a bright signal suggesting an annular tear. The dura does not show any compression, although I need to see axial cuts to check for nerve root compression. The parasagittal image (Figure 6.6d) shows L5 lysis. I need to see T1 sagittal and axial views please.

EXAMINER: Consider them not to add more information. L5 is compressed on axials. What next?

CANDIDATE: I will speak to her about surgery in the form of L5/S1 wide decompression and in situ posterolateral instrumented fusion. Other fusion options include PLIF (posterior lumbar interbody fusion), TLIF (transforaminal lumbar interbody fusion) and ALIF (anterior lumbar interbody fusion). Interbody fusion does lead to increased operative time and more blood loss.

Factors deciding no interbody (posterolateral), TLIF/PLIF or ALIF are [1]:

1. Disc degeneration.
2. Loss of disc height.
3. Segmental lordosis.
4. Reduction of listhesis if planned.
5. Transverse process fusion area.

So, plain posterolateral fusion is usually indicated if there is no disc degeneration, disc height and lordosis is well maintained with a large area of transverse process to ensure fusion. TLIF/PLIF/ALIF if moderate to severe disc degeneration, loss of disc height and segmental lordosis, poor transverse process fusion areas and if planning reduction.

EXAMINER: You mentioned pelvic incidence while describing the X-rays. What do you mean by that and what is its significance?

CANDIDATE: Pelvic incidence (PI) is the angle formed between a line drawn from the centre of the S1 end plate to the centre of the femoral head and a second line drawn perpendicular to the S1 end plate intersecting it at the centre. It is also the sum of pelvic tilt and sacral slope. PI has

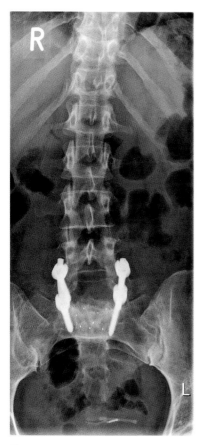

Figure 6.6e Anteroposterior (AP) lumbar spine showing in situ instrumented interbody fusion.

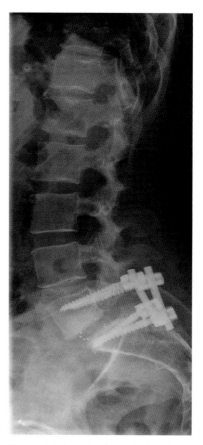

Figure 6.6f Lateral radiograph of lumbar spine showing in situ instrumented interbody fusion.

a direct linear relationship to the severity of spondylolisthesis. PI does not change with posture, unlike other parameters of pelvic morphology. Low pelvic incidence indicates low shear forces at the lumbosacral junction and less lumbar lordosis. A greater pelvic incidence necessitates more lumbar lordosis to maintain sagittal balance. When lumbar lordosis reduces, the pelvis rotates posteriorly, extending the hips. After the hips are maximally extended, further compensation is achieved with knee flexion.

EXAMINER: In low-grade listhesis, would you recommend in situ fixation or reduction?

CANDIDATE: In situ fixation and fusion is still the standard for low-grade listhesis. However, some surgeons prefer reduction via TLIF/PLIF if there is loss of disc height, segmental lordosis or sagittal malalignment.

Reduction for high-grade listhesis (dysplastic, isthmic) remains controversial. Reduction procedures are extremely demanding and potentially dangerous. Reduction does restore sagittal spinopelvic alignment, reduces gait anomalies, the fusion mass is placed in a better biomechanical environment (compression rather than tension or shear) and reduces the risk of postoperative cauda equina as the central canal is restored. The risk of neurological injuries, however, can be as high as 75% [2].

EXAMINER: Please comment on these postop X-rays (Figures 6.6e and 6.6f).

CANDIDATE: AP (Figure 6.6e) and lateral X-rays (Figure 6.6f) of the lumbar spine showing in situ instrumented interbody fusion. This to me looks like TLIF as the facets are missing on the lateral view. The disc height is restored with the use of interbody cages.

145

EXAMINER: This patient now has leg pain postop day one. How would you proceed?

CANDIDATE: I would again start with history, examination, investigations and management. History-wise, I would like to know if it is similar pain to that present prior to surgery. How is it graded on the VAS scale? Any other neurology? Was there any intraoperative incident such as nerve damage or dural tear? Was there prolonged retraction of the nerves? I will examine the patient to make sure the spinal wound is dry. I will do a complete neurological examination to look for any neurology.

Mild pain is expected after surgery like TLIF or PLIF. However, if there is any neurology or significant pain, I will request an urgent CT scan first to look at screw position. Any screw in close proximity to or displacing the nerve will need revision.

EXAMINER: Thank you.

Learning points

1. Oblique view X-ray – discontinuity in the neck of Scotty dog.

2. Pars is the junction between pedicle, lamina and facet.

3. Spondylosis – defect in pars interarticularis.

4. 90% of normal volunteers will show 1–3 mm of translation on flexion–extension lateral radiographs. More than 4 mm is regarded as abnormal.

5. Anterior retroperitoneal approach is sometimes asked for exams.

6. The above scenario can be replaced with degenerative spondylolisthesis. Know that L4/5 is the most common level. Also, it is important to know the nerve root involved, symptoms of canal stenosis and surgical management.

References

1. Bridwell KH. *The Textbook of Spinal Surgery*, 3rd edn. 2011. Lippincott.

2. Sailhan F, Gollogly S, Roussouly P. The radiographic results and neurologic complications of instrumented reduction and fusion of high-grade spondylolisthesis without decompression of the neural elements: a retrospective review of 44 patients. *Spine*. 2006;31(2):161–169.

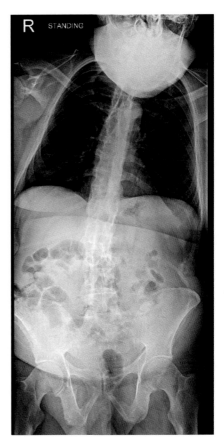

Figure 6.7a Anteroposterior (AP) full spine radiograph.

Structured oral examination question 7

Ankylosing spondylitis

EXAMINER: This is an X-ray of a 25-year-old male referred to your clinic with a history of back pain. Can you please describe this X-ray (Figures 6.7a and 6.7b)?

CANDIDATE: AP and lateral standing X-rays of full spine showing widespread ossification depicting 'Bamboo spine'. AP X-ray shows bilateral sacroiliac ankyloses and early arthritis of both hips. There is positive sagittal balance on the lateral X-rays as the C7 plumb line falls anterior to S1. These findings are suggestive of ankylosing spondylitis.

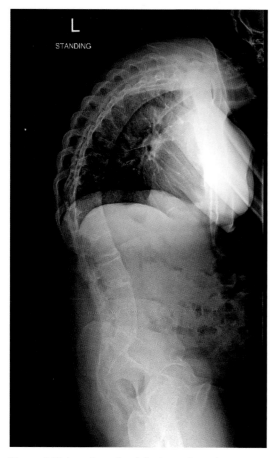

Figure 6.7b Lateral standing full-spine radiograph.

EXAMINER: So, this is an X-ray of a patient with ankylosing spondylitis (AS)?

CANDIDATE: No. To label a patient with AS, *Modified New York Criteria* are helpful. One radiological criterion and at least one clinical criterion are to be satisfied. I need to take a history and examine this patient for obtaining my clinical criteria.

Radiological criterion

Sacroiliitis at least grade 2 bilaterally or grade 3 or 4 unilaterally.

Clinical criteria

- Low back pain and stiffness for more than 3 months that improves with exercise but is not relieved by rest.

- Limitation of motion of the lumbar spine in both the sagittal and frontal planes.
- Limitation of chest expansion relative to normal values correlated for age and sex.

EXAMINER: What are the other X-ray findings of AS?

CANDIDATE: The sacroiliac joints initially show loss of definition of subchondral bone. This is followed by erosions, sclerosis and finally ankyloses.

The earliest sign in the spine is squaring of the vertebral bodies. This is followed by marginal syndesmophytes and finally widespread ankyloses.

EXAMINER: What is the pathology in AS?

CANDIDATE: AS is seronegative (Rh factor negative), autoimmune, chronic, spondyloarthropathy. The exact mechanism is not known, possibly an autoimmune reaction to environmental pathogen in a genetically susceptible individual. There are theories in relation to HLA B27 (90% patients are positive).

EXAMINER: What are the orthopaedic manifestations of AS?

CANDIDATE:

- Bilateral sacroiliitis progressing to frank ankyloses.
- Spine – loss of movements, ankyloses, kyphotic deformity, fractures.
- Hips – flexion contractures, arthritis, ankyloses.
- Other joints (knees, shoulders and ankle) – arthritis, although less likely as it mainly affects the axial skeleton.
- Enthesopathy – inflammation of enthuses or tendon insertion (tendoachilles most commonly affected).

EXAMINER: How do you differentiate between AS and DISH (diffuse idiopathic skeletal hyperostosis)?

CANDIDATE: AS affects young males and has strong predisposition for HLA B27. DISH on the other hand affects older patients who are usually diabetics. The disc and sacroiliac joints are spared in DISH unlike AS. The syndesmophytes are non-marginal in DISH and marginal in AS. Lastly, there is osteopenia in AS but increased radio density in DISH.

147

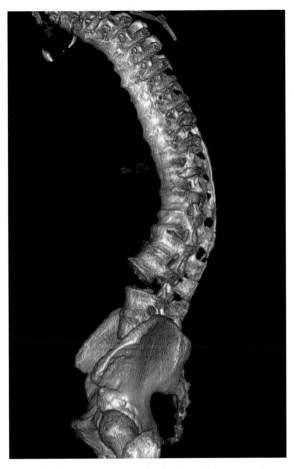

Figure 6.7c CT scan demonstrating fracture dislocation at L3/4.

EXAMINER: How would you go about examining this patient?

CANDIDATE: General examination: cardiac, respiratory (reduced chest expansion, renal and abdomen).

Spine examination: gait, inspection, palpation, movements, neurology (including special tests like Schoeber's, Wall test, chin brow angle).

Rest of orthopaedic examination: sacroiliac joint, hips, knees.

EXAMINER: What are the hip findings in AS?

CANDIDATE: Arthritis, ankyloses, protusio, heterotrophic ossification and severe hip flexion deformities (usually bilateral).

EXAMINER: If patient has concurrent spine deformity and hip deformity needing THR, what surgery would you recommend first?

CANDIDATE: As a general principle, spine deformity is addressed prior to hip. The reason suggested is that dislocation rates are higher in THR that are followed by spine deformity correction.

EXAMINER: How do you manage these patients?

CANDIDATE: This needs a multidisciplinary approach that includes rheumatologist, physiotherapist, occupational therapist, orthopaedician. Medical management includes drugs such as NSAIDS, COX2 inhibitors and TNF alpha inhibitors.

The spine surgeon has a role for correcting deformities or surgical stabilization of fractures.

Deformity correction is correction of kyphosis that can be done lumbar (restore sagittal balance) or cervicothoracic (correction of chin on chest deformity).

EXAMINER: What level are these osteotomies done?

CANDIDATE: Lumbar osteotomy like pedicle subtraction osteotomy is performed usually at L2 or L3 level. This is because the cord ends above this level and this is also the site for the fulcrum of the deformity.

Cervicothoracic osteotomy is performed at C7 T1 level as the vertebral artery is exterior and the canal diameter is also larger at this level.

EXAMINER: This is a CT scan of the same patient presenting with acute-onset back pain after a fall (Figure 6.7c). Please comment.

CANDIDATE: CT scan shows a fracture dislocation at L3/4. Rest of the spine looks ankylosed.

EXAMINER: [Interrupting] Are fractures common?

CANDIDATE: Fractures are not uncommon due to altered biomechanical properties of the spine. The ossified spine creates long lever arms limiting the ability to absorb even small impacts. Besides, there is osteoporosis due to stress shielding, immobility and inflammatory process. These fractures are invariably missed and are associated with high incidence of neurological complications and pseudoarthrosis.

EXAMINER: Thank you.

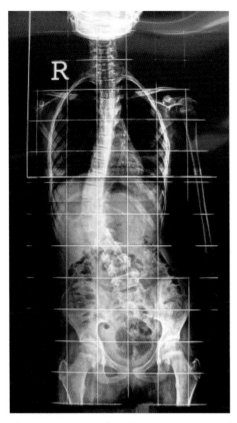

Figure 6.8a Standing frontal posteroanterior (PA) radiograph spine.

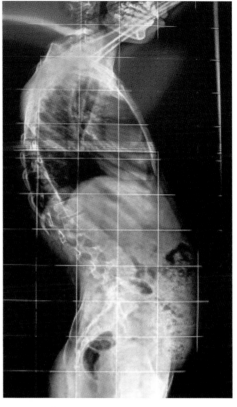

Figure 6.8b Lateral radiograph spine.

Other points

1. Difference between marginal (AS) and non-marginal syndesmophytes (DISH).
2. Non-articular manifestations:
   Eyes: acute anterior uveitis.
   Heart: conduction defects, aortitis, aortic regurgitation or stenosis.
   Respiratory: pulmonary fibrosis.
   Renal: amyloid nephropathy.
   Gastrointestinal: associated with Crohn's disease and ulcerative colitis.
3. Preoperative anaesthesia concerns.
4. Different osteotomies for kyphosis correction.
5. Causes of kyphosis.

Structured oral examination question 8

Idiopathic scoliosis

EXAMINER: Could you please comment on this AP standing X-ray of a 15-year-old female who has come to your clinic with history of spinal deformity (Figure 6.8a)?

CANDIDATE: Standing PA (Figure 6.8a) spine X-ray shows a single right-sided convex thoracic scoliosis with the apex at T12. There is loss of coronal balance with the C7 plumb line falling to the right of the central sacral line. In other words, the curve is unbalanced. The Cobb angle roughly measures around 50°. The pelvis shows Risser's 1 stage based on less than 25% of the calcification of the lateral iliac apophysis.

EXAMINER: What do you mean by Risser's grading?

149

CANDIDATE: Ossification of the iliac apophysis begins laterally (ASIS) and proceeds medially (PSIS) to eventually cap the entire iliac crest. Risser's 1–5 is a measure of skeletal maturity and therefore a predictor of curve progression. Risser's 0 means no ossification centre is visible. Risser 0 and Risser 5 are similar on X-rays with no appearance of ossification centres. However, they are easily distinguished by age with Risser's 0 at 5 years and Risser's 5 after 16 years of age.

It helps in estimating curve progression. So Risser 0 means more growth remaining and more chances of curve progression as the skeleton grows. This translates into more need of surgical intervention. Risser's 5, on the other hand, is less likely to progress as the skeletal maturity has been achieved.

EXAMINER: You mentioned a Cobb angle of 50°. How is this measured?

CANDIDATE: I identified the end vertebra that has the pedicle level with the greatest tilt from the horizontal. These are the end plates with greatest deviation from the horizontal. In this case it seems to be T7 and L2. The Cobb angle is the angle between these two vertebrae.

EXAMINER: Please comment on the lateral X-rays (Figure 6.8b).

CANDIDATE: The lateral spine X-ray shows loss of thoracic kyphosis, but the sagittal balance is well maintained.

EXAMINER: Do you feel this is an idiopathic curve?

CANDIDATE: X-ray findings suggest this is probably an idiopathic curve. But to be certain, I need to take a history, do examination and request investigations if needed.

EXAMINER: How would you go about that?

CANDIDATE: Findings suggestive of a non-idiopathic curve are:

History – symptoms of a generalized syndrome or disorder (e.g. muscular dystrophy of neurofibromatosis), back pain, neurology such as weakness in any limbs, bowel or bladder symptoms.

Examination – asymmetrical reflexes, neurology, foot abnormalities.

Investigations – X-ray findings of atypical left-sided curve, acute angular curve, scalloping of vertebrae or pencilling of ribs. MRI features such as bone and spinal cord anomalies, syrinx, tumour or infection.

EXAMINER: How do you differentiate between flexible and structural curve?

CANDIDATE: A flexible curve normalizes with lateral bending. The structural curve fails to correct.

EXAMINER: What is the role of Adams' forward bending test?

CANDIDATE: After ruling out leg length discrepancy that can be a cause of scoliosis, the patient bends forward at the waist. The examiner looks from behind for the sign of scoliosis which is a prominent rib hump.

EXAMINER: Do you think this curve is likely to progress?

CANDIDATE: This is a Rissers 1 stage of skeletal growth with the curve measuring 50°. Severe curve with skeletal growth remaining is likely to progress.

EXAMINER: Having proved this is idiopathic scoliosis on history and examination in a 12-year-old girl who has not attained her menarche, how do you proceed?

CANDIDATE: I will need to first perform lateral bending views to see if the curve corrects to any degree. This will help decide on the fusion levels.

EXAMINER: Don't you need an MRI?

CANDIDATE: MRI indications would be any clinical features of a generalized syndrome or foot abnormalities pointing towards a non-idiopathic scoliosis. So also, any neurology, abnormal abdominal reflexes, atypical curve such as a left-sided curve, acute angular curve, presence of significant kyphosis would warrant an MRI.

EXAMINER: What next?

CANDIDATE: This is not a curve between 20 and 40° where bracing would be indicated. Observation is indicated for curves less than 20°. This curve being 50° will need surgical correction. Surgical options include posterior spinal fusion, anterior spinal fusion or combined anterior and posterior spinal fusion. Posterior spinal fusion is the surgery most commonly done. Anterior fusion is indicated for thoracolumbar and lumbar curves with normal sagittal profile. Combined anterior and posterior correction is performed for larger curves > 75° or stiff curves and younger patients to prevent the crankshaft phenomenon.

EXAMINER: Thank you.

NOTE: Although it is generally wise to answer to the point and what is asked, it also makes sense to answer in such a manner that it eliminates the need of further questions and depicts a logical thought process on the part of the candidate. This is evident in the last answer with regards to management of the above patient.

Other points

1. Scoliosis is a Cobb angle measure more than 10°. It is a three-dimensional deformity of the spine and rib cage in coronal plane, sagittal plane and abnormal rotation of the vertebrae.

2. Define end vertebrae, stable vertebrae, neutral vertebrae and apical vertebrae.

3. Aetiology of scoliosis:

   Scoliosis is a descriptive term and not a diagnosis.

   (1) Idiopathic: 80% of cases.
       (a) Infantile – 0 to 3 years.
       (b) Juvenile – 3 to 10 years.
       (c) Adolescent – 10+ years.

   (2) Congenital (present at birth):
       (a) Failure of formation – hemivertebrae.
       b) Failure of segmentation – unilateral unsegmented bar.
       (c) Mixed.

   (3) Neuromuscular.
       (a) Upper motor neuron: cerebral palsy.
       (b) Lower motor neuron: polio.
       (c) Muscular weakness: muscular dystrophies.

   (4) Others.
       (a) Syndromes: Marfans, Ehlers Danlos, neurofibromatosis.
       (b) Tumours: osteoid osteoma.
       (c) Trauma.
       (d) Compensatory: leg length discrepancy.

4. Complications of scoliosis surgery.
5. Approaches to spine.

6. Deciding levels of fusion – include levels to correct the sagittal and coronal curvatures. Fusion extends from the caudal end vertebrae to stable vertebrae.

Structured oral examination question 9

Non-idiopathic scoliosis

As stated above, there are many aetiologies for non-idiopathic scoliosis. Clinical pictures or X-rays can pop up for viva stations. For treating scoliosis, certain questions are needed to be answered.

1. Is this idiopathic or non-idiopathic? This is well answered in the previous case.

2. Is the scoliosis part of a syndrome? Look for clues such as Café-au-lait spots, axillary or inguinal freckling, Marfanoid features, scissoring gait of cerebral palsy, etc.

3. Is there any neurology? If yes, investigate with MRI (*MRI is almost always needed for all non-idiopathic scoliosis*) to look for cord tethering, syrinx, diatometamyelia or Arnold Chiari malformation. The treatment for this precedes scoliosis for two reasons. First, as this is the cause, likelihood of recurrence is high. Second, stretching a cord that has a pathology such as tethering during scoliosis correction can lead to high chances of intra- and postoperative neurological deficit.

4. Is the curve structural or non-structural? A non-structural curve normalizes with lateral bending. The structural curve fails to correct less than 25°. This helps in deciding fusion levels.

5. Is the patient fit for anaesthesia? Conservative treatment with a brace for a child not fit for major surgical procedure and anaesthesia.

6. Can this scoliosis be treated with non-surgical management? Non-progressive curves, small Cobb angle, patient compliant to brace. Sometimes, the goal is to delay surgery to an older age. This not only allows growth but reduces the risk of anaesthesia in a very young child. This may not be the case for all aetiology. With some pathologies such as Duchenne's muscular dystrophy, pulmonary function reduces with advancing age.

Congenital scoliosis in the form of unilateral unsegmented bar with contralateral hemivertebrae has the highest chance of curve progression (100%). Hemivertebrae in the lumbosacral region almost always needs surgery as the lumbar spine takes off obliquely from the sacrum leading to a long compensatory curve in the rest of the spine. Surgical treatment involves excision of the hemivertebrae, short or long segment fusion or growing rods. These children may also have other conditions – VACTERL syndrome, Klippel Fiel syndrome, or other systemic anomalies.

For neuromuscular scoliosis (cerebral palsy, muscular dystrophies), surgery is indicated for improvement in seating posture, trunk control or to prevent further deterioration in pulmonary function. Because the musculature is weak, there is a good chance of recurrence if short segment fusion is done. More so, these patients are not physiologically geared for revision surgeries or prolonged anaesthesia. Long segment fusion from T1/T2 to sacrum (pelvic obliquity) is the usual norm for the posterior spinal fusion.

EXAMINER: Please can you comment on these X-rays (Figures 6.9a and 6.9b)?

CANDIDATE: AP (Figure 6.9a) and lateral (Figure 6.9b) X-rays of full spine showing kyphoscoliosis of the thoracolumbar spine. The curve appears balanced on the coronal plane with the convexity towards the left. This is a sharp angulated curve with pencilling of the ribs, enlarged neural foramen on lateral view and vertebral scalloping. These are features of neurofibromatosis. The Cobb angle is about 90°.

EXAMINER: Yes, this is neurofibromatosis (NF). So, what are the orthopaedic manifestations of neurofibromatosis?

CANDIDATE: Spine and extremities are involved in NF. Spinal involvement is the most common with scoliosis, kyphosis and atlanto-axial instability. Extremity involvement is in the form of hemihypertrophy of the limb and pseudoarthrosis of the tibia.

Scoliosis can be of two types. Non-dystrophic scoliosis resembles non-idiopathic scoliosis. Dystrophic scoliosis has features such as short segment with sharp angulation, kyphosis, enlarged neural foramina, vertebral scalloping, pencilling of ribs, similar to the X-rays depicted here.

EXAMINER: How would you confirm this case to be secondary to neurofibromatosis?

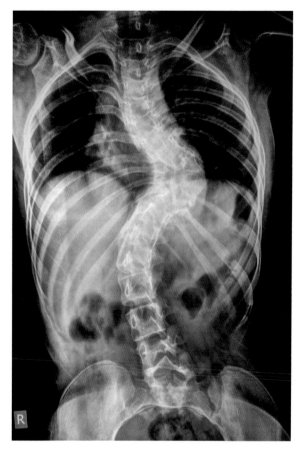

Figure 6.9a Anteroposterior (AP) radiograph of full spine.

CANDIDATE: According to the NIH Consensus Development Conference Statement (1987) the diagnostic criteria for NF-1 are met in an individual if two or more of the following are found:

- Six or more café-au-lait macules over 5 mm in greatest diameter in prepubertal individuals and over 15 mm in postpubertal individuals.
- Two or more neurofibromas of any type or one plexiform neurofibroma.
- Freckling in the axillary or inguinal region.
- Optic glioma.
- Two or more Lisch nodules (iris hamartomas).
- A distinctive osseous lesion such as sphenoid dysplasia or thinning of long bone cortex with or without pseudarthrosis.
- A first-degree relative (parent, sibling, or offspring) with NF-1 by the above criteria is based on presence of both.

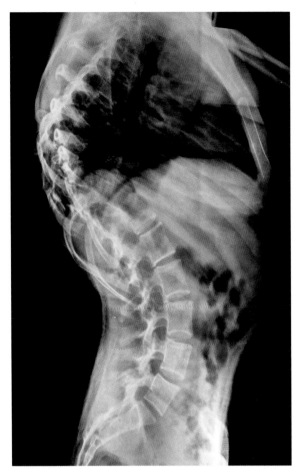

Figure 6.9b Lateral radiograph of full spine.

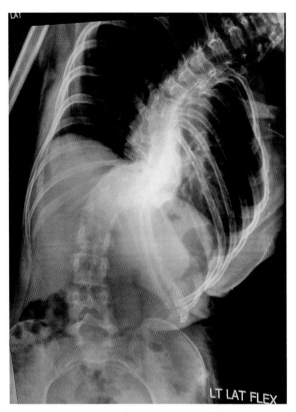

Figure 6.9c Lateral oblique bending radiographic image of lumbar spine (left lateral flexion).

EXAMINER: Consider this to be a case of NF in a 16-year-old female with menarche 3 years ago. The spine is progressive deformity and is the only orthopaedic manifestation. What next?

CANDIDATE: I need to take a history to know the symptoms and examine the child. I need to know what the symptoms are and examine to rule out any neurological deficit. I will also need further investigations.

EXAMINER: If there is neurology, what is the cause?

CANDIDATE: The deformity itself can lead to neurology due to stretching of the neurological structures. So also, neural compromise can be due to tumour (neurofibromata).

EXAMINER: As mentioned, this is a progressive deformity with spine the only concern. There is no neurology on examination.

CANDIDATE: I need further investigations. I need lateral bending X-rays and MRI full spine.

EXAMINER: MRI does not add much. These are the lateral bending X-rays (Figures 6.9c and 6.9d).

CANDIDATE: There is not much correction of the curve on bending views. This being a dystrophic curve will need combined anterior and posterior spinal fusion. There may also be a need of decompression depending on the intraoperative findings. This case will need correction of the coronal as well as the sagittal balance.

EXAMINER: Why do you need combined anterior and posterior fusion?

CANDIDATE: Pseudoarthrosis is very high with PSF alone up to the rate of 40%. Even with the combined approach, the rate is 10%.

EXAMINER: Why not bracing?

CANDIDATE: Bracing is not effective in dystrophic curve. It can be applied to non-dystrophic curves

153

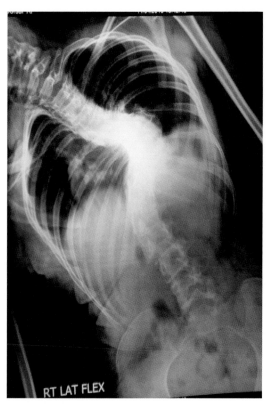

Figure 6.9d Lateral oblique bending radiographic image of lumbar spine (right lateral flexion).

that behave similar to AIS. Also, the magnitude of the curve about 90° is not suitable for bracing.

EXAMINER: You mentioned about sagittal balance. How do you calculate that?

CANDIDATE: Sagittal balance can be found from clinical examination when viewed from the sides, but is best calculated on standing lateral X-rays.

A normal or neutral sagittal balance means a plumb line falling from the centre of C7 should fall on the posterosuperior edge of S1 vertebra. If the C7 line falls in front of S1 then it is positive sagittal balance and if it falls behind S1 then it is negative sagittal balance. The osteoporotic thoracic spine in old patients with previous fractures easily illustrates this. These patients have positive sagittal balance and hence their centre of gravity shifts forward. This in turn predisposes them for further wedge compression fractures with worsening of kyphotic deformity (dowager's hump).

EXAMINER: [Running out of questions] Tell me the blood supply of the spinal cord?

CANDIDATE: Blood supply is provided by:

- Anterior spinal artery – a single artery supplying the anterior two-thirds of the cord that includes both the lateral and ventral corticospinal tract. It originates from branches of the vertebral arteries.
- Posterior spinal arteries – paired on either side and supplying the posterior one-third of the cord (dorsal columns). Originating from the vertebral artery or the posterior inferior cerebral artery.
- Anastomoses between the spinal arteries called arterial vasacorona that supply the peripheral lateral aspect of the cord. These in turn are reinforced by the segmental (radicular) arteries such as the ascending cervical artery, deep cervical artery, posterior intercostal arteries, lumbar arteries and lateral sacral arteries.

The dominant segmental artery is the artery of Adamkiewicz. This arises from the left posterior intercostal artery (originating from aorta) and supplies the lower two-thirds of the spinal cord via the anterior spinal artery. Most often it originates from the left side between T8 and L1 vertebral segments. Damage to this artery can lead to paralysis from spinal cord infarction.

EXAMINER: Thank you.

Structured oral examination question 10

Cervical prolapse disc

EXAMINER: What changes happen in the disc with age?

CANDIDATE: Increasing age is associated with progressive dehydration of the intervertebral disc. Histologically, the boundary between the nucleus pulposus and the annulus fibrosus becomes less distinct. There is a progressive loss of proteoglycan, absolute viable cell number and water. There is an increase in the keratin to chondroitin sulphate ratio.

EXAMINER: Can you tell me the blood supply of the adult intervertebral disc?

CANDIDATE: Adult intervertebral discs are avascular. The nutrition occurs via diffusion across the motor end plates. This can explain discitis after vertebral osteomyelitis in adults. Children, on the

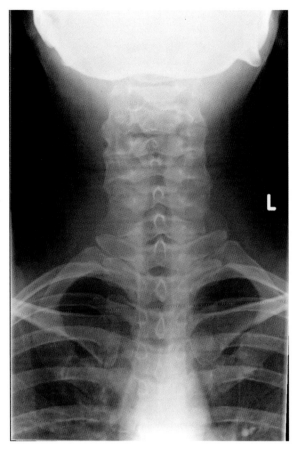

Figure 6.10a Anteroposterior (AP) radiograph of cervical spine.

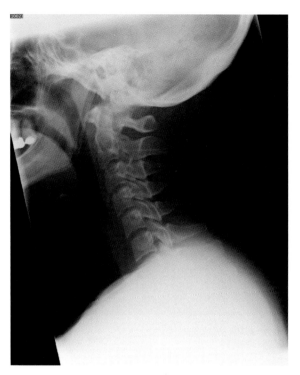

Figure 6.10b Lateral radiograph of lumbar spine.

other hand, have vascular discs, so discitis can occur without vertebral osteomyelitis.

EXAMINER: These are X-rays of a 35-year-old fit and healthy man working at a desk job. Can you please comment on the same (Figures 6.10a and 6.10b)?

CANDIDATE: X-rays AP and lateral of the cervical spine. The lateral X-ray shows loss of cervical lordosis. This lateral X-ray does not show lower cervical levels and is inadequate. The AP X-ray is largely unremarkable. I will need to see a better view of the cervical spine to look for any pathology in the lower cervical spine.

EXAMINER: This man has right upper limb pain with axial neck pain. How would you manage this patient?

CANDIDATE: I will start with history. I would want to know how long he has had these symptoms. Where is the location of the neck pain and arm pain? Does it follow any dermatome? What treatment has he had so far? Expectations?

EXAMINER: His pain is along the right C7 dermatome. He is on over-the-counter analgesics. No other significant history.

CANDIDATE: I will proceed towards examination. General examination, spine examination with neurology, examination of neighbouring joints, especially the shoulders.

EXAMINER: He has reduced neck range of motion. No neurology and no other abnormalities on examination. Reflexes are normal.

CANDIDATE: Spurlings sign?

EXAMINER: How do you perform it?

CANDIDATE: Simultaneous extension, rotation to the affected side, lateral bend, and vertical compression will reproduce symptoms in the ipsilateral arm. This is a provocative test for cervical disc prolapse.

EXAMINER: This sign is positive on one side. What do you do next?

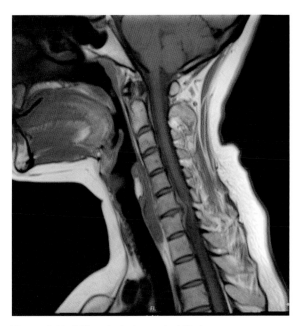

Figure 6.10c MRI cervical spine, sagittal T1 view.

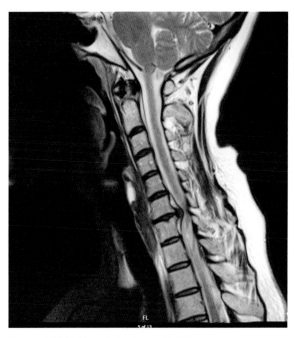

Figure 6.10d MRI cervical spine, sagittal T2 view.

CANDIDATE: So, this patient has radiculopathy most probably due to cervical disc prolapse. I will reassure this patient, provide analgesia and arrange for a follow-up in 4 weeks' time. I will explain to him that this seems to be a prolapsed cervical disc with a good chance of recovery. I will also explain to him that if in the interim he develops any neurology, then he needs to come back and see us urgently.

EXAMINER: Don't you need an MRI?

CANDIDATE: His symptoms are just 4 weeks duration with no neurology or red flags. There is no indication for an MRI at this stage.

EXAMINER: He comes back to you after 4 weeks with persistent symptoms. Now what?

CANDIDATE: I will now request an MRI.

EXAMINER: Please comment (Figures 6.10c and 6.10d).

CANDIDATE: T1 (Figure 6.10c), T2 (Figure 6.10d) and axial (Figure 6.10e) MRI of the cervical spine showing a disc prolapse at C6/7 with compression of the right C7 nerve root. There appears to be some compression of the spinal cord. I will need to make sure this patient has no symptoms and signs of cord compression.

EXAMINER: This patient only has symptoms of radiculopathy with no cord compression. This patient has no change of findings and is now asking questions about surgery.

CANDIDATE: I will continue with non-operative management. I will start the patient on Pregabalin and arrange for physiotherapy if he has not had some already. There is again no indication for surgery at this moment of time. This is as per NICE guidance for management of cervical radiculopathy 2015 [1]. Also, this is a soft disc with high water content and likely to resolve.

The natural history of cervical radiculopathy is favourable with most patients having resolution of symptoms. Lees and Turner in a long-term follow-up of patients with radiculopathy showed that 45% of patients had a single episode of radiculopathy that resolved; 30% had mild symptoms and 25% had persistent or worsening symptoms [2]. It is not common for radiculopathy patients to progress to myelopathy [3].

EXAMINER: What are the surgeries you know for prolapsed cervical disc?

CANDIDATE: Anterior cervical discectomy and fusion, posterior foraminotomy and anterior cervical discectomy with disc replacement. If surgery

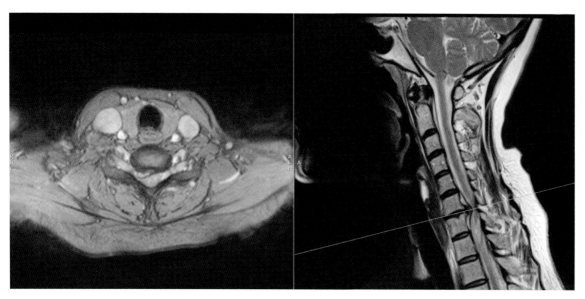

Figure 6.10e MRI cervical spine, axial views.

is indicated for this case, posterior foraminotomy is a good option as this is a soft disc with single-level radiculopathy.

EXAMINER: Is there any role of cervical traction?

CANDIDATE: A Cochrane systematic review aimed to assess the effects of mechanical traction on neck disorders. Graham *et al.* found no statistically significant difference between continuous traction and placebo traction in reducing pain or improving function [4].

EXAMINER: What are the advantages and disadvantages of posterior laminoforaminotomy?

CANDIDATE: Posterior laminoforaminotomy is indicated in patients with radiculopathy with minimal or no neck pain and maintained cervical lordosis. The radiculopathy is due to posterolateral disc herniation or an osteophyte compressing the nerve root. It has minimal patient morbidity and avoids the need of fusion. The disadvantage is that it requires retraction of the nerve root, risking further nerve irritation or injury.

EXAMINER: Is it safe to offer cervical disc replacement (CDR) as compared to fusion if planning anterior surgery?

CANDIDATE: As per the NICE guidance, current evidence on the efficacy of prosthetic intervertebral disc replacement in the cervical spine shows that this procedure is at least as efficacious as fusion in the short term and may result in a reduced need for revision surgery in the long term. The evidence raises no particular safety issues that are not already known in relation to fusion procedures [5].

This patient is an ideal candidate for CDR if contemplating anterior surgery as the compression is mainly anterior with no posterior facet arthrosis as evident on the MRI scan.

EXAMINER: Thank you.

References

1. https://cks.nice.org.uk/neck-pain-cervical-radiculopathy

2. Lees F, Turner JW. Natural history of cervical spondylosis. *BMJ*. 1963;2:1607–1610.

3. Sampath P, Bendebba M, Davis JD, *et al.* Outcome in patients with cervical radiculopathy: prospective, multicenter study with independent clinical review. *Spine*. 1999; 24:591–597.

4. Graham N, Gross A, Goldsmith CH, *et al.* Mechanical traction for neck pain with or without radiculopathy. *Cochrane Database Syst Rev*. 2008;3: CD006408.

5. www.nice.org.uk/Guidance/ipg341

Introduction

A viva examination is like playing a game. The candidate should know the subject well, have a game plan and more importantly should know the opponent. A candidate who manages to answer the higher-order thinking/judgement questions at the end of the viva will make it a rewarding 5 minutes (for both the examiner and candidate) and more importantly will score a 7/8. An examiner relishes a candidate who takes control and makes their life easy.

Again, we must stress the importance of time management in the viva, as you have got only 5 minutes to score either eight or four and time is money! It is important to understand the scenario quickly and progress in the correct direction rather than using guess work. Avoid talking generally about the shoulder conditions to fill the time if your aim is to score well. Wherever possible support your answer by evidence (quoting literature) as this will get you past a basic pass and on to a higher score. Be careful, however, not to quote unnecessary or irrelevant evidence which will not only irritate the examiners and not score you any extra marks but is rather crass and bovine.

The main aim of this chapter is to express the importance of viva techniques and therefore it is not written as a textbook. Analyse the good as well as the poor techniques illustrated in the scenarios and follow the ones you find most useful.

Shoulder

In a shoulder structured oral question try and analyze the question according to its presentation. Broadly, shoulder pathology can be classified as painful, weak, stiff or unstable conditions. Shoulder pathology varies with different age groups and therefore you should have a list of age-related diagnoses clear in your mind, which will be helpful in the viva. There can be overlaps of these conditions, for example a painful stiff shoulder may represent frozen shoulder or acute calcific tendonitis or arthritis. Therefore, candidates should have a list of conditions and one or two classical questions to differentiate one from the other, to lead into the scenario comfortably right from the start.

Some scenarios to remember:

Young patient (less than 30 years of age): instability, SLAP lesions.

Middle-aged patient (30–50): impingement, calcific tendonitis, frozen shoulder, cuff tears.

Elderly patient (> 50): cuff tear, OA, cuff tear arthropathy.

Structured oral examination question 1

Tuberculosis shoulder

EXAMINER: This is a radiograph of the left shoulder of an 84-year-old lady. Describe the radiograph please (Figure 7.1).

CANDIDATE: Well . . . Good morning.
This is the plain radiograph of an 84-year-old lady's left shoulder. Anteroposterior (AP) view. There is evidence of joint destruction with loss of articular anatomy . . .

EXAMINER: What do you think is wrong with this shoulder?

CANDIDATE: Well, to be certain, I need to ask a few questions and examine the patient . . .

EXAMINER: Go on then and ask some questions.

CANDIDATE: Is she right-handed or left-handed?

EXAMINER: Right-handed.

CANDIDATE: How long has she had a problem with this shoulder?

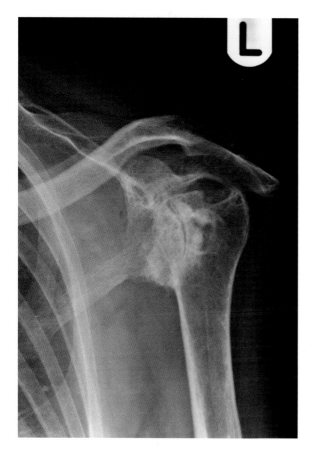

Figure 7.1 Anteroposterior (AP) radiograph of left shoulder.

EXAMINER: 70 years.

CANDIDATE: How did the problem start?

EXAMINER: It started as a painless lump when she was 14 and a few months later she began to have a discharging sinus that required several joint washouts and medication.

CANDIDATE: Does she have an active sinus now?

EXAMINER: No, the sinus healed after she underwent shoulder washouts and started her medication and has never recurred.

CANDIDATE: That is good. What are her current problems?

EXAMINER: Well she has some restriction of movements and therefore visited her GP, who had performed this X-ray and sent her to you for your opinion.

CANDIDATE: Then I would examine the patient.

EXAMINER: She has 60° of abduction and forward elevation and has very restricted rotations.

CANDIDATE: I would like to know the power of her cuff muscles.

EXAMINER: It is not possible to assess the power as she has very restricted range of movements.

CANDIDATE: Now . . .
[Bell]

EXAMINER: Thank you.

Did this candidate do well? Was there a diagnosis? Was there a discussion about the management? Only a 4 or 5 score would be given as the candidate did not even arrive at a diagnosis and missed all the clues/prompts.

A different candidate with the same scenario:

EXAMINER: This is a radiograph of the left shoulder of an 84-year-old lady. Please describe the X-ray.

CANDIDATE: This is an anteroposterior (AP) radiographic view of the shoulder that shows evidence of joint destruction and loss of articular cartilage.

EXAMINER: What do you think is wrong with this shoulder?

CANDIDATE: This appearance suggests several possible causes such as previous joint infection, trauma or a neurogenic cause. May I know how and when the problem started?

EXAMINER: Her shoulder difficulties began as a painless lump when she was 14 years old and after a few months she went on to develop a discharging sinus that required several shoulder joint washouts and medication.

CANDIDATE: The presentation sounds like she had a low-grade joint infection. Was there any microbiological investigation performed at the time of the joint washouts?

EXAMINER: Yes, it was diagnosed as acid-fast bacillus and now what will be your management?

CANDIDATE: Well, I would like to know if she had any reactivation of infection in the last 70 years?

EXAMINER: No.

CANDIDATE: In that case what is the expectation of the patient?

EXAMINER: The patient does not want any surgical treatment. She wants to know if she can have an injection into her shoulder which can prevent the pain at the extremes of movements.

CANDIDATE: I will be cautious about the intra-articular steroid injections as it can trigger the dormant bacillus and rekindle the infection.

EXAMINER: OK, the patient comes back to you after 6 months and wants a shoulder joint replacement as her neighbour had one performed for arthritis a few weeks ago and is now pain-free and doing great with her shoulder. The patient wants the same operation. Will you offer her joint arthroplasty?

CANDIDATE: Again, I would be cautious to do so. I will certainly investigate her in terms of infective and inflammatory markers. I understand the principles of management of this case with the potential risk of recurrence of deep infection. This case will potentially require a biopsy, discussion with a microbiologist as part of an MDT meeting and a staged procedure. If active infection was present a two-stage procedure should be performed. The first stage would involve humeral head resection and insertion of an antibiotic-impregnated cement spacer. Multiple tuberculosis drug therapy for several months. I would biopsy the shoulder again and if it was negative for infection I would proceed with the second stage. I would prefer to use a reverse shoulder replacement in this patient as there is likely to be extensive destruction of the rotator cuff. I would counsel the patient that the surgery was likely to be protracted and drawn out as active TB of the shoulder needs to be eradicated before undertaking the second stage. I would warn her of the risk of further reactivation and reoccurrence of infection in the future.

EXAMINER: Would you offer her a one-stage procedure if active TB infection was present?

CANDIDATE: I am aware of a few case reports in which a primary single-stage cementless hemiarthroplasty has been performed for active TB with satisfactory results reported at 5 years, but I would prefer a more cautious approach and opt for a two-stage procedure [1].

EXAMINER: The patient does not want to take this risk and wants to be left alone. Thank you.

Although the viva questions started in the same manner, this candidate with his/her knowledge took

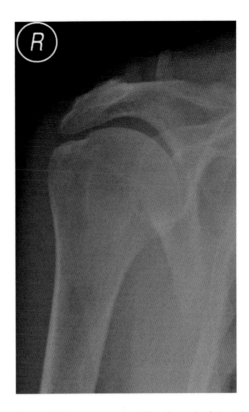

Figure 7.2 Anteroposterior (AP) radiograph of shoulder.

the viva to a good level of demonstration of his/her clinical judgement by asking specific questions and had control over the situation. Certainly, this candidate deserves a good score.

Reference

1. Luenam S, Kosiyatrakul A. Immediate cementless hemiarthroplasty for severe destructive glenohumeral tuberculous arthritis. Case Rep Orthoped. 2013;2013:426102.

Structured oral examination question 2

Rotator cuff tear

EXAMINER: Good afternoon. Can you tell me what is going on in this radiograph of the right shoulder (Figure 7.2)? This patient had anterior dislocation 2 years ago and has ongoing problems.

CANDIDATE: Well, this shoulder is reduced congruently. I cannot see any interposition of bony fragments. And I would like to investigate this shoulder with an MR arthrogram.

EXAMINER: What do you want to rule out?

CANDIDATE: Well, the risk of re-dislocation of the shoulder is much higher with anterior dislocation due to labral detachment in younger patients and it could be treated successfully if identified with MR arthrogram.

EXAMINER: This gentleman is claustrophobic!

CANDIDATE: I would talk to the radiologist and anaesthetist to find out if it could be done under sedation.

EXAMINER: The anaesthetist is not happy! And your radiologist suggests an ultrasound examination of the shoulder.

CANDIDATE: Ultrasound examination is not the gold standard examination for labral pathology.

EXAMINER: Well, the patient only had an ultrasound examination and it shows subscapularis tear!

CANDIDATE: There is then a high risk of having damaged the anterior labrum also ... I think I have to speak to the anaesthetist again ...

Another candidate follows this miserable viva of negotiations between anaesthetist and radiologist in the FRCS ortho exam (by the candidate's own fault). The candidate fails to start with the fundamental questions of age, how and when it happened and current problems and patient expectations, etc. This makes the entire viva go in the wrong direction and leads to a failing scenario.

EXAMINER: Good afternoon. Can you tell me what is going on in this radiograph of the right shoulder? This patient had anterior dislocation 2 years ago and has ongoing problems.

CANDIDATE: Thanks. May I know the age of the patient and the nature of the ongoing problem, please?

EXAMINER: This 76-year-old gentleman dislocated his shoulder 2 years ago. Now has got difficulties in overhead activities and we found out that he is claustrophobic!

CANDIDATE: I suspect rotator cuff tear in this age group following dislocation and also there is a risk of infraclavicular plexus injury following the dislocation; therefore, I would like to assess his cuff muscles clinically.

EXAMINER: He has got weakness on internal rotation and rest of the cuff power is good. Neurologically he is intact.

CANDIDATE: I suspect rotator cuff tear from this clinical assessment and I would investigate this shoulder with an ultrasound examination as he is claustrophobic. Ideally, I would have preferred an MRI scan to look for any fatty atrophy changes in the cuff, which could be detrimental in considering any repair of the cuff tear.

EXAMINER: The ultrasound examination shows full-thickness cuff tear of 4 mm with retraction.

CANDIDATE: I would like to know, what has been done so far? And what are his expectations?

EXAMINER: Nothing has been done so far. He wants to play golf, which he has not been able to do in the last 2 years.

CANDIDATE: Well, I would assess his shoulder clinically to assess for any weakness, stiffness and deltoid muscle compensation before considering any intervention as it's going on for 2 years and he is elderly. Although it could be a traumatic tear secondary to dislocation, quite often it could be over a degenerative tear.

EXAMINER: Would you call this cuff arthropathy as it is going on for 2 years?

CANDIDATE: No. The radiograph does not show any evidence of proximal migration of the humeral head.

EXAMINER: What will you do? How will you manage this patient?

CANDIDATE: I will explain to the patient that options are both non-operative (Deltoid rehab, physiotherapy) or operative management (arthroscopic/mini-open cuff repair – both techniques have equally good results) with caution as evidence suggests/reports up to 30% re-rupture rates in people above 65 years of age.
    [Bell]

This candidate knew the importance of age-related pathophysiology and succeeded well in the viva.

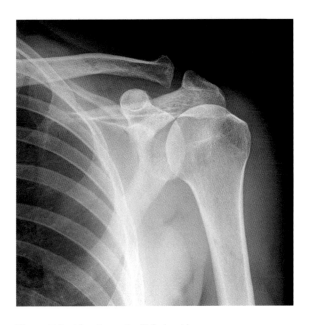

Figure 7.3a AP radiograph of left shoulder.

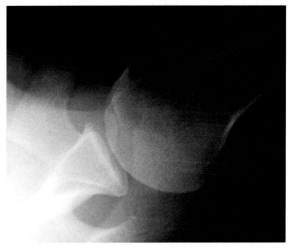

Figure 7.3b Axillary view of left shoulder.

Structured oral examination question 3

EXAMINER: This is a radiograph of the right shoulder of a lady who has got severe pain in her shoulder. Do you find anything interesting (Figure 7.3a)?

CANDIDATE: Well . . . No not really . . . I cannot see any abnormality or disease process in this radiograph. I would like to see a lateral radiograph of her shoulder.

CANDIDATE: I can't see anything abnormal here either.

EXAMINER: She is in your clinic referred by her GP. What would you like to do for her?

CANDIDATE: I want to get the history . . . then examine the patient . . . to decide on the management plan.

EXAMINER: Go ahead.

CANDIDATE: In the history I will first find out her age, job and dominant side . . . and how and when the problem started.

EXAMINER: She is 45, right-hand dominant and does clerical work. The pain started 8 months ago when she was reaching out for the seat belt in her car.

CANDIDATE: The age and history suggest probable frozen shoulder . . . I will proceed with the examination.

EXAMINER: She has got global restriction of her movements.

CANDIDATE: That confirms frozen shoulder. So . . .

EXAMINER: What do you want to do?

CANDIDATE: I would offer intra-articular steroid injection for her shoulder and also advise stretching exercises by physiotherapists.

EXAMINER: She has already had three intra-articular steroid injections and regular physiotherapy from her GP practice.

CANDIDATE: Well in that case I would advise her to have manipulation under anaesthesia (MUA) or arthroscopic arthrolysis.

EXAMINER: What will you specifically offer the patient?

CANDIDATE: mmm . . . MUA.

EXAMINER: The patient wants to know the risks associated with MUA.

CANDIDATE: Well apart from the anaesthetic risks, there is a risk of fracturing the humerus as it can be osteopenic from disuse . . . also the risk of recurrence.

EXAMINER: If the bone fractures, what will be the management?

CANDIDATE: It is like any fracture. Can be treated in a cast or operated.

162

EXAMINER: The patient decides now to leave it alone.

CANDIDATE: I will then convince her to have an injection today and review her situation in 12 weeks.

Do you think this candidate impressed the (patient or) the examiner with this simple shoulder scenario? Before we look at the next candidate, think how you would approach this differently!

EXAMINER: This is a radiograph of the right shoulder of a lady who has got severe pain in her shoulder. Do you find anything interesting?

CANDIDATE: Yes, this radiograph is essentially normal. May I know the age of this patient and does she suffer from diabetes or thyroid-related problems? Was there any history of trauma?

EXAMINER: Well, she is 45 and she has hypothyroidism. Is there anything else would you like to examine other than her shoulders?

CANDIDATE: Yes, I would like to look at her hand to see if she has any evidence of Dupuytren's contracture as it has some association with frozen shoulder.

EXAMINER: She is in your clinic referred by her GP. What would you like to do for her?

CANDIDATE: I want to know the history and examination findings.

EXAMINER: She is right-hand dominant and does clerical work. The pain started 8 months ago when she was reaching out for the seat belt in her car. She has global restriction of her movements.

CANDIDATE: Does this pain affect her sleep? What is the range of her external and internal rotation?

EXAMINER: Yes, she struggles to sleep at night and her ER is only to neutral position and she cannot get her hand to her back to do up her clothes. What would you like to do for her?

CANDIDATE: I want to know what has been done for her so far and what is her expectation.

EXAMINER: She had three intra-articular injections and physiotherapy from her GP practice. She wants to be able to wash and dress herself independently.

CANDIDATE: Well, I would like to offer her either manipulation under anaesthesia or arthroscopic capsular release, explaining the advantages and disadvantages, benefits and risks of both procedures and the importance of immediate postintervention physiotherapy and make her understand the disease process of frozen shoulder so that the patient could have a realistic expectation of the treatment process.

EXAMINER: The patient understands your explanation very well and wants to have the keyhole surgery. What will you do in arthroscopic capsular release?

CANDIDATE: The anterior capsule release especially at the rotator interval, followed by middle gleno-humeral ligament release and the release of the coraco-humeral ligament. The inferior capsule will be stretched by manipulation . . . this is my preference as the arthroscopic release of inferior capsule carries a small risk of damaging the axillary nerve.

EXAMINER: What does the evidence say, which is better – MUA/capsular release?

CANDIDATE: The literature is divided between both treatment modalities. MUA is simple and capsular release is a bit more invasive. There is also hydro-dilatation which some centres perform. The ongoing UK FROST trial (RCT) comparing

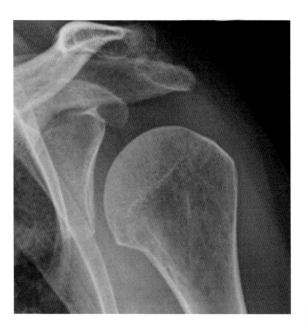

Figure 7.4a Anteroposterior (AP) view of right shoulder.

physio only vs MUA+physio vs MUA+capsular release should enable us to know which modality of treatment is better in the future.

EXAMINER: Thank you.

When the examiner sensed his ability a small extra challenge was given – do you want to examine anywhere else? And the candidate was able to demonstrate his/her knowledge – association with Dupuytren's contracture – the candidate would have been given an extra point for these smart moves and also backed up with evidence of literature and ongoing trials.

Structured oral examination question 4

EXAMINER: This is a radiograph of a 63-year-old gentleman's right shoulder (Figure 7.4a). Proceed.

CANDIDATE: This plain AP radiograph shows normal glenohumeral joint and acromioclavicular joint, well-maintained subacromial space but the under surface of the acromion is sclerotic, suggesting the possibility of him suffering from subacromial impingement. Can I see an axillary view, please?

EXAMINER: Yes (Figure 7.4b).

CANDIDATE: There are deposits of calcium in the supraspinatus tendon . . .

COMMENT: It is important to ask for multiple X-ray views of the shoulder to confirm the diagnosis of calcific tendonitis. The calcification may be missed with one view of the shoulder, particularly with subscapularis involvement, so AP radiographs in internal and external rotation as well as scapular Y and/or axillary views of the shoulder are recommended.

EXAMINER: What is your opinion about his pain in the shoulder?

CANDIDATE: Well, he could be struggling with calcific tendonitis.

EXAMINER: What do you want to do?

CANDIDATE: I would like to know the patient's symptoms, examination findings, the treatments he has had so far and his expectations.

EXAMINER: He is a keen golfer and gradually over the last 2 years he has developed the pain on overhead activities. He has not had any interventions so far. He wants to continue playing golf without pain. He has got positive impingement signs.

CANDIDATE: Well, I would inject his subacromial space with steroid today to relieve the bursitis secondary to the calcific tendonitis, which is causing impingement symptoms, and review him in 8 weeks in clinic with repeat X-rays to assess the calcium deposits.

EXAMINER: Incidentally there is also another X-ray of his right shoulder which was performed 2 years ago when he started to have the pain, which shows the same calcium deposits. Does it change your plan?

CANDIDATE: . . . Well, I would then book him now for arthroscopic excision of the calcium deposits.

EXAMINER: Will you perform any other procedures during the surgery?

CANDIDATE: I will consent him for arthroscopy and proceed . . . so that I can assess the shoulder and perform the necessary at the time of the surgery.

Did he not start well? Did this candidate proceed well – with diagnosis and management plan? Did he pick up the clues from the examiner and correct himself? What will be your scoring for this candidate? Will you diagnose and manage this problem differently like the next candidate?

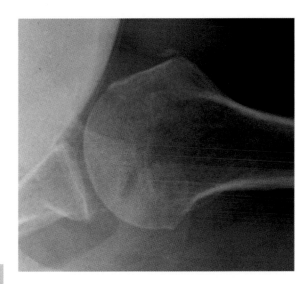

Figure 7.4b Axillary view of right shoulder.

EXAMINER: This is a radiograph of a 63-year-old gentleman's right shoulder. Proceed.

CANDIDATE: This plain AP radiograph shows normal glenohumeral joint and acromioclavicular joint, well-maintained subacromial space but the under surface of the acromion is sclerotic, suggesting the possibility of him suffering from subacromial impingement. Can I see an axillary view, please?

EXAMINER: Yes.

CANDIDATE: There are deposits of calcium in the supraspinatus tendon . . .

EXAMINER: What is your opinion about his pain in the shoulder?

CANDIDATE: Looking at the radiographs, and the duration of his problem . . . (EXAMINER: 2 years) and his age I feel he has got degenerative calcification in his cuff and subacromial impingement.

EXAMINER: What do you want to do?

CANDIDATE: I would like to know the patient's symptoms, examination findings, the treatments he has had so far and his expectations.

EXAMINER: He is a keen golfer and gradually over the last 2 years he has developed the pain on overhead activities. He has not had any interventions so far. He wants to continue playing golf without pain. He has got positive impingement signs.

CANDIDATE: I want to know if he has had any X-rays in the past and would like to assess the status of his cuff with an ultrasound scan/MRI scan.

EXAMINER: This is the X-ray taken 2 years ago – showing the same calcification. The recent ultrasound scan shows intact cuff.

CANDIDATE: Well, I would inject the subacromial bursa today with steroid and review the patient in 8 weeks to see if the injection has helped his pain as a diagnostic test for impingement.

EXAMINER: Suppose his old X-rays do not show any deposits and if it's recent then will you do the same?

CANDIDATE: In which case, this could be recent onset and I would consider sending the patient for ultrasound-guided injection and barbotage if

possible as the current evidence shows it's a good option as non-operative first-line management.

EXAMINER: OK, He comes back in 8 weeks saying the pain was well controlled for 3 weeks and now the pain is back. What will you do?

CANDIDATE: This proves the pathology of subacromial impingement and I am going to talk to the patient about subacromial decompression.

EXAMINER: Will you perform excision of the calcium deposits?

CANDIDATE: No, not necessarily. This degenerative calcification is a chronic one. It is not acute calcific tendonitis. I will perform subacromial decompression and assess his cuff for obvious calcific deposits; if so, I shall clear them during the procedure as long as I don't need to make a big rent/tear in the cuff/tendon which can lead to further weakness and unnecessary repair.

EXAMINER: Thank you.

This second candidate was much clearer about the pathology and management plan, which will be rewarded by a better score. He did not have to be prompted by the examiners regarding the calcium deposit which was there 2 years ago, suggesting the degenerative calcification. The previous candidate failed to understand these prompting clues.

Structured oral examination question 5

EXAMINER: Good afternoon. Can you tell me the findings from this radiograph of the left shoulder of a 76-year-old left-handed fit gentleman (Figure 7.5a)?

CANDIDATE: This anteroposterior view of the left shoulder shows no evidence of glenohumeral joint or acromioclavicular joint arthritis. The subacromial space is narrowed with sclerosis of the under surface of the acromion.

EXAMINER: Would you like any other investigations . . . prior to committing yourself with a diagnosis?

CANDIDATE: I would like to have ultrasound of his shoulder . . . and may I know his symptoms, please?

EXAMINER: The ultrasound which was requested by his GP shows torn subscapularis and supraspinatus

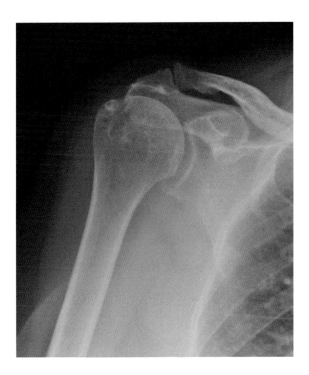

Figure 7.5a Anteroposterior (AP) radiograph of left shoulder.

with massive retraction of the tendons. He has difficulties with overhead activities. Can you tell me what is wrong with this shoulder?

CANDIDATE: From the X-ray ... which shows evidence of impingement by narrowing of the subacromial space, from the ultrasound scan ... which shows evidence of torn subscapularis and supraspinatus tendons and clinically he has got difficulties in overhead activities ...

EXAMINER: Yes, it is a nice summary of the situation [wasting time]

CANDIDATE: I think he has severe subacromial impingement and secondary cuff tear.

EXAMINER: What would you do for this gentleman?

CANDIDATE: Well, first I would perform a steroid injection into his subacromial space.

EXAMINER: Can you tell me the landmarks and how you will perform the injection?

CANDIDATE: Yes, 2 cm inferior and medial to the posterolateral corner of the acromion, I will direct the needle towards the anterolateral corner of the acromion to be specific into the bursa.

EXAMINER: Is it necessary to be specific in this patient ... he has got a massive cuff tear?

CANDIDATE: ??

EXAMINER: Well he comes back to clinic in 8 weeks with no difference to his symptoms. Do you have any management plans?

CANDIDATE: I will then perform an arthroscopic debridement of the cuff and bursa and a subacromial decompression.

EXAMINER: Thank you.

Do you recognize the candidate's mistakes? What would you do differently? Did he treat the patient or the investigations? Did he interpret the investigations appropriately? Now the last candidate of the day arrives for the same scenario.

EXAMINER: Good afternoon. Can you tell me the findings from this radiograph of the left shoulder of a 76-year-old left-handed fit gentleman?

CANDIDATE: This anteroposterior view of left shoulder shows proximal migration of humeral head with narrowing of the subacromial space and there is no evidence of glenohumeral joint or acromioclavicular joint arthritis.

EXAMINER: Would you like any other investigations ... prior to committing yourself with a diagnosis?

CANDIDATE: I would like to have an axillary view of his shoulder.

EXAMINER: Yes, we have axillary view. What are you looking for?

CANDIDATE: I am looking for anteroposterior subluxation of the humeral head in the axillary view ... yes, there is anterior subluxation, suggesting torn anteriorly placed subscapularis and from the AP view, the proximal migration of the humeral head suggesting supraspinatus tear ... this gentleman has got established cuff tear arthropathy.

EXAMINER: What would you do for him?

CANDIDATE: I need to know the patient's symptoms, what has been done for the patient so far and what are his expectations?

EXAMINER: He has got difficulties in overhead activities. He has had three injections by his GP, which have made no difference, and being an

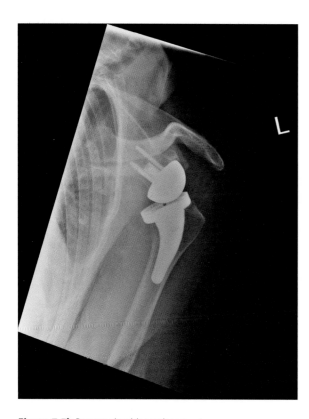

Figure 7.5b Reverse shoulder replacement.

artist he would like to have reasonable ability to abduct his shoulder to reach for the top of the canvas during painting.

CANDIDATE: Could you please tell me if he has any pain associated with his shoulder abduction?

EXAMINER: No . . . not at all.

CANDIDATE: I would start with non-operative management in terms of a deltoid muscle rehabilitation programme to compensate for the cuff deficiency. As he is not in pain and there is no established arthritis, this would be my initial management. If he fails with this treatment regime and is still struggling functionally, I would then offer a reverse-polarity shoulder replacement if he is otherwise healthy and fit for surgery. I will also get a CT scan of the shoulder joint to assess the glenoid bone stock and version as preoperative planning.

I would inform the patient the procedure is performed purely for functional outcome as he is not in pain and go through the benefits and risks and complications associated with such surgery.

EXAMINER: He is very fit. Why do you prefer reverse shoulder to a total shoulder replacement?

CANDIDATE: The reverse shoulder (Figure 7.5b), although non-anatomical, brings the centre of rotation of the glenohumeral joint medially and thereby increases the moment arm of the deltoid, allowing good abduction of the shoulder.

EXAMINER: Would you not try to repair the cuff prior to this major surgery?

CANDIDATE: No. The radiographs show established cuff arthropathy and in this situation it is not possible to reverse the pathology with cuff repair. Also, it would be a difficult cuff repair with a high chance of failure.

EXAMINER: Can you name some complications of the reverse polarity replacement?

CANDIDATE: Short term: infection, dislocation, haematoma formation (due to dead space), nerve injury (axillary, musculocutaneous) and periprosthetic fracture.

Long term: scapular notching, acromion fracture, aseptic loosening, deltoid fatigue and failure.

EXAMINER: Well, we will move on to the next scenario.

Whom do you think played the game well in this scenario? Analyze the candidate's ability to show their knowledge to the examiner. Learn how not to waste time and not to lower the expectations of the examiner. When the examiner's expectations go down, the questions may become simpler and the score drops. Show the knowledge appropriately to please the examiner. Make the game interesting for the examiners and you will walk away with a good score. Treat each scenario as a separate exam to reach a good overall score. Remember: the examiners do not know your previous performance, either good or bad. Therefore, forget the previous performance and move on.

Elbow

Terence Savaridas

Introduction

Practise viva technique in a timed manner and adapt your technique to illustrate your strengths.

The following are viva examples of common clinical scenarios. The suggested reading references are all available to access free online. They provide useful supplementary information to the topic of the viva.

Elbow

Make a list of conditions causing pain, locking, stiffness, flail and unstable elbow. Painful elbow pathology could be best remembered by its anatomical position – anterior, medial, posterior and lateral. Do not forget the nerves around the elbow while making your list.

Structured oral examination question 1

Tennis elbow

EXAMINER: 36-year-old right-hand dominant manual worker, referred by his GP with a painful right elbow. His elbow radiographs are essentially normal. What would you like to do?

CANDIDATE: Well, I need to assess the patient's elbow ... after I had asked the history of his pain.

EXAMINER: Pain is on the lateral side, started gradually 3 months ago ... no history of injury, aggravated by using a hammer and was initially relieved by rest. Now it is constant. He has normal range of movements. The point of tenderness is just around the lateral epicondyle.

CANDIDATE: From history and examination I think he has got tennis elbow ...

EXAMINER: What do you do to confirm the diagnosis?

CANDIDATE: I will test if the pain is reproduced by resisted wrist extension.

EXAMINER: Well, he has more pain on resisted finger extension than wrist extension. Does it make you think more specifically?

CANDIDATE: ...

EXAMINER: Which tendons are involved in tennis elbow?

CANDIDATE: ECRB ...

EXAMINER: Can EDC also be affected?

CANDIDATE: ...

EXAMINER: Well, tell me the pathophysiology of tennis elbow.

CANDIDATE: It's termed as angiofibroblastic hyperplasia, which is ... hyperplasia of the angiofibroblasts ...

EXAMINER: Do you know any other similar pathology around the elbow?

CANDIDATE: Golfer's elbow, which is common flexor tendonitis.

EXAMINER: Why do you say tendonitis? What is the difference between tendonitis and tendonosis?

CANDIDATE: ...

EXAMINER: Going back to the provocation test, if he had tenderness over the lateral proximal forearm on resisted finger extension, what does it tell you?

CANDIDATE: Maybe the disease process is extensive into the common extensor muscle belly.

EXAMINER: We'll move onto the next scenario.

This elucidates a simple scenario where the lack of a pause, to engage a structured taught process, leads to a jumbled poor answer that does not do justice to the candidate's true level of knowledge. Is the candidate a classical example for tennis elbow misdiagnosis? Does the candidate deserve anything above a score of 4? Would you approach this subject differently? Think and analyze before looking into the performance of the next candidate.

EXAMINER: 36-year-old right-hand dominant manual worker, referred by his GP with a painful right elbow. His elbow radiographs are essentially normal. What would you like to do?

CANDIDATE: I want to know the history of his right elbow pain please.

EXAMINER: It is on the lateral side, started gradually 3 months ago . . . no history of injury, aggravated by using a hammer and was initially relieved by rest. Now it is constant.

CANDIDATE: I will proceed with his examination . . . posture of elbow, range of movements especially looking for a lack of full extension and rotation . . . proceed to examine the specific site of tenderness on the lateral aspect.

EXAMINER: He has normal range of movements. The point of tenderness is just around the lateral epicondyle.

CANDIDATE: I would like to know if he has tenderness anterior or posterior to the lateral epicondyle and also any tenderness just distal to the lateral epicondyle.

EXAMINER: What does it tell you?

CANDIDATE: Anterior and distal to lateral epicondyle – ECRB tendinosis.
Posterior and distal to lateral epicondyle – EDC tendinosis.

EXAMINER: It is anterior and distal to lateral epicondyle. Tell me the provocation test for ECRB tendinosis.

CANDIDATE: Pain on elbow extension/forearm pronation/fingers flexion/wrist in extension against resistance.

EXAMINER: What is the test for EDC?

CANDIDATE: EDC tendinosis should have pain on elbow extension/forearm pronation/wrist neutral/fingers extension/long finger extension against resistance.

EXAMINER: Does the EDC provocation test tell you anything else?

CANDIDATE: Yes. If EDC provocation test produces pain over EDC origin, it suggests EDC tendinosis. Pain over radial tunnel – radial tunnel syndrome.

EXAMINER: What do you understand by tennis elbow?

CANDIDATE: It is the tendinosis and not tendonitis of ECRB/EDC tendons.

EXAMINER: Tell me the histological appearance of tendinosis.

CANDIDATE: Histologically, there are no acute inflammatory cells. There is granulation-like tissue consisting of immature fibroblasts and disorganized non-functional vascular elements called angiofibroblastic hyperplasia. It is theorized to result from an aborted healing response to repetitive micro-trauma. There is a lack of extracellular cross-linkage between fibres and fibrils are fragmented with varying length and diameter. Pain arises possibly from tissue ischaemia. Essentially the repetitive tensile overload, which exceeds tissue stress tolerance, causes tissue damage. If the tissue damage occurs at a rate which exceeds the tissue's ability to heal, it causes tissue degeneration.

EXAMINER: Do you know any other tendinosis around the elbow other than golfer's elbow?

CANDIDATE: Yes, the posterior tennis elbow, which is triceps tendinosis.

EXAMINER: Do you know any associated conditions?

CANDIDATE: Cuff pathology, Achilles tendinopathy and CTS.

EXAMINER: Lastly, if you have a refractory tennis elbow what would concern you?

CANDIDATE: I would be worried about the possibility of other diagnoses such as radial tunnel syndrome, radio-capitellar arthritis, posterolateral rotatory instability and radio-capitellar plica.

If you were the examiner, how much would you score for this candidate?

Suggested reading

Vaquero-Picado A, Barco R, Antuña SA. Lateral epicondylitis of the elbow. *EFORT Open Rev.* 2016;1 (11):391–397. http://doi.org/10.1302/2058-5241.1.000049

Key learning points

- Tennis elbow is a degenerative tendinopathic process affecting mainly ECRB within the common extensor origin.

- It is frequently seen in middle-aged individuals (35–50 years) who have excessive and repetitive use of these muscles whereby the rate of tendon damage exceeds the rate of repair.

- Be aware of typical presenting features (local tenderness, poor grip) and be able to describe tennis elbow provocation tests: Maudley's test (resisted third digit extension), Cozen's test, Mills and the 'chair' lift test (lifting the back of a chair with a three-finger pinch (thumb, index and main fingers) and the elbow fully extended).

- Differential diagnosis includes: referred pain, PIN entrapment, lateral column elbow degenerate disease.

- Treatment is essentially non-operative with activity modification in the vast majority of individuals (75–95%): activity modification, physiotherapy, counterforce bracing/wrist splints, ultrasonography, NSAIDs and local cortisone injections.

- Injection technique:
  - Quantity (2–3 cm^3).
  - Location anterolaterally below the extensor tendon, not intratendinous or subdermal.
  - Frequency: no more than three (6–12 weeks apart).
  - BEWARE: subcutaneous fat atrophy.

- Rarely, in recalcitrant cases, surgery is offered.

- Have an awareness of novel therapies: PRP injections, botulinum toxin, high-voltage electrical stimulation and extracorporeal shockwave therapy.

Structured oral examination question 2

Osteochondritis dissecans

EXAMINER: Look at these radiographs of the right elbow of a 33-year-old patient and tell me the findings (Figure 8.1).

CANDIDATE: This plain radiograph of a right elbow shows one loose body in the anterior aspect of the joint.

EXAMINER: What would you like to know if you are allowed to ask only one question?

CANDIDATE: I want to know his presenting symptoms.

EXAMINER: He gets intermittent painful locking symptoms. What is the diagnosis here?

CANDIDATE: Well he has a loose body in the elbow …

EXAMINER: Tell me the conditions which produce loose bodies in a joint.

CANDIDATE: Could be post-traumatic, secondary to osteoarthritis, osteochondritis dissecans (OCD) or synovial chondromatosis.

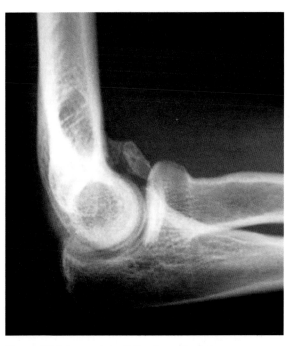

Figure 8.1 Anteroposterior (AP) radiograph of elbow.

EXAMINER: Now again ... What would you like to know if you are allowed one more question?

CANDIDATE: Did he have any injury in the past?

EXAMINER: No, never ... What is your diagnosis here, keeping in mind that there is only one loose body in the elbow?

CANDIDATE: It could be either secondary to osteoarthritis or OCD and I could rule out a post-traumatic cause as he had no injury.

EXAMINER: Can you look at the radiographs again and be more specific? [Showing the X-ray again to the candidate.]

CANDIDATE: I can see only one loose body. There is no calcification in the muscle or capsule.

EXAMINER: What does it tell you?

CANDIDATE: It helps me to rule out myositis ossification and synovial sarcoma.

EXAMINER: I want you to concentrate on the intra-articular pathology and try to narrow down your diagnosis between OCD and osteoarthritis.

CANDIDATE: I would like to know the history of his symptoms and have more investigations to be more specific.

EXAMINER: Well, he had unexplained painful elbow which lasted for about 18 months when he was 17 years of age ... What do you think is going on with this elbow?

CANDIDATE: It sounds like it may not be osteoarthritis ... it could be OCD.

EXAMINER: If you had been consulting him at the time of initial presentation 16 years ago, what would be your concern?

CANDIDATE: I would ...
   [Bell]

Was this a good viva? Did he lack the knowledge of this subject of loose bodies? The candidate appeared to be hesitant and did not display his knowledge in a methodical manner.

EXAMINER: Look at these radiographs of the right elbow of a 33-year-old patient and tell me the findings.

CANDIDATE: These plain radiographs of a right elbow show a well-maintained joint space with evidence of a solitary loose body in the anterior aspect of the joint, most clearly visible in the lateral view.

EXAMINER: What would you like to know if you are allowed to ask only one question?

CANDIDATE: Has this patient had problems with this elbow as a teenager? In particular, whether it impaired his performance in competitive sport that involved repetitive overhead activities such as racquet and throwing sports or frequent axial loading of the elbow as seen in gymnastics or weightlifting.

EXAMINER: Yes, this patient had unexplained painful elbow that lasted for about 18 months when he was 17 years of age ... What do you think is going on with this elbow?

CANDIDATE: Well, I suspect he had osteochondritis dissecans when he was 17, which explains the unexplained pain he had for 18 months and the OCD segment must have separated to form the loose body.

It is anticipated that the prognosis for a full recovery is poor with presentation in older teenagers.

EXAMINER: If you had consulted him at the time of initial presentation of OCD, what would you have done and why?

CANDIDATE: I would have advised him of the importance of activity modification and warned him that he is likely to have ongoing elbow symptoms of lack to full extension with intermittent pain and locking. I would have advised him to return if he had functional restrictions due to his elbow.

It would have been useful to perform an MRI scan to assess lesion size and condition of articular cartilage. In addition, to define and locate the presence of loose bodies. I appreciate that access to MR imaging would have been limited 17 years ago.

EXAMINER: MRI was not widely available then. Are there any other investigations that may have been useful?

CANDIDATE: An elbow arthrogram with contrast would have been an option. However, I suspect that, at the time, there was also limited availability of arthroscopic elbow surgery. Therefore, the value of this invasive investigation would be limited except in a specialist centre. Furthermore, the age at which he presented was not in the favourable range . . . that is after the closure of the physis . . . therefore, I would have followed him clinically more closely with serial plain radiographs and obtained a subspecialist opinion.

EXAMINER: This patient unfortunately had only one X-ray at the start of the presentation and as it did not show any obvious pathology, he was discharged from follow-up. What would you like to do now?

CANDIDATE: I would like to know his presenting symptoms. Has he had any treatment so far and what are his expectations?

EXAMINER: He has had no treatment so far. And can you tell me what would be his presenting symptom?

CANDIDATE: I would expect him to have intermittent painful locking of the elbow with a limitation to full elbow extension.

EXAMINER: Yes, that is his symptom. He wants to have something done to prevent these unexpected painful locking episodes.

CANDIDATE: I would perform an arthroscopic removal of the loose body.

EXAMINER: Can you tell me another cause for one or two loose bodies in a joint?

CANDIDATE: In osteoarthritis the osteophytes can break and present similarly. But the radiograph would show evidence of osteoarthritis.

EXAMINER: If you see multiple loose bodies, what is the diagnosis?

CANDIDATE: Synovial chondromatosis.

This is a good example of using your knowledge appropriately. Compare these two candidates. Candidate 2 has been able to control the viva by processing the information received and providing a thoughtful answer.

Suggested reading

Churchill RW, Munoz J, Ahmad CS. Osteochondritis dissecans of the elbow. Curr Rev Musculoskel Med. 2016;9(2):232–239. http://doi.org/10.1007/s12178-016-9342-y

Key learning points

- OCD in the elbow is frequently an acquired condition affecting the capitellum secondary to repetitive trauma.
- It is frequently seen in adolescent athletes/ gymnasts who participate in repetitive overhead activity or axial loading of the elbow.
- Patients present with pain on exertion. Patients that play through the pain tend to present with higher-grade lesions that may manifest as locking due to an unstable lesion or loose body. Prognosis is poorer when presenting features first occur at a later age, following physeal closure.
- Treatment is essentially non-operative with activity modification in the vast majority of individuals. In high-grade lesion fixation, microfracture or grafting are options.

Structured oral examination question 3

Rheumatoid arthritis elbow

EXAMINER: What do you see in this radiograph of a 67-year-old lady's right elbow (Figure 8.2a)?

CANDIDATE: This radiograph shows extensive erosion of the articular cartilage which has involved both ulnohumeral and radiocapitellar joints. The radial head is dislocated and the elbow articulation is aligned only with ulna and humerus. There is peri-articular osteopenia. There is no subchondral sclerosis or osteophytes.

EXAMINER: What could be the cause?

CANDIDATE: It is characteristic of inflammatory arthropathy and I suspect rheumatoid arthritis.

EXAMINER: Indeed, this lady has had RA for the last 34 years. What would you like to do for her?

CANDIDATE: I want to know her presenting symptoms from this elbow. What has changed for her

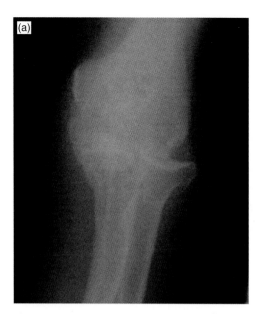

Figure 8.2a Anteroposterior (AP) radiograph of rheumatoid arthritis right elbow.

to seek treatment on this elbow now? What previous treatment has she had? What are her expectations?

EXAMINER: She has many joint problems and recently she is finding lack of strength in her right upper limb to do day-to-day activities. She has had no specific elbow treatments. She wants to do her normal household activities.

CANDIDATE: I would specifically assess her elbow stability and range of movements. And more importantly check her hand function with regards to any tendon ruptures and posterior interosseous nerve function.

EXAMINER: She has no valgus and varus stability but a good range of active and passive movements. Hand function is also good. Now how will you differentiate between PIN palsy and extensor tendon rupture?

CANDIDATE: It is unusual for attritional tendon ruptures to result in loss of wrist extension. A loss of wrist extension is more likely to indicate PIN palsy. The tenodesis test will assess tendon integrity. Well if there is no active extension of the fingers at the MCP joint and the tenodesis test shows no passive finger extension at the MCP

joint on passive flexion of wrist, then the diagnosis is extensor tendon rupture. But I will cautiously assess the other tendons supplied by PIN prior to making the final diagnosis as in RA patients both can exist together.

EXAMINER: What will be your management plan?

CANDIDATE: It is a multidisciplinary approach with re-consultation with rheumatologists and assessment by occupational therapists. I would initially offer her an elbow brace.

EXAMINER: She comes back after 3 months and says the brace has improved her life quality to some extent but finds it difficult as it gets wet in the kitchen and still has difficulties in the shower as she could not wear it in the shower.

CANDIDATE: This lady will likely benefit from a semi-constrained cemented total elbow replacement. I would explain to her that there is a recommended restriction of 5 lb in weight that she is able to lift in the arm post TER. In keeping with the principles of GIRFT (getting it right first time), I would consider referring her on to a high-volume TER surgeon, especially as there is evidence that surgeon volume affects outcome post TER.

The patient will require a preoperative anaesthetic assessment that includes C-spine radiographs to assess the atlanto-axial joint.

EXAMINER: Finally, what happens to juvenile rheumatoid joints?

CANDIDATE: In contrast to adult RA, juvenile RA produces stiff joints.

Who had control in this viva? Did this candidate get the questions he played for? Was his technique good? Did he not manage to get a bonus question? Would you be happy if you were the candidate of this scenario? Would you have played it any better? Now the next candidate approaches this table.

EXAMINER: What do you see in this radiograph of a 67-year-old lady's right elbow?

CANDIDATE: This radiograph shows extensive erosion of the articular cartilage which has involved both ulnohumeral and radiocapitellar joints. The radial head is dislocated and the elbow articulation is aligned only with ulna and humerus.

EXAMINER: What could be the cause?

CANDIDATE: It is characteristic of inflammatory arthropathy and I suspect rheumatoid arthritis. It is a flail elbow.

EXAMINER: Indeed, this lady has had RA for the last 34 years. What features in the radiograph made you rule out osteoarthritis?

CANDIDATE: In osteoarthritis there will be joint space narrowing, subchondral sclerosis, subchondral cysts and osteophytes. This radiograph does not show these features.

EXAMINER: What is the bone quality here?

CANDIDATE: … The bone appears to be osteopenic … could be disuse from pain or the disease process itself.

EXAMINER: Now, what would you do for her?

CANDIDATE: I need to know the history of presenting complaints and I would examine the elbow.

EXAMINER: She recently finds her right upper limb weak affecting her day-to-day activities. In the examination there is valgus/varus instability.

CANDIDATE: It is an unstable elbow from advanced RA. Therefore, I would do a total elbow replacement for her.

EXAMINER: Is there anything you would consider prior to surgery?

CANDIDATE: Well I can try a splint if she is willing to try …

EXAMINER: She comes back after 3 months and says the brace has improved her life quality to some extent but finds it difficult as it gets wet in the kitchen and still has difficulties in the shower as she could not wear it in the shower.

CANDIDATE: Then I will proceed with the total elbow replacement.

EXAMINER: Which nerve specifically would you like to assess in the RA elbow especially prior to total elbow replacement?

CANDIDATE: … Posterior interosseous nerve as it can be affected by the synovial swelling/dislocation of the radiocapitellar joint.

EXAMINER: What would be the findings if she has PIN palsy?

CANDIDATE: There will be no active extension of the fingers at the level of MCP joints.

EXAMINER: Do you know any other cause for the inability to extend MCP joints?

CANDIDATE: Yes, progressive rupture of extensor tendons called Vaughan–Jackson syndrome.

EXAMINER: What if the patient presents with weakness of thumb DIP joint flexion?

CANDIDATE: This could be due to rupture of the flexor pollicis longus (FPL) tendon due to attrition from a bony spur in the carpal tunnel. This can often be seen in rheumatoid patients.

EXAMINER: What name is associated with this?

CANDIDATE: Mannerfelt syndrome.

EXAMINER: Is there any concern regarding this RA patient undergoing general anaesthesia?

CANDIDATE: These patients can have lung fibrosis … apart from this, yes … of course I will perform a C-spine X-ray to see the stability of the atlanto-axial joint.

EXAMINER: Thank you.

Did he answer all the questions? Did he not possess the knowledge of the subject? This candidate answered each question adequately but did not provide any supplementary information to gain control of the viva in order to score a higher mark.

Suggested reading

Ishikawa H. The latest treatment strategy for the rheumatoid hand deformity. *J Orthopaed Sci*. 2017;22 (4):583–592. https://doi.org/10.1016/j.jos. (It is worth a look at figures 2 and 3 which give a pictorial description of the pathological change seen in RA.)

Jenkins PJ, Watts AC, Norwood T, *et al*. Total elbow replacement: outcome of 1146 arthroplasties from the Scottish Arthroplasty Project. *Acta Orthopaed*. 2013;84 (2):119–123. http://doi.org/10.3109/17453674.2013.784658

Key learning points

- RA is managed by a multidisciplinary team. RA is a systemic disorder. Understand its effect on the musculoskeletal system. Be aware of its manifestations in other organ systems especially during the perioperative period.
- The aim of surgical intervention in RA is to maintain patient function.

- Understand the pathology and treatment options in Vaughan–Jackson and Mannerfelt syndrome.

- Develop a method to describe how to distinguish between a nerve palsy and a tendon rupture.

- The semi-constraint, cemented TER (Coonrad–Morrey, Figures 8.2b and 8.2c) is a well-recognized and reliable prosthesis for patients with RA with good long-term implant survivorship.
  - Semi-constrained linking mechanism behaves as a sloppy hinge, allowing some rotational and varus–valgus play.
  - Allows early ROM (anterior flange provides AP and rotational stability).
  - Does not disassemble. The components are linked with a cobalt–chrome axis pin, which articulates with the polyethylene bushings of the ulnar and humeral components.

Structured oral examination question 4

Post-traumatic OA elbow

EXAMINER: Good morning. Here are the radiographs of a right-hand dominant 43-year-old man's right elbow (Figure 8.3a). Tell me the findings.

CANDIDATE: Good morning. These radiographs show narrowing of joint space on both ulnohumeral and radiocapitellar joints with subchondral sclerosis and cysts and medial, anterior and posterior osteophytes suggesting osteoarthritis. Has he had any previous injury to this elbow?

EXAMINER: Well he had a dislocation of this elbow 8 years ago which was reduced in A&E and as he improved to full function in 8 weeks he was discharged from the fracture clinic. Now over the last 3 years he has had problems with this elbow. What would your advice be for this patient?

CANDIDATE: I want to know his present symptoms. How much does it affect his job? What are the treatments he has had so far? And what is his expectation?

EXAMINER: This elbow is affecting his job as he has got restricted movements – flexion

extension from 50° to 110° and supination is only to 40°. He had a few intra-articular injections by his GP. He wants to have more movement in the elbow.

CANDIDATE: He has got post-traumatic osteoarthritis with stiffness. He is not presenting with pain as a main symptom. This patient is young and wishes to have an improved elbow ROM.

This can be achieved either with an arthrolysis and debridement, either performed as an open column procedure or arthroscopically. The column procedure allows for joint arthrotomy, capsular release and excision of osteophytes through a limited lateral approach. My preference would be to perform an arthroscopic procedure as this will likely need to be repeated during this patient's working career. It is anticipated that recovery post-arthroscopy is shorter than open surgery. In addition, he may require a TER in the future and I wish to avoid any surgical scars that may influence the position of a future incision for arthroplasty. However, the patient needs to be counselled that the net gain to ROM following arthroscopic release is likely to be less than that achieved following an open procedure.

It would be reasonable to refer this patient to a dedicated upper limb orthopaedic surgeon who performs elbow arthroscopy more frequently.

EXAMINER: Can you show me the arthroscopic portals in this elbow picture (Figure 8.3b and 8.3c)?

CANDIDATE: [Marking and talking to the examiner.] Portals can broadly be categorized into lateral, medial and posterior portals.

Direct lateral portal: at the centre of a triangle defined by the lateral epicondyle, the radial head and the olecranon. This is one of two frequently used as the initial entry portal to inflate the joint with saline.

Anterolateral portal: 1 cm distal and 1 cm anterior to the lateral epicondyle, between the radial head and the capitellum. This gives good access to the anterior aspect of the joint.

Anteromedial portal: 2 cm distal and 2 cm anterior to the medial epicondyle. This is often created using an 'inside out' technique by cutting down onto the tip of the arthroscope inserted using the antero-lateral portal.

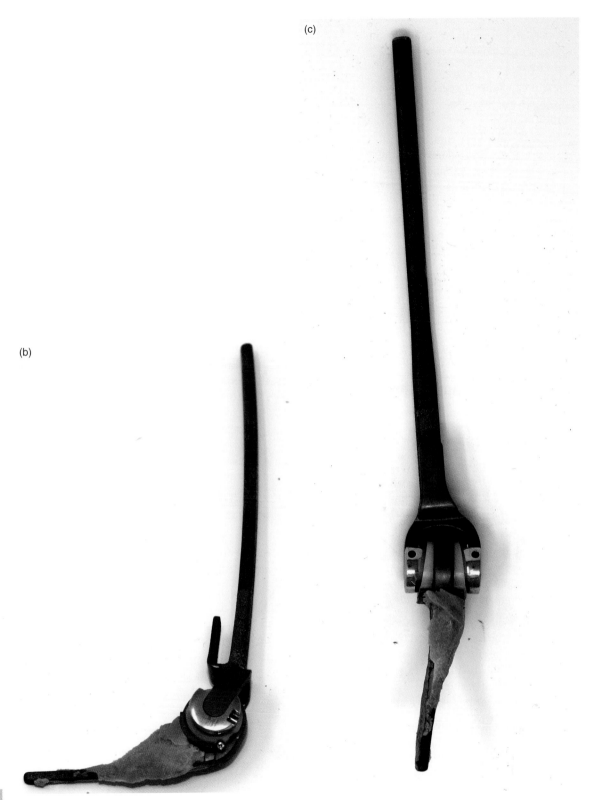

(c)

(b)

Figure 8.2b and 8.2c Coonrad–Morrey linked semi-constrained explanted TER. Humeral component is porous-coated distally. Ulnar component has a plasma-spray metallic coating in its proximal third. Both components should be fixed with polymethylmethacrilate.

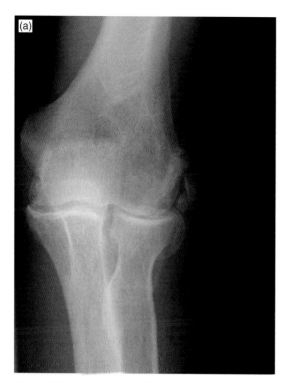

Figure 8.3a Anteroposterior (AP) radiograph of right elbow.

Proximal medial portal: this is often used as the initial entry portal. 2 cm proximal to the medial epicondyle along the anterior surface of the humerus towards the radial head.

Direct posterior portal: 1.5 cm proximal to the tip of the olecranon. Access to olecranon fossae.

Posterolateral portal: access to radiocapitellar joint.

EXAMINER: Is the benefit of the debridement permanent?

CANDIDATE: No, it is not ... and varies between individuals.

EXAMINER: The patient wants to know if there is any procedure that can provide long-lasting benefit.

CANDIDATE: The longer-lasting result can be achieved by a total elbow replacement ... But as this patient is only 43 and he is a manual worker and his dominant elbow is affected with osteoarthritis, I would not advise a total elbow replacement at this moment as TERs do not have a long life expectancy in young osteoarthritic patients.
[Bell]

Would you handle this scenario differently? How much will you score this candidate? Was his knowledge sufficient and well presented? Now a confident-looking candidate approaches the table.

EXAMINER: Good morning. Here are the radiographs of a right-hand dominant 43-year-old man's right elbow. Tell me the findings.

CANDIDATE: The radiographs show advanced osteoarthritis of his dominant elbow.

EXAMINER: Correct. What would be your advice to this patient?

CANDIDATE: It depends on if he has pain, stiffness, difficulty with his job and also depends on his expectations.

EXAMINER: Pain is not a main issue here. This elbow is affecting his job as he has got restricted movements – flexion extension from 50° to 110° and supination is only to 40°. He wants to have more movement in the elbow.

CANDIDATE: I will initially inject his elbow with steroids and send him for stretching physiotherapy.

EXAMINER: The patient has had a few injections already and also physiotherapy from his GP and therefore he prefers to have a more definitive procedure.

CANDIDATE: Well if the injections have been tried without any success, I would advise a total elbow replacement.

EXAMINER: Is there anything you could offer prior to TER?

CANDIDATE: [Suddenly losing confidence ...] Probably an attempt of manipulation under anaesthesia ...

EXAMINER: Is MUA and passive stretching of a stiff elbow good advice?

CANDIDATE: ... perhaps not ... as there is a small risk of myositis ossification.

EXAMINER: In the last 30 years ... the number of implanted TER is in decline. Why?

CANDIDATE: ...

EXAMINER: Well 20–30 years ago the TER was commonly used for which group of patients?

CANDIDATE: Rheumatoid patients and it has declined because rheumatoid patients are better

(c)

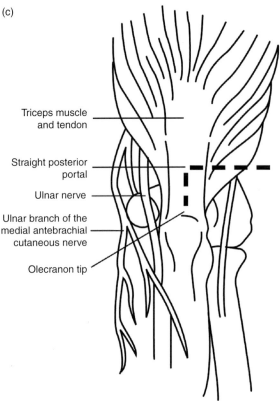

Triceps muscle and tendon

Straight posterior portal

Ulnar nerve

Ulnar branch of the medial antebrachial cutaneous nerve

Olecranon tip

(b)

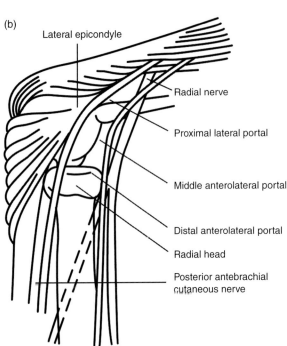

Lateral epicondyle

Radial nerve

Proximal lateral portal

Middle anterolateral portal

Distal anterolateral portal

Radial head

Posterior antebrachial cutaneous nerve

Figure 8.3b and 8.3c Arthroscopic portal sites of the elbow

treated now and we do not see advanced joint pathology in this group of patients . . .

EXAMINER: What is the clinical finding in an advanced RA elbow?

CANDIDATE: Arthritis affects the entire joint, the ligament stability is also lost as RA is primarily a soft tissue problem and the radial head dislocates and the elbow becomes flail.

EXAMINER: Have you seen a flail RA elbow recently?

CANDIDATE: No, I haven't seen any which has progressed to radial head dislocation . . . instead the appearance we see now is more like osteoarthritis.

EXAMINER: Does this modification of disease pathology have anything to do with the declining number of implanted TER?

CANDIDATE: Yes, the TER failed earlier in this group.

EXAMINER: This is because we are treating stable disease-modified osteoarthritic RA elbows, with the implant designed to treat flail elbows.

CANDIDATE: . . .

EXAMINER: Would you like to offer anything else prior to TER for this young manual worker?

CANDIDATE: An arthroscopic wash out?

EXAMINER: Is there any . . .
[Bell]

Did the confident start last long? Was the knowledge adequate to handle this scenario? Would you like to be this candidate on the day of the exam?

Suggested reading

Camp CL, Degen RM, Sanchez-Sotelo J, *et al*. Basics of elbow arthroscopy part I: surface anatomy, portals, and structures at risk. *Arthrosc Tech*.

2016;5(6):e1339–e1343. http://doi.org/10.1016/j
.eats.2016.08.019

Chammas M. Post-traumatic osteoarthritis of the elbow.
Orthopaed Traumatol Surg Res. 2014;100(1 Suppl):S15–24.
http://dx.doi.org/10.1016/j.otsr.2013.11.004

Key learning points

- Clarify patient expectations prior to recommending a treatment option and think about potential disease progression and likely future intervention.
- Know the elbow arthroscopy portals. Accept that elbow arthroscopy is not a common procedure. Not every orthopaedic trainee would have had the opportunity to observe an elbow arthroscopy.

Structured oral examination question 5

Posterolateral rotatory instability of the elbow

EXAMINER: I have a problem with my left elbow. Proceed.

CANDIDATE: Well, I want to know your age, hand dominance, your occupation and the nature of your problem please.

EXAMINER: I am 47, right-hand dominant mechanic and in certain positions my elbow pops with pain.

CANDIDATE: Is the popping sensation on the inner side or outer side of your elbow?

EXAMINER: The outer side ... yes, my thumb side.

CANDIDATE: Have you ever had any problem in your elbow as a child?

EXAMINER: I had problems as a child in my right elbow, but now my right side is fine. My left side although I did not have any problem as a child, 3 years ago I had a simple dislocation.

CANDIDATE: What problem did you have on the right side?

EXAMINER: My older sister pulled me by my right hand and my elbow became painful and the doctor had manipulated my elbow and told my parents not to let anyone pull me by my hand. And he said it was a pulled elbow ... where the radial head pops out.

CANDIDATE: I want to check if you have general joint laxity.

EXAMINER: No, I am rather stiff. What do you think is wrong with my left elbow?

CANDIDATE: I think radial head dislocation ... probably secondary to annular ligament insufficiency secondary to the dislocation. In what position do you get this popping sensation?

EXAMINER: Whenever I push myself off the chair with my arm.

CANDIDATE: ... I would like to perform an X-ray of your elbow to assess the radial head.

EXAMINER: The X-ray is normal. Can you tell me about the ligaments around the elbow?

CANDIDATE: Sure. There are two main groups of ligaments, medial and lateral collateral ligaments. MCL has three bundles: anterior, posterior and transverse bands. LCL has lateral ulnar collateral ligament (LUCL), annular ligament, radial collateral ligament and accessory collateral ligament.

EXAMINER: Have you heard of posterolateral rotatory instability of the elbow?

CANDIDATE: ...

Did the candidate reach the diagnosis? Did he understand the clues given by the examiner? The next candidate arrives.

EXAMINER: I have a problem with my left elbow. Proceed.

CANDIDATE: Well, I want to know your age, hand dominance, your occupation and the nature of your problem please.

EXAMINER: I am a 47, right-hand dominant mechanic and in certain positions my elbow pops with pain.

CANDIDATE: Have you ever injured your left elbow in the past? And in what position are you feeling the popping sensation in the elbow?

EXAMINER: Well, I had a simple dislocation of my left elbow 3 years ago which was reduced in A&E. Now whenever I push myself off a chair using my arm I get this sensation.

CANDIDATE: I would like to assess your elbow.

EXAMINER: What would you like to test?

CANDIDATE: I want to perform the pivot-shift test to assess the lateral ulnar collateral ligament.

EXAMINER: If the pivot-shift test is positive, what is your diagnosis?

CANDIDATE: Posterolateral rotatory instability of the left elbow.

EXAMINER: I had been told that I had 'pulled elbow' on the other side as a child. Could this be the same?

CANDIDATE: No, usually the pulled elbow settles as the child grows and you had a definite injury to the left elbow.

EXAMINER: What could you do for me to prevent these unpleasant episodes?

CANDIDATE: I need to perform an MRI scan to confirm injury to the LUCL and to see if the injury to the ligament is intrasubstance or from the origin to decide on the treatment. Have you had any recent X-rays?

EXAMINER: My X-rays were normal. If the MRI scan shows injury to the LUCL, how will you manage this problem?

CANDIDATE: If the LUCL is avulsed from the origin or insertion and the ligament itself is healthy, it could be reattached to the bone using bone anchors. It may not be possible in your case as the injury was 3 years ago. My main inclination is to reconstruct the LUCL using palmaris longus tendon or triceps fascia.

Did this candidate manage to please the examiner? Which candidate would you prefer to treat your elbow?

Suggested reading

Camp CL, Smith J, O'Driscoll SW. Posterolateral rotatory instability of the elbow: Part II. Supplementary examination and dynamic imaging techniques. *Arthrosc Tech*. 2017;6(2): e407–e411. http://doi.org/10.1016/j.eats.2016.10.012

Englert C, Zellner J, Koller M, Nerlich M, Lenich A. Elbow dislocations: a review ranging from soft tissue injuries to complex elbow fracture dislocations. *Adv Orthoped*. 2013;951397. http://doi.org/10.1155/2013/951397

Key learning points

- Go back to the basics of a thorough history and examination.
- The commonest cause of recurrent instability post elbow dislocation is posterolateral rotatory instability (PLRI).
- Understand the stages of injury that occur in an elbow dislocation.
- Be able to describe the pivot-shift test. An easier test is the push up from a chair. Patients would typically describe being unable to perform this manoeuvre if asked.

Now, the examiner's aim is all about finding out whether this candidate can be allowed to be his or her consultant. As you would like to win the patient's confidence while consulting in the clinics, it is vital to win the examiner's confidence in each and every scenario, showing adequate knowledge expressed with correct technique.

General principles and fracture biomechanics

Roger Walton and Paul A. Banaszkiewicz

Introduction

Fracture biomechanics can be tough-going for most candidates and yet it is definitely an A-list topic. Textbook chapters can be too complicated and detailed to understand whilst short note sections may appear incomplete as biomechanical assumptions have not been fully explained or the brevity of the notes makes them difficult to fully understand, never mind encouraging any higher-order thinking.

We hope this chapter uncomplicates a difficult area of the syllabus that a lot of candidates find offputting.

Structured oral examination question 1

IM nail biomechanics

EXAMINER: This is a radiograph of a broken femoral nail that was used to fix a distal femoral shaft fracture (Figure 9.1). How can you prevent nail breakage?

CANDIDATE 1: I would insert the largest diameter solid nail that is available for use.

COMMENT: Not a good start. The answer isn't particularly well thought out and is not scoring the candidate any marks.

EXAMINER: Why would you use a solid nail? Most nails used in orthopaedics are hollow.

CANDIDATE: Because a solid nail will be stronger than a hollow nail.

COMMENT: This is continuing on with a poor choice of imprecise terms and more importantly the candidate is missing scoring opportunities.

EXAMINER: What do you mean by the term 'stronger'?

CANDIDATE: Strong is the ability of a material to resist deformation.

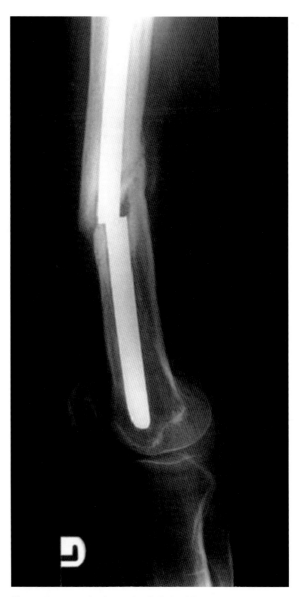

Figure 9.1 Lateral radiograph of left distal femur demonstrating a broken femoral nail.

181

COMMENT: This is an incorrect definition and the viva is going nowhere.

EXAMINER: How does this relate to ultimate tensile strength (UTS)?

COMMENT: UTS is the highest stress observed on the stress versus strain diagram while the failure strength is the stress value at which the material eventually fails.

Strong is an imprecise biomechanical term.

A strong material has a high ultimate tensile strength.

CANDIDATE: [Silence . . .] Can I retract my last few statements and say that the torsional and bending rigidity of a solid nail will be greater than that of a hollow nail?

COMMENT: The candidate is not getting past the opening questions. Better to discuss factors predisposing to nail breakage. This will then lead onto discussions about area and polar moments of inertia, the biomechanical benefits of using larger-diameter nails for long bone fractures, the solid versus hollow nail dialogue, benefits of IM reaming, etc. Another road to journey down is patient factors that could predispose to non union and eventual nail breakage (smoking, alcohol, malnutrition etc)

(Score 4.)

CANDIDATE 2: An unstable fracture pattern (segmental or comminuted) or the use of a small unreamed diameter nail increases the risk of nail breakage.

Distal femoral fractures have a high incidence of intramedullary nail breakage, especially if the fracture has been produced by high-energy trauma and the patient encouraged to weight bear early. Early weight bearing with delayed fracture healing increases the time over which cyclic stress may act to cause fatigue failure and nail breakage.

Technical errors in nail insertion, such as scoring the nail during locking, may weaken the nail or create stress risers. Excessive impaction during nail insertion due to under-reaming of the medullary canal may also weaken the nail.

Intramedullary nails rarely break when no locking screws are used. Statically locked nails can produce high concentrations of stress at the proximal or distal end of the nail, predisposing it to breakage. Nail design changes such as increased material thickness around screw holes, cold

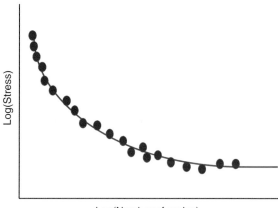

Figure 9.2 S-N curve.

forming which increases material strength reduce risk of nail breakage.

(Score 6.)

EXAMINER: What do you mean by fatigue failure?

CANDIDATE: Failure of a material with repetitive loading below the ultimate tensile strength.

EXAMINER: What do we mean by S-N curves?

CANDIDATE: As mentioned, cyclic loading of an object can result in fatigue failure. An S-N curve gives information about the number of cycles a material can endure for a given stress level.

EXAMINER: Can you draw out an S-N curve?

CANDIDATE: (Figure 9.2)

EXAMINER: What makes fatigue failure more likely?

CANDIDATE: In the presence of stress risers such as a hole, a sharp edge, an indentation, notch or scratch, the loads can go beyond the normal limit that is localized in that area. This can lead to crack propagation.

EXAMINER: Why?

CANDIDATE: Crack propagation.

EXAMINER: What do you mean by this?

CANDIDATE: Sorry, I am not sure.

COMMENT: Score 6.

For a score 8: The applied stress concentrates on residual material beneath a stress riser and means the number of cycles to failure is much lower than the fatigue strength.

All stress risers greatly weaken a structure, stress risers (stress concentrators) produce increased local stresses that may be several times higher than those in the bulk of the material and may lead to local failure. Methods to produce a shorter working length (reaming for larger nail). Using a stainless steel rather than titanium nail (higher Youngs modulus) but long list of pros and cons for each material.

Structured oral examination question 2

Area and polar moment of inertia

EXAMINER: What do we mean by the terms second moment area and polar moment of inertia?

CANDIDATE: The second moment area of inertia provides a measure of how the material is distributed in the cross-section of an object relative to the load applied to it. The further away the material is from the centre of a beam, the greater its bending stiffness.

The polar moment of inertia applies to a cylindrical structure and its ability to resist torsion.

EXAMINER: How do the second moment area and polar moment area differ between a solid and a hollow nail?

CANDIDATE: For a *solid nail* the *second moment area* or *second moment of inertia* is directly proportional to the fourth power of the radius.
$$I = \pi r^4/4$$
For a *hollow nail* the *second moment of area* or *second moment of inertia* is directly proportional to the fourth power of the outer radius minus the fourth power of the inner radius.
$$I = \pi(r_O^4 - r_I^4)/4$$
Nail wall thickness is equal to the difference between r_0 = outer radius and r_1 = inner radius.

Controversial topic

The assumption that if a nail has a thin wall then the inner radius is roughly equal to the outer radius, so the bending rigidity approximates to the third power of the outer radius, is inaccurate.

Hollow orthopaedic implants do not approximate to r_O^3.

In engineering, approximations are made for 'thin' cylinders, which is when the inner radius (r_1) approaches the outer radius (r_0). The $r_O^4 - r_I^4$ term approaches r_O^3 as $r_O \sim r_I$, hence the approximation.

However, in the case of orthopaedic implants, using the r_0^3 approximation is inaccurate. Using a cylinder that thin has no practical use because of the forces it must resist. The wall thickness of a hollow nail must be optimal to be able to withstand bending stress and avoid sudden failing by buckling (local concentrated deformations). The implant also starts behaving as a curved sheet rather than a hollow cylinder .

A Synthes 13 mm nail (6.5 mm radius) has a 1.2 mm wall thickness. r_0 = 6.5 mm, r_1 = 5.3 mm (which is 6.5 – 1.2). So $(r_O^4 - r_I^4)$ = 1785 – 789 = 996. That's the true value of the $(r_O^4 - r_I^4)$ term, the true coefficient for moment of inertia. Approximating r_O^3 is 6.5^3 = 275. 996 is 3.6 × 275, so to estimate a hollow nail to r_O^3 is a 360% underestimate, which is quite significant.[1]

For a *solid nail* the *polar moment of inertia* (polar moment area) varies with the fourth power of its radius.
$$Jo = \pi r^4/2$$
For a *hollow nail* the *polar moment of inertia* varies with the fourth power of the outer radius minus the inner radius.
$$Jo = \pi(r_O^4 - r_I^4)/2$$

EXAMINER: Which type of nail, solid or hollow, biomechanically do we prefer to use?

CANDIDATE: A hollow nail is more efficient as less material can be used for equivalent values of bending and torsional rigidity.

EXAMINER: Why?

CANDIDATE: The further the material is spread away from the neutral axis of the nail, the greater its rigidity against bending and torsional forces.
(For score 7 candidates.)

EXAMINER: Why are spiral fractures of the tibia more common in the lower third of the tibia even though the cortex is much thicker there?

CANDIDATE: The tibia resembles a cylinder. This site has a low polar moment of inertia; even though the cortex is especially thick at this point, it has less resistance against torsional forces because of its smaller radius compared to the upper segment. Under a specific load the lower third segment will deform more than the upper segment of the tibia. The further a material is distributed away from the neutral axis of the structure, the greater the polar moment and therefore greater strength and rigidity against torsional stress.
(For score 8 candidates.)

EXAMINER: What about the bending and torsional rigidity of a hollow nail with an open section?

CANDIDATE: There is very little difference in bending rigidity between a solid hollow nail and an open nail section of the same diameter. For torsional rigidity the situation is different and is a much greater affect. The difference in behaviour of open and closed nails against torsional stress is created by the circumferential discontinuity. Stress is transmitted uniformly through the entire thickness of the cross-section of a closed-section hollow nail without any change in direction. There is a change is stress direction in an open nail when its gap is reached with a significant fall in the magnitude of polar moment (Figure 9.3).

EXAMINER: What about differences between the cross-sectional shape of a nail?

CANDIDATE: A clover leaf cross-section nail improves torsional and bending rigidity compared to a round cross-section.

EXAMINER: Why?

CANDIDATE: I am not sure.

Structured oral examination question 3

IM nail

EXAMINER: What does the picture show (Figure 9.4)?

CANDIDATE: This is a clinical picture showing an intramedullary nail. It looks as though this is a femoral antegrade nail as it has an anterior bow, it has multiple locking options proximally and it is cannulated distally. They are usually made of titanium.

COMMENT: Be able to describe the typical features of an IM nail.

EXAMINER: How does an IM nail function?

CANDIDATE: IM nails stabilize a fracture by acting as internal splints with load-sharing characteristics.

EXAMINER: What do we mean by an internal splint?

CANDIDATE: Splintage is defined as a construct in which micromotion can occur between bone and implant, providing only relative stability without interfragmentary compression. Callus forms at the fracture site.

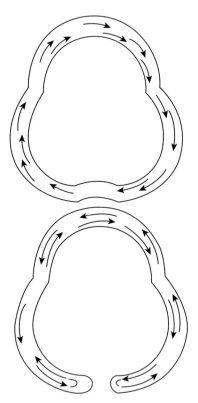

Figure 9.3 With the open-section nail there is reversion of the direction of torsional stress as shown by the arrows. In a closed hollow nail, the nail stress lines are in the same direction because of the continuity and therefore the nail is stronger against torsion.

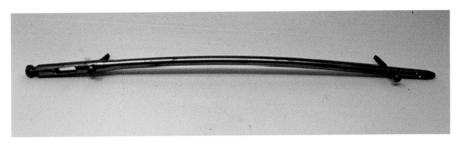

Figure 9.4 Titanium IM femoral nail.

EXAMINER: Do nails always act as a load-sharing device?

CANDIDATE: It depends on how it is used.

COMMENT: Candidate waffle.

EXAMINER: How is it used?

CANDIDATE: [Silence . . .]

COMMENT: In more comminuted fracture patterns that are not axially stable, a nail will have to transmit all the forces applied to the limb, so-called load-bearing.

Ideally, a nail should be used as a load-sharing device, but in certain situations will be used as a load-bearing device.

EXAMINER: Which is stiffer, a solid or a hollow nail?

COMMENT: Be careful with this question as it is poorly explained in some textbooks.

The bending stiffness of a cylindrical cross-section is proportional to the fourth power of its radius as described by the second moment of area.

In the case of a hollow cylinder, the bending stiffness is proportional to the fourth power of the outer radius minus the fourth power of the inner radius. As such, for any given material a hollow cylinder is less stiff than a solid cylinder of the same outer diameter.

If, however, a constant volume of material is used for construction of an IM nail of fixed length, then the use of a hollow nail would allow a greater outer radius to be used, resulting in a stiffer nail.[?]

EXAMINER: When plating a fracture what factors do you need to consider?

CANDIDATE: I would need to decide if I want to achieve primary or secondary bone healing.

If the fracture was significantly comminuted I would ideally choose to plate in bridging mode with fracture healing by indirect or secondary fracture healing with callus formation.

Simple fractures could be treated with interfragmentary compression.

Ideally, plate position should be on the tension side of the fracture. I would need to decide the length of plate itself, the number and relative position of screws needing to be inserted and the type of screws to be used (standard cortical screws, cancellous screws, locking screws, etc.).

The plate length should be 2–3 times higher than the overall fracture length in comminuted fractures and 8–10 times higher in simple fractures.

The plate screw density should be kept below a value of 0.5, indicating that less than half of the plate holes are occupied by screws.

Two screws (monocortical or bicortical) on each main fragment is the minimum number of screws needed to keep the plate bone construction stable. Such a construct will fail if one screw breaks due to overload or if the screw loosens, so it is generally advised to add another screw to each side of the fracture construct.

Plating offers two different fixation concepts – splinting and interfragmentary compression. Comminuted fractures are best treated using a splinting technique, because local bone and soft tissue devascularization can be minimized; while in simple fractures interfragmentary compression is preferred as a stabilization tool.

When nailing the position, the length and diameter of the nail as well as the position of the locking bolts are more or less given and standardized by the local anatomy of the broken bone segment as well as the implant design (Table 9.1).

Table 9.1 Characteristics of fixation.

	Plating	IM nailing
Concept of fixation	Splinting Compression	Splinting
Load transfer	Locking Friction	Locking
Position	Tension side Compression side	Intramedullary
Insertion	Open MIPO	Intramedullary
Length	To decide	Whole length of bone
Dimension	In relation with bone and bone segment	Inner diameter of bone
Number of screws	Minimum 4 Maximum?	Minimum 0 Maximum 6
Position of screws	To decide	Given by nail design
Design of screws	Bicortical	Monocortical Bicortical Self-tapping Self-drilling Standard cortical Locking

EXAMINER: What is the working length of a plate?

CANDIDATE: The working length of a plate is defined as the distance across a fracture site between the two nearest points where the bone is fixed to the plate, e.g. the distance between the two screws closest to the fracture.

EXAMINER: How is the working length of a plate altered?

CANDIDATE: The working length of a plate can be altered by changing screw position. Screws placed close to a fracture create a short working length, which increases a plate's construct stiffness. Screws placed further from the fracture site increase the working length and produce a less-stiff construct that permits more motion at the fracture gap.

EXAMINER: What problems may arise if screws are placed too close to the fracture site?

CANDIDATE: There is the potential to create stress concentration with the risk of plate fracture. Placing screws further from the fracture site can better distribute the stress the plate experiences and decrease the risk for plate fatigue failure.

The addition of more than three screws per fragment does not significantly impact on a plate's construct stiffness in axial loading. Adding an additional screw nearest to the fracture site provides the greatest increase in axial stiffness.

EXAMINER: Why do we want to avoid over-torqueing of screws?

CANDIDATE: Over-torqueing of the screws should be avoided during insertion.

The screw head can be destroyed.

It may cause screw–bone interface failure (i.e. stripping torque).

EXAMINER: What else?

CANDIDATE: As a screw is inserted into bone, the screw head compresses the plate against the bone with a force proportional to the torque applied to the screw.

If the screw is tightened beyond the ultimate strength of the bone–screw interface, the screw threads will lose purchase in the bone and the screw will spin with little resistance. Although pull-out strength is related to the depth of the screw thread and quality of the bone, stripping the screw reduces the pull-out strength of the screw by more than 80%.

EXAMINER: Why do we retighten screws before closure?

CANDIDATE: Before wound closure, all screws should be retightened to allow time for stress relaxation of the screw–bone interface.

Structured oral examination question 4

Biomechanics IM nail

EXAMINER: What is the working length of a nail?

CANDIDATE: Working length is defined as the length of a nail spanning the fracture site from its distal point of fixation in the proximal fragment to its proximal point of fixation in the distal fragment. More simply, it is the distance between the two points on either side of the fracture where the bone firmly grips the metal.

Thus, working length is the unsupported portion of the nail between the two major bone fragments and reflects the length of a nail carrying the majority of the load across the fracture site.

EXAMINER: What is the relationship between the working length of a nail and bending rigidity?

CANDIDATE: The bending rigidity of a nail is inversely proportional to the square of its working length.

EXAMINER: What about torsional rigidity and working length?

CANDIDATE: Torsional rigidity is inversely proportional to a nail's working length.

COMMENT: If all else fails, a shorter working length means the greater the bending and torsional rigidity of a nail, i.e. a stronger fixation.

EXAMINER: What factors affect working length?

CANDIDATE: The working length of a nail can be very variable depending on:

- Type of force (bending, torsion). When the bone bends at the fracture site the nail may become fixed to the bone by 3 point fixation.
- Type of fracture (fracture pattern) and if the fracture is reduced.
- Interlocking. This modifies the working length of a nail and increases torsional stability.
- Reaming. This prepares a uniform canal, allows a larger diameter nail to be used, improves nail/

bone fixation and reduces the working length of the nail.

A nail has a shorter working length in bending with fixation of a transverse fracture than when used to stabilize a comminuted fracture.

EXAMINER: What affects bending rigidity?

CANDIDATE: Bending rigidity is affected by:
1. Material properties (Young's modulus of elastic). A cobalt chromium nail has twice the bending stiffness as that of titanium.
2. Structural properties.
   (a) Length.
   (b) Second moment area (SMA) of the nail, which is a variable that describes the spatial distribution of a material within a structure. The SMA is affected by the organization and shape of the material.

For a solid circular nail, the bending rigidity is proportional to the fourth power of the nail's radius.
    $SMA = \pi.r^4/4$
For a hollow nail the bending rigidity is very roughly proportional to the third power of the nail diameter.

EXAMINER: Are you sure (see above)?

CANDIDATE: It is more accurate to say the bending rigidity is directly proportional to the fourth power of the outer radius minus the fourth power of the inner radius.
    $SMA = \pi. (r^4_0 - r_1^4)/4$ where r_0 is the outer radius and r_1 is the inner radius.

EXAMINER: What affects torsional rigidity?

CANDIDATE:
1. Material properties.
2. Structural properties.
   Torsional rigidity is proportional to the fourth power of the nail diameter.
   A slotted nail has a torsional rigidity of 1/50 that of a non-slotted nail.

EXAMINER: And?

CANDIDATE: A nail with sharp corners or fluted edges resists torsional forces to a greater degree than a smooth-walled nail.

EXAMINER: What is the difference between second area moment and polar moment for a nail?

CANDIDATE: The second area moment and polar moment area represent the relationship between bending and torsional rigidity of a nail and its cross-sectional dimensions.

The greater the material is distributed away from the neutral axis of the structure, the greater is its area and polar moment and thus the strength and rigidity against bending and torsional stress.

COMMENT: This may lead on to the examiners asking about the differences in second area moment and polar moment for a solid and hollow nail (see above). As mentioned previously, this is often poorly or inaccurately described in books or short notes bullet revision texts.

EXAMINER: What happens to polar moment of inertia when a nail has a slot?

CANDIDATE: The polar moment of inertia is greatly reduced.

EXAMINER: What about length of the nail, how does that affect bending rigidity?

CANDIDATE: The length of the nail between the forces working to bend it determines the length of the moment arm and therefore the magnitude of the bending moment. A similar situation applies in cases of torsional forces.

EXAMINER: How is bending and torsional stiffness related to working length?

CANDIDATE: The bending stiffness of a nail is inversely proportional to the square of its working length. The torsional stiffness is inversely proportional to its working length.
   The shorter the working length, the greater is the bending and torsional stiffness (rigidity) of the nail in the construct and the stronger the fixation.

EXAMINER: How does medullary reaming affect working length?

CANDIDATE: Medullary reaming prepares a uniform canal and improves nail–bone fixation towards the fracture, thus reducing the nail's working length.

EXAMINER: What do you mean by stiffness?

CANDIDATE: Stiffness is defined as the slope of the curve in the elastic range on a stress–strain curve.

EXAMINER: Are you sure?

CANDIDATE: Yes.

COMMENT: The slope of the curve in the elastic range on a stress–strain curve is Young's elastic modulus for a material. Stiffness is defined as the slope of a force versus displacement graph. Elastic modulus is the corresponding slope, but of a stress versus strain graph. Load is converted to stress and displacement to strain.

EXAMINER: What material are IM nails made of?

CANDIDATE: They are made of either titanium or stainless steel. IM nails can be solid or hollow.

EXAMINER: How can we reduce the stiffness of a nail?

CANDIDATE: One way of reducing stiffness is to put a longitudinal slot in the wall of a nail. This makes it much more flexible, but does so at the cost of the nail losing overall bending and torsional strength. The slot allows the cross-section to be compressed when inserted into the medullary canal.

Very stiff nails may damage the bone if there is any discrepancy between the shape of the nail and that of the bone.

EXAMINER: What factors alter a nail's axial, bending and torsional rigidity?

CANDIDATE: This can be divided into material and structural properties. Parameters include cross-sectional geometry, nail length, the presence of a longitudinal slot and the elastic modulus of the material.

Structured oral examination question 5

IM nails

Initial questions on area and polar moment of inertia, bending and torsional rigidity (see above).

EXAMINER: How does the presence of a slot affect bending and torsional rigidity of a nail?

CANDIDATE: The presence of a slot reduces both the bending and torsional stiffness of a nail. A slot significantly affects torsional rigidity, but has much less effect on bending stiffness.

EXAMINER: Why do we use slotted nails?

CANDIDATE: It makes the nail easier to insert.

EXAMINER: What else?

CANDIDATE: Err ...

COMMENT: When a solid nail is introduced into the medullary canal it makes room for its entry by

compression of the surrounding bone tissue. Bone tissue exerts an equal and opposite force on the nail (Newton's third law).

EXAMIMER: What about hoop stresses?

CANDIDATE: Sorry?

COMMENT: Hoop (expansion) stresses are generated in the bone when an IM nail is inserted. Hoop stresses are much higher when a solid or closed-section nail is introduced when compared to a slotted nail. If hoop stresses are too high they can cause comminution or splintering of the bone.

EXAMINER: What is the difference between stiffness and rigidity?

CANDIDATE: [Long silence . . .] Sorry, I don't know.

COMMENT: Rigidity and stiffness are very similar concepts often used interchangeably to denote overall performance of a structure. There are however important distinctions between the two.

Stiffness is a material property, a materials ability to resist deformation, force divided by displacement.

Rigidity is a structural property, a structures ability to resist deformation. Depends on a materials stiffness and geometry construct. Rigidity incorporates both the type of material and its shape and size.

EXAMINER: Why do we use interlocking screws (bolts)? What function do they perform?

CANDIDATE: Interlocking screws help control torsion and axial loads placed on the nail. They provide rotational and longitudinal stability.

EXAMINER: Historically, why were they introduced?

CANDIDATE: The use of interlocking screws expanded the indications for use of IM nails to include more proximal, more distal, and more unstable (highly comminuted, segmental) fractures.

EXAMINER: What are the disadvantages of using interlocking screws?

CANDIDATE: Insertion requires reasonable technical skill to place. The holes in the nail act as stress risers. The weakest part of the nail to fatigue is at or just proximal to the most proximal distal locking screw.

There is an increased rate of nail breakage if the fracture is within 5 cm of these screws, or if the screw hole closest to the fracture is left unfilled.

The closer the fracture is to the distal locking screws, the less cortical contact the nail has, which leads to increased stress on the locking screws and greater chance of screw breakage.

The further the distal locking screw is from the fracture site, the more rotationally stable the fracture becomes because of friction of the nail within the medullary cavity and less chance of screw breakage.

Screw holes closer to the end of the nail allow for the fixation of more proximal or distal fractures, but at the expense of stability of the construct.

EXAMINER: When nailing a long bone, how do you decide on how many locking screws to use?

CANDIDATE: The number of interlocking screws used is based on fracture location, amount of fracture comminution, and the fit of the nail within the canal.

Midshaft transverse femoral fractures have the greatest fixation stability because of isthmic cortical contact. Oblique and comminuted fractures rely on interlocking screws for stability, as do very proximal and very distal metaphyseal fractures, where the medullary canal widens and is filled with weaker cancellous bone.

In general, one screw is sufficient for stable fractures.

EXAMINER: How are locking screws (bolts) different to other screws used for fracture fixation?

CANDIDATE: Locking bolts have a wide core diameter and smaller outer thread diameter. The screw functions to reduce torsional stresses acting on the nail and is not designed to maximize pull-out strength.

EXAMINER: What may occur if you place too many screws in multiple planes through a nail?

CANDIDATE: An IM nail allows fracture healing with relative stability even if a nail is statically locked. Minor movements occur between the nail and screw even in a static mode of nail fixation. Placing screws in multiple planes may lead to a reduction of this fragment toggle and hinder fracture healing.

EXAMINER: What is the biomechanical effect of the orientation of the locking screw?

CANDIDATE: There are some studies that suggest oblique tibial locking screws increase the stability of proximal tibial fractures compared to transverse locking screws. Distally, however, there is little difference.

In the femur, studies suggest no difference in biomechanical behaviour with locking screw orientation.

EXAMINER: What effect does multiple locking screw breakage have on fracture stability?

CANDIDATE: Premature failure of locking screws especially with unstable fracture patterns may lead to angulation, shortening, malunion and IM nail migration.

EXAMINER: How can you reduce the risk of locking screw failure?

CANDIDATE: Compared to using a smaller screw a larger screw diameter increases fatigue resistance. A stainless steel screw has a different fatigue life than a titanium screw. Stainless steel is more ductile than titanium.

Thread design and defects from the manufacturing or insertion process can also contribute to breakage.

Some locking screws (bolts) may have surface defects caused by the machining of threads that could act as notches and contribute to the variability of fatigue life by a stress riser effect.

Inserting a screw incorrectly can result in surface defects as well.

EXAMINER: Why not insert the largest locking bolt possible to reduce the risk of locking bolt failure?

CANDIDATE: The largest diameter of locking bolt that can be used is limited by the diameter of the nail. Increasing the diameter of a locking bolt reduces the cross-section of the nail at its hole, thereby predisposing to nail failure. Nail hole size should not exceed 50% of the nail diameter.

Interlocking screws undergo four-point bending loads, with higher screw stresses seen at the most distal locking sites (Figure 9.5). Under axial load, and in the absence of cortical contact, bending of the screw and screw failure may occur.

189

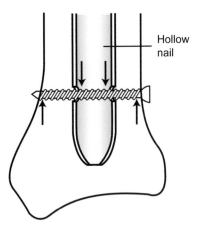

Figure 9.5 Four-point loading on distal interlocking bolts. Four-point loads (arrows) acting on a distal interlocking screw.

Structured oral examination question 6

Plates

The candidate is shown a laminated picture of a plate and asked to describe.

EXAMINER: What is this?

COMMENT: This can be difficult to answer without having a pre-structured approach to the question. With a structure and an earlier rehearsal, it is relatively straightforward.

Think in terms of:

1. Shape (semitubular, one-third tubular).
2. Width of plate (small, narrow, broad).
3. Shape of screw holes (round slots, oval slots).
4. Surface contact characteristics (LCP).
5. Intended site of application (condylar plate).
6. According to the function (locking plate, buttress, neutralisation, bridging, compression).
7. Material (stainless steel, titanium).

EXAMINER: What happens to the moment of inertia if you place a rectangular beam 2 × 4 on its edge rather than on its side?

CANDIDATE: It is 'stronger' in bending when placed on its edge (2″ side) than on its flat (4″) side, yet its cross-sectional area remains constant. A 2″ × 4″ beam on its edge has an area moment of inertia four times greater than on its side and thus demonstrates a fourfold increase in rigidity. More simply put, for a rectangular beam where length, width of thickness is different, the area moment of inertia changes with the change in the orientation of beam with the plane of loading.

COMMENT: In a bending mode of loading, plate strength and stiffness are dependent not only on cross-sectional area but also on the arrangement or distribution of material mass about the neutral axis (shape). The examiner is exploring whether a candidate understands basic biomechanical principles. The practical relevance is that when fixing a fracture, the bone surface chosen to apply a plate can affect mechanical construct stiffness.

CANDIDATE: The bending stiffness of a bone plate is proportional to the thickness of the plate to the third power, whereas the bending stiffness is directly proportional to the width or elastic modulus of the plate. Therefore, changing the plate thickness has more effect upon stiffness than changing the plate width or material.

COMMENT: A plate made of one material can have significantly different properties depending on its width, length, thickness and position of holes.

The *area moment of inertia* (I_a) quantifies the bending resistance (stiffness) of a given cross-section, the larger the area moment of inertia, the greater the bending resistance, the less the stress produced within a structure under a given bending force.

This is expressed as the base (b) times the height or thickness cubed over 12.

$$I_a = bh^3/12$$

Bending stiffness = EI_a, where E is Young's modulus, I_a second moment of area.

COMMENT: Candidates need to understand how the properties of a plate can change depending on its position on the bone, where screws are placed, and the loads it experiences in different areas of the body.

EXAMINER: If you are plating a humerus fracture when would you use a 3.5-mm or 4.5-mm thickness plate?

CANDIDATE: The bending stiffness of a plate is proportional to the thickness of a plate to the third power. Therefore, the bending stiffness of a 4.5-mm plate will be more than twice the bending stiffness of a 3.5-mm plate (3.5 = 42,875, 4.5 = 91,125). Because of the large rotational forces placed on the humerus, it is best to use a 4.5-mm plate.

The 4.5-mm plate is more staggered for screw placement compared to the 3.5-mm plate, which has a narrow area for screw insertion. This reduces the risk of postoperative fracture.

In general, 3.5-mm plates should only be used in the supracondylar region unless the bone size is extremely small and there would be a worry that the screw diameter would be greater than 30% of the bone's diameter of introducing a stress riser that will predispose to a postoperative fracture.

COMMENT: The bone shape of the humerus is not flat and not plate-friendly and it can sometimes be difficult to fit a 4.5-mm plate onto the humerus. However, for examination purposes candidates should err on the side of caution and suggest usage of a 4.5-mm plate.

EXAMINER: What causes a bone to break after fracture fixation?

CANDIDATE: There are two mechanisms. The first is a general difference between the stiffness of the plate and stiffness of the bone, i.e. a mismatch between the plate and bone stiffness. The second reason is that the end of a plate can create an abrupt transition between the metal and bone resulting in a modulus mismatch that can lead to a stress riser. That is why some surgeons prefer to leave the last screw hole in a plate empty. This is particularly concerning if the end of the plate is in a high-stress region such as the subtrochanteric part of the femur. In this situation a longer plate should be used to bypass the high-stress area, especially if bone quality is poor.

EXAMINER. What do we mean by working length of a plate?

CANDIDATE: The distance between the proximal and distal screw in closest proximity to the fracture is defined as the 'working length' of the plate.

EXAMINER: Why is working length important?

CANDIDATE: Plate working length has been shown to influence construct stiffness, plate strain and cyclic fatigue properties of the plate.

EXAMINER: What are the principles of plate fixation?

CANDIDATE: The principle is the conversion of tensile forces to a compression force on the convex side of an eccentrically loaded bone. This is achieved by placing a tension band (bone plate) across the fracture on the tension (or convex) side of the bone. Tension forces are counteracted by the tension band in this position and converted into compressive forces.

The plate should be fixed to the tension side of a long bone to avoid fracture gapping. Plate stresses are significantly increased by gapping at the fracture site and may lead to fatigue failure of the plate.

When a gap is left on the cortex opposite that to which the plate is attached, bending of the plate at the fracture site can cause the plate to rapidly fail.

Gapping may also occur if a plate is not properly contoured during application. Slight prebending of a plate causes the ends of the opposite cortices to be driven together when the plate is applied.

COMMENT: When a prebent plate is used, the inner screws are applied first and then the outer screws.

Torsional and bending stiffness of a fracture construct can be significantly increased, and therefore, plate strain reduced, by increasing the length of the plate itself.

EXAMINER: What about leaving a fracture gap opposite the plate?

CANDIDATE: This makes the plate a fulcrum and leads to increased stress at plate holes.

COMMENT: The candidate has described the principles of tension band plating. As long bones are subjected to eccentric loading, a plate applied to the outer (convex) side counteracts tension forces and provides rigid internal fixation.

EXAMINER: What happens if a plate is applied to the tension cortex, but the opposite cortex is defective?

CANDIDATE: The defective cortex cannot resist compression and the plate will undergo bending stresses and fail under axial load.

EXAMINER: How do plate length and screw number affect the biomechanical stability of a plated construct?

CANDIDATE: The literature is slightly confusing in how plate length and screw number affect the biomechanical stability of a plated construct.

COMMENT: There has been a trend towards fracture fixation using longer plates and fewer screws. Concerns that the plated construct would not provide sufficient construct stiffness and fracture rigidity compared with fixation using shorter plates and more screws have not been realized.

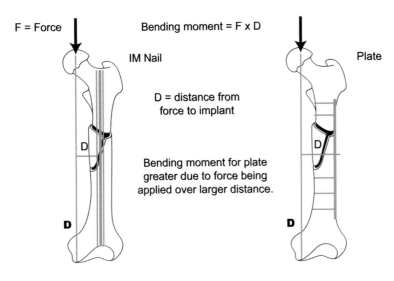

F = Force

Bending moment = F x D

IM Nail

D = distance from
force to implant

Bending moment for plate
greater due to force being
applied over larger distance.

Plate

Figure 9.6 Biomechanical differences between a plate and IM nail. Compared to an IM nail the bending moment (Force × Distance from force to implant) for a plate is greater due to the force being applied over a larger distance.

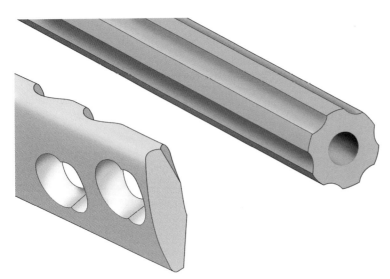

Figure 9.7 Biomechanical comparison of plate vs. IM nail. A nail's cross-section is usually round, resisting loads equally in all directions. A plate's cross-section is rectangular, resisting greater loads in one plane vs. the other.

The use of additional screws to a plated construct has the adverse effects of decreased bone vascularity, increased stress shielding, and possibly an increased risk of stress fracture.

EXAMINER: What are the biomechanical differences between an IM nail and a plate?

COMMENT: This is a very broad question that ideally needs a well-thought out, comprehensive answer.

Start off by first mentioning the function of both an IM nail and a plate. Simplify your answer by sticking to a non-locking plate, otherwise mentioning a locking plate may make your answer too complicated and confusing (Figure 9.6).

A nail's cross-section is round, resisting loads equally in all directions, whereas a plate's cross-section is rectangular, resisting greater loads in one plane compared to another (Figure 9.7).

There are four main types of load acting on an IM nail.

1. Compression.
2. Tension.
3. Torsion.
4. Bending.

Physiologic loading is a combination of all these forces.

The primary function of the plate is to maintain alignment as an internal splint, and to create compression between the fracture ends such that bone can transfer some of the applied loads itself. A compression plate, tension band, or a lag screw does this by generating compression across the fracture.

In fixation constructs in which the plate–bone system can carry load, the compressed fractured bone carries a major part of the load.

EXAMINER: What factors contribute to the overall biomechanical profile of an IM nail?

CANDIDATE: Sorry?

COMMENT: Several factors contribute to the overall biomechanical profile and resulting structural stiffness of an IM nail. These include:
Material properties: most nails are made from either stainless steel or titanium. Titanium nails are less stiff than stainless steel with a lower elastic modulus (closer to bone).
- Cross-sectional shape. Nail diameter affects the bending and torsional rigidity of a nail. For a solid circular nail, the bending and torsional rigidity is proportional to the fourth power of the nail radius. A larger diameter nail with the same cross-section is both stiffer and stronger than a smaller one.
- Diameter curves. Nails are contoured to accommodate IM curvature of long bones. Tibial nails have an 11° bend in the AP direction at the junction of the upper third and lower two-thirds. It is called the angle of Herzog. An anterior bow determines how easily a femoral nail can be inserted as well as bone/nail mismatch that in turn influences the stability of fixation of the nail in the bone. A mismatch in the radius of curvature between the nail and the femur can lead to distal anterior cortical perforation.
- Length and working length (see previous questions).

EXAMINER: What are the benefits of reamed nails?

CANDIDATE: Reaming allows the insertion of a larger-diameter nail that provides more rigidity in bending and torsion.

It reduces the working length of the nail and improves stability.

Reaming increases the contact area between the nail and cortical bone.

EXAMINER: You mentioned IM nails being curved. What is the reason for this?

CANDIDATE: IM nails are contoured to accommodate the curved intramedullary canal of a long bone.

EXAMINER: Anything else?

CANDIDATE: A straight nail if inserted into a curved intramedullary canal will bend and produce stresses that may fracture the bone. Nails should be contoured to accommodate the curves.

EXAMINER: Anything else?

CANDIDATE: A femoral nail is curved in an AP direction to conform to the curvature of the medullary canal. When fully inserted, a femoral nail should fit snugly and not produce any unnecessary stress.

EXAMINER: What happens when you insert a femoral nail into the medullary canal?

CANDIDATE: The nail must bend somewhat to fit the curve of the intramedullary canal. An axial insertional force is necessary to insert the nail and this insertional force is maximal at three-quarters of the insertional length and decreases thereafter as the nail straightens out to adapt to the shape of the medullary canal.

EXAMINER: What about hoop stresses generated when a femoral nail is inserted into the medullary canal?

CANDIDATE: The insertional axial force applied generates hoop stresses within the bone. Excessively large hoop stresses can lead to fracture propagation.

EXAMINER: How do we reduce hoop stresses generated in the femur?

CANDIDATE: Avoid excessive force when impacting the nail into the femur. Introduce the femoral nail in a controlled manner avoiding the use of a hammer if at all possible. Over-reaming the entry hole by 0.5–1 mm and using a slotted nail.

EXAMINER: Anything else?

CANDIDATE: Not sure.

EXAMINER: What about entry point?

CANDIDATE: Not sure.

COMMENT: The most important factor affecting hoop stresses is femoral nail entry point. Avoid an excessive anterior or posterior entry point. If the insertion point is anterior to the central axis of the femur a large insertional force is required for nail insertion. This will generate excessively large hoop (expansion) stresses than can lead to a burst fracture of the femoral shaft. With a posterior entry point there will be loss of proximal fixation and a similar but much less severe increase in hoop stress generation with nail insertion.

IM nails have a straighter (larger) radius than the femoral canal with sometimes a mismatch in radius of curvature. This can lead to distal anterior cortical perforation.

Structured oral examination question 7

Fracture healing

Fracture healing is a definite A-list topic. With a bit of revision and practice candidates should achieve a score 6 without too many difficulties. Most questions are very similar and cover the same material with only occasional deviation into unknown territory midway through a viva.

1. Bone healing: types, types of stability, factors affecting it, cutting cones diagram, different implants for stability, strain theory, what a bridge plating is and how it works.
2. Fracture healing, different types and stages. Absolute versus relative stability options for fracture stabilization, fracture healing, factors affecting it (evidence – did not know!).

EXAMINER: How do fractures heal?

CANDIDATE: Fractures can heal by either direct or primary fracture healing or secondary fracture healing.

COMMENT: The answer needs expanding, as the next obvious question would be to give an example of primary fracture healing.

CANDIDATE: The type of fracture healing that occurs depends on the mechanical stability present at the fracture site. Fractures treated with open reduction in which interfragmentary compression is achieved, such as with a lag screw or with a plate placed in compression mode, will heal by primary or direct fracture healing.

The fracture fixation in this situation provides absolute stability. There is no motion at the fracture site, and no callus is formed. The fracture heals through the formation of osteonal cutting cones and Haversian remodelling of the compressed cortical bone.

Indirect or secondary fracture healing occurs with relative stability and movement at the fracture site. This type of fracture fixation occurs with fractures when treated with a cast or brace, an intramedullary nail, or a plate placed in a bridging mode.

EXAMINER: What do we mean by Perren's strain theory?

CANDIDATE: Perren introduced the concept of strain in fracture healing.

Fracture gap strain is defined as the relative change in the fracture gap (ΔL) divided by the original fracture gap (L). Tissue cannot be produced when strain conditions exceed the tissue strain tolerance.

The strain of cortical bone until it breaks is low, around 2%, while granulation tissue has a high strain tolerance of 100%.

Rigid internal compression fixation, which minimizes strain, will lead to primary or direct fracture healing.

Lamellar bone can tolerate up to 10% strain, and when this relative stability is present, the fracture heals with callus or secondary fracture healing.

Fracture healing will not occur when the strain at a fracture gap exceeds 10%.

EXAMINER: What actually happens at the fracture gap?

CANDIDATE: In a narrow fracture gap, a defined distracting force will disrupt the few cells within it. The same force applied to a wider gap filled with granulation tissue will, however, only deform this tissue and not cause any rupture.

EXAMINER: How does this influence the method of internal fixation you would chose to manage a fracture?

CANDIDATE: In a simple transverse or short oblique fracture, any deforming force is acting very locally on the single fracture gap that corresponds to a high concentration of stress. In a comminuted fracture with multiple fragments the same force will be distributed over a wide range of different fracture fragments or gaps (stress distribution).

Applying Perren's strain theory, a simple fracture type has 'high strain' and is best fixed by a method that produces absolute stability. A more comminuted fracture equates to a low-strain situation and can be managed with fixation that provides relative stability (bridging plate or IM nail).

EXAMINER: So, we can leave large gaps at the fracture site if we are aiming for relative stability?

CANDIDATE: Small gaps can be left at the fracture site in complex fractures managed with relative stability and are usually tolerated. Larger gaps are less well tolerated and may result in delayed or non-union.

EXAMINER: How big a fracture gap?

CANDIDATE: Persistent fracture gaps of over 2 mm in the tibia shaft are associated with delayed healing.
  If you have gone for absolute stability, then any persistent fracture gap should be avoided as this may predispose to non-union.

EXAMINER: What do we mean by a stress riser?

CANDIDATE: A stress riser (concentrator) is a region of an object in which stresses are higher than in the surrounding material.

EXAMINER: What causes crack growth?

CANDIDATE: Crack growth is heightened by stress corrosion, poor bone-to-bone contact at the fracture and if a patient has a large body mass.

EXAMINER: What do we mean by stress corrosion?

CANDIDATE: Stress corrosion combines the effects of local growth of the crack resulting from cyclic loading with galvanic corrosion.

EXAMINER: What is galvanic corrosion?

CANDIDATE: Galvanic corrosion occurs as a result of an electrochemical potential created by the contact of two different metals in an electrochemical medium that causes the release of ions from the metals. Galvanic corrosion can weaken the properties of a plate and screws, causing failure of fracture fixation and possible pain and swelling of the surrounding tissue.

EXAMINER: That's with a plate and screws, but we are discussing an isolated stress concentration propagating and expanding on a plate leading to fatigue failure.

CANDIDATE: In a fixed fracture, the dissimilar materials are the surface of the plate (e.g. stainless steel), which creates an oxide surface coating, and the same material exposed by the fatigue crack that has not yet developed the oxide film. The conductive fluid is saline found in the surrounding tissues.

COMMENT: Galvanic corrosion can accelerate the failure of an implant, even when the implant is loaded well below its yield point, by increasing the rate at which the crack grows. This occurs because in addition to the mechanical propagation at the site of the crack, material at the crack is being removed by the corrosion process.

EXAMINER: Why do we tap before screw insertion?

CANDIDATE: Tapping is required so that the torque applied by the surgeon is converted into compression instead of cutting threads and overcoming the friction between the screw thread and the bone.
  With a pre-tapped hole, around 65% of the torque goes to produce compression and 35% to overcome the friction associated with driving the screw. When the hole is not tapped, only about 5% of the torque is used to produce compression, the rest going to overcome friction and to cut threads in bone.

EXAMINER: So why do we sometimes avoid tapping in cancellous bone?

CANDIDATE: In cancellous bone screw pull-out can become an issue, particularly in osteoporotic bone. Tapping reduces strength in cancellous bone in that running the tap in and out of the hole removes bone, effectively increasing the diameter of the hole and reducing the amount of bone material that interacts with the screw threads.

EXAMINER: What factors affect screw pull-out?

COMMENT: This is a classic predictable screw exam question. Candidates need to have rehearsed and run through their answer beforehand.

EXAMINER: Why is it important to do a final check and tighten all screws at the end of fracture fixation?

CANDIDATE: A screw holds the plate against bone partly by frictional contact, which depends on the frictional force generated between the undersurface of the plate and the bone. If any sliding occurs between the plate and the bone, the bending load will be transferred from the head of the screw into the plate, where screw plate contact occurs.

Bending loads perpendicular to the axis of a screw, along with possible stress corrosion and fretting corrosion, may cause a screw to fail in fatigue.

Structured oral examination question 8

Fracture healing

EXAMINER: How does fracture healing occur?

CANDIDATE: Fracture healing can occur by primary or secondary bone healing.

EXAMINER: What is primary bone healing?

CANDIDATE:

- This requires close anatomical reduction with minimal movement at the fracture site (< 2% strain).
- In the initial stages, osteoblasts differentiate from mesenchymal cells and lay down woven bone in any gaps. Lamellar bone may be laid down directly if there are no gaps.
- Remodelling then occurs across the fracture site, with cutting cones passing across the fracture site.
- Healing is slow.

EXAMINER: What is gap healing?

CANDIDATE: This is a type of primary bone healing.

EXAMINER: And?

CANDIDATE: In this process the fracture site is primarily filled by lamellar bone oriented perpendicular to the long axis, requiring a secondary osteonal reconstruction, unlike the process of contact healing.

The primary bone structure is then gradually replaced by longitudinal revascularized osteons carrying osteoprogenitor cells which differentiate into osteoblasts and produce lamellar bone on each surface of the gap.

EXAMINER: What is contact healing?

CANDIDATE: If the gap between bone ends is less than 0.01 mm and interfragmentary strain is less than 2%, the fracture unites by so-called contact healing.

Under these conditions, cutting cones are formed at the ends of the osteons closest to the fracture site. The tips of the cutting cones consist of osteoclasts which cross the fracture line, generating longitudinal cavities at a rate of 50–100 μm/day.

These cavities are later filled by bone produced by osteoblasts residing at the rear of the cutting cone. This results in the simultaneous generation of a bony union and the restoration of Haversian systems formed in an axial direction.

COMMENT: The answer is a bit out of sync as usually contact and then gap healing is described.

EXAMINER: Can you draw a cutting cone for me, please?

COMMENT: See Chapter 20.

EXAMINER: What is secondary bone healing?

CANDIDATE:

- Secondary healing (by callus) requires some motion at the fracture site (> 2% but < 10%).
- It consists of both endochondral and intramembranous bone healing.
- Hard callus forms under the periosteum at the periphery.
- The callus undergoes a process of progressive stiffening. In the earlier, less stiff, stages it is more resilient to movement at the fracture site, but less good at taking loads or resisting deformation. The strength of the healing fracture does not necessarily correlate with its stiffness.

EXAMINER: What are the stages of secondary fracture healing by callus?

CANDIDATE: The stages of fracture healing include:

- Stage 1: First week. Haematoma formation with invasion of macrophages, leukocytes and lymphocytes. Proinflammatory cytokines (including IL-1 and IL-6 and tumour necrosing factor α), and peptide signal molecules (including BMPs, TGF-β and PDGF) recruit inflammatory cells and promote angiogenesis. Progenitor cells invade. The haematoma coagulates in between and around the fracture ends, and within the medulla forming a template for callus formation. Granulation tissue forms. The acute inflammatory response peaks within the first 24 h and is complete after 7 days.

- Stage 2: 1 week to 1 month. Soft callus forms. In this stage, fibrous tissue, cartilage and woven bone form. Chondroblasts and fibroblasts differentiate and form collagen (mainly type II) and fibrous tissue. Proteoglycans are produced, which suppress mineralization. The chondrocytes then release calcium into the ECM and also protein-degrading enzymes that break down the proteoglycans, thus allowing mineralization to take place.
- Stage 3: 1–4 months. Hard callus forms. The soft callus is invaded by new blood vessels and chondroclasts break down the calcified callus, which is replaced by osteoid (type I collagen) formed by osteoblasts. The osteoid calcifies to form woven bone. The osteoid callus is stiffer than the soft chondroid callus.
- Stage 4: Remodelling – several years. The woven bone is remodelled to lamellar bone. The medullary canal reforms as the bone remodels in response to the stresses placed upon it.

Structured oral examination question 9

Screws[3]

Introduction

This is an A-list 5-minute basic science or trauma viva question. Examiners would expect candidates to be well-versed with the basics of an answer. This material is asked in ST3 interviews and trauma meetings and covered in the mandatory AO Basic Principles of Fracture Management course, and also lots of FRCS (Tr & Orth) revision textbook model answers or on websites.

The examiners usually probe and ask less-obvious questions if candidates have done well and are heading for a good pass (score 7/8). The other alternative is probing because the examiners had been expecting a better performance with greater detail. Lastly probing regardless of how well a candidate is doing as examiners are aware candidates know the routine questions/answers and want to re-invent the topic.

We present an answer outline to be used as a guide only. This is a rather dull topic in print, only really coming to life in a live viva situation observing the to-and-fro questions and answers between examiner and candidate.

A dry run through of the topic is definitely more useful than multiple textbook re-reads of the topic.

COMMENT: Candidates may be asked to draw a screw out or be shown a laminated diagram of a screw and asked to describe the various screw design features (Figures 9.8 and 9.9). Be prepared for both scenarios.

Candidates need to practise drawing and describing out loud the various parts of a screw beforehand, otherwise in the exam if unpractised they can appear quite unrehearsed and amateurish.

EXAMINER: Can you describe the different parts of the screw and their function?

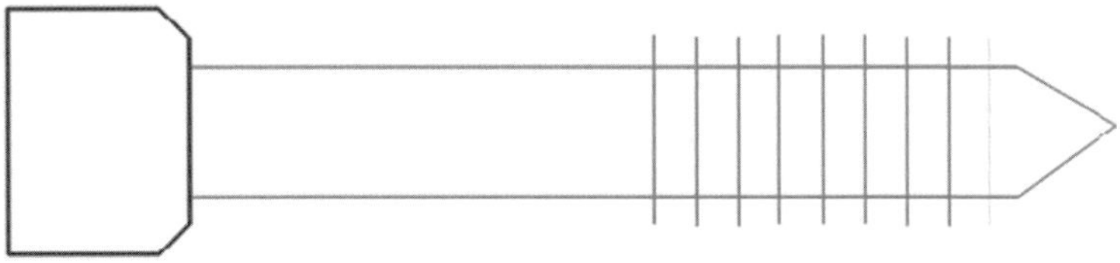

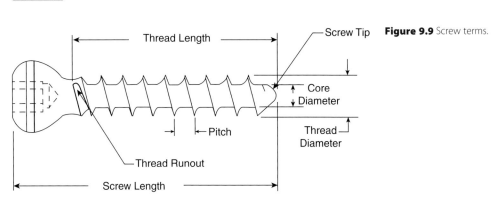

Figure 9.8 Candidate drawing of a screw.

Figure 9.9 Screw terms.

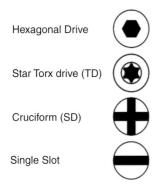

Hexagonal Drive

Star Torx drive (TD)

Cruciform (SD)

Single Slot

Figure 9.10 Slot for screwdriver.

CANDIDATE:

Head

This prevents sinking of the screw into the bone and provides a connection for a screwdriver.

The main slot designs (recess types) for a screwdriver are (1) single slot, (2) cruciate head, (3) Philips, (4) recessed hexagonal head (hex head) and (5) Torx-6 stardriver (Figure 9.10).

A hexagonal head has six points of contact to increase torque, avoid slip and improve directional control. A stardriver maintains the advantage of the hex, but offers better resistance to stripping.

Countersink

The countersink is the undersurface of the head and is either conical or hemispherical.

Run out

Transitional area between shaft and thread. Site of a stress riser and where a screw may break if incorrectly inserted.

Shaft

Smooth link between head and thread. Almost not present in a standard cortical screw.

Thread geometry

Most bone screws have asymmetrical threads, i.e. flat on upper surface and rounded underneath. This provides a wide surface for pulling and little frictional resistance on the underside.

Thread pitch

The pitch is the distance between adjacent screw threads. With each full turn the screw advances by a distance equal to the distance between the threads.

The shorter the distance the 'finer' the pitch, the longer the distance the coarser the pitch. Cortical screws have a fine pitch and therefore a greater number of threads. Cancellous screws have a coarse pitch.

A fine-pitched screw moves a smaller distance linearly for a given angular rotation, offers greater mechanical advantage, producing greater compression, and has more leverage than a coarse-pitched screw.

Thread depth

Thread depth is half the difference between thread diameter and core diameter. The thread depth determines the amount of contact with bone that in turn determines the resistance to pull-out. In cancellous bone a deeper thread is needed to increase the surface area to improve the purchase, as cancellous bone is weaker. This increases resistance to screw pull out.

Thread shape

The shape of thread may be V-thread (more stress at sharp corner), buttress thread (less stress at the rounded corner), reverse buttress or square thread.

Lead

The lead is the linear distance travelled by a screw for one complete (360°) turn of the screw. If a screw is single-threaded, the lead is the same as the pitch. On a double-threaded screw, the lead is two times the pitch. This allows faster screw insertion, but consumes more torsional energy.

Diameters

- *Core diameter:* narrowest diameter in the thread section. Solid section from which the threads project outwards. Also, a weak part of a screw. The size of drill bit used is equal to the core diameter. Torsional strength is proportional to the cube of the core diameter.
- *Shaft diameter:* diameter of shaft where there is no thread.
- *Outer or Thread diameter:* the maximal thread width. The larger the outer diameter, the greater the resistance to pull-out.

Flutes

Channels that provide a route for removal swarf (bone debris).

Tip

Several different designs are available. The tip can be:

- Non-self-tapping screw: smooth, conical tip. Needs pre-drilling of a pilot hole and then use of a tap to create a channel/thread for insertion.
- Self-tapping: needs pre-drilling of a pilot hole, but has cutting flutes for creating its own thread/channel in cortical bone that allows bone cuttings to escape. In general, inferior bone-holding ability.
- Self-drilling and self-tapping: tip will make a drill hole and will cut the channel for the thread.
- Corkscrew tip: used in cancellous screws where the tip clears the pre-drilled hole.

COMMENT: Candidates may be stopped at any stage to be more closely questioned on a particular aspect of screw design.

EXAMINER: What is the biomechanical definition of a screw?

CANDIDATE: There are several definitions.

- A screw is a mechanism that produces linear motion as it is rotated.
- A screw is a device that converts torsional force into an axial force.
- A screw is a mechanical device that converts a rotational movement (torque) into a linear movement (translation).

EXAMINER: What do we mean by a screw's purchase?

CANDIDATE: A screw's hold in bone is referred to as purchase.

EXAMINER: What do we mean by a screw pull-out strength?

CANDIDATE: The axial force required to remove a screw is referred to as its pull-out strength.

EXAMINER: How can you maximize pull-out strength[4]?

CANDIDATE: The pull-out strength of a screw can be increased by increasing the contact surface area (interface) between screw threads and bone. This can be achieved by either:

- Increasing the outer diameter.
- Decreasing the inner (core) diameter.

This effectively increases the width of the threads.

- Increasing the thread density (reducing the pitch).

COMMENT: Enough for a 6 pass. Small-print stuff includes:

- Increasing the number of threads engaged in the bone cortex (increased cortex thickness, bicortical fixation).
- Use a locking screw.

The 'finer' the pitch and the more turns the surgeon needs to make to insert the screw and the more turns of the spiral thread engage in a given depth of cortex. The more threads engaged in the cortex, the greater the pull-out strength (resistance).

EXAMINER: What happens if the pitch is too small?

CANDIDATE: If the pitch is too small there is insufficient bone between individual threads.

EXAMINER: How does the use of a locking screw maximize pull-out strength?

CANDIDATE: With a locking plate failure there is en-bloc pull-out of an interlocking screw system rather than sequential pull-out of conventional screws.

COMMENT: A screw used in a locking plate requires resistance to bending both at the junction between the plate and screw and along the length of the screw. It doesn't require a large pull-out strength. A locking screw as such has a relatively larger core diameter in relation to the thread diameter.

However, in a locking screw fixation, a monobloc effect is produced, with all the screws forcing at the same time. This osteosynthesis method is much sturdier compared to sequential pull-out of conventional screws.

EXAMINER: What surgeon factors can reduce screw pull-out strength?

CANDIDATE:
- Making too large a pilot hole.
- Repeated withdrawal and reintroduction of a screw causing damage to the negative threads in the bone tissue.
- Wobbling of the screwdriver handle during insertion.

COMMENT: Poor technique or technical mistake.

Structured oral examination question 10

A laminated photograph showing different types of screws (usually cancellous, cortical or cannulated) may be shown to a candidate. The candidate is then asked to discuss how the various screws differ in design features.

With the standardized viva format the days of candidates being handed over a screw to describe are over.

EXAMINER: Describe the different types of screw.

CANDIDATE:
- Cortical and cancellous. The main differences relate to:
  - *Pitch*. Cancellous screws have a larger pitch, greater thread depth and a smaller number of threads. Cortical screws have a smaller pitch, a greater number of threads and are designed to have better purchase in cortical bone.
  - *Tip*. Cancellous screw tips are designed as a tapering spiral. These tips create their own threads in cancellous bone. As the tapered spiral advances, it pushes the spongy cancellous bone aside to thread its way into the bone. Cortical screws are usually blunt-ended.
  - *Core to outer diameter*. Higher ratio in a cortical screw.

  COMMENT: Thread depth determines whether a screw is cancellous or cortical. Cortical screws have larger root diameter. Ratio of inner (core) diameter to outer (thread) for a 4.5mm cortical screw is 3/4.5 (66.7%) and for a 4mm cancellous screw is 1.9/4 (47.5%) ~ 2/3rds to 1/2.
- Fully or partially threaded screw. Fully or partial threaded with cancellous. Fully threaded with cortical.
- Locking and non-locking. A locking screw has threads on the head to allow locking into plates and provide angular stability of the plate screw construct, increasing the pull-out strength of the screw. Ideal for use in osteoporotic bone.
- Cannulated and non-cannulated screws. Cannulated screws have a hollow core to allow placement over a guide wire. The hollow core weakens the screw, although clinically this is not often a problem. They are useful for accurate positioning near articular surfaces. Guide wire allows radiological check prior to screw insertion.

EXAMINER: How do the design features of a particular screw relate to its function?

CANDIDATE:
- Cortical screw: a cortical screw is designed to gain maximal purchase in the bone cortices. Cortical bone is usually dense but has limited thickness.

As such, to maximize purchase, cortical screws have a small pitch and their tips are designed to cut into dense cortical bone.
- Cancellous screw: this screw is designed to gain purchase in cancellous bone, most commonly the metaphyses of long bones. Cancellous bone is less dense and spread out compared to cortical bone and to gain maximum purchase cancellous screws have wider threads and larger pitch. The screw threads cut their path in the bone when the screw is inserted (self-tapping screws) with the tip designed to press cancellous bone aside like a snow plough presses aside spread-out snow.
- Locking screw: this has an additional set of threads around the head. It is used in combination with a locking plate that has reciprocal grooves around the plate holes. The locking screw locks into the plate. The plate/screw construct is more rigid than a non-locking construct and provides greater implant stability.
- Cannulated screw: this has a canal through the central core in which a guide wire can be used to guide the position of the screw.
- Locking screw (bolt). This is designed to control torsional and axial loads. A large core diameter (strength of screw and fatigue resistance) and no need for a large thread diameter as pull out resistance is not important.

EXAMINER: What is the technique of lag screw fixation across a fracture site[5]?

CANDIDATE: This involves over-drilling the near-side object to a diameter slightly larger than the thread diameter, creating a gliding hole. The far object is drilled as normal to core diameter and tapped to the thread diameter. The screw thread only gains purchase in the far object, so when the head comes into contact with the near-side object it allows compression of the two objects.

- Drilling large lag (gliding) hole (near cortex).
- Drilling small (threaded) hole (far cortex).
- Countersinking.
- Measuring.
- Taping the far cortex with a protective tap sleeve. Need direction and wobble control.
- Insertion of screw. Reduction forceps should be removed just before final tightening of the screw.

COMMENT: Be sure of your order. For example, if measuring takes place before countersinking then the length of the screw will be too long.

EXAMINER: What about fracture reduction?

CANDIDATE: Normally, the fracture fragments should be reduced before the near cortex is drilled.

EXAMINER: What do you mean by countersinking a screw?

CANDIDATE: When a screw is used without a plate, a countersink hole is created to reduce the risk of fracture as the screw is tightened. This disperses a high pressure over a wider area and reduces the prominence of the screw head.

EXAMINER: What else?

CANDIDATE: Failure to countersink can result in very high stresses at the screw head/bone interface, causing microfractures, leading to screw loosening. Countersinking maximizes the contact between screw and bone to minimize stress.

EXAMINER: What else?

CANDIDATE: Failure to perform proper countersinking causes an eccentric loading and lessens the degree of compression. In a very thin cortex it might also lead to slight displacement of the fragments because of the eccentric force.

EXAMINER: So, what about a small fragment cortical screw, what size is this?

CANDIDATE: A small fragment screw has a thread diameter of 3.5 mm and a core diameter of 2.5 mm.

EXAMINER: What about drill sizes for a lag screw?

CANDIDATE: 3.5-mm drill bit (silver) for the gliding hole and 2.5-mm drill bit (gold) for the thread hole.

EXAMINER: Is that for a large or small fragment cortical screw?

CANDIDATE: Small cortical screw.

COMMENT: For a small cortical lag screw the near cortex is drilled with a 3.5-mm drill before the far cortex is drilled with a 2.5-mm drill, which is tapped with a 3.5-mm tap before inserting a 3.5-mm screw orientated perpendicular to the fracture to obtain compression.

EXAMINER: What about a large fragment screw when it is used as a lag screw?

CANDIDATE: For a large fragment screw this has a thread diameter of 4.5-mm and a core diameter of 3.1-mm. To be used as a lag screw we need two different drill sizes in order to create the gliding hole (near cortex) and a threaded hole (far cortex).

COMMENT: This is score 5/score 6 material. Candidates are not scoring any marks.

EXAMINER: What else?

CANDIDATE: We use a 4.5-mm drill bit for the gliding hole and a 3.2-mm pilot drill bit for the threaded hole.

EXAMINER: What size of tap do we use?

CANDIDATE: The tap is 3.5 mm.

COMMENT: The tap size is 4.5 mm. The screw and tap are the same size. This is basic stuff that is being tested. If a candidate mentions using a 4.5-mm drill and a 3.5-mm tap they are heading for a poor fail (score 4) as they don't understand the principles of lag screw fixation.

EXAMINER: How do we measure the depth of the screw tract?

CANDIDATE: We use a depth gauge.

EXAMINER: How?

CANDIDATE: We just measure the depth.

COMMENT: It is important to engage the hook of the depth gauge against the obtuse edge of the exit hole, not the acute angled edge, otherwise the screw depth will be incorrect. Length reading will be too short. Longest distance allows maximum purchase.

EXAMINER: What about a mini fragment set?

CANDIDATE: These contain cortical screws of size 1.5 mm and 2.0 mm.

EXAMINER: What else?

CANDIDATE: The 1.5-mm screws are used to fix phalangeal fractures while the 2.0-mm screws are used to fix metacarpal fractures.

EXAMINER: Drill bit for gliding hole and threaded hole and tap for a 1.5-mm cortical screw.

CANDIDATE: I don't think they are used as a lag screw.

EXAMINER: They can be used as a lag screw if needed.

COMMENT: For a 2-mm screw it is 2.0 mm for a gliding hole, 1.5 mm for a threaded hole and

⊕ SYNTHES®

Screws, Drill Bits and Taps (Self-tapping and Non-self-tapping Screws)

Screw Diameter (mm)

Thread Diameter	1.0	1.3	1.5	2.0	2.4	2.7	3.5			4.0			4.5			6.5			
Screw Type	Cortex, self-tapping						Cortex	Pelvic Cortex	Shaft	Cortex	Cancellous Non-self-tapping		Cortex	Shaft	Malleolar	Cancellous Non-self-tapping			
	–	–	and Non-self-tapping	and Non-self-tapping	–	and Non-self-tapping	Self-tapping and Non-self-tapping	Self-tapping	Non-self-tapping	Self-tapping	Partial Thread	Full Thread	Self-tapping and Non-self-tapping	Non-self-tapping	Non-self-tapping	16 mm Thread	24 mm Thread	32 mm Thread	Full Thread

Drill Bit and Tap Diameter (mm)

Drill Bit for Gliding Hole	1.0	1.3	1.5	2.0	2.4	2.7	3.5	4.0	–	4.5	4.5 in hard bone

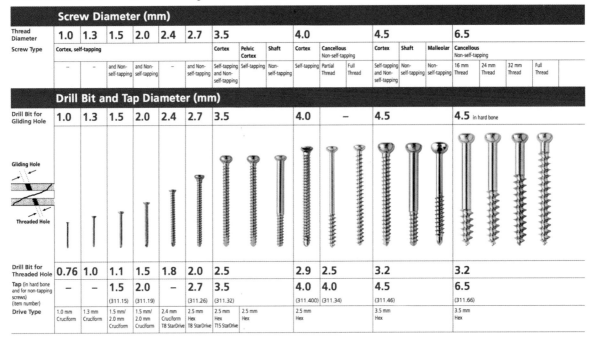

Drill Bit for Threaded Hole	0.76	1.0	1.1	1.5	1.8	2.0	2.5	2.9	2.5	3.2	3.2
Tap (in hard bone and for non-tapping screws) (item number)	–	–	1.5 (311.15)	2.0 (311.19)	–	2.7 (311.26)	3.5 (311.32)	4.0 (311.400)	4.0 (311.34)	4.5 (311.46)	6.5 (311.66)
Drive Type	1.0 mm Cruciform	1.3 mm Cruciform	1.5 mm/ 2.0 mm Cruciform	1.5 mm/ 2.0 mm Cruciform	2.4 mm Cruciform	2.5 mm Hex T8 StarDrive	2.5 mm Hex T8 StarDrive / 2.5 mm Hex T15 StarDrive	2.5 mm Hex		3.5 mm Hex	3.5 mm Hex

Figure 9.11 Screws, drills, bits and taps.

a 2-mm tap. Figure 9.11 gives comprehensive information on thread diameter, drill bit and tap diameter sizes.

EXAMINER: What are the principles of the lag screw technique?

CANDIDATE:
- A lag screw allows compression of two fracture fragments as the screw thread only engages in the far cortex and slides through the near cortex.
- It is a technique, not a type of screw.
- Any screw can function as a lag screw.
- It provides interfragmentary compression.
- It results in absolute stability.
- The lag screw should compress fracture fragments together.

EXAMINER: What are the conditions for interfragmentary compression?

CANDIDATE:
- The screw must glide through the near cortex.
- Threads hold only in the far cortex.
- Screw head should stop at the near cortex.

- The maximum compression occurs at 90° to the fracture.

EXAMINER: When does the lag screw principle fail?

CANDIDATE: Sorry, I am not sure what you mean.

COMMENT: The near cortex needs to be over-drilled as otherwise the threads of the screw will engage both near and far cortex and no fracture compression will occur.

Lag screws should not be used in comminuted fractures. They are ideally suited for simple fractures such as spiral or oblique.

They should be inserted perpendicular to the fracture plane to generate the greatest interfragmental compression and reduce the risk of fracture displacement.

EXAMINER: What are the functions of a screw[6]?

CANDIDATE:
- To produce interfragmentary compression.
- To attach implants to bone by compressing them onto the bone surface.

- To attach implants to bone, producing angular stability.
- To lock an intramedullary nail to the cortices.
- To block movement of a main fragment around an IM nail – Poller screws.

COMMENT: AO teaching.

EXAMINER: OK. Can you name me the different types of screw function?

CANDIDATE: I am not sure.

COMMENT:

- Plate screw: preload and friction is applied to create a force between the plate and the bone.
- Lag compression screw (see above).
- Position screw: holds anatomical parts in correct relation to each other without compression, i.e. thread hole only, no glide. For example, syndesmosis screw.
- Locking head screw: used with locking plate, threads in the screw head allow mechanical coupling to reciprocal threads in the plate and provide angular stability.
- Buttress/antiglide screw: a lag screw may be applied in a buttress function at the tip of the fragment.
- Anchor screw: a point of fixation used to anchor a wire loop or strong suture. For example, K-wire fixation of medial malleolus fracture.
- Push pull screw: a temporary point of fixation used to reduce a fracture by distraction and/or compression.
- Reduction screw: a conventional screw is used through a plate to pull fracture fragments towards the plate, the screw may be removed or exchanged once alignment is obtained.
- Pollar: screw is used as a fulcrum to redirect/guide an IM nail.

Candidates may be quizzed in more detail on each specific function.

Structured oral examination question 11

Screw

The candidate is shown a picture of a cortical screw. What is a screw? What are the parts of the screw? Why

are there different thread diameters? How do you use a lag screw? Why do some screws now have threads in their heads?

COMMENT: Similar question to previous ones, but with a few different twists along the way.

EXAMINER: What is a screw?

CANDIDATE: A screw is a device which converts rotational forces into linear motion [AO definition].

EXAMINER: What are the parts of a screw?

CANDIDATE: A screw has four main functional components.

- Head.
- Shaft. The shaft is the smooth part of the screw between the head and the thread. The run-out is the spot where the shaft ends and the thread begins.
- Thread.
- Tip.

COMMENT: This is your basic score 5/6 answer. Most candidates should aim to give a bit more detail in their answer to make sure of scoring at least a 6. Core diameter, thread diameter, pitch, etc. (see above).

EXAMINER: What is the difference between thread diameter and thread depth?

CANDIDATE: Thread diameter is the maximum diameter of the threads. Thread depth is half of the difference between thread diameter and core diameter. The thread depth determines the amount of contact with the bones, which in turn determines the resistance to pull-out. The size of tap is equal to the thread diameter.

EXAMINER: How do you use a lag screw[7]?

COMMENT: A slightly ambiguous question. Possibly asking about what fractures are best suited for lag screw fixation. Perhaps the question may lead on towards how you perform a lag screw fixation (see above).

EXAMINER: Why do some screws now have threads in their heads?

CANDIDATE: These are locking screws. They increase screw pull-out strength and prevent sequential pull-out failure of a plate.

Structured oral examination question 12

Lag screw

Lag screw, principles, how plates work, how nails work.

Name drill sizes and how to insert a lag screw (3.5 and 4.5 mm cortex lag screw (drill bits, taps, gliding hole and threaded hole)). Types of screw. Draw cross-section of a washer. How does a washer work?

EXAMINER: How do plates work?

CANDIDATE: A bone plate transmits forces from one end of the bone to the other bypassing and therefore protecting the area of fracture.

It also holds the fracture ends together maintaining alignment while the facture heals.

As a screw is tightened against a plate it generates a compressive force between the plate and the bone. A reactionary friction force develops that is equal to the compressive force between the plate and bone.

EXAMINER: What factors determine the success of a bone–plate fixation construct?

CANDIDATE: The success of a bone–plate fixation construct depends on several factors including:

Plate thickness, geometry and material used: a stress on a plate that exceeds the elastic limit will lead to plate bending. Cyclical forces above the fatigue limit will eventually lead to plate failure if the fracture does not heal. A race against time for fracture healing versus hardware failure.

Screw design, material, number and hold in bone: non-locking screws will usually loosen individually by toggling out. Locking screws fail en masse.

Bone mechanical properties and bone health.

Construct-placement of plate and direction of load.

Compression between fragments: always attempt to apply a plate on the tension side of the bone and under compression.

EXAMINER: What determines the strength of a plate?

CANDIDATE: $BH^3/12$

B = base, H = height.

Bending stiffness is proportional to the thickness (h) of the plate to the third power.

EXAMINER: Why do we use a washer?

CANDIDATE: Washers spread the load applied by the head on the underlying cortex and are used to prevent the screw head from breaking through a thin cortex [AO].

Washers can be used with lag screw fixation to optimize compression and reduce the risk of unintentional intrusion of the screw head through cortical bone during screw insertion. They are mainly used in metaphyseal bone or if the bone is osteoporotic.

EXAMINER: Draw a cross-section of a washer.

COMMENT: A washer has two sides, a flat side and a concave side. The flat side of the washer rests on the bone while the concave (countersunk) side matches the undersurface of the screw head.

Structured oral examination question 13

Design features of a screw

You are given a new screw from a rep. How would you appraise it? What would determine if YOU would consider using it or not?

You are given two types of self-tapping screws (one normal, one reverse-cutting as well as self-tapping) – describe these implants. Why would you use a reverse self-cutting screw?

You are given DCS and DHS. What are these implants? Describe their differences. How would you apply them (exactly, with order of screw placement and why)? What are the principles and design specifications of a compression plate?

EXAMINER: You have been given a new screw from a company representative. How would you appraise it? What would determine if YOU would consider using it or not?

COMMENT: This is similar to the 'given a new plate by a rep and asked to evaluate'. This question is designed to test higher-order thinking. It is one level above a candidate talking through the various functional parts of a screw.

What is the material of the screw (titanium, stainless steel, bioabsorbable)?

Titanium: high tensile and yield strengths, reduced stiffness, increased biocompatibility, Young's modulus of elasticity closer to bone, diminished stress shielding MRI compatible, superior strength under the high cycle repeated load stresses. Titanium and titanium alloys are not notch-sensitive, which means that stress raisers have minimal effects on the mechanical properties of titanium implants. Titanium is immune to fretting and local corrosion that is seen with stainless steel implants.

Stainless steel: cheaper and easier to manufacture.

Bioabsorbable: radiolucent, eliminates the need for hardware removal, reduced stress-shielding and allows a gradual load transfer to a healing fracture. Disadvantages include lower mechanical strength, higher cost and in some cases an undesired biological response.

In simple terms, a screw should be made of a strong material that can withstand a heavy load.

What is the size of screw to be used?

Mini fragment, small fragment or large fragment screw.

What *function* will it serve or simply, what is its mechanism of action?

- Conventional bone screw (cortical or cancellous).
- Locking bolt.
- Locking screw.
- Cannulated screw.

Steer the question on to safe territory. Candidates may have a free hand into what screw function they can discuss or be pushed towards one particular direction. Unless you are very confident don't mention small-print stuff such as buttress or anchor screws. Go for something that will allow you to keep talking and scoring marks.

Self-tapping. This is the ability of a screw to advance when turned, while creating its own thread. If a screw is not self-tapping it will generally be necessary to use a tap to cut a thread into the bone before screw insertion.

CANDIDATE: I would want to prevent screw failure and need to consider the following factors.

Tensile strength (resistance to bending): this is directly proportional to the square of its core diameter – core diameter^2.

Torsional strength: proportional to the cube of its core diameter – core diameter^3. A screw can

break during insertion if the applied torsional load exceeds its torsional strength.

Pull-out strength: I would need to decide on the pull-out strength of the screw. This depends on the thread diameter. It is affected by the density of the bone beneath the screw threads.

Core diameter: the core diameter is a weak part of the screw. The smaller the core diameter, the greater the risk to shear off during insertion and removal.

Stripping of the screw head: I would want to avoid stripping of the screw head. Mainly this is caused by the screwdriver incorrectly aligned with the screw axis. This means that the screw driver is not aligned co-linearly with the screw axis and doesn't obtain complete engagement in the screw head. A stardrive recess offers best resistance to stripping. I would certainly want to avoid use of a single-slot head. Titanium screws are more prone to stripping of the screw head than stainless steel.

Countersink: I would want to know the shape of the countersink. A hemispherical undersurface is generally preferred because it allows a screw to be angulated in all directions within a washer or the screw hole of a plate while maintaining concentric contact between the screw and side of the plate.

Score 8: The pull-out strength of a screw increases with increasing screw length, thread diameter, thread depth and bone strength.

$$F = S \times (L \times \pi \times D) \times TSF$$
F = pull out strength
S = ultimate shear strength of bone
L = screw length
D thread diameter

The thread shape factor is defined as 0.5 plus the ratio of thread depth to thread pitch multiplied by a constant

TSF = 05 + thread depth/thread pitch × K (constant)

The TSF and thus screw holding strength increase whenever the thread depth becomes larger (larger threads and smaller root diameter).

EXAMINER: Given two types of self-tapping screws (1 normal, one reverse-cutting as well as self-tapping) – describe these implants. Why would you use a reverse self-cutting screw?

CANDIDATE: Self-tapping screws are produced with sharp cutting flutes at the leading end of the threaded portion of the screw. The flutes are

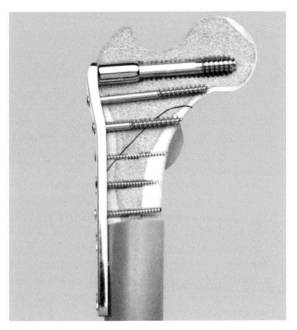

Figure 9.12 DCS plate for stable subtrochanteric fractures.

milled into the thread blank. The flutes cut through bone and facilitate screw insertion.

Tapping is the process of cutting internal threads into the material. Tapping may reduce the torque needed to place the screw threads through dense cortical bone, but in cancellous bone it may decrease the ultimate holding and compressive power of the screw.

Flutes are also milled into the opposite end of the threaded blank. These are called reverse-cutting flutes which allow the thread to cut its way out of the bone after fracture healing.

EXAMINER: Can you give me an example of when to use a reverse self-cutting screw?

CANDIDATE: Reverse self-cutting screws are used to make screw removal easier. The screws are usually self-tapping screws with reverse-cutting flutes. An example would be a paediatric cannulated screw inserted over a guide wire used for a SUFE that will often require removal at a later date.

EXAMINER: Given (shown) a DCS and DHS implant. What are these implants? Describe their differences. How would you apply them (exactly, with the order of screw placement and why)?

What are the principles and design specifications of a compression plate?

CANDIDATE: A DCS plate was initially designed for fixation of distal femoral fractures but can also be used to fix proximal femoral fractures. A DHS implant is the 'gold standard' for intertrochanteric fracture treatment. The main difference between these two implants is the angle of the lag screw with respect to the plate (Figure 9.12).

When used in the proximal femur, the DCS plate can only be used to treat stable fractures; i.e. fractures that can be directly reduced and anatomically reassembled to allow restoration of the bony medial buttress. Because the DCS plate has a 95° barrel angle, it does not allow for controlled compression.

The design of the DCS plate can enhance fixation of selected stable subtrochanteric fractures because it permits stable fixation in the proximal fragment. The DCS plate has a 95° barrel angle, allowing it to enter the femur more proximally than the DHS plate and allowing insertion of independent screws into the calcar. Its two round proximal plate holes permit insertion of two 6.5-mm cancellous bone screws.

Using a 135° DHS plate to treat long oblique subtrochanteric fractures does not always allow fracture compression. With the 95° DCS plate stable fixation can be achieved by lagging the fracture through the plate because controlled collapse is not likely to occur.

Two 6.5-mm cancellous screws are inserted after lag screw insertion and seating of the plate (Figure 9.13).

EXAMINER: What size of drill do we use?

CANDIDATE: We drill a hole in the near cortex with a 4.5-mm drill bit. The 4.5/3.2 drill sleeve is fully seated into the plate hole and a 3.2-mm drill bit is used to drill into the far cortex. Measure, tap and then insert a 6.5-mm cancellous bone screw.

This technique should prevent the drill bit from gliding along the calcar.

EXAMINER: What do you mean by the drill bit gliding along the calcar?

CANDIDATE: Sorry, I am not sure.

COMMENT: If a lag screw technique isn't used the 3.2-mm drill bit will strike the endosteal aspect of the calcar obliquely and be deflected up the neck, where it may break. Over-drilling the outer cortex

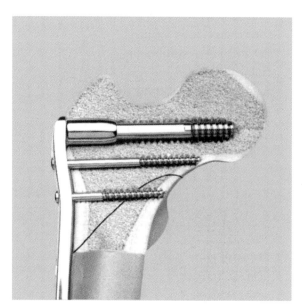

Figure 9.13 Insertion of two 6.5-mm cancellous bone screws through the proximal round holes of the DCS plate.

using a 4.5-mm drill bit and use of the drill sleeve through the hole will guide the 3.2-mm drill and prevent its deviation in the calcar.

The DHS plate is fixed to the femur using 4.5-mm cortical screws. Aim for bicortical fixation and start with the most distal hole.

EXAMINER: When do we use a compression screw?

CANDIDATE: It allows further fracture impaction. It is useful in unstable fractures to prevent disengagement of the lag screw from the plate barrel.

EXAMINER: Are there any concerns with using a compression screw?

CANDIDATE: A compression screw can cause stripping of the lag screw thread in porotic bone. Avoid excessive force and remove the compression screw after use.

EXAMINER: Why?

CANDIDATE: I am not sure.

COMMENT: A recent paper suggested retaining the compression screw as it helped to lessen mechanical failure of the DHS by reducing the peak (von Mises) stress around the connection between the barrel and side plate.[8]

Structured oral examination question 14

Design features of a plate

COMMENT: Plate design needs a bit of thought and pre-planning because if you are hit blind with this topic in a viva you may struggle and not respond well to questions. It gives the examiners the opportunity to focus in and test your knowledge on various subsections of biomechanics.

You need to understand the management principles of your fracture, what you are trying to achieve with your fracture and what your plate is going to do to help you achieve this, and design the plate accordingly.

EXAMINER: Design the perfect plate.

CANDIDATE: Score 4: I use a z plate because I know it well, the company sales representative is very supportive, we use this plate in our hospital and the company have been very competitive in their pricing.

COMMENT: This question is about principles of plate design and is used to test candidates for higher-order thinking skills. Plate implant procurement is usually agreed locally by an orthopaedic department based on many factors including cost, after sales support, educational training, bulk usage discount offered and performance. Stay clear of mentioning specific company implants.[9]

This is in contrast to referring to a cemented Exeter hip implant in a viva. This widely used implant is ODEP 10A rated with 30 years survivorship results and most trainees are familiar with the kit.

It is important to prepare for viva questions, but also important not to over-analyse your answers.

It is also reasonable to mention established local hospital policies such as antibiotic or DVT prophylaxis in a viva. These protocols are usually decided through an appropriate local committee using a best evidence-based approach.

'I would start antibiotics according to my local hospital antimicrobial guideline protocols.' This may even sound quite official, so the examiners may be less likely to challenge you even if you are a little unsure about specifics.

Constructing an answer

Prepare a simple sentence and then divide your answer into various different headings and then work on the headings.

The design of my implant would require consideration of many factors which would include material properties, structural properties, interface fixation and modality of use.

1. Material properties

Candidates may end up discussing:

Youngs modulus.

Yield point.

Toughness.

Hardness.

Material properties are independent of shape.

My ideal material should be bio-inert, reliable, easily manufactured and sterilizable. It should be acceptably priced, have corrosion resistance and provide adequate ductility, toughness and hardness.

2. Structural properties

Bending stiffness.

Torsional stiffness.

Axial stiffness.

3. Interface fixation

Locking vs. non-locking plate.

4. Modality of use

Primary healing vs. secondary healing.

Anatomical reduction versus alignment.

Rigid versus relative fixation.

Load-sharing vs. load-bearing.

Combination.

Straight locking vs. variable angle.

Notes

1. Orthobullets, Ryan Eggers, Comment on structural properties.

2. The key words are 'a constant volume of material for a fixed length.'

3. Take hold of a screw and practise out loud naming its various components until flawless. This may take two or three attempts to become proficient in delivery.

4. The examiners may stop a candidate half-way through their description of a screw and ask this question.

5. Six steps in the lag screw technique.

6. The examiners may drill down for more detail onto a particular function.

7. The question is a bit clumsy. Better phrased as when to use a lag screw rather than how to use a lag screw.

8. Chang C-W, Chen Y-N, Li C-T, Peng Y-T, Chang C-H. Role of the compression screw in the dynamic hip–screw system: a finite-element study. *Med Eng Phys.* 2015;37 (12):1174–1179.

9. Possibly NCB periprosthetic Zimmer system, as its use is very versatile for difficult complex periprosthetic femoral fractures.

Chapter 10

Lower limb trauma I

Rajarshi Bhattacharya and Khaled Sarraf

Introduction

Pointers to candidates

- The mechanism and whether the injury is a high- or low-energy injury should be considered and mentioned at the start of every answer.

- All high-energy injuries should be approached in an ATLS protocol manner.

- The candidate should be very familiar with the latest ATLS guidelines and be ready for the examiner to ignore the orthopaedic injury and go down the ATLS management as this is a trauma viva.

- The candidate should also be very familiar with the BAPRAS/BOA guidelines for the management of open fractures as well as all the BOAST guidelines and base any answer with the support of these guidelines. NICE guidelines are also beneficial to be aware of, e.g. in neck of femur fracture management.

- Always ask for adequate imaging even if it is not provided or not available. This is in the form of X-rays as well as CT scans where appropriate (including angiograms).

- There are always several options to treat a fracture. Always *answer the question*: if the examiner asks '*how would you treat this injury?*' you should state what you would do rather than what options there are. If they want options of treatment they will ask for it.

- Polytrauma patients are also common questions in the viva and the candidate is expected to be very familiar with the principles of damage control orthopaedics vs. early definitive care.

Moran CG, Forward DP. The early management of patients with multiple injuries. *J Bone J Surg Br.* 2012;94B:446–453.

Structured oral examination question 1

Femoral neck fracture in the young

Viva themes
- Timing of surgery.
- Type of reduction.
- Surgical approaches.
- Fixation methods.

EXAMINER: What does the radiograph show (Figure 10.1)?

CANDIDATE: The radiograph is inadequate because it does not show the full pelvis and hips. Otherwise the radiograph shows a displaced subcapital intracapsular neck of femur fracture. I would obtain radiographs in orthogonal views to assess this fracture and consider requesting a CT scan to more fully understand the fracture pattern if necessary.

EXAMINER: Why would you want a CT? You don't normally get CT scans for every hip fracture that presents in casualty.

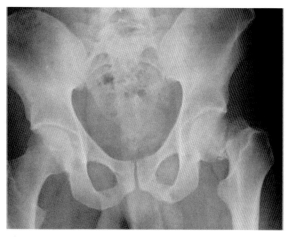

Figure 10.1 Anteroposterior (AP) radiograph of pelvis. Displaced intracapsular fractured left neck of femur.

CANIDATE: A CT could be obtained as part of a pan-trauma series to look for any other associated injuries. A CT can be useful to more accurately classify a fracture pattern to then guide treatment options.

COMMENT: The main role of CT would be in identifying occult femoral neck fractures in a painful hip with normal or equivocal radiographs where MRI is contraindicated or cannot be performed within 24 hours.

EXAMINER: This is the radiograph of a 29-year-old male who fell off his motorbike at 40 mph after slipping on ice. Discuss your management of this patient.

CANDIDATE: This is a high-energy injury and as with any such injury I would assess this patient using an ATLS approach. I would assess distal neurology and pulses.

EXAMINER: What are the key elements in this patient's management?

CANDIDATE: Assessing the pattern of the fracture to ensure and plan for anatomical fracture reduction and fixation. Preservation of the femoral head without developing ON is paramount to avoid future THA.

EXAMINER: What is the blood supply to the femoral head?

CANDIDATE: The majority of the blood supply to the femoral head comes from the medial and lateral femoral circumflex arteries with minimal contribution from the obturator vessels. The medial and lateral femoral circumflex arteries arise from the profunda femoral artery and curl around the trochanteric region before branching proximally to supply the head.

EXAMINER: The patient presented to casualty at 11 pm having sustained the fracture 2 hours beforehand. The SHO has booked the emergency theatre for the fixation to be done straight after a laparotomy as they have been told the risk of ON significantly increases after 6 hours. What will you do?

CANDIDATE: Timing to surgery used to be believed to be very relevant to avoid ON; however, this has recently been refuted in the literature. It is more important to obtain as accurate a reduction as possible including open reduction if needed rather than undertaking emergency hip fixation in the middle of the night. The general scrub staff may be unfamiliar with the trauma kit and it is not the ideal time to be doing this type of surgery. Up to about 10 pm is fine but otherwise I would prefer to put the patient first on the trauma list in the morning when I am at my best so as to reduce the risk of possible surgical errors occurring. The delay also gives me some extra time to more fully explain the risk factors associated with fracture fixation such as non-union, ON and post-traumatic osteoarthritis to the patient.

EXAMINER: If this was not reduced, what method would you do to improve it closed?

CANDIDATE: The Leadbetter is the technique that is described. I have seen it twice, and it has worked on one of those occasions. This is performed under fluoroscopic guidance where the reduction is performed in a non-traumatic manner to avoid causing further injury and damage. The hip is flexed with axial traction, then adducted and brought into abduction and extension. This manoeuvre should not be attempted more than once to avoid the increased risk of ON.

EXAMINER: How would you assess your reduction?

CANDIDATE: I would do so on both the AP and lateral views with fluoroscopy. Garden described the Garden Alignment Index which refers to the angle of the compression trabeculae on the AP and lateral views relative to the longitudinal axis of the femoral shaft. Acceptable reduction is between 155° and 180°, respectively, but ideally 160°. Beyond those ranges the rate of ON is said to increase from 7% to 53%.

EXAMINER: If the hip did not reduce adequately in a closed manner, what would be your next step?

CANDIDATE: I would perform an open reduction via the anterolateral approach and joy-sticking the femoral head into a reduced position followed by three cannulated screws in a triangular configuration. Although biomechanical studies have shown no significant difference between the triangle vs. inverted triangle configuration, I personally prefer having the triangle configuration with two screws along the calcar and compression side of the neck of femur.

EXAMINER: Any other methods of fixation?

CANDIDATE: It is possible to fix the fracture with a two-hole sliding hip screw. Some surgeons believe it is biomechanically more advantageous because it resists shear forces better, particularly in more vertical, higher-energy fracture types. I would temporary stabilize the fracture with a de-rotation K-wire to prevent rotation and go on to use a cannulated derotation screw over the initial K-wire for additional rotational stability. Inserting the cannulated screw can cause the femoral head to rotate stripping the posterior capsular blood supply of the femoral head and increasing the risk of ON.

EXAMINER: What does the literature say?

CANDIDATE: At present there is no clear difference in the literature with clinical outcome for young patients treated with either two-hole DHS or cannulated screw fixation for displaced femoral neck fractures in terms of non-union, ON or the need for revision surgery. The literature would suggest quality of reduction is more important than implant choice.

COMMENT: Biomechanical studies have reported the DHS construct is stronger than CS. A recent paper by Gardner et al. from Boston reported DHS fixation had significantly lower short-term failure rates compared to cannulated screws.[1] Quality of reduction (fair vs. good/ excellent) was an independent predictor of early implant failure. Singh et al. reported a better outcome (less hip pain, better hip function, higher patient satisfaction) in young patients with Pauwels type II and III treated with two-hole DHS fixation but complication rate (re-operation rate, conversion to THA) did not depend on the implant used but quality of fracture reduction.[2]

EXAMINER: Any other approaches that can be considered?

CANDIDATE: Yes, the Smith Peterson approach where you are able to get better direct visualization of the fracture, but it can be challenging in muscular young male patients. This requires two separate incisions, one anteriorly to reduce the fracture and the other laterally to insert the fixation device.

EXAMINER: If you reduced the fracture closed, can you think of a surgical step that can be performed to reduce the rate of ON?

CANDIDATE: Yes, hip decompression by performing a capsulotomy. Although this is controversial it is said to reduce intra-articular pressure which in the acute setting of fracture haematoma can theoretically occlude the trochanteric anastomosis. This has been studied in acute slipped capital femoral epiphysis and shown to reduce ON, so it can possibly be extrapolated to the adult population in a similar fashion. However, there is no good evidence to support this additional step in the literature and it is not something that I would routinely do unless guided by new research supporting its use.

EXAMINER: Apart from ON, what other complication are you concerned about in this patient?

CANDIDATE: The early complications would include wound infection, thromboembolic events and deep infection. In the intermediate to long term I would be concerned about loss of reduction and implant failure, non-union which I would quote in the displaced fractures up to 30%, ON and secondary osteoarthritis, all potentially requiring THA. If using CS, I would touch weight-bear the patient for at least 6 weeks and follow him up closely with radiological monitoring until the 3-year mark to ensure that the femoral head has survived without untoward complications.

EXAMINER: And with a DHS fixation?

CANDIDATE: Weight-bearing status would depend on adequacy of fixation and bone quality.

EXAMINER: So, would you allow full weight-bearing or not?

CANDIDATE: It is unlikely that osteoporosis would be present in a 29-year-old male and a DHS construct has been shown biomechanically to be more robust than CS, so I cautiously partial weight-bear with crutches.

EXAMINER: What does the literature say?

CANDIDATE: I am not sure any difference in outcome has been shown regarding weight-bearing status postoperatively [guess].
[Bell]

EXAMINER: Thank you.

Ly TV, Swiontkowski MF. Treatment of femoral fractures in young adults. *J Bone Joint Surg Am*. 2008;90 (10):2254–2266.

Structured oral examination question 2

Fractured neck of femur in the elderly

Viva themes

- Multidisciplinary management.
- Hip fracture pathway.
- Use a method that allows full weight-bearing.
- Cemented arthroplasty of certain ODEP rating.

EXAMINER: This is an 83-year-old male who fell while gardening, sustaining this injury. He lives with his wife, who he cares for. He mobilized indoors with no aids but uses a stick outdoors. He has a history of hypertension, hypothyroidism and angina. He is a non-smoker and rarely drinks. What does the radiograph show (Figure 10.2)?

CANDIDATE: The AP pelvis radiograph reveals a left sided displaced intracapsular fracture of the neck of femur. There is evidence of osteopenia and a Dorr type C femoral canal. Minimal degenerative changes are present in either hip. I cannot see any evidence of a pelvic or pubic ramus fracture. I would like to see a lateral radiograph of the hip.

EXAMINER: How will you assess this patient and what areas will you ask about?

CANDIDATE: I would clinically assess the whole patient and ensure that this is an isolated injury. I would find out more about his degree of mobility prior to his injury and ask about any comorbidities, systemic illness, red flag signs for any pathological lesion, as well as assess the reason for the

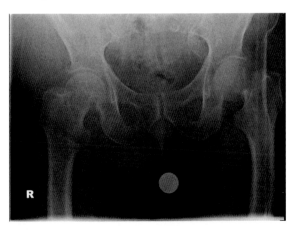

Figure 10.2 Anteroposterior (AP) radiograph of pelvis. Displaced intracapsular fractured left neck of femur.

fall. I would want to establish any preceding symptoms before the fall such as palpitations, chest pain, dizziness, weakness or shortness of breath and if there was a previous history of falls. I would establish if he is oriented in time, place and person, take an AMTS and obtain a collateral history.

EXAMINER: What would you look for in your examination and how would you work the patient up for surgery?

CANDIDATE: I would check the affected leg for shortening and external rotation. Perform a neurovascular examination. I would check the skin and soft tissues surrounding the fracture and proposed incision site. I would very gently confirm pain on movement of the hip. I would also want to perform a cardiovascular and respiratory examination of the patient. I would make sure the patient had a recent chest X-ray and order a new ECG to identify underlying cardiac comorbidities. I would give the patient analgesia for pain and insert a cannula and start IV fluids. Bloods should be sent for FBC, U&E and a group and save. I would want to get an INR/bone profile and stop any anticoagulation that may delay surgery. I would risk-assess warfarin reversal with Vit K.

I would attempt to get the patient as quickly as possible out of the A&E department onto an orthopaedic ward and certainly within 4 hours of admission to the A&E department. I would let the ward doctor know about the admission to ensure a good comprehensive handover with his drug kardex written up. As per NICE guidelines I would liaise with the anaesthetist on call to consider performing a fascia iliaca block as pain management preoperatively can be otherwise difficult to manage with paracetamol and opioids.

EXAMINER: He has well-controlled angina, takes thyroxine for his hypothyroidism and is relatively independent but does have two carers who come and help twice a week. How do you want to treat him?

CANDIDATE: A displaced intracapsular neck of femur requires surgery and, in this case, given the degree of displacement, which seems like a Garden IV (JBJS Garden 1964) I would perform a cemented hip hemiarthroplasty using a polished double-tapered stem with a bipolar head. I would use the lateral approach for my neck of femur

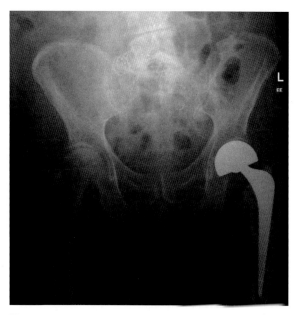

Figure 10.3 Postoperative anteroposterior (AP) pelvis radiograph of cemented bipolar Exeter hip.

fracture surgery as it tends to offer more stability and is not reliant on the soft tissues as much. I prefer an intraosseous abductor repair.

EXAMINER: As you see this was done as per your suggestion (Figure 10.3). Would your management differ if this was an independent and healthy 68-year-old patient who goes for 5-mile daily walks?

CANDIDATE: My initial assessment would be the same, but if the patient is independently mobile I would treat him in accordance with the NICE and the BOAST guidelines and would offer him a total hip replacement. THR offers a better functional outcome in comparison with a hemiarthroplasty, with better survivorship results which is supported by the Swedish registry. My choice would remain a double-tapered polished stem with long-term proven results such as an Exeter stem, with a cemented, highly cross-linked polyethylene cup with a preferably 36-mm head. The NICE guidelines support such practice in a selected population, which include the mentally alert patient with good pre-injury mobility and who is relatively healthy. The patient described seems to comply with the criteria for a THR. I would prefer to perform a fracture neck of femur THR via the lateral approach as opposed to a posterior approach that

I would choose for an arthritic hip. This is to reduce the risk of a dislocation. I would also prefer to use a larger head for that reason. I would aim to restore his leg length and ensure soft-tissue tension is restored.

Postoperatively I would aim for early mobilization with full weight-bearing and discharge back to his usual residence once he has passed physiotherapy and occupational therapy assessment.

Osteoporosis treatment, falls risk assessment and nutritional deficiency should be addressed. The patient's pre- and postoperative care should be carried out via an MDT approach.

EXAMINER: What time would you plan to do this case if the patient arrived in your hospital at 5 pm?

CANDIDATE: This case should not be done after hours and should be done in a scheduled trauma list ensuring the necessary skill, staff and kit is available, especially if a THR is going to be undertaken. The patient should be reviewed by an orthogeriatrician, to be optimized preoperatively, as per national guidelines. The operation should be performed as soon as safe and possible, ideally within 24 hours, but no later than 36 hours as per the national guidelines.

EXAMINER: What are the criteria for best-practice tariffs in patients who have sustained a hip fracture?

CANDIDATE: Best-practice tariff for fragility fractures was introduced to improve patient outcomes, reduce mortality and shorten length of stay. Key features include:
- Surgery within 36 hours of admission.
- Shared care by orthopaedic surgeon and orthogeriatrician.
- Admission using a care protocol agreed by orthogeriatrician, orthopaedic surgeon and anaesthetist.
- Assessment by orthogeriatrician within 72 hours of admission.
- Pre- and postoperative abbreviated mental test score (AMTS) assessment.
- Orthogeriatrician-led multidisciplinary rehabilitation.
- Secondary prevention of falls.
- Bone health assessment.

Other aspects of this question could include:
- *Evidence of THA in NOF fractures.*

213

- *Higher complication rates of THR in NOF vs arthritic hip?*
- *Infection rates.*
- *Thromboprophylaxis.*

Garden RS. Stability and union in sub capital fractures of the femur. *Bone Joint J.* 1964;46B(4):630.

Hoskins W, Webb D, Bingham R, Pirpiris M, Griffin XL. Evidence-based management of intracapsular neck of femur fractures. *Hip Int.* 2017;27(5):415–424.

Structured oral examination question 3

Hip dislocation

EXAMINER: A 23-year-old motorcyclist has been involved in a high-speed head-on collision. He is brought into the A&E department and this radiograph has been taken in the resuscitation bay. Describe the radiograph and explain how you would manage this patient (Figure 10.4).

CANDIDATE: This is an AP radiograph of the patient's pelvis with what appears to be a fracture–dislocation of the left hip.

EXAMINER: Appears or is?

CANDIDATE: Is a fracture–dislocation of the left hip.

There is also a cystogram with a catheter in situ with no evidence of extravasation indicating no bladder injury. With the benefit of the lateral radiographs as well as the mechanism described this is likely to be a posterior dislocation. These injuries are commonly associated with both fractures to the femoral head and/or fracture to the

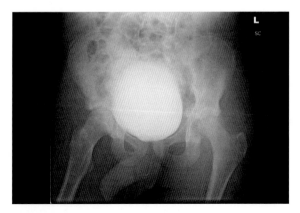

Figure 10.4 Fracture–dislocation, left hip.

acetabular wall, in this case a posterior wall fracture. The sciatic nerve is also at risk and would be a main point of concern. This is a high-energy injury and with such a mechanism there is the possibility of associated visceral and musculoskeletal injuries. This is a trauma call requiring all teams to be ready to receive the patient in the emergency department. I would approach this patient according to the ATLS protocol, ensuring his C-spine is immobilized and making sure no life-threatening injuries are missed.

EXAMINER: That's fine. How would you proceed to manage his hip?

CANDIDATE: I would want to first assess his vascular status and check his pulses throughout his limb, starting with his femoral all the way down to his dorsalis pedis. If I have any concerns I would engage a vascular surgeon, or if one is not available then either plastics or general surgery. I would then assess his neurology as I would be worried about a sciatic nerve injury. Once that has been documented the relevant radiographs would be obtained, which would include a full-length femur and a knee radiograph.

EXAMINER: Why would you get a full-length femur and a knee radiograph – it's a surgical emergency, this will just delay hip reduction?

CANDIDATE: I would want to exclude a coexisting femoral shaft fracture or knee injury which could be missed otherwise. Ideally, I would also get a preoperative hip CT scan if this did not delay the patient's treatment significantly. Assuming there are no large intra-articular fragments requiring urgent open surgery, I would then proceed to attempt a closed reduction, preferably in theatre under GA and with fluoroscopy guidance.

If there would be a significant delay getting into theatre I may consider attempting to reduce the dislocation under appropriate sedation and analgesia in the emergency department. However, these are high-velocity injuries, they can be very difficult to reduce without full muscle relaxation and also have the potential for serious long-term morbidity so I would very much prefer not to go down that route. In theatre, I would perform the reduction with the patient supine on a radiolucent table, with my assistant applying pressure on the pelvis over the anterior superior iliac spines, while I apply longitudinal traction with hip flexion beyond 90°, with adduction and internal rotation, followed by abduction, external rotation and extension. This is known as the Bigelow manoeuvre. Once reduced, I would perform a test of stability. I would then place the patient on skin traction and obtain a postop CT scan, looking at any intra-articular fragments and fractures. As soon as the patient is awake I would repeat the neurovascular observations and document my findings. I would then refer this patient to a pelvic and acetabular surgeon for posterior wall fixation.

EXAMINER: How would your management differ in an anterior dislocation?

CANDIDATE: I would need to perform a reverse Bigelow manoeuvre.

EXAMINER: And if you were unable to reduce it closed?

CANDIDATE: In a posterior dislocation I would have to open via an extended posterior approach (Kocher–Langenbeck) while I would use a modified Smith–Peterson approach in an anterior dislocation.

EXAMINER: How will you manage the CT findings?

CANDIDATE: The aim of the CT is to identify any associated fractures, determine the size of any intra-articular fractures, assess the quality of reduction and identify any loose bodies in the joint. CT is particularly helpful in evaluating any posterior wall fracture and planning surgical management.

EXAMINER: How would you manage a femoral head fracture associated with a dislocation?

CANDIDATE I would use the Pipkin classification as a guide to management (Table 10.1).

Table 10.1 Pipkin classification of femoral head fractures.

Type I: Fracture line inferior to the fovea/ligamentum (small)
Does not involve the weight-bearing portion of the femoral head

Type II: Fracture fragment includes the fovea (larger)
Involves weight-bearing portion of the femoral head

Type III: As types I and II but with an associated femoral neck fracture
High incidence of AVN

Type IV: Any pattern of femoral head fracture with associated acetabular fracture (coincides with Thompson and Epstein's type V)

Pipkin I fractures do not involve the weight-bearing surface of the femoral head and are usually excised. Conservative management is not recommended as fracture fragments may result in a non-congruent joint surface, pain on mobilization and weight-bearing and later osteoarthritis of the joint. Type II fractures involve the weight-bearing surface of the femoral head and are anatomically reduced and fixed usually with headless compression screws. Type III fractures are difficult to reduce and fix and often require primary THA (if unreconstructable) or salvage THA if AVN develops. In type IV fractures the femoral and acetabular fractures should be managed separately, with reconstruction of the acetabulum and fixation of the femoral head fracture as required.

EXAMINER: What surgical approach would you use to manage this injury?

CANDIDATE: The main deciding factors are associated fractures to fix and surgeon familiarity. I am most comfortable performing a posterior approach, which gives good access to areas of injured bone and capsule and is especially useful if a posterior wall fixation needs to be performed. The anterior–inferior part of the head is not well exposed and this can make fixation of the head fracture more difficult. Screw fixation of a large half-head fragment is easier through an anterior approach.

EXAMINER: What complications would you warn the patient of from this injury?

CANDIDATE: The main complication following a hip dislocation is osteonecrosis of the femoral head and secondary osteoarthritis. There can also be concomitant injuries of the sciatic nerve that can be temporary or longstanding. Heterotopic ossification is another common complication in this type of injury whether opened or reduced closed. Indomethacin is given routinely as a preventative measure.

EXAMINER: What would be your diagnosis if the patient woke up in excruciating pain postop with decreased sensation and loss of function distally, following closed reduction?

CANDIDATE: I would suspect that the sciatic nerve has been reduced with the hip and is incarcerated within the acetabulum. This is more common in posterior dislocations due to the position of the head and neck in proximity to the nerve and the method of relocation.

EXAMINER: Would you be worried about any other ipsilateral injury when you are faced with a hip dislocation?

CANDIDATE: Yes, apart from acetabular and femoral head fractures, one can get a neck of femur fracture. Also, an ipsilateral PCL injury can occur, especially with dashboard impaction of the knee.

EXAMINER: Long-term wise, what will you tell the patient?

CANDIDATE: Around 20% of patients will require THA in the first 6 months following a femoral head fracture with a dislocation. Around 55% of patients will have radiographic changes of osteoarthritis at 10 years, although most patients function well.

- Need to be able to discuss fixation of posterior wall fractures including the Kocher–Langenbeck approach.
- Blood supply to the femoral head.
- Definition of nerve injuries (basic sciences).

Structured oral examination question 4

Femoral shaft fracture

EXAMINER: This is a 28-year-old male involved in a motorbike vs. car RTA leading to this injury. Describe what you see (Figures 10.5 and 10.6).

CANDIDATE: This is an AP and lateral radiograph of a comminuted displaced femoral shaft fracture at the junction of the proximal and middle thirds.

EXAMINER: How would you approach this patient?

CANDIDATE: This is a high-energy injury and I would approach the patient according to ATLS protocols to ensure life-threatening injuries are treated first. I would make sure that the C-spine is protected throughout the period of stabilization of airway, breathing and circulatory assessment. I would want to examine the remainder of the limb for injuries, in particular looking for associated injuries of the knee, foot and ankle. I will then want to check sciatic nerve function and distal pulses, and check for any evidence of compartment syndrome. I would order a complete series

Figures 10.5 and 10.6 Anteroposterior (AP) and lateral radiographs of right femur.

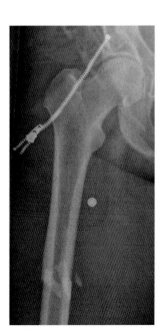
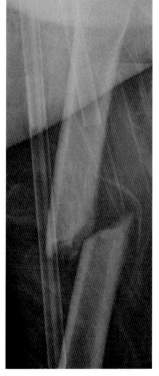

of radiographs to include the ipsilateral hip and knee. I will place the patient on skin traction to give temporary fracture stability until definitive management is performed. Skin traction will reduce pain, realign the fracture, reduce blood loss, may sometimes restore an absent pulse and improve distal perfusion, possibly reduce the risk of fat embolism and reduce any tension on the soft tissues. Distal pulses should be checked before and after application of skin traction.

EXAMINER: If there is a puncture wound, how would you manage it?

CANDIDATE: If there was a puncture wound then this is an open injury Gustillo–Anderson type 1. I would manage this as per the BOA/BAPRAS open fracture guidelines and the adapted BOAST guidelines. This would include antibiotics, picture, saline-soaked gauze and tetanus vaccine administration. I would inform my plastic surgery colleagues, more so if this was a high-energy injury as the zone of injury might be more extensive than the puncture wound area. This would ideally be done in a combined orthoplastics list if available.

EXAMINER: Assuming that this is an isolated limb injury and confirmed that it is only an 'in to out' puncture wound, how would you proceed?

CANDIDATE: I would use a trochanteric entry reamed antegrade cephalomedullary femoral nail. I would place the patient on a traction table and apply sufficient traction to overcome any shortening and aim to achieve a good reduction of the fracture preop. The distal fragment may need to be elevated using a crutch or the proximal fragment lowered using external pressure from a mallet. I would apply firm traction to the leg, making sure that the foot was well padded and correctly applied to the foot stirrup.

I would ensure that I have correct rotational alignment by having assessed the patient's contralateral foot position. The goal is to get an isthmic fit and ream 1.5 mm above the required nail diameter. I would want to make sure that the femoral shaft fracture does not distract, and that the nail does not touch or perforate the anterior cortex due to the variability of the anatomical femoral bow and the bow that is built into the implant. Before I start my nailing, I would address the puncture wound by debriding it and freshening the edges of the skin aiming for primary

closure after a thorough washout. If I had any doubts I would engage the plastic surgeons as a joint orthoplastics case as per the BOA/BAPRAS guidelines.

EXAMINER: What are the advantages of a trochanteric entry point compared to the standard piriformis entry point?

CANDIDATE: The piriform fossa is colinear with the femoral shaft but places the medial femoral circumflex artery at risk, particularly in adolescents, and is technically more difficult to access.

The trochanteric starting point potentially is technical ease, especially in obese patients. The abductor muscles and tendons, branches of the medial circumflex femoral artery and the capsule of the hip joint are less at risk during nail insertion.

A lateral entry position increases the risk of varus malreduction, and an anterior entry position increases the risk of iatrogenic fracture.

EXAMINER: How would you allow this patient to bear weight?

CANDIDATE: With this construct I would get him to fully weight-bear with physiotherapy input.

EXAMINER: OK. Tell me about your choice of implant – in terms of its biomechanics.

CANDIDATE: An intramedullary device is a load-sharing device. The working length of a nail between the most proximal point of fixation in the distal fragment and the most distal point of fixation in the proximal fragment. The unsupported portion of nail is between the bone fragments. Bending stiffness is inversely proportional to the square of the working length. Torsional stiffness is inversely proportional to the working length. For a fracture located within 5 cm of the most proximal distal locking screw, the peak stress around the hole may exceed the endurance limit of the metal. The nail is loaded as a Cantilever beam.

EXAMINER: Any other concerns about this injury?

CANDIDATE: Yes, around 5% of femoral fractures have an undisplaced, often missed neck of femur fracture. Patella fractures and PCL injuries are also not uncommon, especially in dashboard injuries and front seat passengers.

EXAMINER: How would this change your management/choice of implant?

CANDIDATE: Failure to recognize a non-displaced or minimally displaced associated neck fracture prior to fixation of the shaft can lead to displacement, a decrease in neck fixation options, a technically challenging secondary procedure and increased risk of long-term sequelae.

My primary aim would be to first fix the neck of femur fracture as I would be worried about the hip joint and risk of damaging its blood supply leading to AVN.

If the femoral fracture is in the proximal third, then an antegrade cephalomedullary nail can be used to treat both. I would consider placing a temporary wire to hold the reduction of the femoral neck while I insert the nail which I have done in the past. However, if the femoral fracture was distal I would choose to first perform a dynamic hip screw to rigidly fix the femoral neck fracture. I would ensure a closed anatomical reduction before fixation and use a DHS implant rather than cannulated screws as this offers a more stable fixation. I would release traction and follow on with an overlapping retrograde femoral nail. I would leave the last one or two screw holes of the DHS plate empty to allow an overlap of the retrograde nail.

EXAMINER: What about fixing the femoral shaft fracture first. This is more of a danger to life.

CANDIDATE: The femoral neck fracture has to be fixed as well as possible otherwise the patient may go on to develop AVN and require a THA at a very young age. The femoral neck fracture is the more technically demanding of the two procedures and I would prefer to get this out of the way first before tackling the femoral shaft fracture.

EXAMINER: How easy is it to apply traction to the femoral neck fracture if the femoral shaft is broken?

CANDIDATE: Err … Yes it will be difficult and it would be much easier to apply traction to the femoral neck fracture and achieve satisfactory reduction if the femoral shaft fracture is first fixed. However most authors recommend prompt, but not emergent, surgery with priority given to anatomic reduction and stabilization of the neck fracture by either closed or open methods. Fixation of the shaft fracture follows as patient condition allows.

COMMENT: Decide on one or two implants to fix both fractures. Fixing the femoral head fracture first or second is somewhat controversial. There is no right or wrong answer, it is more about presenting your reasoning for the choice that you have made.

EXAMINER: What would you do if the femoral neck displaced during the case?

CANDIDATE: If it cannot be manipulated back then I would have a low threshold to perform an open reduction and get it anatomically fixed, as the key to the outcome is fracture reduction.

EXAMINER: What would your weight-bearing status be?

CANDIDATE: If I am happy with the fixation I allow patients to start weight-bearing as soon as they are happy and able to, with guidance of physiotherapy.

EXAMINER: What are the postoperative complications you would be concerned with?

CANDIDATE: This is a high-energy injury and I would initially be concerned about the risks of RDS, bleeding, compartment syndrome, fat embolism and infection. Later on, I would be concerned with delayed union, non-union, AVN femoral head, post-traumatic osteoarthritis, leg length discrepancy, Trendelenburg gait and continued hip and leg pain.

Bedi A, Ryu RKN. Accuracy of reduction of ipsilateral femoral neck and shaft fractures – an analysis of various internal fixation strategies. *J Orthop Trauma.* 2009;23(4):249–253.

Baumgaertner MR, Solberg BD. Awareness of tip–apex distance reduces failure of fixation of trochanteric fractures of the hip. *J Bone Joint Surg Br.* 1997;79(6):969–971.

Structured oral examination question 5

Distal femur (periprosthetic) fractures

EXAMINER: Tell me about this X-ray of a 65-year-old man who fell at home and sustained this injury (Figures 10.7 and 10.8).

CANDIDATE: These are an AP and lateral radiograph of the left knee and distal femur showing a total knee replacement in place with an associated periprosthetic fracture around the femoral component. The current X-ray view is inadequate, and I would like to see X-rays of the full femur in two orthogonal views, AP and lateral, to ensure there is no other prosthesis further up in the femur like a hip replacement or a neck of femur fracture fixation. (*Do not be afraid to ask for further information including more imaging if you feel it is appropriate.*)

Table 10.2 Classification of knee periprosthetic fractures.[3]

I Undisplaced fracture Prosthesis intact
II Displaced fracture Prosthesis intact
III Prosthesis loose or failing Any type of fracture

The knee replacement looks like a cruciate-scarifying primary implant without patella replacement. It does not appear grossly loose. Overall bone quality appears osteopenic.

EXAMINER: How do you classify these injuries?

CANDIDATE: Periprosthetic fractures around the knee have been classified by Lewis and Rorabeck, but I am unsure of the specifics of the classification system.

COMMENT: There is always some confusion as to whether examiners should be asking classification systems. As a candidate it is helpful to know a classification system, especially if it provides a direct guide to management.

EXAMINER: How would you treat this fracture definitively?

CANDIDATE: If the patient was fit enough to undergo surgery, then my preferred method of treatment would be internal fixation of this fracture. I would like to treat this fracture using plates and screws. I would prefer to use a distal femoral locking plate as I expect the bones around the femoral component to be of poor quality requiring good purchase. (*You can briefly mention ATLS protocol at the start, but do not waste time on this too much if the examiner has talked of definitive fixation.*)

EXAMINER: What do you think of this fixation (Figures 10.9 and 10.10)?

CANDIDATE: The fracture has been fixed using a distal femoral locking plate using a combination of locking and non locking screws and in a bridging mode.

COMMENT: Even if you see any obvious problems in a fixation, try not to be too blunt about it. Although it is very unlikely to be an examiner's own case that he/she is proudly presenting to you, still be discrete and professional. The viva is standardized now, so the same radiographs are similarly presented to different candidates on different viva tables by different sets of examiners.

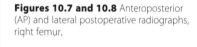

Figures 10.7 and 10.8 Anteroposterior (AP) and lateral postoperative radiographs, right femur,

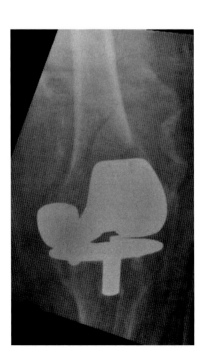
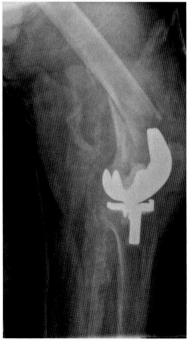

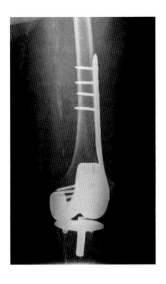 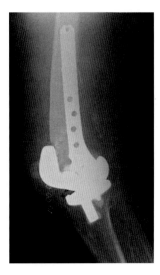

Figures 10.9 and 10.10 Anteroposterior (AP) and lateral postop radiographs, right femur.

EXAMINER: What other ways are there of treating this fracture?

CANDIDATE: Any fracture can be treated non-operatively including this one, although it would be very difficult to control its position here as this is an unstable fracture and this would not be my treatment of choice in this situation. The fracture could also be treated with a retrograde intramedullary nail, provided the femoral component allows a nail to pass through and as long as there are no further implants proximally that could potentially cause a stress riser between that component and the nail. With the new rules introduced for informed consent, all management options would need to be discussed with the patient and their family, including benefits and potential complications, and the discussion fully recorded in the case notes.

EXAMINER: How do you know if the femoral component can allow a nail to pass through?

CANDIDATE: If the total knee replacement has a posterior stabilized component, then the box would not allow a nail to pass through. However, if it is an obvious cruciate-retaining prosthesis then occasionally a nail can be used, although in some cases the femoral components may force the entry point of the nail too posterior to allow proper insertion and therefore cause malreduction of the fracture. Ideally, I would like to know the type of prosthesis that has been used. The paper by Jones et al. describes the commonly used knee implants in the UK that may or may not allow a nail to pass through (Jones et al., 2016). If all else failed I would speak to the company rep as they can make enquiries and can easily find out for you.

Jones MD, Carpenter C, Mitchell SR, et al. Retrograde femoral nailing of periprosthetic fractures around total knee replacements. *Injury*. 2016;47(2):460–464.

Structured oral examination question 6

Knee dislocation

EXAMINER: A 19-year-old female on a bicycle was involved in an accident with a speeding motorbike at a cross-section. The cyclist remained alert and no other injuries were identified. She was taken to the local Major Trauma Centre and this was one of her radiographs (Figure 10.11). Please describe this.

CANDIDATE: This is a lateral radiograph revealing a dislocation of the right knee. An AP radiograph is needed to determine whether this is a posteromedial or posterolateral dislocation. There is also evidence of a bone fragment just anterior to the tibia which indicates an associated fracture – a rim fracture. This is pathognomonic for a more extensive intra-articular injury.

EXAMINER: How can dislocations be classified? (Note: the examiner didn't ask you to classify this injury, but wants to see if you are aware of how this can be classified.)

CANDIDATE: One classification system is based on the tibial displacement. Anterior dislocation is

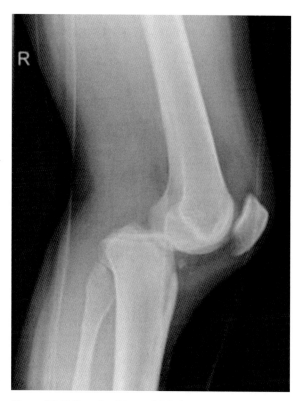

Figure 10.11 Posterior dislocated right knee.

the most common, followed by posterior dislocation as in this case. It can be further classified into medial and lateral displacement. The direction of displacement can indicate the ligaments injured. The Schenk classification describes the dislocation according to the ligaments injured. There are five major injury patterns, with higher Roman numerals having sustained greater trauma.

KD I – multiligamentous knee injury with only one cruciate ligament involved. Seen in sporting injuries and usually low-energy.

KD II – both cruciates ruptured but no other ligamentous injury (rare). Bicruciate injury with functionally intact collateral ligaments.

KD III – both cruciates ruptured, plus either the medial collateral ligament (MCL) or lateral collateral ligament (LCL). Most common injury pattern.

KD IV – both cruciates and both collateral ligaments ruptured (four ligaments injured). Seen in high-energy motor vehicle injuries.

KD V – Multiligamentous injury with periarticular fracture. Fracture/dislocation of the knee.

EXAMINER: What is your initial management of a knee dislocation?

CANDIDATE: Given this is a high-energy injury, the patient should be approached using an ATLS protocol. The history mentions that this was an isolated injury, so our attention can focus on the limb having confirmed that ABC were fine on arrival. Knee dislocations have a considerable incidence of concomitant vascular and/or neurological injury. Vascular injury is reported in the literature at a rate of 22–32%. Neurologic damage involving the common peroneal nerve is estimated to occur in approximately 25% of knee dislocations.

Compartment syndrome is also a risk factor and should be monitored for in the first 24–48 hours. Once the neurological and vascular status of the affected leg has been documented, I would proceed to attempt closed reduction in the emergency department under sedation. This would be with gentle in-line traction on the foot and anterior pressure on the posterior part of the tibia. If successful, I would reassess the limb (neurological and vascular status) and document my findings. If not, I would still document the neurovascular status and plan to take the patient to theatre for a reduction under GA.

EXAMINER: The knee was successfully reduced and remains so, but on your reassessment, there was no palpable pulse. The foot remains warm and pink. What are your next steps?

CANDIDATE: Suspicion of a vascular injury warrants immediate intervention. If time allows and no delay will be caused a CT angiogram would be very useful. I would discuss this with the vascular, plastic or if neither are available then the general surgeons (depending on what services are available at the hospital). I would alert theatres and prepare the patient for a spanning external fixation to stabilize the knee and popliteal fossa arterial exploration ± repair. An on-table angiogram can be performed in theatre. If there was concern about an ischaemic limb then a popliteal shunt would take precedence followed by external fixation and then formal vascular repair or bypass surgery.

EXAMINER: And what if there is a pulse?

CANDIDATE: As this is a high-energy injury, I would discuss this with the radiologist and arrange a CT angiogram. If there is any difficulty in obtaining the CT, I would perform an ankle-brachial pressure index. An index less than 0.9 in the context of this injury warrants surgical exploration. The benefit of the CT in such injuries is that it can detect intimal tears in the popliteal artery which might be masked by a normal pulse. The risk of an unidentified intimal tear is that it progresses, or the artery forms a thrombus leading to ischaemia. If the foot had any signs of ischaemia, prompt vascular intervention is required.

COMMENT: There has been a shift in management from emergency CT angiography in all dislocated knees to selective angiography. Many knee dislocations had intact distal pulses with no hard evidence of vascular damage. Patients with 'hard physical signs of vascular injury' (haematoma, absent pulses, haemorrhage, and bruit) should undergo an immediate intraoperative angiogram. Those without 'vascular injury hard signs' undergo ankle–brachial index (ABI) measurement. In this group, if the ABI is < 0.9, emergent angiography is done. Again, in this group, if the ABI is ≥ 0.90, patients are observed, and pulse checked frequently.

EXAMINER: Which types of dislocations are vascular injuries most commonly seen in?

CANDIDATE: Around 20% of all dislocations have a vascular insult, with 50% being an anterior or posterior knee dislocation. Anterior dislocations generally have an intimal tear from the traction applied on the artery, while posterior dislocations more commonly lead to complete tear of the popliteal artery. This association is due to the anatomical trifurcation of the popliteal artery and its anchorage within proximal and distal soft tissues. Anterior and posterior dislocations lead to the artery tethering at the popliteal fossa. The artery proximally is within a fibrous tunnel at the adductor hiatus and then continues in the fibrous tunnel within soleus.

EXAMINER: What is your order of ligament reconstruction in a multiligament knee injury?

CANDIDATE: It all depends on the ligamentous injuries found on the MRI scan. If I decide to perform early reconstruction I would reconstruct the PLC and PCL primarily (and perform a delayed ACL reconstruction). Neglecting to identify a PLC injury or not reconstructing/

repairing it adequately leads to failure of knee stability. Staged treatment simplifies the operative process and shortens operative time in the acute phase, decreasing the rate of arthrofibrosis compared with acute surgery or repairing or reconstructing all injured ligaments.

EXAMINER: How else can this injury be treated?

CANDIDATE: If the dislocation has been reduced and is relatively stable, and there was no neurological or vascular concert, the knee can be placed in a brace with early rehabilitation. Once the acute injury has settled and the scar tissue has set in, clinical and radiological assessment can be performed. Any areas of instability that remain can be addressed. The commonest complication of knee dislocations (pre- or post-reconstruction) is arthrofibrosis leading to stiffness. In fact, a large proportion of multiligament knee reconstructions require an MUA to improve the range of motion.

COMMENT: Knee dislocations are unusual and therefore not an injury many orthopaedic surgeons will see often. Consequently, the ligament injury pattern and the extent of additional injuries can often be missed. It is important to appreciate the possibility of vascular injury.

Structured oral examination question 7

Open fractures of the lower limb

EXAMINER: A 25-year-old delivery man on a moped gets hit by a car and comes in with this isolated injury (Figures 10.12 and 10.13). His ABC is stable. How would you manage this?

CANDIDATE: These are AP and lateral radiographs of the left tibia showing a multifragmentary fracture of the left tibia and fibula shaft at the junction of the middle and lower thirds. As this is an isolated injury, my initial assessment would be to check for neurovascular status and soft tissues surrounding the injury.

EXAMINER: His neurovascular status is intact. His soft tissues are shown in the picture (Figure 10.14). What would be your management?

CANDIDATE: This is an open fracture of the tibia and I would like to manage this as per the BOAST 4 guidelines. (You must know the BOAST 4

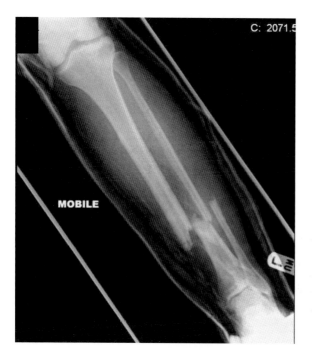

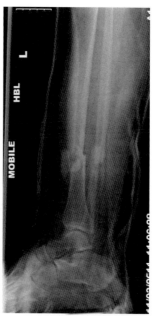

Figures 10.12 and 10.13 Anteroposterior (AP) and lateral radiograph, open left tibial fracture.

guidelines thoroughly.) As per these guidelines, such injuries should be managed jointly by the orthopaedic and plastic team. Initial management in the A&E department will involve removal of gross contaminants administering IV antibiotics and antitetanus, photography, dressing with a saline-soaked gauze and covering the wound with an occlusive film. The fracture should be splinted in an above-knee backslab. If a combined orthopaedic and plastic input is not available, then the patient should be transferred early to an orthoplastic unit for further management. *(Be prepared to be asked about the Gustillo–Anderson classification of open fractures.)*

EXAMINER: What antibiotics should you give and for how long?

CANDIDATE: I would give IV cephalosporins or co-amoxiclav. I would use clindamycin if there was a significant penicillin allergy. Antibiotics should be given as soon as possible after injury, ideally within 1 hour. Antibiotics are continued until definitive wound closure or for 72 hours, whichever occurs soonest.

EXAMINER: When should surgery be done?

CANDIDATE: There is evidence to suggest that the outcomes are better if done in a timely fashion by specialists rather than early surgery by less-

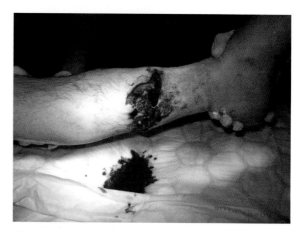

Figure 10.14 Open tibia fracture.

experienced surgeons (Reuss, 2007). The principles should be to 'Extend' (the incision), 'Explore' (the wound properly) and 'Excise' (all dead and devitalized tissue). The medial safe incision is anterior to the posterior tibial artery and its perforators while the safe lateral incision should be away from the lateral (peroneal) perforators.

Debridement should be performed by senior plastic and orthopaedic surgeons working together within 12 hours of the injury for solitary high-energy open fractures and within 24 hours of injury for all other low-energy open fractures. Immediate debridement for highly contaminated wounds such as marine, agricultural or sewage. The 6-hour rule that was previously popular does not apply anymore and the guidelines were modified in December 2017.

EXAMINER: What antibiotics will you give and for how long?

CANDIDATE: In the A&E setting, co-amoxiclav (1.2 g) or cefuroxime (1.5 g) 8-hourly or clindamycin (600 mg), 6-hourly if penicillin allergy; to be continued until wound debridement. At debridement, co-amoxiclav (1.2 g) and gentamicin (1.5 mg/kg) are administered and continued for 72 hours or definitive wound closure, whichever is earlier.

EXAMINER: How will you treat the fracture?

CANDIDATE: If primary closure is possible, and there is no significant bone loss, then my treatment of choice would be a locked intramedullary nailing of the tibia. If primary closure is not possible or there is any concern regarding the wound after primary closure, or if there is large bone defect, I would prefer a temporary external fixation with a view to conversion to definitive fixation in the next few days depending on the wounds. I would consider using a negative-pressure wound dressing if primary wound closure is not possible immediately. Definitive skeletal stabilization and wound cover should be achieved within 72 hours and should not exceed 7 days. If there is bone loss or if the wound requires a flap cover by the plastics team, then I would consider definitive fixation using an external fixator device.

EXAMINER: What other concerns would you have regarding this injury before or after the surgery?

CANDIDATE: As this is a high-energy injury I would be concerned about development of compartment syndrome during the initial period as well as subsequently after surgery, particularly after nailing.

EXAMINER: How would you deal with this?

CANDIDATE: I would be vigilant about this and the diagnosis would be a clinical decision based on examination, although occasionally this can be confirmed with one of the newer available compartment pressure monitors. However, if I was in any doubt about compartment syndrome, I would take the patient to theatre, in conjunction with the plastic surgeon, for a fasciotomy. (*Be prepared to talk about the recommended incisions for fasciotomy.*)

Reuss BL, Cole JD. Effect of delayed treatment on open tibial shaft fractures. *Am J Orthop.* 2007;36:215–220.

Structured oral examination question 8

Tibial plateau fractures

EXAMINER: This 45-year-old gentleman came off his motorbike and sustained the following injury (Figures 10.15 and 10.16). What are your thoughts and how would you manage the patient?

CANDIDATE: These are the AP and lateral view X-rays of a right knee. The most obvious abnormality here is a fracture of the proximal tibia involving both the tibial plateaus. This appears to be a high-energy injury and I would like to manage the patient using standard ATLS protocol. If AB and C are stable I would like to specifically look for and document neurovascular status and also check for the soft-tissue status of the leg, whether it is open or closed, any blisters or degloving. Initial management in the A&E department would involve splinting the fracture in an above-knee backslab, providing pain relief and then planning for fixation.

EXAMINER: This is a closed fracture and neurovascularly intact. What type of fracture is this? What other investigations would you want?

CANDIDATE: This appears to be a type 6 fracture with metaphyseal–diaphyseal dissociation, as per Schatzker's classification from his published series in 1979 (Schatzker, 1979). (*Explain the types of Schatzker fractures and also that Types 4, 5 and 6 usually signify high-energy injuries and are more associated with neurovascular problems.*) I would ideally want to obtain CT scans to define the fracture better and plan for further treatment and possibly also a CT angiogram to ensure there is no damage to the arteries. (*At this point,*

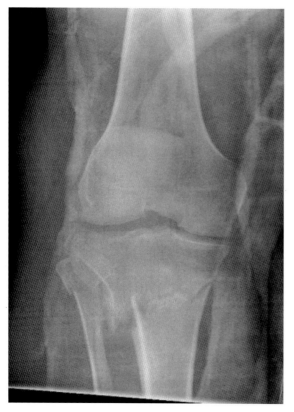 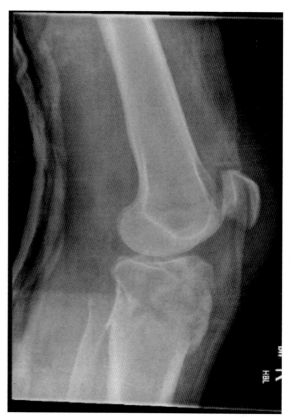

Figures 10.15 and 10.16 Anteroposterior (AP) and lateral radiographs, right knee.

examiner could produce some CT scans to help you plan your management.) (Figures 10.17–10.19).

EXAMINER: How would you like to treat this fracture?

CANDIDATE: He is a young and fit patient with significant joint disruption and displacement of a weight-bearing joint. I would prefer to treat this fracture operatively. As this is a high-energy injury, I would have significant concerns with the soft tissues and therefore I may have to consider staging the surgery through a Span, Scan and Plan approach. This would involve taking the patient to theatre and putting on a spanning external fixator across the knee away from the zone of injury. Following this, I would wait until the soft tissues settle down before planning definitive fixation.

EXAMINER: Where would you place your external fixator pins?

CANDIDATE: I would put two pins in the femur either anteriorly or anterolaterally and two pins in the tibial shaft away from the zone of injury, keeping in mind the skin incisions that would be required for fixation.

EXAMINER: What would be your definitive fixation plans for this fracture?

CANDIDATE: In an appropriately marked and consented patient with all relevant imaging available I would administer IV antibiotics and then apply a thigh tourniquet and inflate. The patient should be positioned supine on the operating table that is broken to allow the knees to flex to 90°. I would like to fix this fracture using a dual-incision approach with an anterolateral and a posteromedial incision. The two incisions should be at least 7 cm apart. The joint capsule is opened through a submeniscal arthrotomy. The meniscus is then lifted out of the way using a stay suture to allow the articular surface to be visualized. I would like to use plates and screws to buttress the posteromedial fragment first and then an anterolateral locking plate for fixation of the rest of the fracture. I would create a window

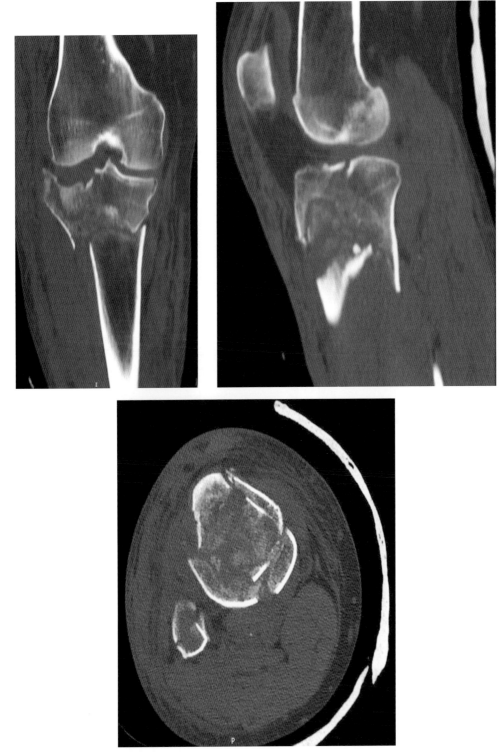

Figures 10.17, 10.18 and 10.19 Coronal, sagittal and axial CT images, right knee.

in the tibia to allow me to use a punch or elevator to restore the articular surface. I would have allograft femoral head on standby in case I needed it to fill in any metaphyseal defect.

EXAMINER: How else could this fracture be fixed?

CANDIDATE: This fracture could also be fixed definitively using external fixator methods like circular frames (Ilizarov, TSF, TL-Hex, etc.). I would have a lower threshold for using a circular frame if the soft tissues were of poor quality and compromised.

EXAMINER: Which treatment method of the two has better results?

CANDIDATE: The Canadian OTS multicentre RCT from 2006 (COTS, 2006) showed that functional results were similar in both groups at 2 years although the ORIF group had more deep infections and unplanned returns to theatre.

EXAMINER: Why would you not use a single mid-line incision?

CANDIDATE: Single midline incisions are known to have poor results in these fractures as they involve a significant amount of stripping of soft tissues. Besides, they do not allow proper access to put a posteromedial plate on.

EXAMINER: How would you rehabilitate this patient?

CANDIDATE: I would treat him postoperatively in a hinged knee brace with controlled range of motion which will be gradually increased to eventually achieve full flexion. He will be non-weight-bearing for 12 weeks. (*Always mention that this would depend on the type of fixation you have achieved, the comminution noted at the time of surgery, other associated injuries, etc. The postoperative regime should be tailor-made for each patient and depends to an extent on the fixation achieved.*)

EXAMINER: What complications could occur?

CANDIDATE: This is a serious injury and I would warn the patient of the possibility of compartment syndrome, infection, delayed union or non-union, malunion, post-traumatic osteoarthritis, arthrofibrosis and peroneal nerve injury.

EXAMINER: What about the final outcome?

CANDIDATE: The key to a good outcome is restoration of the joint line and mechanical axis. In Rademakers *et al.* the overall incidence of osteoarthritis has been reported to be 9% compared to 27% if the axis deviation > 5°.

Schatzker J, McBroom R, Bruce D. The tibial plateau fracture. The Toronto experience 1968–1975. *Clin Orthop Relat Res.* 1979;138:94–104.

Canadian Orthopaedic Trauma Society. Open reduction and internal fixation compared with circular fixator application for bi-condylar tibial plateau fractures. Results of a multi-centre, prospective, randomized clinical trial. *J Bone Joint Surg Am.* 2006;88(12):2613–2623.

Structured oral examination question 9

Tibial plafond fractures

EXAMINER: These are the radiographs of a 54-year-old cyclist who was hit by a van and sustained this injury (Figures 10.20 and 10.21). You are called in to the emergency room via a trauma call. Tell me what you see and your initial management plans.

CANDIDATE: These are AP and lateral X-rays of a right distal tibia and fibula showing a fracture dislocation of the ankle joint. There appears to be a fracture of the distal tibial plafond as well as the fibula. This is a high-energy injury and I would initially manage the patient via ATLS principles. Assuming that this is his only injury, I would check for and document neurovascular and soft-tissue status. If there are no neurovascular problems, I would aim to reduce the fracture–dislocation in the Emergency department using appropriate sedation and muscle relaxant depending on the local protocol. Once I have improved the position, I would splint the lower leg in a below-knee backslab and obtain check X-rays.

EXAMINER: What would you do if there was no pulse at your initial assessment?

CANDIDATE: I would still proceed to reduce the fracture–dislocation, but additionally I would call for the vascular team and plan to take the patient to theatre immediately if the pulse did not return following reduction. If a Doppler was easily available, I would check with a Doppler if there was any signal. I would document my findings in the notes.

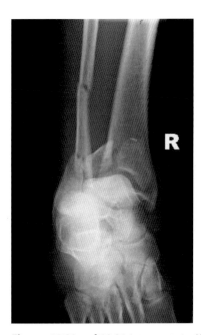
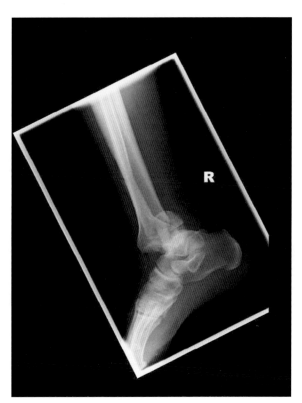

Figures 10.20 and 10.21 Anteroposterior (AP) and lateral radiographs, right distal tibia.

EXAMINER: If you needed to take the patient to theatre, what should be the preferred sequence of intervention?

CANDIDATE: The immediate intervention should be aimed at restoring blood flow. A further check with Doppler may be performed to confirm absence of pulse. An on-table angiogram may also be performed if the facilities are available, but it is best not to delay exploration of the artery if there is no blood supply. The artery should be explored to check for any kinking of the vessels or any damage. If the artery can be unkinked or a primary repair can be achieved promptly then this should be attempted, otherwise a temporary shunt should be inserted to restore blood flow. Subsequent to this, I would aim to apply a bridging external fixator to stabilize the fracture and then the vascular surgeon should restore definitive flow through a primary repair or a graft or bypass.

EXAMINER: What would you do after temporarily stabilizing the fracture and restoring blood flow?

CANDIDATE: I would be observant for compartment syndrome initially. I would base my treatment using a Span, Scan and Plan approach. I would obtain CT scans of the fracture and plan for surgery once the revascularization has become established and soft-tissue swelling has settled.

EXAMINER: What would be your preferred mode of treating this fracture?

CANDIDATE: I would prefer to treat this fracture definitively with an external fixator as there may already be skin incisions that may compromise my approach for internal fixation. The aim would be to restore length, alignment and rotation as well as articular congruity. I may have to use mini-open incisions for this purpose.

EXAMINER: If you were planning to perform internal fixation, how would you plan your surgery?

CANDIDATE: I would take advice from a plastic surgeon with regard to the skin incisions. I would aim to restore the fibular length first and then fix the tibial fracture using a combination of plates and screws, depending on the orientation and placement of the fracture fragments.

EXAMINER: What are the typical fracture fragments that you get in a tibial plafond fracture?

CANDIDATE: The usual fragments are medial, anterior or anterolateral, posterior or posterolateral and occasionally a die-punch fragment.

EXAMINER: What are the complications associated with pilon fractures?

CANDIDATE: There are immediate complications which can be intraoperative or postoperative and there are delayed complications. Immediate intraoperative complications include damage to neurovascular structures and inability to close the wound if performing internal fixation; immediate postoperative complications include DVT, PE, infection, compartment syndrome. Long-term complications include non-union and malunion due to failure of fixation, arthritis, stiffness and pain.

EXAMINER: Is there more incidence of arthritis with internal fixation or external fixation? Which type of fixation has better results?

CANDIDATE: Meta-analysis as well as randomized controlled trials have shown that they have equivalent results with equal incidence of complications including arthritis (Wyrsch, 1996; Wang, 2015) but internal fixation tends to have more severe complications (Wyrsch, 1996).

Wyrsch B, McFerran MA, McAndrew M, *et al.* Operative treatment of fractures of the tibial plafond. A randomized, prospective study. *J Bone Joint Surg Am.* 1996;78 (11):1646–1657.

Wang D, Xiang JP, Chen XH, Zhu QT. A meta-analysis for postoperative complications in tibial plafond fracture: open reduction and internal fixation versus limited internal fixation combined with external fixator. *J Foot Ankle Surg.* 2015;54(4):646–651.

Notes

1. Gardner S, Weaver MJ, Jerabek S, Rodriguez E, Vrahas M, Harris M. Predictors of early failure in young patients with displaced femoral neck fractures. *J Orthopaed.* 2015;12 (2):75–80.

2. Singh M, Sonkar D, Verma R, Shukla J, Gaur S. Comparison of the functional outcome of DHS versus cannulated cancellous screws in Pauwels type II and III fracture neck femur in young adults. *Int J Orthopaed.* 2017;3 (2):745–749.

3. Rorabeck CH, Taylor JW. Classification of periprosthetic fractures complicating total knee arthroplasty. *Orthop Clin.* 1999;30(2):209–214.

Lower limb trauma II

Will Eardley, Mohammed Al-Maiyah and Patrick Williams

Introduction

Alexander Suvorov would have done well in the trauma viva section of the FRCS Tr & Orth. Two citations attributed to him underpin the approach to the exam: *Train hard, fight easy* and *He who is afraid is half beaten*. Approach and strategy is everything and this comes from a combination of practice and knowledge acquisition. It is a time-dependent chess match where every move will be undertaken in a specified time, but in a sequence that is out of your control. Keep this analogy as you attempt different clinical scenarios. It is not only knowing the subject that is important, but also imparting it in an appropriate fashion, flexibly so that you can tell the examiners what they want to hear.

Remember, the examiner does not know you and is basing the standard of your knowledge and patient care on the words that leave your mouth. What they don't hear, they can't score you on. The examiners want a safe and sensible approach of the generalist, not eminence-based practice of someone you may work for.

Treat each question as a chess game that is going to last five minutes.

Structured oral examination question 1

A 35-year-old male lost control on a bend and came off his motorcycle yesterday; he has been fully resuscitated and has an isolated closed injury of the knee (Figure 11.1).

Minute 1

EXAMINER: What do you see?

Here the next minute belongs to the candidate and you can take it whichever way you want to. However, there are essentials to be covered. In the first 30 seconds you are expected to comment on the following:

- Site of radiograph and its suitability – also always ask for two views if only one is given.
- Adult or paediatric skeleton.
- General features: fracture of the proximal tibia with depression of the lateral tibial plateau.

In the next 30 seconds the candidate is expected to comment (without any prompt from the examiner) on the exact nature of the injury, such as Schatzker III fracture with more than 10 mm depression in the articular surfaces, comminuted, concern about the fracture going through the tibial spines and whether the medial side is intact.

The candidate can end these 30 seconds by saying they will assess the soft-tissue envelope, the distal lower limb (palpating the distal pulses and providing a documented assessment of the named nerve function), ensure that a full tertiary survey has been performed and then plan further management of the fracture.

Minute 2

EXAMINER: How would you investigate further?

CANDIDATE: A computed tomography (CT) scan to evaluate the fracture pattern as this helps to plan surgery, particularly with regard to approaches to the fracture and the philosophy of implant choice. (*The examiner is then likely to produce slices of the CT.*)

Don't get carried away at this point. Check the scan is of the same patient and make a basic description of what you see (coronal/sagittal/axial slices, demonstrating . . .). It's vital, in order to score points, that you comment on this constructively, i.e. how what you see may influence your approach/fixation. This is what we actually do – the CT slices are not presented as an abstract diagram, they should be used in your answer to demonstrate that you are used to interpreting them and how they influence your management. End by stating that you would of course discuss the findings of the scan with the patient and use it in the informed consent process.

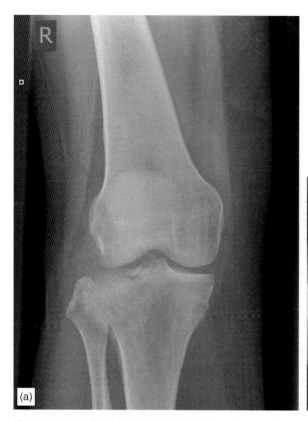

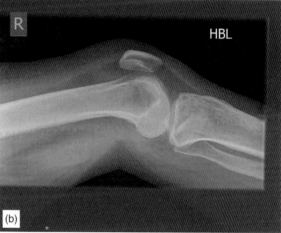

Figure 11.1a and 11.1b Anteroposterior (AP) and lateral radiographs of right knee demonstrating tibial plateau fracture.

You should be at this stage by 90 seconds. Punctuation of the viva is important and helps you stay calm. Having done all this, take a breath and pause. Then, offer to discuss treatment options. Do NOT plough straight in with your plate of choice.

EXAMINER: What are the treatment options?

CANDIDATE: [Take the next 30 seconds to describe operative and non-operative options in the generality. This must be based on the particular patient (recent alignment of consenting processes) and it is critical here that the information will be given to the patient clearly regarding the impact of differing treatment strategies *on that particular patient with that particular injury*.]

Non-operative management would not normally be suitable in this patient. This is due to the articular segment depression, which will impact on overall stability of the joint in addition to the articular congruity and impact on long-term function, as well as the wish to restore joint congruity and stability and avoidance of the generic negative aspects of non-operative

management (such as restricted mobility, prolonged periods of non-weight-bearing, blood clots, etc.). Any operative treatment discussion must be put in the context of the soft tissue envelope and it is important to state that this will influence your decision-making, particularly with regard timing of surgery.

Minute 3

At the two minutes mark you should have committed yourself to offering the patient operative intervention. Before the examiner asks, offer your treatment because it bugs them to keep asking again and again what you will do. Stick with the principles.

The principle of treatment is to restore the articular surface, stabilize and hold the fracture in such a fashion to allow early mobilization. The aim of the treatment is to have a mobile, pain-free and functional joint.

The options of surgical treatment include direct or indirect reduction, percutaneous or open fixation augmented with plate osteosynthesis or external fixation. Before being prompted, suggest your preferred option, which in the authors' opinion is indirect

231

reduction using a cortical window in the proximal tibia, restoration of articular surface with a raft of screws, augmented with a buttress plate. Suggest at that stage you will do assessment under X-ray control for a ligamentous stability and if needed an arthroscopic assessment.

Minute 4 (yes, you are still going …)
The examiner can then take the viva along two routes.

EXAMINER: What is a buttress plate?

CANDIDATE: A plate applied perpendicular to the force that is trying to resist. It is one of the modes of plate uses, along with compression, bridging and tension band, for example.

EXAMINER: What is the role of knee arthroscopy?

CANDIDATE: It is potentially of use in three areas. One, to assess the reduction of the articular surface. Second, to ensure soft tissues (lateral meniscus) are not trapped in the fracture. Third, to assess intra-articular ligament damage. (*Be clear to state that pressure pumps are not to be used in order to avoid iatrogenic compartment syndrome due to extravasation of fluid, as well as the fact that you will use a bladder syringe through the arthroscopy cannula to wash out the haemarthrosis before viewing the joint – this gives the examiner the impression that you have done the procedure before.*)

EXAMINER: What surgical approach will you use?

CANDIDATE: Anterolateral approach with the skin incision being longitudinal and if needed, a reverse L-shaped incision inside. The incision is curved anteriorly over Gerdy's tubercle and is extended distally, 1 cm lateral to the anterior border of the tibia. Proximally the iliotibial band is incised in line with its fibres and the fascia over tibialis anterior divided and elevated bluntly from the tibia distally.

EXAMINER: What about bone graft?

CANDIDATE: I would prefer to use an impacted cancellous femoral head allograft. I realize that cancellous autograft harvested from the iliac crest is probably the gold standard. However, this procedure involves making a separate incision over the iliac crest to obtain the graft, which may result in significant postoperative pain, neuro/vascular injury, haematoma, infection, fractures and cosmetic concerns.

EXAMINER: Anything else you can use?

CANDIDATE: Injectable calcium phosphate bone cement can be used as a buttress in articular cartilage depression. It is thought to reduce the risk of subsidence of the fracture fragments occurring by maintaining articular congruency until the fracture heals.

EXAMINER: What does the literature say?

CANDIDATE: There is some evidence to support the use of bone graft substitutes to fill fracture voids, but a lack of level I evidence.

Minute 5
With one minute left and if the examiner is talking about rehabilitation and weight-bearing status, you know that you are probably winning. Talk about graduated range of motion, protected weight-bearing and the concept that true non-weight-bearing is very difficult for patients and protected weight-bearing 'as able' depending on patient compliance is what is actually going to happen.

Warning: be prepared for an X-ray of metalwork failure with the screws cut out into the articular surface. Stay calm. Assess the patient clinically, radiologically (including CT), rule out infection, soft-tissue problems, patient compliance and then proceed from the start, take out metalwork, align the articular surface, stabilize the fracture and mobilize again, often as a staged process. Key to this is proper work-up and identification of what went wrong and why. It is important not to repeat the same mistakes twice.

EXAMINER: What will you tell the patient about long-term outcome?

CANDIDATE: The reported incidence of post-traumatic radiographic osteoarthritis of the knee following tibial plateau fractures varies from 25% to 45%. Not all patients, however, are symptomatic. The outcome in tibial plateau fractures is more about restoring the mechanical axis rather than accurate reduction of the joint surface. Wasserstein *et al.* reported that regardless of operative fixation, sustaining a tibial plateau fracture requiring surgery increases the likelihood of TKA by 5.3 times.[1] Older patients and those with a more significant fracture were more likely to need TKA.

Evidence base

A 2015 Cochrane review commented that there was insufficient evidence to recommend a specific method of fixation or bone defect replacement technique. They did comment that the evidence does not contradict the idea of minimizing soft-tissue dissection and avoiding donor site morbidity. A review by the EFORT group in 2016 agreed with the above, but also commented on the use of TKA in older patients.

McNamara IR, Smith TO, Shepherd KL, *et al.* Surgical fixation methods for tibial plateau fractures. *Cochrane Database Syst Rev.* 2015;9:CD009679.

Prat-Fabregat S, Camacho-Carrasco P. Treatment strategy for tibial plateau fractures: an update. *EFORT Open Rev.* 2016;1(5):225–232.

Wasserstein D, Henry P, Paterson JM, Kreder HJ, Jenkinson R. Risk of total knee arthroplasty after operatively treated tibial plateau fracture: a matched-population-based cohort study. *J Bone Joint Surg.* 2014;96(2):144–150.

Scott CE, Davidson E, MacDonald DJ, White TO, Keating JF. Total knee arthroplasty following tibial plateau fracture: a matched cohort study. *Bone Joint J.* 2015;97(4):532–538.

Structured oral examination question 2

A 79-year-old woman fell in her garden. She is generally quite independent, has a history of angina which is well controlled and likes meeting her friends at the local social club every Wednesday.

Minute 1

EXAMINER: Please comment on the radiograph (Figure 11.2).

In the first 30 seconds you are expected to comment on the site of radiograph, its acceptability and the general findings it demonstrates.

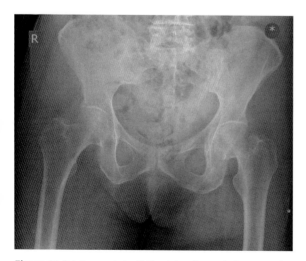

Figure 11.2 Anteroposterior (AP) pelvis radiograph demonstrating intracapsular fractured left neck of femur.

CANDIDATE: The pelvic radiograph shows a displaced left-sided intracapsular neck of femur fracture in the presence of early degenerative changes of the hip joint. (*Always ask for the lateral radiograph.*)

EXAMINER: How will you manage this patient?

CANDIDATE: I would like to assess the whole patient. The degree of mobility prior to injury, comorbidities, 'red flag' features for any pathological lesions, drug history, cause of fall and appropriate investigations. This will include clinical examination of the patient including the left lower limb.

Minutes 2 and 3

EXAMINER: She has well-controlled angina and is otherwise independent.

CANDIDATE: Operative treatment is preferred in this patient group to avoid complications of non-operative management. This will involve a discussion around arthroplasty, either hemiarthroplasty (HA) or total hip arthroplasty (THA). My choice is THA using a well-proven cemented prosthesis provided the patient meets the NICE guidelines of being fit for anaesthesia, not cognitively impaired and able to mobilize independently pre-injury.[1]

EXAMINER: Why do you prefer THA rather than hemiarthroplasty? It is more expensive!

CANDIDATE: A THA has a better functional outcome than HA and has better survivorship results. My choice will be a cemented tapered polished stem of long-term proven results with a cemented, highly cross-linked polyethylene cup using a relatively large head. There are data from a *BMJ* systematic review which suggest better functional outcome and lower re-operation rates in those patients treated with THA. Recent NICE guidelines endorse such practice in a selected population, which includes mentally alert patients with good pre-injury mobility levels and who are relatively healthy. This patient ticks all the criteria and will benefit from THA.

My practice is to use a relatively larger head, such as 32 mm or 36 mm, to counter the increased risk of hip dislocation.[2,3] Surgical technique should focus on the correct orientation of components, good soft-tissue balancing, restoration of hip offset and equalization of leg lengths.

Postoperative management continues with aggressive rehabilitation including early mobilization with full weight-bearing and repatriation to place of usual abode. It also includes addressing any underlying bone abnormalities such as osteoporosis, risk assessment for falls and nutritional deficiency. Ideally, the management should be carried out by a multidisciplinary team. With regards to price and impact on quality of life, THA is considered more cost-effective.[3]

EXAMINER: You keep mentioning NICE guidelines. What is a NICE guideline?

CANDIDATE: NICE clinical guidelines are recommendations for the care of individuals in specific clinical conditions or circumstances within the NHS.

EXAMINER: So why do we use them?

CANDIDATE: NICE guidelines can be used to develop standards to assess the clinical practice of health professionals and can also be used in the education and training of health professionals. They are based on the best available research evidence.

EXAMINER: What's the problem with using NICE guidelines?

CANDIDATE: NICE guidelines do not replace a surgeon's knowledge and skills, they are only guidelines to help a surgeon make an informed decision.

Minute 4

EXAMINER: She arrives at 1800 to your ward. When will you undertake the surgery?

CANDIDATE: The surgery should be undertaken as soon as safely possible and ideally within 36 hours.[4] It should not be rushed in the middle of the night; however, if the patient is fit for anaesthesia then the aim is for surgery on the next morning list with all the theatre staff, kit and consultant cover available. It is important to optimize any correctable medical causes prior to surgery. This should be undertaken in an objective and efficient manner to avoid 'unnecessary' delay.

Minute 5

The examiner can talk about the higher risks of complications of THA in this patient group compared to matched elective controls (9% vs. 4%). This includes

a higher risk of dislocation (7% vs. 1%), leg length discrepancy, cement pressurization side effects such as cement reaction, higher medical complication rate (32% vs. 6%) and higher mortality rate. Length of hospital stay is also increased.

Evidence base

This topic is so common that, yes, you do need to know some numbers:

1. CG 124 – Hip fracture: management (1.6.3).
2. *Injury* volume 47, issue 10, October 2016, pp. 2144–2148: 7% dislocation rate compared to 1%.
3. NIHR HTA volume 15, issue 36: significant increased risk of early dislocation at 1 year (RR 3.98) for THA compared to HA and statistically significant increased risk (RR 2.4) for all follow-up periods up to 13 years.
4. NIHR HTA volume 15, issue 35: cost per QALY $1960 for THA.
5. *Geriatr Orthop Surg Rehabil.* 2014;5(3):138–140.

Structured oral examination question 3

Minutes 1 and 2

EXAMINER: This 49-year-old lady fell on some steps. Her left foot is very painful, bruised, swollen and she can't weight-bear. The junior doctor went to see her in the Emergency Department, but he is not sure what the problem is, what do you think? (Figure 11.3.)

CANDIDATE: These are anteroposterior (AP) and oblique radiographs of the left foot. There is a diastasis between the base of the first and second metatarsals; features suggestive of 'Lisfranc' tarsometatarsal fracture dislocation. There is a small avulsed fragment of bone in that interval. This is an avulsion fracture and could be from the insertion of the Lisfranc ligament (medial cuneiform–second metatarsal) into the base of the second metatarsal ('fleck sign'). Normal alignment on the AP view is demonstrated by examining the lateral borders of the first and second metatarsals, which should line up with the lateral borders of the medial and lateral cuniforms, respectively. The oblique internal rotated view also demonstrates that the medial border of the

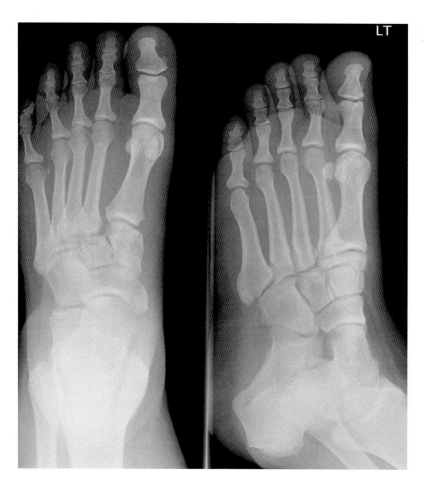

Figure 11.3 Anteroposterior (AP) and oblique radiographs, left foot.

fourth metatarsal lines up with the medial border of the cuboid.

EXAMINER: OK, how will you manage this patient?

CANDIDATE: I would start with the patient's assessment as a whole, following the ATLS (**A**irway and protect cervical spine, **B**reathing, **C**irculation, **D**isability, **E**xposure and environment control) protocol with a focused history including mechanism of injury, patient's general condition, comorbidities, allergies, smoking status as well as occupation and level of function.

I will carry out an examination of the foot noting:

- Soft tissue swelling, pain and ecchymosis.
- Pain on passive abduction/pronation.
- Dorsalis pedis pulse if palpable.
- Compartment syndrome can be a feature of these injuries and I will include this in my differential.

Following assessment, my initial management includes analgesia, elevation and splinting using a below-knee backslab. On admission to hospital I'll arrange for regular, serial examination to detect compartment syndrome.

EXAMINER: What would you do if the radiographs were inconclusive in diagnosing this condition?

CANDIDATE: I would arrange further imaging including oblique and lateral view weight-bearing radiographs if this can be tolerated by the patient. I would arrange a computed tomography scan that should pick up any subtle or occult fractures. MRI scan is useful in allowing direct visualization of the Lisfranc ligament itself, but I would discuss the MRI request with an experience musculoskeletal radiologist beforehand as images can sometimes be difficult to interpret.

Minute 3

EXAMINER: How do you treat Lisfranc tarsometatarsal fracture dislocation?

235

CANDIDATE: This depends on the severity of injury to both the bones and soft tissues and the degree of displacement of the fracture. There is a role for non-operative treatment for an undisplaced stable injury with a cast for 6 weeks with non-weight-bearing and regular clinical and radiological review. However, in the presence of subluxation or dislocation, then accurate reduction and stable fixation is essential. In this case, I would consider open reduction and internal fixation with screws and maybe plating, as required. In the case of a comminuted fracture, then primary arthrodesis of tarsometatarsal joints may be considered, although I would have a full discussion of the treatment options with the patient and record the outcome in the notes.

I would use a dual dorsal incision approach. The first incision is performed between the first and second metatarsals to address the first and second TMT joints. The incision is centred over the TMT joint. The second incision is between the third and fourth metatarsals at the same level.

Minute 4

EXAMINER: What prognosis will you give this patient?

CANDIDATE: This is a serious injury with potentially a poor outcome. Post-traumatic osteoarthritis occurs in over 50% of cases, *even if* operatively treated with open reduction and internal fixation. Residual pain and a stiff foot is a not uncommon complication of this injury. Early identification of the injury is key – up to 20% of tarsometatarsal joint complex injuries are missed on initial examination. The patient must be informed about the length of the recovery period and implications on lifestyle and work in the future.

Minute 5

EXAMINER: If this patient develops compartment syndrome, then how would you manage it?

CANDIDATE: There is no clear evidence regarding the management of presumed compartment syndrome in the foot. In the BOAST guidelines regarding compartment syndrome, it is stated that there is no clear consensus on optimum management. I would discuss the case with the patient and if possible gain a second opinion from a consultant colleague. In general, for low-energy injuries, I adopt a low threshold for decompression in the foot. For high-energy injuries such as following motorcycle trauma or in the intubated patient, my threshold to intervene would be even lower.

EXAMINER: How would you manage the injury if the soft tissues around the foot were very swollen with significant disruption of the bony anatomy but no compartment syndrome?

CANDIDATE: In this situation a prompt reduction of these injuries improves the alignment and relieves the pressure to the surrounding soft tissues, avoids the potential for skin necrosis, helps avert the development of a compartment syndrome, prevents compromise to the neurovascular structures and allows a safe waiting period to be undertaken until the swelling has decreased, re-epithelialization of blisters has occurred and 'wrinkling of the skin' has been noted.

I would be concerned about just applying a backslab and waiting for the swelling to improve as this may leave a malaligned midfoot that may be difficult to reduce once the swelling has subsided.

EXAMINER: So, what are you going to do?

CANDIDATE: I would use an external fixator, applied to one or both sides of the foot to reduce the bony injury and allow the soft tissues to settle before definitive surgery.

Evidence base

The main area of controversy around Lisfranc injuries is whether to treat them with ORIF or ORIF with primary arthrodesis. A systematic review by Smith *et al.* demonstrated a higher rate of hardware removal in patients undergoing simple ORIF. There was no difference between the groups in terms of overall complication rates or PROMs data. ORIF with primary arthrodesis is particularly relevant for purely ligamentous injuries. This relates to the prolonged healing time of a ligamentous injury compared to a bony injury. ORIF has shifted more towards using bridging plates rather than cortical lag screw fixation and K-wires. For further evidence base look through the review article by M. Clare.

Smith N, Stone C, Furey A. Does open reduction and internal fixation versus primary arthrodesis improve patient outcomes for Lisfranc trauma? A systematic review and meta-analysis. *Clin Orthop Rel Res.* 2016;474(6):1445–1452.

Clare MP. Lisfranc injuries. *Curr Rev Musculoskel Med.* 2017;10(1):81–85.

Structured oral examination question 4

A 33-year-old roofer fell 20 feet when scaffolding collapsed under him, landing on his feet and sustaining an isolated injury to his heel.

Minute 1

EXAMINER: This is a radiograph of his foot and ankle (Figure 11.4a). What are your thoughts?

CANDIDATE: This is a lateral radiograph of the left foot. It shows a displaced comminuted intra-articular fracture of the calcaneus with reduced calcaneal height, flattening or even reversal of Bohler's angle, increased angle of Gissane and a fracture of the calcaneal tuberosity.

Regardless of the hindfoot trauma, the patient has had a significant fall, so initially I would assess the patient as a whole following ATLS protocol and screen for potential associated injuries. Vertebral compression fractures (10–15% of cases), fracture of proximal femur, knee (tibial plateau), ankle (pilon fractures) and other foot injures (contralateral calcaneum) must be looked for and excluded.

Minute 2

EXAMINER: Assume that there is no other injury. How would you manage this closed calcaneal fracture?

CANDIDATE: My management plan can be broken down into initial resuscitation followed by further investigation and planning for definitive treatment.

Initial management includes analgesia, splinting, foot elevation and monitoring for compartment syndrome of the foot. The key is managing the soft-tissue envelope, which may require cryotherapy and use of foot pumps to reduce swelling. I would organize a CT scan to assess the fracture personality and plan definitive treatment. Patient factors such as comorbidities (diabetes and peripheral vascular disease) should be considered as well as smoking status, occupation and other functional demands.

EXAMINER: This is the CT scan you requested (Figure 11.4b), what can you see and what would you do next?

CANDIDATE: This CT scan axial section demonstrates shortening, varus deformity and considerable comminution. There is a large sustentacular fragment, depressed middle fragment and blow out of the lateral wall. It also shows considerable heel widening.

EXAMINER: Do you know any classification systems for calcaneal fractures?

CANDIDATE: The Sanders classification is a CT classification based on the number of articular fragments seen on a coronal view at the widest point of the posterior facet (Figure 11.4c).

Type 1: Undisplaced posterior facet (regardless of number of fracture lines).

Types 2, 3 and 4 are displaced fractures.

Type 2: One fracture line (two-part intra-articular fracture). Divided into three subgroups on the basis of fracture line localization.

Fracture line is lateral in Type 2A fractures, central in Type 2B and medial in Type 2C fractures.

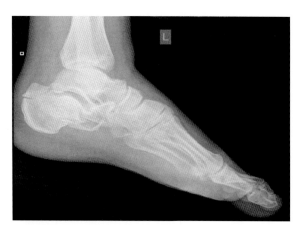

Figure 11.4a Radiograph left lateral foot.

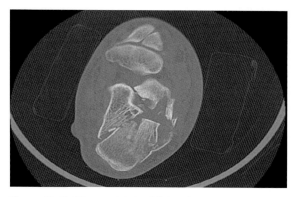

Figure 11.4b CT scan axial view left foot demonstrating calcaneal fracture.

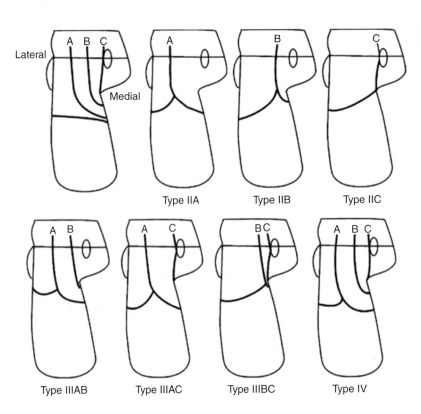

Figure 11.4c Saunders classification of calcaneal fractures.

Type 3: Two fracture lines in the posterior facet (three-part intra-articular fracture).

Type 4: Comminuted fracture with more than three fracture lines in the posterior facet (four or more fragments).

I would discuss treatment options with the patient including open reduction and internal fixation once the soft-tissue envelope is suitably resuscitated. I would base my decision on the fracture pattern, soft-tissue status and patient factors. This fracture pattern will benefit from surgical intervention, but it will depend heavily on several patient factors including smoking, occupation, comorbidities and the expectations of the patient.

Minute 3

EXAMINER: Following discussion with the patient you have decided to proceed with internal fixation. What are the aims/goals of surgery?

CANDIDATE: The aims of surgery are restoration of articular congruity while restoring calcaneal height, length and heel width and minimizing soft-tissue complications.

EXAMINER: How will you fix the fracture?

CANDIDATE: I would take full informed consent, in particular concentrating on the risks and benefits of both operative and non-operative management. The patient will be under general anaesthesia with prophylactic antibiotics, tourniquet and in the lateral decubitus position with fluoroscopy control. I would use an L-shaped lateral incision halfway between fibula and Achilles tendon avoiding damage to the sural nerve. I would employ full-thickness flaps by taking the incision down to the bone and use bent K-wires as retractors. I would take off the lateral wall, manipulate the fracture fragments to restore the length and height of the calcaneum as well as correction of varus deformity, reconstruct the articular surface and then reapply the lateral wall. I would use K-wires for temporary stability and then fixation using a fragment specific plate. My preference is a low-profile lateral calcaneal plate, the size of which depends on the patient's calcaneus and I would contour the plate prior to application. The key is to capture the sustentacular fragment under fluoroscopy.

Postoperatively, the patient would mobilize non-weight-bearing for 6 weeks followed by a further 6 weeks of partial weight-bearing.

EXAMINER: What are the complications from surgery?

CANDIDATE: Complications include wound dehiscence, osteomyelitis, post-traumatic osteoarthritis, increased heel width, subtalar stiffness, peroneal tendinitis, sural nerve injury, persistent heel pain, scar hypersensitivity, tarsal tunnel syndrome and CRPS.

EXAMINER: If the wound got infected, how would you deal with it?

CANDIDATE: I would want to prevent direct extension to bone causing osteomyelitis. This needs aggressive antibiotic therapy and a low threshold for radical debridement. I would attempt to keep in place the plate and screws but would remove the metalwork if the infection was not settling. Soft-tissue coverage with local or free flap involving the plastic surgeons should be considered if the wound is very large. Occasionally amputation may be needed.

EXAMINER: The patient complains of pain.

CANDIDATE: There are many causes of pain which include subtalar incongruity, penetration of screws into the subtalar joint or arthritis. Lateral pain may be caused by lateral impingement or peroneal tendinitis. Anterior pain from talar neck impingement or scar tissue. Subtalar osteoarthritis may require a subtalar arthrodesis.

EXAMINER: What prognosis will you give for this patient?

CANDIDATE: A calcaneal fracture is a significant injury with high incidence of long-term pain and disability. There is about a 40% chance the patient will have long-term chronic pain after a significant intra-articular fracture.

Evidence base

Be careful. Treatment of calcaneum fracture is still a controversial issue and attracts a lot of debate.

A key paper to know is the Griffin article reporting the results of the UK Heel Fracture Trial.[2] This was a multicentre, pragmatic, randomized control trial which demonstrated no difference in patient reported outcomes between operative and non-operative management of intra-articular calcaneal fractures. However, it is important to note that patient selection was based on the idea that patients could be managed by either method. Those patients with clear indications for surgery (see above) were not included and so should still be taken on their own merit.

Another key paper is Buckley et al.[3] In this multicentre Canadian trial over 300 patients with displaced calcaneal fractures were evaluated comparing operative vs. non-operative treatment. The authors found that without stratification of patients, functional results were the same with either non-operative or operative care.

When they looked at subgroups of patients they found that those receiving workers compensation had a worse outcome in general. Women fared better after surgical reduction, as did patients who:

- Were not receiving workers' compensation.
- Were less than 29 years old.
- Had a less severely displaced fracture.
- Had a light workload.
- Had an anatomic reduction.

In a later study, they noted that the overall cost of care of patients was less with surgical care than non-surgical management due to the need for additional surgery for fusion and for the higher disability cost from a longer period of missed work in the non-operatively managed group of patients.

Structured oral examination question 5

A 21-year-old motorcyclist is involved in a road traffic accident. He is fully conscious, alert and following a global assessment using the ATLS protocol, it is revealed that this is an isolated, closed injury (Figure 11.5).

Minute 1

EXAMINER: Tell me how you would manage this injury.

CANDIDATE: These are anteroposterior (AP) and lateral views of the distal tibia and ankle joint. This is a complex intra-articular multifragmentary fracture occurring as a result of high-energy trauma. There is a fracture of the distal tibia involving the ankle joint with articular impaction and comminution extending into the metaphysis, a fractured fibula, a disruption of the syndesmosis and possibly a fractured talus.

239

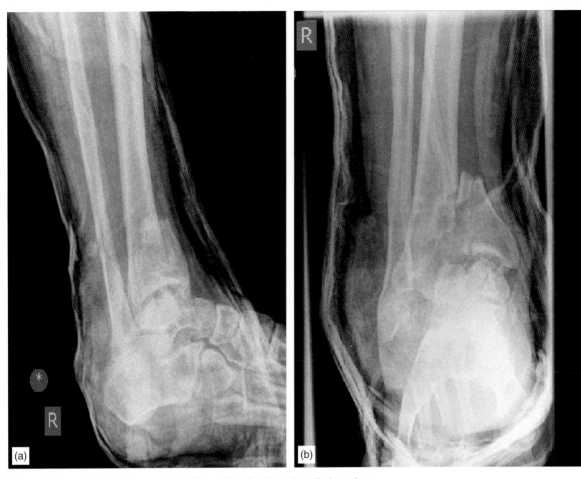

Figure 11.5a and 11.5b Anteroposterior (AP) and lateral radiographs, right lower leg.

I will take a concise history and perform a focused examination. I would enquire about smoking, alcohol consumption, a history of diabetes or peripheral vascular disease, etc. which are important risk factors for soft tissue (and bone) healing. Examination would particularly assess the state of the soft-tissue envelope looking for any skin damage, contusion and fracture blisters. I would also obtain tibial shaft and knee radiographs of the affected limb.

I will ensure the patient is comfortable and splint the limb, realigning the foot into a better position, relieving pressure on the skin to avoid any skin necrosis. I will perform a thorough neurovascular assessment of the involved limb including palpation of the posterior tibial and dorsalis pedis artery as well as examination of capillary refill to check for an adequate vascular supply. I would obtain radiographs of the post

splinted leg to check for adequacy of reduction and commence serial assessment for compartment syndrome.

COMMENT: Isolated closed injury is coded language to say the examiners just want you to focus on the management of this fracture. No need to mention ATLS.

CANDIDATE: Ruedi and Allgower have classified these injuries into three types:

Type 1 Non-displaced fracture cleavage of ankle joint.

Type 2 Displaced fracture with minimal impaction or comminution.

Type 3 Explosive fracture with significant articular comminution and metaphyseal impaction.

EXAMINER: How does this classification system help you?

CANDIDATE: The Ruedi–Allgower classification system is based on the severity of comminution and displacement of the articular surface and offers a rough guide to management.

Minute 2

CANDIDATE: My principle of managing this case is: 'span–scan–plan'. I would prefer a staged management approach for this fracture rather than going for early ORIF. Early ORIF in the face of compromised soft tissues will lead to an increased risk of infection, wound dehiscence, a poor overall clinical outcome and in a worst case scenario may lead to amputation. It is generally thought that a staged management protocol of span, scan and plan is the gold-standard method (first-line intervention) to deal with complex intra-articular fractures, especially in the presence of bruised, swollen, compromised soft tissues. I would consider early involvement of the plastic surgeons if the soft-tissue envelope was very badly compromised and especially so if the fracture was open.

- Span: I will place an external fixator in order to reduce and hold the fracture. This will allow correction of length, restoration of alignment and rotation and allow soft-tissue resuscitation and monitoring. This will also allow us to arrange timely definitive surgery.
- Scan: Following initial stabilization, computed tomography scanning will provide more details of the fracture type and pattern. A CT after EF will illustrate the overall alignment of the tibia, help identify the main fracture fragments, location of fracture lines, amount of articular impaction and comminution. The scan usually influences the surgical approach chosen for definitive fixation.
- Plan: using the CT scan I can then plan the definitive treatment in detail; approach, how to fix fragments, what implant to use, timing of surgery, taking consent from the patient and ensuring all equipment, staff and company representatives are available.

Minute 3

EXAMINER: When are you going to fix this fracture?

CANDIDATE: This is a serious and challenging injury to manage. The soft-tissue envelope needs to be resuscitated until it is in a reasonable condition (this may take up to 10–14 days to settle).

Definitive surgery should be planned on a defined dedicated trauma list involving a surgeon with an interest in managing these complex fractures in order to achieve the best possible outcome.

EXAMINER: How are you going to fix this fracture?

CANDIDATE: The principles of fixation of an intraarticular fracture are anatomical reduction, interfragmentary compression and absolute stability at the fracture site to allow early mobilization.

COMMENT: This is a generic statement that, while correct, isn't using viva time efficiently. It is better for candidates to be more fracture-specific if possible.

CANDIDATE: My goals of treatment are:

- Re-establishment of articular congruency.
- Correction of any mechanical malalignment.
- Management of any bone loss.
- Reduction of the risk of soft-tissue complications.
- Early restoration of motion.

  Ruedi–Allogower specifically recommended four key operative principles:
- Plating the fibula to length.
- Articular reconstruction.
- Bone grafting of metaphyseal defects.
- Medial buttress to the tibia to prevent a late varus deformity.

The approach would be tailored dependent on fracture configuration as corroborated by CT scan prior to and with fluoroscopy during surgery. Looking at the fractures in the radiographs provided, I would favour an anterolateral approach that will allow me to reduce the pilon fracture, and approach the fibula as well as the talus. I would aim for anatomical reduction of the pilon fracture under direct vision and stabilize it with an anterolateral plate and then address the fibula and talus on their own merits. The fracture of the talus may well necessitate extending the approach and a release of the ATFL through a subperiosteal approach. I would anatomically reduce the talus fracture and stabilize it. I would make sure any loose debris is removed from the joint.

EXAMINER: Anything else?

CANDIDATE: Sorry?

EXAMINER: Anything else about the fracture pattern?

CANDIDATE: No, sorry.

241

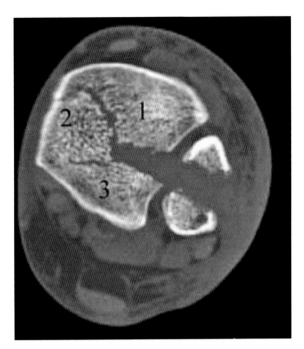

Figure 11.5c Classic articular components of a pilon fracture.

COMMENT: For score 7/8 candidates. There are three classic articular components of a pilon fracture that can be identified on axial CT scan. These are anterolateral (Chaput fragment), medial and posterolateral (Volkmann fragment) (Figure 11.5c).

EXAMINER: How would you perform an anterolateral approach to the ankle?

CANDIDATE: The patient should be supine with antibiotics given and a thigh tourniquet applied. This incision is centred at the ankle joint, parallel to the fourth metatarsal distally, and parallel to and between the tibia and fibula proximally. Dissection through the skin and subcutaneous tissues should proceed sharply with maintenance of full-thickness skin flaps. Because the anterior compartment muscles arise from the anterior fibula, the incision is usually not extended more than 7 cm above the ankle joint. Distally, the incision can extend as far as the talonavicular joint.

Care is taken not to damage the superficial peroneal nerve which lies directly beneath the skin. This nerve crosses the surgical incision proximal to the ankle joint. It should be identified, mobilized, and protected throughout the surgical procedure.

The fascia over the anterior compartment of the distal tibia is then incised sharply, beneath the superficial peroneal nerve. Distally, the extensor retinaculum is incised, and the anterior compartment tendons are all retracted medially. Proximally, the entire anterior compartment musculature, including the peroneus tertius, can then be mobilized and retracted medially. These muscles and tendons are usually easy to mobilize from the underlying anterior tibiofibular ligament, the periosteum of the distal tibia, and the joint capsule.

COMMENT: For score 8 candidates:

EXAMINER: How will you fix the fragments?

CANDIDATE: The articular surface is visualized, and the impacted fragments reduced under direct vision. Reconstruction of the plafond proceeds from posterior to anterior with provisional fixation of fracture fragments using temporary K-wires, and small fragment screws (cannulated and partially threaded) then applied to secure definitive stability. Occasionally if fracture reduction is difficult a distractor can be used to aid fixation. A locking plate is then applied to the distal tibia.

EXAMINER: Any other methods?

CANDIDATE: A circular frame with limited minimally invasive internal fixation is a possible option, but I have no experience with this method of fixation.

Minutes 4–5

EXAMINER: How would you counsel the patient and their family regarding the outcome of pilon fracture?

CANDIDATE: These injuries represent a high-energy axial insult to the lower limb that leads to severe joint comminution, impaction and a large zone of injury. There are considerable risks of complications affecting both bone, joint and overlying soft tissues. Wound breakdown and skin necrosis may lead to late sinus formation or osteomyelitis associated with infected metalwork. Delayed union, non-union, infected non-union and malunion can occur. Post-traumatic osteoarthritis may require arthrodesis or arthroplasty.

EXAMINER: What is Hawkins' sign, is it a good or bad sign?

CANDIDATE: It is the appearance of osteopenia in subchondral bone of the talar dome on the AP view, 6–8 weeks following fracture of the neck of talus. The Hawkins' sign is a good indicator of talus vascularity following fracture – it is therefore a good sign. It indicates that healing will occur without avascular necrosis.

Evidence base

The evidence base here is fairly disparate with no major RCTs. The general consensus is to use the 'span–scan–plan' approach. Fixation can be affected with either a frame or plate osteosynthesis and there is little to say one gives a better outcome than the other.

Structured oral examination question 6

A 50-year-old lady is a front seat passenger involved in a head-on road traffic collision. In the Emergency Department she is diagnosed with dislocation of her native right hip.

Minute 1

EXAMINER: What will be your initial management?

CANDIDATE: A native hip dislocation is a marker of a high-energy injury and I would assess the patient along ATLS principles utilizing an ABCDE approach. I will look to exclude any associated injuries. I would clinically examine her lower limbs looking at alignment, position and neurovascular status in particular that of the sciatic nerve. With the mechanism of injury caused by impact of the dashboard on the knee the hip dislocation is likely to be posterior often with an associated acetabular rim fracture or femoral neck fracture.

EXAMINER: Any clue as to whether it is posterior or anterior clinically?

CANDIDATE: With a posterior dislocation the leg would be shortened and internally rotated while with an anterior dislocation the leg is flexed, shortened, externally rotated and abducted. Anterior dislocations of the hip are rare.

EXAMINER: It appears to be an isolated injury with paraesthesia in the sole of the foot; however, motor function is intact. How will you take it from here?

CANDIDATE: A traumatic hip dislocation is a surgical emergency because of the risks to the vascularity of the femoral head, dangers of chondrolysis as well as pressure effects on the surrounding soft tissues, especially neurovascular structures. The paraesthesia in the foot is an indication of pressure or traction affecting the sciatic nerve. I would arrange for the patient to go to the operating theatre urgently. I would get a CT scan done provided it does not delay transfer to the operating theatre; and of course, inform theatres, anaesthetic team and the ward. I would order baseline blood tests including blood group and save. I would take informed consent for a closed or open reduction under general anaesthesia.

Minute 2

EXAMINER: There is delay in getting the CT scan and you take her to the operating theatre. How will you reduce the hip?

CANDIDATE: I would attempt closed reduction under general anaesthesia. I would position her supine on the table with the table height as low as possible. I would request the anaesthetist to use full muscle relaxant to make it easier to reduce the hip. I would stand on the side of the dislocated hip and have the image intensifier come from the opposite side. My assistant will be on the opposite side towards the head end of the patient to stabilize and hold down her pelvis at the ASISs when I attempt manipulation. I would screen the hip first before attempting reduction to exclude a neck of femur fracture and also assess the acetabulum using Judet views. If it is posterior dislocation, I would apply gentle traction on the hip (inline) and then gradually flex the hip and the knee, maintaining traction. Reduction usually occurs with an audible 'clunk' and I would check reduction under the image intensifier and also check once again for any associated fractures.

Bigelow's technique is with hip flexed to 90°, the affected leg is placed in an adducted and internally rotated position. While an assistant stabilizes the pelvis with downward pressure, traction is applied in line with the femur while abducting, externally rotating and extending the affected hip.

EXAMINER: You manage to reduce the hip and get this radiographic image (Figure 11.6a). What are your thoughts?

COMMENT: In the next 30 seconds you are expected to comment on the name of the patient, site of radiograph and the exact nature of the injury.

CANDIDATE: In this image-intensifier view of the right hip, the femoral head appears to be in the acetabulum but is incongruent; in addition,

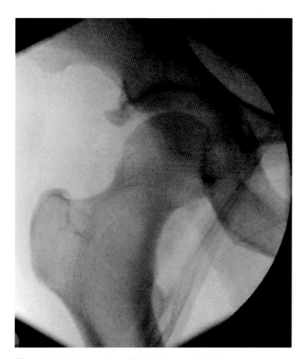

Figure 11.6a Image intensifier (II) image right hip.

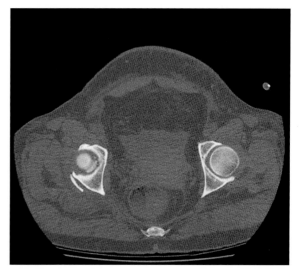

Figure 11.6b CT axial view pelvis.

I would like to confirm this on lateral view. The femoral head is inferiorly subluxed and there appears to be a bony fragment in the hip joint superiorly and another one inferiorly. There is one more fragment on the superolateral lip of the acetabulum. The bony fragments are most likely to be from the acetabulum; however, femoral head fragments need to be ruled out.

Minute 3

EXAMINER: How will you assess this hip further?

CANDIDATE: Peroperatively I would screen the hip in AP and lateral views as well as get Judet views to assess the anterior and posterior walls and columns. In addition, I would carefully assess the hip for stability by screening the hip through a range of motion. I do not want to re-dislocate the hip and cause any further hip damage. A CT scan will be useful to delineate this further, if it has not already been done.

EXAMINER: You get a CT scan done in the morning and this is one of the sections (Figure 11.6b). What do you think?

CANDIDATE: [Note: just comment on what you have rather than ask for more images!]

In this axial section of the pelvis at the level of the hip joints, I note that the femoral head on the injured side is at a different height to the opposite hip. There is a bony fragment trapped in the hip joint as well as a bony fragment lying posterior to the hip. This may represent a fracture dislocation with compromise of the acetabular wall posterosupeiorly. I would, however, need to study the whole CT sequence to ascertain the extent of damage. After obtaining a post reduction CT if I wasn't in an MTC I would discuss the images with the regional acetabular and pelvic reconstruction unit and get their advice.

EXAMINER: What about an MRI scan of the hip?

CANDIDATE: While MRI will demonstrate labral tears and soft-tissue anatomy it has not been shown to be beneficial in the acute evaluation and management of hip dislocations.

EXAMINER: How will you deal with the bony fragment in the hip joint?

CANDIDATE: This depends on a number of factors including the exact original site of the fragment, the size of it, the integrity of the weight-bearing dome and the stability of the hip. The options for a bony fragment trapped in the hip joint are to remove it or to retrieve and fix it. If the fragment is quite small and does not affect the hip stability or the weight-bearing dome, then it can be removed arthroscopically. However, if it compromises the weight-bearing area of the hip or stability then I would retrieve it and fix it. It will have to be an open procedure, although reports of arthroscopic intervention have been published.

(*Note*: If the candidate does not have sound hip arthroscopy knowledge, then the safe option is open procedure and stay clear of hip arthroscopy.)

Minute 4

EXAMINER: You find that it is the posterosuperior lip of the acetabulum. Which approach will you use to fix the fracture?

CANDIDATE: The approach depends on where the bony fragment is arising from. If it is posterosuperior or posterior, I would use a Kocher–Langenbeck approach to the hip. I would position the patient on the fracture table in lateral decubitus. In the posterior approach to the hip I would respect the blood vessels supplying the femoral head and therefore would not take down the quadratus (medial circumflex femoral artery). I would incise the short external rotators at least 1.5 cm from their insertions to again avoid damage occurring to the medial circumflex MCFA. I would retract the gluteus medius superiorly, identify the capsule and dissect superiorly to identify the fractured rim of the acetabulum. I would be careful with the sciatic nerve as it may be closer than realized in the operating field due to the distorted anatomy and could also be bruised from the original injury. I would reduce the fragment anatomically under image-intensifier screening and secure it with 2–3 partially threaded cannulated screws, making sure that the screws do not penetrate the hip joint. If the fragment was large I would consider using a posterior plate one-third small fragment tubular or 3.5 mm reconstruction plate.

If an anterior approach to the hip is needed either an ilioinguinal or Stoppa approach can be used.

Minute 5

EXAMINER: What are the risks of posterior dislocation of the hip?

CANDIDATE: Immediate complications are sciatic nerve injury (10% with posterior dislocation), fractures, and haemorrhage. Intermediate risks are chondrolysis, post reduction neurological damage, avascular necrosis, intra-articular loose bodies, heterotopic ossification, hip instability. Late complications are hip pain and post-traumatic osteoarthritis.

EXAMINER: What other injuries are associated with this injury pattern?

CANDIDATE: This is determined by the direction of forces and may include patella fracture, PCL rupture, femoral shaft fracture, femoral neck and head fractures.

Note: The candidate is smiling as the examiner has run out of questions on his crib sheet!

Evidence base

The evidence base here is largely based on expert opinion and there are no major RCTs.

Structured oral examination question 7

A 78-year-old lady fell out of her bed while visiting friends in another part of the country and sustained this proximal femur fracture. She is in reasonably good health and was independently mobile, able to care for herself and do her own shopping.

Minute 1

EXAMINER: What can you see (Figure 11.7a.)? What are the treatment principles?

CANDIDATE: An AP radiograph of the right hip showing a reverse-obliquity inter-trochanteric fracture with subtrochanteric extension. The lesser trochanter is proximally displaced with associated loss of the posteromedial buttress. I would like to see a lateral view; however, based even on the AP view, it is an unstable fracture pattern.

My management for this patient would start with thorough assessment and optimization of her general condition. We need to consider the possibility of pathological fracture, although the available radiograph shows no evidence of that. I would get adequate radiographs of the full femur. Provided she is fit for surgery, I would aim to treat this fracture operatively and will do this within 36 hours of admission. I would use a cephalomedullary device to fix this fracture. I would do so as a load-sharing implant with a large diameter nail with a shorter, medialized lever arm will afford an enhanced biomechanical environment for this challenging fracture.

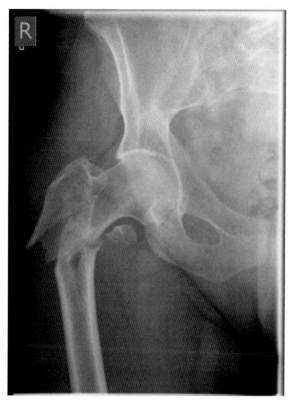

Figure 11.7a Anteroposterior (AP) radiograph of right femur demonstrating inter-trochanteric fracture.

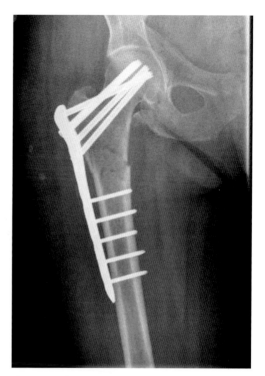

Figure 11.7b Anteroposterior (AP) radiograph, right femur, with fixed locking plate in situ.

Minute 2

EXAMINER: I agree. This lady was treated elsewhere initially with an extramedullary device. She presents 4 months down the line when you are on call with this complication, can you explain what happened (Figure 11.7b and 11.7c)?

CANDIDATE: This lady was treated with a fixed angled locking plate. Two elements of fracture care are perhaps responsible for the implant failure – biomechanics and biology.

Looking at the postoperative radiograph, there is a gap at the fracture site, especially on the medial side. The fixed angled device has been used with locking screws with five screws on either side of the fracture, which will make it a very rigid construct with a very high strain focused across a small fracture working length. This will minimize any micro-motion necessary for callus formation. On the other hand, there is a fracture gap and lack of compression, which will preclude primary bone union. This has resulted in delayed union/atrophic non-union at the fracture site. Essentially this fracture is in a surgical 'no man's land' with none of the requirements of either primary or secondary bone healing.

The implant has been under constant biomechanical load, which had led to the fatigue failure of the implant-grade steel. In this particular design there is a stress riser at the junction of the last proximal locking hole and tapered part of the plate, which dictates the failure point in the implant. In addition, the plating device is applied on the lateral aspect of the femur, increasing the lever arm for the moment of force as compared to a cephalomedullary device, which further puts the fixed angled plating device in this position at a biomechanical disadvantage. In this type of fracture, a cephalomedullary device has better biomechanical stability.

Minute 4

EXAMINER: You fixed it with this nail. What do you think about your check X-ray (Figure 11.7d)?

CANDIDATE: I fixed this?! I'm surprised as there are several fundamental issues with this construct. The screws in the proximal fragment are a bit

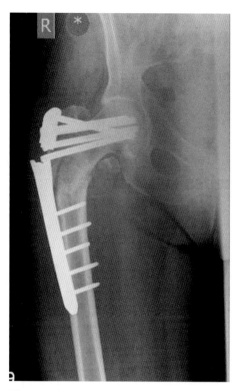

Figure 11.7c Anteroposterior (AP) radiograph, right femur, demonstrating hardware failure, 4 months postoperative.

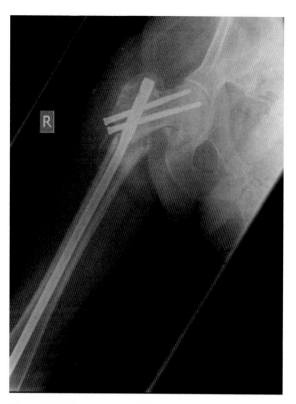

Figure 11.7d Anteroposterior (AP) radiograph demonstrating non-union femoral fracture.

superior to where I'd normally like them to be. The screws are also not absolutely parallel, and I'll study my lateral radiographs carefully to make sure that the screws have not missed the nail while transiting into the head. There is translation of the fragments and the femoral shaft is in varus. None of these features are ideal. In addition, the nail is probably undersized, it looks relatively small for the canal with only limited isthmic fit.

COMMENT: Keep out of the politics of criticizing any suboptimal fixation, especially in the exam. Keep it factually straight down the line with neutral comments.

Minute 5

EXAMINER: How will you follow-up this patient?

CANDIDATE: I would follow-up this patient with clinical reviews and serial radiographs. I would start her weight-bearing as able, ensure she is not on non-steroidal anti-inflammatories or bisphosphonate treatment, counsel against smoking and

do serial radiographs 6 weeks apart. If there is no callus formation at 6 months, I would consider exchanging the intramedullary nail.

Evidence base

A 2014 Cochrane review suggested that there is very poor evidence surrounding cephallomedullary nails and more evidence is required comparing these devices to sliding hip screws.

Queally JM, Harris E, Handoll HHG, Parker MJ. Intramedullary nails for extracapsular hip fractures in adults. *Cochrane Database Syst Rev.* 2014; Issue 9.

While the mechanical benefits of the intramedullary devices may not lead to improved outcomes in patients with a simple intertrochanteric fracture, the more complex unstable patterns such as four-part inter-trochanteric or reverse oblique fractures may be better managed with cephallomedullary nails.

Be prepared to discuss the biomechanical differences between CMN and DHS.

Structured oral examination question 8

A 72-year-old lady, fully independent with good health, was hit by a car when she was walking on a kerb. She was brought to hospital with these two injuries. She was assessed following ATLS protocol, fully resuscitated and her injuries were splinted (Figure 11.8).

Minute 1

EXAMINER: What your thoughts about this patient's management? Do you have any concerns?

CANDIDATE: This 72-year-old lady has multiple high-energy injuries. Although she was enjoying good health prior to this accident, I would be concerned about her physiological response to the trauma. Elderly patients have a limited physiological reserve when compared to younger patients, so she needs to be closely observed, kept well hydrated and her general condition optimized before definitive treatment. Fractured long bones should be stabilized as early as possible for many reasons: pain relief, to reduce the metabolic response to trauma, to allow for early mobilization and rehabilitation as well as a decreased incidence of complications associated with recumbence. The anaesthetic team and orthogeriatricians should be involved early in the plan for her treatment.

Minute 2

EXAMINER: What implants are you going to use to fix these fractures?

CANDIDATE: For the left femur fracture it is an unstable, multifragmentary, supracondylar fracture with femoral shortening. The aim is to reduce the fracture for length, alignment and rotation and then stabilize using a relative stability device. To do this I may need to use a femoral distracter for temporary reduction and then stabilize with either a nail or a plate. Personally, I would use a fixed-angle plate with locking options and a minimally invasive technique. Failure in varus can be a problem for these fractures.

Regarding the tibia fracture it is a distal third fracture that is periprosthetic in nature due to the presence of pre-existing implants from an ankle fixation. I need to employ a technique with minimal soft-tissue stripping and one that enables early weight-bearing. As with the femur I want to achieve reduction for length, alignment and rotation before stabilizing. To this end I would

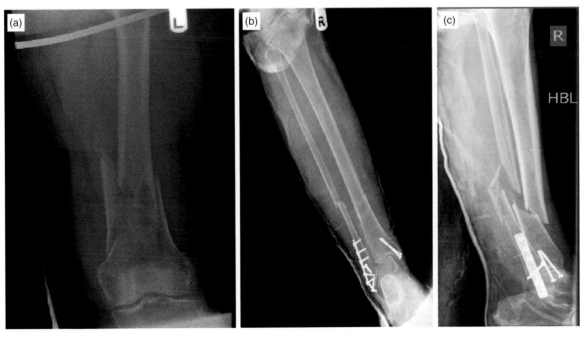

Figure 11.8a, 11.8b and 11.8c Anteroposterior (AP) radiograph, left femur, demonstrating supracondylar fracture femur, and AP and lateral radiographs, right lower leg.

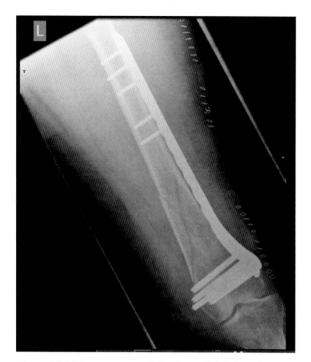

Figure 11.8d Anteroposterior (AP) radiograph, left distal femur with locking plate in situ.

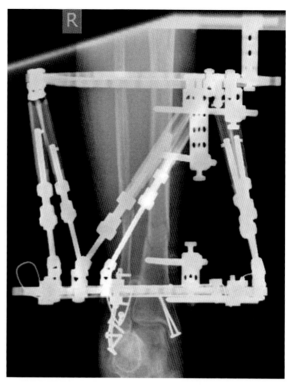

Figure 11.8e Anteroposterior (AP) radiograph, right distal tibia with circular frame in situ.

choose an antegrade, intramedullary, reamed tibial interlocking nail. If the soft tissues were compromised or the canal too narrow to allow nailing, I would consider using a circular frame.

Minutes 3–4

EXAMINER: OK, have look on this radiograph (Figure 11.8d) and explain to me the technique the surgeon used and what the principles of such technique are.

CANDIDATE: The AP radiograph shows a multifragmentary fracture of distal diaphysis/metaphysis of the femur that has been stabilized with a fixed-angle plate, in bridging mode. Examining the skin staples, I can infer that closed indirect reduction and a less-invasive technique was used. This technique was introduced to decrease soft-tissue disruption and preserve blood supply. Length, alignment and rotation of the bone have been restored. Baumgaertel *et al.* introduced the concept of biological plating and proved that indirect reduction and bridge plating was superior to direct fragment reduction and anatomical fixation in respect to bone healing.[4]

EXAMINER: Can you explain why the surgeon put screws on either ends of the plate and missed the middle?

CANDIDATE: The surgeon intended to increase the working length of the implant (the distance between two points on either side of the fracture where the bone is fixed to plate or nail). This produces even distribution of forces over a long segment and decreases (shares) stress between the fracture and the implant.

Minute 5

EXAMINER: You mentioned circular frames – can you tell me the principles of their use?

CANDIDATE: Circular frames consist of fixation elements such as tensioned wires or half pins attached to rings on either side of the fracture. This forms proximal ring blocks and distal ring blocks. Segments of frame can be moved in terms of angulation, rotation, translation and length. Their use has particular worth with poor soft tissues and small segments. They may be definitive or temporary and may also be used in isolation or hybrid with other techniques such as limited ORIF. They allow immediate weight-bearing and therefore are beneficial in the elderly and patients with limited compliance (Figure 11.8e).

Structured oral examination question 9

A 29-year-old female horse rider fell off her horse; she has been fully assessed in the Emergency department and has an isolated closed injury of the foot.

Minute 1

EXAMINER: What are your thoughts (Figure 11.9a)?

CANDIDATE: The radiographs of the left foot, AP and oblique, show a displaced, comminuted fracture of the body of the navicular. There is overlap of the midtarsal bones and I can't exclude fractures of any other tarsal bones. The alignment of the foot is still maintained and there is no varus or valgus deformity.

Given the high degree of ligamentous stability of the navicular this is a serious, high-energy injury. I need to assess the patient as a whole.

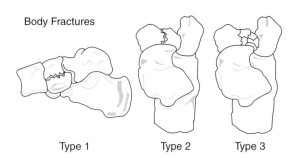

Body Fractures

Type 1   Type 2   Type 3

Figure 11.9b Sangeorzan *et al.* classification of talar body fractures.

I would secure a relevant focused history, clinical examination in general of the patient and in particular of the foot, ruling out compartment syndrome, any neurovascular damage and assessing the soft-tissue envelope of the foot. I would then request further imaging, the modality of choice being a computed tomography scan.

I would initially treat the injured foot in a backslab, with strict elevation and intermittent cryotherapy, adequate analgesia and serial monitoring for any evolving compartment syndrome.

COMMENT: Navicular body fractures are often associated with other injuries of the midtarsal joint often with varying disruption of the talonavicular and cuneonavicular joints.

Sangeorzan *et al.* classified these injuries into three types (Figure 11.9b). This is probably worth knowing, although there is a move away in the exam from pure didactic learning of classification systems to using a classification system as a guide to treatment. It is a useful guide towards difficulty of fracture reduction and eventual clinical outcome.

Type 1 The fracture line splits the navicular into dorsal and plantar segments.
No dislocation occurs.

Type 2 These are the most common injuries.
The fracture traverses from dorsal lateral to plantar medial across the body of the tarsal navicular. The major fragment is dorsal medial, with a smaller, often comminuted plantar–lateral fragment. There is usually medial forefoot displacement.

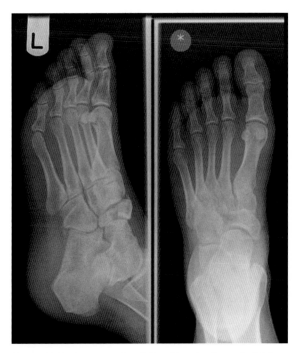

Figure 11.9a Anteroposterior (AP) and lateral radiographs, left foot.

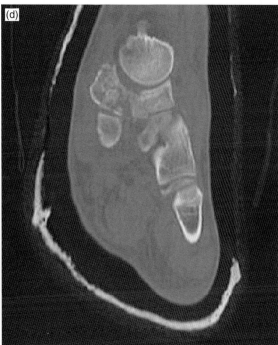

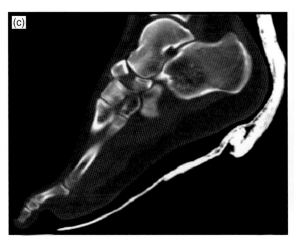

Figure 11.9c and 11.9d CT scan, coronal and sagittal sections of left foot.

Type 3 The fracture is characterized by comminution of fragments and significant displacement. The medial fragment is the major one and the medial border of the foot is often disrupted at the cuneonavicular joint. There is often lateral displacement of the foot. This injury carries the worst prognosis.

Minute 2

EXAMINER: This is the scan you requested, what do you see and how would you manage it (Figure 11.9c and 11.9d)?

CANDIDATE: These are coronal and sagittal sections of the CT scan, and they confirm the radiographic findings of a displaced fracture of the body of navicular bone with comminution. It is an unstable displaced intra-articular fracture and I would therefore favour operative intervention rather than non-operative. The principles of management are to restore the articular surface, stabilize and hold the fracture to allow early mobilization. The aim of the treatment is to have a mobile, pain-free and functional joint. However, sometimes that is not possible due to severe comminution of the articular surface, in which case I may consider primary fusion of the talonavicular joint.

I would discuss the findings, management options, aims of the treatment as well as potential complications with the patient and ensure balanced informed consent is secured before proceeding. I could only proceed once the soft-tissue envelope is satisfactory, however.

COMMENT: Fractures with less than 2 mm articular displacement, no midfoot instability and no loss of bone length can be managed non-operatively. Non-weight-bearing cast for 6–8 weeks. In general, all navicular body fractures with >2 mm displacement require ORIF.

Minute 3

EXAMINER: Can you tell us about any possible complication associated with this case?

CANDIDATE: There are immediate, early and late complications. Immediate complications are in the perioperative period and include iatrogenic injury to structures, compartment syndrome and anaesthetic problems. Early complications

251

include infection, nerve injury (branches of superficial and deep peroneal nerves), vascular injury (dorsalis pedis); and late complications include non-union and loss of medial longitudinal arch support, painful talonavicular joint, post-traumatic osteoarthritis, as well as avascular necrosis and collapse. Late talonavicular fusion may be required as a salvage procedure.

EXAMINER: What are you going to tell the patient?

CANDIDATE: With a good reduction most have a reasonable prognosis, but few are normal.

COMMENT: Sangeorzan *et al.* found that the type of fracture and the accuracy of the operative reduction correlated directly with the final clinical result.[5]

Minute 4

EXAMINER: Why does non-union and avascular necrosis occur in this fracture?

CANDIDATE: The navicular, similar to the talus, has a large articular surface area and for blood supply it relies on the radial arcade of vessels arising from the dorsalis pedis and medial planter arteries, and this could be injured either at the time of the fracture or during surgery, which could lead to AVN, non-union and/or collapse of the bone resulting in a painful midfoot.

EXAMINER: What surgical approach are you going to use?

CANDIDATE: I would use a medial longitudinal approach, between the tibialis anterior and tibialis posterior tendons with minimal dissection to preserve the remaining blood supply as much as possible.

The patient should be positioned supine, I would use a pneumatic thigh tourniquet with IV antibiotics given before inflation and the radiographer should be ready with II in theatre with relevant radiological requests made beforehand to reduce any potential for theatre delays. [*This is all a bit waffly but it is covering the basics. Probably not scoring any real marks but avoids complete silence.*]

It is important to directly visualize the articular surface to ensure accurate reduction of the articular surface. I would stabilize the fracture with cannulated screws from lateral to medial; however, the eventual configuration of screws will depend on the fracture pattern. I would avoid extensive periosteal stripping over the dorsal navicular surface as this

may disturb the tenuous blood supply of the central third portion of the body.

Sometimes a second anterolateral incision is needed to help with reduction of a significantly displaced lateral fragment.

Minute 5

EXAMINER: Take me through your consent process, in general.

CANDIDATE: I follow the General Medical Council guidelines on this subject and broadly run my practice along the lines of the domains of the GMC 'Good Medical Practice'. I work with the patient in partnership to ensure high-quality of care. In particular:

(a) I listen to patients and respect their views about their health.
(b) I discuss with patients what their views about diagnosis, prognosis, treatment and care involve.
(c) I share with patients the information they want or need in order to make decisions.
(d) I maximize a patient's opportunities, and their ability, to make decisions for themselves.
(e) I respect the patient's decisions.

COMMENT: These are quite rare injuries.

Structured oral examination question 10

A 34-year-old male was playing rugby when he made an awkward tackle. He is a right-hand dominant manual worker. He sustained the closed, isolated injury below.

Minute 1

EXAMINER: Talk me through your initial assessment and management of this patient in A&E.

CANDIDATE: I would start with a focused history, making sure to ask about factors that will affect surgery, such as past medical history and allergies, and factors that will potentially affect long-term outcome such as hand dominance, occupation and smoking status. I will then move on to perform an examination. This would include a general examination to ensure fitness for surgery before focusing on the injured limb. Assessing the limb, I would be making sure that this is a closed injury and carefully document the neurovascular status.

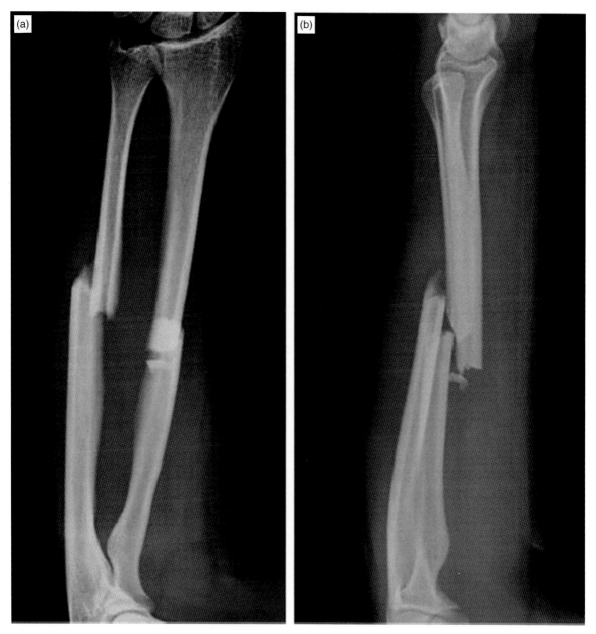

Figure 11.10a and 11.10b Anteroposterior and lateral radiographs, right radius and ulnar.

Following this assessment, I would want to put some simple first aid management steps in place including analgesia and application of a back-slab. I would admit the patient for elevation with a view to surgery on the trauma list the next day. I would also counsel the patient about the risks of compartment syndrome. I would ask nursing staff to conduct serial neurovascular checks.

EXAMINER: How exactly would you assess neurovascular status for this injury?

CANDIDATE: At this level I would be concerned about the function of the small muscles of the hand supplied by median and ulna nerves as well as sensation in the median, radial and ulna nerves. I would assess sensation by comparing light touch between the ulna border of the little finger, radial border of the index finger and dorsal aspect of the first web space to that on the other hand. I would test motor function by resisting abduction of the fingers (ulna nerve) and opposition of the thumb (median nerve).

Vascular status can be tested by palpating the radial and ulna arteries and by checking capillary refill times.

Minute 2

EXAMINER: Despite elevation the patient develops increasing pain in his arm overnight and you are called to see him; how would you proceed?

CANDIDATE: As mentioned earlier, I would be concerned that this gentleman could be developing compartment syndrome. I would want to see him and assess accordingly. I would have a high index of suspicion if he had intractable pain, increasing levels of analgesia requirement and worsening pain on passive stretch. I would also expect to find a swollen forearm and potentially even later signs such as deterioration in neurovascular function.

If, having reviewed the patient, I had a high index of suspicion of forearm compartment syndrome then I would need to think about taking this patient to theatre for fasciotomy.

Prior to doing this, I would need to inform the patient of my findings and diagnosis before explaining possible management options and obtaining informed consent. I would also need to inform the consultant on call, anaesthetics and theatres to find out when there is space to do this emergency case.

Minute 3

EXAMINER: You mentioned informed consent; what specific risks would you mention to this patient?

CANDIDATE: I tend to break surgical risks down by timescale into immediate, intermediate and long-term. For fasciotomies and ORIF the immediate risks would be pain, bleeding, neurovascular injury and anaesthetic risks. Intermediately, he would be at risk of infection, especially given the open wound, DVT/PE and he will need further surgery. Long-term, the risks include mal- or nonunion, stiffness, loss of function and complex regional pain syndrome.

Minutes 4–5

EXAMINER: What are your principles of management in a case like this?

COMMENT: This is your chance to keep talking and tick all the boxes.

CANDIDATE: The aim of surgery is always to ensure the best possible outcome for the patient. There are two main issues facing this patient: compartment syndrome requiring fasciotomies and his forearm fracture which requires stabilization. I would make sure to discuss my plan, in detail, with the theatre team preoperatively and complete a surgical pause as per WHO guidelines prior to starting the case.

The aim of the fasciotomies is to fully release the tension on all three compartments of the forearm, thus allowing maintenance of blood flow through the capillary beds. I would look to complete these fasciotomies through separate dorsal and volar incisions to make sure that all compartments are adequately decompressed. I have found that placing sloops along the periphery of the wound allows me to close the wound more easily further down the line and this is something I do routinely.

The fractures are diaphyseal in nature but due to the requirement for movement throughout the forearm I would treat these fractures as being intra-articular and as such I would be aiming for anatomical reduction and rigid fixation with interfragmentary compression. I would achieve this by means of an open reduction and plate osteosynthesis with DCP type plates. If possible, I would utilize my fasciotomy wounds for this, although I may need a separate incision for the ulna fracture.

Having fixed his fractures and completed his fasciotomies this patient will present another problem: exposed metalwork. To try and mitigate the risk of infection I would put a negative-pressure dressing on the wounds and continue prophylactic IV antibiotics until definitive coverage can be obtained with direct closure or skin grafting.

Evidence base

As stated in the BOAST 10 guidelines there are no RCTs on compartment syndrome and the guideline is based on, predominantly, retrospective studies.

Structured oral examination question 11

A 49-year-old male is bought into the Emergency room having been blasted off his feet by an exploding air cylinder at work.

Minute 1

EXAMINER: How would you initially assess this patient?

CANDIDATE: I would assess this patient utilizing the principles of ATLS. In this particular case I would be concerned about a deteriorating airway due to possible scorching from the explosion. There would also be concerns about thoracic or abdominal injuries due to rapid acceleration and deceleration, which could impact on breathing and circulation. The cervical spine should be immobilized, and ABC assessed using simple monitoring and examination in the first instance. If the patient is conscious I would like to obtain a history and finally assess the limbs for injuries. If the patient is not in extremis, then I would like to consider getting a trauma series CT and plain radiographs of any obviously injured limbs.

Minute 2

EXAMINER: The patient is conscious but muddled. He is maintaining his airway and oxygen saturations. However, the ambulance crew were unable to cannulate him, he is tachycardic at 124 bpm and hypotensive at 90/56. He has a tender abdomen, an open distal tibial fracture with no evidence of major bleeding and a deformed forearm. Pelvic binder is in place. How would you proceed?

CANDIDATE: This patient is demonstrating signs of shock which is likely to be hypovolaemic. Assuming there are no other external sources of blood loss I would assume this is either intraabdominal or pelvic in nature. Initial management would involve gaining access to start replacing lost volume. This can be IV or IO and bloods including FBC, U&E, clotting, group, save and crossmatch should be sent to the lab. I would activate the major haemorrhage protocol and start giving fluid resuscitation with crystalloid solution until

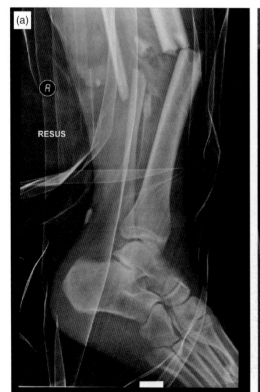
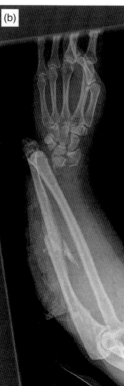

Figure 11.11a and 11.11b Lateral radiograph, comminuted fractured midshaft tibia and fibula, and anteroposterior (AP) radiograph, right radius and ulna.

blood arrives. I would also want to obtain an ABG to look at pH, base excess and lactate levels as these are good surrogate markers of tissue perfusion.

Further to this I would like to give the patient a dose of tranexamic acid (1 g IV), a tetanus booster and a dose of IV antibiotics in line with trust policy for open fractures. I would also check the pelvic binder is positioned correctly.

Minute 3

EXAMINER: Do you still want to send this patient for a CT scan?

CANDIDATE: Yes. Assuming the department is compliant with the Royal College of Radiology guidelines then obtaining a trauma CT should be a quick process and still allow continuing fluid resuscitation. The contrast CT will help identify the source of blood loss as well as any other occult injuries.

Minutes 4–5

EXAMINER: CT scan shows evidence of a ruptured spleen and some blood in the pelvis but no active extravasation here. The patient is transferred back to the emergency where departmental radiographs are obtained of the patient's limb injuries. The general surgeons are intending to take the patient straight to theatre for a splenectomy. How would you proceed?

CANDIDATE: This patient has multiple serious injuries. His splenectomy is life-saving and should take priority. From an orthopaedic point of view he has a confirmed open tibial shaft fracture, a closed forearm fracture and a potential pelvic injury, which is being stabilized by the binder. Further orthopaedic management will be determined by how the patient has responded to his resuscitation. I would use serial ABG measurements to determine whether I should proceed with early total care or move towards damage control orthopaedic surgery.

EXAMINER: What do you mean by damage control orthopaedics?

CANDIDATE: Damage control orthopaedics is an approach to contain and stabilize an orthopaedic injury to improve a patient's physiology.

It is designed to avoid worsening a patient's condition due to the 'second-hit' phenomenon.

Delay definitive surgery until a patient's condition is optimized. It focuses on haemorrhagic control, management of soft-tissue injury and provisional fracture stability.

EXAMINER: Anything else?

CANDIDATE: DCO involves rapid emergency surgery to save life or limb – NOT involving complex reconstructive surgery.
- Control of bleeding.
- Decompress cranium, pericardium, thorax, abdomen and limbs.
- Decontaminate wounds and ruptured viscera.
- Splint fractures.
- Cast, traction, pelvic binder, ex-fix.

Get back to ITU environment ASAP.

Definitive surgery is performed several days later.

EXAMINER: Following his splenectomy the patient has a pH of 7.35, base excess of –3 mmol/l and lactate of 2.0 mmol/l.

CANDIDATE: These values indicate that the patient is currently adequately resuscitated and so I would look to proceed with early total care. I would plan to start with the forearm fracture with the arm extended on an arm table and to be honest with a fracture of this complexity, restoring alignment and performing carpal tunnel decompression with stability through an external fixator would be my plan A. For the tibial fracture, debriding this as a combined case with a consultant plastic surgical colleague to ensure appropriate soft-tissue cover and follow-up will be possible. I would deliver the bone ends through the wound to debride these before reducing the fracture. As a diaphyseal injury I would look to obtain restoration of length, alignment and rotation before stabilizing with a relative stability device. My personal preference here would be an intramedullary nail. If adequate soft-tissue cover was not available, then I would debride as above before using a spanning external fixator to stabilize until the patient was able to better tolerate graft surgery.

EXAMINER: Having dealt with the forearm, a repeat ABG is obtained, this shows a pH of 7.35, base excess of –4.1 mmol/l and lactate of 2.9 mmol/l. Does this change your management?

CANDIDATE: Yes. The patient, while not in extremis, is struggling to cope physiologically, with an early trend for underperfusion showing. As such I would move to a damage control philosophy. This would entail a thorough debridement and then simple external fixation of the tibia. His tibial fracture can be formally stabilized in a planned fashion once his physiology has improved.

EXAMINER: What is SIRS?

CANDIDATE: This is a condition characterized by systemic inflammation, organ dysfunction and organ failure.

EXAMINER: How is SIRS diagnosed?

CANDIDATE:

1. Heart rate > 90/min.
2. Breathing rate > 20/min, hyperventilation with decrease of arterial CO_2 partial pressure ($PaCO_2$) under 32 mmHg.
3. Temperature > 38.8°C or < 36.8°C.
4. Number of leukocytes < 4000/mm^3 or > 12,000/mm^3.

For the definition of SIRS, two or more parameters must be fulfilled. Sepsis is defined as SIRS with detection of bacteraemia or bacterial focus.

COMMENT: Do not forget to mention early appropriate care.

- Accept different patients respond differently to first and second hits.
- Consider severity of initial injury.
- Consider response to resuscitation.
- What further surgery is required?
- Continued reassessment and ability to change from ETO to DCO.

Evidence base

NICE produced a guideline on major trauma in 2016. There is lots of evidence around ETC/DCO and candidates should know some of it. Heather Vallier has published extensively, and the key values lifted from her papers are: pH > 7.25, BE ≥ 5.5 mmol/l, lactate > 4.0 mmol/l. It is also worth knowing about the CRASH-2 trial and use of TXA; make sure you know how TXA works as well.

NICE Guideline No. 39 – Major Trauma: Assessment and Initial Management.

Vallier HA, Moore TA, Como JJ, *et al.* Complications are reduced with a protocol to standardize timing of fixation based on response to resuscitation. *J Orthop Surg Res.* 2015;10:155.

Roberts I, Shakur H, Coats T, Hunt B, Balogun E. The CRASH-2 trial: a randomized controlled trial and economic evaluation of the effects of tranexamic acid on death, vascular occlusive events and transfusion requirement in bleeding trauma patients. *Health Technol Assess.* 2013;17(10):1–79.

Structured oral examination question 12

A 36-year-old lady sustained an open tibial fracture while horse riding. It was treated with wound debridement and closure as well as an intramedullary nail. This is her radiograph at 10 months postop.

Minute 1

EXAMINER: How would you assess this patient?

CANDIDATE: This patient has radiographic evidence of an atrophic non-union. I would start by taking a history. Important factors to draw out include pain, weight-bearing status, postoperative wound issues, completion of antibiotic therapy, comorbidities including diabetes, medication, steroids and smoking history.

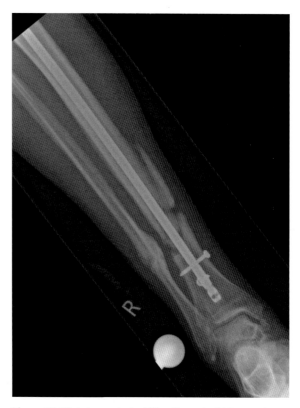

Figure 11.12 Anteroposterior (AP) radiograph, tibial non-union with IM nail in situ.

Table 11.1 Causes for non-union.

Predisposing factors for non-union	Contributing factors for non-union
Mechanical instability	Infection
Inadequate fixation	Nicotine/cigarette smoking
Distraction	Certain medications
Bone loss	Advanced age
Poor bone quality	Systemic medical conditions
	Poor functional level
	Venous stasis
	Burns
	Irradiation
	Obesity
	Alcohol abuse
	Metabolic bone disease
	Malnutrition
	Vitamin deficiencies
Inadequate vascularity	
Severe injury	
Excessive soft tissue stripping	
Vascular injury	
Poor bone contact	
Soft tissue interposition	
Malposition or malalignment	
Bone loss	
Distraction	

I would also examine the patient looking at the wounds and overall condition of the skin, neurovascular status and limb alignment.

Having completed a clinical assessment, I would like to obtain baseline blood tests including CRP, ESR and white cell count to look for any signs of infection.

Minute 2

EXAMINER: The patient is a fit and well, non-smoker who had an uneventful postoperative recovery. She is struggling to weight-bear due to pain at the fracture site. What do you think is the cause of her non-union?

CANDIDATE: Causes of non-union can be broken down into surgeon factors and patient factors. In this case the patient's fracture appears to have been appropriately fixed with good reduction and adequate working length to allow bone healing. There is very little callus formation, which suggests biomechanical stability itself is not an issue here. There are no negative patient factors. I can only assume, therefore, that this is a problem of biology. This is likely to be due to infection or inadequate blood supply to the fracture site.

COMMENT: There are implant factors as well. Distraction at the fracture site at the time of initial nailing may contribute to the development of a non-union.

This is a basic candidate 6 answer, nothing special. On a bad day with more hawkish examiners down to a 5. See Table 11.1 for a more detailed answer.

Minutes 3–4

EXAMINER: The patient's blood tests come back showing a CRP of 29 (< 4), ESR 40 (< 20) and a WCC of 13.4 (< 10.0). You perform a CT which shows no evidence of fracture healing, but there is a fragment of devascularized bone consistent with a butterfly fragment. What management options would you give to the patient?

CANDIDATE: I would counsel the patient that I feel they have an infected non-union and then talk about the broad management strategies of conservative, non-operative or operative management.

Conservative management is unlikely to lead to resolution of symptoms and will most likely lead to hardware failure, making any future surgery more challenging. Non-operative management would involve treatment with suppressive antibiotics to try and allow the fracture to heal despite the infection. This is unlikely to work, as the bone ends are atrophic and therefore the biology of the fracture is unlikely to be favourable for healing even if the infection was suppressed.

My management option of choice would be revision surgery. This would involve removal of the current nail, debridement of the fracture site, removal of all dead bone and reaming of the intramedullary canal. I would want to ensure local elution of empirical antibiotics from an antibiotic loaded nail or by using resorbable beads. The choice would be between exchange nailing and ring external fixation. Reamed tibial exchange nailing has been used successfully to treat infected tibial non-unions, and is thought to promote healing of a non-union by three different mechanisms.[6] Increasing the nail diameter improves mechanical stability and this should stimulate healing. Also, reaming causes a marked increase in periosteal blood flow, which should stimulate the formation of periosteal new bone. Finally, the reaming products are osteoinductive. After primary nailing these products are extruded through the fracture site, but at exchange nailing fibrous tissue will tend to confine the reaming to the medullary canal.

EXAMINER: Are you sure that you are talking about infected tibial non-unions?

CANDIDATE: Pardon?

EXAMINER: I think you may be talking about exchange tibial nailing for aseptic non-union.

COMMENT: The candidate has mixed up the management of infected and aseptic tibial non-unions. A number of authors report that the treatment of choice for tibial diaphyseal fracture non-union is reamed exchange nailing. It is considered to be a relatively simple procedure which does not expose the fracture site and leads to minimal blood loss, low surgical morbidity and a short hospital stay.

However, in the presence of infection it is a more controversial option. There is currently no consensus in the literature with regard to the use of exchange nailing for tibial diaphyseal fracture non-union in the presence of infection.

Simpson *et al.* from Edinburgh looked at a series of tibial non-unions to identify risk factors for failure of exchange nailing.[7] They identified the strongest predictor of failure was infection and suggested that other treatment options such as Ilizarov treatment should be preferred.

CANDIDATE: I would go for an external ring fixator to stabilize the fracture. I would send reamings and bone samples for culture and sensitivity to allow targeting of suppressive antimicrobial therapy in conjunction with my microbiology colleagues.

EXAMINER: What is the role of a circular frame in infected tibial non-unions?

CANDIDATE: Sorry?

EXAMINER: What are the basic requirements for fracture healing?

COMMENT: The examiner has decided to take the viva backwards as he is not sure about the candidate's level of knowledge.

CANDIDATE:

- Mechanical stability.
- Adequate blood supply.
- Bone vascularity.
- Bone-to-bone contact.

These factors may be negatively influenced by the severity of the injury and suboptimal surgical fixation which predisposes to non-union.

EXAMINER: What factors predispose to instability at the fracture site?

CANDIDATE:

1 Mechanical instability, excessive motion at the fracture site

Factors producing mechanical instability include:

- Inadequate fixation (implants too small or too few).
- Distraction of the fracture surfaces (hardware is as capable of holding bone apart as holding bone together).
- Bone loss.
- Poor bone quality (i.e. poor purchase).

If an adequate blood supply exists, excessive motion at the fracture site results in abundant callus formation, widening of the fracture line, failure of fibrocartilage to mineralize, and ultimately failure to unite.

2 Inadequate vascularity

Loss of blood supply to the fracture surfaces may arise because of the severity of the injury or because of surgical dissection.

Open fractures and high-energy closed injuries may strip soft tissues, damage the periosteal blood supply, and disrupt the nutrient vessels, impairing the endosteal blood supply.

Injury of certain vessels, such as the posterior tibial artery, may also increase the risk of non-union.

Vascularity may also be compromised by excess stripping of the periosteum as well as damage to bone and the soft tissues during open reduction and hardware insertion.

Whatever the cause, inadequate vascularity results in necrotic bone at the ends of the fracture fragments.

These necrotic surfaces inhibit fracture healing and often result in fracture non-union.

3 Poor bone contact

Poor bone-to-bone contact at the fracture site may result from soft-tissue interposition, malposition or malalignment of the fracture fragments, bone loss, and distraction of the fracture fragments.

Whatever the cause, poor bone-to-bone contact compromises mechanical stability and creates a defect.

The probability of fracture union decreases as defects increase in size. The threshold value for rapid bridging of cortical defects via direct osteonal healing, the so-called osteoblastic jumping distance, is approximately 1 mm.

Larger cortical defects may also heal, but at a much slower rate and bridge via woven bone.

The 'critical defect' represents the distance between fracture surfaces that will not be bridged by bone without intervention. The critical defect size depends on a variety of injury-related factors.

4 Infection

Infection in the zone of fracture increases the risk of non-union.

Infection may result in instability at the fracture site as implants loosen in infected bone. Avascular, necrotic bone at the fracture site (sequestrum), common with infection, discourages bony union.

Infection also produces poor bony contact as osteolysis at the fracture site results from ingrowth of infected granulation tissue.

EXAMINER: Are there any other investigations you would like to obtain preoperatively?

CANDIDATE: Yes. I would like to obtain blood cultures to look for evidence of bacteraemia which may help guide antimicrobial therapy. I would also like to obtain an echocardiogram, ideally transoesophageal, to rule out endocarditis as a source for bacterial seeding.

Minute 5

EXAMINER: What are the principles of management of an infected non-union?

CANDIDATE: I would need to consider host factors, the microorganism involved, debridement, antibiotic therapy and reconstruction.

Soft-tissue coverage would need to be planned along with bone stabilization and the need for bone grafting.

EXAMINER: What is a biofilm?

CANDIDATE: A layer-like aggregation of cells and cellular products attached to a solid surface or substratum.

An established biofilm structure comprises microbial cells and extracellular polymeric substances (EPS) produced by the microorganisms themselves.

EXAMINER: Have you heard of the Masquelet technique?

CANDIDATE: No, sorry.

COMMENT: This is a method to deal with a large amount of bone loss following radical debridement and excision of infected bone down to healthy bleeding bone. Antibiotic-impregnated cement beads or spacers are used for local antibiotic administration to the soft-tissue bed. In the case of infection following IM nailing the canal should be reamed for debridement and irrigation. A circular external fixator is usually applied to the limb that allows for shortening of any defect if required. The soft-tissue envelope is repaired with vascularized flap transfer if needed. A second stage of bone grafting is performed around 8 weeks after the initial surgery.

An induction membrane should have formed which serves the critical function of preventing graft resorption. It acts like a chamber around the bony defect to contain the bone graft and stimulate bone regeneration. This membrane should be disturbed as little as possible at the time of the second stage.

Structured oral examination question 13

A 33-year-old barrister slips on some ice and sustains an isolated closed ankle fracture. This is his radiograph in the Emergency Department.

Minute 1

EXAMINER: Talk to me about this injury.

CANDIDATE: These are lateral and oblique radiographs of a left ankle showing a complex fracture–dislocation of the ankle such that the talus is almost completely displaced from the mortice and there is considerable rotation seen. The fibula fracture is suggestive of a Weber B injury. It is unclear if there is any syndesmotic widening on these films. Ideally, I would like to see a mortise view of the ankle. This is a serious injury. My first move would be to fully assess the patient quickly and reduce the dislocation to prevent ongoing swelling and compromise to the skin, nerves and blood vessels. The leg should be placed in a below-knee back-slab followed by check radiographs to confirm satisfactory reduction of the ankle mortice. The patient needs to be

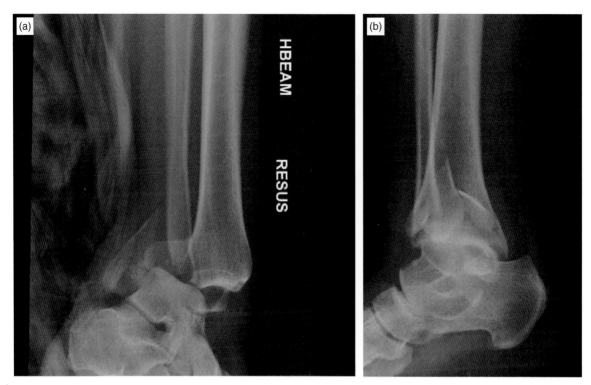

Figure 11.13a and 11.13b Oblique and lateral radiographs, left ankle showing a fracture/dislocation.

admitted to the ward for elevation and a plan for operative intervention worked out.

EXAMINER: OK. He is much more comfortable now and you obtain a good reduction. It is late in the evening and theatres are already busy with emergencies.

Minutes 2–3

CANDIDATE: Timing is important with these injuries due to soft-tissue swelling. I know this may be debatable, but operating through a severely contused and swollen soft-tissue envelope is associated with poor outcomes and as such I would plan to temporize the patient with a spanning external fixator on the theatre list in the morning if soft tissue review is concerning. I would consent the patient for internal fixation and also for external fixation and I would discuss the fact that this is a significant injury with a risk of compromised function in the future.

EXAMINER: What is debatable about operating in the presence of severely contused and swollen soft tissues with marked subcutaneous oedema? This practice would increase the risks of wound

dehiscence, infection, need for plastic surgery involvement, reoperations and adverse outcomes.

CANDIDATE: Some surgeons believe that soft-tissue swelling should not be a contraindication to early operative fixation of ankle fractures. The key point is early fixation within 6–12 hours of injury only. Late presentation of the patient, no availability of theatre time, the presence of general medical comorbidities and more severe concurrent injuries might point to external fixation being used as a temporary method for fracture stabilization. Treatment with a temporary external fixator increases the length of hospital inpatient stay, possibly increases the complication rate and definitely increases the cost of treatment.

The paper from Giannoudis from Leeds in the RCSEng bulletin suggested a fast-track method to get ankle fractures into theatre on the day of injury with the development of a streamlined pathway for early surgery.[8]

COMMENT: The key point is early presentation within a few hours of injury. It is very rare for an ankle to be too swollen to undertake operative

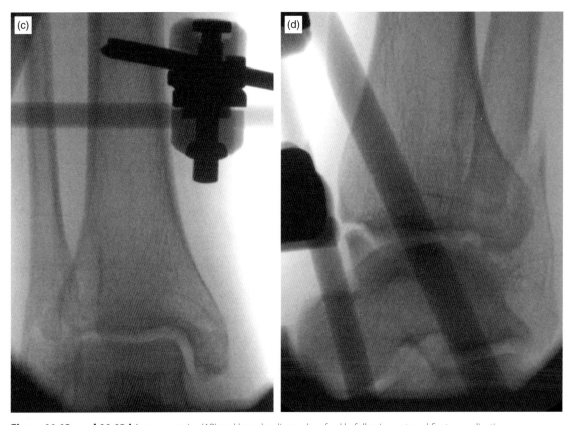

Figure 11.13c and 11.13d Anteroposterior (AP) and lateral radiographs of ankle following external fixator application.

fixation on the day of admission, although each patient's treatment should be decided on an individual basis.[9]

With anything controversial be very clear about what you are actually saying. Stay safe and avoid ambiguity. Perhaps even better to stay clear of any controversy if you are just averaging a straightforward 6.

EXAMINER: OK. You go to theatre and find the ankle too swollen to operate on with significant blistering already present and you achieve a good reduction with the external fixator. Please review the image and tell us what you would do now.

Minute 4

CANDIDATE: The external fixator has been used in a triangular configuration and the reduction is satisfactory. The tension and pressure are now off the soft-tissue envelope, there is improved articular alignment, decreased articular impaction and I can continue the important phase of soft-tissue rest and resuscitation. I will advise the

patient that definitive surgery may occur in about 10–14 days. I would ensure the patient has had a DVT assessment and that the limb is properly elevated. With all complex ankle fractures, when planning reconstruction, 3D cross-sectional imaging is useful and so I would order a CT scan.

COMMENT: On the available radiographs it is not possible to say if the external fixator has been used in a triangular configuration. Try not to make assumptions as sometimes inferences can be wrong.

EXAMINER: What are the concerns with temporary external fixator use?

CANDIDATE: Pin site infections, superficial wound infections and postoperative loss of reduction. In addition, I would want to inspect the skin daily for blistering and as to when the soft tissues are ready for definitive fixation. Patients should be monitored for compartment syndrome and neuropraxia. The affected limb should be elevated.

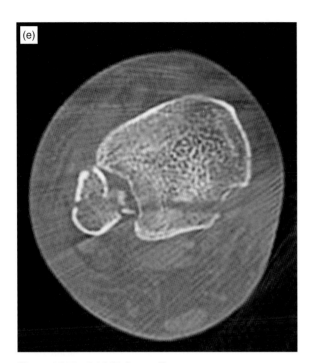

Figure 11.13e Axial CT slices, ankle.

Table 11.2 Haraguchi classification of posterior malleolus fracture of ankle

Type I fracture is an isolated PMF

Type II fracture is either a bi- or trimalleolar fracture associated with a Weber B or C fracture pattern. These are further classified depending on the presence or absence of syndesmotic injury

Type III PMF is associated with an ipsilateral tibial diaphyseal fracture. This is further subdivided based on sagittal or coronal plane instability

EXAMINER: What elements in particular are you interested in evaluating here?

CANDIDATE: Stability in the management of ankle fractures is key. Ligament tension and fracture configuration contribute. The posterior malleolus is important, and I would in particular be interested in the size of the posterior bony chunk, its fracture configuration and its direction. These were classified by Haraguchi *et al.* (2006) as Types I–III and I find this useful to characterize and treat these fractures.

EXAMINER: Here is the axial CT slice – what do you think?

Minute 5

CANDIDATE: This is a Haraguchi Type I as it is 'wedge-shaped' and essentially is a chunk off the posterolateral distal tibia (Table 11.2). The posterior malleolus plays an integral role in ankle joint stability through its anatomical relationship with the posterior tibiofibular ligament (PTFL), which has been shown through cadaver studies to account for 42% of syndesmotic stability. Ankle fractures involving the posterior malleolus are said to have worse clinical outcomes, possibly related to incongruity and the resultant development of post-traumatic arthrosis.

COMMENT: CT is also useful in assessing for syndesmotic injury indicated by widening of the syndesmosis anteriorly or posteriorly on axial scans. A CT would also give information on whether any articular impaction or depression was present.

EXAMINER: How would you fix this fracture?

CANDIDATE: I would fix the lateral malleolar fracture with a lag screw and 3.5 mm one-third tubular plate acting in a neutralizing mode. He is young and has good-quality bone; otherwise, if the patient was elderly and the bone porotic and poor quality I would consider using a locking plate. The posterior fragment can be fixed with lag screws inserted from anterior to posterior.

EXAMINER: Anything else to fix the posterior malleolar fragment?

CANDIDATE: A plate could be used.

COMMENT: Contoured one-third tubular plate acting as in buttress mode. The plate is not contoured, it will contour itself with placement of the initial screw (just proximal to the posterior fracture line), which then helps with fracture reduction.

EXAMINER: How would you put the plate on?

CANDIDATE: Sorry?

EXAMINER: What approach would you use?

CANDIDATE: Standard lateral approach to the fibula.

EXAMINER: Any other approaches you are familiar with?

CANDIDATE: A posterolateral approach.

EXAMINER: Tell me about the posterolateral approach.

CANDIDATE: Ehh?!
[Bell]

263

EXAMINER: Thank you.

COMMENT: Prone position, skin incision midway between the lateral border of the TA and the fibula. Deep dissection between FHL medially and the peroneal tendons laterally. The sural nerve is at risk and needs to be identified and protected.

The posterior surface of the fibula can be reached by retraction of the peroneal tendons laterally, and the plate should be applied posteriorly. The posterior surface of the tibia can be reached by retraction of the FHL and the deep posterior compartment medially.

Evidence base

Solan MC, Sakellariou A. Posterior malleolus fractures. *Bone Joint J.* Published Online: 1 Nov 2017. https://doi.org/10.1302/0301-620X.99B11.BJJ-2017–1072

Notes

1. Wasserstein D, Henry P, Paterson JM, Kreder HJ, Jenkinson R. Risk of total knee arthroplasty after operatively treated tibial plateau fracture: a matched-population-based cohort study. *J Bone Joint Surg.* 2014;96(2):144–150.

2. Griffin D, Parsons N, Shaw E, *et al.* Operative versus non-operative treatment for closed, displaced, intra-articular fractures of the calcaneus: randomised controlled trial. *BMJ.* 2014;349:g4483.

3. Buckley R, Tough S, McCormack R, Pate G. Operative compared with nonoperative treatment of displaced intra-articular calcaneal fractures: a prospective, randomized, controlled multicenter trial. *J Bone Joint Surg.* 2002;84 (10):1733.

4. Baumgaertel F, Buhl M, Rahn BA. Fracture healing in biological plate osteosynthesis. *Injury.* 1998;29:3–6

5. Sangeorzan BJ, Benirschke SK, Mosca V, Mayo KA, Hansen ST Jr. Displaced intra-articular fractures of the tarsal navicular. *J Bone Joint Surg Am.* 1989;71:1504–1510.

6. Banaszkiewicz PA, Sabboubeh A, McLeod I, Maffulli N. Femoral exchange nailing for aseptic non-union: not the end to all problems. *Injury.* 2003;34(5):349–356.

7. Tsang ST, Mills LA, Frantzias J, Baren JP, Keating JF, Simpson AH. Exchange nailing for nonunion of diaphyseal fractures of the tibia: our results and an analysis of the risk factors for failure. *Bone Joint J.* 2016;98 (4):534–541.

8. Kheir E, Charopoulos I, Dimitriou R, Ghoz A, Dahabreh Z, Giannoudis PV. The health economics of ankle fracture fixation. *Bull Roy Coll Surg Engl.* 2012;94(4):1–5.

9. Pietzik P, Qureshi I, Langdon J, Molloy S, Solan M. Cost benefit with early operative fixation of unstable ankle fractures. *Ann Roy Coll Surg Engl.* 2006;88(4):405–407.

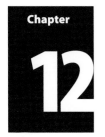

Upper limb trauma I

Matthew Nixon and William Marlow

Structured oral examination question 1

Fracture dislocation shoulder

EXAMINER: A 38-year-old left-hand dominant lady fell on to her right arm when out drinking and attended the accident and emergency department the next day at 4 pm as the pain in the right shoulder had not settled down. These are the X-rays of her right shoulder (Figure 12.1a). What is your diagnosis?

CANDIDATE: Anterior dislocation of the right shoulder with an associated greater tuberosity (GT) fracture. Complete loss of joint congruence is demonstrated on the AP view, while the anterior displacement is best demonstrated on the axial view. There is no visible evidence of fracture through the anatomical neck, although this occurs in about 10% of cases. This pattern of injury is more

in keeping with this patient's age than surgical neck fracture, which is more typically seen in an older demographic.[1]

EXAMINER: How will you manage this condition?

CANDIDATE: Assess the patient according to ATLS protocol and exclude any neurovascular injury because brachial plexus injury is part of a recognized pattern comprising the 'terrible triad' of the shoulder.[2] If there was suspicion of an undisplaced neck fracture, I would obtain an emergency CT to confirm and then plan for open reduction and fixation of both the neck and GT fractures. I would perform a neurovascular examination of the shoulder and document my findings in the case notes before attempting manipulation. I would reduce the shoulder dislocation under sedation using the scapular manipulation technique, as this is the most successful and least painful method with no reported incidences of fracture. This involves the patient lying prone with a weight

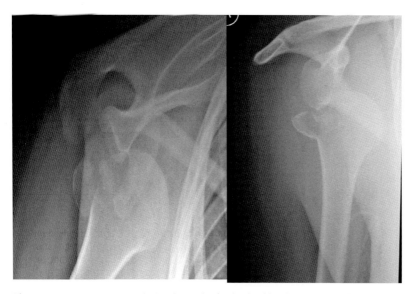

Figure 12.1a Anteroposterior (AP) radiograph of right shoulder demonstrating fracture/dislocation.

applied to the arm while the tip of the scapula is rotated medially and upward. I would immobilize the limb in a shoulder immobilizer. After manipulation I would obtain anteroposterior and axial radiographs and repeat a neurovascular examination of the involved limb.

EXAMINER: What are the risks and complications you anticipate?

CANDIDATE: During reduction there is a risk of displacing an unseen humeral neck fracture or propagating the GT fracture through the neck. Other risks are injury to axillary nerve and artery, brachial plexus and rotator cuff injury.[3]

EXAMINER: Attempted closed reduction in the accident and emergency department has failed and it is 7 pm now. What will you do next?

CANDIDATE: I will take into account availability of space on the emergency list, presence of neurological symptoms, the patient's level of pain and level of anaesthetic risk. If it is safe and within a reasonable time frame, I would take the patient for closed reduction under general anaesthetic. After reduction I would reassess the neurovascular status. If there was a new neurovascular deficit, this may be due to nerve entrapment. In this situation, I would plan for a shoulder surgeon to explore the nerve and perform an open reduction in the morning. If there was going to be a delay in taking the patient to theatre for reduction, as long as there was no neurovascular compromise I would plan for emergent reduction and/or fixation by a shoulder surgeon on the next available list.

EXAMINER: What manoeuvre would you perform to achieve shoulder reduction?

CANDIDATE: Under complete muscle relaxation, I will use the traction/countertraction method given that scapular manipulation has failed. This is the second most effective technique and the associated discomfort will not be felt by the anaesthetized patient.[4] Because failure of reduction may be due to head impaction on the anterior glenoid, this technique also allows controlled external rotation to disengage this.

EXAMINER: What other factors may prevent a closed stable reduction of the dislocation?

CANDIDATE: A large rotator cuff tear or axillary nerve injury may prevent the shoulder from

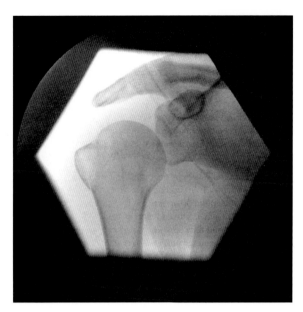

Figure 12.1b II films, relocated right shoulder.

remaining in joint. On occasion, the long head of the biceps may get caught up posterior to the humeral head and prevent reduction. The stability of the joint may also be affected by a structural deficit such as a bony or soft-tissue Bankart lesion or a Hill–Sachs lesion.

EXAMINER: Next day in theatre, closed reduction is achieved (Figure 12.1b). What will you do next?

CANDIDATE: I will assess the greater tuberosity fracture reduction. If it is less than 5 mm superiorly displaced, I will treat it non-operatively with a polysling for 3 weeks with serial X-rays on a weekly basis and if there is no fracture displacement, I will start shoulder mobilization under physiotherapy care.[5]

EXAMINER: X-ray of right shoulder one week later is shown in Figure 12.1c. What will you do?

CANDIDATE: I will arrange a CT scan of the shoulder to assess the degree and direction of displacement as this is useful in borderline cases.[6]

EXAMINER: The CT scan (Figure 12.1d) of the right shoulder shows no humeral neck fracture but significant displacement of the greater tuberosity. What will be your management strategy?

CANDIDATE: If the greater tuberosity fragment has posterosuperior displacement more than 5 mm,[7]

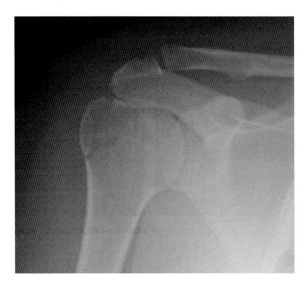

Figure 12.1c Anteroposterior (AP) radiograph, right shoulder with greater tuberosity fracture.

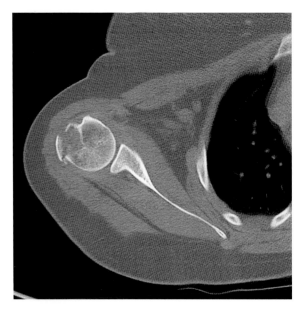

Figure 12.1d CT image, right shoulder.

I would offer the patient reduction and fixation. Arthroscopic fixation with a double row of anchors may be possible – it is less invasive than ORIF and has demonstrated superior postoperative range of motion.[8]

EXAMINER: What are the risks of non-operative management of displaced greater tuberosity fracture?

CANDIDATE: Non-union, malunion, which effectively narrows the subacromial space, leading to mechanical impingement and consequent rotator cuff atrophy.[9]

Structured oral examination question 2

Right wrist fracture

EXAMINER: A 24-year-old man fell down the last few steps of a flight of stairs and sustained an injury to his right wrist. His X-rays are shown in Figure 12.2a. What is this injury?

CANDIDATE: There is a displaced radial styloid fracture, which is classically termed a 'chauffeur's fracture'.[39] In addition, there is radiocarpal dislocation. This is demonstrated by more than 50% of the lunate having subluxed ulnarly from its fossa. This pattern would be classified by AO as type B2.3 and its pathomechanism is suggested to be an avulsion of the styloid by the radioscaphocapitate ligament.[10] On these images there is no visible scaphoid fracture or evidence of scapholunate ligament disruption; however, this would be a common association.

EXAMINER: What other injuries have occurred in addition to the radial styloid fracture?

CANDIDATE: Rupture of volar capsule and radiolunate ligaments, while the radial collateral and volar radiocarpal ligaments are attached to the

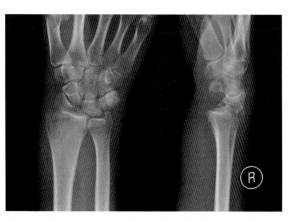

Figure 12.2a Anteroposterior (AP) and lateral radiographs, right wrist.

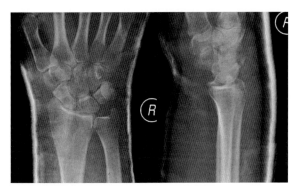

Figure 12.2b Anteroposterior (AP) and lateral post reduction film, right wrist.

fragment, allows subluxation of the radiocarpal joint.[11] The distal part of the brachioradialis insertion is typically 17 mm from the tip; therefore, with this relatively distal fracture, there is no stabilizing force from the brachioradialis.[12]

EXAMINER: How will you manage this injury?

CANDIDATE: Assuming it is an isolated closed injury, I will attempt closed reduction under sedation in casualty, apply a below-elbow moulded dorsal plaster slab, check the distal neurovascular status and get a repeat X-ray of the wrist. Given that this is a type B injury with a high-energy mechanism, I would also arrange a CT to assess for any associated carpal fracture as well as articular reduction.[13]

EXAMINER: Figure 12.2b shows a post reduction X-ray. How will you manage this injury?

CANDIDATE: Post reduction X-rays show that the fracture is well reduced, and the radiocarpal alignment is satisfactory. Given that the CT demonstrated < 2 mm articular disruption, no carpal fracture and radiocarpal congruency, I would treat this in a moulded plaster and weekly radiographic follow-up. If there was evidence of instability, I would offer ORIF of the radial styloid alone, as this should restore radiocarpal stability.[14] If there was evidence of further instability, repair of volar radiocarpal ligaments may be necessary. Neurovascular decompression, joint debridement and management of inter- and transcarpal injuries may also be addressed.

Structured oral examination question 3

Comminuted elbow fracture

EXAMINER: A motor bike rider came off his bike at around 80 miles/hour and has sustained an isolated injury to his right elbow. X-rays in casualty are shown in Figure 12.3a.

CANDIDATE: This X-ray of the right elbow demonstrates a bicolumnar distal humerus fracture. It is intra-articular, complete articular and there is comminution of the articular surface. There is evidence of a well-healed distal humerus diaphyseal fracture which was stabilized with an intramedullary nail. The dressings around the elbow suggest a possible open injury. I will assess the patient according to ATLS protocols and assess neurovascular status. I will also check if it is an open fracture.

EXAMINER: How are these injuries classified?

CANDIDATE: Intra-articular fractures can be divided into partial or complete according to the AO classification. In type B fractures, a single column is involved while the articular surface of the other column remains in continuity with the diaphysis – this is 'partial articular'. In type C fractures, both columns are involved and there is no continuity between any part of the articular surface and the diaphysis – this is 'complete articular'. The severity of these fractures depends on whether their articular and metaphyseal components are simple or multifragmentary.

EXAMINER: This is an open fracture. How will you deal with the wound in casualty?

CANDIDATE: According to BOAST 4 and NICE guidance 37, in conjunction with Orthoplastics input, I will remove gross contamination but not irrigate the wound. I will document and photograph the wound for size and tissue loss then dress with saline-soaked gauze and an occlusive dressing and splint the limb. I will check the patient's tetanus status and give a booster dose if required and analgesia. I will start the patient on intravenous co-amoxiclav which will continue until 72 hours after initial debridement or wound closure.

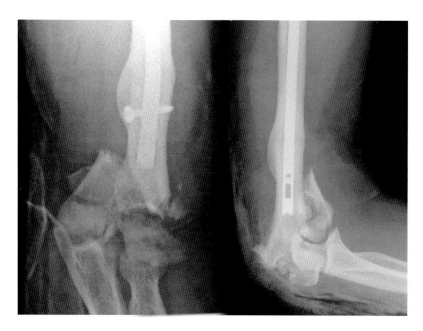

Figure 12.3a Anteroposterior (AP) and lateral radiographs, right elbow, demonstrating comminuted fracture.

EXAMINER: What will be the definitive management and its timing?

CANDIDATE: This will depend upon vascular status and orthoplastics input. If there is vascular compromise, this would necessitate immediate appropriate surgery. If there is evidence of compartment syndrome, this would warrant immediate fasciotomy.

Otherwise, the patient should be taken to theatre by a senior plastic and orthopaedic surgeon on a scheduled trauma list within 24 hours but ideally within 12 hours for high-energy injuries such as this. Initial debridement consists of excising wound edges and extending the wounds in conjunction with plastics to ensure that this will not compromise their plans for soft-tissue coverage. I will deliver the bone ends and excise devitalized bone and ensure the medullary cavity is clean, which in this case may necessitate removal of the humeral nail. I would then irrigate the wound with 6 litres of gravity-assisted normal saline.

If the patient is systemically stable and immediate soft-tissue coverage was possible then I would progress to definitive internal fixation or hemiarthroplasty. Otherwise I would perform limited fixation of the articular fragments, apply a negative-pressure dressing and span the zone of injury with an external fixator.

EXAMINER: If the wound is satisfactory and definitive stabilization is planned, how will you go about it?

CANDIDATE: In an appropriately marked, consented and anaesthetized patient, I would position in a lateral decubitus position. My approach would be posterior under guidance of plastics, likely incorporating the existing defect. An olecranon osteotomy would aid visualization of this intra-articular fracture.

If the nail is still in situ, I would plan my fixation around this, although as the old fracture is well healed, removing the nail is an option if this would make fixation or arthroplasty of the new fracture easier. Principles of fixation are anatomical reduction and rigid fixation of the articular fragments and functional alignment and relative stability of the metaphyseal and diaphyseal sections. According to the principles set out by O'Driscoll,[15] I would initially reduce the articular fragments and stabilize with K-wires. I would use one pre-contoured locking plate on each column.

- Ensure that every screw went through the plate.
- Every screw is anchored in a fragment on the other side.
- As many screws as possible are placed in the distal fragments.
- Screws should be as long as possible.

269

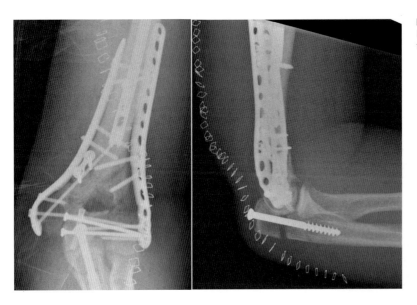

Figure 12.3b Anteroposterior (AP) and lateral radiographs, right elbow, post fixation.

- Distal screws should engage as many fragments as possible.
- Distal screws should interdigitate.
- Plates should apply compression at the supracondylar level.
- Plates should be strong enough to resist breakage.

If there was bone loss, I would shorten the humerus to achieve good bony contact.

EXAMINER: How will you stabilize the olecranon osteotomy?

CANDIDATE: With a traditional apex distal chevron osteotomy, I will use a 6.5-mm partially threaded screw with a washer in a pre-drilled hole as this has been demonstrated to give the highest rate of union and lowest rate of implant removal.[16] However, there is increasing evidence that an extra-articular step-cut osteotomy may produce a more stable construct with a much higher bone contact surface area.[17]

EXAMINER: This is the postoperative X-ray (Figure 12.3b). What will be your postoperative management?

CANDIDATE: There is stable anatomical fixation of the distal humerus. The olecranon osteotomy has been fixed with a partially threaded screw; however, there is a gap at the osteotomy site.

I would allow active assisted mobilization of the elbow and monitor for displacement of the osteotomy. If there were signs of radiological displacement or clinical non-union, I would revise the fixation using a screw with a washer.

I would consider the use of prophylaxis for heterotopic ossification.

EXAMINER: Why not plate the osteotomy?

CANDIDATE: That would be my plan B if the screw and washer failed to achieve compression. I would initially try to avoid plate fixation as there is already a significant amount of metalwork around the elbow.

Structured oral examination question 4

Monteggia fracture

EXAMINER: A cyclist was knocked over by a car and he landed on his elbow. This is an isolated injury. His X-rays are shown in Figure 12.4a.

CANDIDATE: This is a Monteggia fracture–dislocation. The ulna has a comminuted metaphyseal fracture with apex posterior and the radial head is dislocated posteriorly as is seen most commonly in adult injuries. This would be classified by Bado as a Type 2 with disruption at the proximal radioulnar joint. The fracture may extend across the base of the coronoid, although this is undisplaced and the greater sigmoid notch appears to be preserved. A radial head fracture is associated with this pattern of injury and should be carefully examined for.

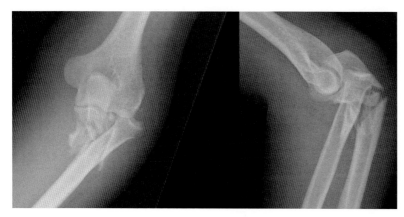

Figure 12.4a Anteroposterior (AP) and lateral radiographs, Monteggia fracture–dislocation, right elbow.

As with all high-energy injuries I would assess the neurovascular status for wounds indicating an open injury.

EXAMINER: How will you manage this?

CANDIDATE: I will reduce the fracture in A&E, apply an above-elbow backslab then reassess the neurovascular status and check position with a plain radiograph. I will then offer the patient open reduction and internal fixation.

EXAMINER: Can this fracture be treated non-operatively?

CANDIDATE: Unless there was an absolute contraindication such as the patient being unfit for surgery or refusing surgery, I would treat this operatively. The fracture is comminuted and is therefore unstable and will allow further dislocation of the joint with limitation of range of motion. There may be loose fragments within the joint which will cause locking. The lateral ulnar collateral ligament is commonly injured with this pattern and may result in instability even if bony alignment is restored. Fixation allows early mobilization and reduced stiffness.

In an appropriately marked and consented patient, I would position the patient lateral decubitus with the arm over a support. I would use the posterior approach and assess for displacement of a coronoid fragment. If this was present I would reduce and stabilize this through a split in the flexor-pronator mass. I would use a pre-contoured locking plate to bridge the comminuted region and restore length and alignment. Stabilization of the coronoid fragment may be achieved via a screw through the plate. I would then assess the range of motion and stability. If the radial head is fractured I would consider fixation or metallic replacement.

EXAMINER: What are the causes for the radial head continuing to sublux after ulna fracture stabilization?

CANDIDATE: Malreduction of ulna fracture – either malalignment or shortening. Capsuloligamentous, coronoid or radial head deficiency. For posterolateral instability, injury to the lateral ulnar collateral ligament is most likely to play a role. Annular ligament interposition is uncommon. If the elbow remained unstable after addressing all of the above, then I would use a temporary static external fixator.

EXAMINER: This is the postoperative X-ray (Figure 12.4b). What will be your postoperative management?

CANDIDATE: I will protect wound healing with a back-slab for 2 weeks then start physiotherapy with active movement as tolerated to prevent stiffness and follow-up the patient to make sure the wound and fracture have healed along with good functional outcome. I would consider the use of prophylaxis for heterotopic ossification as this is common after elbow trauma. I would also monitor for joint subluxation, loss of fixation, non-union and progressive arthrosis.

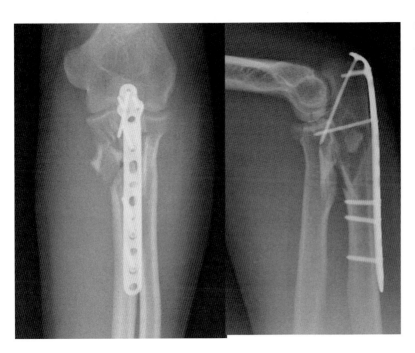

Figure 12.4b Anteroposterior (AP) and lateral radiographs, right elbow, post fixation.

General reading

Wong JC, Getz CL, Abboud JA. Adult Monteggia and olecranon fracture dislocations of the elbow. *Hand Clin.* 2015;31(4):565–580.

Structured oral examination question 5

Galeazzi fracture

EXAMINER: A 23-year-old male while on a night out fell on to his left hand and has come to casualty with pain and deformity. The X-ray of his left distal forearm is shown in Figure 12.5.

CANDIDATE: This is a Galeazzi fracture. There is a diaphyseal fracture of the radial shaft associated with dislocation of the distal radioulnar joint. There is significant shortening of the radius, widening of the DRUJ on the AP view. I will assess the patient with regards to medical conditions, associated injuries, distal neurovascular status and whether it is a closed or open injury.

EXAMINER: This is an isolated closed injury with no distal problems. How will you manage this injury?

CANDIDATE: I will try to reduce the fracture dislocation in casualty under sedation, apply an above-elbow back-slab with the forearm in supination

and get an X-ray of the forearm and wrist. Having said that, these are often quite difficult to reduce closed and reduction may not be possible.

EXAMINER: Check X-ray shows no change in position, it is 9 pm. What will you do?

CANDIDATE: If there are no signs of any neurovascular deficit, I will prioritize the patient in the next day's trauma list for open reduction and stabilization of radial fracture with stabilization of the distal radioulnar joint, if required. Overnight, the arm will be kept elevated and frequent neurovascular assessment will be made.

EXAMINER: How will you fix this fracture?

CANDIDATE: I would use a dynamic compression plate of the radius through a volar Henry's approach, aiming for absolute stability. Bone healing will be primary. There is no need to use a locking plate in this situation as he is a young patient with good bone quality.

EXAMINER: What are the prerequisites for primary osteonal fracture healing?

CANDIDATE: Absolute stability at the fracture site with a strain environment less than 2%, perfect reduction with the bone ends touching so that the cutting cones can pass across the fracture site and viable bone end.

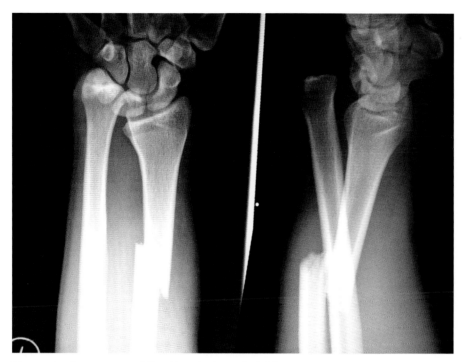

Figure 12.5 Anteroposterior (AP) and lateral radiographs, left forearm.

EXAMINER: During surgery the radius fracture is stabilized, but the distal radioulnar joint is still dislocated. What are the causes for this?

CANDIDATE: The radius fracture may have been fixed in either a shortened or angulated position. There may be soft-tissue interposition (most commonly the ECU tendon) or a bony fragment in the distal radioulnar joint. There may be disruption of the TFCC allowing redislocation of the DRUJ.

EXAMINER: Radius fracture reduction is satisfactory and there is no interposition, but the joint is dislocated. How will you deal with it?

CANDIDATE: This implies that the TFCC is defunctioned. This may be due to an ulnar styloid fracture – if so, I would open this, reduce it and fix using a tension band technique. Otherwise, I would explore the DRUJ via a dorsal approach and repair the TFCC and other soft-tissue restraints. Following stabilization, I would protect the repair using two K-wires just above the sigmoid notch with the forearm in neutral.

EXAMINER: What will be your postoperative protocol?

CANDIDATE: If the DRUJ was stable I would mobilize this patient early after a couple of weeks of immobilization; however, as the TFCC has had to be repaired, I will keep the arm immobilized for longer. He will need the arm in an above-elbow plaster (to immobilize the DRUJ) for around 4 weeks, at which point the K-wires can be removed and he can be put into a splint. A sugar tong splint would protect the DRUJ while allowing some elbow movement.

Topic reference

Giannoulis FS, Sotereanos DG. Galeazzi fractures and dislocations. *Hand Clin.* 2007;23(2):153–163.

Structured oral examination question 6
Humeral shaft fracture

EXAMINER: A 58-year-old man sustained an injury to his arm when he fell from standing height. He is right-handed, suffers from hypertension and has a sedentary lifestyle. His X-rays are shown in Figure 12.6a.

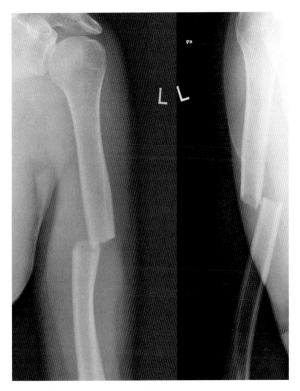

Figure 12.6a Anteroposterior (AP) and lateral radiographs, transverse fractured left humerus.

CANDIDATE: The X-rays show a simple transverse fracture of the right humeral shaft in the middle third, distal to the deltoid tubercle. There is 100% translation; however, the bone ends are in contact, there is no evidence of shortening and there is less than 20° of angulation in either view.

I will check for other injuries, neurovascular status and whether it is a closed or open fracture.

EXAMINER: It is a closed fracture with no associated problems. How will you manage it?

CANDIDATE: In casualty, I will apply a U-slab, then check for distal neurovascular status and get a check X-ray. The majority of patients can be successfully managed with a functional brace applied after the swelling starts to settle and gentle mobilization. Internal fixation would allow earlier mobilization and is one of the indications for surgery.

EXAMINER: What will you do once the humeral brace is applied?

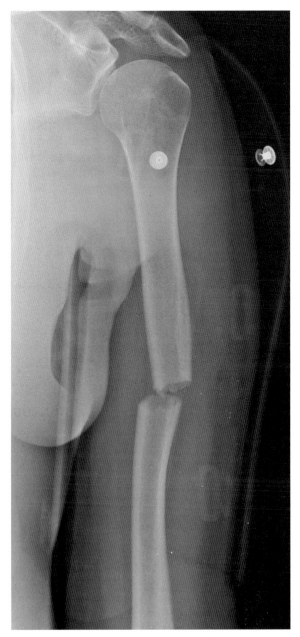

Figure 12.6b Anteroposterior (AP) radiograph, distracted left humerus fracture.

CANDIDATE: I will encourage pendulum exercises and active hand and wrist movements. I will get a check X-ray to ensure the fracture has not displaced, then I will monitor the position with weekly serial radiographs for 3 weeks. I will advise the patient to adjust the tension of the brace twice-weekly.

EXAMINER: At 2 weeks the repeat radiograph (Figure 12.6b) shows some distraction at the fracture site, what will you do?

CANDIDATE: This may imply interposed tissue with a potential for non-union. I will explain that the rate of non-union may be as high as 20% with non-operative and 10% with fixation. The fracture is transverse, the contact area is small; therefore, this fracture may be at a higher risk of non-union. I would mention that we can continue with conservative treatment, but also give the patient the option of surgery.[18]

EXAMINER: The patient does not want to wait and see. He is in a lot of pain and is struggling with the humeral brace. He is keen for fixation. What will you do?

CANDIDATE: I will discuss with the patient the advantages and risks involved in operative fixation of humeral fractures. The rate of non-union may be reduced, the rate of malunion is certainly reduced and the rate of nerve injury does not appear to be increased in using plate fixation. There are, however, risks of iatrogenic radial nerve injury, infection, stiffness, implant failure and CRPS.

EXAMINER: What operative intervention will you undertake?

CANDIDATE: Plate or nail fixation is possible, but I would offer plate fixation using a large fragment DCP as this has been demonstrated to have a lower risk of shoulder impingement than intramedullary nailing.

EXAMINER: This is the X-ray at 3 months (Figure 12.6c). What will you do?

CANDIDATE: My first aim will be to rule out infection. I will check the patient for systemic illnesses, like fever, chills, shivering, loss of appetite/weight. I will also perform blood tests – FBC, CRP.

EXAMINER: The patient has no symptoms and is happy with progress with physiotherapy. Why do you suspect infection?

CANDIDATE: In a plate fixation, absolute stability is the aim. This means that the fracture will heal by primary intention. In the presence of callus formation, I will suspect infection or aseptic implant loosening.

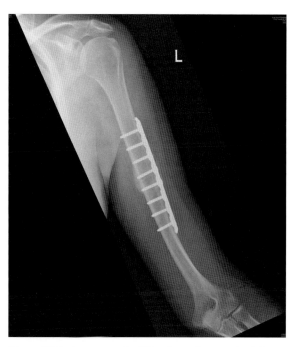

Figure 12.6c Anteroposterior (AP) radiograph, non-union left humerus fracture post-plate fixation.

COMMENT: This last question is about primary healing in rigid/stiff fixation. When there is callus formation in these 'rigid fixations', especially of transverse or oblique fractures, then the possibility of either early plate loosening of grumbling infection should be kept in mind. Although external callus can occur in plate fixations, in these circumstances the stiffness of the construct is lower and is flexible enough to allow secondary fracture healing as the working length is longer.

A perfectly plated Swiss fracture does not go through endochondral repair.

Structured oral examination question 7

Clavicle fracture

EXAMINER: A 70-year-old female falls awkwardly on to her left side and presents with pain and bruising to her shoulder.

CANDIDATE: This is an AP radiograph of the left clavicle – it demonstrates a mid-shaft clavicle fracture (Figure 12.7). There is evidence of a butterfly fragment, and there is overlap of the

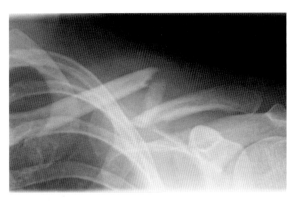

Figure 12.7 Anteroposterior (AP) radiograph, mid-shaft fractured left clavicle.

bone ends indicating shortening. I would assess for any neurovascular deficit and assess the skin for any skin tenting.

EXAMINER: How would you manage this patient?

CANDIDATE: I would discuss the pros and cons of conservative vs. surgical management. The potential advantages of surgery being lower rate of non-union, earlier mobilization, pain control and better outcome scores at one year.[19]

EXAMINER: What factors are predictive of a poor outcome with conservative management?

CANDIDATE: Smoking is the most strongly associated factor along with comminution and displacement. Robinson has demonstrated that the risk of non-union can be predicted according to independent risk factors of comminution and displacement in an older female.[20] More recently, elevated PROMs at 6 weeks have also been demonstrated to be predictive of non-union.[21] This information is invaluable in helping patients to decide whether to opt for surgery. By selecting out those at a particularly high risk, the number needed to treat to prevent non-union can be reduced – in preventing non-union, an improvement in DASH scores can be seen. Shortening has previously been suggested as an indicator for surgery, and although recent evidence argues against this in the short term,[22] it may have a functional effect in the longer term.

EXAMINER: How would you fix this fracture?

CANDIDATE: I would use plate fixation as this has been demonstrated to have a lower rate of non-

union than intramedullary fixation in comminuted fractures.[23] In an appropriately marked and consented patient, I would position them in a beach chair position with the arm prepped. I would use a 'necklace' incision as this provides a more satisfactory scar. I would use an anteroinferior plate in the middle third of the clavicle as there is evidence that this produces a quicker operation, less blood loss and the plate is significantly better tolerated. I would use a superior plate if involving the medial third due to close proximity of the subclavian vessels posteriorly in this region.

Structured oral examination question 8

ACJ dislocation

EXAMINER: A 25-year-old rugby player landed heavily onto the tip of his shoulder and is now complaining of pain on moving his shoulder – what can you see (Figure 12.8)?

CANDIDATE: This is an AP radiograph of the shoulder demonstrating superior subluxation of the lateral end of the clavicle relative to the acromion. There is complete loss of articulation between them – i.e. the acromioclavicular joint (ACJ) is dislocated. I would classify this as type 3 according to Rockwood, although the interobserver reliability of this system is limited.[24] Therefore, it is important to assess stability clinically – the

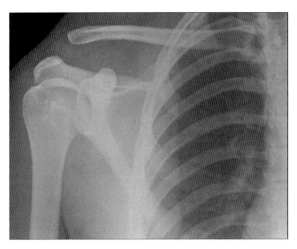

Figure 12.8 ACJ dislocation. There is marked widening of the ACJ space with the distal clavicle positioned superior to the superior border of the acromion and a marked increase in the coraco-clavicular distance.

cross-arm adduction (scarf) test may demonstrate painful posterior instability and this is an indication for surgery.

EXAMINER: What is the sequence of pathoanatomy in ACJ injuries?

CANDIDATE: Initially there is a sprain of the AC ligaments. Next the AC ligaments rupture and there is a sprain of the coracoclavicular (CC) ligaments allowing subluxation of the joint. If the CC ligaments rupture, this will allow complete dislocation. The clavicle can then displace posteriorly through the trapezius muscle or superiorly if the deltoid and trapezius become completely detached. Rarely, the clavicle can also displace inferiorly.

EXAMINER: How would you manage this patient?

CANDIDATE: As previously mentioned, it is important to assess stability. In a stable injury I would manage this patient conservatively with a sling for 2 weeks followed by mobilization. The natural history for type 3 injuries has demonstrated that although there may be a permanent cosmetic step-off (although this needs to be balanced with a surgical scar), the functional deficit is minimal and well tolerated in the majority of patients.[25] Recent systematic reviews and multicentre randomized controlled trials have demonstrated no difference in outcomes between conservative and operative management;[26] however, the most common operative intervention in these studies is clavicular hook plate fixation.

EXAMINER: What are the other surgical options and how do their outcomes compare?

CANDIDATE: The modified Weaver–Dunn technique has largely been superseded by anatomical reconstruction techniques, of which multiple studies have demonstrated superior PROMs data and a lower loss of reduction.[27] I would use a loop suspensory fixation technique as this is straightforward and allows early mobilization when compared to hook plate techniques.

EXAMINER: What are the indications for operative intervention?

CANDIDATE: There are few absolute indications for surgery such as skin-tenting or an open injury. Otherwise, the consensus is that types 4, 5 and 6 should be managed operatively in order to reduce the ACJ where the clavicle may have button-holed through fascia or lie subcutaneously.[28] The art of managing these injuries is differentiating between type 3 and type 5 injuries, which may have very similar radiographs. Although the general belief is that patients participating in overhead sports or occupations benefit from operative intervention, there is little clear published data.

EXAMINER: Have you heard about LARS reconstruction?

CANDIDATE: LARS is a synthetic ligament augmentation and reconstruction device. It acts as a reinforcement to allow the coracoclavicular ligament to heal and grow into the synthetic device. The fixation is via two tunnels and not an over-the-top approach, thus reducing clavicular erosions. Two tunnels are drilled in the clavicle either side of the coracoid process. A LARS ligament is passed under the coracoid and through the tunnels in the clavicle. The clavicle is then aligned with the acromion and titanium screws are placed in the tunnels. The ends of the ligament are trimmed flush to the clavicle in order to avoid any irritating projections.

Structured oral examination question 9

Proximal humerus fracture

EXAMINER: This 65-year-old lady has fallen onto her right side and sustained the following injury (Figure 12.9).

CANDIDATE: This is an AP radiograph of the left shoulder demonstrating a two-part, varus displaced, surgical neck of humerus fracture. I would take a history and examine the patient, looking for evidence of neurovascular deficit – particularly in the axillary nerve. I would rule out other injuries and look for any signs in the history that this could be pathological, although this is not evident on this radiograph. This fracture could be classified according to Neer, although the reliability and clinical relevance of this system has been demonstrated to be limited. More recently, a pathomorphologic system assessing qualitative elements has been demonstrated to have a stronger reliability and good correlation with indication for surgery.[29] I would consider a CT if the pattern was unclear.

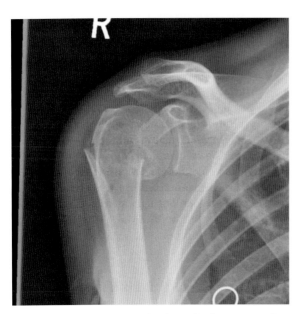

Figure 12.9 Anteroposterior (AP) radiograph of varus proximal humerus fracture.

EXAMINER: What other factors affect the prognosis of these fractures?

CANDIDATE: Hertel has demonstrated a strong association between several radiological factors and avascular necrosis. These are a medial metaphyseal extension less than 8 mm, medial hinge displacement more than 2 mm and fracture patterns involving the anatomic neck.

EXAMINER: What is the blood supply of the humeral head?

CANDIDATE: The classical understanding of the vascularity was that the anterior circumflex artery was the dominant supply via the arcuate artery. However, a recent MRI study has suggested that the posterior circumflex artery is dominant.[30]

EXAMINER: How will you manage this patient?

CANDIDATE: I would discuss the options with regards to the fracture pattern, the patient's comorbidities and functional expectations. Although the recent PROFHER trial has suggested that surgical fixation is no better than conservative management in managing these fractures, there are significant limitations in these conclusions.[31] The first is that many patients who were felt to have a 'clear indication for surgery' were excluded, producing a subjective selection bias. The number of cases per surgeon was quite low and the subspecialization of the surgeons is unknown, leading to suggestions that management by a shoulder specialist may provide better results with surgery. In addition, the fracture patterns were categorized according to Neer rather than pathomorphology, and therefore it is difficult to differentiate whether there is a subgroup which would benefit from surgery.

It is accepted that fracture morphology influences the decision whether to operate.[32] Given that a residual varus deformity is associated with poor functional outcomes,[33] I would give this patient the option of ORIF.

EXAMINER: What if you take this patient for ORIF and find that it is difficult to reconstruct?

CANDIDATE: There are a number of techniques to manage this fracture – conservative, fixation, hemiarthroplasty and reverse-polarity arthroplasty. In a fit and active 65-year-old patient, I would persist with fixation given that arthroplasty doesn't have fantastic outcomes, and, in this age group, is likely to require revision; there is also evidence that reverse arthroplasty after failed ORIF still has reliable outcomes.[34] If it was decided that a similar fracture was not reconstructable then arthroplasty should be considered. Although this is a contentious issue, with ongoing multicentre randomized trials like SHERPA, a recent meta-analysis suggests a reverse may be superior to a hemiarthroplasty.[35]

Structured oral examination question 10

EXAMINER: A man presents to your fracture clinic complaining of pain in the antecubital fossa of the elbow and weakness of his biceps 4 weeks after injuring it at the gym. What is the likely diagnosis and how would you assess the patient?

CANDIDATE: This is a likely distal biceps tendon rupture. I would assess for localized bruising and tenderness and if there is a palpable gap in the biceps tendon. In addition, I would assess the neurovascular status of the arm and perform a hook test. I would take a history looking for risk factors such as anabolic steroid use and smoking.

EXAMINER: Why might the hook test be difficult to interpret, and the muscle belly retraction be minimal?

CANDIDATE: The distal biceps has distinct insertions of the long and short heads at the radial tuberosity; therefore, there may be an incomplete rupture. In addition, the lacertus fibrosus may tether the tendon. In this situation, I would request an MRI to clarify the diagnosis and assess for tendon retraction.

EXAMINER: The MRI demonstrates a partial tear.

CANDIDATE: I would review the patient's functional demands and expectations. Non-operative management is an option in this situation; however, in the active patient, pain symptoms may be persistent. If there is failure of conservative management, I would proceed to surgical treatment – completing the tear and anatomically repairing it. There is a high rate of satisfaction reported for this approach.[36]

EXAMINER: How would you approach this?

CANDIDATE: I would use a single-incision technique to relocate and fix the distal biceps tendon to the radial tuberosity. A number of fixation techniques are described, although a cortical button has demonstrated lower complication rate than suture anchors or transosseous screws.[37] In this case, I would use a transverse incision over the elbow, with the potential to extend the incision in line with Henry's approach to the forearm to allow greater access in light of the delayed presentation in case there is any retraction and scarring requiring release. I would not anticipate significant retraction because the rupture is not complete.

EXAMINER: What complications are seen with this procedure?

CANDIDATE: Nerve injury is most commonly seen. The lateral antebrachial cutaneous nerve is most frequently affected followed by the posterior interosseous nerve and the superficial radial nerve. The majority of these are transient neuropraxias. Also seen are problems resulting from errors in the cortical button deployment and heterotopic ossification.[38]

Notes

1. Kim E, Shin HK, Kim CH. Characteristics of an isolated greater tuberosity fracture of the humerus. *J Orthop Sci.* 2005;10(5):441–444.

2. Groh GI, Rockwood CA. The terrible triad: anterior dislocation of the shoulder associated with rupture of the rotator cuff and injury to the brachial plexus. *J Shoulder Elbow Surg.* 1995;4(1):51–53.

3. Alkaduhimi H, van der Linde JA, Willigenburg NW, van Deurzen DF, van den Bekerom MP. A systematic comparison of the closed shoulder reduction techniques. *Arch Orthop Trauma Surg* 2017;137(5):589–599.

4. Alkaduhimi H, van der Linde JA, Willigenburg NW, van Deurzen DF, van den Bekerom MP. A systematic comparison of the closed shoulder reduction techniques. *Arch Orthop Trauma Surg.* 2017;137(5):589–599.

5. Rouleau DM, Mutch J, Laflamme GY. Surgical treatment of displaced greater tuberosity fractures of the humerus. *J Am Acad Orthop Surg.* 2016;24(1):46–56.

6. Janssen SJ, Hermanussen HH, Guitton TG, van den Bekerom MP, van Deurzen DF, Ring D. Greater tuberosity fractures: does fracture assessment and treatment recommendation vary based on imaging modality. *Clin Orthop Rel Res.* 2016;474(5):1257–1265.

7. Verdano MA, Aliani D, Pellegrini A, Baudi P, Pedrazzi G, Ceccarelli F. Isolated fractures of the greater tuberosity in proximal humerus: does the direction of displacement influence functional outcome? An analysis of displacement in greater tuberosity fractures. *Acta Bio Medica Atenei Parmensis.* 2014;84(3):219–228.

8. Liao W, Zhang H, Li Z, Li J. Is arthroscopic technique superior to open reduction internal fixation in the treatment of isolated displaced greater tuberosity fractures. *Clin Orthop Rel Res.* 2016;474(5):1269–1279.

9. Verdano MA, Aliani D, Pellegrini A, Baudi P, Pedrazzi G, Ceccarelli F. Isolated fractures of the greater tuberosity in proximal humerus: does the direction of displacement influence functional outcome? An analysis of displacement in greater tuberosity fractures. *Acta Bio Medica Atenei Parmensis.* 2014;84(3):219–228.

10. Alkaduhimi H, van der Linde JA, Willigenburg NW, van Deurzen DF, van den Bekerom MP. A systematic comparison of the closed shoulder reduction techniques. *Arch Orthop Trauma Surg.* 2017;137(5):589–599.

11. Reichel LM, Bell BR, Michnick SM, Reitman CA. Radial styloid fractures. *J Hand Surg.* 2012;37(8):1726–1741.

12. Koh S, Andersen CR, Buford WL, Patterson RM, Viegas SF. Anatomy of the distal brachioradialis and its potential relationship to distal radius fracture. *J Hand Surg.* 2006;31(1):2–8.

13. Komura S, Yokoi T, Nonomura H, Tanahashi H, Satake T, Watanabe N. Incidence and characteristics of carpal fractures occurring concurrently with distal radius fractures. *J Hand Surg.* 2012;37(3):469–476.

14. Ilyas AM, Mudgal CS. Radiocarpal fracture–dislocations. *J Am Acad Orthop Surg.* 2008;16(11):647–655.

15. O'Driscoll SW. Optimizing stability in distal humeral fracture fixation. *J Shoulder Elbow Surg.* 2005;14(1):S186–194.

16. Woods BI, Rosario BL, Siska PA, Gruen GS, Tarkin IS, Evans AR. Determining the efficacy of screw and washer fixation as a method for securing olecranon osteotomies used

in the surgical management of intraarticular distal humerus fractures. *J Orthop Trauma.* 2015;29(1):44–49.

17. Zumstein MA, Raniga S, Flueckiger R, Campana L, Moor BK. Triceps-sparing extra-articular step-cut olecranon osteotomy for distal humeral fractures: an anatomic study. *J Shoulder Elbow Surg.* 2017;26(9):1620–1628.

18. Clement ND. Management of humeral shaft fractures; non-operative versus operative. *Arch Trauma Res.* 2015;4(2): e28013.

19. Canadian OT. Nonoperative treatment compared with plate fixation of displaced midshaft clavicular fractures. A multicenter, randomized clinical trial. *J Bone Joint Surg Am.* 2007;89(1):1.

20. Robinson CM, McQueen MM, Wakefield AE. Estimating the risk of non-union following nonoperative treatment of a clavicular fracture. *J Bone Joint Surg.* 2004;86 (7):1359–1365.

21. Clement ND, Goudie EB, Brooksbank AJ, Chesser TJ, Robinson CM. Smoking status and the Disabilities of the Arm Shoulder and Hand score are early predictors of symptomatic nonunion of displaced midshaft fractures of the clavicle. *Bone Joint J.* 2016;98(1):125–130.

22. Goudie EB, Clement ND, Murray IR, *et al.* The influence of shortening on clinical outcome in healed displaced midshaft clavicular fractures after nonoperative treatment. *J Bone Joint Surg* 2017;99(14):1166–1172.

23. Chan G, Korac Z, Miletic M, Vidovic D, Phadnis J, Bakota B. Plate versus intramedullary fixation of two-part and multifragmentary displaced midshaft clavicle fractures – a long-term analysis. *Injury.* 2017;48:S21–26.

24. Ringenberg JD, Foughty Z, Hall AD, Aldridge JM, Wilson JB, Kuremsky MA. Interobserver and intraobserver reliability of radiographic classification of acromioclavicular joint dislocations. *J Shoulder Elbow Surg.* 2018;27(3):538–544.

25. Schlegel TF, Burks RT, Marcus RL, Dunn HK. A prospective evaluation of untreated acute grade III acromioclavicular separations. *Am J Sports Med.* 2001;29 (6):699–703.

26. Mah JM. General health status after nonoperative versus operative treatment for acute, complete acromioclavicular joint dislocation: results of a multicenter randomized clinical trial. *J Orthop Trauma.* 2017;31(9):485–490.

27. Kocaoglu B, Ulku TK, Gereli A, Karahan M, Türkmen M. Palmaris longus tendon graft versus modified Weaver–Dunn procedure via dynamic button system for acromioclavicular joint reconstruction in chronic cases. *J Shoulder Elbow Surg.* 2017;26(9):1546–1552.

28. Li X, Ma R, Bedi A, Dines DM, Altchek DW, Dines JS. Management of acromioclavicular joint injuries. *J Bone Joint Surg.* 2014;96(1):73–84.

29. Gracitelli ME, Dotta TA, Assunção JH, *et al.* Intraobserver and interobserver agreement in the classification and treatment of proximal humeral fractures. *J Shoulder Elbow Surg.* 2017;26 (6):1097–1102.

30. Hettrich CM, Boraiah S, Dyke JP, Neviaser A, Helfet DL, Lorich DG. Quantitative assessment of the vascularity of the proximal part of the humerus. *J Bone Joint Surg.* 2010;92(4):943–948.

31. Handoll H, Brealey S, Rangan A, *et al.* The ProFHER (PROximal Fracture of the Humerus: Evaluation by Randomisation) trial – a pragmatic multicentre randomised controlled trial evaluating the clinical effectiveness and cost-effectiveness of surgical compared with non-surgical treatment for proximal fracture of the humerus in adults. *Health Technol Assess.* 2015;19(24):1.

32. Gracitelli ME, Dotta TA, Assunção JH, *et al.* Intraobserver and interobserver agreement in the classification and treatment of proximal humeral fractures. *J Shoulder Elbow Surg.* 2017;26(6):1097–1102.

33. Südkamp NP, Audigé L, Lambert S, Hertel R, Konrad G. Path analysis of factors for functional outcome at one year in 463 proximal humeral fractures. *J Shoulder Elbow Surg.* 2011;20(8):1207–1216.

34. Shannon SF, Wagner ER, Houdek MT, Cross WW, Sánchez-Sotelo J. Reverse shoulder arthroplasty for proximal humeral fractures: outcomes comparing primary reverse arthroplasty for fracture versus reverse arthroplasty after failed osteosynthesis. *J Shoulder Elbow Surg.* 2016;25 (10):1655–1660.

35. Shukla DR, McAnany S, Kim J, Overley S, Parsons BO. Hemiarthroplasty versus reverse shoulder arthroplasty for treatment of proximal humeral fractures: a meta-analysis. *J Shoulder Elbow Surg.* 2016;25(2):330–340.

36. Behun MA, Geeslin AG, O'Hagan EC, King JC. Partial tears of the distal biceps brachii tendon: a systematic review of surgical outcomes. *J Hand Surg.* 2016;41(7):e175–189.

37. Watson JN, Moretti VM, Schwindel L, Hutchinson MR. Repair techniques for acute distal biceps tendon ruptures: a systematic review. *J Bone Joint Surg.* 2014;96(24):2086–2090.

38. Panagopoulos A, Tatani I, Tsoumpos P, Ntourantonis D, Pantazis K, Triantafyllopoulos IK. Clinical outcomes and complications of cortical button distal biceps repair: a systematic review of the literature. *J Sports Med.* 2016;2016.

39. Lund F. Fractures of the radius in starting automobiles. *Boston Med Surg J.* 1904;151:481–483.

Upper limb trauma II

Chapter 13

Sarah Kleinka and Matthew Jones

Structured oral examination question 1

Lunate dislocation

EXAMINER: What do these radiographs (Figures 13.1a and 13.1b) show?

CANDIDATE: These are PA and lateral radiographs of a wrist showing a lunate dislocation.

EXAMINER: What signs are there on the radiographs which point to this diagnosis?

CANDIDATE: There is disruption of Gilula's lines on both views. The lunate can be seen sitting palmarly in the carpal tunnel.

EXAMINER: What do you suppose was the mechanism of injury?

CANDIDATE: This is usually caused by high-energy trauma such as a road traffic collision or a fall from a height.

EXAMINER: Why do you infer that?

CANDIDATE: This is a hyperextension injury in ulnar deviation: a Mayfield stage 4. Lower-energy hyperextension injuries might result in scapholunate ligament injury. In order to dislocate the lunate, this patient must have torn the scapholunate ligament, dislocated the lunocapitate joint, torn the lunotriquetral ligament and the dorsal

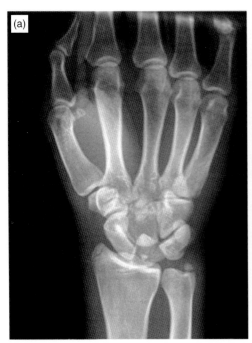
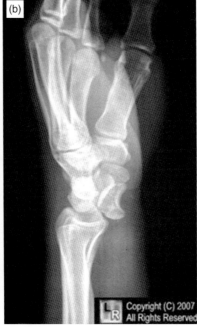

Figure 13.1a and 13.1b Posteroanterior (PA) and lateral radiographs, lunate dislocation.

281

radiolunate ligament. The only remaining ligamentous attachments are the strong volar radiocarpal ligaments.

EXAMINER: How will you manage this injury?

CANDIDATE: This patient has sustained high-energy trauma, so first I would treat any life-threatening injuries. As regards the wrist, this is an emergency as the median nerve is likely stretched over the dislocated lunate. This needs an emergent reduction in A&E.

EXAMINER: How will you reduce it?

CANDIDATE: Before reduction I would assess and document the neurovascular status of the hand with particular attention to the median nerve. The patient needs to be relaxed and sedated. I would apply traction to the limb to stretch the soft tissues; this is best achieved using gravity and finger traps. I would then hyperextend the wrist and push the lunate back onto the radius with my thumb. Then, leaving my thumb on the lunate to prevent displacement, I would distract and flex the wrist to lift the capitate back onto the lunate. I would then reassess and document the neurovascular status, apply a below-elbow plaster backslab and obtain plain radiographs to confirm reduction.

EXAMINER: What if you can't reduce it?

CANDIDATE: If I cannot reduce this in A&E then the patient will need to go to theatre for reduction. Ideally this should be done by someone who can proceed to definitive fixation, but reduction should not be delayed for this as it is imperative that the dislocation is reduced to protect the neurovascular structures. I would attempt a closed reduction under general anaesthetic in theatre with an image intensifier, then proceed to open the wrist if I cannot achieve reduction.

EXAMINER: How will you open the wrist?

CANDIDATE: Palmarly first. I would do an extended carpal tunnel release which should relieve pressure on the median nerve and should enable me to reduce the dislocation, which is my main objective. If I still cannot reduce the dislocation, I will open the dorsum of the wrist. This is done with a midline longitudinal incision centred on Lister's tubercle. I would incise the third extensor compartment, lift EPL from its bed, then dissect into compartments 2 and 4 to reveal the dorsal carpal

ligaments. I would then use a Berger flap to open the wrist joint.

EXAMINER: Can you describe the Berger flap?

CANDIDATE: This is a ligament-preserving technique for opening the dorsum of the wrist. The incision splits the dorsal intercarpal ligament and radiotriquetral ligament in line with the fibres to form a radial-based triangular flap. When elevating the flap, it is important to protect the intrinsic carpal ligaments, particularly the scapholunate ligament which is most significant dorsally, although in this case I expect it to be torn.

EXAMINER: OK, so let's assume you are a hand surgeon and are prepared to manage this definitively. How will you proceed?

CANDIDATE: I would first reduce the carpus, by direct means if necessary, and assess the damage. I expect the scapholunate ligament and lunotriquetral ligaments to be torn. I would need to stabilize the carpal bones in their normal orientation using K-wires as joysticks and further K-wires to transfix the carpus. Once the bony anatomy is restored, I would repair the scapholunate ligament, with a bone anchor if necessary, then return to the volar wrist wound where I would pull the contents of the carpal tunnel to the radial side to protect the recurrent motor branch of the median nerve. I would anticipate a rent in the volar capsule in conjunction with a volar lunotriquetral ligament tear which I would repair directly with sutures. I would apply a backslab postoperatively and emphasize the importance of elevation as these injuries tend to swell a lot.

EXAMINER: What are the long-term outcomes of this injury?

CANDIDATE: This is a severe injury and the wrist will never be normal. As long as it was treated promptly, I would expect the median nerve to make a full recovery, although this is not guaranteed and depends on the degree of primary injury. Further surgery is required to remove the K-wires at 8 weeks, then intensive physiotherapy will be required to optimize function. The wrist will likely be quite stiff (about 50% normal movement) but should be stable and strong enough to return to most kinds of work. As the joint has been injured, there is a risk of degenerative change in the long term which may require salvage surgery.

References

Capo JT, Corti SJ, Shamian B, *et al*. Treatment of dorsal perilunate dislocations and fracture–dislocations using a standardized protocol. *Hand (NY)*. 2012;7(4):380–387.

Berger RA, Bishop AT, Bettinger PC. New dorsal capsulotomy for the surgical exposure of the wrist. *Ann Plast Surg*. 1995;35(1):54–59.

Structured oral examination question 2

Jersey finger

EXAMINER: This 15-year-old boy noticed that he couldn't flex the end of his ring finger after a rugby match. What does the radiograph (Figure 13.2) show?

CANDIDATE: This is a lateral radiograph of a finger with a small avulsed fragment of bone sitting volar to the proximal phalanx. This is consistent with an avulsion of the FDP from the distal phalanx known as jersey finger.

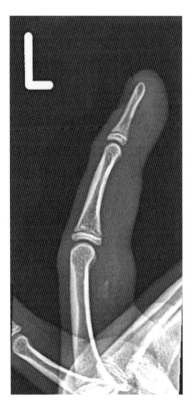

Figure 13.2 Lateral radiograph, ring finger.

EXAMINER: What is the typical mechanism of injury?

CANDIDATE: An extension force is applied to the finger while in active flexion. This is typical of a hand that is grasping a rugby jersey which is jerked from the patient's grip.

EXAMINER: What is the anatomy of the flexor mechanism to the ring finger?

CANDIDATE: There are two flexor tendons. The FDP originates from a common muscle belly on the ulna and interosseous membrane and inserts distally into a broad footprint at the base of the distal phalanx. The FDS has its origin from the medial elbow and the radius. Each tendon has its own muscle belly. The tendon splits into two and inserts into the base of the middle phalanx. The FDP passes from deep to superficial through the two slips of FDS at Camper's chiasm.

EXAMINER: What is the innervation of these muscles?

CANDIDATE: In the ring finger, the FDP is ulnar innervated and the FDS is median innervated. The median nerve supplies all FDS and, via the AIN, the radial two FDPs. The ulnar nerve supplies the ulnar FDPs.

EXAMINER: How would you classify this injury?

CANDIDATE: According to Leddy and Packer this is a grade 2 injury. Grade 1 retracts to the palm, grade 2 to the PIPJ, grade 3 involves a large fragment which sticks at the DIPJ, and grade 4 involves an avulsed fragment of bone which dissociates from the tendon, a so-called 'double avulsion'.

EXAMINER: In this grade 2 injury, what is preventing further proximal migration of the fragment?

CANDIDATE: The vinculae.

EXAMINER: How will you treat this young man?

CANDIDATE: I would recommend surgery to repair the avulsed tendon and restore active flexion. I would counsel him that there is a prolonged recovery period involving splintage and physiotherapy for around 3 months. Alternatively, he may opt for non-operative management and rehab the finger with physiotherapy, accepting that active flexion will remain absent at the DIPJ. If he later finds the DIPJ unstable, he could have this fused.

EXAMINER: What other possible sequel is there of treating this non-operatively?

CANDIDATE: He may develop a lumbrical plus finger.

EXAMINER: What does that mean?

CANDIDATE: The origin of the lumbrical is on the FDP tendon. The function of the lumbrical is to flex the MCP joint and extend the IP joints. If the origin of the lumbrical migrates proximally such as in FDP avulsion, this applies an extension moment at the IP joints. The patient cannot actively flex the DIP joint due to the avulsion, but also struggles to flex the PIP joint with FDS due to the intrinsic tightness.

EXAMINER: What technique would you use to repair his tendon?

CANDIDATE: After proper consent and a regional or general anaesthetic, I would open the finger with a Brunner incision. I would identify the avulsed tendon and deliver it through the pulley system back to the footprint. I expect I may need to vent the pulley system and would probably need to fully release A3 but would take care not to release all of either A2 or A4 as these are the key restraints to prevent bowstringing. I would ensure that the anatomy of the chiasm is correct and that the FDP is appropriately passing between the FDS slips. I would take care to handle the tendon as little as possible and would site my core Bunnell suture early and use this to deliver the tendon through the pulley system.

EXAMINER: How would you anchor the tendon to the bone?

CANDIDATE: The bony fragment is too small to fix directly, but I wouldn't excise it as it may improve the healing potential at the insertion site. There are various techniques described for anchoring the tendon, but the one I use is to drive two hollow needles though the phalanx from volar to dorsal, distal to the lunula, and pass the sutures through them and tie them over a button on the nail plate.

EXAMINER: What is the quadregia effect?

CANDIDATE: The FDP tendons share a common muscle belly. If the FDP to the operated finger is repaired too tight, as the patient attempts to make a fist, the operated finger contacts the palm first. The other fingers are unable to

achieve maximal flexion as they are prevented from contracting any further.

EXAMINER: How would you rehab the patient after his tendon repair?

CANDIDATE: He needs early hand therapy with an early active motion protocol. This is to protect the repair and prevent adhesions forming.

EXAMINER: Do you know of any evidence showing superiority of early active motion over static or passive protocols?

CANDIDATE: There was a systematic review by Star et al. published in the American Journal of Hand Surgery in 2013. They reported a higher risk of finger stiffness in the passive protocols and a higher risk of tendon rupture in early active motion protocols. Despite this, they suggested that modern improvements in surgical technique, materials, and rehabilitation now allow for early active motion rehabilitation that can provide better postoperative motion while maintaining low rupture rates.

References

Khor WS, Langer MF, Wong R, Zhou R, Peck F, Wong JK. Improving outcomes in tendon repair: a critical look at the evidence for flexor tendon repair and rehabilitation. Plast Reconstr Surg. 2016;138(6):1045e–1058e.

Starr HM, Snoddy M, Hammond KE, Seiler JG, Flexor tendon repair rehabilitation protocols: a systematic review. J Hand Surg Am. 2013;38(9):1712–1717.

Structured oral examination question 3

Scaphoid fracture

EXAMINER: This gentleman slipped on ice and fell onto his outstretched hand. What do the radiographs show (Figure 13.3)?

CANDIDATE: These scaphoid views demonstrate a fracture of the proximal pole of the scaphoid.

EXAMINER: What position do you expect the wrist was in when the bone fractured?

CANDIDATE: Extended and radially deviated.

EXAMINER: What would you expect to find on examination?

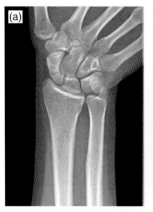
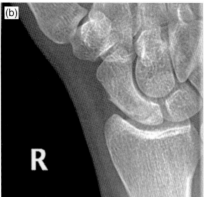
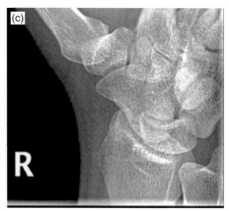

Figure 13.3a, 13.3b and 13.3c Right scaphoid series.

CANDIDATE: I would expect pain on the radial side of the wrist, with tenderness over the scaphoid tubercle and in the anatomical snuffbox. There may also be swelling on the radial side of the wrist.

EXAMINER: So, if he had presented as you describe but with normal scaphoid views, would you assume there was no fracture?

CANDIDATE: I would be suspicious of a scaphoid fracture as they are not always visible on plain radiographs acutely. I would manage him in a below-elbow plaster and see him again in 1–2 weeks for further clinical assessment. If he was still tender, I would repeat the plain films and if no fracture was seen I would arrange an urgent MRI scan.

EXAMINER: You work in a unit where it takes 6 weeks to get an urgent MRI scan. Would a CT scan suffice?

CANDIDATE: A CT scan would detect most scaphoid fractures, but the sensitivity for acute fractures is not as good as MRI. MRI will show bone oedema in the presence of an acute fracture. A CT scan can miss a fracture as the slices could be aligned with the fracture.

EXAMINER: OK, so back to our original scenario with an acute proximal pole fracture. How will you manage him?

CANDIDATE: Fractures of the proximal fifth of the scaphoid have a very high non-union rate approaching 100%. I would advocate surgery to fix the fracture to reduce the risk of non-union and avascular necrosis. I would warn the patient that, even with surgery, there is still a fairly high non-union rate.

EXAMINER: Why is there such a high non-union rate with proximal fractures?

CANDIDATE: The blood supply to the proximal pole is tenuous. It comes via the dorsal carpal branch of the radial artery in a retrograde direction.

EXAMINER: How would you fix the fracture?

CANDIDATE: Following appropriate consent and anaesthesia, I would utilize a dorsal approach to the scaphoid. I recognize that this can be done purely percutaneously, but in my hands, I would use a mini-open approach. I would make a straight incision starting at Lister's tubercle and extending distally for about 4 cm. I would incise the third compartment to expose EPL and retract it radially with the ECRB and ECRL tendons. I would then incise the dorsal wrist capsule from the distal edge of the radius up to the dorsal intercarpal ligament. I would maximally flex the wrist over a large bolster to reveal the proximal pole and inspect the fracture to ensure I can identify the centre of the small fracture fragment. I would then place a guidewire through the centre of the fracture fragment and fix it to the main body of the scaphoid with a differential pitch screw to apply compression.

EXAMINER: It's now 6 months later and the patient is still in some pain and has difficulty using the wrist in his work as a postman. The plain films show no signs of union. What will you do?

285

CANDIDATE: I'll order a CT scan to assess for any evidence of union. If there is none I would consider revision surgery with a vascularized bone graft.

EXAMINER: Why is it important to achieve union with a scaphoid fracture?

CANDIDATE: In this case, the patient is still symptomatic and is struggling to work. In any case, if the fracture does not unite there is a high risk of the patient developing symptomatic degenerative changes in the wrist known as scaphoid non-union advanced collapse or SNAC.

EXAMINER: What if the CT showed partial union of the scaphoid?

CANDIDATE: I would allow the patient to mobilize but to avoid contact sports. I would arrange a follow-up CT in 3 months' time to confirm union. Singh *et al.* published a study in 2005 in which a group of patients with partially united scaphoid fractures went on to unite.

References

Strauch RJ. Scapholunate advanced collapse and scaphoid nonunion advanced collapse arthritis – update on evaluation and treatment. *J Hand Surg Am*. 2011;36 (4):729–735.

Singh HP, Forward D, Davis TR, Dawson JS, Oni JA, Downing ND. Partial union of acute scaphoid fractures. *J Hand Surg Br*. 2005;30(5):440–445.

Structured oral examination question 4

Mallet finger

EXAMINER: This 34-year-old lady presents to you with an injury to the tip of the middle finger sustained when she was struck on the end of the finger by a basketball during a game. What does the photograph (Figure 13.4a) show?

CANDIDATE: This is a clinical photograph showing the fingers of the left hand viewed from the ulnar side. There is an apparent flexion deformity at the DIPJ of the index finger consistent with a mallet finger.

EXAMINER: What is a mallet finger?

CANDIDATE: This is when the extensor mechanism to the distal phalanx has been disrupted. This can

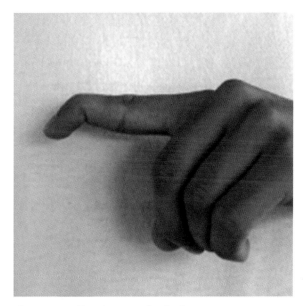

Figure 13.4a Clinical picture of mallet finger.

be due to a purely tendinous rupture, or to a bony avulsion from the base of the distal phalanx.

EXAMINER: How would you differentiate the two?

CANDIDATE: Clinically, the purely tendinous rupture tends to be much less painful than the bony avulsion, but I would obtain radiographs to differentiate the two and to characterize any fracture.

EXAMINER: Why do you need to differentiate the two?

CANDIDATE: This would affect my management. The soft-tissue mallet needs to be immobilized for much longer than the bony mallet due to the relatively poor blood supply and healing rate of the tendon. Also, if there is a bony mallet it is important to establish whether there is any subluxation of the joint which would indicate surgery.

EXAMINER: Here is a radiograph of this lady's finger (Figure 13.4b). What does it show?

CANDIDATE: It shows a small bony avulsion from the distal phalanx dorsally, a flexion deformity at the DIPJ and subluxation of the DIPJ palmarly.

EXAMINER: How would you manage this injury?

CANDIDATE: Assuming it is closed, isolated and neurovascularly intact, I would fit a splint such as a Stack splint to maintain slight extension at the DIPJ and then repeat the radiographs. If the joint

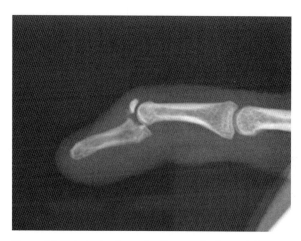

Figure 13.4b Lateral radiograph of bony mallet finger deformity.

congruity is restored, I would X-ray her weekly for 3 weeks to ensure the reduction was maintained. I would insist that the joint be kept in passive extension at all times. Assuming it doesn't slip, I would leave it in a splint constantly for 4 weeks, then at night and during risky activities for a further 4 weeks.

EXAMINER: What if you couldn't achieve a satisfactory reduction?

CANDIDATE: I would advocate reducing the joint and maintaining the reduction surgically. I would use the Ishiguro technique of a dorsal blocking wire to prevent proximal migration of the fracture fragment, followed by closed reduction and trans-fixation of the DIPJ with an axial K-wire. I would leave these wires proud for removal in clinic 4 weeks later.

EXAMINER: Do you know any classification systems for this injury?

CANDIDATE: Doyle's classification. Type 1 is a closed tendinous injury with or without a flake of bone. Type 2 is open. Type 3 is open with skin and tendon loss. Type 4 is a mallet fracture such as this one. Type 4 is subdivided into (A) physeal fractures in children, (B) fractures 20–50% articular surface and (C) more than 50% joint surface. This would be a C.

EXAMINER: What are the potential complications of this injury?

CANDIDATE: An extensor lag is common but rarely significant enough to cause symptoms. The patient

may develop degenerative change and require later fusion. The patient could develop a swan neck deformity which may require correction.

Reference

Sheth U. Mallet finger. Retrieved from www.orthobullets.com/hand/6014/mallet-finger

Ishiguro T, Itoh Y, Yabe Y, Hashizume N. Extension block with Kirschner wire for fracture dislocation of the distal interphalangeal joint. *Tech Hand Upper Extrem Surg.* 1997;1:95–102.

Structured oral examination question 5

Animal bite

EXAMINER: A lady presents to you with a cat bite on the index finger that was sustained when she was breaking up a fight between two cats. There are puncture wounds over the palmar and dorsal surface of the index finger, which is swollen and red (Figure 13.5). What key findings are you looking for on examination?

CANDIDATE: I would look for signs of injury to the neurovascular and tendinous structures of the finger and for signs of flexor sheath infection.

EXAMINER: How would you diagnose flexor sheath infection clinically?

CANDIDATE: I would look for Kanavel's signs. These are: a flexed attitude to the finger, pain on passive extension, tenderness along the flexor sheath and sausage-shaped swelling.

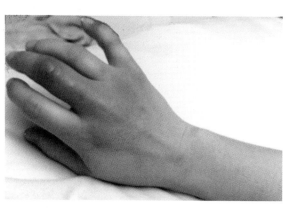

Figure 13.5 Cat bite.

EXAMINER: What is the classic organism that causes infection with cat bites?

CANDIDATE: *Pasteurella multocida* is classically associated with cat bites.

EXAMINER: Let's say you find convincing signs of flexor sheath infection. How would you manage this?

CANDIDATE: This is a surgical emergency. The patient needs to go to theatre as soon as possible, ideally within 6 hours, for a washout of the flexor sheath. I would immediately elevate the limb in a Bradford sling. As long as theatre is not delayed and the patient not septic, I would hold off antibiotics until I have a sample of pus for microbiological assessment.

EXAMINER: Talk me through your surgical technique.

CANDIDATE: After appropriate consent and regional or general anaesthesia, I would elevate the limb in theatre and inflate an arm tourniquet. I would not exsanguinate the limb for fear of driving infection proximally. I would open the region of the A1 pulley with an oblique incision in the palm, retract the neurovascular structures, open the flexor sheath proximally and take a sample of pus or fluid from the sheath. I would then make a transverse incision in the DIP joint skin crease palmarly, open the distal end of the flexor sheath and irrigate the sheath from proximal to distal via a cannula in the proximal window. I would leave the proximal wound open for drainage. I would keep the patient on IV antibiotics and elevation and take them back to theatre for a second look and closure at 24–48 hours.

EXAMINER: Which antibiotic would you start empirically?

CANDIDATE: In my hospital, I would use co-amoxiclav for animal bites as per the local antibiotic guidelines. I would then await the sensitivities from microbiology and adjust my therapy accordingly.

EXAMINER: What are the consequences of missing a flexor sheath infection?

CANDIDATE: Locally, adhesions form between the tendon and the flexor sheath resulting in a very stiff finger. The infection can spread into the palm and up the limb and the patient can become septic. The tendon or a pulley can rupture.

EXAMINER: A slightly different scenario now. Let's say there are no Kanavel signs. How would you manage this cat bite now?

CANDIDATE: This still needs to be treated aggressively as there is a high risk of infection developing and there is potential contamination of the flexor sheath which may give rise to infection here. I would admit the patient for elevation and plan to open and washout the wounds. If there were signs of flexor sheath contamination intraoperatively I would wash this out too. If the patient can go to theatre within 6 hours and is not septic, I would hold off antibiotics until samples can be taken. If not, I would commence empirical co-amoxiclav IV.

References

National Institute for Health and Care Excellence. Clinical Knowledge Summary Scenario: Managing a cat or dog bite. 2015. Retrieved from https://cks.nice.org.uk/bites-human-and-animal#!scenario:2.

Structured oral examination question 6

Boxer's fracture

EXAMINER: This gentleman punched a wall during a night out. He presents to you the next day with a painful, swollen hand. What do these radiographs (Figures 13.6a–c) show?

CANDIDATE: These are AP, lateral and oblique radiographs of the left hand showing a fracture at the neck of the little finger metacarpal. This is angulated palmarly. This is commonly known as a boxer's fracture as it is typically sustained from a punch.

EXAMINER: What do you need to assess clinically?

CANDIDATE: I need to see if there is any wound associated with the injury. If there is any full-thickness break in the skin, there is a high likelihood of the MCP joint being open. There is a risk of contamination from whatever the patient struck, which may have been another person rather than a wall. This is known as a 'fight bite'. I would also need to assess rotation as this will not remodel and can result in functional difficulties if it malunites.

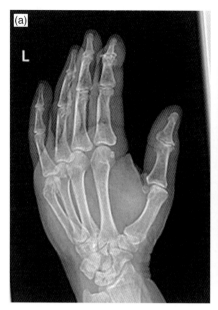
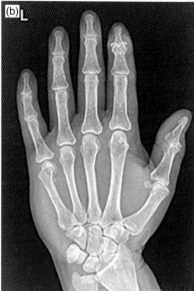
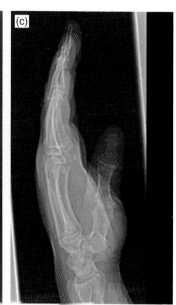

Figure 13.6a, 13.6b and 13.6c Anteroposterior (AP), oblique and lateral radiographs, left hand.

EXAMINER: What if you are not sure that there is a full-thickness wound to the skin?

CANDIDATE: I would rub the skin with a saline-soaked swab to hopefully reveal whether this was just an abrasion. If I was still unsure I would treat this as an open joint injury or open fracture. I would admit the patient for elevation, IV antibiotics and surgical washout and debridement.

EXAMINER: How will you ensure intraoperatively that the joint is not open?

CANDIDATE: I would first confirm whether the skin was indeed broken by attempting to pass a narrow blunt instrument through it, such as one limb of a non-toothed forceps. Assuming the skin is broken, I would then open the skin sufficiently to inspect the extensor tendon and dorsal capsule. This would need to be approximately 2–3 cm. As the finger was flexed when the injury was sustained, it is important to assess the tendon intraoperatively with the finger flexed. If this is not done, any rent in the tendon may migrate proximal to the incision and be missed.

EXAMINER: Let's say this is a closed injury and there is no rotational malalignment. How will you manage it?

CANDIDATE: I would strongly recommend conservative management to the patient. This would involve mobilization of the finger with the aid of a Bedford splint or neighbour strapping. I would explain that these injuries almost always will malunite, resulting in a pain-free hand with normal function. I would explain that any extensor lag will improve with time as the muscle shortens. I would explain that, when the patient makes a fist, the little metacarpal head will always appear depressed, but this will not be painful or affect function.

EXAMINER: What if the fracture were more proximal, let's say in the shaft of the metacarpal?

CANDIDATE: Malunion here is less well tolerated than in the neck. I would advise the patient that this ought to be reduced and held somehow to improve long-term function and cosmesis. This can be achieved by manipulation and plastering, but with a significant risk of displacement. Personally, I would stabilize the fracture with an intramedullary wiring technique according to Foucher.

Reference

Foucher G. 'Bouquet' osteosynthesis in metacarpal neck fractures: a series of 66 patients. *J Hand Surg Am.* 1995;20(3 Pt 2):S86–90.

Structured oral examination question 7

Fight bite

EXAMINER: Please describe this clinic photograph (Figures 13.7a and 13.7b).

CANDIDATE: This is a clinical photograph showing a wound on the dorsum of the left hand between the ring and middle metacarpal heads. It appears slightly erythematous, but there is no gross swelling or pus exuding.

EXAMINER: What do you suppose is the mechanism of injury?

CANDIDATE: This type of injury is commonly sustained by punching someone or something. I would be concerned that the patient has punched someone in the mouth and has sustained a fight bite injury.

EXAMINER: Why is a fight bite injury a significant problem?

CANDIDATE: The metacarpophalangeal joint is very superficial and located very near to the wound. It is likely that the wound may communicate with the MCP joint, predisposing the patient to septic arthritis. This could make the

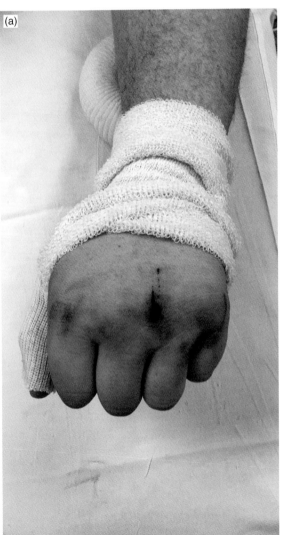

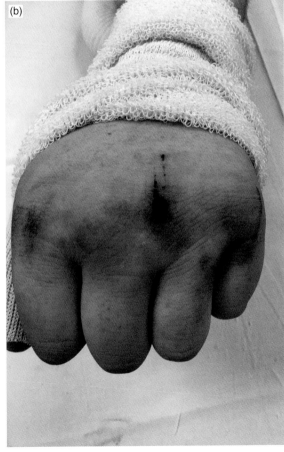

Figure 13.7a and 13.7b Clinical picture of a 21-year-old male presenting to accident and emergency department with a painful left hand following an injury.

patient quite ill, but could also result in significant damage to the joint, with long-term stiffness and dysfunction.

EXAMINER: How does infection cause joint damage?

CANDIDATE: Metalloproteases are released by inflammatory cells which destroy the articular cartilage.

EXAMINER: How will you determine whether the wound has breached the dermis?

CANDIDATE: It is often very difficult to assess this, especially if the presentation is delayed. I would attempt to clean the skin with a saline-soaked swab to see if this was just an abrasion or a full-thickness wound. I would have a very low threshold for treating this as a full-thickness wound as I find it quite difficult to be sure that the dermis has not been breached.

EXAMINER: So how would you treat this patient?

CANDIDATE: This is a significant injury. I would admit the patient for IV antibiotics and high elevation in a Bradford sling. My local hospital protocol for animal and human bites is to use co-amoxiclav 1.2 g IV tds. I would arrange plain X-rays to check for signs of fracture or foreign body. I would plan for surgery as soon as reasonably possible. I would not normally take such a case to theatre in the night, but would operate same day if possible, or next morning if not.

EXAMINER: What operation would you do?

CANDIDATE: Under GA or regional block, I would excise the wound edges and extend the wound as far as necessary to access the extensor mechanism and MCPJ. If there is any pus I will send a swab for microbiology. I will carefully assess the integrity of the extensor mechanism and joint. It is important to note that the rent in the extensor hood will migrate proximally when the fingers are extended, so one must be mindful of this as it may disguise a deeper injury. When the finger is passively flexed into a fist, the zone of trauma becomes clearer. It is important to assess the joint capsule to determine whether this has been breached. Often it is and the joint will need washing out. I would assess the status of the articular cartilage and comment upon any defect. I would washout the wound thoroughly with saline and loosely tack the skin only to prevent drying out of the tendon.

I would plan to return to theatre for a second look and formal closure in layers at 48 hours, assuming the wound was clean at that stage, otherwise a third operation may be needed.

EXAMINER: And what would be your postoperative instructions?

CANDIDATE: After the first surgery I would continue IV antibiotics and elevation. Whether to mobilize at this point is controversial, but I would splint the hand in the Edinburgh position for comfort. After the definitive closure I would allow the patient home on oral antibiotics and elevation. Unless I had to repair a divided tendon, I would mobilize the fingers with the help of physio to avoid stiffness. I would see the patient again in clinic a few days later to check that the infection was subsiding and further surgery was not indicated.

EXAMINER: What is the characteristic organism that causes infection with human bites?

CANDIDATE: Eikenella corrodens is the classic organism with human bites, but the most common infective agents are Streptococcus viridans and Staphylococcus aureus. These are generally sensitive to co-amoxiclav, but I will be guided by local antibiotic guidelines and by sensitivities on tissue and pus samples.

EXAMINER: OK, let's assume that you treat a particularly bad case which presented late, and although you were able to save the finger, the joint was destroyed and you see the patient 5 years later with a very stiff, painful, arthritic middle MCP joint. What can you offer him?

CANDIDATE: In many ways I would treat him much like any other osteoarthritis of the MCPJ. I would explain that there are a number of treatment options and recommend conservative treatment in the first instance. This would be painkillers, splintage and lifestyle modifications. If I were to consider invasive treatment I would want to be sure the infection had fully resolved. I would check inflammatory markers and for features in the history suggestive of infection. If conservative measures failed and I was happy there was no residual infection, I would offer X-ray or ultrasound-guided steroid injection. If this was ineffective I would consider surgery in the form of fusion or replacement. For most young adult patients, I would recommend fusion, but only if conservative measures fail.

EXAMINER: Why would you recommend fusion over replacement?

CANDIDATE: Fusion is a reliable way of relieving pain, but at the cost of stiffness. In a young adult I feel that silastic replacement is unlikely to tolerate heavy use or provide longevity. Anatomic MCPJ replacements are available and are a motion-preserving option, but come with risks of infection, wear and loosening. Medium-term results are encouraging. Professor Dias has presented his 5-year results in 13 joints. He had one revision for infection and three joints with evidence of loosening. The range of motion and patient reported outcome scores were good. If a patient was very keen to preserve motion, I would refer them on to a hand surgeon experienced in this technique for discussion about suitability.

Reference

Singh H, Dias J. Surface replacement arthroplasty of the proximal interphalangeal and metacarpophalangeal joints: the current state. *Indian J Plast Surg*. 2011;44 (2):317–326.

Pelvic trauma

Paul Middleton and Gunasekaran Kumar

Introduction

There are several areas of pelvis/acetabulum that candidates need to be familiar with and other areas that are within a subspecialty interest.

Acetabular/pelvic radiology is usually discussed at the beginning of a viva and should be slickly and quickly answered so as to move on and to get onto the main testing area of the viva.

A basic appreciation of the various surgical approaches to fix an acetabular fracture is reasonable, but it is unlikely candidates will need to know this in great detail. Management of the open-book pelvis and the resuscitation around this is an A-list topic.

Familiarize and pattern-recognize various acetabular/pelvic fractures from either a large trauma book or website (usually radiology based) and be able to effortlessly describe out loud the pertinent/salient features.

Know the various classification systems, as although there is less emphasis on them these days, the viva invariably ends up at some point with the opportunity for a candidate to discuss them.

Structured oral examination question 1

EXAMINER: A 25-year-old professional motorbike racer came off his bike at more than 60 miles/hour speed. His only area of pain is his left hip. This is an X-ray of his pelvis. What does it show (Figure 14.1a)?

CANDIDATE: Anteroposterior pelvis radiograph of a skeletally mature adult marking out the iliopectineal and ilioischial lines (representing landmarks of the anterior and posterior columns) . . . [Silence]

COMMENT: Keep talking about the acetabular lines. The candidate has stopped too soon. They should have continued on and mentioned that the iliopectineal line represents the anterior column and the ilioischial line the posterior column.

The medial aspect of the acetabulum is represented by the teardrop and the weight-bearing dome by the sourcil.

EXAMINER: [Candidate prompt] Tell me about pelvic anatomy. What acetabular lines do you know and are any disrupted?

COMMENT: Practise out loud describing disrupted acetabular lines on pelvic radiograph until it all comes together. Big-volume trauma books or internet image searches are the best sources. The aim is to get through this info in the first minute rather than getting bogged down and stuck as a candidate is losing scoring opportunities in not getting to the next stage of the viva.

CANDIDATE: The posterior wall is larger, more lateral and more easily visualized than the smaller, more medial anterior wall. The acetabular dome appears intact; Shenton's line is intact. My concern is a possible posterior wall injury. The right sacroiliac joint appears wider than the left. There is a

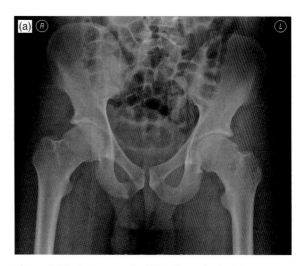

Figure 14.1a Anteroposterior (AP) radiograph of pelvis.

small bony avulsion in the pubic symphysis area. Both hip joints appear concentric.

EXAMINER: What will you do next?

CANDIDATE: This is a high-energy injury and the patient should be assessed according to ATLS protocols so that life-threatening injuries are not missed. As per ATLS protocols I will reassess the patient, performing primary and secondary surveys to identify any other injuries than the left hip. I will assess the range of movements in the left hip joint, distal neurovascular status and examine the left knee and left ankle. I will check the pulse rate, blood pressure and respiratory rate trend.

COMMENT: In the initial lead in question the examiner has implied that the injury is an isolated closed injury and doesn't want the ALTS talk. However, the candidate isn't assuming anything as the examiner hasn't made this point absolutely crystal clear.

If, however the ATLS talk has already been done in the previous viva question then a candidate should default to 'Assuming the injury is an isolated closed injury and ATLS protocols have been performed I will assess range of movements in the left hip joint . . . etc.'

If exam tactics are really not your strong point, then if all things fail at least you should avoid mentioning the 'ATLS talk' for all six of the trauma viva topics – now that will really annoy the examiners who are looking for an excuse to moan!

EXAMINER: Left hip movements are limited to a jog of movements by pain; the rest of the examination is unremarkable. What is the next step?

CANDIDATE: I will ensure the patient has adequate analgesia and frequent neurovascular assessment of the left leg. I will request a CT scan of the pelvis and both hips.

EXAMINER: Would you order a CT scan in the middle of the night?

CANDIDATE: The timing of the CT scan would depend on the timing of the injury, the admitting hospital's facilities and any associated injuries. If the injury occurred during the day it should be fairly straightforward in most hospitals to obtain an urgent CT scan that day. If the injury presents in the middle of the night, say 2 a.m., it could wait until the following morning, as the

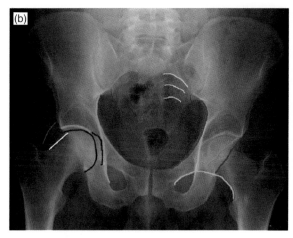

Figure 14.1b Iliopectineal line (red); ilioischial line (light green); sacral arcuate lines (yellow); Shenton arc (light blue); line of Klein (white); gluteal fat stripe (purple); acetabular roof (pink); medial acetabular wall (dark green); anterior acetabular wall (orange); posterior acetabular wall (dark blue); femoral head line (black).

scan does not need to be performed immediately. If a CT scan is required for some other area of concern such as to exclude an abdominal injury, then it may be reasonable to also include the pelvis and both hips rather than have to rescan again in the next day or so.

COMMENT: This question tests real-life decisions and the rationale (and evidence) behind your choice – what you will do in an actual situation with a real patient in front of you. The question is examining higher-order judgement in the real world and not facts from a book. This is the highest level of knowledge the examination sets out to test. This is the score 7 and 8 opportunity that if a viva gets stuck down on competency questions the candidate will never get to.

EXAMINER: These are axial CT scans of both hips and SI joints. Describe the injury (Figures 14.1c and 14.1d).

CANDIDATE: The axial section of the left hip shows an intra-articular fragment, marginal impaction of the posterior wall, and loss of concentricity of the hip joint. There is no subluxation of hip or evidence of femoral head/neck injury. There is also a cystic lesion in the femoral head that looks benign.

Both SI joints appear symmetric and there are no other injuries that I can identify.

EXAMINER: What is the definitive management of this injury?

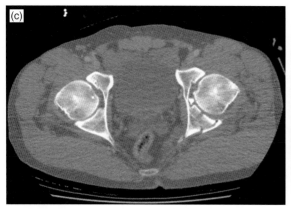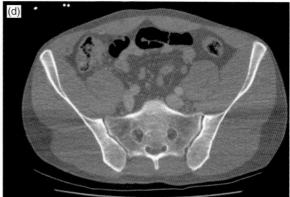

Figure 14.1c and 14.1d CT scan of pelvis and SI joints.

CANDIDATE: Non-operative management is not recommended due to the intra-articular fragment. This will result in early degenerative changes and post-traumatic osteoarthritis. The aims of operative management are to remove intra-articular fragments, reduce the marginal impaction, bone graft the bony defect if needed, then buttress plate fixation of the posterior wall. The amount of comminution could make fracture reduction difficult.

EXAMINER: When will you operate?

CANDIDATE: The surgery should be performed by an orthopaedic surgeon with interest in pelvic and acetabular fracture fixation. Surgery should be performed ideally within 5 days as per BOAST guidelines.

COMMENT: It is much better if a candidate avoids pure recitation of the BOAST text and actually thinks about the problem they have in front of them.

EXAMINER: What are BOAST guidelines?

CANDIDATE: British Orthopaedic Association Standards of Trauma guidelines.

Pelvic fractures

First line of management is control of haemorrhage – pelvic binder, blood transfusion, pelvic packing or embolization.

Look for genitourinary tract injury and open fractures – wounds in perineum, rectum or vagina.

Surgical treatment of these injuries as soon as possible.

Early CT scan of pelvis.

Transfer images to local referral unit within 24 hours.

Once haemodynamic and skeletal stabilizations are achieved, the patient should be transferred to a specialist unit for surgery within 5 days if possible.

Acetabular fractures

Urgent reduction of dislocated hips, skeletal traction should be applied. CT scan within 24 hours and images should be transferred to the specialist unit.

Surgery if needed should be performed within 5 days, ideally.

EXAMINER: What approach will you use? What are the significant risks and complications of the approach?

CANDIDATE: Posterior Kocher–Langenbeck approach. This allows access to the posterior wall and posterior column of the acetabulum.

EXAMINER: Take me through this approach.

CANDIDATE: This is a proximal extension of the posterior approach to the hip, which allows access to the posterior column, posterior wall and dome of the acetabulum. The patient is positioned either prone or in the lateral decubitus position.

Bony landmarks include: (1) posterior superior iliac spine, (2) greater trochanter, (3) shaft of femur.

The skin incision begins 5 cm anterior to the PSIS, curves over the greater trochanter and runs parallel to the shaft of the femur for 15–20 cm.

The superficial dissection involves incision of the fascia lata and gluteus maximus muscle.

295

The deep dissection involves exposing the insertion of the piriformis tendon, the gemelli and the internal obturator muscle. These muscles may have been damaged at the time of injury and their identification may be difficult.

The piriformis is divided through its tendon 1–2 cm from its femoral insertion after a stay suture has been passed through it. The tendons of obturator internus, superior and inferior gemelli muscles are tagged, divided 2–3 cm from their femoral insertion and then retracted. Subperiosteal dissection along the retroacetabular surface is performed. The lesser sciatic notch is exposed.

It is important to leave a cuff of tissue around the external rotators and avoid dissecting into quadratus femoris in order to preserve the ascending branch of the medial femoral circumflex artery.

The gluteus maximus insertion into the femur is released which aids retraction and reduces the stretch on the sciatic nerve.

EXAMINER: Would you prefer to position the patient in the lateral position or prone?

COMMENT: This question is testing higher-order thinking about what a surgeon would do in real life and what are his/her justifications for a particular decision.

CANDIDATE: Higher rates of infection and revision surgery are reported in the prone group. Lateral positioning is more common with most surgeons because it allows easier manoeuverability of the limb and avoids the unfamiliarity of operating in the prone position.

The main disadvantages of the lateral position are:

- Difficulty applying manual traction.
- Potential for sciatic nerve injury.
- Difficulties achieving reduction due to persistent posterior column displacement as the result of gravity that cannot be eliminated in this position.
- Access through the greater sciatic notch for palpation or clamp placement is impaired.

The prone position is particularly indicated for transverse or T-type fractures. It offers the main advantage of gravity elimination and aids in the reduction of the posterior column. The leg can be held flexed at the knee and extended at the hip to avoid traction on the sciatic nerve, greatly reducing the chance of nerve injury. Controlled lateral traction can also be applied to help visualize the joint surface through the window of the posterior wall fracture after the posterior column has been reduced.

The posterior column should be fixed first as it provides a stable surface to reduce the posterior wall fracture.

EXAMINER: What are the significant risks and complications of the approach?

CANDIDATE: Important blood supply to the femoral head is from medial femoral circumflex artery that passes close to the insertions of short external rotators of the hip. During surgery the short external rotators should be divided at least 1 cm from their insertions to protect this artery and avoid avascular necrosis of femoral head.

The sciatic nerve should be identified and protected.

The superior gluteal nerve and vessels are vulnerable during dissection of the superior border of the greater sciatic notch.

It is important to make sure no screws are penetrating the joint using II or intraoperative radiographs.

Other risks include infection, DVT, PE, loss of fixation, heterotropic ossification and secondary osteoarthritis.

EXAMINER: Can you think of any technical difficulties that you may encounter when fixing the fracture?

CANDIDATE: It is important to use a specialized pelvic traction table that allows controlled traction to be applied. Traction is very important in allowing fracture reduction. Traction unloads the joint allowing better joint visualization and assists direct manipulation of the fracture fragments. Manual methods of applying traction are unpredictable and usually difficult.

Bone graft may be needed to fill in any fracture gaps.

EXAMINER: Does this injury have a good or a bad prognosis, historically?

CANDIDATE: Posterior wall fractures have in general poor prognosis due to the damage to articular surface, impaction and difficulty in achieving anatomic reduction.

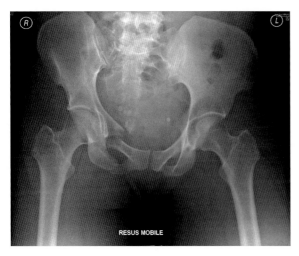

Figure 14.2a Anteroposterior (AP) radiograph of pelvis.

EXAMINER: What will be your postoperative rehabilitation protocol?

CANDIDATE: I will start hip range of movement
exercises from day one and continue with non-
weight-bearing for 3 months.

Structured oral examination question 2

EXAMINER: A 23-year-old professional dancer is
involved in a road traffic accident at 5 pm (motorbike rider vs. car). The patient is brought to
casualty with GCS of 15, BP 110/70 mmHg, PR
90/min. The patient is complaining of pain
around the right buttock area.

Fifteen minutes after arrival the patient's BP
dropped to 70 mmHg systolic. What will you do?

CANDIDATE: As per ATLS protocols I will perform
primary and secondary survey making sure two
large-bore cannulae are introduced and blood
taken for FBC, U&E, cross-match 6 units of
blood. I will apply a pelvic binder and reassess
the chest, abdomen, long bones and look for any
open wounds that are bleeding.

EXAMINER: The patient's blood pressure stabilized
at 110/70 mmHg and 2 units of blood are being
transfused.

X-ray of pelvis was performed. Describe the
injury (Figure 14.2a).

CANDIDATE: This is a vertical shear-type pelvic
fracture involving the right hemipelvis with fractures through both superior and inferior pubic

rami and through right sacral alae and possibly
neural foraminae.

EXAMINER: Is there a spur sign?

CANDIDATE: No, I can't see one.

COMMENT: The 'spur' sign represents the edge of
intact ilium adjacent to the fracture, and is
pathognomonic of a both-column fracture.

EXAMINER: Is there any obturator ring disruption?

CANDIDATE: No.

EXAMINER: Is there a fracture of the transverse
process of L5?

CANDIDATE: I didn't see one.

EXAMINER: Why is this important?

CANDIDATE: A fracture of the transverse process of
L5 in the presence of a pelvic fracture is associated
with an increased risk of instability of the pelvic
fracture.

EXAMINER: You mentioned vertical shear, how can
you classify pelvic injuries?

CANDIDATE 1: [Silence . . .]

CANDIDATE 2: Judet and Letournel classification.

EXAMINER: I think you are mixing up acetabular
and pelvic classification system names.

CANDIDATE 3: Pelvic fracture can be classified
based on the stability of the pelvic ring.

EXAMINER: Do you know a name?

CANDIDATE: Young and Burgess (Table 14.1).

EXAMINER: How does this classification guide your
management?

CANDIDATE: This classification is based on the
mechanism of injury and the severity of pelvic
trauma. Fractures are divided into one of four
categories based on the mechanism of injury,
two of which are further subdivided according to
the severity of injury.

EXAMINER: What is the typical mechanism of
injury for a lateral compression fracture?

CANDIDATE: [Long silence . . .]

EXAMINER: What are the radiological landmarks/
lines you assess for a pelvic fracture? Show them
on the normal side.

Table 14.1 Young and Burgess classification.

	Grade I	Grade II	Grade III
Anterior posterior compression	Symphyseal diastasis – slight widening ± sacroiliac joint. Intact anterior and posterior ligaments	Symphyseal diastasis – widening of SIJ, anterior ligaments disrupted, posterior ligaments intact	Complete hemipelvis separation without vertical displacement. Symphyseal disruption and complete disruption of sacroiliac joint, anterior and posterior ligaments
Lateral compression	Anterior transverse fracture of pubic rami plus ipsilateral sacral compression	Plus – crescent (iliac wing) fracture	Plus – contralateral anterior posterior compression injury
Vertical shear	Vertical displacement, anterior and posterior through sacroiliac joint		
Combined mechanical injuries	Combination of other injury patterns: lateral compression/vertical shear or lateral compression/anterior posterior compression		

CANDIDATE: For pelvic fractures I start looking at the pubic symphysis, pubic rami, iliac wing, sacroiliac joints, sacral alae, neural foraminae, sacral bodies, transverse processes of lower lumbar vertebrae, sacral spinous processes. I will also look for associated acetabular fracture by looking at ilioinguinal, ilioischial lines, acetabular dome, anterior and posterior walls, obturator foramen and teardrop.

EXAMINER: What is this view?

CANDIDATE: This is a Judet view. An iliac oblique view. It demonstrates the anterior rim of the acetabulum and the posterior ilioischial column.

EXAMINER: Can you identify the lines for me?

CANDIDATE: I am not sure.

EXAMINER: Have a try.

CANDIDATE: Line one is ilioischial line, line 4 is the iliac crest.

EXAMINER: How is this radiograph taken?

CANDIDATE: This is obtained on a supine patient with the injured side of pelvis rotated anteriorly at 45°. The X-ray beam is directed vertically toward the affected hip.

EXAMINER: That is the other Judet view, the obturator view.

COMMENT: The obturator oblique view is obtained on a supine patient with the injured side of pelvis rotated anteriorly at 45°. The X-ray beam is directed vertically toward the affected hip. It is useful to assess the obturator ring, anterior column (iliopectineal line) and posterior wall of the acetabulum.

The iliac oblique view is obtained on a supined patient with the unaffected side of the pelvis rotated anteriorly at 45°. The X-ray beam is directed vertically toward the affected hip. It is useful to assess the posterior ilioischial column and anterior wall. The iliac wing 'flatten' out on the image should be well demonstrated.

EXAMINER: How will you manage the patient now?

CANDIDATE: I will assess both lower limbs and distal neurovascular status followed by assessment of both upper limbs. I will also look for any open wounds around the perineum, groin, buttocks, vagina, rectum to rule out an open fracture. Until the spine is assessed the patient will have to be logrolled and the neck should be triple immobilized.

EXAMINER: The patient has altered sensation in the S1 nerve root area of the right foot, but no motor deficit was noted. What do you do?

CANDIDATE: I will obtain CT scan of cervical spine, chest, abdomen and pelvis to assess for associated injuries and look specifically for any evidence of S1 nerve root injury due to the pelvic fracture.

Then, I will perform distal femoral pin traction once I have ruled out any femoral fracture.

EXAMINER: CT scan does not show any other visceral or vascular injuries. No urethral or perineal injuries were identified. What will be the definitive management and the timing?

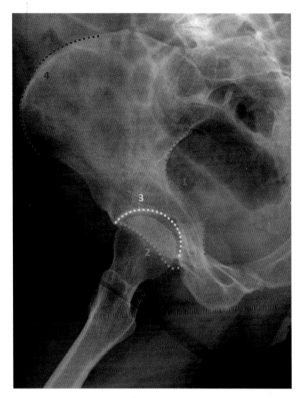

Figure 14.2b Radiograph of Iliac oblique view. 1, ilioischial line (posterior column); 2, anterior acetabular wall; 3, roof of acetabulum; 4, iliac crest.

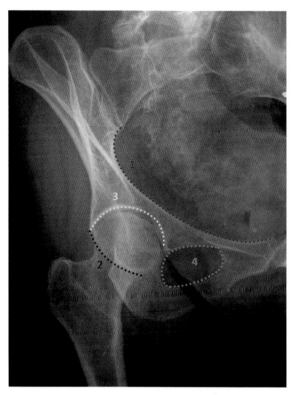

Figure 14.2c Obturator oblique view. 1, iliopectineal line; 2, posterior acetabular wall; 3, acetabular roof; 4, obturator foramen.

CANDIDATE: The images and patient details should be sent to the local specialist unit for a decision on transfer of the patient. Definitive management principles include reduction of the vertical shear, usually by skeletal traction, sacral fixation with sacroiliac screws, pubic ramus fixation with percutaneous ramus screw fixation or open reduction and plate fixation. If the fixation is still tenuous then external fixation could be used to augment the fixation.

EXAMINER: What are the specific risks involved?

CANDIDATE: Closed reduction of vertical shear may not be possible. If so, then open reduction of the sacral fractures can be performed with patient prone and stabilization with sacroiliac screws followed by pubic ramus stabilization. The L5 nerve root is at risk during sacroiliac screw insertion.

Other risks include infection, DVT, PE, failure of fixation and persistent low back pain.

Structured oral examination question 3

EXAMINER: A 75-year-old gentleman who lives in a hostel, independently mobile, not on any medications, sustained a fall while coming down stairs. He used to smoke 30 cigarettes a day and drinks 'a lot'. This is an X-ray of his pelvis. Describe the injury (Figure 14.3a).

CANDIDATE: This is a right acetabular fracture with medialization of femoral head. Both ilioinguinal and ilioischial lines are broken. Acetabular dome, anterior and posterior wall are also involved.

EXAMINER: How will you manage this patient initially?

CANDIDATE: I will examine the patient as per ATLS protocols and make sure that there are no other injuries or any distal neurovascular deficits. I will apply distal femoral pin traction after making sure there is no femoral fracture. CT scan of pelvis

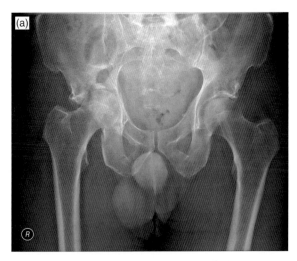

Figure 14.3a Anteroposterior (AP) radiograph of pelvis.

including both hips should be done as soon as possible. The images will be transferred to a local specialist unit along with patient details for consideration towards surgical management.

EXAMINER: Why do you want a CT scan? What is a CT scan going to tell you that a plain X-ray will not? Plain films were good enough 30 years ago before CT scanners were invented.

CANDIDATE: Although radiographic examination is the first-line investigation for acetabular classification, CT is extremely helpful in visualizing complex fracture patterns.

It also depicts soft-tissue complications, such as involvement of the sciatic nerve and the superior and inferior gluteal arteries.

It is good at picking up subtle or non-displaced fractures and sacral or quadrilateral surface fractures.

EXAMINER: What info will a CT provide that will change your management?

CANDIDATE: It will help you to identify the degree of fracture displacement more accurately.

EXAMINER: CT scan axial views are shown in Figures 14.3b–14.3d. What type of fracture is it? How can you classify acetabular fractures?

CANDIDATE: Acetabular fractures can be classified by the Judet and Letournel classification. There are five elementary fracture patterns:

- Posterior wall.
- Posterior column.
- Transverse.
- Anterior column.
- Anterior wall.

There are also five associated patterns, which are a combination of the elementary patterns:

- Posterior wall and posterior column.
- Transverse and posterior wall.
- T-shaped.
- Anterior wall/column and posterior hemitransverse.
- Bilateral column.

This fracture involves both anterior and posterior columns. There is an area of intact acetabular dome. Based on the image shown, this fracture looks like anterior wall and column fracture with a posterior hemitransverse fracture.

It is more common in older age groups due to associated osteoporosis. Hence, these fractures are

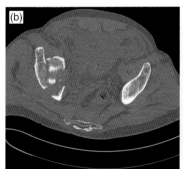
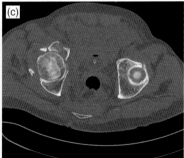
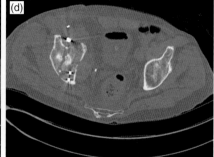

Figure 14.3b–14.3d CT scan axial views of pelvis.

often due to low-energy injuries, such as a fall from standing height.

EXAMINER: What is your definitive management?

CANDIDATE: Definitive management includes non-operative and operative management. Non-operative management accepts some degree of malunion and if this becomes symptomatic a total hip replacement can be performed. Skeletal traction for 6 weeks followed by a further 6 weeks of non-weight-bearing but hip range of movements are started.

Operative management could be either just internal fixation with plate and screws or internal fixation and total hip replacement.

EXAMINER: What are the advantages and disadvantages of just ORIF versus ORIF and THA?

CANDIDATE: ORIF means the native hip joint can be salvaged. However, a patient has to be non-weight-bearing for 3 months. Risk of failure of fixation is higher due to osteoporosis. Even if fixation does not fail, due to the increased risk of secondary osteoarthritis, a patient could still face a relatively big second operation. Technically, total hip arthroplasty could be performed with relative ease as the fracture should have healed and will provide a stable base for the acetabular cup.

ORIF and THA avoid the risks of fixation failure and secondary osteoarthritis. Also, the patient could potentially start weight-bearing earlier. However, it is a larger procedure associated with increased risks of dislocation and infection.

Structured oral examination question 4

EXAMINER: A 48-year-old man known to have mental health issues jumped off a bridge from a height of 30 feet, landing on a concrete pavement. In A&E his injuries identified are all orthopaedic injuries. Lumbar spinal fractures at L2, L3 burst fractures, pelvic and hip injuries as shown in this X-ray (Figure 14.4a), fracture of left radius and ulna, closed intra-articular pilon fracture of left distal tibia. How do you manage this patient?

CANDIDATE: This patient has sustained multiple significant injuries. As per ATLS protocols I will perform primary and secondary surveys. Closed reduction of left hip as soon as possible and distal femoral pin traction.

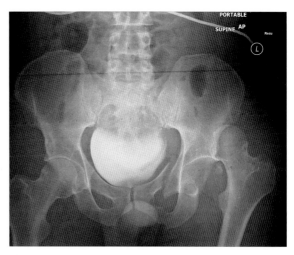

Figure 14.4a Anteroposterior (AP) radiograph of pelvis.

Logrolling, neurological assessment, triple immobilization.

Soft-tissue status of pilon fracture.

Below-knee backslab and below-elbow backslab application.

Adequate analgesia.

Regular neuro observations, haemodynamic status.

Once haemodynamic stability is achieved, CT scan of neck, chest, abdomen and pelvis is performed to rule out other injuries and better identify the fracture patterns.

EXAMINER: What are his injuries on X-ray?

CANDIDATE: Posterior dislocation of left hip with possible fracture, cannot say where the bony fragment has come from. Pubic rami fractures on left side. Both sacroiliac joints, right hip joint, obturator foramen, pubic symphysis appear normal. Cystogram has been performed which does not show any extravasation of dye.

EXAMINER: Axial CT scans of pelvis are shown in Figures 14.4b and 14.4c. What do they show?

CANDIDATE: This view shows bilateral sacral alae and neural foraminal fractures. In conjunction with the pubic rami fractures, this is an unstable pelvic fracture.

EXAMINER: What other reconstruction view is essential to look at?

CANDIDATE: The sagittal view of the sacrum will show whether there are any transverse sacral

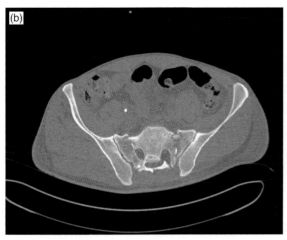

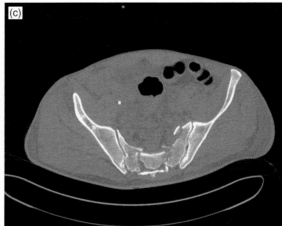

Figure 14.4b and 14.4c CT scan axial views of pelvis.

fractures. If there is also a transverse sacral fracture, then the fracture pattern is 'H'-shaped and it is a spino pelvic dissociation.

EXAMINER: What is the definitive management plan for this pelvic fracture and its timing?

CANDIDATE: Once the patient is stable enough for surgical fixation the left hip is stressed under fluoroscopy to decide whether it is stable. The pelvic fracture fixation is with spino pelvic stabilization with pedicle screws and a rod system connecting the fifth lumbar vertebra and posterior iliac spines followed by pubic ramus fracture fixation with plate and screws or percutaneous screw fixation.

Structured oral examination question 5

EXAMINER: A 65-year-old lady front-seat passenger of a car involved in an RTA is brought to A&E complaining of pain in her pelvic area and abdomen. GCS is 15, observations are stable. She is obese, suffers from hypertension, NIDDM, has had several laparatomies for diverticulitis, adhesions, total hysterectomy. This is a reconstruction of a CT scan of her pelvis (Figure 14.5a). What is the fracture pattern?

CANDIDATE: There are pubic rami fractures in the left hemipelvis along with comminuted fracture of left sacral foraminae and alae. There is also vertical displacement along with fractures of left

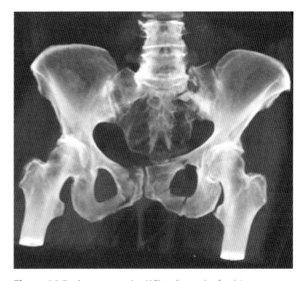

Figure 14.5a Anteroposterior (AP) radiograph of pelvis.

transverse process of fourth and fifth lumbar vertebrae. This is a vertically unstable fracture.

EXAMINER: What are you looking for in examination of this patient?

CANDIDATE: As per ATLS protocols, I will perform primary and secondary surveys. I will look for any associated chest and abdominal injuries, distal neurovascular status.

EXAMINER: This is a CT scan axial view (Figure 14.5b). Describe the injury.

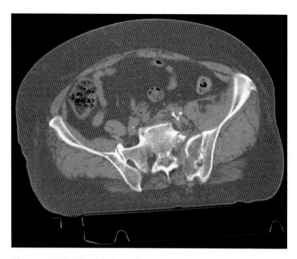

Figure 14.5b CT axial view of pelvis.

CANDIDATE: There is a fracture of the left half of the sacrum along the neural foraminae that is displaced.

EXAMINER: Do you know of any classification for sacral fractures?

CANDIDATE: Yes, Denis classification.

Type I – sacral ala fracture.

Type II – fracture through neural foraminae.

Type III – fracture medial to neurol foraminae.

This fracture is Type II.

EXAMINER: What is your management plan?

CANDIDATE: Adequate analgesia.

Left distal femoral pin traction.

Regular assessment of left leg neurological status.

Transfer of images and patient information to specialist unit.

EXAMINER: What are the options for managing the pelvic injury?

CANDIDATE: Iliosacral fixation with percutaneous screws after closed reduction with traction or posterior transiliac rods. Anterior stabilization with plate and screws via Pfannesteil approach.

EXAMINER: What perioperative difficulties do you anticipate?

CANDIDATE: If posterior transiliac rods fixation is planned, then positioning the patient may be difficult.

Intraoperative fluoroscopic images will be suboptimal due to obesity.

Poor bone quality with poor bone purchase of screws.

Due to previous abdominal procedures, exposing pubic ramus and symphysis may be difficult due to adhesions of bowel and urinary bladder.

Structured oral examination question 6

EXAMINER: A 16-year-old male pedestrian was hit by a car at about 40 miles/hour speed. GCS at scene was 5–6. Hence, he was intubated at scene. Systolic blood pressure is around 90 mmHg, PR 100/min and peripheral pulses are well felt. Trauma series show no chest or neck injury, but pelvic X-ray has been taken. Describe the injury (Figure 14.6a).

CANDIDATE: There is a posterior dislocation of the left hip with associated acetabular fracture and anterior dislocation of right hip with associated acetabular fracture. Iliac apophysis is still open.

EXAMINER: CT scan of head, neck, chest, abdomen, pelvis was done. It showed cerebral oedema, fluid in the abdomen and the injury to both hips as seen in Figures 14.6b–14.6d. How will you manage the orthopaedic injuries?

CANDIDATE: Both hip dislocations require urgent reduction and regular check of distal vascular status.

EXAMINER: What are you worried about?

CANDIDATE: The right femoral head is probably very close to the external iliac artery and could

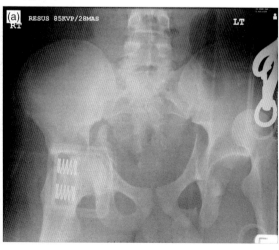

Figure 14.6a Anteroposterior (AP) radiograph of pelvis.

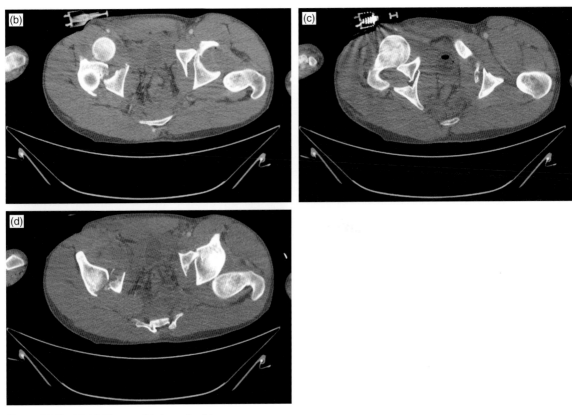

Figure 14.6b–14.6d CT scan axial views of pelvis.

compress it along with compressing or stretching the femoral nerve.

EXAMINER: After closed reduction of both hips what will you do?

CANDIDATE: I will assess distal vascular status. I will perform distal femoral pin traction for both lower limbs, organize a CT angiogram to confirm the patency of the external iliac artery even if there are good pulsations distally. There is collateral circulation possible that will provide distal blood supply even if there is external iliac artery blockade.

EXAMINER: What will be your definitive management?

CANDIDATE: I will transfer the images to the local specialist unit. When the patient is safe for transfer, patient will undergo open reduction and internal fixation of both acetabular fractures either in the same sitting or as a staged procedure.

Structured oral examination question 7

EXAMINER: A 29-year-old male cyclist has been admitted to casualty after being hit by a car. A trauma call has been put out. He has had pelvic radiographs taken by the A&E team involved with his initial care (Figure 14.7a). What do they show?

CANDIDATE: This is an AP pelvic radiograph which shows an open-book pelvis fracture with diastasis of the pubic symphysis. This is a significant injury usually sustained through high-energy trauma and is often associated with other severe injuries. I would immediately ask for the patient to be transferred to the Resus room of the Emergency department and I would assess with the other members of the trauma team according to ATLS principles and apply a pelvic binder.

EXAMINER: What are the ATLS principles?

CANDIDATE: ATLS is a system used by the trauma team to assess and treat multiply-injured patients

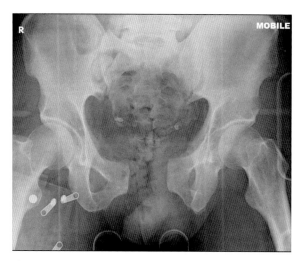

Figure 14.7a Anteroposterior (AP) pelvic radiograph demonstrating open-book pelvis.

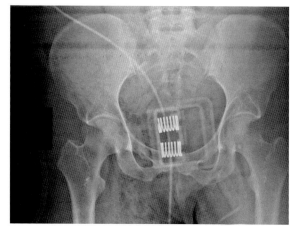

Figure 14.7b Radiograph of pelvic binder in situ. Candidates should be able to recognize binder placement on a pelvic radiograph and if in correct position.

in a consistent manner. It involves a primary and secondary survey.

The primary survey involves:

(1) Assessment of airway with cervical spine control.
(2) Breathing and ventilation.
(3) Circulation with haemorrhage control.
(4) Disability/neurologic assessment.
(5) Exposure of the patient.

The secondary survey is a 'head to toe' evaluation of the patient including full history, examination and reassessment of all vital signs.

COMMENT: The first time you mention an ATLS evaluation you should describe it in detail unless asked not to do so. In subsequent questions it is not necessary to go through ATLS in detail unless told otherwise.

EXAMINER: Who would you want to be in the trauma team? Who should lead the team?

CANDIDATE: The trauma team is a multidisciplinary team consisting of doctors and nurses from different specialties. The team leader should ideally be an Accident and Emergency Consultant. Furthermore, we would require an A, B and C doctor focusing on Airway, Breathing and Circulation, respectively. The Airway doctor should be someone competent in difficult airway management, usually an anaesthetist. These doctors should each have a nurse assisting them.

EXAMINER: You mentioned a pelvic binder earlier, how would you apply this?

CANDIDATE: The pelvic binder is positioned at the level of the greater trochanters and is tightened at this level.

EXAMINER: What could you do if one is not available?

CANDIDATE: If a pelvic binder is not available, a sheet wrapped around the patient at the level of the greater trochanters can be used in conjunction with internally rotating the legs. The aim of this or the binder is to splint the bony pelvis and reduce haemorrhage from venous disruption.

EXAMINER: The patient is found to be profoundly hypotensive despite fluid resuscitation. It is felt the patient is bleeding into their pelvis and it is suggested that the major haemorrhage protocol is activated. What do you know about this protocol?

CANDIDATE: The major haemorrhage protocol varies slightly from hospital to hospital but is activated when a patient is identified who would benefit from a large-volume blood transfusion. The protocol is activated by a senior member of the trauma team. By activating the protocol, it ensures the rapid availability of blood products which include red blood cells, platelets and FFP. These should be transfused in a 1:1:1 ratio to prevent coagulopathy following large-volume transfusion. In addition to these, tranexamic acid can be administered.

EXAMINER: Is your hospital 1:1:1?

CANDIDATE: I think my own hospital is 2:1:1 and I think most hospitals, unless an MTC, are 4:4:1.

EXAMINER: How does tranexamic acid work?

CANDIDATE: It acts as an antifibrinolytic by reversibly binding to lysine receptor sites on plasminogen. This prevents plasmin from binding to and subsequently degrading fibrin.

The CRASH trial showed that it reduced mortality.[1]

EXAMINER: How much tranexamic acid?

CANDIDATE: 1 g IV loading dose within 3 hours of injury followed by a second dose 1 g over 8 hours.

The CRASH trial showed that it reduced mortality if given within 3 hours, but if given after this time mortality was increased.[2]

EXAMINER: What about crystalloids and vasopressin?

CANDIDATE: I would avoid using them.

EXAMINER: Why?

CANDIDATE: Because they interfere with the resuscitation process.

EXAMINER: How?

CANDIDATE: I am not sure.

COMMENT: Large amounts of early high-dose crystalloids can cause an imbalance of coagulation haemostasis. This may increase hydrostatic pressure in injured vessels, dislodge haemostatic blood clots (loss of the first clot), induce dilutional coagulopathy with an acceleration of haemorrhage and also result in hypothermia.

Giving blood early is a better alternative and a move away from the traditional ATLS teaching of 2 l of crystalloids stat.

EXAMINER: What is permissive hypotension?

CANDIDATE: This refers to managing trauma patients by restricting the amount of resuscitation fluid and maintaining blood pressure in the lower than normal range if there is continuing bleeding during the acute period of injury.

EXAMINER: Do you know any common complications from massive transfusion?

CANDIDATE: Hypothermia, thrombocytopaenia from dilution, metabolic alkalosis and hypocalcaemia due to citrate from the transfused RBCs binding calcium are all recognized complications.

EXAMINER: Despite this, the patient continues to remain hypotensive. There are no other obvious injuries apart from the pelvis injury. How would you manage this patient now?

CANDIDATE: The patient still appears to be bleeding into the pelvis. There are two options. The patient could either be taken to theatre and pelvic packing performed in order to tamponade the bleeding. The alternative is angiographic embolization performed by an interventional radiologist. The choice between the two would depend on resource availability and surgical experience.

EXAMINER: Selective or non-selective embolization?

CANDIDATE: I would definitely prefer selective embolization.

EXAMINER: Why?

CANDIDATE: Non-selective embolization may lead to an increased risk of wound-healing complications, increased risks of hip ON, fracture non-union peripelvic soft-tissue necrosis and infection. You shotgun the internal iliac artery and are causing a wide ischaemic insult to the surrounding soft tissues with an increased risk of severe sepsis occurring. One hopes a well-perfused collateral circulation will compensate, but non-selective angiography is not without its consequences.

EXAMINER: What about genitourinary injury?

CANDIDATE: Widening of the symphysis pubis and sacroiliac joint may predict bladder injury while fractures of the inferior and superior pubic rami are more commonly associated with urethral injuries.

Clinical examination may reveal bleeding from the urethral meatus. Where there is suspicion of a urethral or bladder injury a cystourethrogram should be performed. Traumatic urethral injuries also result in strictures, recurrent infection, erectile dysfunction and infertility.

[Bell]

Structured oral examination question 8

EXAMINER: You are called to the Resus department to see this 23-year-old who has been hit by a bus while drinking on a night out. His pelvic radiograph is shown here (Figure 14.8a). What does it show?

CANDIDATE: This AP pelvis radiograph shows a lateral compression (LC) type pelvis fracture, with fractures to the pubic rami and ipsilateral posterior ilium. LC results from side impaction and causes inward rotation of the hemipelvis and rotational instability.

EXAMINER: What are your priorities for this patient?

CANDIDATE: I would want a warm, oxygenated and well-perfused patient. I would want to make sure they had a safe, secure airway, were well-ventilated and had good oxygen saturation.

COMMENT: This is the ATLS talk but in a subtler, less obvious manner.

EXAMINER: What else?

CANDIDATE: I would activate the trauma team.

EXAMINER: Who is in the trauma team?

CANDIDATE: The trauma team is a multidisciplinary team consisting of doctors and nurses from different specialties (see previous question).

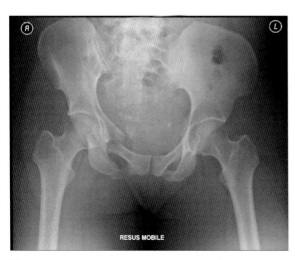

Figure 14.8a Anteroposterior (AP) radiograph pelvis demonstrating lateral compression injury.

EXAMINER: It should be consultant-led because this saves lives.

EXAMINER: What is a sterile handover?

CANDIDATE: This is where the ambulance crew hand over the patient to the trauma team.

EXAMINER: What else?

CANDIDATE: The ambulance crew provide a detailed handover of the patient in a quiet area of casualty and the trauma team refrain from treating the patient unless there is an impending airway problem or visible catastrophic haemorrhage. All the team needs to be attentive and focused. It doesn't really need to take that long as long as everyone is on the same page.

EXAMINER: What do we mean by ATMIST?

CANDIDATE: This stands for:

Age.

Time of incident.

Mechanism of injury.

Injuries top to toe.

Vital signs.

Mode of **t**ransport.

EXAMINER: Typically, what other injuries are associated with this type of fracture?

CANDIDATE: Lateral compression fractures are typically associated with head, chest and abdominal injuries.

This differs to open-book AP compression type fractures which are typically associated with urethral and bladder injuries and pelvic vascular injuries.

EXAMINER: You arrive in the emergency department and his observations are: pulse 120, BP 95/55 with a capillary refill time of 3 seconds and feels cool peripherally. He is confused and agitated. What are your thoughts?

CANDIDATE: The patient is haemodynamically unstable. He appears to be in shock. Shock is inadequate perfusion of tissues and is an emergency. His confusion and agitation may be due to hypoperfusion of the brain secondary to his hypovolaemic state, or it may be due to an associated head injury.

My priorities are the management of immediate life-threatening injuries. I would want to rapidly assess his physiology and prevent hypoxia, acidosis, coagulopathy and hypothermia.

I may wish to consider a definitive airway and want to stop the bleeding.

EXAMINER: How can shock be classified?

CANDIDATE: Shock can be classified by its underlying cause. Haemorrhagic shock is the most important cause of shock in trauma patients. Haemorrhagic shock can be divided into four classes depending on the volume of blood loss. Classes 3 and 4 are life-threatening and require blood product transfusion.

Other causes of shock include neurogenic shock, septic shock and haemodynamic shock from causes such as cardiac tamponade and tension pneumothorax.

EXAMINER: An ABG is carried out and his lactate is found to be 4.1 mmol/l. What is the significance of this?

CANDIDATE: This shows that the patient is inadequately resuscitated. The lactate level acts as an indicator for the amount of anaerobic metabolism by the body and is a good measure for the adequacy of resuscitation. Lactate levels below 2.5 mmol/l are generally accepted to show adequate resuscitation.

Lactate values are important in multiply-injured patients in deciding whether to proceed with damage control orthopaedics. Anything above 4 mmol/l would be an indication for damage control orthopaedics (DCO) while between 2.5 and 4 mmol/l the patient needs to have a period of resuscitation before considering surgery. Below 2.5 mmol/l is usually good for surgery, but this is based on a trend.

COMMENT: No need to discuss lactate and DCO. The candidate is out of date with latest developments. The term 'early appropriate care' has superseded DCO and early total care. Early appropriate care focuses on the physiological state of the patient and the success of the resuscitative effort.

In particular, no single physiological parameter or blood marker can as yet be used to guide intervention, but the accepted level of 2.5 mmol/l for lactate is likely too conservative and is being superseded by a more comprehensive and patient-centred approach, focusing on physiological improvement and reversal of acidosis reflected by a lactate < 4.0 mmol/l, pH $\geq$ 7.25, or BE above 5.5 mmol/l.

EXAMINER: On the same ABG the patient's O_2 saturation was 91%. What is the significance of this?

CANDIDATE: Oxygen saturation is the percentage of haemoglobin molecules that are saturated by oxygen. A normal value in an individual with no underlying lung disease is above 96%. At levels below 96%, due to the sigmoid shape of the oxygen dissociation curve, the pO_2 drops quickly for a decreasing oxygen saturation reading. This will mean there is the potential for inadequate end-organ oxygenation and further anaerobic metabolism.

EXAMINER: You have given him 2 units of blood, his pulse is 120, BP 95/60, O_2 saturations 94% on high-flow oxygen. What now?

CANDIDATE: I would want to secure a definitive airway and apply a pelvic binder, I would give him tranexamic acid, trigger the massive transfusion protocol. I would want to identify any injuries directly related to the pelvic fracture.

EXAMINER: Why are you applying a pelvic binder? It isn't an open-book pelvis. Will it help you with resuscitation of the patient?

CANDIDATE: Pelvic binders control bleeding by compressing and stabilizing fractures, not by significantly reducing pelvic volume. Binders may be used in all fracture patterns and not just open-book injuries. They are indicated for use in haemodynamically unstable patients with a mechanically unstable pelvis.

EXAMINER: What about worsening an injury when a pelvic binder is applied?

CANDIDATE: As a fracture pattern is often unknown before pelvic binder application, it is possible to exacerbate certain injury patterns if excessive force is applied. This is particularly true of severe lateral compression or vertical shear injuries.

EXAMINER: What are the characteristics of the ideal binder?

CANDIDATE: The ideal pelvic binder:

- Should be light and easily applied.
- Allows access to the abdomen for laparotomy, and to the groins for angioembolization.

- May need to stay on for 24 hours or more and thus should be of a soft material that will be comfortable and not induce pressure ulceration.
- Should not limit access to the perineum and anus for examination.
- Must fit various sizes of patients (including children).
- Should be washable or cheap enough to be disposable.

EXAMINER: How long would you leave a pelvic binder on for?

CANDIDATE: Up to 24 hours.

EXAMINER: That is probably too long. One would be worried about pressure sores and skin abrasions.
   What is the function of the pelvic binder?

CANDIDATE: [Silence . . .] To stop bleeding.

EXAMINER: To allow the unhindered formation of clot which will stop the bleeding. If you disturb the clot re-bleeding will occur. In our hospital we aim to have released the pelvic binder by 8 hours.
   We would make sure the patient is normothermic, haemodynamically stable and any metabolic acidosis corrected. All imaging should have been completed and the fracture should have been fully characterized, and we have a definitive plan of action in place for management if the patient becomes unstable once more.

COMMENT: The examiner wouldn't necessarily volunteer any of this info unless it was a mock examination.

EXAMINER: How do you determine if there is a coagulation issue?

CANDIDATE: I would check full blood count, U&Es and coagulation screen.

EXAMINER: Anything else?

CANDIDATE: Ensure patient warming, avoid acidosis and perform an INR.

EXAMINER: Have you heard of thromboelastography (TEG) and rotational thromboelastometry (ROTEM)?

CANDIDATE: No.

COMMENT: The candidate isn't scoring well in the viva (possibly 4 or 5). TEG allows real-time assessment of clotting and may be a valuable adjunct in acute resuscitation and guide transfusion of blood products different from a standard 1:1:1 ratio.

EXAMINER: What next?

CANDIDATE: I would consider obtaining a CT angiogram to investigate for ongoing sources of bleeding.

EXAMINER: What type of CT angiogram?

CANDIDATE: A triple-phase CT contrast angiogram is my modality of choice. The three phases are arterial, portal venous and delayed phase.

EXAMINER: You don't have access to a CT angiogram as it wouldn't be ready for at least 2 hours as the vascular list has overrun.

CANDIDATE: As the patient is haemodynamically unstable he will need to go to theatre for more definitive pelvic stabilization and for pelvic packing. He may have associated extrapelvic injuries (thoracoabdominal or extremity trauma) or injuries to structures within the pelvis (bladder, rectum, vasculature). We would liaise with the general surgeons so that all teams were available and ready to go.

EXAMINER: What type of pelvic packing?

CANDIDATE: Extraperitoneal.

EXAMINER: What else?

CANDIDATE: The vast majority of pelvic bleeding originates from the presacral venous plexus and fracture sites – sources that will stop with tamponade – while only 10–20% is related to major arterial injury.

EXAMINER: How do you perform pelvic packing?

CANDIDATE: I have never seen it performed, but the packing is into the preperitoneal pelvic packing.

COMMENT: General candidate advice is that in the exam (it is said that) if you haven't done a procedure, don't say you would do it.

EXAMINER: What incision would you use?

CANDIDATE: A vertical incision is preferred to a Pfannenstiel incision.

EXAMINER: Why?

CANDIDATE: [Silence . . .] No, not sure.

COMMENT: For PPP, a vertical midline incision is made from the pubic symphysis extending up 6–8 cm. If a laparotomy is necessary, the two incisions should remain separate or effective tamponade of the pelvic space will be difficult. The laparotomy incision may extend from the xiphoid to just below the umbilicus while the PPP incision is approximately 6 cm away in the suprapubic area.

The pelvic haematoma often dissects the space to be packed and is encountered upon entry through the midline fascia.

Packs need to be removed after 48 hours.

Notes

1. A bland, throw-away statement that doesn't score a candidate any points.

2. Much better and more strategic than 1.

15

Spinal trauma

Jonathan A. Clamp and David J. Bryson

Structured oral examination question 1

Bifacet dislocation

EXAMINER: A 53-year-old man was involved in a road traffic accident. He was driving the car and was wearing a seat belt. This is the radiograph obtained in casualty (Figure 15.1a). What does it show?

CANDIDATE: This is a plain lateral radiograph of the cervical spine that shows anterior translation of the C6 vertebra on C7. This translation is more than 25% so this is likely a bifacet dislocation. The inferior facets of C6 can be seen to lie anterior to the superior facets of C7. This is a bifacet dislocation. The C7/T1 border is not clearly seen and therefore this is an inadequate radiograph. Further imaging is required, and a CT would be my choice in this patient. There is no obvious anterior soft-tissue swelling or any associated fractures of the facets, laminae or spinous processes.

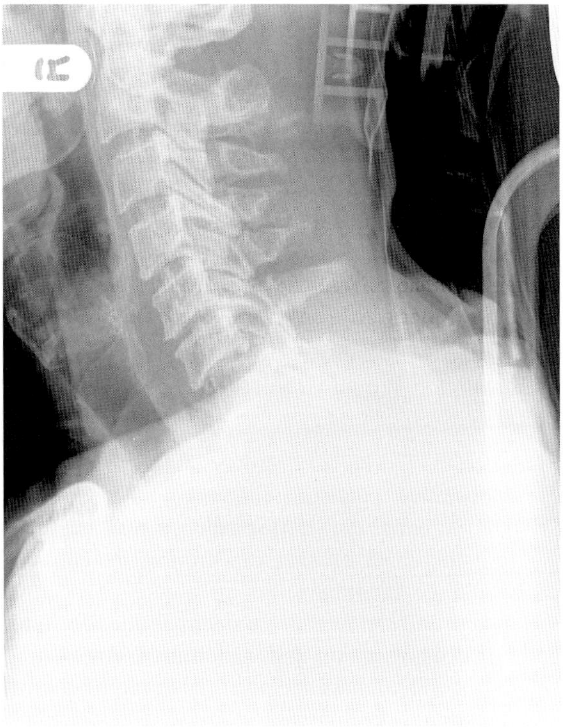

EXAMINER: Assume there is no injury at C7/T1. How will you manage this patient?

CANDIDATE: I will manage this patient according to ATLS guidelines. I will perform a primary survey to identify and treat immediately life-threatening injuries, carrying out any emergency treatment and stabilization of the patient as required.

I would then proceed with a secondary survey to identify and treat potentially life-threatening injuries; spinal assessment is part of this. The aim is to protect the cord and maintain cord perfusion. I would ensure adequate fluid resuscitation, supplementary oxygen and catheterize the patient. I am mindful that 10% of patients have a fracture elsewhere so maintaining the patient supine on a spinal board with triple spine immobilization (rigid collar, sandbag, tape) and log-rolling is required. The incidence of neurological deficit with a bifacet dislocation is 50% so a full neurological assessment is required. I would want to assess for any neurological injury and obtain an ASIA grading. Given the mechanism of injury and the injury identified I would obtain a trauma CT series (head, cervical spine, thoracic/lumbar spine, chest, abdomen and pelvis) to exclude any associated injuries (Figure 15.1b) [1].

I would want to make an early referral to the local spinal injuries unit for transfer of the patient for more specialized surgical management of this injury.

Figure 15.1a Lateral radiograph demonstrating C6 on C7 facet dislocation.

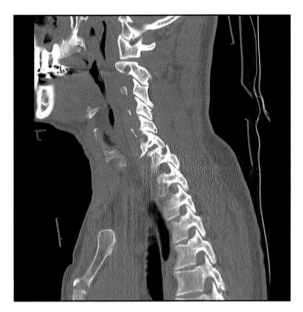

Figure 15.1b C6 7 facet dislocation parasagittal CT.

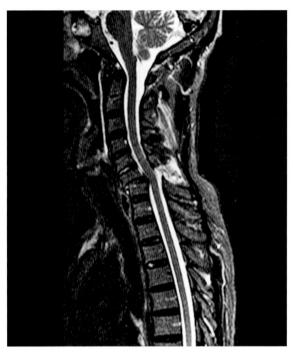

Figure 15.1c Parasagittal MRI stir of C6 on C7 facet dislocation.

COMMENT: This is a highly unstable injury result-ing from hyperflexion of the cervical spine with a high risk of associated spinal cord damage. The patient may present with spinal shock includ-ing bradycardia and hypotension unresponsive to fluid resuscitation. This is due to loss of vasomo-tor sympathetic tone. Candidates should be able to safely deal with the initial management of this injury in casualty and get past the initial ques-tions. This will allow them to then move on to discuss more definitive management of the injury (score 6). If a candidate is doing very well (score 7–8) they may discuss the more controversial areas of management (i.e. MRI versus no MRI prior to reduction (score 7) with evidence (score 8)). If a candidate is struggling with A&E manage-ment (score 4–5) they may not get past the initial management of the patient in the A&E department.[1]

EXAMINER: Assume the patient is being managed in an appropriate spinal injuries unit.

CANDIDATE: I will then need to reduce and stabi-lize the spine.

EXAMINER: How will you reduce the dislocation?

CANDIDATE: The dislocation can be reduced closed with traction or open with an anterior surgical approach.

EXAMINER: Well of course all options apply, what would you do?

CANDIDATE: I would take the patient immediately to theatre and apply halo traction. I would add 5 kg weight initially and increase steadily in 2 kg increments, observing carefully the neurological function and the reduction of the spine using an image intensifier. Once the vertebral bodies and facet joints have been realigned traction can be reduced and a collar applied (Figure 15.1d –h) [2].

EXAMINER: Would you not organize an MRI scan first?

CANDIDATE: This is controversial [3]. In an awake cooperative patient this is not required. The potential risk is displacing a disc fragment into the canal causing catastrophic deficit. This would be identifiable in an awake cooperative patient and can be addressed with immediate ante-rior decompression and stabilization. An existing deficit will not have the potential to improve until the spine is realigned and an MRI delays this.

EXAMINER: Are you telling me you would never get an MRI first?

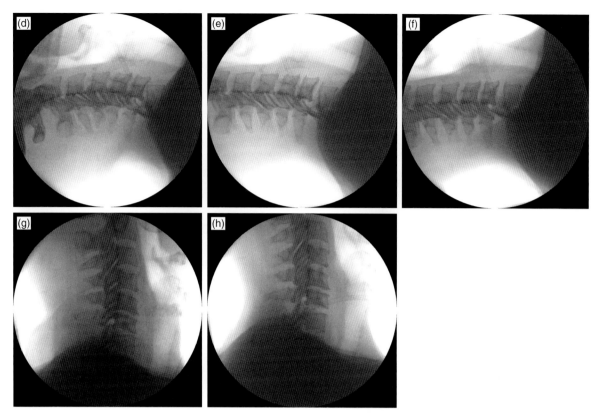

Figure 15.1d–h Image intensification views of closed reduction of C6 on C7 facet dislocation.

CANDIDATE: If it were a unifacet dislocation with only nerve root injury I would organize an MRI first as there is no urgent requirement to reduce the dislocation. If the patient were obtunded or uncooperative and not able to cooperate with serial examinations during reduction manoeuvres I would organize an MRI scan first [4]. I would also do so if they were neurologically intact (Figure 15.1c).

EXAMINER: How would you stabilize this injury?

CANDIDATE: An anterior cervical discectomy and fusion (ACDF). This can be done with a cage and plate or tricortical iliac crest graft (harvested with a small sagittal saw) and a plate. I would prefer the latter as autograft will more reliably achieve fusion. These injuries may also require instrumented stabilization posteriorly depending on the degree of soft-tissue injury and instability. This can be done as a delayed procedure or at the same time. ACDF with plating gives the injury a degree of stability before a patient is turned prone and the cord should not be in danger.

EXAMINER: What would you do if closed reduction failed?

CANDIDATE: If a closed reduction fails, an anterior or posterior approach should be performed to reduce the locked facet dislocation. This is usually via a posterior approach.

Key Points

Cervical disc herniation can occur with facet dislocations. When reduction occurs the disc herniation can be displaced posteriorly into the spinal canal, causing catastrophic deficit. This is rare. An MRI scan can be performed as follows:

1. Before reduction.

   a. Advantage – allows identification of disc herniation, which then provides an argument for proceeding with open discectomy rather than closed reduction.

b. Disadvantage – delays treatment which in the presence of neurological deficit might adversely affect outcome as cord is compressed for longer.

2. After reduction.

a. Advantage – allows identification of disc herniation that might dictate surgical approach, e.g. herniation behind vertebral body may require corpectomy.

b. Disadvantage – time-consuming and often these herniations are not clinically significant so should not affect treatment which is ACDF.

3. Not performed.

a. Advantage – facilitates more rapid reduction by avoiding delay. Studies suggest that closed reduction can be safely performed, provided that serial neurological examination is possible during this procedure. Studies report the incidence of herniated disc material is higher after successful closed reduction than before but without increase in neurological injury, i.e. is not clinically relevant.

b. Disadvantage – very small risk of worsening deficit by displacing disc herniation.

It is generally accepted that an MRI scan should be performed before reduction if the patient is neurologically intact and in the patient that is obtunded or non-cooperative. In an awake cooperative patient with deficit this has little chance of improving until cord compression is alleviated by reduction and the incidence of disc herniation is higher after closed reduction, but the incidence of neurological deficit is not, i.e. these herniations don't appear to be clinically significant.

References

1. Arnold PM, Brodke DS, Rempersaud YR, *et al.* Differences between neurosurgeons and orthopaedic surgeons in classifying cervical dislocation injures and making assessment and treatment decisions: a multicenter reliability study. *Am J Orthop.* 2009;38: E156–E161.

2. Vaccaro AR, Falatyn SP, Flanders AE, *et al.* Magnetic resonance evaluation of the intervertebral disc, spinal ligaments and spinal cord before and after closed traction reduction of cervical spine dislocations. *Spine.* 1999;24:1210–1218.

3. Grant GA, Mirza SK, Chapman JR, *et al.* Risk of early closed reduction in cervical spine subluxation injuries. *J Neurosurg (Spine).* 1999;90:13–18.

4. Hart RA, Vaccaro AR, Nachwalter RS. Cervical facet dislocation: when is magnetic resonance imaging indicated? *Spine.* 2002;27:116–118.

Structured oral examination question 2

Incomplete cord injury

EXAMINER: A 75-year-old female presents with abnormal neurological findings having fallen onto her face. What does the MRI scan show (Figure 15.2a)?

CANDIDATE: The MRI scan (sagittal T2 sequence) demonstrates multilevel central canal narrowing most notable at C4/5 and C5/6. The narrowing is due to a combination of anterior disc/osteophyte complex and posterior ligamentum flavum infolding. At C4/5 where the narrowing appears severe (but requires axial cuts for proper assessment) there is focal high signal change in the cord, which is either myelomalacia (spinal cord damage due to compression) or oedema (due to the acute injury).

EXAMINER: What pattern of injury do you expect?

CANDIDATE: It is likely that the pattern of injury is one of central cord syndrome. It is the most common incomplete spinal cord injury. The history is characteristic, often an elderly person with a hyperextension injury. The pathophysiology is one of anterior osteophytes and posterior infolded ligamentum flavum compressing the cord. There is a pre-existing cervical degenerative disc disease that may well have been asymptomatic. There may be forehead/facial bruising.

EXAMINER: What do you think the clinical features will be?

CANDIDATE: There will be weakness affecting the upper and lower limbs. The upper limbs are affected to a greater extent, with the motor deficit especially apparent in the hand.

EXAMINER: What is the pathophysiology of the condition?

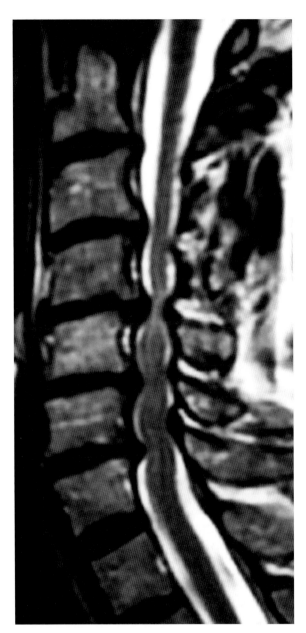

Figure 15.2a T2 sagittal MRI scan, cervical spine. C5–7 hyperintense signal.

CANDIDATE: The cord is usually injured as a result of posterior pinching by a buckled ligamentum flavum or from anterior compression by osteophytes. There is usually cord contusion with stasis of axoplasmic flow and/or Wallerian degeneration of the corticospinal tracts. The original description of the condition was based on postmortem studies that demonstrated a destructive haematomyelia, but more frequently this is absent, and the injury caused by oedema alone.[2] If haemorrhage is present this has been correlated with a worse injury and limited neurologic recovery.

EXAMINER: How will you manage this person?

CANDIDATE: Initial management of such an injury in the emergency department would include a full ATLS work-up. I would want to take a full history and perform a thorough clinical examination including a full neurological examination and document my findings in the notes. The spine should be fully immobilized, systolic blood pressure maintained, a urinary catheter passed, and careful fluid resuscitation undertaken. A digital rectal exam should be performed and an American Spinal Injury Association (ASIA) score should be obtained.

It is also important to perform serial neurological examinations especially to check for any deterioration in function, as this is a strong indication to consider surgical decompression.

EXAMINER: Would you give steroids?

CANDIDATE: Administration of methylprednisolone for the treatment of acute spinal cord injury (SCI) is no longer recommended. I am not sure of the specifics of the literature, but there is very little hard evidence to support the clinical benefit of steroids in the management of acute SCI, but plenty of evidence documenting their harmful side effects.

EXAMINER: What about prognosis?

CANDIDATE: Central cord syndrome has a good prognosis although full functional recovery is not likely. It is usual to see significant early neurological recovery. In the absence of spinal instability, I would manage this condition non-operatively. The typical recovery sequence begins with the lower limbs, followed by bladder and bowel function, the proximal muscles of the upper extremity and finally the hands are the last to recover function. Typically, the patient is ambulatory at final follow-up. If there is a plateau in recovery with MRI-proven cord compression, or if there are signs of instability, surgical decompression and stabilization should be considered [1].

315

EXAMINER: What surgical approach would you use?

CANDIDATE: The optimal surgical approach is a matter of debate. As a general rule, the ideal surgical approach should target the site of predominant compression of the spinal cord: anterior, posterior, or combined. Usually, if the compression is restricted to one or two levels, the anterior approach is preferred; if more than two levels are involved, the posterior approach may be more advantageous.

EXAMINER: Are you aware of any other incomplete cord syndromes?

CANDIDATE: Anterior cord syndrome affects the anterior two-thirds of the spinal cord via anterior spinal artery lesions. It is a vascular phenomenon. It causes profound motor weakness due to involvement of the corticospinal tracts. Proprioception and vibratory sense (both carried in the dorsal, unaffected, columns) are preserved. This condition has the worst prognosis.

Brown–Sequard syndrome is a hemi-section of the spinal cord, seen with a penetrating trauma. There is ipsilateral loss of motor function, proprioception and vibratory sense; there is contralateral loss of pain and temperature sensation.

COMMENT: If a candidate is progressing well with the viva, they may be asked to draw out the spinal cord tracts and spend more time discussing anterior cord and Brown–Sequard syndromes.

Key Points

Central cord syndrome has a reasonable prognosis. Historically, non-surgical treatment was advocated for CCS.

Early surgery is indicated if there is instability from a co-existing fracture that requires stabilization [2]. In this situation it would be reasonable to describe the case as neurological deficit as a result of a fracture, which is therefore by definition unstable, and perform early stabilization. If the cause of the CCS is a large central disc protrusion, early surgery is supported.

The Surgical Timing in Acute Spinal Cord Injury Study (STACIS) suggests decompressive surgery should be performed within 24 hours if there is a neurological deficit or 12 hours if the neurological deficit is deteriorating [3].

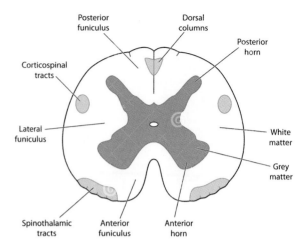

Figure 15.2b Cross-section of spinal cord.

References

1 Samuel AM, Grant RA, Bohl DD, *et al*. Delayed surgery after acute traumatic central cord syndrome is associated with reduced mortality. *Spine*. 2015;40:349–356.

2. Fehlings MG, Vaccaro A, Wilson JR, *et al*. Early versus delayed decompression for traumatic cervical spinal cord injury: results of the Surgical Timing in Acute Spinal Cord Injury Study (STASCIS). *PLoS ONE*. 2012;7:e32037.

3. Anderson KK, Tetreault L, Shamji MF, *et al*. Optimal timing of surgical decompression for acute traumatic central cord syndrome: a systematic review of the literature. *Neurosurgery*. 2015 77:s15–s32.

Structured oral examination question 3

Thoracolumbar burst fractures

EXAMINER: What does this X-ray (Figures 15.3a and 15.3b) show?

CANDIDATE: There is a fracture of the T12 vertebral body (it is reasonable to say a vertebral body at the thoracolumbar junction but L5/S1 not visible so exact level difficult to be sure) with greater than 50% loss of the vertebral body height. There is retropulsion of the posterosuperior corner of the vertebral body. On the AP view there is widening of the interpedicular distance. This is a burst fracture. It does not involve the inferior end plate, so it is an incomplete burst fracture.

EXAMINER: What is a stable spine?

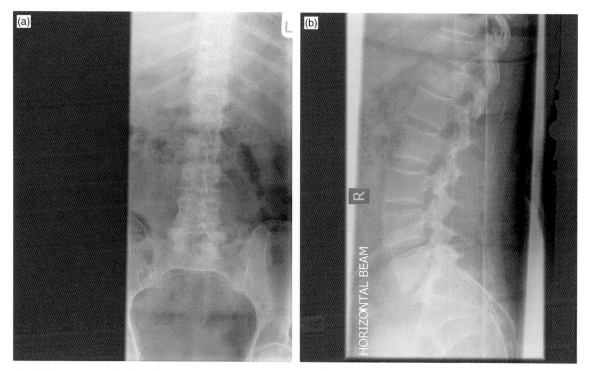

Figure 15.3a and 15.3b AP and lateral radiograph burst thoracolumbar fracture.

CANDIDATE: I will be honest, I don't know.

COMMENT: Under physiological load the spine is sufficiently stable to prevent significant pain, neurological deficit and progressive deformity.

EXAMINER: So, is this fracture stable?

CANDIDATE: At the thoracolumbar junction a fracture with this much loss of height is likely to become progressively kyphotic, so no, it is not stable.

EXAMINER: What is your management?

CANDIDATE: I would manage the patient according to ATLS principles. This will ensure optimal cord perfusion. This combined with maintenance of neutral spinal alignment aims to prevent secondary injury. There may be other treatment priorities identified, e.g. concurrent abdominal trauma. The initial aim is to prevent secondary injury by protecting (neutral spinal alignment) and perfusing (appropriate resuscitation) the cord.

A full neurological examination is undertaken, and the presence of sacral sparing documented (which is suggestive of a better prognosis). The neurological examination is repeated (frequently if a deficit is identified) in order to ascertain whether there is a progressive neurological deficit.

I would assess the patient for signs of neurogenic shock.

EXAMINER: Do you mean neurogenic shock?

CANDIDATE: Neurogenic shock is a loss of sympathetic tone. It is a *vascular* phenomenon. Typically, the patient will be hypotensive but bradycardic. It is important to exclude other causes of hypotension, however (10–15% of patients with spinal injuries have visceral injuries), before attributing hypotension to neurogenic shock.

EXAMINER: So, is this likely here?

CANDIDATE: The majority of sympathetic innervation has come off the cord before T12, so no. Spinal shock is possible. This is a *neurological* phenomenon. It is a temporary loss of spinal cord function and reflex activity below the level of the injury. It is typically characterized by diaphragmatic breathing (if cervical/high thoracic), paralysis, absent reflexes, erection, urinary retention and an absent bulbocavernosus reflex.

317

EXAMINER: What is the importance of spinal shock and how do you know when it's over?

CANDIDATE: The importance of spinal shock is that one cannot evaluate the neurologic deficit until the spinal shock phase has resolved. Resolution is determined by the return of the bulbocavernosus reflex – squeezing the glans penis elicits an anal sphincter contraction. It can also be performed by tugging the catheter, which is the best way to perform the assessment in a female.

EXAMINER: Is there any further imaging you would obtain?

CANDIDATE: A CT scan would be helpful to more fully assess fracture morphology.

EXAMINER: You have just told me the fracture is unstable, we are going to treat it as an unstable injury, so is a CT really needed, are you not just using up limited NHS resources?

COMMENT: This is testing higher-order judgement and the appropriate reasoning for use of musculoskeletal imaging.[3] The ICB place a lot of importance on these types of questions as they deal with the real-life world of NHS clinical practice rather than just reading facts from a book for an exam.

CANDIDATE: The majority of orthopaedic units would request a CT scan. Kyphotic and translation injuries can be visualized on sagittal and coronal reconstructions. The scan would demonstrate any degree of canal compromise. Vertebral body height, disc spaces, interpedicular distances and interspinous process intervals can be seen and compared between injured and the non-injured levels.

EXAMINER: Would an MRI not be better?

CANDIDATE: CT scans have a limited role in demonstrating associated soft-tissue injuries. An MRI scan is better at picking up disc herniations, epidural or subdural haematomas, ligamentous injuries and spinal cord parenchymal injury.

MRI and CT are complimentary imaging modalities that provide different information. In the absence of neurological deficit, it is usual to request a CT. I would request an MRI in addition if there is neurological deficit.

EXAMINER: So how would you manage this fracture?

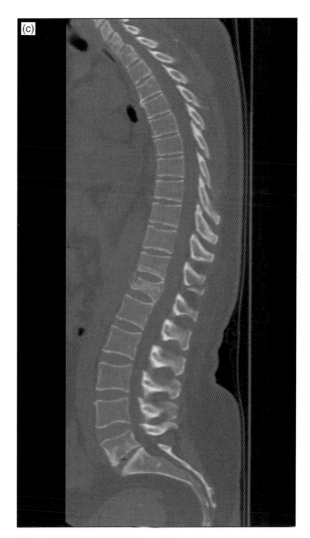

Figure 15.3c Sagittal CT T12 burst fracture.

CANDIDATE: The fracture is unstable. I would advocate posterior stabilization with pedicle screws and rods [1]. The fracture can be reduced using the principle of ligamentotaxis.

Key Points

Protecting the cord and perfusing the cord to prevent secondary injury are paramount. Lumbar burst fractures (L3–L5) without neurological deficit are usually treated conservatively. Lumbar burst fractures with neurological deficit are by definition unstable (see definition of stability above) and are treated surgically.

There is no general consensus on how to treat neurologically intact thoracolumbar burst fractures (T10–L2), which can be treated with extension orthoses or with surgery [2]. In the long term some progression of deformity and back pain is expected in neurologically intact patients despite adequate bracing; therefore, follow-up radiographs should be obtained at regular intervals to assess the angle of kyphosis and vertebra height loss.

References

1. Wood K, Butterman G, Garvey T, *et al.* Operative compared with non-operative treatment of a thoracolumbar burst fracture without neurological deficit. A prospective, randomized study. *J Bone Joint Surg Am.* 2003;5:773–781.

2. Siebenga J, Leferink VJM, Segers MJM, *et al.* Treatment of traumatic thoracolumbar spine fractures: a multicenter prospective randomized study of operative versus nonsurgical treatment. *Spine.* 2006;25:2881–2890.

Structured oral examination question 4

Odontoid peg fractures

Introduction

The management of type II odontoid fractures in the elderly is controversial for several reasons. The literature is unclear, with a lack of randomized control trials and high-quality literature.

There is supportive evidence of successful outcomes for both non-surgical and surgical management. With surgical stabilization there is a lack of agreement as to the optimal surgical procedure. There is uncertainty regarding the consequences of non-union, with some authors arguing that a stable fibrous union in an asymptomatic patient > 65 years is acceptable. However, for an independent active elderly patient there would be a risk of catastrophic neurological injury with subsequent falls or the late onset of a progressive myelopathy.

It would be expected that candidates should be able to describe radiographic features and discuss the Anderson and D'Alonzo classification system [3]. The score 6 material is being able to discuss the

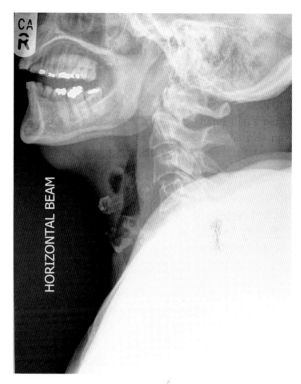

Figure 15.4a Lateral cervical spine radiograph demonstrating odontoid peg fracture.

pros and cons of the four possible separate treatment options available: (1) rigid and (2) non-rigid immobilization, (3) anterior screw fixation of the odontoid and (4) posterior fusion of the C1/2 motion segment.

EXAMINER: What does this X-ray (Figure 15.4a) show?

CANDIDATE: This is a lateral radiograph of the cervical spine. The most obvious abnormality is a fracture through the base of the odontoid peg (process) of C2 with posterior angulation. I would ideally like see an AP and odontoid peg (open mouth) view and obtain a CT scan.

EXAMINER: Yes, are you aware of any classification systems for this type of injury?

CANDIDATE: I am familiar with the Anderson and D'Alonzo classification. This classifies fractures according to their location within the peg. Type I fractures (< 5% cases) affect the tip of the odontoid and are caused by avulsion of the alar ligaments. They are rare. Type II injuries (> 60%) run through the base of the odontoid peg. They have a high ratio of cortical to cancellous bone and so

319

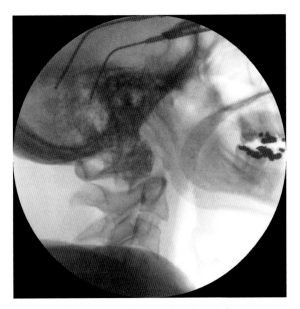

Figure 15.4b Image intensifier view, lateral cervical spine radiograph demonstrating odontoid peg fracture.

have a higher rate of non-union than other fractures. Type III injuries (30%) involve the vertebral body; they run through the metaphyseal bone of the vertebral body. As these fractures have a higher proportion of cancellous to cortical bone and a greater surface area they are more likely to heal than Type II injuries.

EXAMINER: So how does this classification guide your management?

CANDIDATE: Type I injuries, which are rare, are usually managed in an Aspen collar.

EXAMINER: Is this always the case?

CANDIDATE: Type I avulsion fractures can indicate occipito-cervical instability. If there were evidence of distraction on CT imaging occipito-cervical stabilization would be appropriate.

EXAMINER: And the other types?

CANDIDATE: Type III injuries are likely to heal and so I would treat them conservatively. Immobilization can be with a halo jacket or a hard collar. The complication rate and associated morbidity and mortality are high in patients over the age of 80 treated with a halo jacket so I would avoid them in this age group. Type II injuries are more likely to go on to non-union and so they are

the injuries for which I would consider fixation as an option as opposed to conservative treatment.

EXAMINER: So, do you normally operate on Type II peg fractures?

CANDIDATE: They usually occur on older patients (> 65) and so I would prefer to manage them non-operatively in an Aspen collar.

EXAMINER: Are there any factors with Type II injuries that would make it more likely that they would go on to non-union to guide your decision?

CANDIDATE: Yes. If there is more than 5–6 mm fracture displacement, if there is angulation > 10°, posterior displaced fractures (non-union rate > 70%), smokers, delay in diagnosis and patients over the age of 65. These all make it more likely that there will be a non-union and guide the decision towards surgery.

EXAMINER: What will you do if the patient finds the Aspen collar difficult to wear and he wants to take it off as it is too uncomfortable?

CANDIDATE: First, I would make sure the collar is the correct size and is fitted in the correct manner. If we still had difficulties I would arrange an early outpatient follow-up appointment by the spinal team to give further reassurance and assistance. If I was worried he was going to take the collar off I would counsel him that it would be very dangerous to do so and could result in paralysis or death [2].

EXAMINER: What are the surgical options for treatment of a Type II fracture?

CANDIDATE: The two options are posterior C1/C2 fusion (either Magerl transarticular screws or Harms C1 lateral mass/C2 pedicle screws) or direct anterior single- or double-screw osteosynthesis of the dens of C2 [4]. The benefit of C1/2 fusion is that it is a reliable operation that is not dependent on the fracture configuration, is biomechanically more secure but results in loss of rotation. The patient would need to be prone and dissection involves the risk of brisk bleeding from the C1/2 venous plexus or injury to the C2 nerve. Additionally there is risk of injury to the vertebral artery.

C2 osteosynthesis gives the benefit of retaining the rotational movement that occurs at the atlanto-axial joint but can cause airway or swallowing issues from local trauma due to the approach. With anterior screw fixation in the elderly, comminution at the fracture site and stiffness of the cervical spine can prevent ideal screw positioning, leading to a poor result.

EXAMINER: What factors would guide your choice of surgery?

CANDIDATE: If there is a fracture of the peg that courses from anterior inferior to posterior superior, parallel to the lag screw trajectory, then this will lead to poor fixation with a tendency to displacement. In this situation I would choose to perform a C1/2 fusion instead. Relative contraindications to screw fixation include large BMI, fracture older than 3 weeks or poor bone quality.

EXAMINER: Yes, let's move on.

Key Points

Type I odontoid peg fractures are rare. They are usually treated conservatively. Type III fractures generally heal and are also treated conservatively. Type II fractures in the young are treated with a halo jacket unless there are risk factors for non-union, when surgery is advocated.

Type II fractures in the elderly are usually treated with an aspen collar. The risks of surgery are significant and halo jacket treatment has a high complication rate including pin-site infections and loosening, skin breakdown, pneumonia or respiratory insufficiency, facet joint stiffness, and loss of spinal reduction. A number of elderly patients find Aspen collars uncomfortable to wear, made worse by the fact they need to be worn for several weeks.

Complications from surgery include postoperative haematoma, dysphagia, hoarseness, damage to the vertebral artery, and neural injuries.

Complications of non-operative treatment include the risk of non-union, catastrophic neurological injury with subsequent falls or late-onset progressive myelopathy.

Progressive myelopathic changes may occur in patients who develop a non-union. However, a stable pseudarthrosis is often adequate in the elderly low-demand patient and late translation is unusual.

Many elderly patients have significant comorbidities so the risk of catastrophic neurological injury with non-operative treatment is less than the morbidity and mortality associated with surgery.

Table 15.1 Anderson and D'Alonzo classification of peg fractures according to fracture location.

- Type I – Avulsion fracture of the tip of the dens
- Type II – Fracture between the base of the transverse ligament and the body of the vertebrae
- Type III – Fracture running through the body of the vertebrae

References

1. Koivikko MP, Kiuru MJ, Koskinen SK, Myllynen P, Santavirta S, Kivisaari L. Factors associated with non-union in conservatively treated type II fractures of the odontoid process. *J Bone Joint Surg Br.* 2004;86(8):1146–1151.

2. Kuntz CIV, Mirza SK, Jarell AD, Chapmen JR, Shaffrey CI, Newell DW. Type II odontoid fractures in the elderly: early failure of non-surgical management. *Neurosurg Focus.* 2000;8(6):e7.

3. Anderson LD, D'Alonzo RT. Fractures of the odontoid process of the axis. *J Bone Joint Surg Am.* 1974;56:1663–1674.

4. Grauer JN, Shafi B, Hilibrand AS, *et al.* Proposal of a modified, treatment-oriented classification of odontoid fractures. *Spine J.* 2005;5:123–129.

Structured oral examination question 5

Hangman's fracture

EXAMINER: What does this X-ray (Figure 15.5) show?

CANDIDATE: It is a lateral radiograph of the cervical spine. The most obvious abnormality is an anterior subluxation of C2 on C3.

EXAMINER: Do you know what we call this fracture?

CANDIDATE: It is a traumatic spondylolisthesis of C2, also known as a hangman's fracture.

EXAMINER: What is the mechanism of injury?

CANDIDATE: The injury usually occurs due to rapid deceleration in a motor vehicle accident when the patient is thrown forward with the head striking the windscreen. The accident is usually a head-on collision with another vehicle or with a fixed object such as a lamppost. It is a hyperextension injury.

EXAMINER: How do these fractures present?

CANDIDATE: It is relatively unusual for these fractures to present with a neurological deficit unless

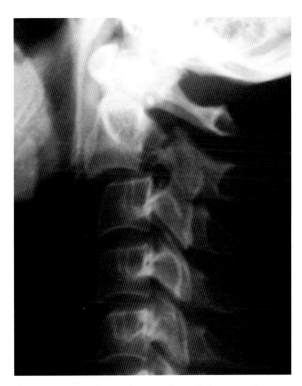

Figure 15.5 Lateral cervical spine radiograph demonstrating hangman's fracture.

there has been gross displacement due to the large diameter of the spinal canal at this level.

EXAMINER: Do you know any classification systems for this injury?

CANDIDATE: Yes, I am aware of the Levine classification. It grades the injury as Type I with bilateral pars interarticularis fractures and no displacement. Type II injuries involve anterior translation (Type II) or significant angulation and widening of the disc space posteriorly indicating an intervertebral disc injury (Type IIA). Type III injuries also involve C2/3 facet joint dislocation.

EXAMINER: Did you say Levine?

CANDIDATE: Yes.

EXAMINER: It was originally described by Effendi, whose classification system was revised as you describe by Levine and Edwards.

How would you manage a patient with a hangman's fracture?

CANDIDATE: Levine and Edwards suggest in their paper that Type I injuries are essentially stable due

to the intact ligamentous restraints (principally C2/3 disc) and are likely to heal with external immobilization in a hard collar.

Type II fractures have an intact anterior longitudinal ligament. They can be treated in a halo jacket. If there is a failure to reduce the fracture or maintain the reduction, then stabilization will be required.

The Type IIA fracture more commonly involves an injury to the disc. They are treated with immobilization, often with a halo jacket or stabilized surgically.

Type III fractures are inherently unstable and require urgent reduction of the facet dislocation. These are very unstable injuries and the majority will require early fixation.

Key Points

There has been much debate over management of these fractures over the years with no clear management that is shown to be appropriate for all cases. Levine and Edwards put forward their management protocol as described above. This has had support from the literature.

Two reviews that have been published regarding the management of these fractures have similar ideas [1,2]. These reviews support the use of external immobilization for Type I and II fractures, requiring only a rigid hard neck collar for Type I and some stable Type II fractures.

Types IIA and III fractures are much more unstable than the first two types. If they can be adequately reduced and held with a rigid external orthosis, then they may be managed non-operatively and closely monitored. Otherwise these injuries require stabilization (C2 direct osteosynthesis – transpedicular screw fixation). If the C2/3 disc integrity is compromised, C2/3 fusion is required, which can be done anteriorly with a discectomy and bone graft (or posteriorly).

References

1. Li XF, Dai LY, Lu H, Chen XD. A systematic review of the management of hangman's fractures. *Eur Spine J.* 2006;15(3):257–269.

2. Greene KA, Dickman CA, Marciano FF, Drabier JB, Hadley MN, Sonntag VK. Acute axis fractures: analysis of management and outcome in 340 consecutive cases. *Spine.* 1997;22(16):1843–1852.

Structured oral examination question 6

Chance fractures

Chance type fractures of the thoracolumbar junction are becoming increasingly common, with seat belts increasing survival from high-speed road traffic collisions. They account for approximately 15% of all thoracolumbar injuries and are most commonly seen at the thoracolumbar junction.

EXAMINER: What does this picture show (Figure 15.6a)?

CANDIDATE: This is a clinical photograph of a lady's abdomen. There is gross bruising in a horizontal configuration across the lower anterior abdominal wall.

EXAMINER: What do you think has happened to her?

CANDIDATE: I would imagine that she has been involved in an RTC restrained by a seat belt.

EXAMINER: Yes, that's right. So how would you assess this lady in the emergency department?

CANDIDATE: I would follow ATLS principles and identify and treat any immediately life-threatening injuries (primary survey) and then any potentially life-threatening or limb-threatening injuries (secondary survey).

EXAMINER [interrupting]: Yes, all right, but what injuries would you expect to find?

CANDIDATE: I would expect this lady to have intra-abdominal injuries due to the blunt trauma. With this mechanism, which is flexion distraction, I would suspect a transverse bicolumn injury that is either bony (Chance fracture) or soft-tissue type injury. I would want to examine the patient neurologically and would need to consider non-contiguous injuries.

EXAMINER: Tell me about Chance fractures (Figure 15.6b).

CANDIDATE: These are flexion–distraction injuries affecting the thoracolumbar spine. It involves an injury to both the anterior and posterior columns (B-type injury according to the AO classification system) [1]. It can be purely bony, which is a Chance fracture, purely ligamentous or mixed. Typically, the anterior column fails in compression whereas the posterior columns fail in tension.

EXAMINER: So how would you investigate this person in the Emergency department?

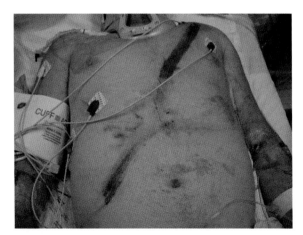

Figure 15.6a Clinical photograph demonstrating gross abdominal bruising.

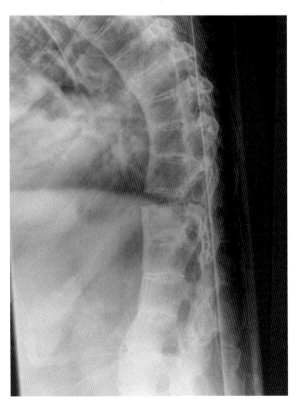

Figure 15.6b Lateral radiograph of thoracic spine demonstrating Chance fracture.

CANDIDATE: The patient would often have a trauma CT scan that will include the injured spine. This can be reformatted in the sagittal and coronal planes to quantify the injury. It is important to ensure the whole spine has been imaged to rule out non-contiguous injuries.

EXAMINER: What would you expect to see?

CANDIDATE: If there was a bony injury then you could see the pattern of the fracture running through the vertebral body and the posterior elements. If it was a ligamentous injury, then there may be some widening of the interspinous space.

EXAMINER: Would you do any further investigations?

CANDIDATE: If there was no bony injury and I suspected a flexion–distraction type injury (or AO B-type injury) then I would also request an MRI scan to assess the integrity of the posterior ligamentous complex (PLC) [2,3].

EXAMINER: How would you manage these injuries?

CANDIDATE: If the patient was neurologically normal and there was no displacement this could be managed non-operatively. If it was a bony injury, it would be managed in a brace and would be monitored very closely. These fractures are often managed operatively to prevent progressive displacement and deformity and to allow the patient to return to normal function faster.

EXAMINER: What if this was a soft-tissue Chance, i.e. a ligamentous flexion–distraction injury?

CANDIDATE: These heal less reliably so would require surgical management with a posterior construct to recreate the tension band [4].

EXAMINER: What if they were to have a complete injury? Is there a role for surgery then?

CANDIDATE: The role of surgery in a complete spinal cord injury is to facilitate rehabilitation by providing a stable and pain-free spine.

EXAMINER: Would you use steroids?

CANDIDATE: There is no convincing evidence that steroids make any difference to the outcome of spinal cord injury. They do cause potential problems, e.g. gastrointestinal ulceration. They are not used in my institution.

EXAMINER: OK, let's move on.

Spinal injuries can be classified by a number of different systems. The AO system identifies two columns. The anterior column includes the vertebral bodies, intervertebral discs and the anterior and posterior longitudinal ligaments, while the posterior column includes the neural arch and the posterior elements. There are three different mechanisms of injury. A-type injuries (compression) may be unstable, B-type injuries (flexion–distraction or hyperextension) are often unstable and C-type injuries (translation or rotation) are always unstable.

Associated injuries

As well as there being a need for awareness regarding diagnosis of the soft tissue element of these injuries, intra-abdominal injuries are extremely common. They have been seen on 40% of scans in a recent study and must be actively sought out at the time of presentation. This can be a classic exam question posed in a number of different ways. You could be presented a picture of a seat-belt contusion and asked about likely injuries. It could also be shown as a treated Chance fracture with a delayed deterioration from a perforated viscus. Alternatively, the surgeons may have identified the intra-abdominal injury but failed to recognize the association with spinal injuries.

The other injury that must be assessed for is neurology. These injuries commonly occur at the thoracolumbar junction in the region of the conus. Any neurological deficit or worsening neurological function is an indication for surgery.

Management

The management of these injuries largely depends on the pattern of the injury and associated injuries from the patient. If we treat the spinal injury in isolation, worsening neurological function requires stabilization and decompression. Bony injuries may heal if they can be reduced and adequately held in an extension brace but will require close monitoring. Those which have soft-tissue injuries alone are unlikely to heal without stabilization procedures due to the poor healing potential of ligamentous structures. There are, however, advocates of operating on all Chance fractures due to the unstable nature of the fracture and the vast improvements in surgical instrumentation. They believe that pedicle screw constructs can restore the posterior tension band and allow earlier, more reliable mobilization. However, this remains controversial, and there is clearly a role for non-operative management in select patients.

References

1. Chapman JR, Agel J, Jurkovich GJ, Bellabarba C. Thoracolumbar flexion–distraction injuries: associated morbidity and neurological outcomes. *Spine*. 2008;33 (6):648–657.

2. Groves CJ, Cassar-Pullicino VN, Tins BJ, Tyrrell PN, McCall IW. Chance-type flexion–distraction injuries in the thoracolumbar spine: MR imaging characteristics. *Radiology*. 2005;236(2):601–608.

3. Bernstein MP, Mirvis SE, Shanmuganathan K. Chance-type fractures of the thoracolumbar spine: imaging analysis in 53 patients. *AJR Am J Roentgenol*. 2006;187 (4):859–868.

4. Ramieri A, Domenicucci M, Cellocco P, Raco A, Costanzo G. Effectiveness of posterior tension band fixation in the thoracolumbar seat-belt type injuries of the young population. *Eur Spine J*. 2009;18(Suppl 1):89–94.

Structured oral examination question 7

Incomplete spinal injury

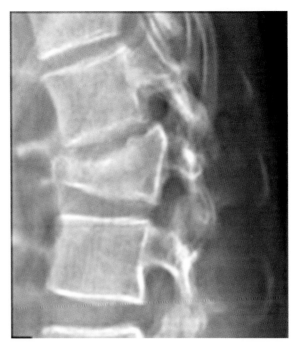

Figure 15.7 Thoracolumbar injury.

EXAMINER: We have a young girl who was paragliding and fell down around 20 meters sustaining a high-energy injury. This is her vertebral fracture at the thoracolumbar junction.

No other injuries, isolated unstable injury.

Physical examination is ASIA C.

CANDIDATE: This is an incomplete spinal injury with a neurological lesion.

COMMENT: A person is ASIA C if they have any preserved motor function below the neurological level, but more than half of the key muscles have a muscle grade of 3 or less.

EXAMINER: How will you manage this injury?

CANDIDATE: I would want to get an MRI.

COMMENT: 'No other injuries, isolated unstable injury' is coded language for no ATLS chitchat, as this will not score you any marks. Although this is a high-energy injury the examiners want you to concentrate on the injury only as otherwise you will waste viva scoring opportunities.

Perfuse the spine; prevent secondary cord injury, urinary catheterization, IV fluids, etc. Thorough inspection of the spine should be performed after a careful log-roll manoeuvre to look for abrasions, tenderness, local kyphosis and a palpable gap in between spinous processes. Perform a thorough neurological assessment that follows standard American Spinal Injury Association (ASIA) guidelines and record this in the patient's notes.

An MRI will be needed, but the patient needs to be first evaluated following the basic principles of trauma assessment. Candidates will score 4 (poor fail), as they need to resuscitate and stabilize the patient first and before thinking about obtaining scans.

EXAMINER: How do you classify these thoracolumbar fractures?

CANDIDATE: There are some stable fractures and some that are unstable.

COMMENT: The Thoracolumbar Injury Classification and Severity (TLICS) Scale is a guideline for the management of thoracolumbar injuries. It is a composite scoring system based on three injury components: (1) integrity of the posterior ligamentous complex, (2) radiographic injury morphology, and (3) neurological status of the patient.

Other systems include modified *AO classification*.

Type A: Compression injuries.

Type B: Distraction injuries.

Type C: Displacement or dislocation.
Each type then has further subtypes.

EXAMINER: What are the goals of surgery. What are you trying to achieve?

CANDIDATE: You would want to stabilize the fracture and decompress the neural elements either directly or indirectly, usually indirectly.

EXAMINER: Regarding medical treatment, do you think these patients would benefit from using steroids?

CANDIDATE: Yes, I would give steroids.

EXAMINER: Do you think there is clear evidence, literature evidence? Where is the controversy?

CANDIDATE: [. . . Silence]

EXAMINER: You don't know.
    Where is the controversy?
    Do you think there is a controversy (leading question)?
    Are you using steroids in your place (institution)?

CANDIDATE: Yes [. . . long silence]

EXAMINER: OK. This is a 37-year-old woman who . . .
    [Candidate debrief]

COMMENT: Where can we begin? The candidate was having a bad viva for whatever reason and would have scored a 4.

The candidate should have known the arguments for and against steroid use much better. A specific direct question on the use of steroids. If you cannot answer this, you are down to a 6.

Key Points

It is generally accepted that the spine has two columns, anterior to resist compression and posterior a tension band. Counting the number of columns injured to determine stability can be misleading. A lumbar burst fracture is a single-column injury (lamina split if present not considered significant) and may be unstable, requiring fixation. An undisplaced Chance fracture (two-column injury) may be treated conservatively if felt to be suitably stable. The 'column concept' helps to guide treatment: is my anterior column competent – if not how do I make it so? Is my posterior tension band intact? If not, I need to address this.

Reference

Sethi MK, Schoenfeld AJ, Bono CM, Harris MB. The evolution of thoracolumbar injury classification systems. *Spine J.* 2009;9(9):780–788.

Structured oral examination question 8

Application of a halo

EXAMINER: How do you apply a halo?

CANDIDATE: My indications for applying a halo would be:
- Temporary or definitive stabilization following cervical spine trauma.
- Need for additional postoperative external stabilization.
- Paediatric trauma patient [1].

EXAMINER: I asked how you apply a halo, not indications.[4]

CANDIDATE: I would first explain to the patient what I am going to do and why.
    I would choose the appropriate halo ring size by measuring the skull circumference. The halo ring must provide 1–2 cm clearance circumference around the head. It is preferable to be constructed of graphite/titanium to be MRI-compatible.

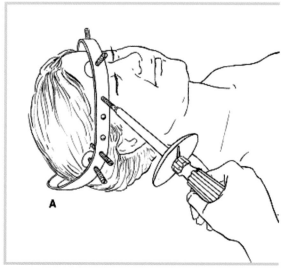

A

Figure 15.8 Halo traction.

Typically, three people are required to apply a halo, with one person maintaining alignment and the remaining two applying the halo.

After antiseptic preparation and using local anaesthetic infiltration to the scalp, four pins are applied to the adult skull (eight in the paediatric population) and tightened with a torque-limiter (8 inch-pounds; 2–4 inch-pounds in the paediatric skull).

The pins are placed equidistant and symmetrically in order to allow for stability of the construct.

Care should be taken to prevent damage to important structures: the superficial temporal artery and vein, the supraorbital nerves and the sinuses.

The anterior pins are placed 1 cm above the lateral one-third of the eyebrow (supraorbital ridge) *with the eyes tightly closed*. This is lateral to the supraorbital nerve [2].

EXAMINER: Why should the patient close their eyes?

CANDIDATE: If not, the periorbital tissues may be tented and limit eye closure.

The posterior pins are placed 1 cm above the ear.

Pins are advanced through the skin (without an incision) perpendicular to the skull.

Skin release around the pin sites may be needed to avoid tenting.

An appropriately sized jacket is then applied (or traction as may be necessary).

A radiograph is obtained to ensure correct reduction. Radiographs are required at regular intervals to ensure reduction is maintained.

The patient should be instructed to return at 24–48 hours to have the pins retightened and should be educated on pin hygiene.

EXAMINER: How do you ensure correct pin placement and why is it important?

CANDIDATE: Correct pin placement relies on an appreciation of relevant surgical anatomy and attention to detail. Correct pin placement is important to minimize the risks of direct neural or vascular injury, inner calvarial penetration and pin migration while providing adequate strength of fixation [3].

EXAMINER: What are the potential complications?

CANDIDATE: Loss of position or reduction, pin-site infection and loosening, pain, nerve (sixth cranial nerve[5]) or vessel injury. One-fifth of patients also complain of pain, which can be managed by loosening. Pressure sores. Restricted ventilation and pneumonia (elderly). Dysphagia due to over-extension of the neck. Rarely there is a complication of dural puncture (1%).

Protocols have been developed for managing pin-site infections. Pin-site care twice daily. Inspection for crusting, redness, drainage or swelling.

COMMENT: A halo vest provides the best immobilization of the cervical spine of all external immobilization methods. In children a proper fit with a prefabricated halo vest is seldom achieved and the use of a custom moulded halo vest is a better option.

References

1. Bono CM. The halo fixator. *J Am Acad Orthop Surg.* 2007;15(12):728–737.

2. Botte MJ, Byrne TP, Abrams RA, *et al.* Halo skeletal fixation: techniques of application and prevention of complications. *J Am Acad Orthop Surg.* 1996;4:44–53.

3. Garfin SR, Botte MJ, Waters RL, *et al.* Complications in the use of the halo fixation device. *J Bone Joint Surg Am.* 1986;68:320–325.

Structured oral examination question 9

Cauda equina syndrome

EXAMINER: You review a 42-year-old lady in your elective spinal clinic. She attends with her three children. She was referred by her own GP with troublesome unilateral L5 radicular symptoms. She briefly mentioned that she had a single episode of urinary incontinence. Does this worry you?

CANDIDATE: I would be worried with her presentation of a single episode of urinary incontinence with unilateral L5 radicular symptoms. However, I would like to take a detailed history and clinical examination of this patient. I would like to know the chronicity of the unilateral leg pain, its distribution, treatment and medications to date, any previous imaging, aggravating and relieving factors. I would also like to know more of the episode of urinary incontinence, such as urge or stress incontinence, the timing from it happening to her presentation to clinic and whether she's able to feel

327

when voiding. I would also like to know about her obstetrics and gynaecology history. Clinical examination would involve palpating the abdomen for a distended bladder and would include a per rectum examination testing for perianal sensation and the presence of voluntary sphincter contraction. Clinical examination also includes tests for both lower limb power, reflexes and sensation.

EXAMINER: This does not sound like a dramatic presentation, but what is your concern?

CANDIDATE: I am concerned about cauda equina syndrome based on her clinical presentation. That's the reason I would like to take a detailed history and clinical examination. I would have a low threshold to arrange for an urgent MRI for this patient if the history is potentially consistent with cauda equina syndrome provided she has no contraindications for MRI scan. I would keep the patient nil by mouth and admit her to the ward for monitoring of neurological progression until the MRI is done.

EXAMINER: I had an MRI scan report on my desk yesterday reporting cauda equina compression in a patient who is 75 years old with spinal stenosis. Do I need to act urgently?

CANDIDATE: Spinal claudication due to spinal stenosis is a slowly progressive compression of the cauda equina over a long period of time. The pathology is different, and the sacral roots usually accommodate so the patients have cauda equina compression but not cauda equina syndrome. It is the syndrome which requires urgent attention. However, I would bring the patient back to the next available review clinic for further clinical evaluation as the patient may benefit from early decompression of spinal stenosis if he remains symptomatic.

EXAMINER: Tell me more of cauda equina syndrome (CES).

CANDIDATE: Cauda equina syndrome is typically bilateral radiculopathy with reduced perineal sensation (S3–S5 dermatomes), disturbance of bladder and/or bowel and/or sexual function. The potential for permanent bowel and bladder dysfunction as well as sexual dysfunction contributes to the associated psychosocial distress and enhanced medicolegal profile of this condition. It often presents on a spectrum between simple

radiculopathy with no bladder, bowel or perineal sensory symptoms and CES with the full complement of symptoms. The nearer it is to the simple end of the spectrum, the more suspicion required to identify it.

The pathophysiology of CES includes compression of the cauda equina within the lumbosacral region [1]. The causes can be divided into:
- Traumatic: disc herniation, epidural haematoma, retropulsion from bony fragment.
- Tumours: intramedullary or extramedullary.
- Infective: epidural abscess.
- Degenerative: spinal stenosis.

EXAMINER: Do you know the subtypes of CES?

CANDIDATE: Subtypes of CES include:

CES incomplete (CESI): patient has objective evidence of CES – commonly impaired perineal sensation and some parasympathetic disturbance. They have preserved voluntary control of initiating and stopping micturition and bowel emptying but may exhibit some degree of disturbance (for example, might need to strain heavily or manually contribute pressure to aid emptying of the bladder).

CES with retention (CESR): patient has a paralyzed, insensate bladder with painless urinary retention. This progresses to urinary incontinence secondary to overfilling. However, it is important to note that there may not be complete loss of cauda equina function.

EXAMINER: You managed to arrange an urgent MRI of lumbosacral spine after discussing with the radiologist on call. The radiologist phoned you at 5 pm and reported that the MRI scan showed radiological evidence of caudal equina syndrome. What would you do now?

CANDIDATE: As the patient has been admitted and kept nil by mouth, I would go to the ward, re-examine the patient and discuss the diagnosis with her. I would explain to her that this requires emergent decompression; this is conventionally with a generous midline decompression and discectomy. The operation should be carried out on an emergency basis within 48 hours of symptom onset [2]. It should be done as soon as it is practically safe to do so to prevent further complications such as bowel and/or bladder and/or sexual dysfunction. I would aim to operate within the same evening after the diagnosis has been made provided it's safe to proceed. Meta-analysis has shown that the patient has better outcome in terms of bladder and bowel function if decompression surgery is performed within 48 hours of symptom onset.

EXAMINER: How would you perform a decompression for cauda equina syndrome?

CANDIDATE: The patient will be positioned prone for this procedure with particular attention being paid to the airway and access to surgical site. I would use the image intensifier in theatre to identify the level of decompression after prepping the patient. I would approach the lumbar spine through posterior midline approach utilizing the internervous plane between two paraspinal muscles (erector spinae). After dissecting superficially through the fat and fascia, I would elevate the erector spinae muscle subperiosteally and continue dissecting down to lamina. Deep dissection involves performing a laminotomy of the proximal lamina until lamina has been resected above the ligamentum flavum insertion on its underside. The ligamentum flavum is then resected from proximal to distal before the laminotomy of the distal lamina is performed by undercutting it. When the decompression is full width the lateral edge of the dura is identified, and the nerve root can be retracted to access the disc and remove it. Some literature suggests laminectomy for CES while other literature highlights no clear evidence to support one single strategy and decompression can be tailored to the disc level. The strategy is to ensure adequate decompression of the cauda equina at the end of the operation.

EXAMINER: What are the complications of the operation?

CANDIDATE: The complications of this operation can be divided into local or general.

Local complications: damage to dura, nerve roots and incomplete decompression.

General complications: deep vein thrombosis, pulmonary embolism, loss of airway during operation, stroke and myocardial infarction.

MARKING
4: urinary frequency, bilateral sciatica.
5: Hx +Exam.
6: MRI findings.
7: decompression.
8: literature.

References

1. Ahn UM, Ahn NU, Buchowski JM, Garrett ES, Sieber AN, Kostuik JP. Cauda equina syndrome secondary to lumbar disc herniation – a meta-analysis of surgical outcomes. *Spine*. 2000;25(12):1515–1522.

2. Gleave JRW, Macfarlane R. Cauda equina syndrome: what is the relationship between timing of surgery and outcome? *Br J Neurosurg*. 2002;16(4):325–328.

Structured oral examination question 10

Spinal trauma assessment

EXAMINER: You are asked to review a patient with suspected spinal injury after a high-speed road traffic accident. The patient was stabilized in the Emergency department resuscitation bay but has persistent hypotension. What are your thoughts?

CANDIDATE: I have high suspicion of spinal injury in this patient who has been involved in a high-speed road traffic accident. The hypotension is likely hypovolaemic shock secondary to blood loss, which is the most common after such an injury. I would assess the patient as with any other patient using the Advanced Trauma Life Support (ATLS) principles. The patient should have a patent and safe airway with in-line triple immobilization of cervical spine using hard collar, blocks and tape. The ATLS principles would then move on to breathing, circulation, disability and exposure. Once life-threatening injuries are excluded, I would then proceed to secondary survey to look for any other associated injuries.

EXAMINER: You suspected spinal injury in this patient. How are you going to assess this patient?

CANDIDATE: Assuming ATLS principles have been applied in the initial management of this patient and life-threatening injuries have been excluded, I would proceed to assess the cervical, thoracic and lumbar spine. I would like to take a detailed history and examination from the patient. I would like to know the mechanism of injury, allergies, medications, past medical history and when the patient last ate. The patient needs to be log-rolled with full protection of the cervical spine during clinical examination of the thoracolumbar spine looking for swelling, bruising, deformity and focal

Patient Name _____

Examiner Name _____ Date/Time of Exam_____

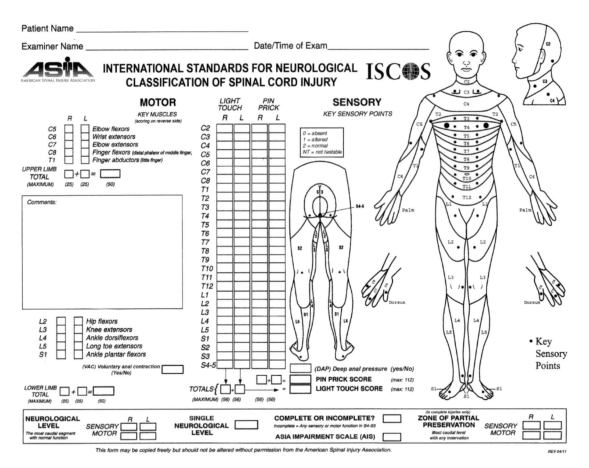

Figure 15.9 ASIA chart.

---

pain on palpation of the thoracolumbar spine, which may indicate posterior spinal column injury. I would also perform per rectum examination while the patient is being log-rolled to assess for perianal sensation and anal tone. The cervical spine is then examined with in-line immobilization looking for tenderness and deformity on palpation. I would complete the examination by performing a complete neurological examination of each dermatome and myotome using the American Spinal Injury Association (ASIA) chart (Figure 15.9) [1]. Assessment of the neurological status of the patient would need repeating frequently to monitor for any deterioration in neurological status that would require immediate intervention.

EXAMINER: What investigations would you request?

CANDIDATE: I would like to have a computed tomography scan of the cervical, thoracic and lumbar spine. However, I assume that this patient would have had a complete body CT scan performed as major trauma protocol. Reformat in three planes of the cervical, thoracic and lumbar spine would be available for viewing as part of the whole-body CT scan and early report by the duty radiologist would influence the initial management of this patient. This is now a routine practice in all major trauma centres in the UK.

EXAMINER: What do you understand by the term neurogenic shock?

CANDIDATE: Neurogenic shock occurs due to disruption of the sympathetic pathways in the spinal cord with resultant peripheral vasodilation, a decrease in peripheral vascular resistance and drop in blood pressure. Depending on the level of the spinal cord injury there may also be bradycardia present due to loss of sympathetic cardiac innervation. Patients are often warm. This contrasts with hypotension due to hypovolaemic shock in which the patient is shut down, clammy and tachycardic. Often neurogenic and hypovolaemic shock can co-exist and when dealing with a trauma patient one must always assume that any hypotension is due to blood loss.

EXAMINER: What do you understand by the term spinal shock?

CANDIDATE: Spinal shock is a neurological phenomenon. It is a temporary loss of spinal cord function and reflex activity below the level of the injury. It is typically characterized by diaphragmatic breathing (if cervical/high thoracic), paralysis, absent reflexes, erection, urinary retention and an absent bulbocavernosus reflex.

EXAMINER: What is the importance of spinal shock and how do you know when it's over?

CANDIDATE: The importance of spinal shock is that one cannot evaluate the neurologic deficit until the spinal shock phase has resolved. Resolution is determined by the return of the bulbocavernosus reflex – squeezing the glans penis elicits an anal sphincter contraction. It can also be performed by tugging the catheter, which is the best way to perform the assessment in a female.

EXAMINER: So, what are you going to do with this spinal problem?

CANDIDATE: The management depends upon spinal stability. If the spine is sufficiently stable under physiological load to resist deformity, with no significant pain and neurological deficit, the injury is considered stable and can be managed conservatively; 10% of spinal fractures will have non-contiguous injuries elsewhere, so these need to be excluded with imaging.

EXAMINER: How will you decide if it is stable?

CANDIDATE: This is decided by recognizing patterns of injury. Those insignificant, e.g. isolated transverse process, fractures require no further treatment. If it is not clear, then further information may be required, e.g. a standing X-ray to see if there is progressive collapse which would justify surgical treatment. Clearly unstable fractures, e.g. rotational or translation injuries, are likely to require surgical management. This decision should be made by someone with appropriate experience in spinal injury, such as the spinal surgeon.

Reference

1. Dodwad SN, Dodwad SJ, Wisneski R, Khan SN. Retrospective analysis of thoracolumbar junction injuries using the thoracolumbar injury severity and classification score, American Spinal Injury Association class, injury severity score, age, sex, and length of hospitalization. *Clin Spine Surg.* 2015;28(7): E410–416.

Notes

1. The candidate is stuck in the A&E department and can't get to theatre for the surgery.

2. Haematomyelia haemorrhage centrally causing mass effect on MRI imaging.

3. Vaccaro AR, Kim DH, Brodke DS, *et al.* Diagnosis and management of thoracolumbar spine fractures. *J Bone Joint Surg.* 2003;85(12):2456–2470.

4. There are no absolutes and we think it is at least worth trying to sneak these in.

5. Abducens nerve responsible for causing contraction of the lateral rectus muscle to abduct (i.e. turn out) the eye.

Chapter 16

Paediatric trauma

John Davies and Clare Carpenter

Structured oral examination question 1

EXAMINER: This 10-year-old boy was hit by a car while crossing the road and sustained a closed head injury with GCS 8/15. He has been intubated because he is combative. A secondary survey has revealed this associated limb injury (Figure 16.1).

CANDIDATE: I can see a shoulder trauma series with an AP and an attempted shoot-through or trans-scapular view. It's not quite a lateral Y-view I'm suspecting as the radiographer couldn't get the correct projection. There's a transverse fracture of the metaphysis, which is angulated medially due to the pull of the pectoralis major. If he was conscious I would specifically look at the axillary nerve function. I'd also document the vascular status of the arm.

EXAMINER: Assume that there is no associated neurovascular deficit. How are you going to manage this patient?

CANDIDATE: My concern is that the fracture fragments are completely translated with no bony contact and the distal fragment is being pulled medially into the axilla. As he has a closed head injury of unknown prognosis, he may not be able to be nursed upright for some time. I would consider surgical intervention in this child for ease of nursing.

When the child was stable, I would plan to take him to theatre after appropriately counselling the parents, marking the child and the WHO checklist. I would screen with the image intensifier to

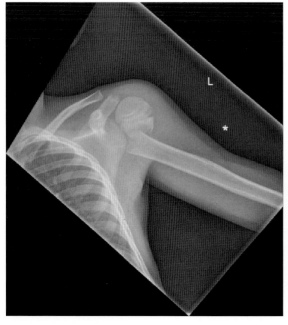
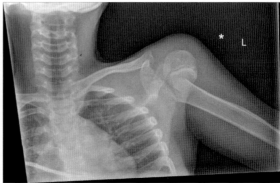

Figure 16.1a and 16.1b Displaced proximal humerus fracture.

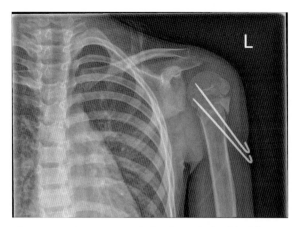

Figure 16.1c Anteroposterior (AP) radiograph, shoulder following K-wire fixation.

check the shoulder is in joint and realign the fracture with gentle traction.

EXAMINER: What if it doesn't reduce closed?

CANDIDATE: I would ask the anaesthetist to give muscle relaxant for the MUA. If the fracture doesn't reduce closed I would do a limited open reduction through a deltopectoral approach (internervous plane: axillary and the medial and lateral pectoral nerves). In terms of the fracture, I would stabilize this with retrograde K-wires from the lateral side through a mini-incision. The long head of the biceps can sometimes get interposed in the fracture, blocking reduction.

The major structure at risk from percutaneous K-wires is the axillary nerve. Its surface landmark is 5 cm from the lateral edge of the acromion. The nerve is a branch of the posterior cord, and travels through the quadrangular space with the posterior circumflex vessels before going anterior around the surgical neck, underneath the deltoid.

EXAMINER: What do you think about this postop radiograph (Figure 16.1c)? I thought these fractures were usually managed conservatively?

CANDIDATE: I can see the fracture is reduced and held with K-wires from the lateral side obliquely into the medial metaphysis. One of them is crossing the growth plate, and on this view, there's no penetration of the surface of the head. The reduction is in slight varus, but overall, it's well aligned. I would be careful about allowing the patient to mobilize before the wires come out at 4 weeks; I'd anticipate there might be limited hold

in the metaphysis. Taking the wires out will need another GA as they are threaded, and you could screen it at the time to check it was united.

For proximal humerus fractures in young children, almost any level of deformity is acceptable, for instance, bayonet apposition, as the remodelling potential is so great. Typically, these are managed conservatively in a sling for a short time.

In children older than 13 with little growth remaining there is an argument for accepting less deformity, such as < 30° angulation or < 50% translation, although there's no consensus in the literature about what level of deformity is an absolute indication for fixation, and there is a higher incidence of stiffness compared to patients treated non-operatively [1].

Structured oral examination question 2

EXAMINER: This 7-year-old child fell from swings in the park sustaining a closed injury (Figure 16.2a and 16.2b).

CANDIDATE: I can see AP and lateral radiographic views of the left elbow. I'm assuming this is an isolated injury and I would like to get additional views of the wrist. My initial priority is to assess the neurovascular status and splint the limb. This is a Monteggia injury where there is a displaced and volarly angulated ulna fracture in addition to an anterior dislocated radial head.

EXAMINER: Let's assume there is available time to do this on the trauma list and you are taking the child to theatre. What are the principles of treating this injury? What would be your surgical plan?

CANDIDATE: By restoring the ulna length this should reduce the radial head. I would initially attempt a closed reduction by traction. If length, alignment and rotation were correct and with restoration of the radiocapitellar alignment, I would stabilize the ulna with an elastic nail. If I had any doubts about the reduction, I would plate it.

EXAMINER: How do you perform an elastic nailing? What problems do you anticipate arising if you try to use a nail for this?

CANDIDATE: Patient is positioned supine, arm board, bipolar (diathermy), tourniquet and

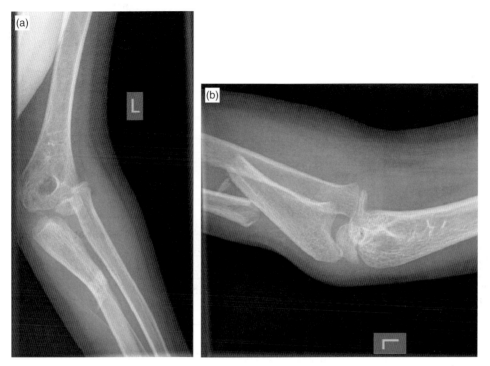

Figure 16.2a and 16.2b Anteroposterior (AP) and lateral radiographs, left elbow.

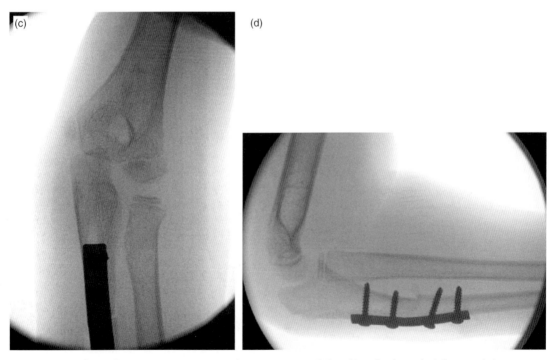

Figure 16.2c and 16.2d Intraoperative image intensifier anteroposterior (AP) and lateral radiographs, left proximal ulna.

image intensifier screen positioned within unrestricted view.

Initially I'd screen (with the image intensifier) and mark the physis and the fracture with a skin marker. The nail is sized according to one-third diameter of the isthmus. By prebending, the nail has elastic recoil, which exerts a force in the intramedullary canal to reduce the fracture.

Elastic nails are best suited to diaphyseal fractures. This is metaphyseal and near the entry point for the nail, so I'd have a low threshold for open reduction and plate fixation with a one-third tubular plate or LCP.

EXAMINER: Let's say the nail doesn't work. Even when you plate the ulna, the radial head does not reduce. What do you do?

CANDIDATE: I'd recheck I had properly reduced the fracture. In some cases, the ulna is plastically deformed, so you have to osteotomize it, but I don't think that's happening here.

In this case I would suspect that the annular ligament is either torn or interposed, blocking reduction of the radial head.

I'd open the radiocapitellar joint via a Kocher's approach (between the anconeus and ECU). It is possible to reconstruct the annular ligament with a fascial sling. This fascia can be obtained from a number of sites within the upper limb, e.g. triceps fascia.

Structured oral examination question 3

EXAMINER: This 6-year-old child is a new referral to the fracture clinic, please look at and describe these radiographs (Figures 16.3a and 16.3b).

CANDIDATE: These are AP and lateral radiographic views in plaster. There is a displaced lateral condyle fracture which is easiest to see on the AP. This looks like a Milch type 2 and the fracture line extends from the trochlear groove into the metaphysis. Because it's extending from the medial side

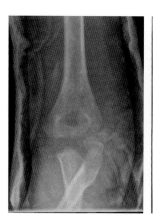
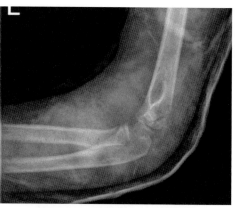

Figure 16.3a and 16.3b Anteroposterior (AP) and lateral radiographs, left elbow.

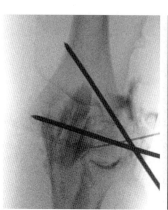
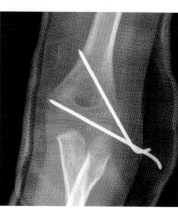

Figure 16.3c and Figure 16.3d Intraoperative arthrogram of left elbow, and postop radiograph in cast.

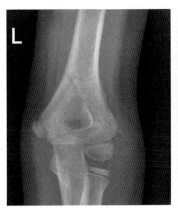
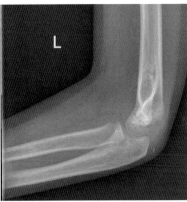

Figure 16.3e and 16.3f Anteroposterior (AP) and lateral radiographs, left elbow after healing.

of the lateral ridge of the sulcus, the ulnohumeral articulation is unstable.

A Milch type 1 is lateral to the ulnohumeral articulation: going through the capitellar physis into the metaphysis. This is the equivalent of a Salter Harris type IV. A more recent and practical classification by Jakob describes three types. Type 1: under 2 mm of displacement, indicating the presence of a cartilaginous hinge. Type 2: where there is between 2 and 4 mm of displacement with intact intra-articular cartilage on arthrogram. Type 3: greater than 4 mm of intra-articular displacement.

EXAMINER: What problems can you foresee with this fracture?

CANDIDATE: These are intra-articular fractures and have a higher incidence of specific complications:

- Non-union due to synovial interposition from the joint surface, causing persistent elbow instability.
- Fishtail deformity from a fracture gap between the condyles, central area of avascular necrosis or physeal bar.
- Apparent cubitus varus due to lateral periosteal overgrowth, after the fracture heals, causing a cosmetic deformity.
- Cubitus valgus occurs from physeal arrest of the lateral capitellar physis, which can cause a tardy ulna nerve palsy.

In undisplaced fractures, assessing the intra-articular component of the fracture can be difficult on plain radiographs, as the distal humerus is cartilaginous. In these cases, an MRI or EUA and arthrogram may be useful to assess the fracture further.

EXAMINER: How do you surgically manage displaced fractures?

CANDIDATE: The aim is to restore articular congruity. For those fractures where the arthrogram demonstrates an articular hinge or mildly displaced (< 2 mm) fractures, the fracture can be stabilized with percutaneous divergent wires.

For those fractures that are displaced, visualizing the articular surface is required. This can be achieved with a lateral approach to the elbow. Avoid dissecting around the posterior aspect of

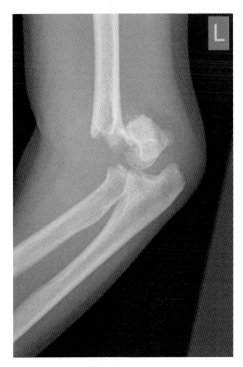

Figure 16.4a Lateral radiograph, left elbow.

the capitellar fragment as this can devascularize the fragment. Reduce the fracture and hold with at least two divergent K-wires. These can either be buried or left outside of the skin.

Structured oral examination question 4

EXAMINER: This 7-year-old boy was waiting for his dinner and fell outside in the back garden (Figure 16.4a).

CANDIDATE: This is a lateral radiograph in a skeletally immature patient, which demonstrates a displaced supracondylar fracture. Typically, the mechanism is a fall with the elbow extended and axial loading. My first priority is assessment of the child and limb. I'm assuming this is an isolated injury?[Yes.] I would check vascularity by checking the radial and ulna pulse, capillary refill and ensuring the hand is warm and well perfused. I would check the

motor and sensory function of the median, radial and ulna nerves. I would examine the antecubital fossa to see if the skin was under threat: such as a pucker sign due to buttonholing through brachialis. I would splint in a position of comfort after intranasal diamorphine.

EXAMINER: The child has a pink hand that's perfused but no palpable radial pulse. There is no motor or sensory deficit.

CANDIDATE: While the evidence is a pink, perfused hand without any neurological deficit, it can be elevated and observed [2,3]: if the child is fasted and I can get him to theatre at a reasonable time, my preference is to operate on him that evening.

EXAMINER: He's fasted, consented and ready. Explain what you are going to do.

CANDIDATE: I would warn the vascular surgeons. Set-up is key: the child is supine, with head ring and shoulder at the level of the arm table extension. I would have the C-arm from the foot-end of the

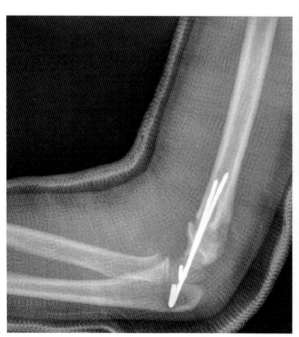
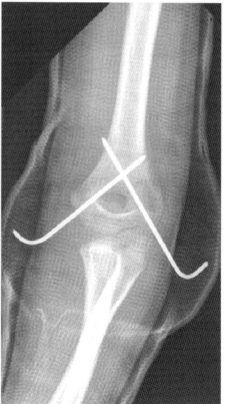

Figure 16.4b and 16.4c Lateral and anteroposterior (AP) radiographs in cast.

table: for access for AP and lateral views. The image intensifier screens are opposite me, on the other side of the table. I would prep and drape with a high tourniquet applied but not inflated. After the WHO checklist, I'd ask the anaesthetist to give muscle relaxant and antibiotics.

I would reduce this by traction with the elbow in slight flexion. I would first check the AP to see I've got it out to length and correct for medial or lateral translation. I then flex the elbow with my thumb pushing on the olecranon, and depending on which best reduces the fracture, the forearm is either supinated or pronated. If the child's fingers can touch their shoulder: this indirectly shows the fracture is reduced. I would check the medial and lateral columns are restored by taking oblique column views and a lateral X-ray.

I put my lateral side wires in first. I do this by laying a 2.0-mm K-wire on the skin and marking with a skin marker. I make a small stab, place the wire free-hand on the entry point and tap it in a bit with a toffee hammer before driving it with the wire driver under image guidance. I aim for bicortical fixation, engaging both distal and proximal fragments. Either lateral divergent wires or a crossed configuration is biomechanically stable, with maximal spread and avoiding crossing at the fracture site. On the medial side, I would extend the elbow to take the ulna nerve away from the epicondyle, then make a mini-incision to see the bone before placing and driving the medial wire in. I would screen the fixed construct under real-time imaging to check stability.

I'd recheck pulse and circulation before applying a backslab. If there are any doubts about the pulse, a hand-held Doppler can be used. If the hand remained pink, it may take a few hours for the palpable radial pulse to return.

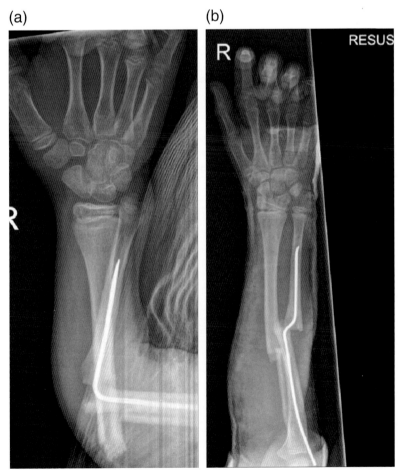

(a)

(b)

Figure 16.5a and 16.5b Anteroposterior (AP) radiographs, right forearm.

EXAMINER: You find the hand is white when you recheck his circulation!

CANDIDATE: I'd reduce flexion on the elbow to see if that restored circulation. If it didn't, I'd screen to see if there was a gap at the fracture site, indicating the brachial artery was interposed or tethered. If I thought this was the case I'd remove the wires, place him on straight longitudinal traction and call the vascular surgeon, who would do an on-table angiogram and explore the brachial artery through an anterior approach.

Structured oral examination question 5

EXAMINER: This 13-year-old boy had a previous forearm injury which healed, and he was due to have an operation to remove the metalwork. He was involved in exuberant play and pushed over (Figures 16.5a and 16.5b). The injury is closed and neurovascularly intact.

CANDIDATE: I can see an initial radiograph and a repeat view, probably in A&E resus, after procedural sedation with his forearm reduced into a straighter position. There is an elastic nail in the ulna with a double bend, with mid-shaft re-fractures of both bones.

EXAMINER: Could he be taken to theatre and have it manipulated, and a cast put back on it?

CANDIDATE: As he's 13 years old, there isn't much remaining growth. The mid-shaft position of the fracture also implies that this will have poor remodelling potential. At his age, I would not accept any deformity with this fracture pattern.

I think trying to manipulate his forearm closed and achieve an adequate reduction of both bones is unlikely to work. My plan would be to either remove the ulna nail and then insert elastic nails into both bones or open the fractures and plate them.

EXAMINER: Are there any technical problems you anticipate while doing this?

CANDIDATE: Trying to remove the bent nail may be a problem, in which case I would open the fracture site and cut the nail. It's then possible to capture each half of the nail with the pliers and pull it out.

EXAMINER: Is it necessary to remove metalwork? Do you know any evidence?

There is divided opinion on the necessity for routine metalwork removal. Children have exuberant periosteal bone formation and thereby metalwork can get buried when placed at a young age. Assuming there are no further complications then they can be left in situ. With the risk of subsequent periprosthetic fracture and the difficulty of excavating metalwork,

(c)   (d)

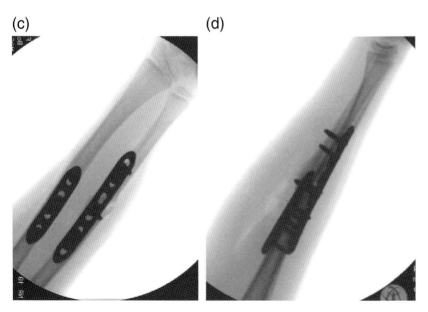

Figure 16.5c and 16.5d
Anteroposterior (AP) and lateral intraoperative images.

some surgeons have a low threshold to remove paediatric metalwork.

There is morbidity associated with metalwork removal, which includes a 40% complication rate when removing forearm plates that is related to the seniority of the surgeon doing the procedure [4].

Structured oral examination question 6

EXAMINER: This 8-year-old boy has had multiple previous fractures which have healed but left him with clinical deformities of the long bones (Figure 16.6a). He had an innocuous fall which caused this injury (Figures 16.6b and 16.6c).

CANDIDATE: I can see a pre-injury radiograph of a right femur with a significant anterior bow and appearances of Park Harris growth arrest lines. On the right-hand side AP and lateral, there is an oblique fracture through the distal third of the femur with a Thomas splint. It's translated and in varus, but the fracture is approximately out to length in his traction. The cortices are thin and

(a)

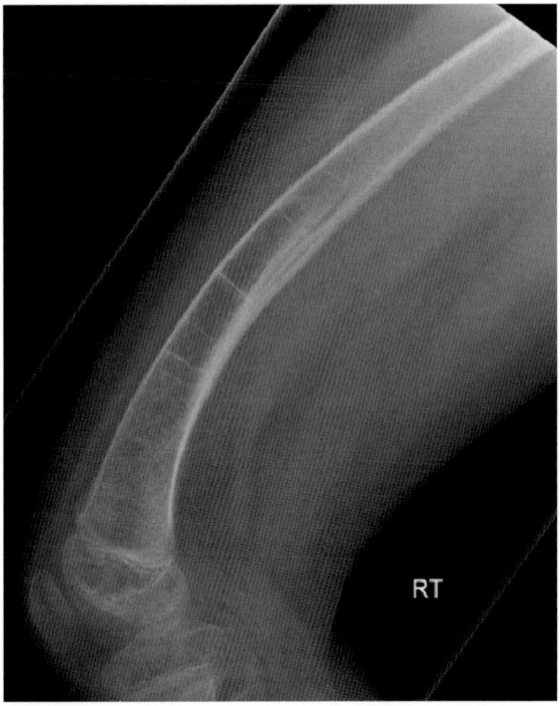

Figure 16.6a Lateral radiograph, femur.

bone quality is osteopenic. Does the child have an underlying metabolic bone disease? I would take a history and ask about inherited conditions in his family.

EXAMINER: What are Park Harris growth arrest lines?

CANDIDATE: Park Harris lines are transverse sclerotic lines in the metaphysis which correspond to stress or an insult to the bone and then resumption of growth. A similar appearance can occur with bisphosphonate treatment.

EXAMINER: Do you know of any paediatric orthopaedic conditions where we use bisphosphonates?

CANDIDATE: Osteogenesis imperfecta.

EXAMINER: His sclera are blue and dad is affected. What type of OI does he have?

CANDIDATE: Likely Type 1 (according to Sillence): as they have blue sclera and the condition is autosomal dominant.

EXAMINER: What is the treatment for this fracture? Are there any technical considerations?

CANDIDATE: I would discuss with a tertiary centre because of his pre-existing OI, but essentially the principles of management are to restore alignment and correct pre-existing deformity. The options are limited due to the anatomical abnormality and background osteopenia. An intramedullary device offers the strongest biomechanical option; however, due to the age of the child this needs the capacity to grow with the child and not damage either the physis or the vascularity to the proximal femur.

I am aware of the use of growing telescopic rod systems. The rods have a trochanteric entry point with male and female sliding components. The proximal and distal ends are threaded to anchor in the epiphysis. As the nails are straight, there may be a requirement for sequential osteotomies (Shish–Kebab/Sofield procedure) in pre-existing bony deformities to allow tension-free passage of the nails.

Postoperatively I will liaise with his physician about the commencement of bisphosphonate therapy.

(b)

(c)

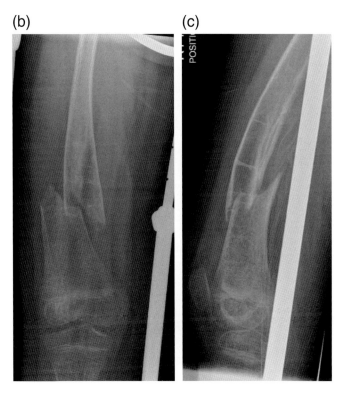

Figure 16.6b and 16.6c Anteroposterior (AP) and lateral radiographs, femur.

(d)

(e)

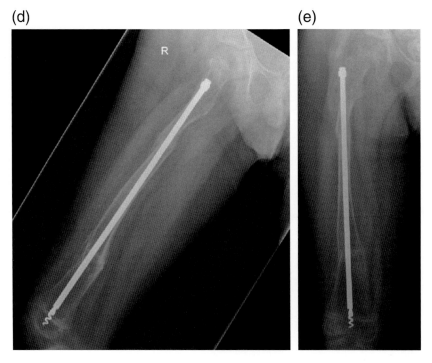

Figure 16.6d and 16.6e Lateral and anteroposterior (AP) postoperative radiographs, femur.

Structured oral examination question 7

EXAMINER: This 8-year-old girl sustained an injury walking home from school when she was hit by a car at low speed, pedestrian versus car (Figures 16.7a and 16.7b).

CANDIDATE: These are AP radiographs in a Kendrick traction splint used by paramedics at the scene as well as in a Thomas splint. I can see a short, oblique fracture of the femoral diaphysis, at the junction of the proximal and middle thirds. I would initially assess the patient according to ATLS protocol: prioritizing the resuscitation and treatment of life- and limb-threatening injuries.

From the point of view of this injury: I would want to check the condition of the skin, ensure the foot is warm and well-perfused with intact pedal pulses, and the patient is moving the toes actively with no motor or sensory deficit. Is this a closed, isolated injury?

EXAMINER: Yes. On secondary survey, you are happy this is an isolated injury and the patient is physiologically suitable for an operation, if you think it appropriate.

CANDIDATE: I would be inclined to treat this by elastic nails. This pattern of injury is length-stable. It's a fracture in a paediatric femur with an appropriate size of canal for elastic nails: typically, a child between 5 and 10 years of age. The nails should each be one-third the diameter of the canal at the narrowest point. As a rough estimate, I would measure canal diameter using the PACS system to check this.

My set-up would be a Jackson table with my assistant applying traction on the leg. I would check alignment and rotation with fluoroscopy. I would use retrograde nails via medial and lateral entry points about 2.5 cm above the distal physis. The nails are pre-bent, so the apex is at the fracture site. The biomechanical principle is of 'double arc secant in equilibrium': the bending

Figure 16.7a and 16.7b Anteroposterior (AP) radiographs, femur.

(a)

(b)

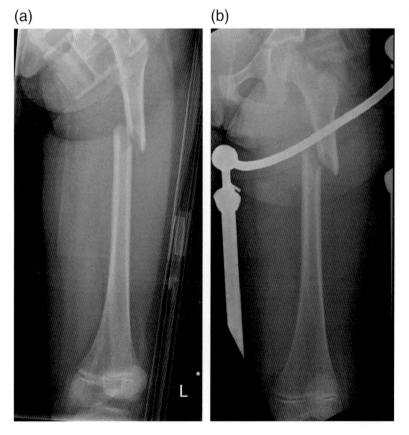

(c) (b)

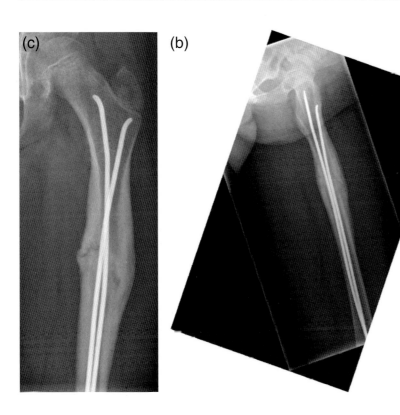

Figure 16.7c and 16.7d
Anteroposterior (AP) and lateral postoperative radiographs, femur.

moments of two nails counteract each other with an equal and opposite force to create a stable construct.

EXAMINER: Stable? What does that mean? Is it rigidly fixed? What type of bone healing occurs?

CANDIDATE: Fracture healing occurs by secondary bone healing with callus formation; this is a relative stability technique. The nails are far from rigid. They especially do not resist torsion: I'd be observant for rotational malalignment on follow-up in clinic. Loss of alignment is particularly seen with nails that have unequal curves, different size nails and when the fracture is comminuted. End caps have been advocated by some to increase the stiffness of titanium elastic nails, although the evidence for this is in biomechanical studies only as far as I'm aware. In children greater than 50 kg bodyweight, stainless steel flexible nails can be used to increase the nail strength and have been shown to have a lower rate of malunion compared to titanium elastic nails [5].

Structured oral examination question 8

EXAMINER: This 14-year-old boy was a trauma call from an RTA. He has sustained multiple rib fractures and a lung contusion on the same side as this closed injury to his leg. He's had a pan-CT scan in A&E resus (Figure 16.8a) and is awake and stable on paediatric HDU. The general surgeons have said his liver laceration can be managed conservatively without the need for laparotomy and CT has excluded a pelvic injury.

CANDIDATE: I'm assuming he's had a primary survey according to ATLS protocol by the trauma team. My priority would be the secondary survey on HDU. I would check him head to toe for additional injuries. I would have a high index of suspicion for a spinal injury or an injury to the hip. I would speak to the ITU team to see if they have been happy with his monitoring, and to make a plan for theatre. His lactate on blood gas and urine output are indicators of organ perfusion and whether he is physiologically safe to proceed.

343

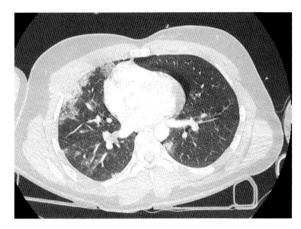

Figure 16.8a Axial CT, chest.

From the point of view of assessment of the distal femur fracture: I would check pulses in his leg, the condition of the skin, neurological status and for signs of impending compartment syndrome.

EXAMINER: The ITU team says you can proceed, what is your plan?

CANDIDATE: My plan would be to fix his femur using a distal femoral locking plate. He's almost an adult, with an adult pattern of injury in terms of the butterfly fragment and comminution. The capital femoral physis on his AP pelvis appears almost shut down in terms of remaining growth. The distal physis is open. To control this would be difficult using a paediatric lateral entry nail, because it is at the junction of the diaphysis and metaphysis. A retrograde nail is not an option. He's also had a significant lung injury and there are risks from reaming in terms of fat embolus. I would approach this using a lateral approach, being careful around the blood supply to the physis. It might be possible to do a submuscular technique and slide the plate up: I'd have a low threshold for opening it to check reduction was adequate in terms of length and rotation.

EXAMINER: Do you foresee any problems after this has been fixed? What do you warn him and his parents?

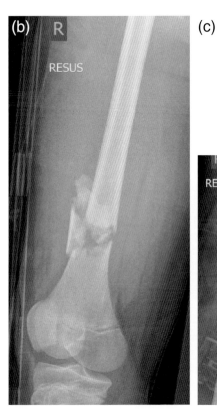

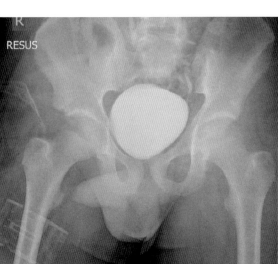

Figure 16.8b and 16.8c Anteroposterior (AP) radiographs, right femur and pelvis trauma series.

(d)

(e)

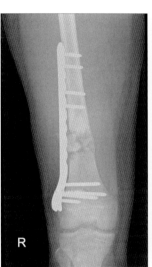

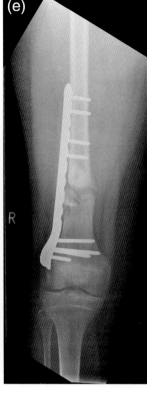

Figure 16.8d and 16.8e Anteroposterior (AP) postoperative radiographs, right femur.

CANDIDATE: An injury near the distal femoral physis has a potential for growth disturbance. Although this injury was in the metaphyseal region, I can see on later radiographs his physis is starting to shut down. I would check to see if clinically he had signs of a significant leg length discrepancy and obtain standing alignment views. There is an incidence of valgus deformity associated with plating of femoral shaft fractures close to the physis and I would warn the parents we would monitor him for this during follow-up. As he's almost at maturity I would not expect there to be a significant angular deformity or length discrepancy.

Structured oral examination question 9

EXAMINER: This 13-year-old boy sustained this injury playing football (Figures 16.9a and 16.9b).

CANDIDATE: I can see an AP and lateral plain radiograph of an adolescent knee showing a comminuted tibial tubercle avulsion fracture. This is typically due to eccentric quadriceps contraction with a flexed knee, such as jumping and landing on a bent knee. On examination, I would expect to find swelling, bruising and the patient would be unable to straight-leg raise. I would check for impending compartment syndrome as there is a risk of injury to a branch of the recurrent anterior tibial artery, which bleeds into the anterior compartment. Initial management is splintage, admission for elevation and planned definitive fixation. There is a Watson-Jones classification modified by Ogden. This looks like a comminuted Type II: where the apophysis is avulsed from the metaphysis.

EXAMINER: Tell me about the Watson-Jones classification as modified by Ogden.

CANDIDATE:

- Type I is a fracture of the tibial tubercle apophysis (secondary ossification centre where the patella tendon inserts). It is *distal to the junction* of the ossification centres of the apophysis and epiphysis. IA is undisplaced. IB is a displaced avulsion, with the fragment hinged anteriorly.
- Type II is *at the junction* of the apophysis and epiphysis. IIA is undisplaced. IIB is comminuted

345

(a)　　　　　　　　　　　　　(b)

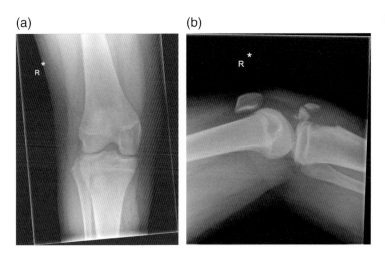

Figure 16.9a and 16.9b Anteroposterior (AP) and lateral radiographs, knee.

(c)　　　　　　　　　　　　　(d)

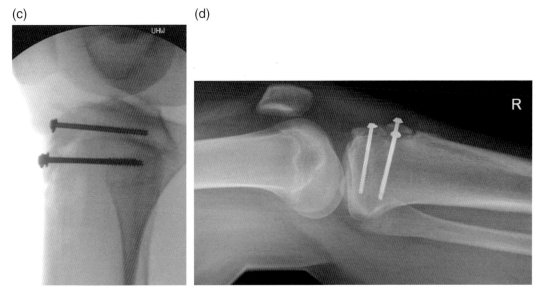

Figure 16.9c and 16.9d Intraoperative and postoperative lateral radiographs, right knee.

and the apophysis is displaced by the pull of the patella tendon.

- Type III is *above the junction*, where the fracture extends into the knee joint through the epiphysis. IIIA is where the apophysis and epiphysis are a 'composite' or single fragment. IIIB is where they are comminuted and separated.

EXAMINER: What is your management plan?

CANDIDATE: This needs operative fixation to restore the integrity of the extensor mechanism. My preference is to use 4-mm partially threaded cannulated screws. I would have a tourniquet and a sterile gown rolled up under the calf as a bolster to hyperextend the knee. I would make an incision anteriorly over the fracture: pull out any interposed periosteum and then pass my guidewires from anterior to posterior, while avoiding crossing the physis and being mindful of the neurovascular structures within the popliteal fossa. After passing the screws I would screen the knee to check the fixation was stable when flexing to 90°. Postop I would mobilize the patient touch weightbearing with a hinged brace initially locked in extension, and then allow progressively more flexion over 6 weeks.

EXAMINER: This boy is an elite sports person. Are there any future problems you need to warn his parents about?

CANDIDATE: He may require removal of the metalwork after the fracture has united if it is prominent or causes a bursitis and anterior knee pain. There is a risk of genu recurvatum from decreased tibial slope after premature closure of the anterior physis in younger children. I'd anticipate, as he has little remaining growth before his physes fuse, that this is not likely to be an issue, but I would follow him up to watch for this. If there were any signs this was starting to develop, I would do an epiphysiodesis to complete the growth shut down and he may then require a corrective osteotomy.

Structured oral examination question 10

EXAMINER: This 12-year-old girl attended A&E and was told she had a sprain after a trampoline injury (Figures 16.10a and 16.10b). She was allowed to weight bear with an ankle stirrup, although is struggling with pain when you see her in the fracture clinic.

CANDIDATE: I can see AP and lateral radiographs of a skeletally immature patient. There's evidence of an effusion within the joint and I can see a fracture line in the distal tibial physis exiting

into the plafond. At this age, I'd be concerned about a triplane or transitional type of injury and obtain a CT scan.

EXAMINER: What do you mean by transitional?

CANDIDATE: Closure of the distal tibial epiphysis occurs in adolescents at 12–15 years of age, over an 18-month period. This is an injury when they are transitioning to skeletal maturity. The growth plate closes asymmetrically: first centrally then anteromedially, posteromedially and finally the lateral distal tibial physis is the last to close.

EXAMINER: Is this a triplane fracture (Figures 16.10c–16.10e)? What is the management?

CANDIDATE: A triplane injury involves fracture lines in the sagittal, transverse and coronal planes, traversing the physis and entering the ankle joint. On the lateral X-ray typically, there is a Salter Harris II and a Salter Harris III on the AP, corresponding to the displaced anterolateral part of the physis.

The CT confirms a triplane pattern of injury. The principles of management are to restore the articular surface by anatomical reduction, and fixation using absolute stability. Any displacement > 2 mm at the articular surface is an indication for surgical intervention. In this case, I would see if I could obtain a closed reduction and percutaneously fix it with a partially threaded 4-mm cannulated screw from a lateral to medial direction. I would use a large reduction clamp to aid reduction if

(a)

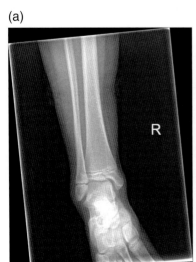

(b)

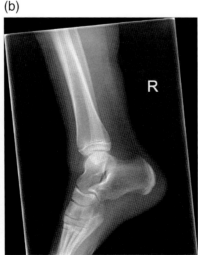

Figure 16.10a and 16.10b
Anteroposterior (AP) and lateral radiographs, right ankle.

(c)   (d)   (e)

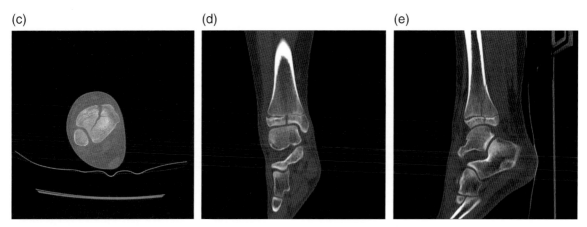

Figure 16.10c–16.10e Sagittal, coronal and axial CT slices, respectively, right ankle.

(f)   (g)

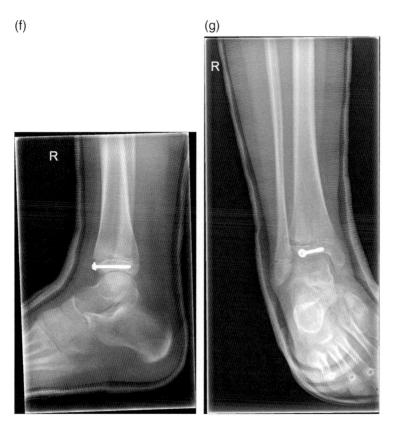

Figure 16.10f and 16.10g Postoperative lateral and mortise/anteroposterior (AP) radiographs, right ankle in cast.

necessary. If there was movement of the Thurston Holland fragment on screening, I would also use metaphyseal screws in an anterior to posterior direction. If I could not obtain reduction by closed means, I would openly reduce the articular surface with an incision over the fracture line to remove any potential soft-tissue interposition.

References

1. Pahlavan S, Baldwin K, *et al.* Proximal humerus fractures in the pediatric population: a systematic review. *J Child Orthop.* 2011;5:187–194.

2. Mangat KS, Martin AG, Bache CE. The 'pulseless pink' hand after supracondylar fracture in children: the predictive value of nerve palsy. *J Bone Joint Surg Br.* 2009;91(11):1521–1525.

3. Scannell BP, Jackson JB, *et al.* The perfused, pulseless supracondylar humeral fracture: intermediate-term follow-up of vascular status and function. *J Bone Joint Surg Am.* 2013;95 (21):1913–1919.

4. Langkamer VG, Ackroyd CE. Removal of forearm plates. A review of the complications. *J Bone Joint Surg Br.* 1990;72(4):601–604.

5. Wall EJ, Jain V, *et al.* Complications of titanium and stainless steel elastic nail fixation of pediatric femoral fractures. *J Bone Joint Surg Am.* 2008;90(6):1305–1313.

Chapter

17

Hand and upper limb

John W. K. Harrison and Kim Weng Chan

Structured oral examination question 1

Distal radius fracture and malunion

EXAMINER: Please describe the radiographic findings (Figure 17.1a and 17.1b).

CANDIDATE: These are posteroanterior (PA) and lateral radiographs of the wrist that show an extra-articular distal radius fracture. On the PA view, the radial height and inclination are maintained. On the lateral view, there is dorsal comminution with dorsal angulation of the distal radius. The radiographs also showed thumb carpometacarpal arthritis.

EXAMINER: These are the radiographs of an 83-year-old lady. What are the acceptable parameters for conservative management of distal radius fracture post manipulation in A&E?

CANDIDATE: There are several parameters that I would use to judge the adequacy of reduction

for distal radius fracture radiologically. I would look at the overall alignment of the distal radius including less than 10° dorsal angulation of the distal radius articular surface; if this was an intra-articular fracture then less than 2 mm gap or step off, radial length within 2 mm of the ulna length, radial inclination of 21°, and no secondary carpal malalignment.

EXAMINER: The on-call registrar has kindly reduced this fracture in A&E under haematoma block. The position in below-elbow plaster post closed reduction at 1 and 2 weeks follow-up in the fracture clinic was acceptable. Please comment on these radiographs taken at 6-week follow-up in the fracture clinic following conservative management of the distal radius fracture (Figure 17.1c and 17.1d).

CANDIDATE: These are posteroanterior (PA) and lateral radiographs of the wrist in a plaster that show extra-articular distal radius fracture. On the PA view, there is loss of radial height and inclination. On the lateral view, there is dorsal angulation of the distal radius with a carpal malalignment.

(a)

(b)

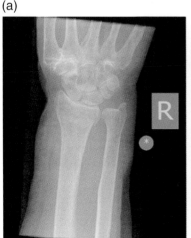
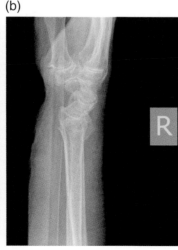

Figure 17.1a and 17.1b Posteroanterior (PA) and lateral radiographs of extra-articular distal radius fracture.

(c)

(d)

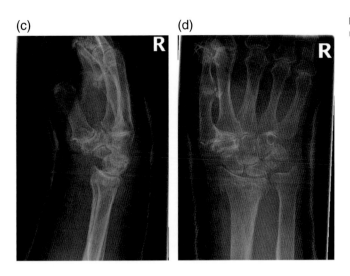

Figure 17.1c and 17.1d Posteroanterior (PA) and lateral radiographs of malunited distal radius fracture.

EXAMINER: What would you do now?

CANDIDATE: I would inform the patient that the fracture has slipped and healed in a less-than-ideal position. I would warn her that there may be some reduction in range of wrist movement and possible activity-related wrist pain. Despite this setback, we would be hopeful she would make a good recovery from her injury. I would arrange urgent physiotherapy in order to maximize her rehabilitation. I would review her progress in clinic in 6 weeks with repeat radiographs.

EXAMINER: The patient asks why the fracture wasn't fixed surgically.

CANDIDATE: I would explain that the fracture has been in an acceptable position but unfortunately moved, possibly as the swelling in the hand subsided. I would emphasize that conservative management where possible is the best treatment option as it avoids the risks of both anaesthetic- and surgical-related complications. I would mention to the patient the complications that could occur with volar locking plate fixation including infection, painful scar, tendon rupture/irritation, injury to neurovascular structures such as the median nerve and radial artery, screw cut out and hardware failure, carpal tunnel syndrome, secondary fracture displacement and chronic regional pain syndrome (CRPS).

COMMENT: Don't forget to mention CRPS as a possible complication from any type of hand surgery undertaken.

EXAMINER: That's assuming you would have treated this fracture with a volar locking plate and not K-wire fixation, but we'll not go there.

COMMENT: The management of displaced distal radius fractures is controversial. A recent meta-analysis showed no significant difference between patients who underwent internal fixation and conservative management for displaced distal radius fractures (UK DRAFFT). Several other studies have demonstrated no difference in outcome between K-wire fixation and volar locking plate fixation. The aim of the viva was to focus on the management of a complication from trauma, i.e. painful distal radius malunion, and the examiner didn't wish to take the viva in the direction of discussing the evidence for different treatment options for distal radius fixation.

EXAMINER: The patient comes back in 8 weeks and now complains of difficulty performing her daily tasks due to the wrist deformity. What would you offer her at this stage?

CANDIDATE: I would like to take a detailed history and examination of the wrist. If the patient had ulnar-sided wrist pain and due to shortening from the distal radius malunion, I would offer her a correction osteotomy of the distal radius using a volar locking plate through an extended flexor carpi radialis (FCR) approach. The fixation is supplemented with an autologous bone graft from the iliac crest. The FCR approach utilizes the interval between the radial artery and the FCR tendon. An incision is made (e)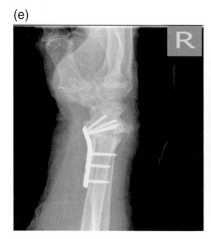

(f)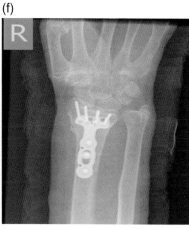

Figure 17.1e and 17.1f Posteroanterior (PA) and lateral radiographs of the wrist showing correction osteotomy with autologous bone graft.

directly along the tendon sheath of the FCR followed by ulnar retraction of the FCR to protect the median nerve. The pronator quadratus muscle is then elevated subperiosteally from the radial volar cortex, and brachioradialis insertion released. I would use an image intensifier throughout the procedure to ensure adequate correction of the deformity. I would immobilize the wrist in a short arm plaster for 2 weeks for wound healing. At 2 weeks I would change it to a future-type wrist splint to allow mobilization of the wrist once the plaster is removed, 4 times a day, and take a check X-ray at 6 weeks to confirm bony union (Figure 17.1e and 17.1f).

COMMENT: Another scenario: a patient with distal radius fracture treated non-operatively came back at 8 weeks with persistent pain, swelling and erythema. Radiographs show the fracture has united in a satisfactory position, but osteopenia is noted in the distal radius.

EXAMINER: How would you approach this patient?

CANDIDATE: I would like to take a thorough history and examination of the wrist. My main concern for this patient is development of chronic regional pain syndrome.

EXAMINER: What is chronic regional pain syndrome?

CANDIDATE: Chronic regional pain syndrome (CRPS) is contingent on the presence of regional pain combined with autonomic dysfunction, atrophy and functional impairment affecting musculoskeletal, neural and vascular structures. CRPS is divided into two types:

Type 1 – initiated by trauma with no identifiable peripheral nerve injury.

Type 2 – associated with identifiable peripheral nerve injury after trauma (causalgia).

EXAMINER: How do you confirm the diagnosis?

CANDIDATE: CRPS is principally a clinical diagnosis based on the patient's history and physical examination. There are no specific tests to confirm CRPS. The clinical presentations of CRPS can be divided into acute and chronic.

Acute – intolerance to cold, swelling, stiff and painful limb, sensitivity to slightest touch (allodynia).

Chronic – trophic changes in which the skin is shiny and smooth, brittle nails, Sudek's osteoporosis.

EXAMINER: How are you going to treat the patient?

CANDIDATE: After confirming the diagnosis of CRPS, I would manage this with a thorough explanation of the diagnosis and likely treatment course. I would ensure adequate analgesia, urgent physical and psychotherapy. I will make an urgent referral to the pain team. Other treatments that may be considered include sympathetic nerve block and medical treatment (local anaesthesia, anti-epileptics and anti-depressants).

References

Ng CY, McQueen M. What are the radiological predictors of functional outcome following fractures of the distal radius? *J Bone Joint Surg Br.* 2011;93(2):145–150.

Costa ML, Achten J, Plant C, *et al.* UK DRAFFT: a randomised controlled trial of percutaneous fixation with Kirschner wires versus volar locking-plate fixation in the treatment of adult patients with a dorsally displaced fracture of the distal radius. *Health Technol Assess*. 2015;19(17).

Leung F, Kwan K, Fang C. Distal radius fractures: current concepts and management. *Focus on series, Bone Joint*. 2013.

Structured oral examination question 2

Extensor pollicis longus (EPL) tendon rupture

EXAMINER: What does the photograph (Figure 17.2a) show?

CANDIDATE: This is a clinical photograph of the right hand with the thumb in an abnormally flexed posture at the interphalangeal (IP) joint.

EXAMINER: The patient has recently come out of plaster for a distal radius fracture. What is the likely pathology?

CANDIDATE: This is usually caused by rupture of the extensor pollicis longus (EPL) tendon at the level of the Lister's tubercle in the third dorsal extensor compartment at around 6–8 weeks. EPL rupture usually occurs after an undisplaced or minimally displaced distal radius fracture. The severity of the fracture is not indicative of the likelihood of EPL rupture. It occurs in about 1% of cases secondary to either attrition or ischaemia. Callus formation around the healed fracture site leaves a roughened surface over which the tendon attrition occurs, leading to rupture.

The other theory is microvascular disturbance secondary to increased pressure present in the non-ruptured tendon sheath with compromised blood supply to the tendon causing degeneration and rupture. It can be thought of as a type of compartment syndrome occurring in the tendon tunnel from fracture bleeding leading to interruption of tendon blood supply, nutrition and eventual rupture. With a more extensive fracture the tendon tunnel is breached and there is no build up of pressure.

EXAMINER: How would you test for EPL rupture?

CANDIDATE: The patient would be unable to extend the IP joint of the thumb.

EXAMINER: I would not rely on testing for thumb IP extension as the EPB tendon inserts into the extensor apparatus of the thumb at varying levels and may be able to extend the IP joint of the thumb. Any other tests you would perform?

CANDIDATE: I would ask the patient to lift their thumb off a table, which is not possible without an intact EPL tendon.

EXAMINER: Can you describe the extensor tendon compartments at the wrist?

CANDIDATE: There are six compartments in which the extensor tendons cross the dorsum of the wrist with contents as below:

First dorsal compartment (site of De Quervain's tenosynovitis):
- Extensor pollicis brevis (EPB) – attaches to base of proximal phalanx.
- Abductor pollicis longus (APL) – attaches to thumb metacarpal.

Second dorsal compartment (intersection syndrome):
- Extensor carpi radialis brevis (ECRB) – attaches to middle finger metacarpal.
- Extensor carpi radialis longus (ECRL) – attaches to the index finger metacarpal.

Third dorsal compartment (passes around Lister's tubercle):
- Extensor pollicis longus (EPL) – passes around Lister's tubercle of radius and inserts on distal phalanx of thumb.

Fourth dorsal compartment (contains PIN on the floor of this compartment):
- Extensor indicis proprius (EIP) – lies deep to EDC tendon.
- Extensor digitorum communis (EDC) – no direct attachment to proximal phalanx, attaches to the extensor expansions.

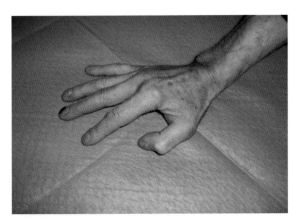

Figure 17.2a Clinical picture of a hand.

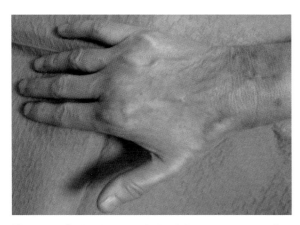

Figure 17.2b Clinical picture of a hand showing restoration of thumb extension following reconstruction of EPL. Note the three incisions used.

Fifth dorsal compartment (approach to DRUJ through floor of the fifth compartment):

- Extensor digiti minimi (EDM) – attaches to extensor expansion of little finger.

Sixth dorsal compartment:

- Extensor carpi ulnaris (ECU) – attaches to base of little finger metacarpal.

EXAMINER: How do you manage EPL rupture as in this case?

CANDIDATE: I would like to take a full history and perform a clinical examination. I would like to perform a functional assessment of the affected hand to determine the functional loss and deformity from the EPL rupture. If the patient has significant functional loss or deformity from the EPL rupture (reduced span or finds thumb catches when grasping objects), then I would request an ultrasound to confirm the diagnosis and check clinically for an intact EIP. At this stage I would refer the patient to a hand surgeon for surgical reconstruction. The EPL would have retracted and would not be repairable. This would need reconstruction with tendon transfer, normally extensor indicis proprius to restore extension movement of the thumb.

EXAMINER: What is the role of ultrasound scan in EPL rupture?

CANDIDATE: Sonography is to confirm the diagnosis of an EPL tendon rupture.

EXAMINER: You are the hand surgeon, how many incisions would you use? Can you show it on my hand?

CANDIDATE: Three incisions are needed – a 1-cm transverse incision dorsal to the index finger metacarpal head (EIP lies ulnar to the EDC tendon), a 3-cm midline dorsal incision proximal to the wrist to bring the divided EIP tendon proximal to the extensor retinaculum, a zig-zag incision over the thumb metacarpal to identify EPL tendon distal to the rupture. The extensor indicis is sutured to the remnant of the EPL tendon distally using the Pulvertaft weave technique (Figure 17.2b).

EXAMINER: How do you test for extensor indicis preoperatively?

CANDIDATE: Point the index finger with the middle to little fingers fully flexed (this prevents EDC acting).

EXAMINER: What are the basic principles of tendon transfer?

CANDIDATE: Principles when deciding on tendon transfers are:

1. The donor tendon must match the muscle strength.
2. The force of donor tendon should be proportional to muscle cross-sectional area.
3. Work capacity = force × amplitude.
4. Amplitude should be proportional to length of the muscle.
5. Motor strength will decrease one grade after transfer.
6. Appropriate tensioning of the donor tendon.
7. Appropriate excursion of donor tendon (can adjust with pulley or tenodesis effect).

The other requirements include patient compliance, no joint contractures, no active infection and grade 5/5 power on MRC scale (this will drop one grade after transfer).

COMMENT: The other variant of this question is if an extensor tendon rupture has occurred following volar locking plate fixation. Typically, this would be a comminuted displaced intra-articular fracture treated with volar locking plate. Tendon rupture occurs possibly due to screw or drill penetration of the third extensor compartment. One of the locking screws could be overlong, penetrating the dorsal cortex.

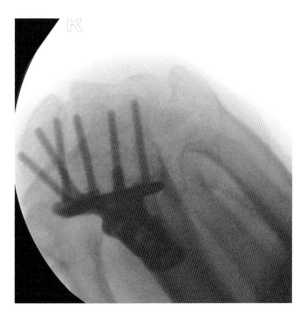

Figure 17.2c Skyline view distal radius taken during a volar locking plating with wrist maximally flexed. Note: the most radial peg has probably just penetrated through the cortex.

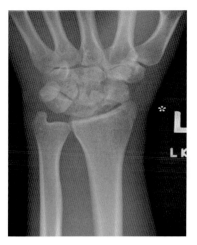

Figure 17.3a Posteroanterior (PA) wrist view demonstrating transscaphoid perilunate fracture–dislocation.

EXAMINER: How will you minimize the risk of extensor tendon rupture following volar locking plate fixation?

CANDIDATE: The surgeon should choose the appropriate length of screw to avoid penetration of the far cortex causing tendon irritation and rupture. The use of smooth locking pegs or tines rather than sharp-tipped self-tapping screws can also decrease the risk of tendon rupture. A 'skyline' view can be taken to confirm appropriate locking peg length (Figure 17.2c).

EXAMINER: Are there any other causes of EPL rupture?

CANDIDATE: EPL rupture can occur secondary to rheumatoid arthritis, bony spur developing after a scaphoid fracture, misplaced external fixator pin and steroid injection.

Structured oral examination question 3

Transscaphoid perilunate fracture–dislocation

EXAMINER: Please describe this X-ray (Figure 17.3a).

CANDIDATE: This is a posteroanterior view of the left hand showing transscaphoid perilunate fracture–dislocation. There are breaks in Gilula's lines, and fractures of the radial styloid and scaphoid. I would like to confirm my radiological diagnosis with a lateral view of the wrist.

EXAMINER: Here it is (Figure 17.3b).

CANDIDATE: This lateral radiograph shows a perilunate dislocation with dorsal dislocation of the carpus. This is a greater arc injury and stage III on the Mayfield classification. Mayfield classification has divided this injury into four sequential stages.

Stage I – scapholunate dissociation.

Stage II – lunocapitate disruption (capitate dislocates).

Stage III – lunotriquetral disruption ('perilunate').

Stage IV – lunate dislocation from lunate fossa (usually volar).

This classification describes the stages of disruption of the lunate found when the wrist is hyperextended, pronated and ulnar deviated. Initially, the radioscaphocapitate ligament and the scapholunate interosseous ligament rupture, then the capitolunate joint dislocates as the injury progresses. This is followed by lunotriquetral interosseous ligament rupture and finally the lunate dislocates through the space of Poirier. This is a greater arc injury with bony involvement of the radial styloid and/or scaphoid. Lesser arc injuries refer to purely ligamentous wrist injuries.

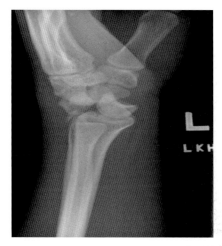

Figure 17.3b Lateral wrist view demonstrating transscaphoid perilunate fracture–dislocation.

EXAMINER: What is the difference between perilunate dislocation and a transscaphoid perilunate dislocation?

CANDIDATE: A perilunate dislocation is where there is dorsal displacement of all carpals except the lunate which stays in place. A transscaphoid perilunate dislocation is the same injury but with an associated scaphoid fracture.

EXAMINER: How would you like to proceed with this patient?

CANDIDATE: Assuming that ATLS has been performed in the initial management and life-threatening injuries have been excluded, I would like to proceed and take a thorough history including hand dominance, occupation and mechanism of injury. I would examine the hand, looking for deformity, swelling, open wound, perfusion status and check for median nerve symptoms. This would need to be reduced as an emergency in theatre with an image intensifier as prolonged dislocation increases swelling to the area and is associated with a higher rate of nerve injuries. Chinese finger traps can be used to help in the reduction by applying longitudinal traction. The sequence of reduction is by extending the wrist, applying direct pressure onto the lunate with the thumb and then palmar flexing the wrist to complete the reduction. I would confirm the reduction with image intensifier and apply a short arm plaster afterwards. I would admit the patient for high elevation with Bradford sling and hourly monitoring for compartment syndrome.

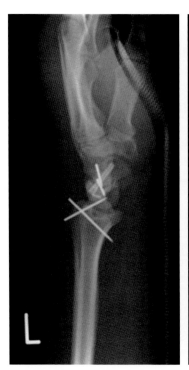
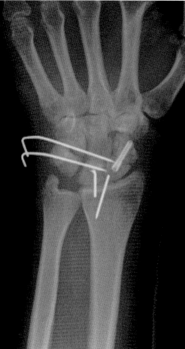

Figure 17.3c Postoperative radiographs showing ORIF of the scaphoid and repair of capitolunate and lunotriquetral ligaments (note the bone anchor in the lunate) and temporary K-wire stabilization of the carpus, all done through a dorsal approach.

EXAMINER: You have been successful in performing the closed reduction. How would you proceed now?

CANDIDATE: I would request an MRI scan to confirm the extent of injury as part of preoperative planning. The patient would need to have open reduction and internal fixation of the scaphoid and reconstruction of the scapholunate and lunotriquetral ligaments through a volar or dorsal wrist approach. This should preferably be performed by a hand surgeon.

The dorsal approach is favoured by many as it provides access to the midcarpal joints so that intrinsic ligaments can be repaired. The incision is centred over the Lister's tubercle. A V-shaped flap is created along the edge of the dorsal intercarpal ligament and the dorsal radiocarpal ligament. This can be satisfactorily closed post fixation.

The volar approach is via an extended carpal tunnel approach. The benefit of this approach is that it allows fixation of the volar capsule and decompression of the carpal tunnel. However, it does not allow the same exposure as found in the dorsal approach. A combined approach can also be undertaken. K-wire fixation is still routinely used. Scaphoid fractures are generally fixed with a headless compression screw. Stabilization of the lunate and reconstruction of the scapholunate ligament are frequently performed using suture anchors (Figure 17.3c).

EXAMINER: What is the expected outcome following this injury?

CANDIDATE: Patients should be counselled following this injury that there is a high risk of long-term problems of pain, stiffness and post-traumatic arthritis (36%). Carpal instability is also linked with this injury. Scapholunate instability and chronic perilunate dislocation can be treated with proximal row carpectomy or total wrist arthrodesis. Both of these result in reduced range of movement in the wrist, which can be unsatisfactory for the active patient.

EXAMINER: What is the normal scapholunate angle?

CANDIDATE: The average scapholunate angle is 45° (abnormal if < 30° or > 60°).

EXAMINER: What is the 'spilled tea-cup sign' (Figure 17.3d)?

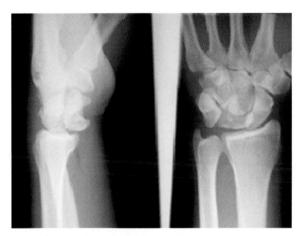

Figure 17.3d PA and lateral radiographs demonstrating a lunate dislocation (spilled tea-cup sign).

CANDIDATE: The spilled tea-cup sign describes abnormal volar displacement and tilt of a dislocated lunate on a lateral radiograph of the wrist. The convexity of the lunate is no longer congruent with the lunate fossa of the distal radius, while the concavity is no longer in articulation with the capitate head on a lateral wrist radiograph. It is an important sign to help differentiate lunate dislocation from perilunate dislocation. In perilunate dislocation, the lunate remains in articulation with the distal radius and therefore does not appear to 'spill' forward.

Structured oral examination question 4

Scaphoid fracture

EXAMINER: You saw a 44-year-old patient in the fracture clinic with the above radiographs 2 days following an injury. Please comment on these radiographs (Figure 17.4a and 17.4b) and how you would manage this patient.

CANDIDATE: The radiographs taken show a scaphoid waist fracture. I would take a thorough history and examination of the hand and wrist. I would like to know the handedness, occupation, hobbies and previous similar injury in the history. I would like to examine the wrist for swelling and tenderness over the anatomical snuffbox and see further lateral and oblique views. If these confirmed the fracture was undisplaced, I would manage this non-operatively in

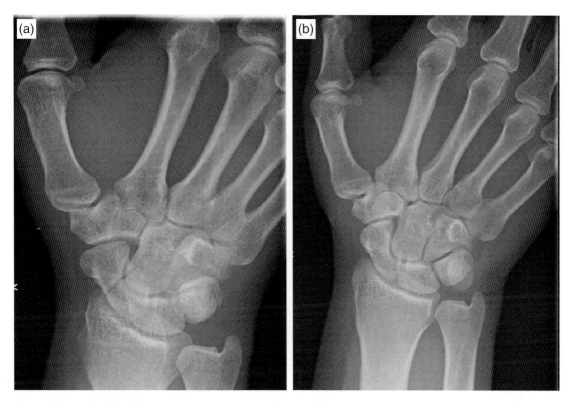

Figure 17.4a and 17.4b Radiographs demonstrating waist of scaphoid fracture.

a short arm cast without thumb immobilization for 6 weeks initially. A randomized prospective study published by Dias *et al.* has shown no evidence to support thumb immobilization in the treatment of scaphoid fracture [1]: 292 patients with scaphoid fracture were randomized to receive either Colles cast (forearm gauntlet) or scaphoid cast incorporating the thumb as far as its interphalangeal joint in the study. The incidence of non-union at 6 months follow-up is independent of type of cast used. The healing rate for conservative treatment is 80–90% for undisplaced waist of scaphoid fracture.

EXAMINER: What is the blood supply to the scaphoid?

CANDIDATE: The major blood supply of the scaphoid bone is distally based derived from branches of the radial artery entering the dorsal ridge. Between 70% and 80% of the intraosseous vascularity and the blood supply to the entire proximal pole enters this way with no blood vessels penetrating the cortex of the proximal pole

separately, explaining the higher rate of avascular necrosis with proximal pole fractures [2,3].

EXAMINER: What are the indications for internal fixation of the scaphoid?

CANDIDATE: The indications for internal fixation of scaphoid fracture include displacement of more than 1 mm, intrascaphoid angle > 20° (humpback deformity), delayed union, proximal pole fracture or scaphoid fracture associated with perilunate dislocation.

The indications for internal fixation of the scaphoid remain debatable. A systematic review and meta-analysis performed in 2010 concluded that there is currently insufficient evidence to make definitive conclusions on the indications for, or effectiveness of, operative versus non-operative management of acute scaphoid fractures [4]. Some evidence does suggest acute fixation of minimally displaced or undisplaced fractures in high-level athletes and manual workers to have a better functional outcome in the short term [5,6].

(c)   (d)

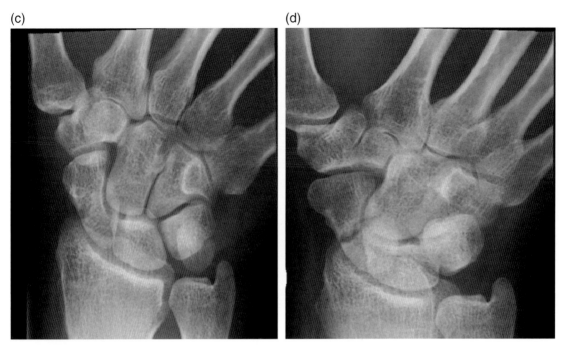

Figure 17.4c and 17.4d Radiographs demonstrating non-union scaphoid.

EXAMINER: These are the patient scaphoid radiographs at 4 months follow-up in the fracture clinic (Figure 17.4c and 17.4d). He remains symptomatic. What would you do?

CANDIDATE: The scaphoid radiographs shown non-union of the waist of scaphoid fracture with sclerosis at the fracture site. If the patient remains symptomatic, I would offer the patient surgical fixation of this non-union. I would like to request a computed tomography (CT scan) to confirm the diagnosis of non-union, which forms part of preoperative planning. I would offer the patient bone grafting and surgical fixation with a headless compression screw through either a volar approach if the CT scan confirms a humpback deformity, or the dorsal approach if there was no carpal malalignment. The ideal position for a headless compression screw should be down the central axis of the scaphoid for maximal compression and fixation.

The volar approach to the scaphoid utilizes the FCR as an anatomical landmark with incision extended 2 cm proximal to the scaphoid tubercle with the distal incision directed towards the base of the thumb. The FCR sheath is then opened as distally as possible and retracted ulnarly to protect the radial artery and retracted radially to expose the

capsule. Capsulotomy is then performed through a longitudinal incision from the volar lip of the radius to the proximal tubercle of the trapezium to expose the scaphoid. The capsule and intracapsular ligaments are carefully divided and reflected off the scaphoid. The capsule needs to be preserved as it contains the radioscaphocapitate ligament, which needs to be repaired if possible at the end of the procedure. The bone graft can be harvested either from the distal radius or iliac crest.

The dorsal approach is the preferred technique for proximal pole scaphoid fractures. The dorsal approach to the scaphoid utilizes Lister's tubercle as an anatomical landmark with an incision over it and extended distally as desired. The structure at risk is the superficial radial nerve branch. The extensor retinaculum is identified and incised, taking care to protect the EPL. The EPL is then retracted radially to expose the capsule. Capsulotomy is then performed to expose the scaphoid.

EXAMINER: The patient has heard about percutaneous fixation techniques. What will you say to the patient?

CANDIDATE: Percutaneous fixation techniques are suitable for minimally displaced or undisplaced scaphoid fractures that allow earlier mobilization without adverse effects on healing. Haddad reported the results of 15 patients with minimally displaced or non-displaced scaphoid fractures treated percutaneously using a volar approach, traction and a cannulated screw [7]. The early rigid fixation of scaphoid fractures allows early mobilization, patients were allowed movement soon after operation. Union was achieved in all at a mean of 57 days. The range of movement after union was equal to that of the contralateral limb and grip strength was 98% of the contralateral side at 3 months. Patients were able to return to sedentary work within 4 days and manual work within 5 weeks. Results of the study showed percutaneous scaphoid fixation permitted a rapid functional recovery.

EXAMINER: What are the complications of percutaneous fixation techniques?

CANDIDATE: The complications of percutaneous fixation techniques can be divided according to the approach being used, either the volar or dorsal approach. The complications through the volar approach include damage to the FCR, radial artery and suboptimal position of screw placement (the trapezium tends to block the path of the guide wire). The complications of the dorsal approach include damage to the PIN, EPL and EDC. Possible complications for both approaches include guide wire breakage, prominence of the screw (through the subchondral bone), bleeding, infection and chronic regional pain syndrome.

EXAMINER: If the fracture fails to unite after a period of conservative management and goes into nonunion, what are the other surgical options?

CANDIDATE: The surgical options for non-union depend on the blood supply to the proximal pole and the presence or absence of osteoarthritis. Magnetic resonance imaging (MRI) of the scaphoid may help in preoperative planning to determine the vascularity and avascular necrosis (AVN) of the scaphoid. Open reduction internal fixation with a headless compression screw using a corticocancellous bone graft can be used in the absence of AVN and higher success rates are seen in more distal fractures [8]. Where AVN is present, a vascularized bone graft can be considered. There are various options available for revascularizing the proximal pole, including a vascularized pedicled bone graft or potentially a vascularized periosteal patch onlay graft,

although this technique has demonstrated disappointing union rates [9].

References

1. Clay NR, Dias JJ, Costigan PS, *et al.* Need the thumb be immobilised in scaphoid fractures? A randomised prospective trial. *J Bone Joint Surg (Br).* 1991;73B (5):828–832.

2. Dawson JS, Martel AL, Davis TR. Scaphoid blood flow and acute fracture healing: a dynamic MRI study with enhancement with gadolinium. *J Bone Joint Surg (Br).* 2001;83B:809–814.

3. Gelberman RH, Menon J. The vascularity of the scaphoid bone. *J Hand Surg Am.* 1980;5:508–513.

4. Suh N, Benson EC, Faber KJ, MacDermid J, Grewal R. Treatment of acute scaphoid fractures: a systematic review and meta-analysis. *Hand.* 2010;5:345–353.

5. Patel PD, Richard MJ. Scaphoid fracture: open reduction internal fixation. *Oper Tech Sports Med.* 2010;18:139–145.

6. Modi CS, Nancoo T, Powers D, *et al.* Operative versus nonoperative treatment of acute undisplaced and minimally displaced scaphoid waist fractures – a systematic review. *Injury.* 2009;40:268–273.

7. Haddad FS, Goddard NJ. Acute percutaneous scaphoid fixation: a pilot study. *J Bone Joint Surg (Br).* 1998;80:95–99.

8. Ramamurthy C, Cutler L, Nuttall D, *et al.* The factors affecting outcome after nonvascular bone grafting and internal fixation for non-union of the scaphoid. *J Bone Joint Surg (Br).* 2007;89B:627–632.

9. Thompson NW, Kapoor A, Thomas J, Hayton MJ. The use of a vascularised periosteal patch onlay graft in the management of non-union of the proximal scaphoid. *J Bone Joint Surg (Br).* 2008;90B:1597–1601.

Structured oral examination question 5

Scaphoid fracture (proximal pole)

EXAMINER: An apprentice joiner has fallen on his hand at work. Please describe this radiograph (Figure 17.5a).

CANDIDATE: This posteroanterior (PA) radiograph of the wrist shows an undisplaced proximal pole scaphoid fracture. I would like to confirm this further with other scaphoid views.

EXAMINER: What is the relevant anatomy?

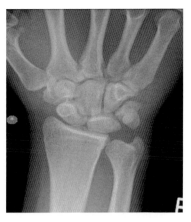

Figure 17.5a Posteroanterior (PA) radiograph of the wrist showing an undisplaced proximal pole scaphoid.

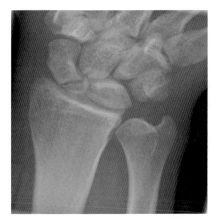

Figure 17.5b Posteroanterior (PA) radiograph of the same wrist at 4 weeks showing an undisplaced proximal pole scaphoid.

CANDIDATE: The proximal pole blood supply is from distal to proximal. A proximal 1/5 fracture

has a non-union rate of 80–100% when treated non-operatively.

EXAMINER: How do you manage this injury?

CANDIDATE: Open reduction and internal fixation with a screw placed from a proximal entry point through a dorsal incision.

EXAMINER: In this case, the fracture was treated non-operatively. This is an X-ray at 4 weeks after immobilization in a plaster cast (Figure 17.5b). Please comment.

CANDIDATE: The fracture ends appear sclerosed with some cyst formation around the edges, suggesting this is progressing to a non-union. At this stage, the proximal segment appears normal density, suggesting no loss of vascularity.

EXAMINER: How would you manage the patient now?

CANDIDATE: I would offer the patient open reduction and internal fixation through a dorsal approach with a vascularized bone graft using a 1, 2-intercompartmental supraretinacular artery (1, 2-ICSRA) pedicle [1] (Figure 17.5c and 17.5d).

EXAMINER: What is the natural history of a scaphoid non-union?

CANDIDATE: This will progress to a scaphoid non-union advanced collapse (SNAC wrist). The stages of SNAC wrist:

Stage I – arthritis between radial styloid and distal scaphoid.

Stage II – radioscaphoid fossa involvement.

Stage III – capitolunate arthritis.

Stage IV – generalized wrist arthritis.

(c)

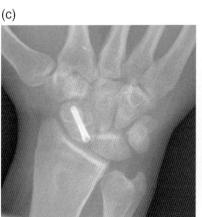

(d)

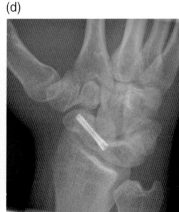

Figure 17.5c and 17.5d Anteroposterior (AP) and oblique radiographs showing union at 8 weeks postoperatively (note the lucency in the distal radius where the graft has been taken from).

EXAMINER: Why does the arthritis affect the radial styloid and distal scaphoid initially?

CANDIDATE: With a non-union, the distal scaphoid typically flexes, leading to incongruity between the distal scaphoid and radial styloid, whereas the proximal pole of the scaphoid behaves as a ball and socket joint and is not affected by being extended.

Reference

1. Zaidemberg C, Siebert JW, Angrigiani C. A new vascularized bone graft for scaphoid nonunion. *J Hand Surg Am.* 1991;16(3):474–478.

Structured oral examination question 6

Rheumatoid hand

EXAMINER: Please describe the X-ray of a 52 year old lady that was seen in your hand clinic (Figure 17.6).

CANDIDATE: This is a posteroanterior X-ray of both hands showing a symmetrical polyarthropathy typical of a rheumatoid hand and characterized by radial deviation of the wrist, ulnar drift and subluxation of the metacarpophalangeal joints (MCP).

EXAMINER: What other features are associated with rheumatoid hand?

CANDIDATE: Other hand features include Swan-neck and Boutonnière's deformities, Z-thumb deformity, swelling of the joints secondary to synovitis, muscle wasting and surgical scars.

EXAMINER: What do you mean by a Swan-neck and Boutonnière's deformity? [This is more likely to be a quick question in the clinicals rather than a detailed viva question.]

CANDIDATE: Hyperextension of the PIP joints with flexion of the DIP joints (Swan-neck deformity).

Flexion of the PIP joints and hyperextension of the DIP joints (Boutounnière deformity).

COMMENT: The viva scenario may then lead into a detailed classification of each deformity. If 'thought block' mention they can be classified as a flexible or fixed deformity.

Factual rote-learned classification systems that do not necessarily help in planning management have fallen out of favour as viva questions. It is more important to understand and apply general management principles.

EXAMINER: What would be your management options in this patient?

CANDIDATE: I would like to take a thorough history and examine both hands. I would be particularly interested in hand dominance, pain and any functional loss, asking specifically about ADLs such as doing up buttons, writing, handling coins, etc. I would also perform a functional assessment of the hand in the clinic. The patient may also be concerned about cosmesis of both

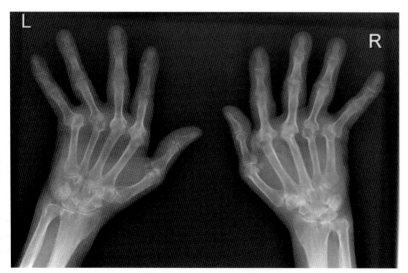

Figure 17.6 Radiographs of hand demonstrating features of rheumatoid arthritis. Erosions MCP and PIP joints. Bilateral symmetrical involvement. Never the DIP joint. Destructive changes at the wrist. Look for periarticular osteopenia, uniform joint space loss, bone erosions and soft-tissue swelling. Joint subluxation and subchondral cysts, ulnar deviation MCP joints.

hands. I would also address the realistic expectations from operative intervention of the hands.

If the patient is struggling with pain I would offer her MCP joint replacements using silastic implants. I would explain surgery aims to correct the ulnar deviation of the fingers, improve any pain from those joints and the appearance of the hand, and possibly the ability to pinch (the range of movement and grip strength are unlikely to improve).

EXAMINER: You have decided to put the patient on the waiting list for MCP joint replacement. Any challenges you could foresee in this case?

CANDIDATE: Rheumatoid arthritis is a systemic autoimmune disease, which involves cell-mediated immune response against soft tissues, cartilage and bone. The challenges can be divided into pre-, intra- and postoperative. Preoperatively, the patient would need to be seen in high-risk anaesthetic preassessment with close involvement of a rheumatologist regarding medications and biological agents. The challenges intraoperatively include skin condition, soft-tissue release and correct balancing and osteopenic bone. The challenges postoperatively include wound healing, risk of infection and postoperative splinting and hand therapy.

EXAMINER: What about medications in the rheumatoid arthritis patient?

CANDIDATE: I would enquire about steroid usage that would need covering perioperatively. Methotrexate can be continued as there is no evidence to suggest increase in infection risk [1]. However, newer biological factors such as etanercept and infliximab should be discontinued for 1 week and 6 weeks, respectively, to reduce risk of infection postoperatively [2].

EXAMINER: What are the complications of MCP joint replacement?

CANDIDATE: I would divide the complications into early and late complications. Early complications include joint infection, stiffness, implant dislocation and incomplete correction of deformity. Late complications include recurrence of ulnar drift, prosthesis wear and breakage, loosening, implant subsidence and silicone synovitis [3].

References

1. Grennan DM, Gray J, Loudon J, Fear S. Methotrexate and early postoperative complications in patients with rheumatoid arthritis undergoing elective orthopaedic surgery. *Ann Rheum Dis*. 2001;60:214–217.

2. Scanzello CR, Figgie MP, Nestor BJ, Goodman SM. Perioperative management of medications used in the treatment of rheumatoid arthritis. *HSS J*. 2006;2 (2):141–147.

3. MP joint arthroplasty. www.wheelessonline.com/ortho/ mp_joint_arthroplasty

Structured oral examination question 7

Thumb carpometacarpal (CMC) joint arthritis

EXAMINER: Please describe the X-ray findings (Figure 17.7a).

CANDIDATE: This is a posteroanterior (PA) view of the right hand showing joint space narrowing over the thumb carpometacarpal (CMC) joint with subchondral sclerosis. I would like to have true AP and lateral views of the thumb to further confirm this. A Robert's view, which is a true AP view of the thumb CMC joint, is taken with the elbow extended, the forearm fully pronated and the thumb abducted. This is shown in the X-ray below (Figure 17.7b).

EXAMINER: Do you know any classification system for thumb CMC joint arthritis?

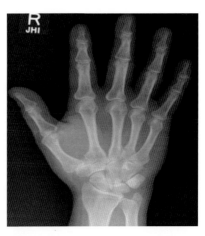

Figure 17.7a Posteroanterior (PA) radiograph, wrist.

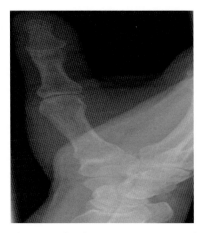

Figure 17.7b Robert's view (true AP view of the thumb CMC joint).

CANDIDATE: I would classify thumb CMC joint arthritis using the Eaton and Littler classification. This is a radiological classification.
Stage I: slight widening of the joint (2° effusion or ligament laxity), Pre-arthritic joint. Normal articular contours.
Stage II: slight joint space narrowing with sclerosis, osteophytes < 2 mm, < 1/3 metacarpal base subluxation.
Stage III: complete loss of CMC joint space with osteophytes > 2 mm, cystic changes, increased sclerosis.
Stage IV: pan-trapezial arthritis.

EXAMINER: These X-rays belong to a 65-year-old lady with a painful thumb for the past 2 years. How would you proceed?

CANDIDATE: I would like to take a thorough history and examination. I would ask about hand dominance, night pain, effect on ADLs and treatment to date. I would ask her where the pain is. Pain can be either diffuse or radial wrist pain up to the thumb MCP joint.

I would also examine the thumb, looking for squaring-off at the base of thumb and performing a grind test to confirm pain is localized at the base of thumb CMC joint.

I would consider and exclude other differential diagnoses such as:
- De Quervains (more radial styloid).
- Intersection syndrome (tender proximal to the styloid).
- STT arthritis (X-ray).
- SLAC/SNAC wrist (X-ray).

- Trigger thumb (clicking, volar pain and swelling).
- Concomitant CTS (high volume of patients in hand clinics have both CTS and basal thumb OA).

The management of thumb CMC arthritis includes non-operative and operative. Non-operative includes analgesia, activity modification, thumb splint and therapeutic injection of local anaesthesia into thumb CMC joint (as per NICE guidelines on osteoarthritis).

COMMENT: Candidates can apply the general NICE guidelines on managing osteoarthritis to different clinical situations. This quality standard covers diagnosing, assessing and managing osteoarthritis in adults. It includes treatment and support, and referral for joint surgery.

EXAMINER: What would YOU perform?

CANDIDATE: I would offer the patient simple trapeziectomy if all non-operative management has failed [1]. Prof. Davis et al. published their study in 2012 with a minimum 5 years follow-up of 153 thumbs with trapeziometacarpal osteoarthritis randomized into three groups to undergo either simple trapeziectomy, trapeziectomy with palmaris longus interposition or trapeziectomy with ligament reconstruction and tendon interposition (LRTI) using 50% of the flexor carpi radialis tendon [2]. The study showed no benefit to tendon interposition or ligament reconstruction in the longer term compared to trapeziectomy alone in regard to thumb pain, function and strength. A Cochrane review in 2015 reported low-quality evidence to guide management, with insufficient evidence to suggest LRTI had additional benefit. LRTI patients experienced more adverse events.

EXAMINER: Which ones?

CANDIDATE: Sorry, my mind has gone blank.
I would explain preoperatively this is mainly a pain-relieving procedure, she would require hand splinting for 5–6 weeks postoperatively and is likely to have some loss of grip strength on a permanent basis.

EXAMINER: What are the complications of trapeziectomy?

CANDIDATE: Complications of trapeziectomy can be divided into early and late complications.

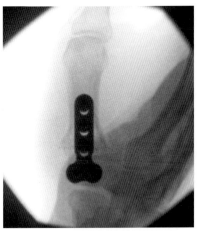 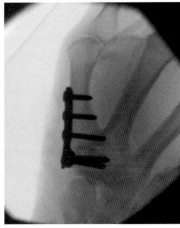

Figure 17.7c Radiographs demonstrating fusion CMC joint, as this possibly allows improved grip strength in a manual worker, but has a higher incidence of complications such as non-union.

Early – infection, haematoma formation, and injury to the superficial sensory nerves.

Late – pain, collapse of trapezial space with pain and instability, tender scar and chronic regional pain syndrome.

EXAMINER: What would you offer if this is a 34-year-old male manual worker?

CANDIDATE: I would offer the patient thumb CMC joint fusion if he is a young manual worker. A fusion may allow improved grip strength in a manual worker. However, I would also counsel the patient that fusion has a higher incidence of complication such as non-union (Figure 17.7c).

EXAMINER: You mentioned the grind test. Show me how you do it on my hand.

CANDIDATE: I would stabilize your wrist with my left hand then hold your thumb metacarpal with my right hand, and compress and rotate the metacarpal base at the CMC joint. The test is positive if this causes pain and then the pain goes with rotation and distraction.

EXAMINER: How would you try to address the adduction deformity of the thumb?

CANDIDATE: The adduction of the thumb is related to the radial subluxation of the metacarpal base and may be associated with soft-tissue contracture. A complete excision of the trapezium will shorten the radial column and may improve the deformity. However, if there is ongoing deformity and unacceptable reduction in hand span following trapeziectomy, then I would consider an extension osteotomy of the thumb metacarpal.

EXAMINER: How would you try to address the hyperextension at the MCP joint?

CANDIDATE: The hyperextension is greater than 30° and therefore if left untreated may cause a secondary swan-neck deformity of the thumb. The options for treatment are either soft-tissue procedures such as volar capsulodesis or EPB tendon transfer or a fusion of the MCPJ. I would treat this with a volar capsulodesis using a suture anchor.

References

1. Davis TR, Brady O, Barton NJ, Lunn PG, Burke FD. Trapeziectomy alone, with tendon interposition or with ligament reconstruction? *J Hand Surg Br*. 1997;22 (6):689–694.

2. Gangopadhyay S, McKenna H, Burke FD, Davis TR. Five- to 18-year follow-up for treatment of trapeziometacarpal osteoarthritis: a prospective comparison of excision, tendon interposition, and ligament reconstruction and tendon interposition. *J Hand Surg Am*. 2012;37(3):411–417.

Structured oral examination question 8

Flexor tendon sheath infections

EXAMINER: Please describe the clinical picture (Figure 17.8).

CANDIDATE: This clinical picture shows diffusely swollen and erythematous fingers, right hand. The fingers are held in flexion.

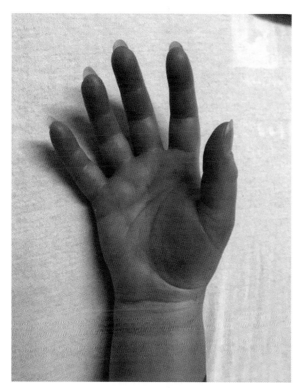

Figure 17.8 Flexor sheath tenosynovitis. There is diffuse swelling of the fingers. The fingers are flexed.

EXAMINER: What's your main concern and how would you approach this patient?

CANDIDATE: My main concern is flexor sheath tenosynovitis. I would like to take a thorough history and examine the hand. In the history, I would like to know the hand dominance, duration of swelling, pain and other associated systemic symptoms. I would examine the hand to look for any other wounds, collection and tenderness along the flexor sheath on palpation. I would then request white cell count, CRP and ESR to look for raised inflammatory markers. I would also request a plain X-ray of the digit involved to exclude the presence of foreign bodies.

EXAMINER: Who and how is this underlying condition classically described?

CANDIDATE: The classic description of flexor sheath tenosynovitis is by Kanavel [1]. He was credited with describing four cardinal signs of flexor sheath tenosynovitis, although his original paper described three – fusiform swelling,

tenderness along the flexor sheath and flexed position of the digit. Pain on passive extension of the digit was discussed in subsequent reports. Pain with passive stretching of the involved digit is perhaps the most sensitive test.

EXAMINER: You have made the diagnosis of flexor sheath tenosynovitis. How would you manage this patient?

CANDIDATE: This is an orthopaedic emergency. I would like to counsel and consent the patient for incision and drainage of the flexor sheath. I would speak to the anaesthetist and take the patient to theatre on an emergency basis. Once in theatre, I would position the patient supine with a tourniquet over the arm with the hand lying on an arm board. I would use a two-incision technique for incision and drainage of flexor. I would place my proximal incision over the A1 pulley at the distal palmar crease with complete release of this structure to gain access to the flexor sheath. A second oblique incision is made over the region of the A5 pulley, taking care to avoid injury to the neurovascular bundle. The flexor sheath is then opened up proximally and distally. Cultures are obtained and a small rigid catheter (use a venflon with the metal trochar removed) is passed into the flexor sheath for irrigation. The sheath is copiously irrigated with a minimum of 500 ml normal saline but avoiding excessive fluid extravasation into the digit because this can result in necrosis of the digit. Wounds should be left open. Postoperatively, the hand should be splinted, elevated, discussion with the microbiologist regarding appropriate intravenous antibiotics continued for 5–7 days until the redness and inflammation has subsided. Early hand therapist input plays an important role in the recovery of the patient.

EXAMINER: Is there any role in continuous catheter irrigation postoperatively?

CANDIDATE: A retrospective review comparing the intraoperative incision, drainage and irrigation with or without postoperative continuous catheter irrigation demonstrated no difference in outcomes between the two groups [2].

EXAMINER: What are the complications if this condition is not treated promptly?

CANDIDATE: The complications include early skin loss, tendon necrosis and rupture, tendon

367

adhesions, deep palmar space infection, septic arthritis, osteomyelitis and hand stiffness. The need for amputation is a known complication, especially in patients with diabetes, peripheral vascular disease and chronic renal disease.

EXAMINER: What about an open approach for flexor sheath irrigation for acute pyogenic flexor tenosynovitis?

CANDIDATE: The approach uses longitudinal midaxial or a volar zig-zag Brunner's incision with direct drainage of any purulent material. The midaxial approach is possibly preferable as there is less concern about skin coverage postoperatively. The thumb and small finger are approached from the radial side; the other digits are approached from the ulnar side. The incision begins just distal to the distal flexion crease and is extended proximally to the web space. The incision is kept dorsal to the neurovascular bundle. There is an increased risk of tendon necrosis, increased scarring and stiffness and significant morbidity. The procedure usually requires secondary procedures and prolonged rehabilitation.

EXAMINER: When would you use an open approach?

CANDIDATE: Some surgeons would prefer to use an open approach with an atypical mycobacterium infection or for chronic infections. There is some evidence to recommend open treatment of stage III infections (necrosis of the tendon, pulleys or tendon sheath).

EXAMINER: You have mentioned stage 3 infection.

CANDIDATE: The extent of infection can be graded by the Michon classification scheme.
Stage 1: serous exudate.
Stage 2: purulent fluid, granulomatous synovium.
Stage 3: necrosis of the tendon, pulleys or tendon sheath.

References

1. Kanavel A. *Infections of the Hand: A Guide to the Surgical Treatment of Acute and Chronic Suppurative Processes in the Fingers.* London: Balliere, Tindall and Cox; 1939.

2. Lille S, Hayakawa T, Neumeister MW, *et al.* Continuous postoperative catheter irrigation is not necessary for the treatment of suppurative flexor tenosynovitis. *J Hand Surg (Br).* 2000;25(3):304–307.

Structured oral examination question 9

Flexor tendon injury

EXAMINER: Can you describe this clinical photograph and what it represents (Figure 17.9)?

CANDIDATE: This is a clinical photograph of the right palm showing the five zones of flexor tendon injury.
Zone 1 – flexor digitorum profundus distal to insertion of flexor digitorum superficialis.
Zone 2 – insertion of flexor digitorum superficialis to proximal edge of A1 pulley (no man's land).
Zone 3 – proximal edge of A1 pulley to distal edge of carpal tunnel.
Zone 4 – within the carpal tunnel.
Zone 5 – proximal to the carpal tunnel.

EXAMINER: When would you consider repairing a lacerated tendon?

CANDIDATE: I would consider repairing a lacerated tendon if involving more than 60% of cross-sectional area. Studies have shown that a lacerated

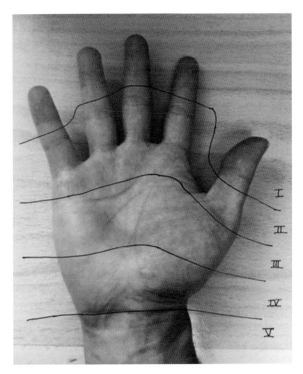

Figure 17.9 Flexor tendon injury zones.

tendon with less than 60% cross-sectional area involvement can be managed without repair, but with debridement and early mobilization. This has resulted in better tendon excursion as well as increased tendon strength compared to tendons that were repaired or immobilized [1].

EXAMINER: What is the goal of tendon repair and how would you perform it?

CANDIDATE: The goal of tendon repair is to maintain sufficient strength to avoid rupture with either passive or active movement during mobilization. I would repair the tendon using a modified Kessler technique with epitenon reinforcement to decrease gap formation across the repair site and reduce friction. I would aim for a minimum of four strands as core sutures as the strength of tendon repair is directly proportional to the number of core sutures across the tendon repair site. Circumferential epitenon suture has also been shown to significantly increase the resistance of the tendon repair to gap formation as well as adding 20% to the ultimate tensile strength of the repair [2].

EXAMINER: What is the significance of Zone 2 flexor tendon injury?

CANDIDATE: Bunnell referred to this area as no man's land because the initial results of the tendon here were so poor. This zone has the highest probability of developing adhesions and the poorest prognosis. There are two flexor tendons, FDP and FDS, within the flexor tendon sheath and compounded by the fact that FDP travels through the FDS tendon at Champer's chiasm, creating another adhesion surface. The advances in suture techniques, better understanding of the tendon morphology and its biomechanics as well as early active mobilization rehabilitation protocols have resulted in better outcomes in Zone 2 flexor tendon repair.

EXAMINER: What is the postoperative rehabilitation following flexor tendon repair?

CANDIDATE: Postoperative rehabilitation aims to mobilize early (48 hours postoperatively) to prevent adhesions. Most patients will be put into an active 'place and hold' regimen rather than traditional passive range of motion regimen. This was supported by a randomized controlled trial by Trumble *et al.* in 2010 which showed that active motion had significantly fewer flexion contractures, better satisfaction scores and improved

range of motion than passively rehabilitated patients. Importantly, there was no difference in the tendon re-rupture rate [3].

References

1. Bishop AT, Cooney WP 3rd, Wood MB. Treatment of partial flexor tendon lacerations: the effect of tenorrhaphy and early protected mobilisation. *J Trauma.* 1986;26(4):301–312.

2. Pruitt DL, Manske PR, Fink B. Cyclic stress analysis of flexor tendon repair. *J Hand Surg (Am).* 1991;16 (4):701–707.

3. Trumble TE, Vedder NB, Seiler JG 3rd, *et al.* Zone-II flexor tendon repair: a randomised prospective trial of active place-and-hold therapy compared with passive motion therapy. *J Bone Joint Surg (Am).* 2013;38:1800–1802.

Structured oral examination question 10

Enchondroma

EXAMINER: Please describe the clinical picture of a 10-year-old girl who fell onto her left hand a few hours ago (Figure 17.10a).

CANDIDATE: I noticed swelling over the proximal phalanx left middle finger with no associated bruising or rotational deformity. There is widening of the interspace between the index and middle fingers.

EXAMINER: How would you manage this patient?

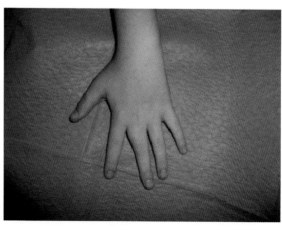

Figure 17.10a Clinical picture of an 11-year-old's hand.

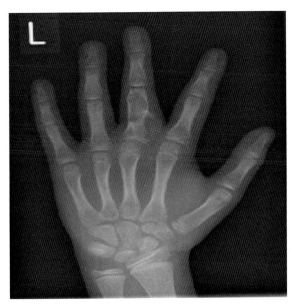

Figure 17.10b Radiograph of the child's hand.

CANDIDATE: I would take a detailed history and examination of the affected hand and finger. I would look for any swelling, bruising or rotational deformity of the middle finger on clinical examination. I would provide adequate analgesia for the patient and arrange an X-ray of the middle finger to exclude fracture.

EXAMINER: Please describe the X-ray of the left middle finger of this patient (Figure 17.10b).

CANDIDATE: This is a posteroanterior (PA) view of the left hand of a skeletally immature patient. The radiograph shows a pathological fracture through the cystic lesion affecting the proximal phalanx of the middle finger. The proximal radial cortex is markedly thinned and expanded to the radial side, causing widening between the middle and index fingers. The X-ray finding is highly suggestive of enchondroma (benign cartilage tumour of bone). I would confirm this further with lateral and oblique views of the middle finger.

EXAMINER: How would you manage this fracture?

CANDIDATE: As discussed earlier, I would take a detailed history and examination of the affected finger. History includes rapid increase in size or pain over the middle finger. I would also look for swelling elsewhere in the contralateral hand and body. Enchondroma has been associated with multiple enchondromatosis (Ollier's disease) and haemangiomas (Mafucci's disease). I would explain this is a benign tumour that has been present prior to the injury.

I would manage this fracture conservatively with buddy strapping for 2 weeks provided there is no rotational deformity. I would also arrange a contralateral hand X-ray to look for associated enchondroma. I would review them at 6 weeks and then annually. If it continued to increase in size, I would refer to a hand surgeon for partial excision and bone grafting [1].

EXAMINER: What are you going to tell the parent who is concerned regarding this lesion?

CANDIDATE: I would discuss and reassure the patient and parent that this is a benign cartilage tumour of bone that is mostly asymptomatic. Most patients present with incidental findings on X-ray after trauma. Most enchondromas do not require any surgical intervention unless symptomatic. The malignant risk with a single lesion is low but the risk increases to 20–30% for Ollier's disease and near 100% for Mafucci's disease. I would reassure the parent that this lesion simply requires further follow-up to make sure it doesn't increase in size.

References

1. O'Connor MI, Bancroft LW. Benign and malignant cartilage tumours of the hand. *Hand Clin.* 2004;20 (3):317–323.

2. Athanasian EA. Bone and soft tissue tumours. In DP Green, RN Hotchkiss, WC Pederson *et al.* (Eds.), *Green's Operative Hand Surgery*, 5th ed. Philadelphia: Churchill Livingstone; 2005: pp. 2211–2263.

Structured oral examination question 11

Wrist ganglion

EXAMINER: Please describe this clinical picture (Figure 17.11a).

CANDIDATE: This clinical picture of a clenched right fist shows a swelling over the dorsoradial aspect of the wrist, suggestive of ganglion.

EXAMINER: How would you confirm your diagnosis?

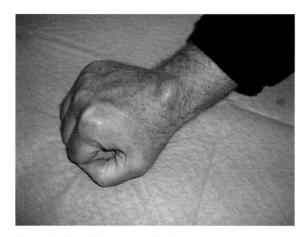

Figure 17.11a Clinical picture of wrist.

CANDIDATE: I would take history from the patient, specifically asking about any fluctuation in size. Clinically this would be a firm smooth swelling attached to deep structures that classically transilluminates. I would request radiological investigations such as ultrasound or magnetic resonance imaging (MRI) to confirm my diagnosis.

EXAMINER: This is the investigation that has been performed. Please comment (Figure 17.11b).

CANDIDATE: This is a T2-weighted MR scan showing a well-circumscribed, focal, multiloculated lesion overlying the lunate and capitate dorsally on the sagittal view of the wrist. The MR scan confirms the diagnosis of ganglion that is likely to have arisen from the scapholunate ligament.

EXAMINER: What is the aetiology of this condition?

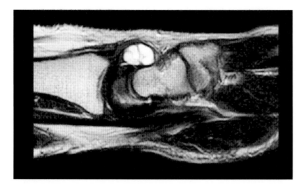

Figure 17.11b Imaging of the same wrist.

CANDIDATE: Ganglion is a mucin-filled synovial cyst with no true epithelial lining that arises from the tendon sheath or joint capsule.

EXAMINER: How would you manage this?

CANDIDATE: I would counsel the patient that this is a benign condition. As long as there is no history of increasing size or pain, this can be treated with observation only. If there is pain affecting function, especially with forced wrist extension, then aspiration or surgical excision may be offered.

EXAMINER: What complications can occur with aspiration?

CANDIDATE: Haematoma, bruising, infection and reoccurrence.

EXAMINER: What is the incidence of reoccurrence following aspiration?

CANDIDATE: The reoccurrence rate following aspiration is 50%.

EXAMINER: What would you do if the ganglion reoccurs after aspiration?

CANDIDATE: If the ganglion reoccurs after aspiration and the patient remains symptomatic, I would offer the patient surgical excision, taking into consideration the reoccurrence rate of 5%. I would perform surgical excision through a transverse incision, taking into consideration the location of the ganglion and structures at risk.

EXAMINER: What complications can occur with surgical excision?

CANDIDATE: Haematoma, bruising, infection, neurovascular damage and reoccurrence.

EXAMINER: What is the second most common hand swelling?

CANDIDATE: A giant cell tumour or xanthelasma.

EXAMINER: Correct.

Structured oral examination question 12

Dupuytren's disease

EXAMINER: Please describe the clinical photograph of a 45-year-old with this problem in the non-dominant hand (Figure 17.12a).

371

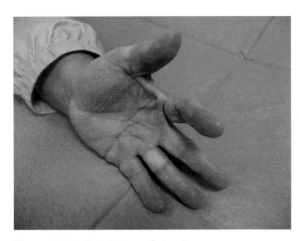

Figure 17.12a Clinical picture of a hand.

CANDIDATE: The clinical picture shows a thick cord crossing the first webspace of the left hand, causing a web space contracture, and fixed flexion at the metacarpophalangeal (MCP) and proximal interphalangeal (PIP) joint of index finger. The appearance is very suggestive of Dupuytren's disease. The cord seen is known as the commissural band, usually associated with Dupuytren's diathesis.

Dupuytren's diathesis is the aggressive form of the disease related to features such as bilateral multiple digits involvement; young age < 50 years old, male and positive family history. Other features include ectopic lesion such as Garrod's pad, Peyronie disease, Ledderhose disease and frozen shoulder. The degree of diathesis is considered important in predicting recurrence and extension of Dupuytren's disease after surgical management [1].

EXAMINER: What is the primary cell involved?

CANDIDATE: The primary cell involved in Dupuytren's disease is the myofibroblast. They are probably derived from fibroblasts and contain smooth muscle actin which leads to contracture of the cord.

EXAMINER: What other risk factors are associated with this disease?

CANDIDATE: Other risk factors for Dupuytren's disease include diabetes, epilepsy, high alcohol intake, smoking, COPD, liver disease, positive family history, tuberculosis and HIV/AIDS.

EXAMINER: What structures make up a spiral cord and how does it affect the neurovascular bundle?

CANDIDATE: The pretendinous, lateral and spiral bands and Grayson's ligament make up the spiral cord. A spiral cord displaces the neurovascular bundle centrally and superficially and places it at risk during cord excision.

EXAMINER: How do you classify the disease?

CANDIDATE: The British Society for Surgery of the Hand (BSSH) classifies Dupuytren's disease as:

Mild – no functional problems, no contracture or metacarpophalangeal joint contracture of less than 30°.

Moderate – functional problems, metacarpophalangeal joint contracture of 30–60°, proximal interphalangeal joint contracture of less than 30°, or first web contracture.

Severe – severe contracture of both metacarpophalangeal joint (greater than 60°) and proximal interphalangeal joint (greater than 30°).

EXAMINER: What are the management options?

CANDIDATE: Management can be divided into non-operative and operative. Non-operative management includes observation ± night splintage, and collagenase injections.

Operative intervention includes fasciotomy (division of the cord), fasciectomy (excision of the cord) and dermofasciectomy (cord and

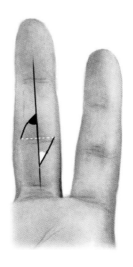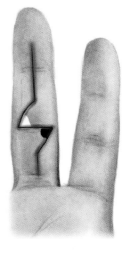

Figure 17.12b How to draw a Z-plasty. 1. Draw perpendicular (white dotted line) to longitudinal incision. 2. Mark flaps (white and black angles are at 60°). 3. Cross over flaps as shown.

overlying skin excised) and skin grafting. Occasionally, amputation would be indicated in a multiply operated digit.

EXAMINER: What is a Z-plasty? Can you draw it?

CANDIDATE: It is a technique to manage skin deficiency. Angles should be made at 60° to the incision to achieve a 75% increase in length (Figure 17.12b).

EXAMINER: How would you consent for a fasciectomy?

CANDIDATE: The operation will be carried out under general anaesthetic (you will be put to sleep) or an axillary bock (nerves to your arm are numbed by an injection in your armpit), and as a day case procedure. The aim is to restore lost movement. You will wake up with your hand in a heavy bandage and allowed home once you are comfortable. You will be seen at 10 days for removal of your sutures. You will then have physiotherapy to help with scar management and regaining finger movement and may need a splint. Complications include the following [2]:

Early infection, bleeding and haematoma formation, arterial or nerve injury, necrosis of digit leading to amputation, tendon injury and delayed wound healing.

Late joint stiffness, recurrence (50% recur but most do not require further surgery) and reoperation, incomplete correction of deformity and complex regional pain syndrome.

EXAMINER: Do you know any new treatments for Dupuytren's contracture?

CANDIDATE: Collagenase (Xiapex®) injections are now licensed in Europe for a Dupuytren's contracture. Two randomized controlled studies of 374 patients comparing Xiapex to placebo have shown benefit with 60% showing correction to 5° of full extension [3]. The patient has an injection at three points along the cord and returns the next day for a finger extension procedure. The technique is appropriate treatment for a patient with single-digit involvement and contractures limited to the palm and MCP joint. The patient can receive up to a maximum of three injections per cord, limited to two digits (one at a time) at 4-week intervals. The usage of collagenase is of limited benefit in patients with multiple digit involvement. The complications of this treatment include swollen lymph nodes, itching, pain, swelling, injection site bleeding, tenderness and bruising.

References

1. Hindocha S, Stanley JK, Watson S, Bayat A. Dupuytren's diathesis revisited: evaluation of prognostic indicators for risk of disease recurrence. *J Hand Surg Am.* 2006;31 (10):1626–1634.

2. Hayton MJ, Gray ICM. Dupuytren's contracture: a review. *Curr Orthop.* 2003;17:1–7.

3. Hurst LC, Badalamente MA, Hentz VR, *et al.* Injectable collagenase *Clostridium histolyticum* for Dupuytren's contracture. *N Engl J Med.* 2009;361(10):968–979.

Structured oral examination question 13

Kienbock's disease

EXAMINER: Please describe this X-ray (Figure 17.13a).

CANDIDATE: This is a posteroanterior radiograph of a left hand showing sclerosis of the lunate with some cyst formation and partial collapse. There are no radiological arthritic changes to the surrounding joints. The radiograph is suggestive of Kienbock's disease (avascular necrosis of the lunate).

EXAMINER: What are the predisposing factors for Kienbock's disease?

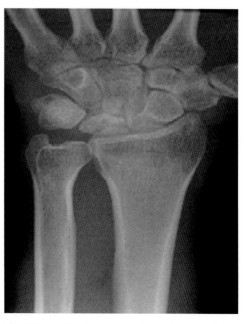

Figure 17.13a Posteroanterior (PA) radiograph of left hand.

CANDIDATE: Predisposing factors include ulnar minus variant – this is thought to lead to increased loading on the lunate, poor intraosseous anastomosis and a single extraosseous nutrient vessel.

EXAMINER: What are the patterns of intraosseous blood supply for lunate?

CANDIDATE: Gelbermann described the various patterns of intraosseous blood supply for lunate – Y pattern (60%), I pattern (30%) and an X pattern (10%) – in his paper in 1980. Single or repetitive microfractures can result in disruption of the blood supply to the lunate. Recurrent compression of the lunate between the capitate and distal radius can also disrupt the intraosseous structures. The I-pattern as described by Gelbermann is a single blood supply to the lunate and is most susceptible to AVN from repetitive microfractures as compared to X and Y patterns. As such, a patient with I-pattern lunate blood supply is more susceptible to AVN.

EXAMINER: What classification do you know for Kienbock's disease?

CANDIDATE: Lichtman, which is a radiological classification. The stages as described by Lichtman are as follows:

Stage I – plain radiographs normal (changes seen on MRI). Clinical findings are similar to a wrist sprain.
Stage II – lunate sclerosis seen on plain radiographs. The overall size, shape and relationship to the carpal bones are not altered. Clinically the patient complains of recurrent pain, swelling and wrist tenderness.
Stage IIIA – fragmentation and collapse of lunate without fixed scaphoid rotation (derangements or instability).
Stage IIIB – fragmentation and collapse of lunate with fixed scaphoid rotation, decreased carpal height and ulnar migration of the triquetrium. Clinically the patient will complain of progressive wrist weakness, stiffness, pain along with clicking and clunking.
Stage IV – radiocarpal and midcarpal arthritis, degenerative wrist changes. Clinically the patient has degenerative arthrosis of the wrist.

EXAMINER: What is the role of MRI in Kienbock's disease?

CANDIDATE: MRI is particularly useful in the early stages of the disease when clinical findings are suggestive of the disease, but radiographs are normal. MRI will show decreased signals on T1- and T2-weighted images.

EIXAMINER: What's the differential diagnosis?

CAINDIDATE: The differential diagnosis includes post-traumatic arthritis, rheumatoid arthritis, synovial-based inflammatory diseases, ulnar abutment syndrome, fracture and carpal instability.

EXAMINER: What are the management options for Kienbock's disease?

CANDIDATE: This depends on the patient's symptoms, functional demands, stage of the disease and patient factors. Conservative treatment with a period of time in splintage can be discussed. However, in symptomatic patients with Stage I/II/IIIA disease and if ulnar minus, I would offer a joint levelling procedure, either a radial shortening or less commonly an ulnar lengthening. I would prefer a shortening osteotomy because the incidence of non-/delayed union is less. If ulnar neutral or plus, I would consider a procedure aiming to reduce loading on the lunate – either a partial carpal arthrodesis (scaphotrapezium-trapezoid or scaphocapitate) or a capitate shortening. Other options are a vascularized bone graft with 4, 5-ICSRA, core

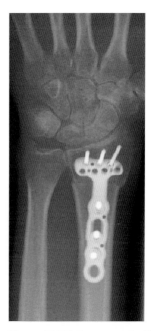

Figure 17.13b Posteroanterior (PA) radiograph demonstrating a joint levelling procedure (radial shortening).

decompression of the distal radius or a distal radial osteotomy. Surgical options for Stage IIIB/IV disease include a neurectomy, or salvage procedures such as a proximal row carpectomy or a wrist arthrodesis.

EXAMINER: How would you manage this case?

CANDIDATE: I would confirm these were true length films for ulna variance – i.e. a wrist PA view with the shoulder forward flexed 90°, elbow 90° and forearm midprone. If these were, the wrist appears to be ulnar minus and I would offer a joint levelling procedure with a radial shortening using a volar locking plate (Figure 17.13b).

Reference

1. Gelberman RH, Bauman TD, Menon J, Akeson WH. The vascularity of the lunate bone and Kienbock's disease. *J Hand Surg Am*. 1980;5(3):272–278.

Structured oral examination question 14

Ulnar collateral ligament (UCL) injury of thumb

EXAMINER: What test is being done here (Figure 17.14a)?

CANDIDATE: This is a stress test being performed for ulnar collateral ligament (UCL) injury of the thumb. The test is done by stabilizing the thumb metacarpal and applying a valgus stress to the thumb MCP joint with the thumb flexed at 30°. The test is positive when the metacarpophalangeal (MCP) joint opens up 20° or more compared to the contralateral side.

EXAMINER: Tell me about ulnar collateral ligament injury. What is a Stener lesion and its significance?

CANDIDATE: Acute ulnar collateral ligament injury is known as skier's thumb and chronic injury is known as a gamekeeper's thumb. A Stener lesion occurs when the UCL avulses from its insertion to the base of the proximal phalanx, folds proximally and the adductor aponeurosis becomes interposed between the torn UCL and the MCP joint preventing its healing. A Stener lesion requires surgical intervention.

EXAMINER: How would you differentiate between complete and incomplete tear?

CANDIDATE: Clinical examination should differentiate between complete and incomplete lesions. Incomplete lesions have a definite end point to collateral ligament testing. There are two components to the ulnar collateral ligament, the proper and accessory UCL. Instability of the MCPJ in flexion suggests an isolated proper UCL injury whereas instability in extension suggests the accessory ligament is involved.

Plain radiographs would not demonstrate any joint widening on the ulnar border of the MCPJ in

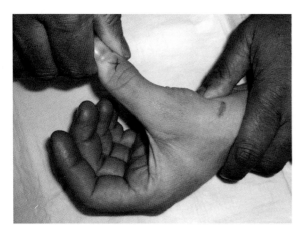

Figure 17.14a Clinical picture of stress testing ulnar collateral ligament (UCL).

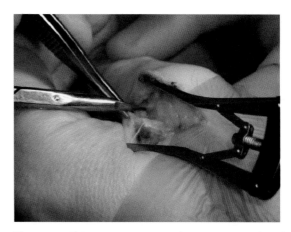

Figure 17.14b Intraoperative picture showing an approach to the medial side of the thumb MCP joint for an ulnar collateral ligament repair. The scissor tips are pointing at the bare insertion of the ligament to the base of the proximal phalanx. This is a chronic case and the scarred proximal ligament is lying bunched up over the metacarpal head.

an incomplete lesion. Ultrasound scanning is useful.

EXAMINER: When would you decide to operate on UCL injury?

CANDIDATE: I would opt to operate if there's more than 20° of opening on radial stressing of an acute UCL injury or the presence of a Stener lesion. The UCL can be repaired with direct suture repair, suture anchor or small screw fixation if there is a large avulsed bony fragment (Figure 17.14b).

EXAMINER: How does a chronic UCL injury present?

CANDIDATE: Patients will complain of pain mainly on the inner side of the thumb when stressing the thumb with activities like gripping or pinching. In addition, they complain that the thumb feels weak on pinching.

EXAMINER: How would you manage a chronic UCL injury?

CANDIDATE: In a symptomatic chronic UCL injury, this would need reconstruction using the palmaris longus tendon as a graft. In longstanding cases, patients can develop arthritic changes and, in this situation, MCP fusion would be indicated.

Structured oral examination question 15

Boutonnière deformity

EXAMINER: A rugby player has injured his finger during a game. He has pain and swelling and attends casualty where radiographs are taken. Describe what you see and the likely diagnosis (Figure 17.15a).

CANDIDATE: The radiographs show flexion at the PIP joint of the little finger and hyperextension at the DIP.

EXAMINER: How would you manage this?

CANDIDATE: I would test the central slip of the extensor mechanism by Elson's test – the PIP joint is flexed to 90° over the edge of a table, and the patient is asked to extend the finger against resistance (the examiner presses on the middle phalanx). A positive test shows weakness of extension of the PIP joint with hyperextension of the DIP joint due to recruitment of the lateral bands.

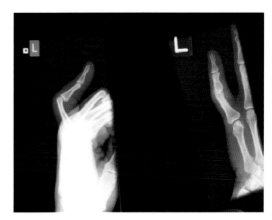

Figure 17.15a Anteroposterior (AP) and lateral radiographs of a little finger.

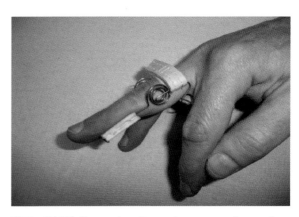

Figure 17.15b Picture of a splint used to manage a Boutonnière deformity.

A closed central slip rupture if left may lead to a Boutonnière deformity. I would offer a dynamic splint – a Capener – to keep the PIP joint passively extended but allow active flexion (Figure 17.15b). This needs to be worn for 6 weeks. I would explain that a mild flexion deformity is likely even with treatment.

Structured oral examination question 16

Swan-neck deformity

EXAMINER: These are clinical pictures of a 60-year-old lady complaining of difficulty making a full fist with her left hand (Figure 17.16).

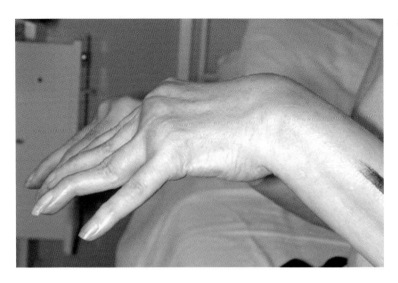

Figure 17.16 Swan-neck deformity, fingers.

CANDIDATE: The photograph shows hyperextension at the proximal interphalangeal joint (PIPJ) and flexion at the distal interphalangeal joints (DIP) of the left middle and ring fingers.

EXAMINER: What deformity is this and what is the pathophysiology of it?

CANDIDATE: This is swan-neck deformity. These deformities occur due to volar plate laxity or an imbalance of forces on the PIP joint.

COMMENT: Candidate should have followed through and said the picture was highly suggestive of swan-neck deformity in keeping with a picture of a generalized symmetrical polyarthropathy, most likely rheumatoid arthritis. The patient is unable to make a full fist due to the hyperextended posture of the PIP joint.

EXAMINER: What is the classification system associated with this deformity?

CANDIDATE: Swan-neck deformity in a rheumatoid hand is classified according to PIPJ mobility and radiographic appearances:
Type I – PIP joint flexible in all positions.
Type II – PIP joint motion limited only by tenodesis effect (tight intrinsics).
Type III – fixed PIP joint contracture, X-ray preserved joint space.
Type IV – arthritic changes with loss of active and passive motion at PIPJ.

EXAMINER: What are the causes of this deformity?

CANDIDATE: Swan neck deformity has several different aetiologies. The primary pathology is a lax volar plate; this may be caused by rheumatoid arthritis, trauma or generalized ligamentous laxity. The secondary pathology is an imbalance of hand intrinsic muscles. This may occur at different sites such as at MCP, PIP or DIP joints.

MCP joint volar subluxation seen in RA causes intrinsic and central tendon tightness leading to volar subluxation and flexion at the MCP joint.

PIP joint FDS rupture with unopposed PIPJ extension resulting in intrinsic contracture. There is tethering of the lateral bands by the transverse retinacular ligament as a result of PIPJ hyperextension. The excursion of the lateral bands is restricted; therefore, the extension force is not transmitted to the terminal tendon. The extension force is transmitted to the PIP joint instead.

DIP joint Mallet injury. The DIP joint extension force is transferred to the PIPJ central slip.

EXAMINER: What are the surgical treatments for swan-neck deformity?

CANDIDATE: The patient's hand function and expectations must be fully assessed. The surgical treatment depends upon the site of the lesion (DIPJ, PIPJ or MCPJ), where the deformity originated from and whether the deformities are fixed or flexible. Flexible deformities can be treated with soft-tissue procedures, whereas fixed deformities require bony procedures such as arthrodesis or arthroplasty. The surgical intervention is tailored in addressing the primary pathology of the swan-neck deformity. I would divide the surgical procedures according to the joints involved such as below:

MCP joint problems can be addressed with synovectomy and MCP joint arthroplasty. A lateral tenodesis can be performed using the ulnar lateral band which is mobilized at the MCP joint. The band is passed volar to Cleland's ligament and fixed to itself around the A2 pulley attachment (as for FDS tenodesis).

PIP joint problems, FDS tenodesis can be performed with a single slip of the FDS being passed around the A2 pulley sewn to itself holding the PIP joint flexed. This position can be maintained with a temporary K-wire. A dorsal release may also be necessary using a curvilinear incision over the PIP joint. The extensor expansion including lateral bands and collateral ligaments is released with removal of osteophytes and with a synovectomy if required, ensuring full PIP joint range of movement. Particular attention should be paid to the central slip to ensure that it's not damaged during surgery.

DIP joint problems can be addressed with a DIP joint fusion or possibly a dermodesis.

EXAMINER: What are the complications of surgery?

CANDIDATE: I would divide the complications of surgery into those related to the actual surgical procedures, those related to the systemic disease of rheumatoid arthritis or those related to anti-rheumatoid medications.

Complications related to surgery

Soft-tissue procedure infection, wound breakdown, failure to correct deformity, recurrence of deformity, overcorrection of deformity, neurovascular damage, scar pain, stiffness and CRPS.

Arthrodesis procedure non-union, malunion, implant failure or prominence metalwork (additional to the complications of soft-tissue procedure).

Arthroplasty procedure implant failure, fracture, dislocation, loosening, stiffness, osteolysis, tendon/ligament damage, failure to relieve symptoms.

Complications related to medications

Medications should be managed in conjunction with a rheumatologist. Patients taking corticosteroids undergoing surgery may need corticosteroid coverage perioperatively. Coverage should be provided if the patient has been on 10 mg of prednisolone per day for 1 week or more within the last 6 months. This is usually given in the form of hydrocortisone IM or IV. The exact regime depends upon the amount of surgical stress expected.

Aspirin/NSAIDs use affects platelet function and bleeding during and after surgery. NSAIDs can also increase the risk of GI bleeds and renal impairment perioperatively.

Anti-TNF and other biological medications may affect wound healing and increase the risk of infection postoperatively. Speak to a rheumatologist preoperatively. It is considered safe to continue methotrexate during the operative period, with most studies showing no increase in infection rates.

Complications related to systemic diseases

Cervical spine cervical spine disease is common in patients with RA. This must be fully assessed clinically and radiologically preoperatively. Atlantoaxial subluxation or basal invagination is a possible complication of RA and the C-spine anaesthetist should make a full assessment preoperatively.

Cardiac disease mostly not related to RA, but some cardiac disease can be secondary to RA such as pericarditis, conduction blocks secondary to granulomas or nodules, left-sided heart failure and disease of the myocardium or valves.

Airway disease along with cervical spine pathology, cricoarytenoid RA and laryngeal oedema can make management of airway difficult.

Lung disease: pleurisy, pleural effusion, rheumatoid nodules and mild fibrosing alveolitis. More severe lung disease such as interstitial pneumonitis or fibrosis and bronchiolitis can affect operative risk. These may be secondary to rheumatic drug therapy such as gold, penicillamine or methotrexate.

Bone disease can lead to osteoporosis and care should be taken when handling these patients.

Vasculitis can lead to non-healing ulcers and neuropathy.

Renal disease: the kidneys may be affected by vasculitis or amyloidosis (chronic disease). Pharmacological treatments may also damage the kidneys.

Haematological RA patient may have anaemia or neutropenia (Felty's syndrome).

Infection patients with RA may have an increased susceptibility to infection postoperatively. This may be related to the disease process or secondary to medications (anti-TNF).

Children's orthopaedics

Mohamed Hafez and Sattar Alshryda

Introduction

Feedback from candidates who did the FRCS exam showed that the pediatric viva section has certainly changed since the introduction of the first edition of this book. The paediatric viva section seems to contain the followings three areas:

1. One of the big paediatric topics such as DDH, septic hip, SUFE, clubfoot or knee deformities, during which in-depth knowledge is expected from candidates.
2. A common significant paediatric trauma such as elbow/supracondylar fracture, forearm fractures, femur fractures, NAI or paediatric ankle fractures. Again, the candidate is expected to have a solid knowledge about these subjects.
3. The last area is about common conditions that could face orthopaedic surgeons in any subspecialty such as bone cyst, multiple hereditary exostosis, tarsal coalition, pes cavus, osteochondritis dissecans.

In this section, we follow the exam format with a simple question around a clinical picture, X-ray or a video clip, followed by increasingly difficult questions to explore candidate depth and breadth of knowledge. Some of the questions are made deliberately difficult and beyond average candidate level, some are easy and the majority are average. We also support some of the answers with clinical photographs to create mental images to aid recall information during the exam. The online version of this book will have more cases, videos and discussion. This section complements the first edition of this book, the postgraduate paediatric orthopaedic book (the green book) [1] and the third edition of the parent book. Candidates are strongly encouraged to read all of them to have a better overview of the paediatric section of the exam.

Candidate 1

EXAMINER: This is a clinical photograph of a child (Figure 18.1) who tripped and fell, hurting his knee. He was seen in the A&E department and referred to your fracture clinic. Describe what you see. How would you approach him?

CANDIDATE: My approach is to take a detailed history, perform a thorough examination and order the appropriate investigations guided by my examination and provisional diagnosis. The left image shows a child standing with two crutches, wearing a knee splint on the left lower limb. The left leg is externally rotated and may be short. My first impression is that this child may have a slipped upper femoral epiphysis (SUFE).

EXAMINER: How can you confirm your diagnosis?

CANDIDATE: History, examination and radiological tests to confirm my diagnosis. History of previous pain in the hip before the fall is an important clue. He stands with crutches (if he has a slip, it is probably a stable type). Hip examination may reveal limited internal rotation or even obligatory external rotation on flexing the hip (Drehmann sign). I also request pelvis X-ray (AP and cross-table lateral views of both hips). I do not prefer frog lateral as it may worsen the severity in unstable slips; however, it is reasonable to request in a stable slip.

EXAMINER: This is his pelvis X-ray (Figure 18.2). What can you see?

CANDIDATE: This is a plain X-ray of the pelvis (AP view only) showing both hips. The most obvious abnormality is the slipped upper femoral (capital) epiphysis on the left side. The head remained in the socket while the neck moves anteriorly and superiorly. Trethowan's sign is positive; a line (often referred to as Klein's line) drawn on the superior border of the femoral neck on the AP view should pass through the femoral head.

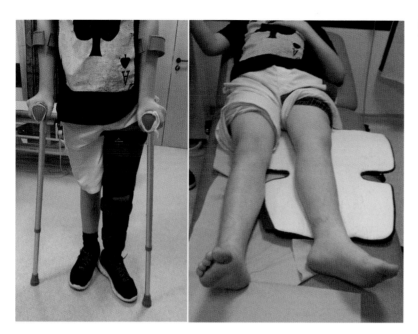

Figure 18.1 Twelve-year-old boy who tripped and fell.

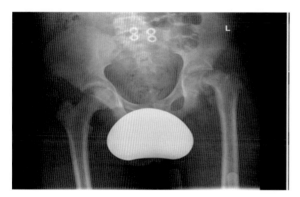

Figure 18.2 Pelvis X-ray of 12-year-old child with knee pain shown in Figure 18.1.

In SUFE, the line passes over the head rather than through the head. There are remodelling changes of the neck with sclerotic, smooth superior part of the neck and callus formation on the inferior border. This indicates the slip is not acute and has been subclinical for a while.

EXAMINER: What other radiological signs might you see in SUFE?

CANDIDATE: Several radiological signs are described to aid diagnosing SUFE (particularly subtle ones). These are not present in every case of SUFE, such as Trethowan's sign that I just mentioned; widening and irregularity of the growth plate (early sign); decreased epiphyseal height as the head slipped

posteriorly behind the neck; remodelling changes of the neck and increased distance between the teardrop and the femoral neck metaphysis. Capener's sign: normally, on the AP pelvis the posterior acetabular margin cuts across the medial corner of the upper femoral metaphysis. In SUFE, the entire metaphysis is lateral to the posterior acetabular margin. Steel's blanch sign, which is a crescent shape dense area in the metaphysis due to superimposition of the neck and the head.

EXAMINER: What if this child's X-ray was normal?

CANDIDATE: Normal X-ray does not exclude SUFE (it may be in the preslip stage); therefore, I would request an MRI scan but also, I would consider other possible diagnoses.

EXAMINER: Can you grade the severity?

CANDIDATE: I measure the severity using either Wilson grading on the AP views or the Southwick angle on the lateral views. I consider that this is a severe slip as the head almost slipped by more than two-thirds of the physis width.

EXAMINER: Can you draw for me how these two classifications measure the severity of the slip?

CANDIDATE: Radiological grading of the severity of the slip has been based on either the degree of

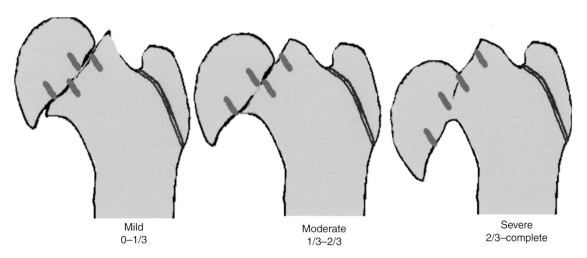

Mild
0–1/3

Moderate
1/3–2/3

Severe
2/3–complete

Figure 18.3 SUFE radiological grading.

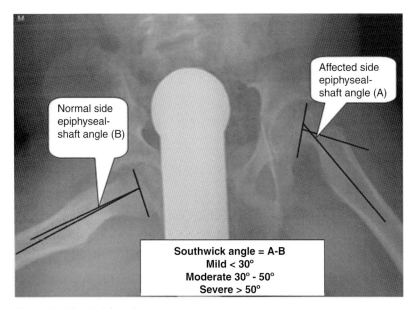

Normal side epiphyseal-shaft angle (B)

Affected side epiphyseal-shaft angle (A)

Southwick angle = A-B
Mild < 30°
Moderate 30° - 50°
Severe > 50°

Figure 18.4 Southwick angle.

displacement of the head relative to the neck (Wilson), or by degree of the angulation of the head relative to the shaft (Southwick). Wilson recognized three grades on the AP view: mild slip (grade I) is one where the displacement of the head as a proportion of neck (physis) width is less than a third, moderate slip (grade II), displacement is between a third and a half of the neck width and severe slip (grade III) has displacement of greater than half of the neck width (Figure 18.3).

Southwick graded the severity on the frog lateral view by measuring the Southwick angle, which is the difference between the lateral epiphyseal shaft angle of the slipped and the non-slipped sides (Figure 18.4). Mild slip (grade I) has an angle difference of less than 30°, moderate slip (grade II) has an angle difference of between 30° and 50° and severe slip has a difference of over 50°. If both sides slipped, Southwick angle is calculated by subtracting 12° from the corresponding lateral epiphyseal shaft angle.

381

EXAMINER: You mentioned that the slip is stable. Why?

CANDIDATE: Randall Loder [2] classified SUFE into two types:

I. Stable slip: child is able to weight bear.
II. Unstable slip: child is not able to weight bear on the affected side even with crutches.

This classification has been shown to be of prognostic value. The risk of AVN is high in an unstable SUFE and low in a stable one. In Loder's original paper the AVN rate was 47% in unstable SUFE and 0% in stable ones. Similar findings were shown in other centres [3,4].

There has been some confusion about the exact meaning of 'able to weight bear' in Loder's original paper. 'Ambulation' may be a better term to describe slip stability. So, to me the slip is unstable if the child cannot weight bear and ambulate even with crutches. This child is standing and even if he does not put weight on the affected limb, there must be enough stability to allow him to stand. That is why I said it is a stable slip.

EXAMINER: How would you treat this child?

CANDIDATE: This child has grade III stable slip. My options are:

1. Pinning in situ to stabilize the slip and prevent further progression until physis closure.
   I anticipate that he would have impingement symptoms that may require future surgery if remodelling is not enough, which is the case in most cases with such severity.
2. Primary open reduction and internal fixation. Several techniques have been described and currently the Ganz surgical dislocation is the preferred option. It is technically demanding and better performed in specialized centres that do it on a regular basis.

EXAMINER: Do you think you can pin this SUFE?

CANDIDATE: Yes, although it will not be easy and the worse the deformity is the more difficult the pinning in situ will be.

EXAMINER: Take me though how you would pin it.

CANDIDATE: Before I perform any operation, I will make sure that my patient is as fit as can be for surgery. I review their health records, investigations and obtain an informed consent for surgery.

I will make sure that all the required equipment and implants are available. The operation is done under general anaesthetic (GA). Intravenous antibiotic is given at induction.

The patient is positioned supine on a fracture table (without traction). The other limb can be placed in abduction or flexed and abducted on stirrup to allow for imaging. Optimum visualization of the femoral head before the procedure is essential.

(In bilateral stable slip, a radiolucent table is preferred over the fracture table because it reduces the chance of worsening the contralateral slip by overenthusiastic positioning. This also reduces the time for re-positioning and re-draping the contralateral side. The stability is usually adequate to obtain a lateral view of the femoral neck by gentle flexion of the hip.)

The trajectory of my screw is identified and marked using a free guide wire placed on the skin overlying the proximal part of the femoral neck and head, crossing the physis in a perpendicular fashion in the AP and lateral views (Figure 18.5).

The guide pin is advanced freehand where the lines intersect through the soft tissues to engage the anterolateral femoral cortex. The position and angulations of the guide pin are adjusted under fluoroscopic guidance, to obtain the proper alignment before the guide pin is advanced into the bone. The entry point is usually quite anterior. It is essential to screen the hip to ensure there is no protrusion of the guide pin in the joint; particularly in the blind spot (Figure 18.6). For unstable slips, a second guide wire is useful to provide some rotational stability and can be used for the insertion of a second cannulated screw if desired.

After the appropriate screw length has been determined, the femoral neck and epiphysis is drilled using the cannulated instruments while periodically checking that the guide wire position is not advancing into the hip.

I prefer to use a 7.3- or 6.5-mm fully threaded, reversed cutting cannulated screw. The screw position should be carefully checked (using the withdrawal technique) to ensure there is no protrusion. If available, 3D C-arm is valuable for this purpose. Several other methods have been proposed for the same reason, but none is without limitations.

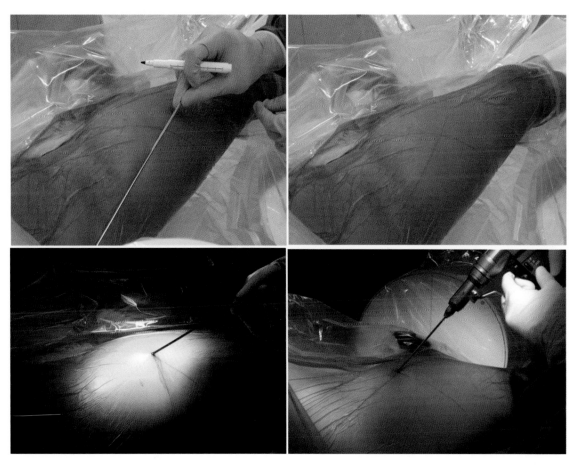

Figure 18.5 Pinning in situ.

The patient is allowed touch weight-bearing with the use of crutches and gradually advances to full weight-bearing as tolerated. Follow-up is until physeal closure.

EXAMINER: Would you pin the other side?

CANDIDATE: I would consider pinning the other side in the following situations:

1. Age of the child (< 10 years is associated with a higher risk of bilaterality).
2. Slips associated with renal osteodystrophy and endocrine disorders (a high incidence of bilaterality approaching 95%).
3. Poor compliance of the child and family.
4. The nature of the current slip (a very bad slip occurring over a very short period of time may justify pinning the other side).

The quoted risk of contralateral slip varies from 18% to 60%. Prophylactic PIS is not devoid of risk and should be weighed against the benefit. The proponents and opponents have some evidence to support their views [5].

Some radiological markers have been proposed to aid decision-making about pinning the other asymptomatic side in patients with SUFE, such as the posterior sloping angle and the modified Oxford bone age [6,7]. Both of these markers are not perfect and do not have 100% positive or negative predictive value. I would have a low threshold to prophylactically pin the other side if the posterior sloping angle is more than 14° as research has shown that the risk of contralateral slip would be around 83%.

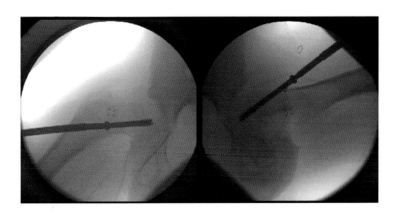

Figure 18.6 Blind spot.

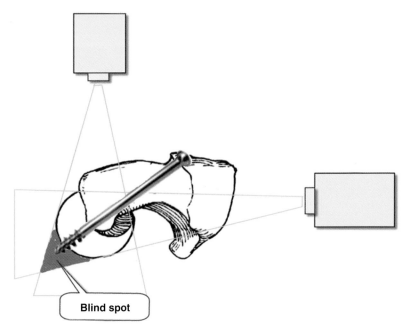

Blind spot

EXAMINER: Can you draw the posterior slip angle?

CANDIDATE: The posterior sloping angle (PSA) is measured by a line (A) from the centre of the femoral shaft through the centre of the metaphysis; a second line (B) is drawn from one edge of the physis to the other, which represents the angle of the physis. Where lines A and B intersect, a third line (C) is drawn perpendicular to line A. The PSA is the angle formed by lines B and C posteriorly, as illustrated in Figure 18.7.

Authors' note: 1

SUFE is a very important topic for the exam. Excellent knowledge is expected. The above scenario is typical; however, the examiners may wish to explore the following (this is a good sign indicating that you have done well to reach these areas):

1. When pinning in situ:
   a. Radiolucent table vs. fracture table.
   b. Single or double screws for unstable severe slips: double screws offer 66% stiffer construct

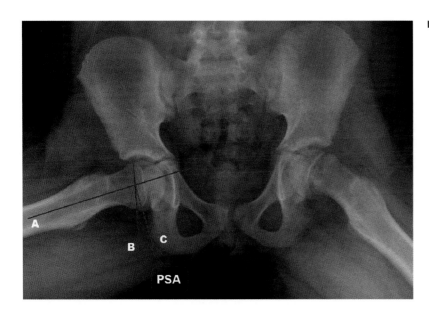

Figure 18.7 Posterior sloping angle.

than single screws, but the risk of intra-articular penetration increases from 4% to 20% with double screws.

c. Fully threaded vs. partially threaded.

d. Would you remove screws routinely?

2. Management of grade III slips; open reduction with or without surgical dislocation: both can be used as long as there is no undue pressure on the retanicular blood vessels. Parsch [8] reported 4.7% AVN with open reduction without surgical dislocation while Ganz [9] reported no AVN with surgical dislocation. In a systematic review and meta-analysis we compared all treatment options and risk of AVN, and surgical dislocation has 3% AVN but better patient satisfaction rates whereas PIS has 1.5% AVN rate and lower satisfaction rates [3,10].

3. If you do well, you may be asked about the technique of surgical dislocation or the Parsch technique.

4. Treatment of residual deformity (corrective osteotomies, arthroscopic osteochondroplasty).

5. AVN (and its medical and surgical treatments).

EXAMINER: This is a clinical photograph of the elbow of a 5-year-old child who fell off a monkey bar (Figure 18.8). How would you manage this child?

CANDIDATE: The photograph shows wrist and elbow swelling, deformity and bruises. There may be skin puckering in front of the elbow. This child most likely has wrist and supracondylar fractures of the humerus (SCH#).

I always follow the ATLS protocols in assessing and managing traumatic injuries in children. Primary survey, then secondary survey and followed by AMPLE history. AMPLE stands for Allergies, Medication, Past medical history, Last food and drinks and Events around the accident.

EXAMINER: You perform primary and secondary surveys and find that this is an isolated upper limb injury.

CANDIDATE: Then I perform a thorough assessment of that limb. Optimum analgesia is extremely helpful to calm the child and makes my assessment pleasant. I look for obvious swelling, bruises, wounds, colour of the hands and fingers,

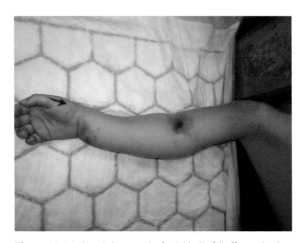

Figure 18.8 A clinical photograph of a child who fell off a monkey bar.

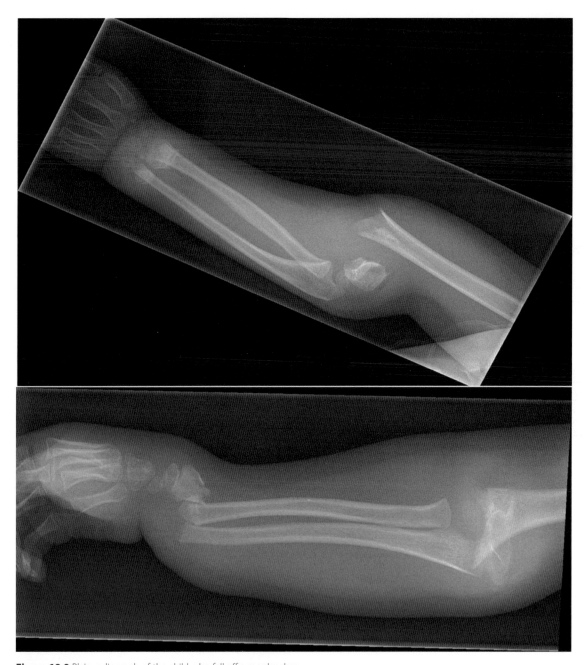

Figure 18.9 Plain radiograph of the child who fell off a monkey bar.

etc. in that limb. I feel for skin temperature, pulses and tenderness. I assess the movement of the joints that are not involved to ensure that there are no unexpected problems. I would not move the elbow joint at this stage as it is expected to be painful. I assess the neurovascular status of the limb using special tests to test for nerve injuries.

EXAMINER: You find the hand warm and relatively well perfused but there was no radial pulse.

CANDIDATE: What about the neurological status?

EXAMINER: The child was not cooperative and you could not assess him optimally despite your best effort.

Table 18.1 Modified Gartland classification

Extension type	Type I	Undisplaced. In the absence of a clear bony injury, a posterior fat pad sign is an important sign of an occult intra-articular or supracondylar fracture	Can be treated with above-elbow cast and collar and cuff splint for 3–4 weeks. X-ray within a week to ensure no displacement
	Type II	Angulated with intact posterior cortex. (IIA = angulation only, IIB = with rotation)	It is usually treated with closed reduction and K-wires. Supported with above-elbow cast or backslab and collar and cuff sling This type is technically easier to reduce and fix and it is ideal for trainees to do it with the senior surgeon unscrubbed
	Type III	Complete displacement (IIIA = posteromedial, IIIB = posterolateral)	It is usually treated with closed reduction (may require open reduction) and K-wires. Then above-elbow back slab and collar and cuff sling This type can be technically demanding and some experience is required
Flexion type		As the name implies, the distal fragment flexes. This indicates that the thin posterior periosteum has been disrupted rendering the fracture very unstable.	As in type III, but even with three wires this type can still be unstable

1. Low and high SCH fractures (below and above the olecranon fossa), flexion type and medial comminutions are radiological signs that predict technically difficult surgery – be prepared.
2. Collar and cuff is part of the stabilization and should be worn 24/7. It is not for comfort as in forearm or wrist fractures.

CANDIDATE: This is not an uncommon scenario. I would document this accurately (i.e. warm hand with no radial pulse) and I could not assess his neurological status (because of the pain and the lack of cooperation). I would like to confirm the diagnosis by requesting an X-ray.

EXAMINER: This was his X-ray.

CANDIDATE: The radiograph confirms my thoughts that this child has supracondylar humeral and distal radius fractures. Both are displaced. The supracondylar humerus fracture is an extension type (Gartland type III) injury with the distal fragment displaced posteriorly and rotated externally. It is not very clear from the X-ray, but there may be some comminution of the lateral column.

This is a limb-threatening injury and requires an immediate intervention. I would like to take the patient to theatre to reduce and stabilize the fracture. A vascular surgeon or a plastics surgeon (with microvascular skills) must be consulted before taking patients to theatre in case hand perfusion becomes worse after the reduction.

EXAMINER: How did Gartland classify these fractures?

CANDIDATE: Gartland classified this fracture into three types: Type I (undisplaced), type II angulated and type III complete displacement.

The classification has undergone several modifications as more knowledge developed.

EXAMINER: How do you fix this fracture?

CANDIDATE: Preoperative planning and thoughtful preparation are key to successful outcome. I obtain an informed consent for surgery. I inform theatre about the child and the urgency of surgery. I liaise with my anaesthetist and vascular colleagues. The fracture pattern is extension type (Gartland type III), there may be some comminution. There is significant elbow swelling and there may be tethering. There is a wrist fracture distally which complicates things further. The risk of compartment syndrome is high. I still think closed reduction and percutaneous pinning (using two or three 2-mm K-wires) will be successful; however, an open reduction may become necessary.

After the WHO check, the child will have a GA and IV antibiotic. I position the child supine on the operating table and his hand is stretched on a hand table. The child's head should be placed in a position close to the hand table, so it will not fall off the main table. The C-arm should come parallel to the main table to allow viewing the AP and lateral of the elbow without changing the elbow position.

I will gently check how easily I can reduce both fractures. Reduction is usually achieved by a gentle traction in line with the humerus, with the elbow in slight flexion. Traction in full extension may cause tethering of neurovascular structures over the proximal fragment. I will use the mid-forearm part for applying the traction to avoid traction damage to the distal neurovascular structures crossing the wrist fracture. If the proximal fragment has pierced through the brachialis muscle, a 'milking' manoeuvre over the brachialis can help untethering of the muscle off the bone. Traction usually takes between 1 and 3 minutes to allow for the muscle to relax and the soft tissue to stretch. Successful traction should allow the visibility of the fracture without overlapping of the proximal and the distal fragments on the AP screening. Then medial or lateral translation is corrected by pushing the distal fragment medially or laterally. An important precaution here is not to cause varus or valgus deformities. It should be pure translation. I then flex the elbow while keeping traction. This makes reduction more stable because the main pull vector of the triceps muscle becomes the fracture compressor (or even flexor) rather than the extensor. In words, the triceps muscle force changes from a deforming force into a stabilizing force. Successful completion of this step is marked by the fact that the child's fingertips can touch the shoulder easily.

Fluoroscopic assessment to confirm reduction using AP and two oblique views at 90° (lateral and medial oblique views). A lateral view can be taken either by carefully rotating the elbow if the fracture is stable enough or by rotating the X-ray machine if not. After flexing the elbow, there will be overlapping of the proximal ulna and radius over the fracture site (Jone's view) but it is still possible to assess the continuity of the medial and lateral columns and Baumann's angle (see Figure 18.10).

Once the fracture is reduced, it needs to be held in the reduced position until stabilized. There are two methods that I use depending on the fracture stability and the experience of my assistant (Figure 18.11). If the fracture is stable and I do not have an experienced assistant, I would tape the limb (hand to shoulder as in Figure 18.11) to keep it reduced; otherwise, I will rely on my assistant to hold it reduced during the procedure. In this child, I cannot use the taping method as there is a wrist fracture.

Then I prepare the skin using antiseptic solution and drape the upper limb. I use two smooth K-wires (size 2 mm unless the child is very small, when I use a smaller size). I pass the first wire through the capitellum in a superomedial direction through the olecranon fossa and the medial cortex (holding up to six cortices – this is not always possible depending on the site and direction of the fracture). I pass the second wire through the distal fragment with maximal spread at the fracture site from the first wire. The wires should not be crossed inside the bone (or even worse, at the fracture site). I check the wires on the AP and lateral views to ensure optimum positioning. Then I test the fracture stability; if it is stable, I will do the wrist, but if not, I may supplement with a third wire or I may use the medial wire. The latter requires a small incision to visualize the ulnar nerve.

EXAMINER: This is what has been done. Any thoughts?

CANDIDATE: The images showed a good reduction of the humeral fracture. There may be a slight lateral translation on the AP view. This needs careful follow-up. The positions of the wires are perfect. The medial wire is passing through the capitellum, olecranon fossa and as low as possible through the medial cortex. This gives good purchase to the bones as it passes through six cortices. The lateral wire is going through the lateral column and is not crossing with the medial wire. On the lateral they are both in good position. The same can be said about the wrist.

EXAMINER: Was the second wire in the wrist necessary?

CANDIDATE: I think so, although it is not always possible to correctly judge the stability of a fracture from a static 2D picture. Moreover, the risk of compartment syndrome is high in this patient, and it is important to obtain a stable fixation in anticipation of cast splinting or even removal if compartment syndrome happens or if the vascular surgeon decides to explore and repair a blood vessel in this case. So, I think the surgeon was right to use two wires in the wrist.

EXAMINER: Fair enough. You stabilized the fracture but the radial pulse did not return. What would you do?

CANDIDATE: BOAST guidelines suggest that a well-perfused limb does not require brachial artery exploration, whether or not the radial pulse is

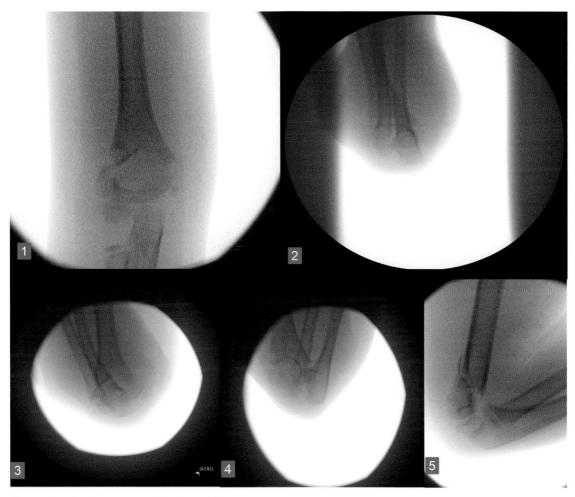

Figure 18.10 Reducing supracondylar humeral fracture.

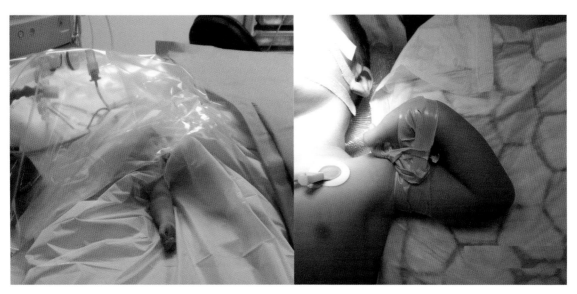

Figure 18.11 Supracondylar methods of fixation.

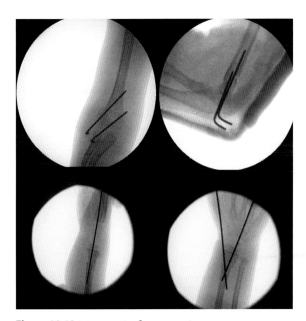

Figure 18.12 Intraoperative fluoroscopy images.

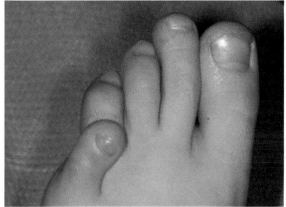

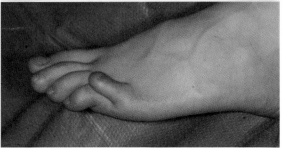

Figure 18.13 A child with the little toe deformity.

present. However, if the upper limb remains ischaemic (pale, cold, delayed capillary refill and pulseless limb) after fracture reduction, a surgeon competent to perform small vessel vascular repair should explore the brachial artery and that is why I informed them before taking the child to surgery [11].

Authors' note: 2

Fractures around the elbow are commonly featured in the exam as they have diagnostic, therapeutic and prognostic challenges which are ideal to explore high-level thinking of candidates. Try to master them. Always practise with your colleagues and seniors the five 'whys' questions until you become confident to tackle any potential questions in these areas.

Candidates must also know the following topics in equivalent detail:

1. Gunstock deformity.
2. Lateral condyle fracture.
3. Medial condyle fracture.

EXAMINER: This young boy presented with the above toe deformity. What is your thought?

CANDIDATE: The pictures show a typical overlapping fifth toe. It is a congenital deformity of the fifth toe which overlaps the fourth. Children and parents seek advice for either cosmetic reasons or problems with footwear. The toe is usually adducted and externally rotated and the MTPJ is dorsiflexed. The nail is sometimes smaller than the contralateral normal toe. I usually advise non-operative treatment in the form of passive stretching, neighbour taping and shoe modifications. If this fails I would offer a modified Butler's procedure if they cannot cope with the symptoms.

EXAMINER: How do you perform Butler's procedure?

CANDIDATE: The essence of the surgery is to lengthen all the tight structures at the back and pull the toe into the correct place using the dermodesis principle.

I perform a double racket incision then release the extensor digitorum longus and release the dorsal capsule. Then I close the skin (Y in V at the plantar aspect and V in Y at the dorsal aspect) (see Figure 18.14).

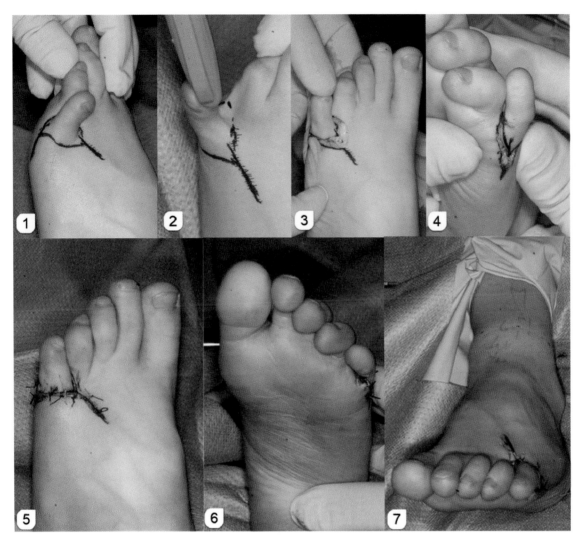

Figure 18.14 Butler's procedure.

Candidate 2

EXAMINER: This is a clinical photograph of newly born foot (Figure 18.15). What can you see?

CANDIDATE: This photograph shows typical features of a clubfoot (congenital talipes equinovarus (CTEV)) deformity. This is often summarized as (CAVE) deformity: **C**avus (high arched foot due to tight intrinsic foot muscles, FHL, FDL); **A**dductus of forefoot (tight tibialis posterior); **V**arus (tight tendoachillis, tibialis posterior, tibialis anterior); **E**quinus (tight tendoachillis).

It looks severe. There are two classifications in use to assess the severity: Pirani score and Dimeglio scoring system. The former is more popular in the UK.

EXAMINER: How does Pirani score club feet?

CANDIDATE: The Pirani score is simple and reproducible. It uses six clinical signs to quantify the severity of each hind foot and mid foot deformity. Each component is scored as 0 (normal), 0.5 (mildly abnormal) or 1 (severely abnormal) (Table 18.2).

The six clinical signs are divided equally between the hind foot and midfoot as follows:

Hind Foot Contracture Score (HFCS) 0–3

1. Equinus.

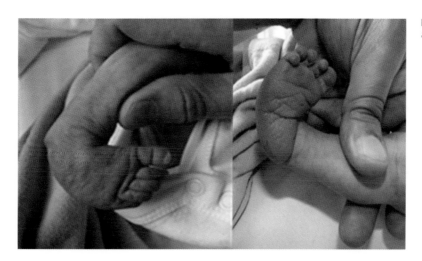

Figure 18.15 A newly born child with a foot deformity.

2. Deep posterior crease.
3. Empty heel.

Midfoot Contracture Score (MFCS) 0–3
4. Curved lateral border.
5. Medial crease.
6. Lateral head of talus.

Total Score (TS) 0–6

EXAMINER: What causes club feet?

CANDIDATE: The cause in the majority of cases is unknown (idiopathic). A few theories have been postulated to explain the aetiology.

1. The neuropathic theory [12]: biopsies were taken from the posteromedial and peroneal muscle groups in 60 patients mostly under the age of 5 years. Evidence of neurogenic disease was seen in most instances and was more obvious in the older patients.

2. The myopathic theory [13]: a histochemical analysis was made of 103 muscle biopsies taken from 62 patients with idiopathic club feet. Authors noticed the muscles in patients aged under 6 months contained 61% Type 1 fibres in the affected legs compared to 44.3% in normal legs.

3. Genetic theory: it is common in certain races such as Polynesian and rare in the Japanese race. There is a 10% risk if a first-degree relative is affected; combination of environmental/genetic [14]. Twenty-five per cent have a family history. Recent link to PITX1, transcription factor critical for limb development.

4. Arrested development of the growing limb bud.
5. Congenital constriction annular band.
6. Viral infection.
7. Mechanical moulding theory.
8. Multifactorial.
   a. Common in Polynesian race and rare in the Japanese race.
   b. Not more common in consanguinity.
   c. 10% risk if a first-degree relative is affected: combination of environmental/genetic [14].
   d. 25% have a family history.

Several associated conditions have been identified and these need to be excluded. These include the following:
1. Neurological causes: spina bifida (myelomeningocele), polio, CP.
2. Sacral agenesis.
3. Foetal alcohol syndrome.
4. Congenital myopathy.
5. Down's syndrome (may include vertical talus).
6. Arthrogryposis.
7. Hand anomalies (Streeter dysplasia/constriction band syndrome).
8. Diastrophic dwarfism.
9. Prune belly syndrome.
10. Opitz syndrome.
11. Larsen syndrome.
12. Anterior tibial artery hypoplasia or absence is common.
13. Tibial hemimelia.

EXAMINER: How would you manage this child?

Table 18.2 Pirani score for club feet.

	Deformity	0	0.5	1
Hind Foot Contracture Score	Equinus (images 1–3)	No equinus contracture	Can reach plantigrade (0°)	Unable to reach plantigrade (in the minus range)
	Deep posterior crease (images 4–6)	Several fine creases is scored 0, and a single, 1	A single crease where you can see the bottom (disappears on passive dorsiflexion)	A deep crease where you cannot see the bottom
	Empty heel (images 7–8)	Easy to palpate the calcaneus, which is not far under the skin (like touching your own chin)	The calcaneus is palpable, which is just felt through a layer of flesh (like touching the tip of your nose)	Calcaneus is deep under a layer of tissue and very difficult to feel (like touching the soft part of your palm below the base of your thumb)
Mid Foot Contracture Score	Curved lateral border (images 9–11)	The lateral border of the foot (excluding the phalanges) is straight and without deviation	The lateral border deviates at the level of the metatarsals	The lateral border of the foot deviates at the calcaneo-cuboid joint (image 15)
	Medial crease (images 12–14)	The presence of several fine creases	A single crease where you can see the bottom (disappears on passive stretching)	A single, deep crease where you cannot see the bottom (image 15)
	Lateral head of talus (Palpate the head of the talus with the foot uncorrected) (image 15)	The talus head is completely covered under the navicular	The talus head is covered partially	The talus head is fixed and cannot be covered by the navicular

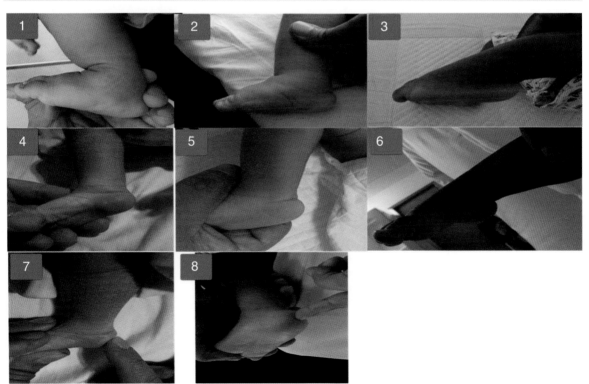

Table 18.2 (cont.)

Deformity	0	0.5	1

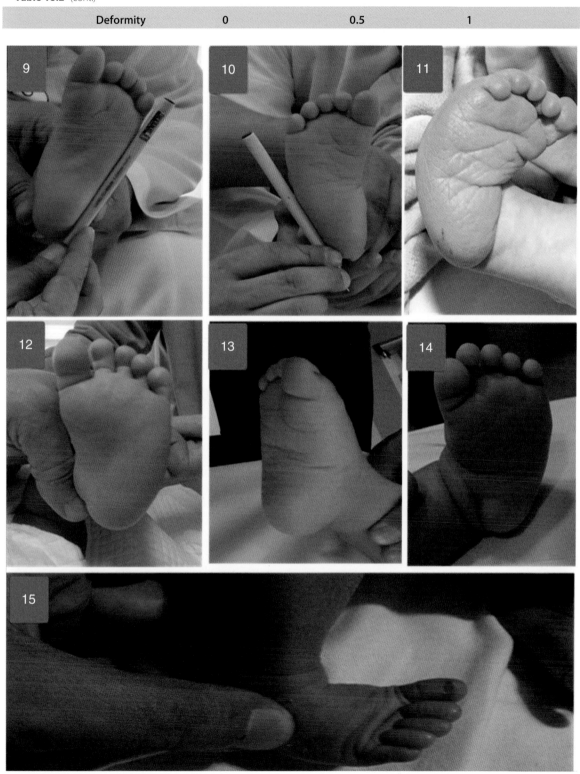

Pictures courtesy of Dr Sattar Alshryda.

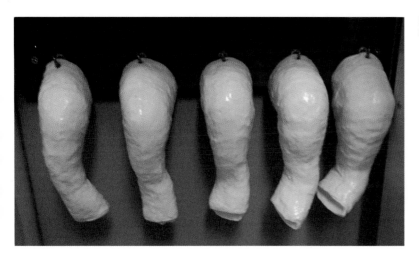

Figure 18.16 The classic shapes of casts in Ponseti weekly serial casting.

CANDIDATE: Most club feet are diagnosed prenatally in the 20-week scan and management and counselling starts before birth. Prenatal counselling is usually focused on the accuracy of diagnosis (65–90%) [15], potential associated conditions (see above) and treatments.

Having established the diagnosis of idiopathic club feet, I recommend the Ponseti serial casting [16,17] (Figure 18.16). The treatment should be started as early as possible; the severity of the deformity is quantified using the Pirani score, then serial casting weekly for an average of 4–6 cast changes. This usually corrects all deformities (CAV) with the exception of equinus, which requires a tendoachillis tenotomy in more than 90% of the cases.

Sequence of deformity corrections follows the deformity pattern which is (CAVE):

1. Cavus (high medial arch) is due to the pronation of the forefoot in relation to the hindfoot. This is corrected by positioning the forefoot in a proper alignment with the hindfoot. The cavus is supple in newborns and requires only elevating the first ray of the forefoot to achieve a normal longitudinal arch of the foot. The foot usually looks worse in the first cast as the forefoot is facing inward.

2. Adduction of the forefeet and varus of the heel are corrected concomitantly using the talus head (not the cuboid) as a fulcrum. This is achieved while keeping the foot in equinus.

3. Equinus of the heel correction starts in the serial casting stage, but often requires tendoachillis tenotomy for full correction in

90% of patients. The timing to start correction of the equinus is critical. Premature correction could lead to midfoot break and rocker bottom foot. Three signs indicate the right time to start equinus correction:

   i. The ability to palpate the anterior process of the calcaneus as it abducts out from beneath the talus.
   ii. Forefoot abduction of approximately 60° in relationship to the frontal plane of the tibia.
   iii. Neutral or slight valgus heel.

Tendoachillis tenotomy is performed when the residual equinus is about 0–5°. It is performed under local anaesthetic, then the final cast applied for another 3 weeks.

Successful correction is followed by a regime of using Denis Browne (DB) splint (Figure 18.17) on a full-time basis for 3 months, after which the splint will be used at nap and nighttime until the age of 4–5 years. The splint consists of open-toe straight shoes attached to a bar. The bar should be of sufficient length so that the heels of the shoes are at shoulder width. This can be adjusted using the sliding clamp in the middle. The bar should be bent 5–10° to hold the feet in dorsiflexion. For unilateral cases, the brace is set at 60–70° of external rotation on the clubfoot side and 30–40° of external rotation on the normal side. In bilateral cases, it is set at 70° of external rotation on each side.

EXAMINER: This is another child who was referred to you with a clubfoot (Figure 18.18). Have a look at the picture and tell us what your thoughts are.

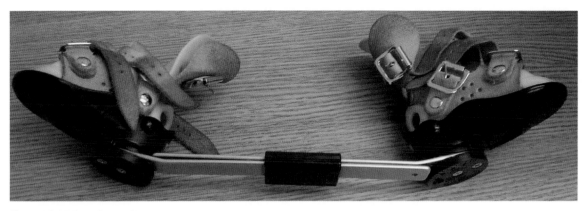

Figure 18.17 Denis Browne boots.

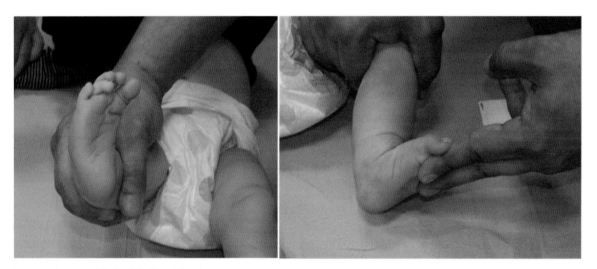

Figure 18.18 A child with right foot deformity.

CANDIDATE: This clinical photograph of the right foot shows a marked foot deformity with forefoot adducted; however, there is no convincing equinus or varus deformity. My thoughts are that the child has a metatarsus adductus and not a clubfoot. I need to examine the child to confirm my thoughts.

EXAMINER: Tell me more about metatarsus adductus (MA)?

CANDIDATE: As the name implies, the metatarsus (forefoot) is adducted in relation to the hind foot. It is as common as club feet (1 in 1000 births), no sex predominance and bilateral in approximately 50% of cases. It is widely considered as a foetal packaging disorder (that is why it is common in late pregnancies, first pregnancies, twin pregnancies and oligohydramnios). For the same reasons,

MA is linked to DDH (15–20%), torticollis and plagiocephaly. It can be part of a more complex foot deformity such as clubfoot and skew foot.

Bleck classified the severity using the heel bisector line into mild, moderate and severe (Figure 18.19). Normally, the heel bisector line passes through the second and third toe web space. In a mild MA, the heel bisector line passes through the third toe; in a moderate MA the line passes through the third and fourth toe web space and in a severe MA, it passes through the fourth and fifth toe web space.

EXAMINER: How would you treat metatarsus adductus?

CANDIDATE: Isolated MA is a benign condition that resolves by the age of 5 years (or even earlier). I would advise serial stretching by parents if the

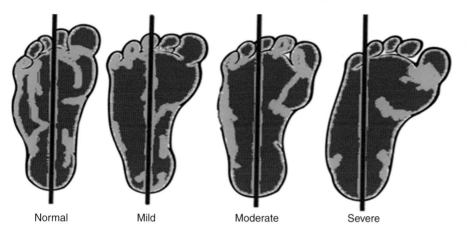

Figure 18.19 Bleck classification of metatarsus adductus severity.

Normal   Mild   Moderate   Severe

MA is flexible and can be actively or passively corrected to midline, whereas a rigid deformity with medial crease requires serial casting.

Surgery is rarely indicated (and often unnecessary) before the age of 5. However, persistent and symptomatic MA after the age of 5 may warrant lateral column shortening if the foot is long or medial column lengthening if the foot is short. Lateral column shortening is done with cuboid closing wedge osteotomy. Medial column lengthening includes a cuneiform opening wedge osteotomy with medial capsular release and abductor hallucis longus recession.

EXAMINER: How do you know whether the foot is long or short?

CANDIDATE: By comparing it to the standard growth charts.

Authors' note: 3

Clubfoot is another A-list topic in the paediatric section. It should be an area where you get a full mark. The above scenario is a typical example for a straightforward pass performance. The candidate answered all the questions in a comprehensive and correct matter and clearly talked more than the examiner. He did not need prompting and supplemented some evidence.

Our advice is that you should aim for more than a pass by considering the following:

1. The Ponseti vs. the French method.
2. Complications of treatments.
3. Relapse and its treatment.
4. Potential operative intervention:

a. Posteromedial soft-tissue release and tendon lengthening.
b. Medial column lengthening or lateral column-shortening osteotomies.
c. Talectomy (in severe, rigid recurrent clubfoot in children with arthrogryposis).
d. Gradual correction using a circular frame.

Clubfoot, metatarsus adductus and congenital vertical talus are completely different conditions and clear understanding of these three conditions and their treatment is essential. Make sure that you do not confuse them in the exam (and real life!).

EXAMINER: The below is a photograph of a child with a thumb deformity (Figure 18.20). What is the diagnosis?

CANDIDATE: The right thumb IPJ looks in a fixed flexion deformity; the likely diagnosis is a congenital trigger thumb; however, without a proper examination, I cannot be certain. I need

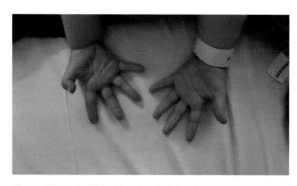

Figure 18.20 A child with a thumb deformity.

to see that the IPJ can be flexed further, I would like to feel the mobile lump at the base of the thumb. Sometimes, the deformity can be corrected with a palpable (and even visible) clunk.

EXAMINER: You are correct. This is a trigger thumb. What would you tell the parents?

CANDIDATE: I would tell them about the condition and the known reason behind it. I will explain the management options including conservative (observation, exercises, splinting) and surgical (open A1 pulley release or percutaneous A1 pulley release). In my practice, if conservative treatment fails, I would offer the child open A1 pulley release. It is a small operation, with low comorbidity and a high success rate.

Unfortunately, the natural history of congenital trigger thumb is not very well studied, and the evidence accumulated is predominantly level III and IV. Many of the study interpretations are vulnerable to bias [18].

Candidate 3

EXAMINER: You have been called to see an 8-year-old boy who presented to the A&E with limping on the right leg. How would you approach this child?

CANDIDATE: Limping is one of the commonest reasons why parents seek medical advice. The list of causes for a limping child is long and ranges from trivial conditions that require just reassurance such as minor trauma to the most serious conditions that require admission, investigations and urgent surgery, such as infections and tumours.

A thorough history and examination are essential to narrow the list to a few working diagnoses. It is essential not to miss important diagnoses even if they are not common (such as infections or tumours), as delay may jeopardize the outcome.

EXAMINER: What do you want to know in the history?

CANDIDATE: I would like to know whether there is a history of trauma (trauma or SCFE), temperature (infection), upper respiratory tract infection or earache (transient synovitis), constitutional symptoms and weight loss (tumour or infection).

I would like to know about the onset of symptoms, precipitating and relieving factors, impact on his daily activities.

EXAMINER: There was no history of trauma, no temperature and no recent URTI or contact with an unwell child. He has never had this problem before and there are no swollen joints.

CANDIDATE: I will proceed with my examination, I would start with general signs and walking, then I examine his lower limbs, back and upper limbs. I will look, feel, move his joints and perform special tests relevant to particular joints and what I am looking for.

EXAMINER: You examined him and he was walking with obvious limp, he was holding his leg in a position of rest and there was a reluctance to move the right hip.

CANDIDATE: This is important information to know as I can now focus on hip causes of limping and I can investigate accordingly. I would like to obtain a pelvic X-ray and request some blood tests (FBC, ESR, CRP).

EXAMINER: Your junior has already requested these as well as rheumatoid factor (RF) and serum uric acid (UA).

CANDIDATE: That is OK. I would not recommend checking RF and UA at this stage. Juvenile rheumatoid arthritis and gout are rare in children and these are not at the top of my list at this stage unless there are clear signs to indicate the contrary, such as gouty tophi or the patient being on cytotoxic medicines. My investigations are guided by what I want to rule in and rule out at this stage of presentation. When I want to find the diagnosis ASAP, I do not want to miss or delay important diagnosis such as infection. Therefore, I requested the above blood tests to estimate the probability of infection in this child using Kocher's criteria.

EXAMINER: What are Kocher's criteria?

CANDIDATE: These are criteria to help differentiate between transient synovitis and septic arthritis, as both have a similar early presentation. The criteria include:
1. Fever (> 38.5°C).
2. Inability to weight-bear.
3. ESR > 40.
4. WBC > 12,000/mm^3.

In Kocher's original paper, the predicted probability of septic arthritis with one positive predictor was 3%, two predictors 40%, three predictors 93% and four predictors 99.6%.

EXAMINER: What about the CRP that you requested?

CANDIDATE: CRP is more sensitive to infection than ESR (although it was not mentioned in the Kocher criteria). It usually rises within 6 hours after an insult (whether infection or injury). Caird and colleagues [19] noted that CRP (> 20 mg/l) was a further independent predictor of septic arthritis. However, the fact that CRP can be elevated after injury (including surgery) precludes its diagnostic value.

Procalcitonin (PCT) is another infection marker that has become increasingly popular. PCT has even greater specificity than ESR and CRP in identifying patients with infection. It is still expensive and not widely available [20,21].

Authors' note: 4

The FRCS exam is about safe and high-standard practice. This should be based on evidence. There is a myth that candidates should not quote published evidence. You can pass the exam without quoting a paper; however, quoting papers and published evidence will enhance your performance. It is even more impressive if you know the evidence, its strength and weakness and how you would utilize this evidence in your practice knowing its limitations. The above candidate scored high by quoting a well-recognized paper and showed that he kept updated with recent advances in the field (the PCT value in diagnosing septic arthritis). He could have emphasized the limitation of the evidence that he quoted, for example by saying, 'It is important to appreciate that even when all Kocher's criteria are negative, the risk of infection is still present ranging from 0.3% to 17%'.

As this area is extremely important, we summarize the evidence below.

In a study of 282 patients, Kocher and colleagues [22] identified the above four independent predictors to differentiate between transient synovitis and septic arthritis: They put the patients into three groups: confirmed septic arthritis, presumed septic arthritis and transient synovitis.

The diagnosis of true septic arthritis which occurred in 38 patients was assigned when a patient had one of the following:

1. A positive finding on culture of joint fluid.
2. WCC ≥ 50,000 cells per cubic millimeter with positive findings on blood culture.

The diagnosis of presumed septic arthritis (44 patients) was assigned when a patient had WCC ≥ 50,000 cell per cubic millimeter in the joint fluid with negative findings on culture of joint aspirate and blood.

The diagnosis of transient synovitis (86 patients) was assigned when the patient had WCC < 50,000 cells per cubic millimetre in the joint with negative findings on culture, resolution of symptoms without antimicrobial therapy, and no further development of a disease process as documented in the medical record.

The group with septic arthritis (88 patients) included both groups with confirmed and presumed septic arthritis. Predicted probability of septic arthritis with one predictor was 3%, two predictors 40%, three predictors 93% and four predictors 99.6%.

Kocher validated his criteria prospectively in another study of 154 patients [23]: 24 had true septic arthritis, 27 were presumed to have septic arthritis, 103 had transient synovitis. He had slightly different findings (see Table 18.3).

Table 18.3 Predictors for septic arthritis.

No. of predictors	Predicted probability of septic arthritis (%)		
	Kocher 1999 [22]	Kocher 2004 [23]	Caird 2005 [19]
0	0.2	2	16.9
1	3	9.5	36.7
2	40	35	62.4
3	93.1	72.8	82.6
4	99.6	93	93.1
5			97.5

Caird et al. noted that CRP (> 20 mg/l) was a further independent predictor in a study of 53 patients with 34 patients who had confirmed septic arthritis of the hip [19]. Caird indicated a much higher risk of septic arthritis (16.9%) when all predictors are negative, something many practitioners would disagree with.

The CRP did not perform as well as PCT in a systematic review and meta-analysis by Zhao [21]. The review included 10 studies (838 patients) and found that the overall sensitivity of serum PCT levels for the diagnosis of septic arthritis was 0.54 (95% CI, 0.41–0.66), and the specificity was 0.95 (95% CI, 0.87–0.98). The sensitivity and specificity of CRP were 0.45 (95% CI, 0.35–0.55) and 0.079 (95% CI, 0.0.021–0.25), respectively.

EXAMINER: The blood tests that you requested came all within normal. This is the X-ray that you requested.

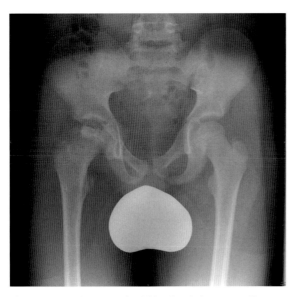

Figure 18.21 Pelvis X-ray of a child with right hip pain and limping.

CANDIDATE: This AP pelvis radiograph (unlabelled) shows obvious abnormality of the right femoral head, the epiphysis is small, denser (whiter in colour) and there is some fragmentation. Several possibilities can cause such a picture. On the top of my list is Legg Calves Perthes disease (LCPD), but there are others such as:

1. Infections (normal blood does not exclude septic arthritis or osteomyelitis).
2. Multiple epiphyseal dysplasia (MED. as the name implies, there will be involvement of the other side and other joints).
3. Spondyloepiphyseal dysplasia (similar to the MED but with spinal involvement).
4. Sickle cell disease (history and family history).
5. Eosinophilic granuloma (other lesions of the skull, radiological feature, biopsy).
6. Gaucher's disease.
7. Hypothyroidism.
8. Meyer's dysplasia.

EXAMINER: How do you confirm your diagnosis?

CANDIDATE: The history, examination and initial investigations indicate that the likely diagnosis is LCPD. However, if I am still in doubt, other investigations can rule out other possibilities.

Joint aspiration and MRI scan could largely exclude joint and bone infection. Thyroid function test to rule out hypothyroidism, sickling test or HB electrophoresis to rule out sickle cell diseases, etc.

Every test that I may use to confirm my top diagnosis (LCPD) has some limitation and the eventual diagnosis will have some uncertainty.

EXAMINER: You did all these tests and you are convinced that this child has LCPD. How would you treat him?

CANDIDATE: My first line of treatment for all children with LCPD is to treat their symptoms and educate them and their parents about the disease itself. Rest, analgesia, anti-inflammatory, temporary non-weight-bearing with crutches and I may consider admitting for a short period of gentle traction if his hip is very stiff. Physiotherapy plays an important role in improving range of motion. Several types of braces have been advocated, but their values have been contested and compliance is a real issue in this age group.

EXAMINER: How would you educate them?

CANDIDATE: I would explain the condition to them verbally and I would also provide them with a written leaflet about the condition. I would explain that LCPD is a unique disease that is not fully understood. The disease is caused by interruption of blood supply to the femoral head. We do not know why this happens. There are a few theories suggested to explain the reasons, but none has been proven. The blood supply is restored spontaneously over a period of 2–4 years. During this period the femoral head passes through distinctive stages (Figure 18.22):

1. Initial (also called necrotic or avascular necrosis stage).
2. Fragmentation (or resorption stage).
3. Healing (re-ossification or reconstitution stage).
4. Remodelling stage.

Each stage lasts 6 months on average (range 3–18 months). There is overlap between these stages. Some areas of the femoral head may start healing while other parts are still fragmenting. The child's symptoms tend to get worse as the disease progresses into the fragmentation stage regardless of the types of treatment that the child gets.

Several radiological classifications have been advised to grade the severity of the disease. The most popular is the lateral pillar classification (by Dr Herring). The classification depicts that the femoral head is made of three equal pillars (medial, middle and lateral). The severity is divided into

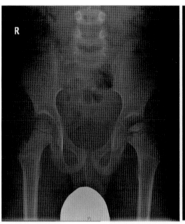

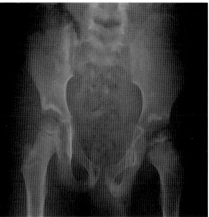

Figure 18.22 LCPD stages.

Initial (avascular necrosis stage)

Fragmentation stage

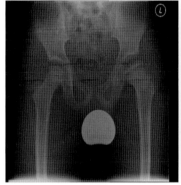

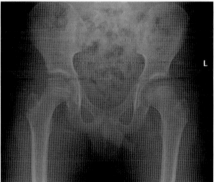

Healing (re-ossification) stage

Remodelling stage

four groups based on the height of the lateral pillar or third on the AP film at the beginning of the fragmentation stage (Figure 18.23). The groups are:

Group A: Normal height of the lateral third of the head is maintained.

Group B: More than 50% of the original lateral pillar height is maintained.

Group C: Less than 50% of the original lateral pillar height is maintained.

Group B/C: Less than 50% of the original lateral pillar height is maintained but the lateral pillar is higher than the central segment.

I would also explain that when LCPD is fully healed, there are other classification systems that can help us predict how well the child's hip would do in the future. I personally prefer the modified Stulberg classification (Figure 18.24). It consists of three groups: Group A hips have a spherical femoral head, group B have an ovoid (or mushroom-shaped) femoral head and group C have a flat femoral head. Group A usually do

well. Group C do not usually do well, and they would require total hip replacement in their fifties. Group B usually run a course between groups A and C.

There are some clinical and radiological factors that help predict which hip would do well and which does not. The following are not good signs (often referred to as the FOOBS):

1. Females.
2. Older children (older than 6 years).
3. Overweight.
4. Bilateral hip involvement.
5. Stiffness of the involved hip.

EXAMINER: So which Herring group would you think this child belongs to?

CANDIDATE: I would classify this as group B. The lateral pillar is more than 50% (compared to the other side).

EXAMINER: Would you consider surgery?

401

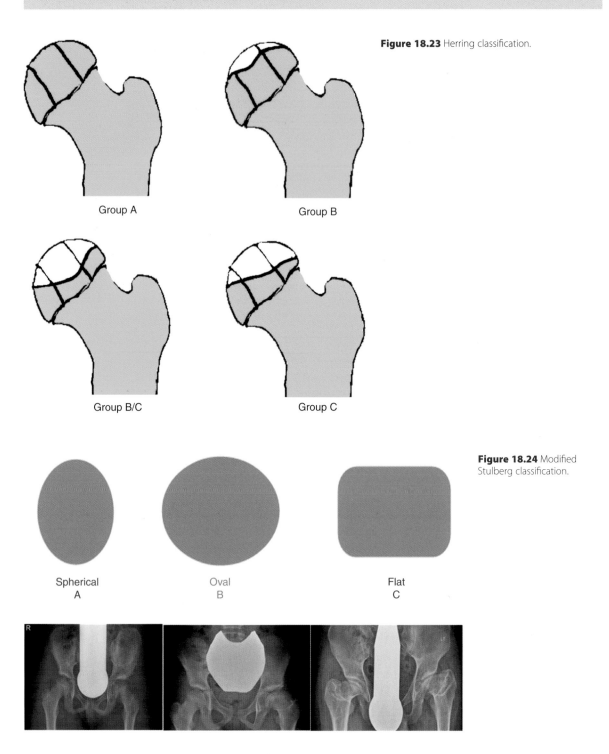

Figure 18.23 Herring classification.

Group A

Group B

Group B/C

Group C

Figure 18.24 Modified Stulberg classification.

Spherical
A

Oval
B

Flat
C

CANDIDATE: Yes, I would consider containment surgery (femoral varus derotation osteotomy, Salter osteotomy or both). My preferred option is femoral varus derotation osteotomy. The evidence shows that containment surgery is beneficial in patients with lateral pillar B and B/C stages who are 8 years or older [24,25]. It increases the number of patients with Stulberg A by 30%.

EXAMINER: Have you done or seen femoral varus osteotomy for LCPD? Can you take me through it?

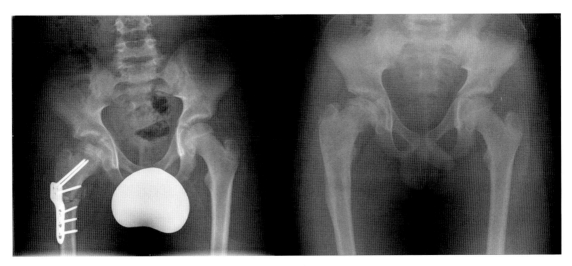

Figure 18.25 Varus osteotomy of patient with LCPD and a few years later.

CANDIDATE: Yes.

Preoperative planning is essential. It is important to ensure that there is a good hip abduction to compensate for the varisation of the femur. We can also estimate how much varus is required to achieve good containment by obtaining a plain radiograph, in the neutral position and abduction (in neutral rotation). This step can be done in theatre using fluoroscopy.

The patient is positioned supine on the operating table and surgery is performed under GA. The lower limbs are prepared and draped free. Adductors release may be required if there is significant tightness.

I use the lateral subvastus approach. The periosteum is incised and elevated with a Cobb elevator. I prefer the paediatric proximal locking plate, I use the size which is appropriate for the patient weight (3.5 mm for those under 35 kg and 5 mm for those above). I set my guiding jig based on the plate angle and the desired amount of varisation.

Jig angle = plate angle + the desired amount of varisation

So, if I want a varisation of 30°, I will use 110° plate and I set my jig to 140°.

I fix the plate proximally then I remove it (so that it will be ready to be re-fixed again after the femoral osteotomy). It is important to mark rotation before performing the femoral osteotomy. Several techniques have been used. I use two K-wires; one above and one below the osteotomy, using the hockey stick (a small curved spanner on the paediatric locking plate that looks like a hockey stick) to identify the level of the femoral osteotomy.

I perform femoral osteotomy using an oscillating saw. Gentle soft-tissue releases around the osteotomy site to aid varisation. I fix the plate proximally then distally. Depending on the femoral head damage, I may add some internal rotation or extension for better containment. I wash out the wound and close it in layers.

EXAMINER: Would you do the same if this child has lateral pillar type C?

CANDIDATE: The evidence shows that surgery does not improve the outcome in this group. However, I may consider other options such as rest, traction, adductor release and Petri if there are significant stiffness and lateral extrusion.

EXAMINER: Would you do the same if this child has lateral pillar type A?

CANDIDATE: For the best result, surgery should be performed in the earliest stage of the disease; maybe even before being able to classify the severity. There is uncertainty whether type A is a genuine type or will progress to type B or even C.

If all children older than 8 years were to be offered surgical treatment, the group A and C hips would not likely benefit. These groups combined represent only 13% of hips presenting at age older than 8, and this approach may be justified [26].

Authors' note: 5

LCPD is another A-list topic. The ability to discuss the findings and differential diagnosis is a must to pass the exam. Treatment is very controversial and there is a paucity of evidence to support treatment. There are only two level II evidence for intervention and they are worth reading:

Herring *et al.* [24] reported on the results of the Legg Perthes Study Group. Thirty-nine surgeons from 28 centres took part in a prospective study. Each surgeon agreed to apply a single treatment method to each patient who met the study criteria. All patients were between 6 and 12 years of age at the onset of the disease, and none had had prior treatment. The treatment groups were no treatment, range of motion treatment in which the patient did exercises once a day, Atlanta brace treatment, femoral varus osteotomy and Salter osteotomy.

The study showed that age, lateral pillar grading and treatment methods were significantly related to outcome.

In group B hips with an age at onset of more than 8 years, 73% of the operated hips had a Stulberg I or II result compared with 44% of the non-operated hips (*P* = 0.02). In the group B hips with onset at 8 years or younger, there was no advantage demonstrated for the surgical group. The group C hips were not shown to benefit from surgical or non-surgical treatments.

Wiig [25] reported on a nationwide prospective study. Twenty-eight hospitals in Norway were instructed to report all new cases of LCPD over a period of 5 years.

A total number of 368 with unilateral disease were included in the study. For patients over 6 years of age at diagnosis with more than 50% necrosis of the femoral head (152 patients), the surgeons at the different hospitals had chosen one of three methods of treatment: physiotherapy (55 patients), the Scottish Rite abduction orthosis (26) and proximal femoral varus osteotomy (71). The study showed that the strongest predictor of poor outcome was femoral head involvement of more than 50% (modified Catterall classification) followed by age at diagnosis, then lateral pillar grades. In children over 6 years at diagnosis with more than 50% of femoral head necrosis, proximal femoral varus osteotomy gave a significantly better outcome than orthosis or physiotherapy. There was no difference in outcome after any of the treatments in children under 6 years.

It is worth knowing more details about Stulberg classification and its modification. The original classification is based on sphericity of the head and congruency of the hip joint.

A modified version of the Stulberg classification is becoming more popular. It consists of three groups: group A hips (Stulberg I and II) have a spherical femoral head, group B (Stulberg III) have an ovoid femoral head and group C (Stulberg IV and V) have a flat femoral head.

Other small studies showed the benefit of shelf acetabuloplasty as a salvage operation for extruded head [27,28]; valgus osteotomy in hinged abduction [29]; and trochanteric growth arrest or advancement when there is overgrowth.

Soft-tissue release and articulated hip distractor in treating late-onset LCPD (even severe ones) have shown promising results [30,31]. Segev and colleagues studied 16 children with late-onset and type C LCPD. Fourteen patients had a saddle-shaped subluxating femoral head with hinge abduction. They found that soft-tissue release and articulated hip distraction produced good results, including the disappearance of the saddle-shaped femoral head in 10 of the 14 patients.

Table 18.4 Stulberg grading.

Sphericity and congruency	Class	Description	Modified Stulberg classification
Spherical congruency	I	Normal spherical head	A
	II	Spherical head, coxa magna/Breva, steep acetabulum	A
Aspherical congruency	III	Ovoid or mushroom-shaped head	B
	IV	Flat head on flat acetabulum (may hinge on abduction)	C
Aspherical incongruency	V	Flat head but normal acetabulum	C

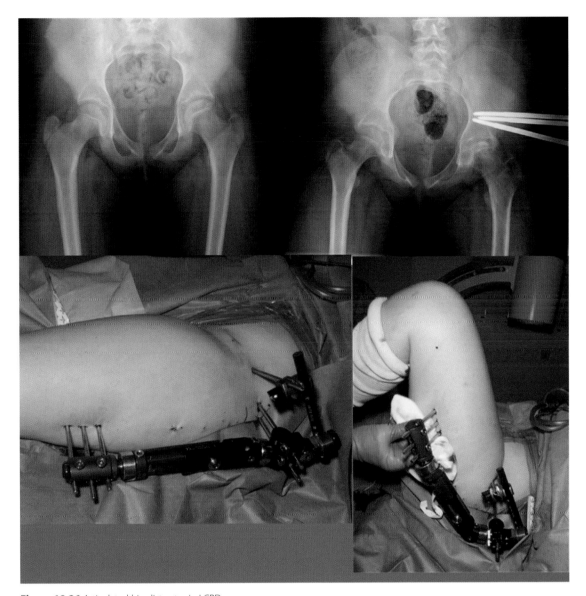

Figure 18.26 Articulated hip distractor in LCPD.

Candidate 4

EXAMINER: This is a clinical photograph of a 2-year, 8-months-old girl who was brought to you by her parents because they are concerned about the bent legs that she has (Figure 18.27). What are your thoughts?

CANDIDATE: This is a clinical photograph of a standing child. There is an obvious asymmetry of leg alignment, with the right leg more varus than the left, which looks almost straight.

I anticipate a child of this age has almost straight knees (or slight valgus) as depicted by the Salenius curve.

EXAMINER: Tell me more about the Salenius curve.

CANDIDATE: Salenius and Vankka reported on the development of the tibiofemoral angles in 979 children from Finland. They showed that the tibiofemoral angle (coronal alignment for the knee) follows a distinct pattern. Newborn babies were born with an average knee varus of

10–15°. As children started standing and walking, the knee became straight at around 18 months of age. This was followed by a progression into valgus of an average of 10° around the age of 4. Thereafter, knee valgus gradually reduced to the adult valgus of about 6° over the next several years (Figure 18.28). The standard deviation (SD) of the above-quoted angles was 8° (more in boys (10°) and less in girls (7°)).

EXAMINER: How would you approach this patient?

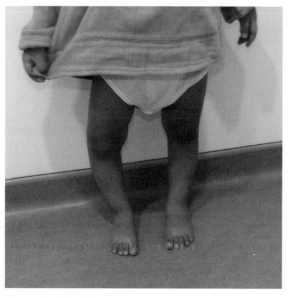

Figure 18.27 A child with bent legs.

CANDIDATE: I would like to take a detailed history and perform a thorough examination. I want to know when they noticed the deformity, is it getting worse or better, are there any symptoms, did they have any treatment? I want to know whether there is any history of trauma or previous infection (growth arrest). Any family history of similar conditions, joint diseases, congenital or genetic disorders.

I would perform a general examination looking for any signs to explain the deformity. Overweight children from Afro-Caribbean backgrounds (Blount's disease), other limb deformities (growth arrest, congenital disorders), widened metaphysis and rachitic rosary (Rickets). Is there a lateral knee thrust or rotational lower limb deformity on walking?

Then I would examine the lower limbs (looking, feeling, moving and special tests). I will look for any obvious abnormalities, feel for swellings, tenderness or abnormal sounds (clicking, clunking or crepitus), I will check joint movements (active and passive) then I will do relevant special tests. The cover-up test is a useful screening test to assess this child's lower limb alignment. A positive test (bowing in the upper tibia) or a neutral test (a straight thigh–upper leg axis) is an indication for radiographic evaluation. A negative test (slight valgus at the upper tibia) indicates physiologic bowing. A positive cover-up test has a high sensitivity; a negative cover-up test has a high specificity and negative predictive value [32].

Figure 18.28 Salenius curve of tibiofemoral angle.

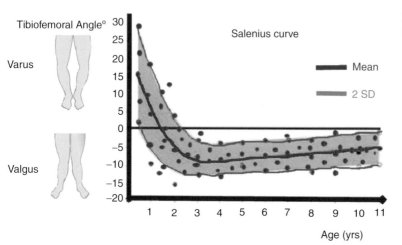

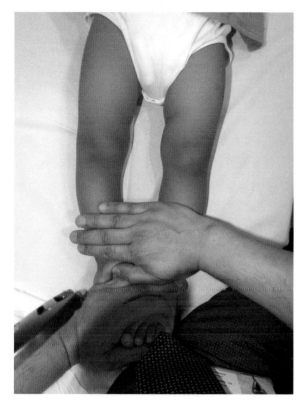

Figure 18.29 Cover-up test (positive on the right and neutral on the left – both are indication for X-ray).

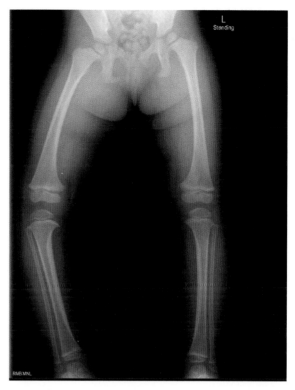

Figure 18.30 A long legs alignment view in a child.

EXAMINER: The below clinical photograph (Figure 18.29) shows the cover-up test. What do you think?

CANDIDATE: I think the child has a positive cover-up test on the right and neutral on the left and I would request a long legs alignment view.

EXAMINER: This is the X-ray that you have requested (Figure 18.30). Tell me what you can see.

CANDIDATE: The X-ray shows most of the lower limbs. Ideally, I would like to see the top of the iliac crest and the heels. I also noted the X-rays are not fully labelled (names, dates, time, etc.) so I have to bear this in mind when I make my decision. It confirms my clinical impression that there is an asymmetry of the lower limb alignment. There are features that are suggestive of Blount's disease (stage I) with a varus deformity of the knee and medial beaking of the metaphysis. I would like to draw and measure some angles and distances to confirm my suspicions and predict the probability that the deformity may progress.

EXAMINER: OK; go ahead. Show us what angles you measure and how.

CANDIDATE: I usually measure the tibiofemoral angle (TFA), mechanical axis deviation (MAD), metaphyseal–diaphyseal angle of Levine and Drennan (MDA)[33], epiphyseal–metaphyseal angle (EMA), femoral–metaphyseal–diaphyseal angle (FMDA) of O'Neill and MacEwen [34] and femoral–tibial ratio of McCarthy (FTR) [35] and tabulate them comparing right and left.

The TFAs show bilateral varus with the right side worse. The right side is probably more than 2 SD of the average predicted by the Salenius curve; however, the left side is still within the expected range. This is also reflected by the MAD, which is more than the normal value (0 ± 3 mm from the centre of the knee). MAD is valuable to monitor progression of the disease.

The other angles help to differentiate between physiological and pathological genu varum. As with any test, they are not 100% sensitive or specific and clinical judgement is often required when the values fall in the grey zone. In general, when the EMA < 20°,

407

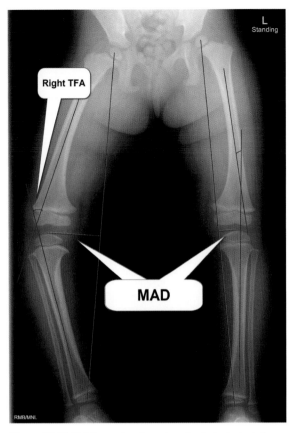

Figure 18.31 Tibiofemoral angle and mechanical axis deviation. The TFA is the angle the femoral and tibial mid-diaphyseal. MAD is the distance between the mechanical axis and the centre of the knee.

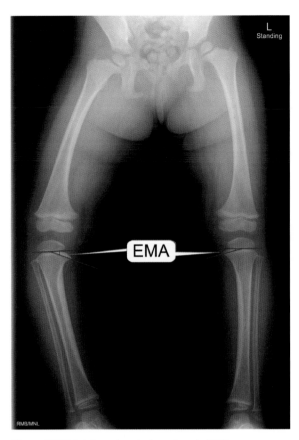

Figure 18.32 Epiphyseal–metaphyseal angle (EMA). The EMA is the angle formed by the epiphyseal line (a line through the proximal tibial physis parallel to the base of the epiphyseal ossification centre) and a line connecting the midpoint of the base of the epiphyseal ossification centre with the most distal point on the medial beak of the proximal tibial physis.

TMDA < 10°, TFA < 10° and the FTR > 1.4 Blount's disease is very unlikely, whereas if EMA > 20°, TMDA ≥ 16° and FTR < 0.7 Blount's disease is likely. The grey zone is when the values are between this range.

EXAMINER: So, what is Blount's disease?

CANDIDATE: Blount's disease is an uncommon paediatric knee condition in which there is a growth disorder of the medial aspect of the proximal tibial physis. This is probably caused by a combination of excessive compressive forces on the proximal medial physis of the tibia. There are two recognized types:

1. Infantile (0–4).
2. Adolescent (> 10 years).

In the infantile tibia vara, patients generally start to walk early (9–10 months; it is more prevalent in females, blacks and those with marked obesity.

It is bilateral in approximately 80% of cases and associated with a prominent metaphyseal beak, internal tibial torsion and LLD. The deformity is usually painless.

In the adolescent type, patients complain of pain at the medial aspect of the knee. These patients are normally similar to the SUFE type of patient with more incidences in overweight Afro-Caribbean males and unilateral involvement in 80% of cases.

Langenskiold recognized six radiological stages of the disease (Figure 18.34). Spontaneous resolution according to Langenskiold is common for stages 1–2, possible for stages 3–4, while stages 5 and 6 are associated with recurrence and permanent deformity even after mechanical realignment.

EXAMINER: So, what do you advise parents?

Table 18.5 Angle measurements around the knee.

Angles	Right	Left
Tibiofemoral angle (TFA)	34°	10°
Mechanical axis deviation (MAD)	57 mm	20 mm
Epiphyseal–metaphyseal angle (EMA)	35°	25°
Metaphyseal–diaphyseal angle (MDA) (also called TMDA where T stands for tibial)	10°	3°
Femoral–metaphyseal–diaphyseal angle (FMDA)	13°	10°
Femoral–tibial ratio of McCarthy (FTR)	1.3	3.3

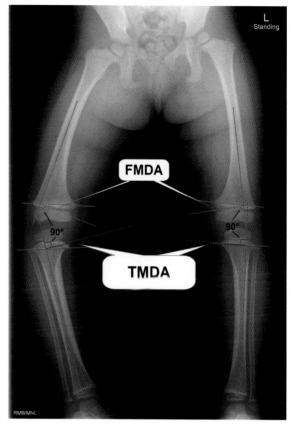

Figure 18.33 Metaphyseal–diaphyseal angles.
The MDA is the angle formed by a line connecting the most distal point on the medial and lateral beaks of the metaphysis (distal femur in FMDA and proximal tibia in the TMDA) and a line perpendicular to the anatomic axis (or lateral cortex) of the bone. The femoral tibial ratio (FTR) is defined as the FMDA divided by the TMDA.

CANDIDATE: My advice is that bowed legs are common (in fact, the norm) before the age of 2 years. I get concerned when I see it after the age of 2 years or if there is asymmetry, which is the case with this child.

This may resolve spontaneously; however, there are several predictors against spontaneous resolution. My options are either start treatment now or observe it for another 4–6 months. If things improve, observation will continue; otherwise, I will treat with a brace.

EXAMINER: Do you think the brace will help?

CANDIDATE: There is evidence that braces can improve deformity in younger than age 3 or prior to Langenskiold stage II. An elastic Blount brace provides valgus force in conjunction with a medial upright, with drop locks to increase corrective force during weight-bearing [36]. Bracing schedules vary from full-time to day or night only, with frequent adjustment of the medial upright every couple of months to provide a continuous valgus force. Compliance is an issue. The success of the true bracing effect is confounded by the benign natural history of physiologic bowed legs treated as Blount's disease. One study limited to patients with Drennan's angles over 16° showed 86% success. Bracing failure was more likely with ligamentous instability, body weight exceeding the 90th percentile, or late initiation [37]. Another study demonstrated 70% success in Langenskiold stage II disease, although this was mainly in unilateral disease. Seventy percent of patients with bilateral involvement required surgical management [38].

Authors' note: 6

Genu varum, valgum and Blount's disease are favourite exam topics. The former is very common in clinical practice (and exams) and the latter, although rare, is closely related to the genu varum and it has become the favourite linked topic to genu varum.

Please master these topics. They are easy, and you can score high marks!

The proximal tibial and distal femoral morphology is typical. Several angles have been advocated to differentiate physiological and Blount's disease (Table 18.7).

Table 18.6 Langenskiold classification of Blount's disease.

Stages	Descriptions	Treatment
Stage 1	Medial beaking, irregular medial ossification with protrusion of the metaphysis	Orthotic for < 3 years
Stage 2	Cartilage fills depression. Progressive depression of medial epiphysis with the epiphysis sloping medially as disease progresses	Failure of full correction or progression to type III → surgery
Stage 3	Ossification of the inferomedial corner of the epiphysis	Surgery
Stage 4	Epiphyseal ossification filling the metaphyseal depression	
Stage 5	Double epiphyseal plate (cleft separating two epiphyses)	
Stage 6	Medial physeal closure	

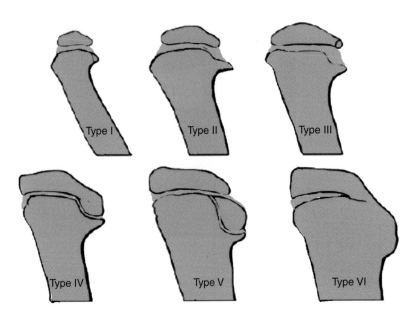

Figure 18.34 Langenskiold classification of Blount's disease.

Type I Type II Type III Type IV Type V Type VI

Candidate 5

EXAMINER: The clinical photograph (Figure 18.35) is for a newborn child who was referred to you with a left foot deformity; the referrer thinks the baby may have a congenital vertical talus (CVT)? What do you think?

CANDIDATE: The clinical photograph shows features that are very suggestive of congenital calcaneovalgus foot, which is a benign soft-tissue contracture of the foot secondary to intrauterine foetal packaging. There is an excessive dorsiflexion of the foot to the extent that the dorsum of the foot touches the frontal aspect of the leg. The deformity is usually passively correctable. Although it may look similar to CVT for the inexperienced, the differences are clear: in CVT

the hindfoot is a rigid equinus/valgus (not a flexible calcaneovalgus) (see Figure 18.36).

EXAMINER: How would you manage it?

CANDIDATE: It is important to rule out similar deformities (CVT and neurologic foot deformities) and associated conditions (posteromedial bowing and dislocated hips).

In a classical flexible congenital calcaneovalgus foot the diagnosis is usually obvious and further investigations are not required. However, radiographs can be useful to exclude CVT and posteromedial bowing, and US to exclude DDH.

I usually reassure parents and advise them on simple stretching manoeuvres and it usually resolves over 6 months. In resistant cases serial casting may be used to expedite correction

Table 18.7 Differences between Blount's disease and physiological varus

Angles	Blount's disease	Physiological varus
Tibiofemoral angle (TFA)	28 ± 11°	22 ± 8°
Mechanical axis deviation (MAD)	NA	NA
Epiphyseal–metaphyseal angle (EMA)	> 20°	< 20°
Metaphyseal–diaphyseal angle (MDA) (also called TMDA where T stands for tibial)	17 ± 4°	8 ± 4°
Femoral–metaphyseal–diaphyseal angle (FMDA)	7.4 ± 5°	14 ± 5°
Femoral–tibial ratio of McCarthy (FTR)	0.48 ± 0.4	2.6 ± 3

Know the differences between infantile and adolescent Blount's disease.

Table 18.8 Comparison between infantile and adolescent tibia vara.

Characteristic	Infantile Blount's disease	Adolescent Blount's disease
Incidence	More common	Less common
High BMI	Correlates with magnitude of deformity	Higher than early onset, correlates with deformity when BMI > 40
Low vitamin D level	Both	Both
Gender	Male predominance	Higher male predominance
Laterality	Bilateral (can be unilateral)	Unilateral (can be bilateral)
Proximal tibial varus	Higher magnitude	Lower magnitude
Distal femur varus	Not present	More often present (20%)
Internal tibial torsion	More prominent	Less prominent
Procurvatum	More prominent	Less prominent
Radiographic changes	Medial metaphyseal beaking	Medial proximal tibial physiolysis (widening)
Advanced bone age	Average 26 months	Average 10 months
Efficacy of bracing	Successful in early stages when initiated before age 3	Ineffective and poorly tolerated

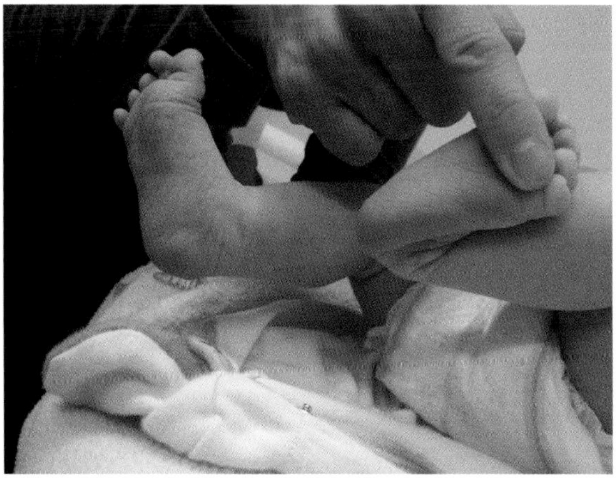

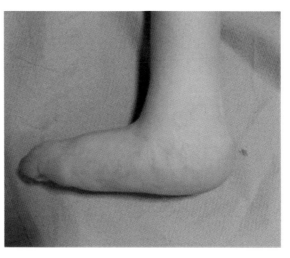

Figure 18.35 A newborn with left foot deformity.

(particularly if the foot cannot be plantar flexed beyond neutral).

EXAMINER: This is a radiograph of another child with the same condition (Figure 18.37). Any comments?

CANDIDATE: This clinical photograph shows a posteromedial bowing of the tibia (the apex of the deformity is pointing posterior and medial). It is often called physiologic bowing of tibia and it is thought to be a result of intrauterine foetal packaging. It is often associated with congenital calcaneovalgus foot. The two conditions may occur together or independently. In most cases

Figure 18.36 Rocker bottom foot in congenital vertical talus.

411

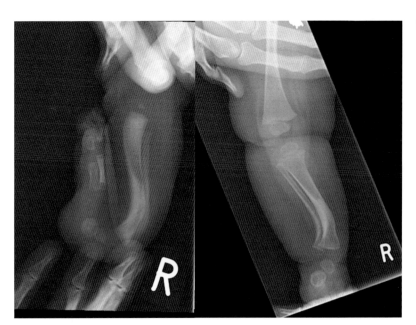

Figure 18.37 Lower limb radiograph.

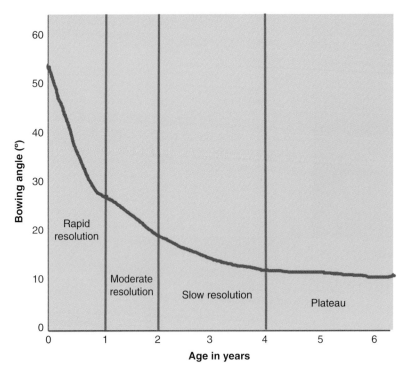

Figure 18.38 Resolution of posteromedial bowing.

the bowing resolves spontaneously over 3–5 years (Figure 18.38). However, it needs to be followed up, as LLD is not uncommon.

EXAMINER: You followed-up this patient and these are his X-rays over the last 3 years (Figure 18.39–18.41) (see also Table 18.9).

CANDIDATE: The X-rays show gradual improvement of the deformity (as expected), but there is still residual deformity and LLD as evident by the pelvic tilt. I would like to measure the LLD and the angular deformity. I would like to have lateral views as well.

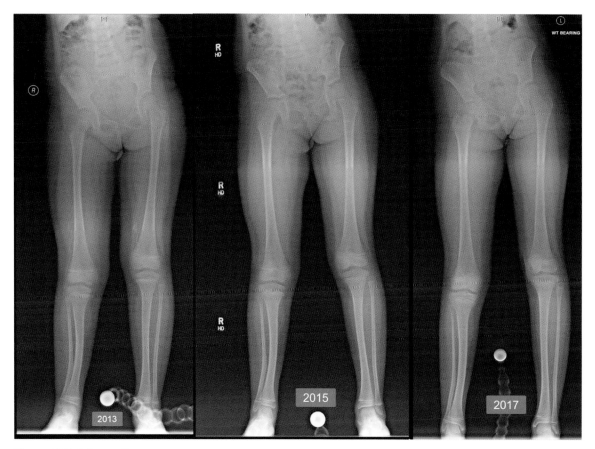

Figure 18.39 Follow up X-rays.

EXAMINER: Show me how you would do your measurement.

CANDIDATE: My measurements indicate that there is a LLD of 4 cm (mainly from tibia 3.4 cm) and a coronal angular deformity (valgus) of 15° at the junction between the distal and middle third of the tibia. I do not have lateral views to measure how much deformity there is at the sagittal plane.

I would like to take a full history to know the child's age, height, any comorbidity, expectations and previous consultations and treatments. I also need to check her skeletal age.

EXAMINER: She was 8 years and 10 months when she had the X-ray in 2017, her height was 134 cm, she is fit and healthy. She and her parents will be guided by your advice.

CANDIDATE: OK, I need to estimate her height and the LLD at maturity, then plan my management. I use the multiplier app on my phone to do so, but I also double-check it with the charts to ensure they give comparable results (Figure 18.42, 18.43) (see Authors' note).

So, her estimated height at maturity would be 166 cm, which is just above the 50th centile. The estimated full LLD would be 5.1 cm, whereas the tibia LLD would be 4.3 cm.

I expect almost equal results using a different method; for example, the rule of thumb method (Menelaus method). There is an increase in the full LLD of 6 mm and tibial LLD of 5 mm every 2 years from the table above or 3 and 2.5 mm every year. On average, girls finish growth at 14 years of age, so she has 5 years and 2 months of growth. Simple calculation reveals a full LLD of

5.5 cm and tibia LLD of 4.5 cm, which are very close to the multiplier methods.

EXAMINER: What will be your management plan?

CANDIDATE: My objectives are to correct all deformities. In this child, this includes LLD and the distal tibia deformity.

As for the LLD, I want to achieve equal leg lengths at skeletal maturity without excessive risk, morbidity or height reduction. My options are:

1. Shoe raise.
2. Epiphysiodesis of the long side.
3. Limb lengthening of the short side.
4. A combination of all.

Given the significant LLD and the deformity of the distal tibia (15° of valgus), my preferred option will be lengthening of the short leg with gradual correction of the leg deformity using a circular frame. I will use a double-stack frame with two osteotomies; one to correct the deformity and another at the proximal tibial metaphysis.

EXAMINER: What is your rationale for this? Why not correct and lengthen at the deformity site?

CANDIDATE: I could but the bone healing at the site of deformity in this condition is not ideal for lengthening and may end in delayed union and poor regeneration.

EXAMINER: The radiograph below shows what has been done (Figure 18.44). Any criticism?

CANDIDATE: The surgeon chose to slow the growth of the left leg. It is a small operation, revisable and given the remaining few years of growth, it is potentially able to equalize the leg. It is a good option; however, it has drawbacks. The child will be shorter and the distal tibial deformity has not been addressed.

Authors' note: 7

Limb reconstruction in general and lengthening in particular is an important topic not only in the paediatric section but in the adult section as well. The viva started with a simple case of congenital calcaneovalgus foot, which all candidates must recognize and come with a sensible plan. The viva progressed into a more complicated area of posteromedial tibial bowing and subsequent deformity and LLD. The candidate was doing very well and he clearly had a good understanding of how to manage LLD and deformity with a very good pass.

Table 18.9 Leg length discrepancy table.

Dates	Segments	Right	Left	Δ
2013	Total	51.7	54.4	2.7
	Femur	31.0	31.2	0.2
	Tibia	20.7	23.2	2.5
2015	Total	56.5	59.9	3.4
	Femur	34.2	34.6	0.4
	Tibia	22.3	25.4	3.0
2017	Total	69.7	73.6	4
	Femur	41.2	41.5	0.6
	Tibia	28.5	31.9	3.4

He was not derailed when he realized that the patient did not have what he had suggested. He pointed out the pros and cons of what had been done and explained why he would have chosen a different plan.

Please be objective and sensitive when you criticize other people's operation and do not be very negative, even if you think the choice of operation or the technique was completely wrong.

We recommend you familiarize yourself with the multiplier app. You can download it from:

https://itunes.apple.com/us/app/multiplier/id460335161?mt=8

Try to practise using the Mosley chart method (Figure 18.45) to do the calculation for the above patient.

More information is available on the following website: www.pedipod.com/Chapters/StepByStep.asp#

Candidate 6

EXAMINER: These are AP and lateral views of a 13-year-old child (Figure 18.46) who was brought in after a football injury. How would you manage such an injury?

CANDIDATE: I always approach these types of injuries according to ATLS protocols. It is very tempting to start with the ankle fracture or the deformed limb and it is important to resist this temptation.

EXAMINER: You did your primary and secondary survey, and this is the only injury that this child has.

CANDIDATE: I ensure adequate analgesia on board when I assess this child with substantive trauma. I look for obvious swelling, bruises, wounds, colour of the foot and toes. The X-ray indicates the

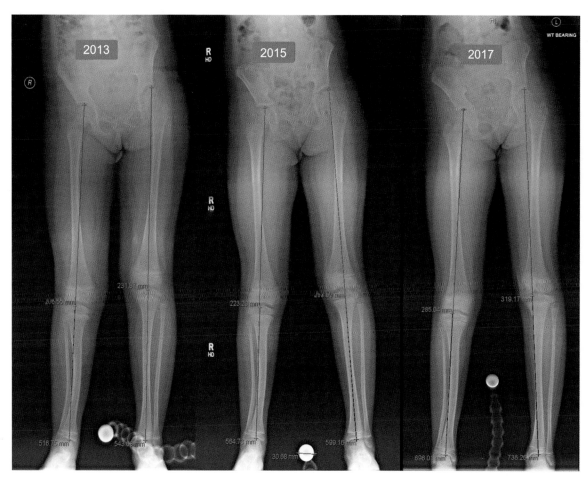

Figure 18.40 LLD following posteromedial bowing.

skin on the medial side of the ankle might be overstretched and there may be impending skin breakdown that requires immediate fracture reduction. I feel for skin temperature, pulses, tenderness. I assess the movement of the joints that are not involved to ensure that there are no unexpected problems. I would not move the ankle joint at this stage as it is expected to be painful. I assess the neurovascular status of the limb using special tests to test for nerve injuries.

EXAMINER: Indeed, you have found the skin over the medial malleolus is overstretched, white and about to tear.

CANDIDATE: Then we need to reduce the fracture immediately to prevent this fracture from becoming an open fracture, which has more comorbidity. If theatre space is immediately available, I will take the patient to the operating room; otherwise,

I may need to do it in the emergency room under sedation or Entonox.

EXAMINER: Theatre is available, but the patient had food an hour ago.

CANDIDATE: I think this a limb-threatening condition and justifies a rapid sequence induction anaesthesia (to prevent aspiration). I will discuss this with my anaesthetic colleague and we should proceed to perform the procedure. Of course, other preoperative preparation and consenting should be done appropriately and timely to prevent any delay in performing surgery.

These physeal injuries are usually stable after reduction and they need closed reduction and a well-moulded cast application.

EXAMINER: This is what has been done (Figure 18.47), any thoughts?

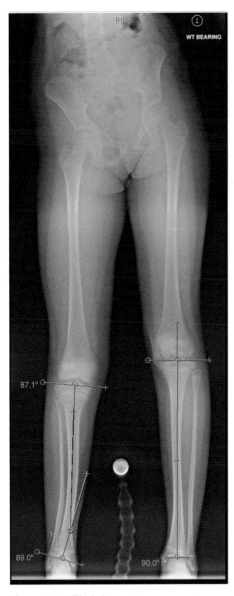

Figure 18.41 Tibial alignment measurements.

CANDIDATE: The surgeon reduced the fracture nicely and stabilized with a single K-wire crossing the physis. As I mentioned, my experience with these fractures is that they are relatively stable, and K-wire is not usually required unless the fracture is not stable. The concern is that the K-wire may cause physeal damage.

EXAMINER: What would you do next?

CANDIDATE: My postoperative instruction is to keep the foot elevated on a Braun frame, to mobilize non-weight-bearing. I would like to check the skin and the wound in 48 hours or so to ensure the skin is healing well. The patient will be discharged when deemed safe and I would like to see him in a week's time for wound check and X-ray. If everything is satisfactory, I will plan to remove the K-wire in 6 weeks' time. As the risk of growth plate disturbance is high in these fractures, I would like to follow this patient until I am sure that there is no growth arrest.

EXAMINER: This is the ankle X-ray after 8 months (Figure 18.48).

CANDIDATE: It is difficult to be certain, but I think the patient is developing a growth arrest on the right. I cannot see the growth plate very clearly and there is more valgus around the ankle. I would like to get more imaging (CT scan or MRI scan).

EXAMINER: There was no CT scan or MRI scan but there are long legs alignment views and some measurements (Figure 18.49).

CANDIDATE: The long leg alignment views confirm my initial suspicions that there is a growth arrest which led to a shortening of almost 1 cm and distal tibial valgus deformity of at least 10°. How old is the patient now?

EXAMINER: 15 years old.

CANDIDATE: So, he still has two years or more to go. A hand X-ray to establish his skeletal age will be valuable. My thought is to do bilateral distal tibial and fibular epiphysiodesis to stop the deformity and the LLD from getting worse.

EXAMINER: Would you consider correcting the distal tibial deformity?

CANDIDATE: If he is asymptomatic and there is a good subtalar join movement I probably would not; however, if he is symptomatic and there is a limited subtalar joint movement that does not compensate for the deformity then I would.

EXAMINER: The patient underwent left distal tibia and fibular epiphysiodesis and right distal tibial medial hemiepiphysiodesis. These are his pictures a year after (Figure 18.50), any thoughts?

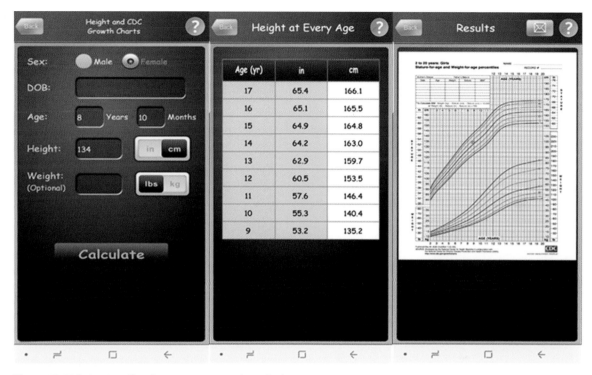

Age (yr)	in	cm
17	65.4	166.1
16	65.1	165.5
15	64.9	164.8
14	64.2	163.0
13	62.9	159.7
12	60.5	153.5
11	57.6	146.4
10	55.3	140.4
9	53.2	135.2

Figure 18.42 Estimation of height at maturity using the multiplier app.

CANDIDATE: I think this is a very good idea and it seems to have worked. The LLD reduced and the deformity was reduced. I thought about it; however, I was not sure whether the right distal tibia physis is still reliable to correct deformity.

Authors' note: 8

Physeal injuries are common in children. They are relatively stable after reduction; however, this is not always true. Instability is far more dangerous than a small wire crossing the physis. The above fracture was unstable and using a smooth K-wire to stabilize was the right thing to do. K-wire rarely causes growth arrest (take the supracondylar fracture as an example). Several technical tips can even reduce the risk further, such as using the smallest possible size, smooth wire, burst driver mode rather than continuous, cooling the heat generated by friction, etc...

EXAMINER: These clinical photographs (Figure 18.51) are for an 18-month-old child who is about to have surgery. Could you tell me what the pictures show and what the surgery involves?

CANDIDATE: The clinical photographs show the lower parts of a child's body. The surgeon tries to demonstrate the limited right hip abduction and the Galeazzi sign (the apparent shortening of the right femur) and the abnormal skin crease on the left proximal femur. All are signs of hip dislocation. In an 18-month-old child, I anticipate the surgery will be hip adductors release, open reduction, pelvic osteotomy (with or without femoral osteotomy) and application of hip spica.

EXAMINER: This is a plain pelvis X-ray of the above baby (Figure 18.52). What can you say about the X-ray?

CANDIDATE: The radiograph confirms my initial thought that the baby has a left hip dislocation. The femoral nucleus is smaller on the left side and has created a false acetabulum. The true acetabulum is shallow and not very well formed when compared to the other side. If I draw

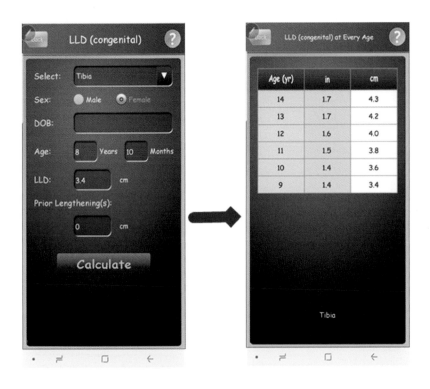

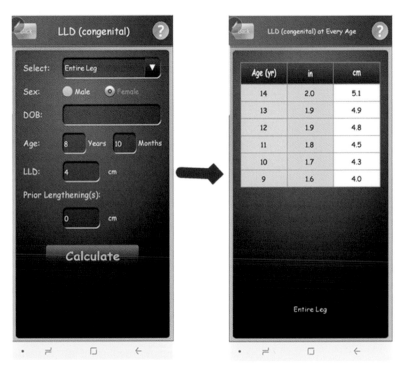

Figure 18.43 Estimation of LLD at maturity using the multiplier method.

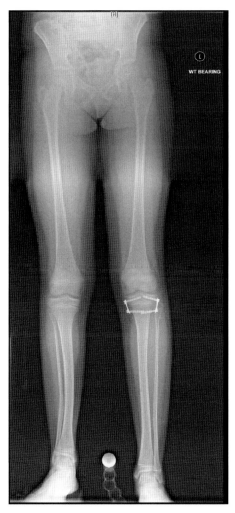

Figure 18.44 Proximal tibia epiphysiodesis using eight plates.

Hilgenreiner and Perkin lines, the head will be sitting in the upper lateral quadrants. There is a break in the inferior and lateral Shenton lines (Figure 18.53).

EXAMINER: What would you do if you were the surgeon?

CANDIDATE: He is 19 months old. I will be surprised if this hip can be reduced closed. However, there is always a patient who does not follow the rule. So, I would perform EUA and trial of closed reduction. If it is reduced, stable and has a large zone of safety, I would perform a hip arthrogram to assess how good my reduction is.

EXAMINER: Tell me what you mean by zone of safety?

CANDIDATE: This term was coined by Ramsey and associates [39] and refers to the range of motion in which the hip remains reduced in comparison to the maximum range of motion. The wider the range, the better. Two important facts are to be considered:

1. The average movement of the hip in a hip spica is 15°; so, it is important to keep the hip away from the line of dislocation by about 20° to reduce the risk of dislocation inside the spica.

2. The risk of AVN increases with the hip put at the maximum range of motion so it is safe to be 20° inside the maximum range of motion.

So, the safety zone is the range of motion (cone of motion) within 15–20° of the maximum range of motion and dislocation range. The maximum range of motion can be increased by adductor (to increase abduction) and psoas (to increase extension) tenotomy. These are not needed in all cases (Figures 18.54 and 18.55).

EXAMINER: You tried to reduce it closed and did a hip arthrogram. Figure 18.56 shows the arthrogram. Do you want to comment on the findings?

CANDIDATE: The arthrogram nicely shows the full size of the femoral head, which is much bigger than the ossified nucleus. The femoral head is not reduced in any of the below images and it remained articulating with a false acetabulum on the ileum. The capsule is distended and has the classical hourglass shape. This happens because as the head grows the femoral side becomes bigger while the isthmus of the capsule remains small. The isthmus is further constricted by the Chinese trap effect as well as by pressure from the iliopsoas tendon (visible in pictures 2 and 6). The ligamentum teres is thickened and elongated (pictures 2–6). None of the pictures demonstrate a reduced hip and there is significant medial dye pool. So, I believe this hip is not reducible.

EXAMINER: What prevents reduction?

CANDIDATE: There are several anatomical structures that can prevent reduction. These can be summarized as:

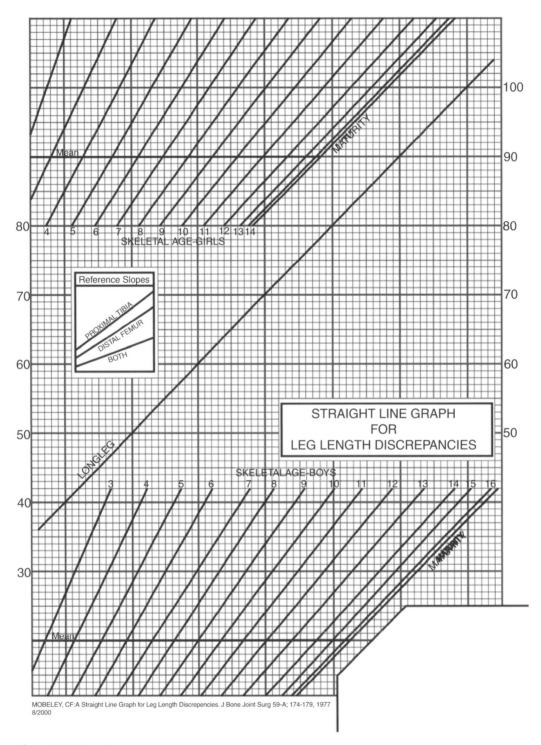

MOBELEY, CF:A Straight Line Graph for Leg Length Discrepencies. J Bone Joint Surg 59-A; 174-179, 1977
8/2000

Figure 18.45 Blank Mosley chart.

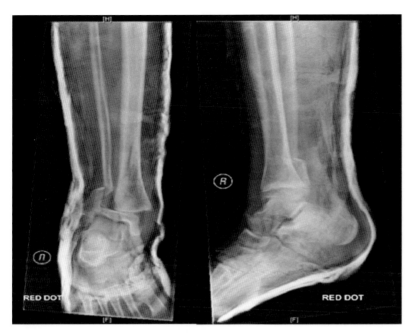

Figure 18.46 Ankle injury.

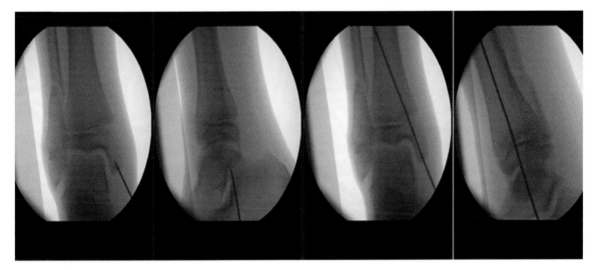

Figure 18.47 Ankle facture fixation.

A. Extra-articular structures:
   1. Iliopsoas tendon.
   2. Capsular constriction.
B. Intra-articular (2 ligaments + 2 pathological structures):
   1. Elongated ligamentum teres.

2. Thickened transverse acetabular ligament giving the acetabular cartilage the classic horse-shoe structure.
3. Pulvinar (fibro-fatty tissues filled the acetabulum).
4. Inverted limbus.

421

Figure 18.48 Eight months postoperative.

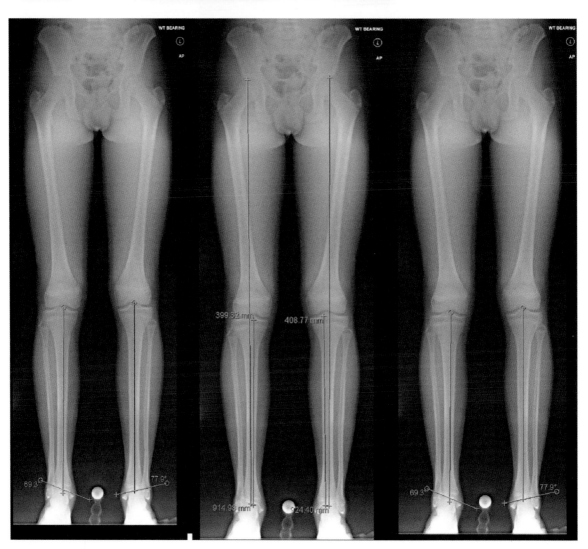

Figure 18.49 Long leg views measurements.

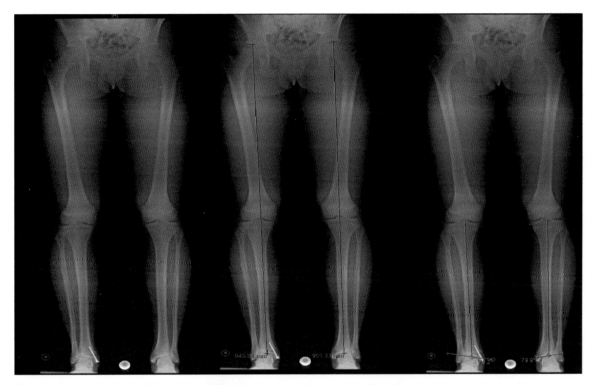

Figure 18.50 Postoperative left distal tibia and fibula hemiepiphysiodesis and right distal tibia medial hemiepiphysiodesis.

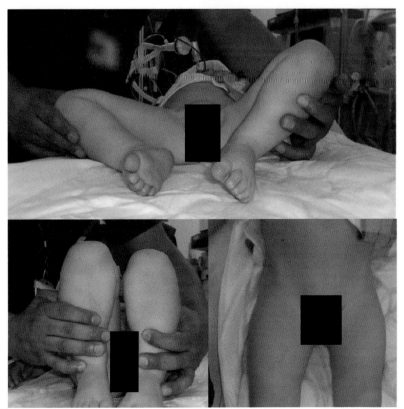

Figure 18.51 Clinical photographs of 18-month-old child.

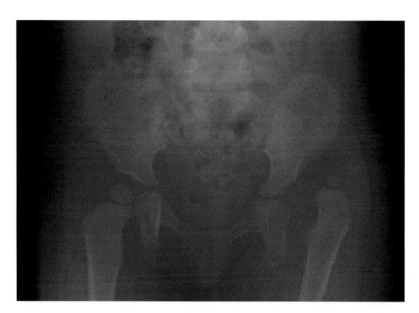

Figure 18.52 Plain pelvic X-ray.

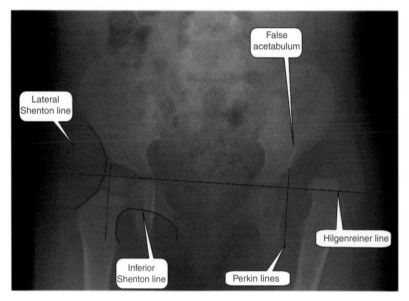

Figure 18.53 Plain pelvis X-ray of the hip of an 18-month-old child.

EXAMINER: What is the limbus?

CANDIDATE: There is no anatomical structure called limbus (or neolimbus), but it is the name given to the deformed and moulded labrum with the attached cartilaginous roof of the acetabulum pushed into the acetabulum preventing the femoral head reduction.

EXAMINER: So, what would you do in the above situation?

CANDIDATE: I would proceed to open reduction of the hip through the anterior hip approach (Smith Peterson). This is combined with adductors tenotomy and over the brim psoas muscle release. Pelvic osteotomy is often needed and femoral osteotomy may be needed as well.

EXAMINER: Take me through how would you do open reduction through an anterior hip approach?

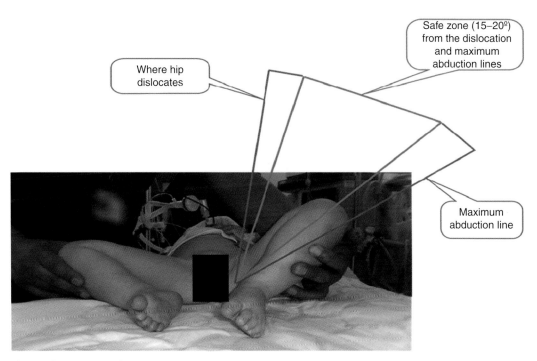

Figure 18.54 Coronal safe zone.

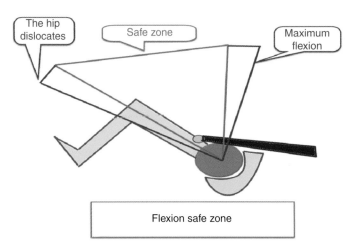

Figure 18.55 Sagittal safe zone.

Authors' note: 9

DDH is one of the commonest paediatric topics that have been featured in the exam. It is not the candidates' favourite, particularly if they have not done a paediatric orthopaedic job. The topic is nicely covered in the postgraduate paediatric orthopaedic book and the relevant section in the third edition.

You do not need to know all the ins and outs of the topic as long as you know the principles. Treatment options depend on the age of child at presentation, reducibility of hip, stability after reduction and amount of acetabular dysplasia.

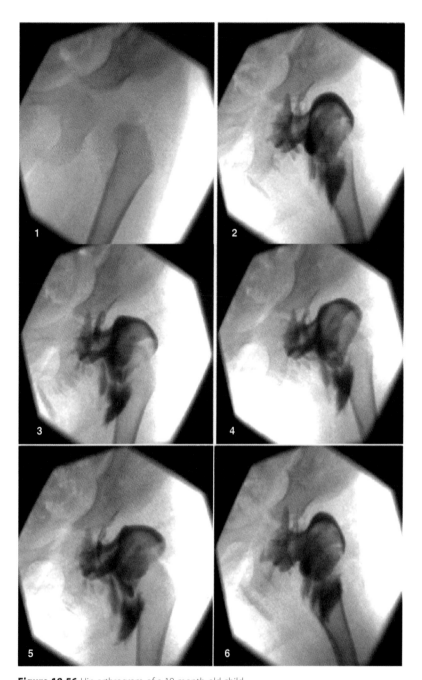

Figure 18.56 Hip arthrogram of a 19-month-old child.

Authors' note: 10

The FRCS (Trauma and Orthopaedic) exam is easy to pass, but ironically it is also easy to fail. Having helped hundreds of candidates to pass their exam, we find it is all about preparation:

'If you fail to prepare, then prepare to fail'.

Core knowledge and skills are important, but what is most important is how to present them clearly and confidently. This will come with practice.

The Postgraduate Orthopaedic faculty wish you all the best for your exam.

Table 18.10 Dislocated hip management.

Age groups	Treatment
< 6 months	Pavlik harness
6–18 months	Tenotomy, closed reduction and hip spica. Sometimes open reduction is required. Controversy about medial open approach. It has fallen out of favour because of high AVN rates (controversial).
18–36 months	Tenotomy, open reduction, pelvic osteotomy and hip spica. Femoral osteotomy may be required. Femoral osteotomy is becoming more common.
36–96 months	Tenotomy, open reduction, pelvic and femoral osteotomies and hip spica.
> 96 months	Reconstruction (tenotomy, open reduction, pelvic and femoral osteotomies and hip spica) vs. Leave it unreduced.

Have some answers about controversial points, including:

• Routine screening: currently in the UK all infants have clinical exam and only patients at risk/with abnormal exam will have an ultrasound scan.

• Traction before closed reduction: different units follow different protocols. Supporters suggested that traction reduces the need for open reduction and decreased AVN rate, other studies show similar results with and without traction mainly due to better understanding of treatment principles, which encourage gentle reduction, the use of the human position to maintain reduction, and avoiding extreme positions for immobilization.

• Medial vs. anterior approach for open reduction.

• Pelvic osteotomy types and indications.

• Reconstructive: must have concentric reduction.

A. Redirectional: Salter, Pemberton, double (Sutherland), triple (Steel) and periacetabular (Ganz/PAO).

B. Reshaping: Dega and Pemberton (Pemberton osteotomy mainly directional but can change the shape as well).

• Salvage: Shelf and Chiari.

References

1. Alshryda S, Jones S, Banaszkiewicz P. *Postgraduate Paediatric Orthopaedics: The Candidate's Guide to the FRCS (Tr and Orth) Examination.* Cambridge: Cambridge University Press; 2014.

2. Loder RT, Richards BS, Shapiro PS, Reznick LR, Aronson DD. Acute slipped capital femoral epiphysis:

the importance of physeal stability. *J Bone Joint Surg Am.* 1993;75(8):1134–1140.

3. Alshryda S, Tsang K, Chytas A, *et al.* Evidence based treatment for unstable slipped upper femoral epiphysis: systematic review and exploratory patient level analysis. *The Surgeon.* 2018;16(1):46–54.

4. Alshryda S, Tsang K, Ahmed M, Adepapo A, Montgomery R. Severe slipped upper femoral epiphysis; fish osteotomy versus pinning-in-situ: an eleven year perspective. *The Surgeon.* 2014;12(5):244–248.

5. Jerre R, Billing L, Hansson G, Wallin J. The contralateral hip in patients primarily treated for unilateral slipped upper femoral epiphysis. Long-term follow-up of 61 hips. *J Bone Joint Surg Br.* 1994;76(4):563–567.

6. Phillips PM, Phadnis J, Willoughby R, Hunt L. Posterior sloping angle as a predictor of contralateral slip in slipped capital femoral epiphysis. *J Bone Joint Surg Am.* 2013;95(2):146–150.

7. Stasikelis PJ, Sullivan CM, Phillips WA, Polard JA. Slipped capital femoral epiphysis. Prediction of contralateral involvement. *J Bone Joint Surg Am.* 1996; 78(8):1149–1155.

8. Parsch K, Weller S, Parsch D. Open reduction and smooth Kirschner wire fixation for unstable slipped capital femoral epiphysis. *J Pediatr Orthop.* 2009;29 (1):1–8.

9. Ziebarth K, Zilkens C, Spencer S, Leunig M, Ganz R, Kim Y-J. Capital realignment for moderate and severe SCFE using a modified Dunn procedure. *Clin Orthop Relat Res.* 2009;467(3):704–716.

10. Naseem H, Chatterji S, Tsang K, Hakimi M, Chytas A, Alshryda S. Treatment of stable slipped capital femoral epiphysis: systematic review and exploratory patient level analysis. *J Orthop Traumatol.* 2017;18:469.

11. British Orthopaedic Association. *BOAST11.* Supracondylar fractures of the humerus in children. 2014.

12. Isaacs H, Handelsman JE, Badenhorst M, Pickering A. The muscles in club foot – a histological histochemical and electron microscopic study. *J Bone Joint Surg Br.* 1977;59B(4):465–472.

13. Gray DH, Katz JM. A histochemical study of muscle in club foot. *J Bone Joint Surg Br.* 1981;63B(3):417–423.

14. Wynne-Davies R. Genetic and environmental factors in the etiology of talipes equinovarus. *Clin Orthop Relat Res.* 1972;84:9–13.

15. Sharon-Weiner M, Sukenik-Halevy R, Tepper R, Fishman A, Biron-Shental T, Markovitch O. Diagnostic accuracy, work-up, and outcomes of pregnancies with clubfoot detected by prenatal sonography. *Prenat Diagn.* 2017;37(8):754–763.

16. Ponseti IV, Morcuende JA. Current management of idiopathic clubfoot questionnaire: a multicenter study. *J Pediatr Orthop*. 2004;24(4):448.

17. Ponseti IV, Smoley EN. Congenital club foot: the result of treatment. *J Bone Joint Surg Am*. 1963;45(A(2)):261–344.

18. Huntley JS. What is the best treatment for paediatric trigger thumb (acquired thumb flexion contracture)? In S Alshryda, JS Huntley, P Banaszkiewicz (Eds.), *Paediatric Orthopaedics: An Evidence-Based Approach to Clinical Questions*. Cham: Springer; 2016.

19. Caird MS, Flynn JM, Leung YL, Millman JE, D'Italia JG, Dormans JP. Factors distinguishing septic arthritis from transient synovitis of the hip in children. A prospective study. *J Bone Joint Surg Am*. 2006;88(6):1251–1257.

20. Maharajan K, Patro DK, Menon J, *et al*. Serum procalcitonin is a sensitive and specific marker in the diagnosis of septic arthritis and acute osteomyelitis. *J Orthop Surg Res*. 2013;8:19.

21. Zhao J, Zhang S, Zhang L, *et al*. Serum procalcitonin levels as a diagnostic marker for septic arthritis: a meta-analysis. *Am J Emerg Med*. 2017;35(8):1166–1171.

22. Kocher MS, Zurakowski D, Kasser JR. Differentiating between septic arthritis and transient synovitis of the hip in children: an evidence-based clinical prediction algorithm. *J Bone Joint Surg Am*. 1999;81(12):1662–1670.

23. Kocher MS, Mandiga R, Zurakowski D, Barnewolt C, Kasser JR. Validation of a clinical prediction rule for the differentiation between septic arthritis and transient synovitis of the hip in children. *J Bone Joint Surg Am*. 2004;86A(8):1629–1635.

24. Herring JA, Kim HT, Browne R. Legg–Calve–Perthes disease. Part II: Prospective multicenter study of the effect of treatment on outcome. *J Bone Joint Surg Am*. 2004;86A(10):2121–2134.

25. Wiig O, Terjesen T, Svenningsen S. Prognostic factors and outcome of treatment in Perthes' disease: a prospective study of 368 patients with five-year follow-up. *J Bone Joint Surg Br*. 2008;90(10):1364–1371.

26. Wright JG. *Evidence-Based Orthopaedics. The Best Answers to Clinical Questions*, ed. J. Wright. Philadelphia: Saunders; 2009.

27. Daly K, Bruce C, Catterall A. Lateral shelf acetabuloplasty in Perthes' disease. A review of the end of growth. *J Bone Joint Surg Br*. 1999;81(3):380–384.

28. Domzalski ME, Glutting J, Bowen JR, Littleton AG. Lateral acetabular growth stimulation following a labral support procedure in Legg–Calve–Perthes disease. *J Bone Joint Surg Am*. 2006;88(7):1458–1466.

29. Bankes MJ, Catterall A, Hashemi-Nejad A. Valgus extension osteotomy for 'hinge abduction' in Perthes' disease. Results at maturity and factors influencing the radiological outcome. *J Bone Joint Surg Br*. 2000;82(4):548–554.

30. Segev E, Ezra E, Wientraub S, Yaniv M, Hayek S, Hemo Y. Treatment of severe late-onset Perthes' disease with soft tissue release and articulated hip distraction: revisited at skeletal maturity. *J Child Orthop*. 2007;1(4):229–235.

31. Laklouk MA, Hosny GA. Hinged distraction of the hip joint in the treatment of Perthes disease: evaluation at skeletal maturity. *J Pediatr Orthop B*. 2012;21(5):386–393.

32. Davids JR, Blackhurst DW, Allen Jr BL. Clinical evaluation of bowed legs in children. *J Pediatr Orthop B*. 2000;9(4):278–284.

33. Levine AM, Drennan JC. Physiological bowing and tibia vara. The metaphyseal–diaphyseal angle in the measurement of bowleg deformities. *J Bone Joint Surg Am*. 1982;64(8):1158–1163.

34. O'Neill DA, MacEwen GD. Early roentgenographic evaluation of bowlegged children. *J Pediatr Orthop*. 1982;2(5):547–553.

35. McCarthy JJ, Betz RR, Kim A, Davids JR, Davidson RS. Early radiographic differentiation of infantile tibia vara from physiologic bowing using the femoral–tibial ratio. *J Pediatr Orthop*. 2001;21(4):545–548.

36. Herring JA (Ed.). *Tachdjians Pediatric Orthopaedics*, Vol. 1. Philadelphia: Saunders Elsevier; 2008.

37. Raney EM, Topoleski TA, Yaghoubian R, Guidera KJ, Marshall JG. Orthotic treatment of infantile tibia vara. *J Pediatr Orthop*. 1998;18(5):670–674.

38. Richards BS, Katz DE, Sims JB. Effectiveness of brace treatment in early infantile Blount's disease. *J Ped Orthopaed*. 1998;18(3):374–380.

39. Ramsey PL, Lasser S, MacEwen GD. Congenital dislocation of the hip: use of the Pavlik harness in the child during the first six months of life. 1976. *J Bone Joint Surg Am*. 2002;84A(8):1478; discussion 1478.

Anatomy and surgical approaches

Tom Symes and Kiran Singisetti

Introduction

It is important to spend time learning surgical approaches and anatomy. At least two questions in the exam will be drawn from these areas in either the trauma and/or basic science vivas. Anatomy is fairly straightforward for the FRCS(Tr & Orth), either it's learnt and known well for the exam, allowing candidates to score easy marks, or it hasn't been learnt and the viva quickly unfolds, losing scoring opportunities for the candidate. The skill is anticipating which questions are more likely to appear in the exam than others and adjusting your revision time accordingly to take this into account.

If candidates are not expecting to be questioned in any great detail on basic anatomy, then it will become quite difficult as anatomy for most purposes just needs to be known.

The WHO Safer Surgery checklist has to be known. This has become important for patient safety and the prevention of system failure,

Structured oral examination question 1

Approach to hip for total hip arthroplasty

The candidate is shown a radiograph of THA (Figure 19.1a).

EXAMINER: What approach do you use for THA?

CANDIDATE: The posterior approach to the hip joint.

COMMENT: This is probably the most common approach you will be asked to describe. You could mention any of the hip approaches, but the most common approaches used in the UK are the posterior and the anterolateral (Hardinge).

Talk about the approach that you know and use routinely. If you try to describe something that you have only read in a book, you will probably struggle to explain the details, including any technical tips or how to enlarge the approach. Read up

on your favoured approach beforehand, especially the neurovascular intervals and structures at risk.

EXAMINER: What approach would you use for a THA operation done for fracture neck of femur?

CANDIDATE: The posterior approach. I am aware that many surgeons use an anterolateral approach for this indication to reduce the risk of dislocation. The NICE guidance for hemiarthroplasty prefers an anterolateral over a posterior approach, but no such differentiation is suggested with THA. I would use a posterior approach in this situation, as this is the approach I am more familiar with using in THA.

COMMENT: Candidates should be able to describe some rationale in using their preferred approach for the procedure.

EXAMINER: Describe the approach from skin, fat, fascia, bursa, and muscular interval if relevant to the joint.

CANDIDATE:

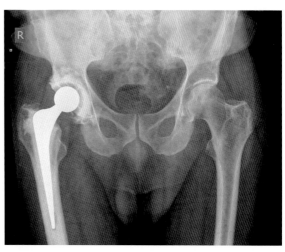

Figure 19.1a Anteroposterior (AP) pelvic radiograph demonstrating cemented right Exeter THA.

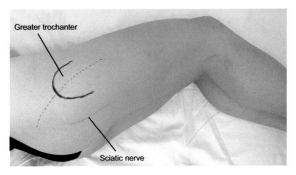

Figure 19.1b Skin incision for posterior approach hip. Landmarks: greater trochanter. Incision: a curvilinear incision starting 10 cm distal to the PSIS extended distal and laterally parallel to the fibres of the gluteus maximus to the posterior margin of the greater trochanter and then direct the incision 10 cm distally parallel to the femoral shaft. The sciatic nerve enters the lower limb in the gluteal region and passes inferiorly midway between two major palpable bony landmarks: the greater trochanter and the ischial tuberosity.

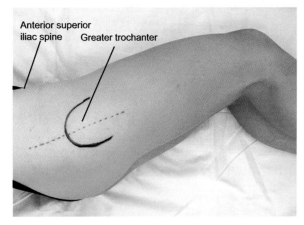

Figure 19.1c Skin incision for a lateral approach to the hip (Hardinge). Landmarks: greater trochanter and anterior superior iliac spine. Incision: longitudinal incision centred over the tip of the greater trochanter in the line of the femoral shaft.

Posterior

Position: Lateral decubitus. Supports placed anteriorly over ASIS, and posteriorly over the sacrum.

Landmarks: Greater trochanter.

Incision: The skin incision is 15–20 cm centred over the posterior aspect of the greater trochanter, curving posteriorly.

Superficial dissection: Incise fat and deep fascia in line with the skin incision. Insert Charnley retractors under the fascia/tensor muscle to allow visualization of the posterior aspect of the hip and trochanter.

Deep dissection: Sweep fat of the short external rotators (ER) at the posterior aspect of the hip joint. Identify and tag the piriformis tendon, which can be difficult to identify if flimsy. Divide the piriformis, gemelli obturator tendons and quadratus femoris muscle off the trochanter from just below the trochanteric ridge. Release of the gluteus maximus insertion distally into the linea aspera may be necessary when greater mobilization of the femur is required, such as complex primary, resurfacing and revision. Consider partial release in unfavourable primary THA situations such as large BMI, inexperienced scrub assistant or during the surgery learning curve. Divide the capsule, dislocate the femoral head posteriorly. Excise the femoral head using a saw. Place a large retractor at the anterior edge of acetabulum at 2–3 o'clock rim, releasing incision inferior capsule, place

Charnley spike or Judd pin posterior to the acetabular wall and an additional retractor inferiorly (Hohmann) just below the transverse acetabular ligament to overall give a 360° view/exposure of the acetabulum.

> *EXAMINER:* Some surgeons do not routinely detach the piriformis.
>
> *CANDIDATE:* I generally do so unless I am particularly worried about instability – but I would go anterolaterally if this was the case.
>
> *COMMENT:* Candidates may be asked origins/insertions and nerve supply of the short external rotator muscles hip.

Lateral (Hardinge)

Position: Lateral decubitus position with supports.

Landmarks: ASIS, GT and femoral shaft.

Incision: Longitudinal midlateral incision centred over the GT tip and distally in line with the femoral shaft.

Internervous plane: No true plane.

Superficial dissection: Incise fat and fascia in line with the skin. The greater trochanter should come into view. The tensor fascia lata is retracted anteriorly and the gluteus maximus posteriorly (Figure 19.1c).

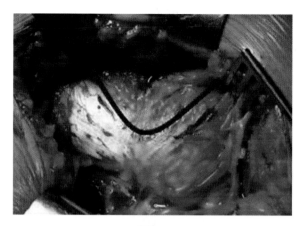

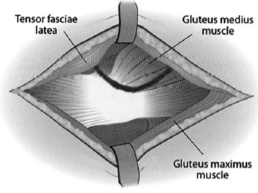

Figure 19.1d Omega incision into the gluteus medius tendon. Modified Hardinge approach maintaining two-thirds of the medius and releasing towards the lesser trochanter and not vertically downwards, maintains the medius–lateralis tension band as well as exposes the acetabulum and the femoral shaft necessary for standard THA.

Deep dissection: The gluteus medius is incised, extending from the uppermost end of the ridge of vastus lateralis, curving around the greater trochanter in an omega-shaped incision, until it reaches the apex of the greater trochanter, where it is extended proximally between the fibres of the gluteus medius. Distally the incision is extended into the vastus lateralis in line with its fibres, elevating the anterior third in continuity with the medius tendon.

Avoid taking the dissection too far proximally (injury to the superior gluteal nerve). Perform an H- or inverted T-shaped capsulotomy and then dislocate the femoral head.

Anterolateral (Watson-Jones approach)

This approach avoids the need to cut the gluteus medius muscle, but involves considerable pulling

(traction) on the gluteus medius and TFL muscles and potentially on the superior gluteal nerve. If used for THA it often requires additional division of the gluteus medius and minimus which lie over the anterior capsule for adequate exposure, which may lead to a Trendelenburg gait. This approach is not often used in the UK for primary THA, although a minimally invasive anterolateral approach hip (modified Watson-Jones) using special retractors, patient positioning devices, and offset reamers has gained some popularity recently.

Position: Supine position with a sandbag under the buttock and the buttock hanging slightly over the edge of the table.

Landmarks: ASIS and greater trochanter.

Incision: Incision is started 2 cm posterior and distal to the ASIS. It curves distally and posteriorly to the apex of the greater trochanter to extend longitudinally down about 6 cm distally along the shaft of the femur.

Internervous plane: No true internervous plane as tensor fascia lata and gluteus medius share the same nerve supply (superior gluteal nerve).

Superficial dissection: Subcutaneous tissue and fascia lata are incised in the same line as the skin. The interval between the gluteus medius and the tensor fascia lata is often difficult to delineate. However, it can be found more easily by beginning the separation midway between the anterior superior iliac spine and the greater trochanter before the tensor fascia lata blends with its fascial insertion. The incision is continued proximally along the posterior border of tensor fascia lata and the inferior branch of the superior gluteal nerve innervating the TFL is often seen.

Deep dissection: The tensor fascia with tensor fascia lata is retracted anteriorly and the gluteus medius posteriorly, exposing the fatty tissue covering the anterosuperior aspect of the hip capsule. The vastus lateralis is sometimes needed to be reflected from the proximal femur distal to the greater trochanter.

Structures at risk: Superior gluteal nerve.

Extension of approach: The fibres of the vastus lateralis may be split longitudinally to expose the upper part of the femoral shaft.

EXAMINER: What nerve is at risk in each approach and when?

CANDIDATE: Posterior: sciatic nerve during approach. Femoral nerve during retraction/exposure of the anterior acetabulum. Obturator nerve: during inferior acetabulum retraction.

Lateral: Superior gluteal nerve (3–5 cm above the upper border of the greater trochanter) during the approach through the abductors, femoral nerve, artery and vein (retractors); transverse branch of lateral circumflex femoral artery (as vastus lateralis is mobilized).

EXAMINER: What is the consequence of damage in terms of sensory loss, weakness?

CANDIDATE: Sciatic – most commonly affects peroneal branch; therefore, foot drop and sensory loss dorsum of the foot.

Femoral – weak knee extension and loss of sensation over the medial border of the leg and foot.

Superior gluteal nerve – abductor weakness, Trendelenburg gait.

COMMENT: You must know your peripheral nerve lesions and sensory dermatomes for many different topics, e.g. spinal injuries, ATLS assessment, brachial plexus.

EXAMINER: Which approach is more extensile for revision hip surgery?

CANDIDATE: The posterior.

COMMENT: It is acceptable to mention another approach if you can justify it.

EXAMINER: What manoeuvres can be performed to improve exposure of the acetabulum?

CANDIDATE: Release piriformis, anterior capsule, reflected head of rectus femoris, psoas tendon.

EXAMINER: What manoeuvres can be performed to facilitate removal of cement and/or a femoral stem which are difficult to remove?

CANDIDATE: Extended trochanteric osteotomy.
Trochanteric osteotomy/slide.
Window in femur.

EXAMINER: Describe how you would perform an ETO.

CANDIDATE: Ideally preoperative planning in which the osteotomy length is determined from the tip of the greater trochanter.

I would expose the lateral femur by elevating the vastus lateralis off the linea aspera with due care to identify the perforating vessels. Then mark out the osteotomy line using cautery planning for a posterior to anterior longitudinal cut and a short distal transverse cut. Then two or three osteotomes are used to elevate the osteotomy fragment with a muscular hinge anteriorly. I use a prophylactic cerclage cable distal to the osteotomy site.

EXAMINER: What are your indications for ETO?

CANDIDATE:
1. Improved exposure during approach.
2. Removal of femoral cement (especially infection).
3. Removal of well-fixed uncemented femoral prosthesis.
4. Removal of cement plug, poor bone stock, high risk of perforation (varus malformation).
5. Abnormalities of the proximal femur.

Structured oral examination question 2

Approach to the hip for drainage

A radiograph of a child's hip is shown (Figure 19.2).

EXAMINER: A 5-year-old boy presents to A&E with a 2-day history of fevers, off legs, c/o painful hip and knee. This is his X-ray. After taking a history and examination, what tests would you perform (likelihood of hip sepsis)?

CANDIDATE: FBC, CRP, ESR, USS, MRI.

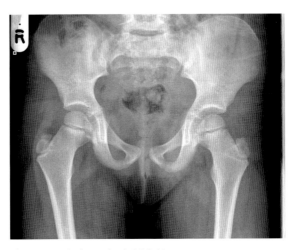

Figure 19.2 Radiograph of child's hip.

COMMENT: Hip sepsis in children is a common question at several points in the exam and needs to be known well. There are studies that have produced prediction of the likelihood of septic arthritis depending on blood markers and clinical features. If the viva station is progressing well it should be relatively easy to throw in Kocher's criteria for a child with a painful hip:

- Raised CRP.
- Raised white cell count.
- Inability to bear weight.
- Pyrexia.

Four of the criteria are 99% sensitive for septic arthritis; three are 93% sensitive; two are 40% sensitive; and one is 3% sensitive.

Reference

Kocher MS, Zurakowski D, Kasser JR. Differentiating between septic arthritis and transient synovitis of the hip in children: an evidence-based clinical prediction algorithm. *J Bone Joint Surg Am.* 1999;81(12):1662–1670.

EXAMINER: The candidate is presented with test results (increased WBC, CRP, ESR, effusion on X-rays and USS). What is the management?

CANDIDATE: Open washout and drainage.

COMMENT: Some surgeons may argue that you should perform a USS-guided drainage to identify pus or a positive culture but the examiners in this situation want you to describe the approach, so will make it a barn door case.

EXAMINER: Which approach is recommended to perform open drainage and washout of a child's septic hip and why?

CANDIDATE: Anterior (Smith Peterson) because the main blood supply to the femoral head is posterior.

COMMENT: You must know this approach for the basic science and also the paeds viva.

EXAMINER: Describe the layers and nerve supply.

CANDIDATE: Supine position.
Incision (use part of this) following anterior half of iliac crest to ASIS then curved down vertically 4–5 cm towards lateral side of patella.
Externally rotate the leg, identify the gap between the sartorius (femoral nerve) and the tensor fascia lata (superior gluteal nerve) about

5 cm below the ASIS, avoid the lateral femoral cutaneous nerve which pierces the deep fascia near the interval, incise the fascia medial to the TFL and retract it downwards and laterally, retract the sartorius upward and medially.

Ligate the ascending branch of the lateral femoral circumflex artery (which crosses the gap between the sartorius and tensor fascia lata), then develop the plane between the rectus femoris (femoral nerve) and the gluteus medius (superior gluteal nerve). Detach the two origins of the rectus femoris (AIIS and superior lip of acetabulum), retract the rectus femoris and the iliopsoas medially and the gluteus medius laterally to expose the hip capsule, capsulotomy (longitudinal or T-shaped) and then wash out the hip joint.

COMMENT: This is a pass–fail question and must be known.

Structured oral examination question 3

Henry's/anterior approach to arm

EXAMINER: Describe this radiograph (Figure 19.3).

CANDIDATE: It is an X-ray of the right forearm of an adult. There are transverse fractures of the mid shaft of both radius and ulna. They are completely displaced.

COMMENT: You must be able to quickly and concisely describe a fracture as if you were talking to your consultant on the end of a phone and so he can easily imagine the fracture pattern.

EXAMINER: How would you describe the displacement concisely?

CANDIDATE: They are off-ended.

EXAMINER: What is the generally accepted surgical treatment for this injury?

CANDIDATE: Plating of both bones with dynamic compression plates.

EXAMINER: If you were to approach the fractured radius anteriorly, how would you do it?

COMMENT: The anterior approach to the radius was first described by Henry and his name is usually associated with it. Henry's approach can

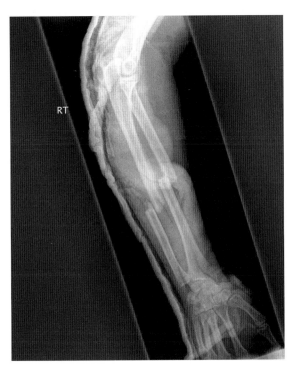

Figure 19.3a Forearm fracture.

be divided into a proximal internervous plane between the brachioradialis muscle (radial nerve) and the pronator teres (median nerve) or a distal approach between brachioradialis (radial nerve) and the flexor carpi radialis muscle (FCR) (median nerve). The internervous planes are the same throughout the forearm, but the muscles encountered are different proximally and distally.

The deep surgical dissection is divided into thirds (proximal, middle and distal third).

CANDIDATE:

    Landmarks: Biceps tendon, brachioradialis (part of the mobile wad), lateral epicondyle of humerus and styloid process of radius.

    Incision: Incise the skin over the FCR aiming towards the biceps insertion. Develop the plane between the brachioradialis (radial nerve) and the FCR (median nerve) distally and retract the FPL.

I would approach the distal radius through the bed of the FCR. The sheath of FCR is incised and the tendon freed and retracted in an ulnar direction to protect the median nerve. Next, the floor of the FCR sheath is incised. Directly beneath the sheath is the belly of the flexor pollicis longus (FPL). The muscle is bluntly swept to the side to expose the deep fibres of the pronator quadratus. The radial portion of the pronator quadratus is incised and dissected off the distal radius using a combination of sharp dissection and a periosteal elevator with an L-type incision. A small cuff of tissue is left for later repair. Often there is partial disruption by the fracture fragments in high-energy injuries.

COMMENT: The candidate for whatever reason has described the anterior volar approach to the distal radius. The radiograph demonstrates a mid-third radius fracture and as such the examiner should have guided the candidate back onto the mid-third radius approach.

    The superficial muscular dissection is similar for all three parts of Henry's anterior approach: the interval between the brachioradialis (mobile wad) and the flexor carpi radialis (FCR) muscle. The radial artery lies deep to the brachioradialis in

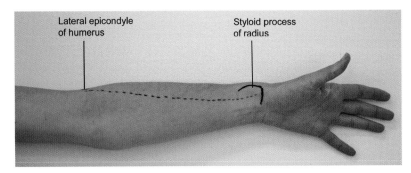

Figure 19.3b Anterior approach to the radius. Landmarks: biceps tendon, brachioradialis, lateral epicondyle humerus and styloid process of radius. Incision: a longitudinal incision from the elbow flexor crease lateral to the biceps tendon down to the radial styloid.

the middle part of the forearm and between the tendons of the brachioradialis and the FCR distally. It is identified by its two venae comitantes that run alongside it.

The middle third of the radial shaft is covered by the pronator teres (PT) and the flexor digitorum superficialis (FDS) muscle. The arm is pronated to expose the insertion of the PT onto the lateral radial shaft. The insertion is detached, and the muscle stripped off in an ulnar direction, which also detaches the origin of the FDS.

EXAMINER: How would you position the patient?

CANDIDATE: I would position the patient supine with an arm board and upper arm tourniquet. I would elevate the arm but not exsanguinate it so as to keep the veins engorged. This helps with identification of the venae comitantes of the radial artery. I would perform a surgical time-out before inflating the tourniquet, undertaking skin preparation and draping.

COMMENT: Go through a set standard routine for each approach. This question is about how you set the patient up for surgery. Ideally, the candidate should have initially mentioned this.

EXAMINER: What do you mean by a surgical time-out?

CANDIDATE: This is the final step before the start of the surgical procedure where the patient, surgical procedure and side/site are reviewed by the surgical team.

COMMENT: This is a classic approach and anecdotally candidates have been failed for not knowing it! Some approaches have quirks or peculiarities, and this is one of them – the need to change the position of the limb depending on the fracture location.

Try to have a mental picture of the origins and insertions on the radius from proximal to distal when describing this approach.

EXAMINER: How would you extend the exposure proximally?

CANDIDATE: This approach can be extended across the elbow into an anterolateral approach to the humerus, but this is rarely required.

EXAMINER: How would you extend the exposure distally?

CANDIDATE: The approach can be extended distally into the wrist with a carpal tunnel-type incision.

EXAMINER: What are the structures at risk (SAR)?

CANDIDATE: PIN: this travels through the body of supinator and can be damaged when exposing the proximal third of the radial shaft. Fully supinate the forearm when dissecting the supinator muscle off the radius as this moves the PIN away from the operative field. A subperiosteal dissection stripping the muscle from bone rather than splitting the muscle thereby leaving the PIN in the substance of the muscle. Ensure full supination and avoid using a retractor on the posterior radial neck to avoid potential injury.

Superficial radial nerve (SRN): this runs down the forearm underneath the brachioradialis muscle. It is vulnerable when the mobile wad of three is mobilized and retracted laterally. The nerve can be damaged with vigorous retraction. The SRN is notorious in developing a painful neuroma second to innocuous injury.

Radial artery: runs down the middle of the forearm under brachioradialis. A leash of vessels from the radial artery supply the brachioradialis and they need to be ligated in order to mobilize the brachioradialis. The radial artery is vulnerable during mobilization of the brachioradialis and is

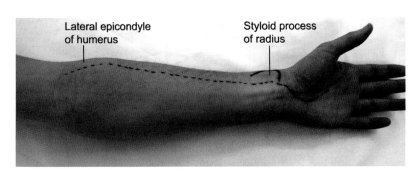

Lateral epicondyle of humerus

Styloid process of radius

Figure 19.3c Anterior approach to the radius. How to enlarge the approach proximally and distally.

often retracted medially to expose the deeper muscular layers.

For score 7/8

EXAMINER: What are the relative advantages and disadvantages of a volar compared to a dorsal approach to the radius?

CANDIDATE: While a volar approach is the standard and preferred method for a fracture of the distal half of the radius, the approach for its proximal half is controversial.

Henry's anterior approach to the radius is an extensile approach and offers full exposure of the radial shaft if required. As mentioned, the structures at risk in this approach include the PIN, radial artery, superficial radial nerve, lateral cutaneous nerve of forearm and recurrent leash of Henry.

In the dorsal approach, access to the bone is easier and the posterior or tension surface of the bone is in full view. The plate is applied to the tension dorsal side of the radius, which is biomechanically more favourable. The PIN is more vulnerable to injury in this approach, but injury to the nerve can occur whatever approach is used, and great care is needed during surgical dissection of the supinator muscle.

Plating on the anterior surface may cause impingement on the bicipital tuberosity and the biceps tendon.

COMMENT: The AO website has excellent intraoperative drawings and tips on surgical technique.

EXAMINER: What plate size would you use?

CANDIDATE: 3.5 DCP.

COMMENT: This may lead on to a discussion of what is a plate, what is a screw, what are the features of a screw. You should be able to describe all these pieces of orthopaedic hardware.

Structured oral examination question 4

Posterior approach to the knee

EXAMINER: A patient is admitted with the above isolated injury [candidate is shown a radiograph of a knee dislocation].
Describe your initial steps in management.

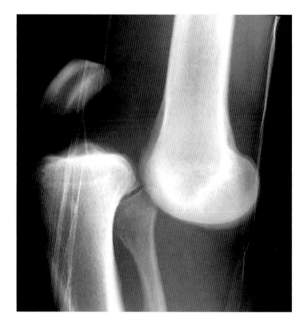

Figure 19.4a Lateral radiograph of anterior knee dislocation.

CANDIDATE: This is a high injury and as such I would want to manage according to ATLS principles. It is important to perform a neurovascular assessment.

COMMENT: The examiners have mentioned this is an isolated injury, so they do not want a great deal of detail about ATLS assessment, they want to get to the orthopaedic stuff.

EXAMINER: The patient has a cold foot, no peripheral pulse and altered sensation.
What is the management?

CANDIDATE: I would reduce the knee in theatre if possible under II control with the option of applying a spanning external fixation if needed to maintain reduction and provide stability. If there are major delays getting into theatre I would consider reducing the knee in casualty under sedation.

EXAMINER: Now what?

CANDIDATE: I would reassess the neurovascular status.

EXAMINER: The patient's foot is still cold with possibly a faint pulse.
Any other tests you want to do?

CANDIDATE: ABPI – you need to know what ratio is good/bad (> 0.9 rules out significant arterial injury).

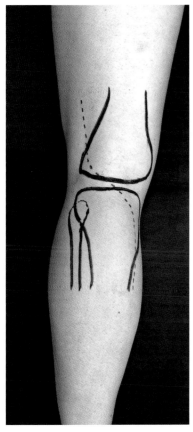

Figure 19.4b Posterior approach to the knee. Curved incision, starting laterally over the biceps femoris, obliquely across the popliteal fossa, downwards over the medial gastrocnemius.

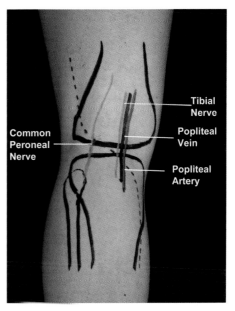

Figure 19.4c Posterior approach to knee. The popliteal vein lies between the tibial nerve and the popliteal artery.

EXAMINER: Arteriogram – would you delay surgery if imaging will take longer than 2 hours?

CANDIDATE: I would obtain an urgent vascular review.

COMMENT: There is some debate about whether all patients should have an arteriogram, but several papers have demonstrated good outcomes using clinical assessment and selective arteriography. Obtaining an arteriogram should not delay the emergency treatment of an obvious vascular injury.

Try to have evidence to back up your answer, if you can quote a paper such as the one below you will be on your way to a 7.

Reference

Stannard JP, Sheils TM, Lopez-Ben RR, McGwin G Jr, Robinson JT, Volgas DA. Vascular injuries in knee dislocations: the role of physical examination in determining the need for arteriography. *J Bone Joint Surg Am* 2004;86A(5):910–915.

EXAMINER: The vascular surgeon is 1 hour away. He wants you to start the posterior approach to the popliteal fossa.

COMMENT: In reality, it would be very rare to have to perform this approach, but it is known to be one of the most commonly asked approaches in the vivas.

EXAMINER: How do you position the patient?

CANDIDATE: Prone position.

EXAMINER: Anything you might do before positioning to make your life easier?

CANDIDATE: Apply a tourniquet.

EXAMINER: What landmarks do you use for the skin incision?

CANDIDATE: The two heads of the gastrocnemius muscle from the posterior femoral surface just above the medial and lateral condyles. Semimembranous and semitendinous on the medial border of the popliteal fossa. Curvilinear incision centred over the popliteal fossa starting laterally over the biceps femoris and distally over the medial head of the gastrocnemius. To prevent skin necrosis I would avoid an acute incision angle when

437

transitioning from the vertical to the transverse portion of the incision.

EXAMINER: What about the internervous plane?

CANDIDATE: There is no true internervous plane. The approach exploits the fossa between the medial and lateral heads of the gastrocnemius.

COMMENT: The candidate should have volunteered this without the need for it to be teased out of them.

EXAMINER: What structures are you looking for to guide you in this approach?

CANDIDATE: I would identify the short saphenous vein; on the lateral side of the vein is the medial sural cutaneous nerve; I would trace the nerve to its origin from the tibial nerve in the apex of the popliteal fossa.

At the apex the common peroneal nerve separates from the tibial nerve; I would identify and protect this. The popliteal artery and vein lie deep and medial to the tibial nerve.

EXAMINER: Where is the artery in relation to the vein?

CANDIDATE: The popliteal vein lies medial to the artery as it enters the popliteal fossa from below. Then it curves, lying directly posterior to the artery while in the fossa. Above the knee joint, it moves to the posterolateral side of the artery. The tibial nerve enters the popliteal fossa from its superior edge, lateral to the popliteal artery. In the middle of the popliteal fossa, the tibial nerve crosses posterior to the artery to its medial aspect and remains at that location.

The deep dissection involves retracting the muscles that form the boundaries of the popliteal fossa to expose the posterior knee joint capsule. The medial and lateral heads of the gastrocnemius can be released to increase exposure, but this should be avoided if possible.

EXAMINER: What are the structures at risk?

CANDIDATE: Structures at risk include the medial sural cutaneous nerve, tibial nerve, common peroneal nerve and popliteal vessels (the vein is posterolateral to artery at the apex, crosses posteriorly behind the knee and then lies medial). I would use blunt dissection when handling the neurovascular bundle. Care must be taken to avoid injuring the tibial nerve, which is the most superficial portion of the neurovascular bundle.

Because of anatomic variation it is important to take care to avoid injuring any unusual branching patterns of the nerve or blood vessels.

EXAMINER: How can you extend this approach?

CANDIDATE: There is no useful extension.

Structured oral examination question 5

Posterolateral approach to the ankle

EXAMINER: Describe this fracture (Figure 19.5).

CANDIDATE: These are AP and lateral views of a right ankle demonstrating a trimalleolar ankle fracture. There is talar shift, dislocation of the ankle and significant displacement of the posterior malleolus.

EXAMINER: What classification systems do you know to describe ankle fractures?

CANDIDATE: The Weber system.

EXAMINER: Please expand on this.

CANDIDATE: The Weber classification describes the fracture in relation to the syndesmosis between the tibia and fibula.

Weber A fractures occur below the syndesmosis.

Weber B fractures occur at the level of the syndesmosis.

Weber C fractures occur above the syndesmosis.

EXAMINER: Do you know of another classification system based on mechanism of injury?

CANDIDATE: That would be the Lauge Hansen system.

EXAMINER: How would you classify this fracture and what is the sequence of injury to the ankle?

CANDIDATE: This is a supination external rotation injury.

The first injury is to the anterior tibiofibular ligament, then a fracture of the fibular, followed by rupture of the posterior tibiofibular ligaments and then injury to the medial side, either a fracture of the medial malleolus or rupture of the deltoid ligament.

EXAMINER: What direction is the fracture of the fibula?

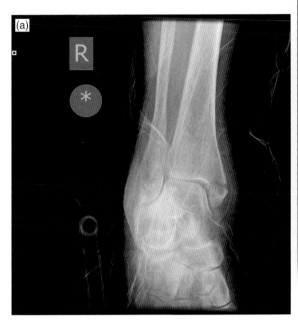

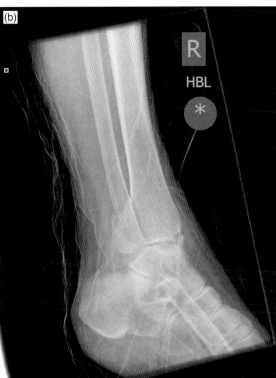

Figure 19.5a and 19.5b Anteroposterior (AP) radiograph of a trimalleolar fractured ankle with a large displaced posterior malleolar fragment.

CANDIDATE: I don't know.

COMMENT: It is important to recognize that the direction of the fibular fracture in a SER injury is distal anterior to proximal posterior. In the pronation external rotation injury, the fracture line runs proximal anterior to distal posterior.

EXAMINER: How would you fix this fracture?

CANDIDATE: Answer options.
1. Reduce and fix the fibula. If the post malleolus reduces, fix PM with AP screws.
2. Reduce the PM through fracture site. Fix with AP screws.
3. Reduce and fix the PM through the posterolateral approach.

EXAMINER: The posterior malleolus does not reduce when the fibula is reduced; therefore, you decide to perform a posterolateral approach to the ankle to reduce and fix the fragment under direct vision.

COMMENT: You could say that you are not familiar with this approach and you would prefer to use one of the other approaches above, which is acceptable as long as you know it well and how to reduce and fix the fracture using this approach.

EXAMINER: Describe the steps and neurovascular interval.

CANDIDATE: The position can be prone or lateral. I prefer the prone approach because I am more familiar with it.

Tourniquet.

Landmarks: Fibula and lateral border of Achilles tendon.

Skin incision half-way between the fibular and the Achilles tendon, from the tip of the fibular to 10 cm proximal. Mobilize identical skin flaps.

Identify, preserve and protect the sural nerve and short saphenous veins that run just behind the lateral malleolus. Incise the deep fascia and identify the peroneal tendons, retract these laterally and anteriorly.

Incise the fibres of the flexor hallucis longus over its lateral border and retract it medially, incise the periosteum longitudinally to reach the fracture site.

439

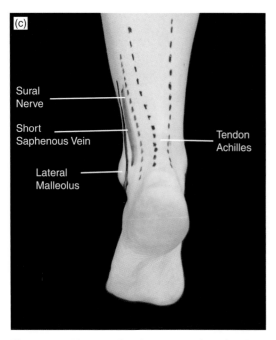

Figure 19.5c The posterolateral incision is performed on the medial side of the posterior edge of the fibula. The short saphenous vein and sural nerve run close together and should be preserved as a unit.

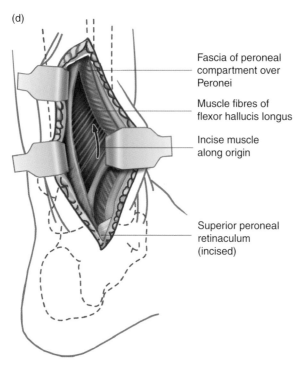

Figure 19.5d Deep dissection. A longitudinal incision is made through the lateral fibres of the flexor hallucis longus as they arise from the fibula.

EXAMINER: What internervous plane are you utilizing?

CANDIDATE: This is between the peroneal tendons laterally (superficial peroneal nerve) and the flexor hallucis longus medially (tibial nerve).

EXAMINER: Can you extend this approach proximally?

CANDIDATE: Yes, by extending the skin incision and then developing the interval between the peroneal muscle laterally and the gastrosoleus complex medially.

EXAMINER: What are the structures at risk?

CANDIDATE: The sural nerve. The nerve crosses the incision at its midpoint so is at particular risk in this area. If injured a painful neuroma can develop.

Short saphenous vein.

Score 7

EXAMINER: What are the advantages of fixing the posterior malleolar fracture by this method compared to anteroposterior screws?

CANDIDATE: Although AP screw fixation is less invasive than the direct posterolateral approach, it does not allow direct visualization of the fracture fragments and does not allow removal of any interposed periosteum or removal of organized blood clots. It is a real internervous plane and allows muscle tissue between the hardware and skin. Gravity will help with intraoperative reduction, rather than being a deforming force, when the patient is placed in the supine position. Another advantage is that the hardware with the posterolateral approach is deep in the ankle, with good soft-tissue coverage and no irritation to the patients. Reported minimal major wound complications and need for reoperation. A major advantage is that a buttress plate can be applied rather than using one or two screws, which provides better biomechanical fixation.

EXAMINER: What about the fibula fracture?

CANDIDATE: The peroneal tendons are retracted medially, which gives excellent access to the posterior distal fibula.

Score 8

EXAMINER: How do you fix the fibula?

CANDIDATE: Direct visualization for posterior antiglide plating of the fibula is one of the most valuable aspects of the approach.

Although posterior plating of the fibula may be performed through the lateral approach, retraction of the peroneals, supine patient positioning and direct anterior to posterior screw placement is more difficult. The approach enhances the ability to position the antiglide plate without those factors impeding optimal plate placement as well as facilitating posterior malleolus fracture fixation.

EXAMINER: What are the disadvantages?

CANDIDATE: Fixation of the medial malleolus can be difficult using the posterolateral approach. Unfamiliarity of the approach.

Structured oral examination question 6

Anterior approach to the cervical spine

A radiograph of a normal cervical spine is shown (Figure 19.6a).

EXAMINER: A patient presents with an 8-week history of severe and worsening pain radiating from his neck down his arm into his hand. He has pins and needles affecting his thumb and index finger.

What nerve root is probably affected?

CANDIDATE: C6.

EXAMINER: What weakness might you expect to find?

CANDIDATE: Weakness in wrist extension.

EXAMINER: OK. What muscles are weak?

CANDIDATE: ERCL and ERCB.

EXAMINER: Where is the most reliable place to test for C6 sensory change?

CANDIDATE: I'm not sure, on the back of the hand?

COMMENT: The back of the hand is not precise enough. The American Spinal Injury Association Guidelines and the ATLS guidelines are that the most reliable place is on the dorsal surface of the proximal phalanx of the thumb.

EXAMINER: An MRI scan shows a cervical disc prolapse. What is the standard surgical procedure for treatment of intractable pain resulting from this condition?

CANDIDATE: Anterior discectomy and fusion.

EXAMINER: What is the approach to the anterior cervical spine?

COMMENT: This is another approach that unless you are going to be a spinal surgeon you are unlikely to come across; however, it is another classic approach and you should at least know the intervals.

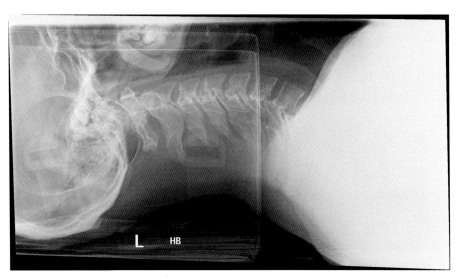

Figure 19.6a Lateral radiograph of a normal cervical spine.

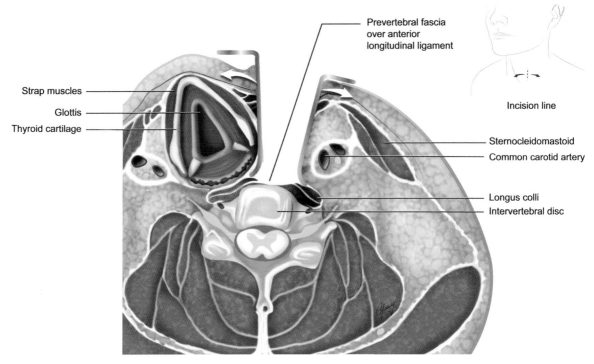

Strap muscles

Glottis

Thyroid cartilage

Prevertebral fascia over anterior longitudinal ligament

Incision line

Sternocleidomastoid

Common carotid artery

Longus colli

Intervertebral disc

Figure 19.6b Anterior approach to the cervical spine. The sternocleidomastoid and carotid sheath are retracted laterally and the strap muscles, trachea and oesophagus medially. The longus coli and pretrachial fascia are exposed.

CANDIDATE: Position: Beach chair with head in ring. Sandbag between shoulder blades, turn head away from planned incision site, neck extended.

Landmarks

C2/3: mandible.

C3: hyoid.

C4/5: thyroid cartilage.

C6: cricoid cartilage and carotid tubercule.

Skin incision: Transverse incision at the level of pathology (see levels above) from posterior border of sternocleidomastoid (SCM) (spinal accessory nerve) to the midline. If more than three levels are approached, then use a longitudinal incision.

Internervous plane: There is no true internervous plane during the anterior approach to the cervical spine.

Superficial dissection: Incise fascia over platysma in line with the skin and split the fibres of the platysma (cranial nerve VII) longitudinally.

Identify the anterior border of SCM and incise the fascia immediately anterior to it.

Retract the SCM laterally and the strap muscles (C1, C2, C3) medially.

The carotid sheath can now be identified.

Develop a plane between the medial side of the carotid sheath and the midline structures (thyroid, trachea and oesophagus) by cutting the pretracheal fascia on the medial side of the sheath.

Watch for the superior and inferior thyroid arteries, which run transversely and may limit dissection above C3/4.

Deep dissection: Develop a plane behind the pretracheal fascia and behind the oesophagus. The prevertebral fascia and longus coli muscle should now be seen and after splitting them longitudinally the anterior longitudinal ligament and the cervical vertebra can be identified.

EXAMINER: What structures are at risk during this approach?

CANDIDATE: The carotid sheath and its contents. Be careful with using self-retaining retractors in this area.

The vertebral artery lies in the costotransverse foramen on the lateral portion of the transverse processors and should not be visible unless the plane of the operation strays well away from the midline.

The recurrent laryngeal nerve (RLN) may be injured during the deeper dissection of the approach.

The sympathetic chain may be damaged, causing Horner's syndrome. It should be protected by making sure dissection onto the bone is subperiosteal from the midline.

Poorly placed retractors may damage the trachea or oesophagus.

EXAMINER: What is the result of damage to the recurrent laryngeal nerve?

CANDIDATE: If one side is damaged the patient develops a hoarse voice; if both sides are damaged the patient can be left aphonic and have breathing difficulty.

EXAMINER: Left- or right-sided approach?

CANDIDATE: The course of the RLN is more variable on the right, but dissection is easier for a right-handed surgeon. Studies have suggested the risk to the RLN is similar on both sides so surgeons should go for the side that they find easiest to do.

Structured oral examination question 7

Shoulder fracture dislocation

EXAMINER: How would you treat a shoulder fracture dislocation?

CANDIDATE: In an appropriately consented patient, I would prefer to reduce the fracture under anaesthesia with image-intensifier screening due to the risk of fracture propagation. I would explain to the patient that an open reduction may have to be considered if the closed reduction technique fails to reduce the shoulder.

COMMENT: A candidate's description of any surgical approach should begin with a brief gambit on preparing the patient for surgery. It may seem a bit forced and contrived, but you just need to offer it up. If the examiners want to probe you further on this then that is their prerogative. In general, they want to get onto the main thrust of the question, which is the surgical approach.

EXAMINER: What approach would you use for open reduction of shoulder?

CANDIDATE: A deltopectoral approach.

EXAMINER: Describe the deltopectoral approach to the shoulder joint.

CANDIDATE: Position: I would position the patient in a beach chair with a sandbag between the spine and scapula. The patient is sat up at 45° with two pillows under the knees and the head supported in a head ring reinforced with tape. I would make sure the anaesthetist is happy with the airway and neck position. Before scrubbing I would check the

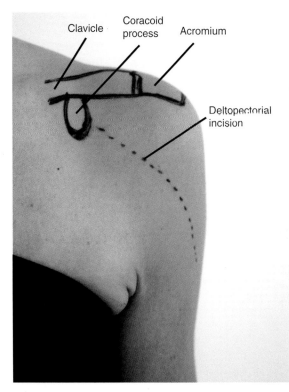

Figure 19.7a Surface landmarks: coracoid process and deltopectoral groove. Incision: straight incision from the tip of the coracoid process along the deltopectoral groove to the deltoid insertion.

II visualizes the shoulder with ease. I would particularly want to avoid any obstructed views from the operating table attachments and make sure swinging the II into position did not compromise or any interfere with the scrub set up or sterility.

COMMENT: Again, this is how 'YOU YOURSELF' actually position and set up the patient in real life so as to perform the surgery. These little details are often forgotten or not thought about, but are very important to the smooth flow of the operation. If the examiner is not wanting to probe you on this, they will quickly move you on.

Landmarks

The surgical landmarks (Figure 19.7a) are:
- Coracoid process.
- Deltopectoral groove (cephalic vein).
- Lateral border biceps brachii.

Skin incision: I would make a skin incision in the line of the deltopectorial groove from just above the coracoid process along the deltopectorial groove to the deltoid insertion.

EXAMINER: Internervous plane?

CANDIDATE: Between the axillary nerve (deltoid) and the medial/lateral pectoral nerves (pectoralis major).
    Superficial dissection:
- The interval is between the deltoid (axillary nerve) and the pectoralis major (medial and lateral pectoral nerves).
- The cephalic vein lies in a layer of fat and is used to identify this interval. The vein can be taken either medially or laterally.

EXAMINER: Make up your mind. Is it medial or lateral?

CANDIDATE: In most situations it is usually taken lateral as the tributaries come from the lateral side. In practice it is whatever ends up being easiest to do.
    This superficial dissection can bleed considerably, and I would make sure haemostasis is achieved before moving on to deep dissection.

EXAMINER: Anything you can do to lessen bleeding in this area?

CANDIDATE: I have seen some surgeons infiltrate the area with local anaesthetic combined with adrenaline, but this is something I personally would prefer to avoid doing.

EXAMINER: Why?

CANDIDATE: I prefer to know if a structure is bleeding, so I can secure haemostasis rather than risk it is bleeding postoperatively when the adrenaline wears off, causing a wound haematoma.
    Deep dissection:
- I would identify the short head of the biceps and coracobrachialis (both musculocutaneous nerve) and retract it medially and the deltoid laterally.

The other option is to perform a coracoid osteotomy.

EXAMINER: How do you do a coracoid osteotomy?

CANDIDATE:
- Drill and tap before the osteotomy, if you are planning to fix it back with a screw.
- Avoid abduction of the arm, as this will bring the axillary sheath closer to the coracoid during the osteotomy.
- Stay lateral to the coracoid to avoid damage to the neurovascular structures on the medial aspect of the coracoid.

EXAMINER: How many centimetres below the coracoid does the musculocutaneous nerve enter the coracobrachialis?

CANDIDATE:
- 5–8 cm distal to the coracoid.
- Stay lateral to the muscle during deep dissection.
- Damage to the musculocutaneous nerve causes paralysis of the elbow flexors.

Identify the subscapularis tendon and externally rotate the arm to put the subscapularis under tension. A vertical capsulotomy is performed.

EXAMINER: What are the structures at risk during the deltopectoral approach?

CANDIDATE:
- Musculocutaneous nerve.
- Axillary nerve – this is at risk during the release of the inferior part of the subscapularis; external rotation of the arm puts the subscapularis at stretch and takes the point of incision away from the axillary nerve.
- Cephalic vein.
- Anterior circumflex humeral artery.

EXAMINER: Describe the quadrangular and triangular spaces in the shoulder.

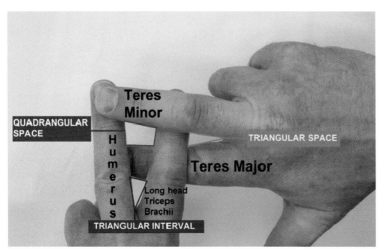

Figure 19.7b Spaces of the shoulder using finger arrangement.

CANDIDATE:

Quadrangular space:

Borders:

Superior: teres minor.

Inferior: teres major.

Medial: long head of triceps brachii.

Lateral: humeral shaft.

Contents:

Axillary nerve and posterior circumflex humeral artery.

Triangular space (this is the space between the two teres muscles. It has two sides, a base and an apex):

Borders:

Superior: lower border of teres minor.

Inferior: teres major.

Base (lateral boundary): long head of triceps.

Apex: meeting point of teres minor and major muscles.

This can be pointed to on the lateral border of the scapula.

Contents:

Scapular circumflex artery and vein.

Triangular interval (this lies below the quadrangular space. It is formed due to the teres major muscle cutting across the long head of triceps brachii to reach its insertion. It has two sides, a base and an apex):

Borders:

Superior (base): teres major.

Lateral boundary: humerus shaft or lateral head of the triceps.

Medial boundary: long head of triceps.

Apex: meeting point of the medial and lateral boundaries.

Contents:

Profunda brachii artery.

Radial nerve.

Both structures pass through the lower triangular space to reach the spiral groove on the shaft of the humerus.

Structured oral examination question 8

Compartment syndrome of leg

A postoperative patient develops severe lower leg pain overnight following intramedullary nailing of the tibia. The pain hasn't improved much even after administering intravenous morphine.

EXAMINER: What is the most likely diagnosis and how would you treat this patient?

CANDIDATE: Compartment syndrome of the lower leg. I would treat this with a two-incision technique for fasciotomy making sure that all four compartments of the lower leg are decompressed adequately.

EXAMINER: What is compartment syndrome?

CANDIDATE: It is defined as 'elevation of the interstitial pressure in a closed osseofascial compartment that results in a microvascular compromise' (Mubarak and Hargens 1983). Compartment syndrome can occur at sites where muscle is surrounded by fascia. Common sites for compartment syndrome are the leg, forearm, hand, foot, thigh, buttock and paraspinal muscles.

COMMENT: The initial questions are usually for setting the scene (definition, causes, pathophysiology, etc.). The questions are likely to lead to discussion onto the surgical anatomy of the lower leg compartments.

EXAMINER: Describe the compartments of the lower leg. Draw a cross-section diagram of the middle third of the lower leg and describe the compartments.

CANDIDATE: Anterior compartment: tibialis anterior, extensor hallucis longus, extensor digitorum longus, peroneus tertius.

Lateral compartment: peroneus longus, peroneus brevis.

Deep posterior compartment: tibialis posterior, flexor digitorum longus, flexor hallucis longus.

Superficial posterior compartment: gastrocnemius, soleus, plantaris.

COMMENT: The description of compartments of lower leg by a cross-sectional diagram comes across as a much better answer compared to listing the names of muscles in each of the compartments. Practise an easy and quick way of drawing the lower leg compartments.

EXAMINER: What is/are the incisions used for fasciotomy of the lower leg?

COMMENT: While there are several described techniques of lower leg fasciotomy, describing the two-incision technique is the non-controversial and safe answer in an exam.

CANDIDATE: I would use a two-incision approach. The anterolateral incision is 2 cm lateral to the anterior border of the tibia midway between the tibia and the fibula. This decompresses the anterior and lateral compartments.

EXAMINER: How long is the incision and what are your landmarks?

CANDIDATE: Around 15–20 cm. The proximal landmark is approximately 3 cm distal to the level of the tibial tuberosity. The fibula head is another useful landmark. The distal landmark is the lateral malleolus.

These landmarks are often difficult to palpate if the leg is grossly swollen.

The posteromedial incision is 1–2 cm posterior to the medial border of the tibia. This is a longitudinal incision the entire length of the gastrocnemius–soleus complex. It decompresses the superficial and deep posterior compartments.

EXAMINER: How do you actually decompress the compartments?

CANDIDATE: For the anterolateral decompression I would perform a subcutaneous dissection to expose the fascia overlying the anterior and lateral compartments. I would identify the intermuscular septum between the anterior and lateral compartments. I would make a small transverse fascial incision at least 1 cm either side of the intermuscular septum at the midpoint of the incision. I would then longitudinally extend these incisions using scissors proximally aiming for the lateral border of the patella and distally the centre of the ankle joint. The sural nerve is at risk as it pieces the deep fascia (around 10–15 cm proximal to the lateral malleolus).

EXAMINER: How do you actually know if you have decompressed the anterior compartment?

CANDIDATE: Identification of the deep peroneal nerve and/or the anterior tibial vessels would confirm this.

With the posteromedial incision the superficial posterior compartment is dissected off the posteromedial border of the tibia. It is important to proximally release the soleus bridge from the back of the tibia to ensure adequate release of the deep posterior compartment. The fascia is incised along the whole length of the tibialis posterior and flexor digitorum muscle if needed. The posteromedial incision must be anterior to the posterior tibial artery in order to avoid injury to the perforating vessels that supply the skin used for local fasciocutaneous flaps. It is essential to preserve the perforators and avoid incisions crossing the line between them.

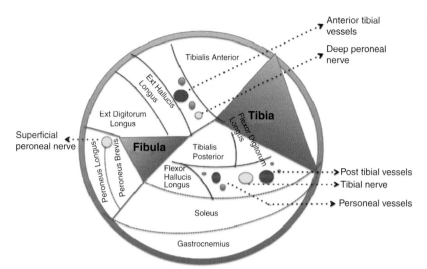

Figure 19.8a Muscle compartments of the lower leg.

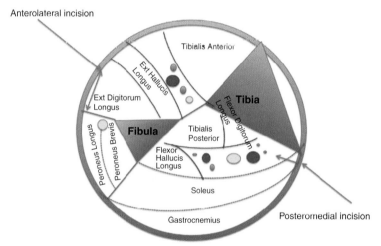

Figure 19.8b Fasciotomy incisions for compartment syndrome.

EXAMINER: What do you mean by the soleus bridge?

CANDIDATE: The soleus muscle attaches to the medial edge of the tibia and dissecting these fibres (the 'soleus bridge') completely free from and exposing the underside of the tibia ensures entry into the deep posterior compartment.

Further reading

www.boa.ac.uk/wp-content/uploads/2015/01/BOAS T-10.pdf

www.bapras.org.uk/professionals/clinical-guidance/open-fractures-of-the-lower-limb#Full Guide

EXAMINER: What are the structures at risk during fasciotomy?

CANDIDATE: The posteromedial incision should be placed anterior to the course of the posterior tibial artery to avoid damaging the perforators that supply the skin used for local fasciocutaneous flaps. Also, care should be taken to protect the saphenous nerve and vein.

The anterolateral incision should be placed with care taken to identify and protect the superficial peroneal nerve.

Accurate skin incisions are important and need to be planned and marked out beforehand, especially if the leg is grossly swollen.

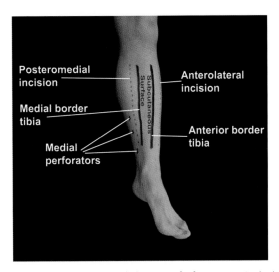

Figure 19.8c Recommended incisions for fasciotomies in the leg. The medial incision is used to decompress the superficial and deep posterior compartments and the lateral incision is used for decompression of the anterior and peroneal compartments. Margins of subcutaneous border of the tibia are marked in black, access incisions are marked in green and perforators arising from the medial side are marked as red crosses.

A lateral incision inadvertently placed over the fibula will expose the periosteum and extending the incision too far distally may expose the peroneal tendons. Exposure of bone or tendons increases the risks of delayed healing, infection and, ultimately, amputation.

As mentioned, the medial incision must be anterior to the posterior tibial artery, but placement too anteriorly leads to exposure of the tibia and any underlying fracture.

Structured oral examination question 9

Anatomy of tarsal tunnel

EXAMINER: What is medial tarsal tunnel syndrome?

CANDIDATE: The medial tarsal tunnel syndrome is a compression neuropathy of the tibial nerve or its terminal branches, the medial and lateral plantar nerve. Impingement occurs within the boundaries of the fibro-osseous tarsal tunnel or as it passes into the abductor hallucis muscle.

EXAMINER: What is the tarsal tunnel?

CANDIDATE: It is an osseo-fascial tunnel on the posteromedial aspect of ankle with the following boundaries:
Flexor retinaculum.
Calcaneus (medial).
Talus (medial).
Abductor hallucis (inferior).

EXAMINER: Where does the tarsal tunnel begin and end?

CANDIDATE: It begins a few centimetres proximal to the tip of the medial malleolus where the crural fascia starts to condense forming an unyielding 'roof', the flexor retinaculum (laciniate ligament). It ends where the medial and lateral plantar nerves enter or pass deep to the abductor hallucis.

COMMENT: It is a descriptive space with ill-defined limits.

Figure 19.9 Contents of tarsal tunnel.

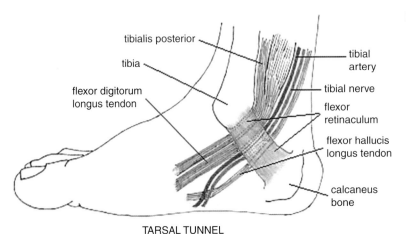

TARSAL TUNNEL

EXAMINER: What are the contents of the tarsal tunnel (Figure 19.9)?

CANDIDATE: Tibial nerve, posterior tibial artery, FHL tendon, FDL tendon, tibialis posterior tendon.

EXAMINER: What are the branches of the tibial nerve following its exit from the tarsal tunnel?

CANDIDATE: The tibial nerve has three distal branches: medial plantar, lateral plantar and medial calcaneal.

EXAMINER: What is the Baxter nerve?

CANDIDATE: It is the first branch of the lateral plantar nerve. This nerve has been implicated as one of the causes of heel pain, which can be similar to plantar fasciitis. The Baxter nerve provides motor innervation for the abductor digiti minimi.

Structured oral examination question 10

Extensor compartments of wrist

A 62-year-old lady presents with not being able to extend the thumb after non-operative management of a distal radius fracture.

EXAMINER: What is the likely diagnosis?

CANDIDATE: Rupture of the extensor pollicis longus (EPL) tendon.

EXAMINER: Where is the EPL tendon at the dorsal aspect of the distal radius? Can you name the contents of the extensor compartments at the wrist?

CANDIDATE:

1. Abductor pollicis longus (APL) and extensor pollicis brevis (EPB).
2. Extensor carpi radialis longus (ECRL) and extensor carpi radialis brevis (ECRB).
3. Extensor pollicis longus (EPL).
4. Extensor digitorum communis, extensor indicis proprius, posterior interosseous nerve.
5. Extensor digiti minimi (EDM).
6. Extensor carpi ulnaris (EDU).

EXAMINER: What is Vaughn-Jackson syndrome?

CANDIDATE: It is seen in rheumatoid hand/wrist conditions with rupture of the extensor tendon noted from the ulnar to the radial aspect. Attritional rupture of the extensor tendons

occurs due to DRUJ instability and carpal subluxation, thereby resulting in dorsal ulnar head prominence. EDM is typically the first extensor tendon ruptured in this condition.

EXAMINER: Which compartment is involved in De Quervain's tenosynovitis?

CANDIDATE: First extensor compartment comprising of APL and EPB.

Structured oral examination question 11

Anatomy of carpal tunnel

A 40-year-old lady with known hypothyroidism presents with intermittent paraesthesias of thumb, index and middle fingers.

EXAMINER: What could be the potential causes of this patient's symptoms?

CANDIDATE: Carpal tunnel syndrome, cervical nerve impingement.

EXAMINER: Describe the boundaries of the carpal tunnel.

CANDIDATE: It is an osseo-fibrous canal situated in the volar aspect of the wrist. The boundaries are as follows:

Ulnar: hook of hamate and pisiform.

Radial: scaphoid tubercle and trapezium.

Roof (palmar): transverse carpal ligament.

Floor (dorsal): proximal carpal row.

EXAMINER: Describe the contents of the carpal tunnel.

CANDIDATE: In addition to the medial nerve, the carpal tunnel contains nine tendons: the flexor pollicis longus, the four flexor digitorum superficialis and the four flexor digitorum profundus (Figure 19.10a).

EXAMINER: What are the branches of median nerve around the carpal tunnel? What are the structures at risk during carpal tunnel release?

CANDIDATE: The palmar cutaneous branch of the median nerve lies between the palmaris longus and the flexor carpi radialis at the level of the wrist. It arises about 5 cm proximal to the wrist joint level and provides sensory innervation to the thenar skin.

449

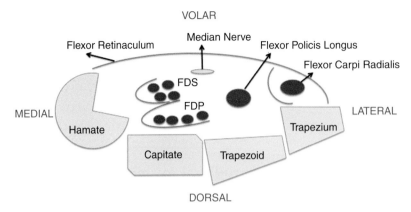

Figure 19.10a Anatomy, carpal tunnel.

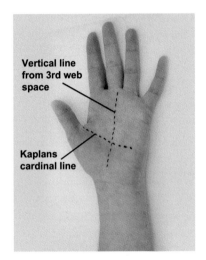

Figure 19.10b Skin markings. Vertical line drawn from the third interdigital space to the wrist crease on the palm. Horizontal line drawn joining the radial aspect of the thumb to the styloid process (Kaplan's cardinal line).

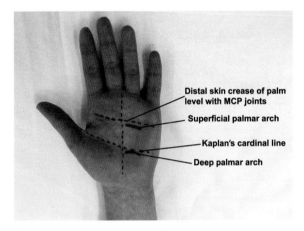

Figure 19.10c Vascular anatomy. The transverse palmar crease is the landmark for the superficial palmar arch. This is formed by the ulnar artery and the superficial palmar branch of the radial artery. Kaplan's cardinal line is the landmark for the deep palmar arch. The deep palmar arch is formed mainly by the terminal part of the radial artery and the deep palmar branch of the ulnar artery.

The recurrent motor branch of the median nerve has a variable course – 50% extraligamentous, 30% subligamentous and 20% transligamentous. The transligamentous course of recurrent motor branch can be at risk of unrecognized injury during carpal tunnel release. Hence, release on the ulnar aspect of the carpal tunnel reduces the hazard of this inadvertent injury.

EXAMINER: What muscles does the median nerve innervate in the hand?

CANDIDATE: 'LOAF' muscles in the thenar eminence including Lateral two lumbricals, Oppenens pollicis, Abductor pollicis and Flexor pollicis brevis.

EXAMINER: Are you aware of any anastomotic anomaly that occurs between median and ulnar nerves?

CANDIDATE: Martin-Gruber anastomosis is a communication between the median and ulnar nerves in the forearm.

Riche-Cannieu anastomosis is a communication between the median and ulnar nerves in the hand.

EXAMINER: Describe how you would do a carpal tunnel release?

CANDIDATE: I am aware there are several techniques of carpal tunnel release including endoscopic, open and mini-open techniques. My preferred technique is an open carpal tunnel release under local anaesthesia. The incision is placed longitudinally from the distal wrist crease in line with the radial border of the ring finger. The distal extent of the incision is the Kaplan's line, which is a transverse line from the distal border of the abducted thumb to the hook of the hamate (Figure 19.10b). The Kaplan's line is an external reference for the deep palmar arch (Figure 19.10c).

Following the skin incision, I would go through the fibres of the superficial palmar fascia to expose the transverse carpal ligament. Occasionally, palmaris brevis muscle fibres may need to be cleared to expose the transverse carpal ligament. The transverse carpal ligament is released on the ulnar side under direct vision, protecting the median nerve. I would ensure that releasing the transverse carpal ligament both proximally and distally adequately decompresses the median nerve.

Chapter 20

Structure and function of connective tissue

Paul A. Banaszkiewicz

Introduction

Section 2 of the basic science (Tr & Orth) syllabus is a large topic, difficult to grasp at face value as it appears quite removed from the average orthopaedic surgeon's practice. However, it pervades many aspects of clinical practice and therefore must be understood.

It contains large sections of A-list topics that just need to be learnt as well as possible, otherwise marks will be thrown away.

Candidates may be asked very general questions or questions in more detail, so you need to cover both bases. Esoteric or un-Googleable questions are also fairly common in this section.

Candidates will need to double time on this section to both understand the topics and then work through viva practice sessions to home in on the target answers.

This section was generally well received in the first edition viva book and we have kept and updated the majority of previous viva questions. As such, in certain sections there is a rough marking scheme, so you can judge your level.

1. Bone structure and function

This is an A-list topic. The topic is large with a number of subtopics within the main topic that the examiners can easily focus in on.

Structured oral examination question 1

EXAMINER: What is bone?

CANDIDATE: Bone is a dynamic composite form of specialized connective tissue composed of cells (10%) and matrix (90%). The matrix has inorganic (60%) and organic (40%) components . . .

COMMENT: The viva could start off awkwardly with a definition that may catch the unsuspecting candidate off-guard. Go for an uncomplicated, non-controversial answer that allows you to continue talking if you feel confidently able to do so.
   Or

CANDIDATE: Bone is an organ.

EXAMINER: What is an organ?

CANDIDATE: [Pause] I am not sure.

COMMENT: Make sure you know the definition of an organ.[1] Try to avoid giving an answer that will lead you up a blind alley.
   An organ is composed of multiple tissue types. For bone these include:

- Bone tissue (a.k.a. osseous tissue).
- Fibrous connective tissue.
- Cartilage.
- Vascular tissue.
- Lymphatic tissue.
- Adipose tissue.
- Nervous tissue.

EXAMINER: What are the functions of bone?

CANDIDATE: The three main functions of bone are:

1. As a reservoir for calcium.
2. As a source of haematopoietic cells such as erythrocytes, leucocytes and platelets.
3. A mechanical role in supporting the body's tissues, providing attachment for muscles and protecting internal organs.

COMMENT: There are other minor functions, but again, keep it simple.

EXAMINER: Describe the structure of bone.

CANDIDATE: There are two main macroscopic types of bone, either (1) lamellar or (2) woven. The structure of lamellar bone can be either

Table 20.1 Lamellar bone versus woven bone.

Property	Woven bone	Lamellar bone
Definition	'Primitive', immature	'Mature' bone, remodelled woven bone
Found in	Immature (embryonic/neonatal skeleton, metaphyseal region fracture healing)	Cortical compact
	Pathological bone (pagetic bone, tumour)	Cancellous trabecular
Composition	Dense collagen fibres, varied mineral content, greater turnover, more cells per unit volume	Formed by intramembranous or endochondral ossification, contains collagen fibres
	No lamellae	
Organization	Randomly arranged collagen fibres, disorganized	Highly ordered, stress-orientated collagen fibres
Response to stress	Isotropic: independent of direction of applied forces	Anisotropic: mechanical behaviour differs according to direction of applied force
		Bone's greatest strength is parallel to its longitudinal axis
Biomechanics	Weaker, more flexible, more easily deformed	More stiffness and strength

High-yield orthopaedics: Differentiating features of woven vs. lamellar bone. No lamellae, isotropic.

cortical compact or cancellous trabecular bone. Woven bone can be either immature (fracture callus) or pathological.

COMMENT: Candidates may be pressed in a bit more detail about the differences between woven and lamellar bone, especially at the beginning of a viva, because it is basic information candidates would be expected to know.

Woven bone
- Has a random arrangement of collagen, there are no lamellae, it is weaker and more flexible than lamellar bone.
- More cellular (×8 lamellar bone).
- More metabolically active with increased turnover.
- Variable irregular mineral content.
- It is found in the embryonic skeleton and the metaphyseal region of growing bones. It is also present in early hard callus and found in pathological bone such as tumours, osteogenesis imperfecta and pagetic bone.
- It is found where bone needs to be laid down rapidly.

Lamellar bone
- This is mature adult bone that is subdivided into cortical or cancellous bone.

- Osteoblasts lay down collagen matrix in microscopic thin, layered sheets called lamellae.
- Collagen fibres are orientated more parallel to each other.
- Low number of cells.
- Slow deposition/turnover.
- Stronger and less flexible than woven bone.
- Anisotropic.

EXAMINER: What is the difference between cortical and cancellous bone (Table 20.2)?

CANDIDATE: Cortical bone is compact with a high matrix mass per unit volume, low porosity and is subjected to bending, torsional and compressive forces. It is usually found in the diaphysis of long bones. The basic structure is the osteon or Haversian system.

Cancellous bone is found in the metaphysis or epiphysis of long bones. It has an architecture of 3D lattice rods and plates, high porosity with large spaces between trabeculae and predominantly subjected to compressive loads.

EXAMINER: What do we mean by the term isotropic?

CANDIDATE: Isotropic refers to uniform properties in all directions, independent of the direction of load application.

EXAMINER: So, which type of bone is isotropic?

CANDIDATE: Woven.

453

Table 20.2 Cortical bone versus cancellous bone.

Property	Cortical bone	Cancellous (trabecular bone)
Description	Dense or compact bone	Spongy or cancellous bone
Location	Diaphysis (outer layer of long bone)	Metaphysis or epiphysis (long bone)
Architecture	Basic structure is the osteon	3D lattice rods and plates
		Rods (thin trabeculae), plates (thick trabeculae)
		Loose network of struts
Porosity	Low porosity (10%)	High porosity (50–90%)
		Large spaces between trabeculae
	Compactness	Softer, more elastic
	Higher Young's modulus of elasticity	
Mechanical stress	Subjected to bending, torsional and compressive forces	Predominantly subjected to compressive forces
	High matrix mass per unit volume	Reduced matrix mass per unit volume

High-yield orthopaedics: cancellous bone.

No osteons – has a 3D lattice of rods and plates high porosity.

EXAMINER: So, what about lamellar bone. Is this isotropic?

CANDIDATE: No.

EXAMINER: Why?

CANDIDATE: I am not sure.

COMMENT: These are fairly straightforward questions but may catch the unprepared candidate out. Lamellar bone has stress-orientated collagen fibres and has anisotropic features. The mechanical behaviour differs according to the direction of applied force: the bone's greatest strength is parallel to the longitudinal axis.

EXAMINER: What is the structure of bone?

CANDIDATE: The main structural unit within cortical bone is the Haversian system (osteon) with its central neurovascular channels enclosed within concentric lamellae.

Lying in between intact osteons separated by cement lines are incomplete lamellae called interstitial lamellae. These fill the gaps between osteons and are remnants of bone remodelling.

Neither collagen nor canaliculi cross cement lines, forming areas of relative weakness.

Each osteon or Haversian system consists of five to seven concentric layers (lamellae) of bone matrix.

Volkmann's canals run perpendicular to the long bone axis carrying blood vessels to and from the Haversian systems to the outer surfaces of the bone.

COMMENT: The viva may just begin by candidates being shown a diagram of the bone Haversian system and being asked to talk through the diagram. Less likely but still possible is for candidates to be asked to draw out the bone Haversian system.

CANDIDATE: Bone compromises cells (10%) and extracellular matrix (90%).

The cells include osteoblasts, osteocytes, osteoclasts and bone lining cells.

The matrix has organic (collagens, mainly type 1) and inorganic (calcium phosphate, osteocalcium phosphate) constituents.

EXAMINER: What are the main types of bone cells and what are their functions?

CANDIDATE: The main types of bones cells, and their function, are as follows:

1. Osteoblast: bone-forming cells.
2. Osteoclast: bone-resorbing cells, multinuclear irregular giant cells.
3. Osteocyte: maintains bone, important for calcium and phosphate homeostasis.
4. Osteoprogenitor cell: precursors to osteoblasts that line the Haversian system and can be stimulated to differentiate into osteoblasts and form new bone.
5. Bone lining cells: inactive osteoblasts.

COMMENT: Some textbooks mention only three or four types of bone cells, usually omitting osteoprogenitor cells and sometimes bone lining cells.

The osteoprogenitor cells originate from mesenchymal stem cells and line the Haversian canals, endosteum and periosteum. They can quickly differentiate into osteoblasts if needed.

EXAMINER: How do osteoblasts and osteoclasts differ?

CANDIDATE: Osteoblasts are derived from undifferentiated mesenchymal cells; they are bone-forming and lay down osteoid (type 1 collagen) as well as activating osteoclasts to resorb bone via the receptor activator of nuclear factor κβ (RANK) and its ligand (RANKL) system. RANKL is expressed by macrophages and osteoblasts, and functions as an activator of RANK. RANK, expressed on osteoclast precursors, is a key regulator of osteoclastogenesis.

These processes are controlled by cytokines, growth factors and bone morphogenic protein (BMP).

Osteoclasts are derived from a haemopoietic monocyte cell lineage. They are multinucleated giant cells that resorb bone and are characterized by a cytoplasm that has a homogeneous foamy appearance due to a high concentration of vesicles and vacuoles. These vacuoles include lysosomes filled with acid phosphatase.

They can sit in small pits called Howship's lacunae, on the bone surface, or lead cutting cones that tunnel through the bone. Under their ruffled brush border, with an increased surface area, they create a low pH microenvironment that dissolves inorganic apatite crystals. Enzymes are released (tartrate resistance acid phosphatase, TRAP) and proteases then break down the organic matrix components. This process is controlled via the RANKL system (inhibited by osteoprotegerin) of activated osteoblasts.

Osteocytes are osteoblasts that have become trapped in bone matrix (comprising up to 90% of the cells in bone). They have an important role in the homoeostasis of calcium and phosphate metabolism.

EXAMINER: What is Wolff's law?

CANDIDATE: Wolff's law states that bone will adapt to the loads placed through or across it. It is the result of the close coupling within bone remodelling units consisting of osteoblasts, osteoclasts and supporting stromal tissues. If loading on a particular bone increases, the bone will remodel itself over time to become stronger to resist that sort of loading.

COMMENT: Bone models and remodels in response to the mechanical stresses it experiences, resulting in a minimal-weight structure that is adapted to its applied stresses.

EXAMINER: Can you give me an example of Wolff's law?

CANDIDATE: The racket-holding arms of tennis players are stronger than the other arm. There is thicker cortical bone alongside hypertrophy of the muscle attachment sites. The arm is about a third bigger in size (35%).

The femoral neck width of obese people changes to accommodate the added weight. In this case the width of the femoral neck has increased to dissipate weight throughout the bony area by increasing surface area and strength through redistribution of bone.

The reverse is true: if loading on a bone decreases, the bone will become less dense and weaker due to the lack of stimulus required for continued remodelling.

EXAMINER: What is the Hueter–Volkman law?

CANDIDATE: Remodelling occurs in small packets of cells known as basic multicellular units (BMUs). Compressive forces inhibit longitudinal growth; tension stimulates it. This law suggests mechanical factors influence longitudinal growth, bone remodelling and fracture repair. The underlying mechanisms remain unclear.

EXAMINER: What controls the differentiation of osteoblasts?

CANDIDATE: Two transcription factors are important for osteoblastic differentiation.

1. Osterix (Osx) is an osteoblast-specific transcription factor essential for osteoblast differentiation and bone formation.
2. Runx2 is a multifunctional transcription factor that induces differentiation of multipotent mesenchymal cells into immature osteoblasts.

EXAMINER: What are transcription factors?

CANDIDATE: Transcription factors are proteins involved in the process of converting, or

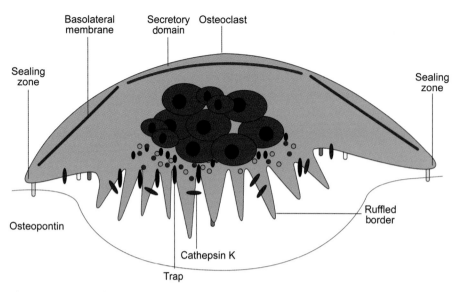

Figure 20.1 Activated osteoclast. The osteoclast plasma membrane is divided into multiple domains. At the ruffled border, the osteoclast secretes acid and lysosomal enzymes that digest the mineral and protein components of the underlying bone. The degradation products of collagen and other matrix components are endocytosed, transported through the cell and exocytosed through a functional secretory domain.

transcribing, DNA into RNA. Transcription factors include a wide number of proteins, excluding RNA polymerase, that initiate and regulate the transcription of genes.

EXAMINER: What is this cell line?

COMMENT: A picture was shown of an osteoclast in Howship's lacuna (Figure 20.1).
CANDIDATE: This is an activated osteoclast.

EXAMINER: How do osteoclasts resorb bone?

CANDIDATE: Osteoclasts resorb bone by binding to the bone surface using integrin anchor proteins and secreting hydrogen ions into the sealed area produced with a carbonic anhydrase system allowing dissolution of hydroxyapatite mineral matrix. They also secrete proteolytic lysosomal enzymes that hydrolyze the organic cellular components. The ruffled border greatly increases the surface area osteoclasts.

EXAMINER: What do you understand by the term remodelling? Describe the process.

CANDIDATE: Remodelling is the process whereby the structure of bone is transformed from disorganized, haphazard immature bone to organized lamellar bone by osteoclast cutting cones. The osteoclasts dissolve the inorganic

matrix by acid secretion and as they move forwards the resorption cavity is occupied by osteoblasts that lay down osteoid before it is calcified.

EXAMINER: Can you please draw an osteoclastic cutting cone for me?

COMMENT: Learn to draw a cutting cone and be able to describe how this functions to remodel bone as you go along (Figures 20.2 and 20.3).
EXAMINER: How and from where does bone derive its blood supply?

CANDIDATE: The blood supply to bone is derived from three sources.
(a) **High-pressure nutrient artery system**. The nutrient arteries are branches of the systemic circulation and enter the bony mid-diaphysis through the nutrient foramen passing to the medullary canal before branching into ascending and descending vessels and arteriolar branches supplying the inner two-thirds of the diaphyseal cortex (endosteal circulation).
Remember that the end arterioles run in the Volkmann canals which drain into the Haversian system and finally drain back into the central venous sinus and out via the nutrient vein.

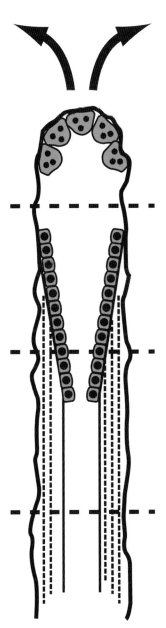

Figure 20.2 Osteoclastic cutting cone. Candidate drawing. The cutting filling cone has a head of osteoclasts that cut through the bone, and a tail of osteoblasts that form a new secondary osteon.

(b) The **low-pressure periosteal system circulation**. This supplies the outer third of the bone cortex and consists of an extensive network of capillaries covering the length of the diaphysis. The normal direction is centrifugal; however, following endosteal damage this system is reversed to centripetal. This is the dominant

system in children, which allows their circumferential growth.

(c) **Metaphyseal–epiphyseal system** is the periarticular vascular complex that penetrates the cortex and supplies the metaphysis, physis and epiphysis with end arterioles.

EXAMINER: What is the direction of blood flow within a long bone?

CANDIDATE: Arterial flow in mature bone is centrifugal (inside to outside), which is the net effect of the high-pressure nutrient artery system and the low-pressure periosteal system.

When a fracture disrupts the nutrient artery system, the periosteal system pressure predominates, and blood flow is centripetal (outside to inside).

Flow in immature, developing bone is centripetal because the highly vascularized periosteal system is the predominant component.

Venous flow in mature bone is centripetal.

EXAMINER: Describe the structure of the periosteum.

CANDIDATE: The periosteum consists of an outer layer of fibroblasts and an inner layer of osteoblasts. The outer fibrous layer is structural, less cellular and continuous with the joint capsule, while the inner cambial layer is vascular, osteogenic and contributes to bone growth and fracture healing. With age, the periosteum thins and has less osteogenic capability.

EXAMINER: What are the functions of the periosteum?

CANDIDATE: Functions of the periosteum include:

• Medium through which muscles, tendons and ligaments are attached.

• Forms a nutritive function.

• Can form bone when required.

• Forms a limiting membrane that prevents bone tissue from 'spilling out' into neighbouring tissues.

EXAMINER: What is the structure of collagen in bone?

CANDIDATE: Collagen is type 1 in bone. The structural unit of type 1 collagen is called tropocollagen and is a trimer composed of three polypeptide chains. Two chains are α1 chains and the third chain is α2. The three chains form a distinctive unit in which the polypeptide chains wrap around

457

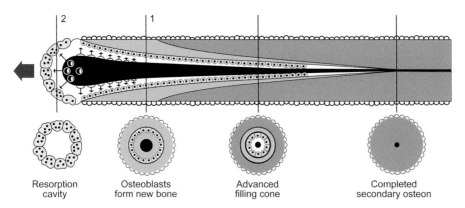

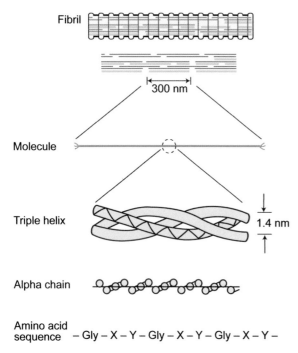

Figure 20.3 Osteoclastic cutting cone. At its tip, osteoclastic resorption takes place while in the latter parts of the cone osteoblasts deposit osteoid with subsequent mineralization. Reversal refers to a 1- to 2-week interval between completion of resorption and initiation of bone matrix formation. The structure terminates as a closing zone in which osteoblasts close the newly excavated osteon by adding centripetal layers of lamellar bone inward from the cement line boundary.

Figure 20.4 Several tropocollagen molecules are aggregated in an organized head-to-tail fashion into a structure called a collagen fibril. These collagen fibrils can be seen with an electron microscope and exhibit a 67-nm D-period banded appearance due to staggered gaps between the heads and tails of the molecules in each row.

each other for most of their length, forming a tight triple helical braid.

Each polypeptide chain is a left-handed helix, but the triple helix is a right-handed superhelix (i. e. the opposite way around) (Figure 20.4).

The triple helical structure is not the same as the α helix that is formed by a single polypeptide chain and is the defining feature of all collagen. Collagen is secreted as an oversized molecule, procollagen, with specialized enzymes removing the N and C terminal propeptides leaving a triple helix with short non-triple helical stubs at the amino and carboxyl terminal chain ends. These non-helical regions are denoted telopeptides and they play a role in the registering of collagen α chains and cross-linking.

It is a fibril-forming collagen.

EXAMINER: How is collagen assembled?

CANDIDATE: Collagen biosynthesis and assembly is a complex process that involves several steps. Intracellular events include post-translational hydroxylation of proline and lysine and subsequent glycosylation. Procollagen is secreted out of the cell. Extracellular events include terminal peptide cleavage and cross-linkage and self-assembly of collagen fibrils.

EXAMINER: What do we mean by osteoclastogenesis?

CANDIDATE: Osteoclastogenesis refers to the process of osteoclast differentiation and function. It is regulated by receptor activator of nuclear factor κB (RANK), RANK ligand (RANKL) and osteoprotegerin (OPG). RANK is expressed on the surface of osteoclast precursors and mature osteoclasts.

Osteoblasts secrete receptor activator of nuclear factor κβ ligand (RANKL) and macrophage colony-stimulating factor (M-CSF) to activate osteoclasts.

Stromal cell/Osteoblast

Figure 20.5 Osteoblast/osteoclast coupling.

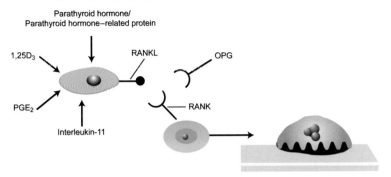

Osteoclast precursor   Osteoclast

RANKL is a potent inducer of osteoclast formation.

With RANK activation, specific genes are switched on and the osteoclast becomes programmed to resorb bone. OPG acts as a decoy receptor, blocking RANKL binding and subsequent activation of the RANK system, thus inhibiting osteoclast differentiation and bone resorption.

EXAMINER: What are osteotropic factors?

CANDIDATE: Osteotropic factors include 1,25-dihydroxyvitamin D3, parathyroid hormone, prostaglandin E2, and interleukin 11.

They induce the formation of osteoclasts by upregulating RANKL expression on the surface of marrow stromal cells and immature osteoblasts (see Figure 20.5).

EXAMINER: What is an osteoclastic cutting cone?

CANDIDATE: An osteoclastic cutting cone is a mechanism to remodel cortical bone by osteoclastic tunnelling (cutting cones). Osteoclasts at the front of the cutting cone remove bone and are followed by layering of osteoblasts and successive deposition of layers of lamellae after the cement line has been laid down.

The tunnel size narrows to a Haversian canal.

The head of the cutting cone is made up of osteoclasts (which bore holes through hard cortical bone).

Behind the osteoclast front are capillaries followed by osteoblasts (which lay down osteoid to fill the resorption cavity).

EXAMINER: Can you draw a cutting cone out?

COMMENT: [Figure 20.3] Remember to keep the diagram simple.

EXAMINER: Draw me the structure of bone.

COMMENT: Again, keep the diagram simple. Use the orthopaedic 20-second diagram. Candidates should discuss the structure of bone as they draw paying particular attention to Haversian systems (Figure 20.6).

EXAMINER: What is bone composed of?

CANDIDATE: Bone consists of cells (10%) and extracellular matrix (90%). The extracellular matrix has organic (40%) and inorganic (60%) components.

- Organic (40%).
  - Collagen (type I) 90%.
  - Proteoglycans.
  - Matrix proteins (non-collagenous).
    - Osteocalcin, osteonectin, osteopontin.
  - Growth factors and cytokines.

- Inorganic (60%).
  - Primarily hydroxyapatite $Ca_5(PO_4)_3(OH)_2$.

EXAMINER: What type of collagen is present in bone?

CANDIDATE: Type 1 [Remember – **BONE**].

EXAMINER: Draw me some collagen.

CANDIDATE:

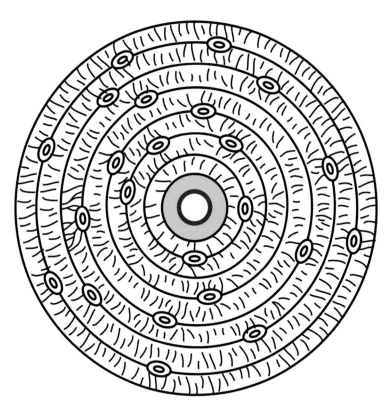

Figure 20.6 Structure of bone. Candidate drawing.

COMMENT: Figure 20.7(a) focuses on the triple helix. Figure 20.7(b) is more complicated, but allows candidates more opportunity to focus on the hierarchical collagen arrangement.

EXAMINER: What do you know about the collagen structure in osteogenesis imperfecta (OI)?

CANDIDATE: Collagen is type 1 in bone. The structural unit of type 1 collagen is called tropocollagen and is a trimer composed of three polypeptide chains. Two chains are α1 chains and the third chain is α2. The three chains form a distinctive unit in which the polypeptide chains wrap around each other for most of their length, forming a tight triple helical braid.

The collagen triple helix forms because both the α1 and α2 chains contain repeat sequences of amino acids (-gly-X-Y), where gly is glycine, X is proline and Y is usually hydroxyproline.

This arrangement results in a constrained structure that imparts a tight kink in the polypeptide chain with the glycine chain preventing steric hindrance that would otherwise impair wrapping of the helical band.

With OI the majority of identified mutations are single nucleotide substitutions that result in alteration of glycine codons within the triple helical domain of either of the chains of type I procollagen (Figure 20.8). These substitutions for glycine within the triple helix are severely destabilizing and interrupt the triple helix. One-fifth of glycine substitutions in α2(I) are lethal, whereas nearly one-third of all glycine substitutions in α1 (I) are lethal.

EXAMINER: What is the gene coding for OI?

CANDIDATE: COL1A1 and COL1A2 are the genes that encode the two chains pro α1(I) and pro α2 (I), respectively, of type I procollagen.

EXAMINER: What about qualitative versus quantitative collagen deficiencies in osteogenesis imperfecta (OI)?

CANDIDATE: OI is a group of disorders with broad variations in clinical severity. Inheritance can be autosomal dominant or recessive. Quantitative defects are often heterozygous, with one copy not producing any collagen. Qualitative defects

(a)

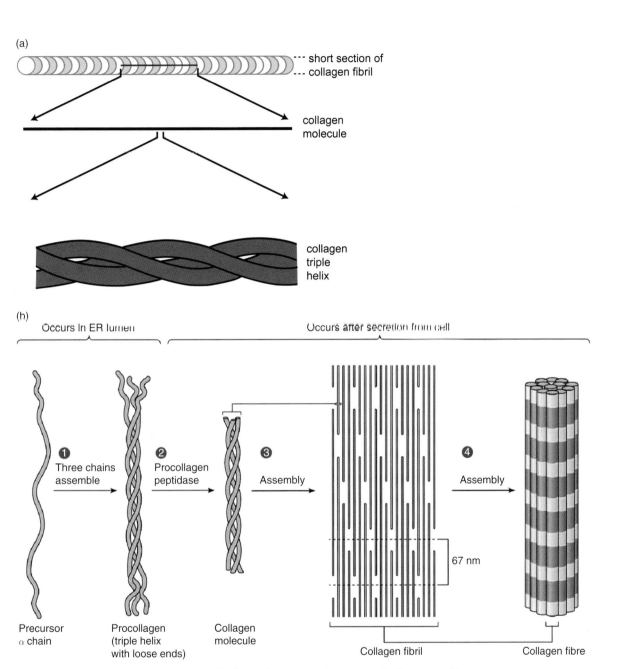

short section of collagen fibril

collagen molecule

collagen triple helix

(b)

Occurs in ER lumen | Occurs after secretion from cell

❶ Three chains assemble

❷ Procollagen peptidase

❸ Assembly

67 nm

❹ Assembly

Precursor α chain

Procollagen (triple helix with loose ends)

Collagen molecule

Collagen fibril

Collagen fibre

Figure 20. 7 (a) Candidate drawing. Structure of collagen. (b) More complex drawing of collagen assembly.

are usually errors in substitution or deletion leading to abnormal, less effectual collagen.

EXAMINER: What about compression and tension of bone?

CANDIDATE: An eccentrically loaded bone has a compression and tension side. When bending occurs, one side of the bone is in tension, the other side is in compression. Bone resists compression better than tension and the side with tension will fracture first. Whenever feasible, any internal or external fixation device should be applied to the tension side to provide maximum stability.

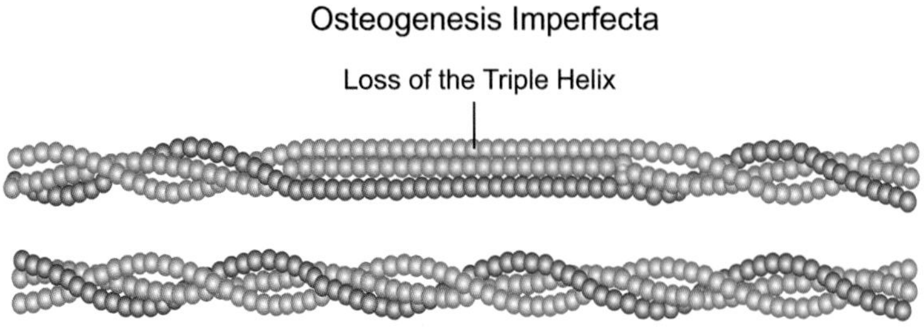

Osteogenesis Imperfecta

Loss of the Triple Helix

Figure 20.8 Collagen structure in osteogenesis imperfecta. Triple helix steric hindrance.

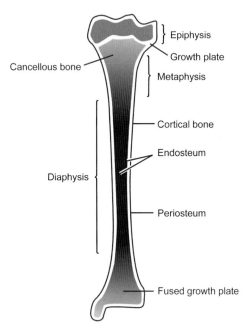

Figure 20.9 Drawing of a typical long bone.

EXAMINER: Draw me a longitudinal cross section of a long bone and tell me the areas (Figure 20.9).

EXAMINER: Where are the cells? Where are the osteoblasts? Where are the osteocytes?

CANDIDATE: Osteoblasts are responsible for laying down new bone and are found in the growing portions of bone such as the periosteum and endosteum.

Osteocytes occupy lacunae that are contained within the calcified matrix of bone between lamellae. Osteocytes are derived from osteoblasts and are essentially osteoblasts surrounded by the products they secrete (Figure 20.10).

EXAMINER: What do you know about skeletal dysplasias?

CANDIDATE: Skeletal dysplasias are a large group of rare, complex, heterogeneous disorders that involve

cartilage and bone. Rubin's classification of bone dysplasia is based on the type of abnormality (hypo-/hyperplasia) and the site involved in the bone: (1) epiphyseal, (2) physeal, (3) metaphyseal, (4) diaphyseal location.

Structured oral examination question 2

EXAMINER: Draw me the structure of cortical bone (Figure 20.11a and 20.11b).

COMMENT: The cross-section of a long bone was quickly drawn, but we then almost immediately moved on to discussing the structure of compact bone.

EXAMINER: What runs in a Haversian canal?

CANDIDATE: Haversian canals contain blood vessels, lymphatics and nerves and are enclosed by closely packed concentric lamellae of bone. These canals branch into large transverse Volkmann canals that provide circulation to the cortical bone.

EXAMINER: What is the Haversian system?

CANDIDATE: The Haversian system, or osteon, is the basic structural unit of cortical bone and lies parallel to the long axis of the bone.

The osteon consists of a central Haversian canal that transmits a neurovascular bundle; surrounding this canal are at least five concentric lamellae of collagen. Within each lamella, collagen fibres lie in parallel but perpendicular to those fibres of adjacent lamellae. Volkmann's canals run transversely to the bone's long axis and permit communication between the outer vessels of the periosteum and the Haversian canals. Cement lines separate osteons.

EXAMINER: Where do osteocytes originate from?

CANDIDATE: Osteocytes are trapped osteoblasts located within lacunae between lamellae,

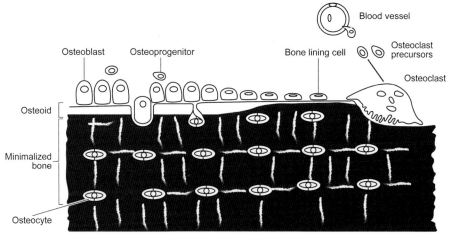

Figure 20.10 Bone remodelling. The origins and locations of bone cells.

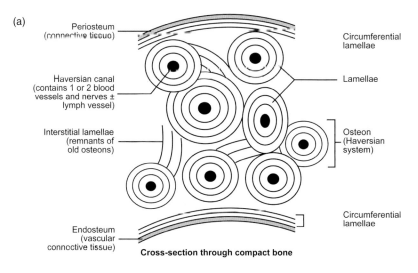

(a)

Cross-section through compact bone

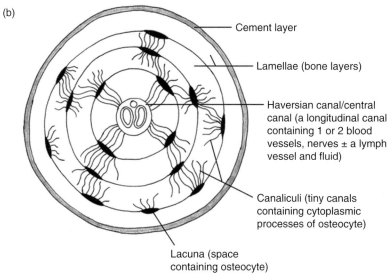

(b)

Figure 20.11 Candidate drawing. Cross-section of (a) long bone and (b) osteon.

communicating with adjacent osteocytes via cytoplasmic processes that travel through canaliculi.

EXAMINER: What do canaliculi do?

CANDIDATE: Canaliculi are the spaces or 'canals' occupied by osteocyte cell processes. They connect the lacunae together within the cortical bone. Canaliculi are thought to modulate the response of bone to mechanical stimuli.

COMMENT: Simple basic questions on the structure of bone, but in the viva situation they usually appear much more than straightforward.

EXAMINER: How do bisphosphonates work?

CANDIDATE: Bisphosphonates are a class of anti-resorptive agents used to treat diseases characterized by osteoclast-mediated bone resorption.
There are two classes of bisphosphonates.
1. Nitrogen-containing bisphosphonates (etodronate).
2. Non-nitrogen-containing (alendrolate, zoledronate, risedronate).

They act differently to diminish bone resorption.
Non-nitrogen-containing BPNs are metabolized into non-functioning ATP analogues, which cause eventual osteoclast apoptosis.

Nitrogen-containing BPNs act by inhibiting farnesyl pyrophosphate synthase (FPPS), resulting in decreased prenylation of small GTPases. These small GTPases are signalling proteins that regulate a number of cell processes such as membrane ruffling, cytoskeletal organization and trafficking of vesicles, which are required for osteoclast function.

EXAMINER: Can you tell me some clinical uses of bisphosphonates?

CANDIDATE: Clinical uses would include osteoporosis, hypercalcaemia of malignancy, Paget's disease, solid tumours and metastatic bone disease, AVN and stress fracture. With children they can be used in fibrous dysplasia, osteogenesis imperfecta and Perthes' disease.

Structured oral examination question 3

Bone healing, primary vs. secondary. Including cellular signalling pathways. Draw an osteonal cutting cone.

EXAMINER: What do we mean by primary bone healing?

CANDIDATE: Primary bone healing is a direct attempt by the cortex to re-establish the Haversian structure after a fracture but without fracture callus formation. Primary bone healing is led by osteonal cutting cones that consist of osteoclasts at the front of the cone that ream out a tunnel in the bone into which a blood vessel grows. This is followed by trailing osteoblasts that lay down new bone across the gaps to form a secondary osteon.

Primary bone healing occurs only under low interfragmentary movement (rigid fixation). There is direct osteonal remodelling and healing without external callous formation.

Primary bone healing can be further divided into gap and contact healing.

EXAMINER: What is contact healing?

CANDIDATE: Contact healing occurs if bone fragments have direct appositional contact and the gap between bone ends is less than 0.01 mm with an interfragmentary strain of less than 2%.

Osteons are able to grow parallel to the long axis of the bone by tunnelling osteoclastic activity.

Osteons traverse the fracture line.

EXAMINER: And gap healing?

CANDIDATE: Gap healing occurs when a small stable fracture gap less than 1 mm is present between bony fragments.

The fracture site is initially filled with transverse lamellar bone without intermediate fibrous or cartilage precursors. The bone is initially deposited perpendicular to the long axis of the bone prior to later osteonal remodelling along the lines of functional stress.

COMMENT: Contact healing – essentially no or minimal fracture gap. Direct osteonal remodelling. Absolute stability.

Gap healing – small stable fracture gap.

EXAMINER: What is secondary bone healing?

CANDIDATE: Secondary bone healing involves the formation of fracture callus. There is:
1. Haematoma formation with devascularization of the bone ends.
2. An inflammatory phase with local accumulation of macrophages, MSC, cytokines. Delivery of osteoprogenitor cells from the periosteal cambium layer and osteoclasts starting to remove necrotic bone. Coagulation and fibrin formation.

3. Primary soft callus formation. New blood vessels invade the haematoma, fibroblasts from the periosteum colonize the haematoma and produce collagen fibres. Granulation tissue gradually differentiates into fibrous tissue and afterwards fibrocartilage.

4. Callus mineralization (hard callus). Osteoblasts lay down woven bone at the periphery (intramembranous ossification) and fibrocartilaginous callus bridges the fracture site, chondroid matrix calcifies, new woven bone is laid down (endochondral ossification).

5. Remodelling. According to Wolff's and Heuter–Volkmann's laws: remodelling occurs with motion at the fracture site. Cartilage is found during the early stages of healing replaced by woven bone laid down by osteoblasts.

COMMENT: Primary and secondary bone healing comes up repeatedly in the viva exam and candidates need to be very clear about the distinction between them. Key points are as follows:

Primary bone healing

- Requires anatomical reduction and interfragmentary compression.
- Absolute stability.
- This system will not tolerate strain.
- Be clear about the differences between gap and contact healing.
- Be able to describe and draw a cutting cone.

Secondary bone healing

- Relative stability.
- Endochondral and intramembranous ossification.
- Fibrocartilage develops at the bone ends and this is subsequently calcified and replaced by woven bone or osteoid.
- Haematoma, inflammation and cellular proliferation, soft callus (chondrogenic and osteogenic proliferation), hard callus and remodelling.

EXAMINER: What is Perren's strain theory?

CANDIDATE: Perren introduced the importance of strain in fracture healing. Fracture gap strain is defined as the relative change in the fracture gap (ΔL) divided by the original fracture gap (L).

Tissue cannot be produced when strain conditions exceed the tissue strain tolerance. Cortical bone can only tolerate 2% strain. Rigid internal compression fixation, which minimizes strain, will lead to primary fracture healing. Lamellar bone can tolerate up to 10% strain, and when this relative stability is present, the fracture heals with callus or secondary fracture healing. Fracture healing will not occur when the strain at a fracture gap exceeds 10%. Comminuted fractures can tolerate more motion than simple fractures, because in a comminuted fracture the overall motion is shared among many fracture gaps.

CANDIDATE: [At the very end of the topic after discussing primary and secondary bone healing, Perren's strain theory] There was a very well-written important paper published recently that discussed fracture healing. This paper mentioned Perren's strain theory and introduced some exciting new ideas on fracture healing to challenge our traditional views on these complicated healing mechanisms.

EXAMINER: Which paper is that?

CANDIDATE: It was a paper published in the JBJS.[2]

EXAMINER: What did the paper say?

CANDIDATE: I haven't had time to read it fully, so I am not too sure, but it's a really well-written paper that everyone keeps mentioning and I am going to sit down and read it when I have more time.

COMMENT: The candidate should have kept quiet, they have ruined an otherwise good performance (score 7) and would probably be marked down to a 6. Candidates should refrain from mentioning a paper they haven't fully read and struggle to say anything sensible about.[3]

Elliott et al. consider the whole fracture to be a 'bone-healing organ' that works as a functional unit and responds to biological and mechanical stimuli. They combined Wolff's law, Perren's strain theory, and Frost's 'mechanostat' model to create their own model of bone homeostasis, healing and non-union (BHN conceptual model).

Using BHN, the behaviour of a 'bone-healing organ' was determined with respect to the mechanical strain applied to the organ. In BHN, the bone is in homeostasis when under tolerable strain (much less than 2%). For strains greater than 2% and less than 100%, a fracture occurs and is considered to be the beginning of the 'bone-healing organ'. Finally, for strains above 100%, the 'bone-healing organ' stops and fails to heal, leading to non-union.

Structured oral examination question 4

EXAMINER: Which cells reside in bone?

CANDIDATE: Osteoblasts, osteoclasts, osteocytes, bone lining cells and osteoprogenitor cells.

COMMENT: Do not forget osteoprogenitor cells that are derived from primitive mesenchymal cells and are located in the inner cellular layer of the periosteum, the endosteum and the lining of osteonic canals (Figure 20.10).

EXAMINER: What do they all do?

CANDIDATE: Osteoblasts are large cells responsible for the synthesis and mineralization of bone during both initial bone formation and later bone remodelling. Osteoblasts form a closely packed sheet on the surface of the bone, from which cellular processes extend through the developing bone. Osteocytes lie within the substance of fully formed bone. They lie within a small space called a lacuna, which is contained in the calcified matrix of bone. Osteocytes are derived from osteoblasts, or bone-forming cells, and are essentially osteoblasts surrounded by the products they secreted. Cytoplasmic processes of the osteocyte extend away from the cell toward other osteocytes in canaliculi. These canaliculi allow nutrients and waste products to be exchanged to maintain the viability of the osteocyte. [*Examiner cut me off, as he realized I would sit and regurgitate the whole book!*]

EXAMINER: Where are osteoclasts derived from?

CANDIDATE: Osteoclast precursors are a member of the monocyte/macrophage family, and, although the resorptive cell can be generated from mononuclear phagocytes of various tissue sources, the principal precursor resides in the marrow. RANKL is produced by osteoblasts, binds to immature osteoclasts and stimulates differentiation into active mature osteoclasts and macrophage colony stimulating factor (M-CSF). Osteoprotegerin inhibits bone resorption by binding and inactivating RANKL.

COMMENT: A lot of candidates get confused in this section.

EXAMINER: Tell me about mesenchymal stem cells.

CANDIDATE: MSCs are multipotent stem cells that can differentiate into a variety of cell types. Cell types that MSCs have been shown to differentiate in vitro or in vivo include osteoblasts, chondrocytes, myocytes and adipocytes.

EXAMINER: What types of cartilage do you know about?

CANDIDATE: There are three types of cartilage: hyaline cartilage, fibrocartilage and elastic cartilage.

COMMENT: Elastic cartilage exists in the epiglottis and the eustachian tube.

EXAMINER: Draw a cross-section of articular cartilage (Figure 20.12).

COMMENT: Draw and talk about the different layers. This is one of the commonest questions to get asked in the basic science viva, know it well! Fail to draw this diagram at your peril! Practise the drawing and discussion of it at least 10 times.

EXAMINER: What are the differences between articular cartilage and meniscus?

CANDIDATE: Articular cartilage is 68–85% water, 10–20% (type II) collagen and 5–10% proteoglycans. Meniscus is 60–70% water, 15–25% (type II) collagen and 1–2% proteoglycans.

COMMENT: It's easy to get confused with these facts.

EXAMINER: Can you draw a picture of collagen and proteoglycans?

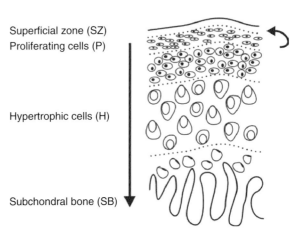

Superficial zone (SZ)
Proliferating cells (P)

Hypertrophic cells (H)

Subchondral bone (SB)

Figure 20.12 Articular cartilage layers.

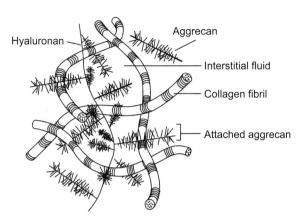

Figure 20.13 Collagen and proteoglycan arrangement in articular cartilage.

COMMENT: Draw the standard picture seen in many text books (Figure 20.13).

EXAMINER: What's the importance of water?

CANDIDATE: 30% of the total water exists between the collagen fibres and this is determined by the negative charge of the proteoglycans which lie within the collagen matrix. Because the proteoglycans are bound closely, the closeness of the negative charges creates a repulsion force that must be neutralized by positive ions in the surrounding fluid. The amount of water present in cartilage depends on the concentration of proteoglycans and the stiffness and strength of the collagen network. The proteoglycan aggregates are basically responsible for the turgid nature of the cartilage and in articular cartilage they provide the osmotic properties needed to resist compressive loads. If the collagen network is degraded, as in the case of OA, the amount of water in the cartilage increases because more negative ions are exposed to draw in fluid. The increase in fluid can significantly alter the mechanical behaviour of the cartilage.

COMMENT: That is a very specific question, but a common theme.

EXAMINER: Bearing in mind what we have discussed, what do you want to talk about next?

CANDIDATE: Growth plates.

EXAMINER: Correct answer! Tell me about any classifications you know of specific to the growth plate.

CANDIDATE: Salter–Harris fractures are classified from types I to V in the order of prognosis, with Salter–Harris Type V having the poorest prognosis and the greatest impact on potential deformity. SH I is a slipped growth plate, II the fracture lies metaphyseal, III is epiphyseal, IV both metaphyseal and epiphyseal and in V the physis suffers a compression injury. Salter–Harris Type II fractures are the most common. When all types of Salter–Harris fractures are considered, the rate of growth disturbance is approximately 30%. However, only 2% of Salter–Harris fractures result in a significant functional disturbance.

The fracture types described later, also less common, include:

- Type VI (injury to the perichondral structures – rare).
- Type VII (isolated injury to the epiphysis only).
- Type VIII (isolated injury to the metaphysis).
- Type IX (an injury to the periosteum which could interfere with membranous growth).

COMMENT: I would not mention any of this unless you get asked. You may end up speaking to an orthopaedic paediatric professor!

EXAMINER: Draw me a growth plate.

CANDIDATE: [I drew a simple schematic like Figure 20.14]

Zone I is the reserve or resting zone with low rates of proliferation, proteoglycan synthesis and type IIB collagen. These cells have a high lipid body and vacuole content which is involved with storage for later nutritional requirements. This is not a germinal layer of 'mother cartilage cells'.

Zone II is the upper proliferative or columnar region. The function of the proliferative zones is matrix production and cell division that results in longitudinal growth. Chondrocytes are flat and are arranged longitudinally. The zone is the true germinal layer of the growth plate and Type II collagen synthesis is increased.

Zone III is the mature proliferating zone, morphologically similar to zone II, but with less DNA synthesis.

Zone IV is the hypertrophic zone, where cell size increases, and the columnar arrangement is less regular. Metabolic activity is high, with matrix synthesis approximately threefold compared to the proliferative zone; the main matrix components synthesized are types II and X collagen and aggrecan.

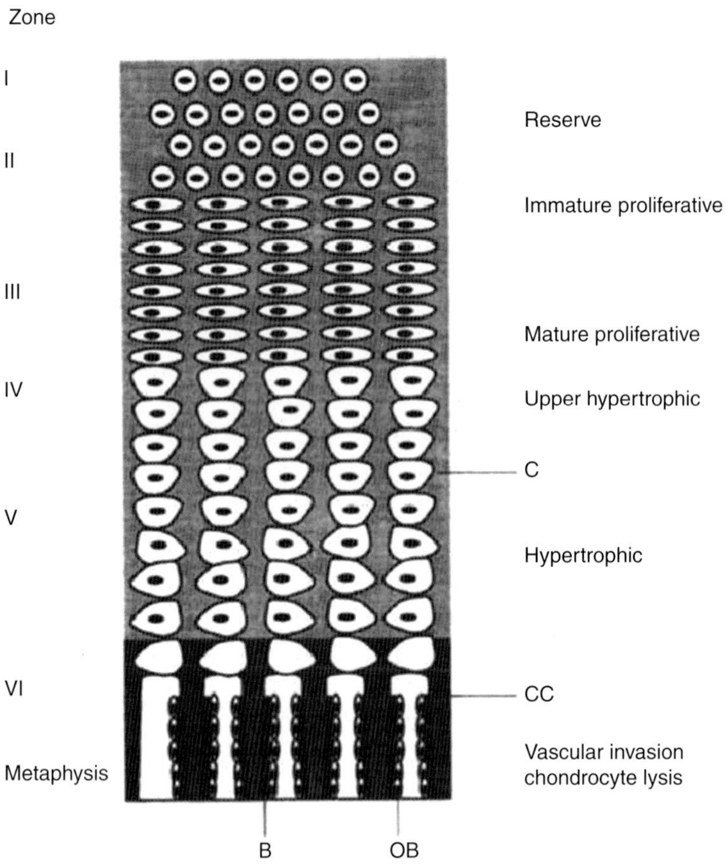

Zone

I

II — Reserve

Immature proliferative

III

Mature proliferative

IV — Upper hypertrophic

C

V

Hypertrophic

VI — CC

Vascular invasion
chondrocyte lysis

Metaphysis

B   OB

Figure 20.14 Diagram of a growth plate. B, bone; OB, osteoblast; CC, calcified cartilage; C, cartilage matrix.

[I got stopped at this point but will continue for completeness]

Zone V is the zone of the matrix calcification as this calcified matrix becomes the scaffolding for bone deposition in the metaphysis. High levels of alkaline phosphatase synthesis of type X and type II collagen cell death by hypoxia.

Zone VI is the junction of the growth plate with the metaphysis, the region where the transition from cartilage to bone occurs. Type I collagen, a marker of the osteoblast phenotype, is immunolocalized to this area.

COMMENT: There are a lot more facts in many textbooks, but if you know roughly about each zone that will be fine for a pass, more detailed knowledge will equal a good pass.

The zones of the growth plate can be confusing as many textbooks use a variety of differing names, some referring to cell function, others to cell morphology.

A non-controversial standard textbook zone description would be: (1) reserve zone, (2) proliferating zone, (3) hypertrophic zone which can be subdivided into (a) maturation zone, (b) degenerative zone, (c) zone of provisional calcification, (4) metaphysis subdivided into (a) primary spongiosa and (b) secondary spongiosa.

EXAMINER: How is the growth plate regulated?

CANDIDATE: The growth plate is regulated by growth factors, hormones and vitamins. Growth factors include insulin-like growth factor, which is one of the most potent GF for skeletal tissue, previously known as somatomedins. They have significant effects on the growth plate chondrocytes, and IGFs retained in bone matrix are important in the regulation of bone remodelling. IGFs stimulate osteoblast and chondrocyte proliferation, induce differentiation in osteoblasts and maintain the chondrocyte phenotype.

Transforming growth factors (TGFs) have an important role in skeletal tissue, particularly certain members of the TGF-b gene family which includes the bone morphogenetic proteins involved in morphogenesis and regulation of endochondral ossification and in bone remodelling. BMPs are the only molecules so far discovered capable of independently inducing endochondral ossification in vivo.

COMMENT: Urist 1965 is the paper to quote.[4] Be able to mention something about BMP2 and BMP7.

Key message[5]

Over 50 years ago, Urist made the key discovery that demineralized bone fragments implanted either subcutaneously or intramuscularly in animals induced bone formation.

The extracellular matrix of bone contains substances that can stimulate new bone formation when implanted into extraskeletal sites in a host. These substances were later identified as bone morphogenetic proteins (BMPs).

Both BMP2 and BMP7 are approved for use in acute tibial fractures and complex non-unions.

They increase the local signals needed to initiate the cascade of bone healing. Both BMP2 and BMP7 have been shown to induce ectopic bone formation. At present, the use of BMP2 is preferred as studies suggest it may be more effective than BMP7 at promoting healing and it is also less costly.

Study outcomes can be highly variable according to indication, implying that more rigorous prospective studies are needed to precisely identify the fracture population, timing and delivery mechanism via which BMP can be used to optimize bony healing.

Fibroblast growth factor stimulates proliferation of mesenchymal cells in the developing limb that leads to limb outgrowth. This group is also involved in later stages of bone growth.

Platelet-derived growth factor plays a role in bone development and growth, being important in the regulation of bone and cartilage cells, although little is currently known of their role in normal endochondral ossification.

Tumour necrosis factors stimulate bone and cartilage resorption and division, and reversibly inhibit ectopic bone formation in animal models.

If you get to this stage it's a good pass. Other growth factors to think about are: interleukin I,6,8, interferons, colony-stimulating factors, parathyroid hormone-related peptide and calcitonin gene-related peptide.

2. Structure and function of cartilage: (a) articular

Introduction

This is an A-list basic science viva topic that almost always appears with each diet of exams. In practical terms this means a candidate has a 1 in 4 or 25% chance of being asked this topic.

In the past, there was a predictable line of questions the examiners would ask. However, most candidates are now more aware of A-list topics than ever before and have pre-learnt their answers. As such the challenge for the Intercollegiate Board is to avoid asking the same questions each and every exam sitting.

To make the subject less predictable the topic focus can be changed mid viva onto different more detailed areas within this large topic such as proteoglycan structure and function.

The flip side is that regular examiners become more familiar with the topic and on occasion may ask esoteric questions to stretch you out to see if you are a possible score 7/8 candidate. What is the function of the tidemark and what insets into it, etc.

One word of caution with A-list topics is that candidates can continue to read further and further into a subject and end up concentrating on unfocused minutia details that have no relevance to any possible viva question likely to be asked.[6] This is very different to reading extra details, but being able to apply these details into higher-order thinking to better answer a question. However, it is sometimes a thin line between the two.

Props

Candidates may immediately be handed a laminated photograph of articular cartilage at the start of the viva or be asked a couple of warm-up questions before being asked to draw out the structure of articular cartilage. Articular cartilage is definitely on the top 10 list for 'must-know' how-to-draw diagrams.

Structured oral examination question 1

EXAMINER: What are the functions of articular cartilage?

CANDIDATE: The two main functions are:

- To provide a smooth, low-friction, lubricated surface for joint motion (lubrication).

- The surfaces roll or glide during motion.
- Hyaline cartilage should be thought of as a fluid-filled wear-resistant surface.
- It reduces the coefficient of friction down to 0.0020, which is 30 times superior to the best performing artificial joint.

- To resist the compressive forces encountered across the joint under loading (shock absorber).

COMMENT: These are the two main functions of articular cartilage, although some textbooks mention other minor roles.[7] There is some controversy as to the relative importance of articular cartilage as a shock absorber. Some authors have suggested that because it is a very thin structure it has negligible shock-absorbing capacity compared to the surrounding muscle and bone. Again, we suggest stay simple and don't mention this standpoint unless it comes up in discussion (very unlikely).[8]

EXAMINER: Can you draw the histological appearance of articular cartilage?
[Draw the structure of articular cartilage.[9]]
What are the articular cartilage layers?

COMMENT: This is one of the commonest diagrams candidates will be asked to draw in the basic science viva. Fail to master this diagram at your peril. Candidates should be able to draw the various layers of articular cartilage without hesitation. Candidates may then be asked to explain why the layers appear like this, with reference to the three-dimensional ultrastructure.[10]

CANDIDATE: The histological appearance of articular cartilage is structured into zones . . .:

COMMENT: Take the examiner sequentially through the layers. Focus your discussion on (1) the differing orientation of type II collagen fibrils, (2) orientation and cellular features of the chondrocytes.
Why is there a different pattern of collagen orientation through the layers of cartilage?
How does the differing pattern of collagen affect its properties?
You 'the candidate' should explain this as you draw out articular cartilage and not allow the examiner to get in and ask you these questions.[11,12]

Structure. The histological structure can be divided into four zones.

1. **Superficial (tangential/gliding) zone**: 10–20% of thickness.
   - Collagen fibres are arranged parallel to the joint surface, forming a dense mat.
   - The most superficial part is called the lamina splendens,[13] providing a very low-friction lubrication surface. It contains no cells, a clear film of collagen fibrils with little proteoglycan. This dense collagen arrangement reduces leakage of proteoglycans from the articular surface and protects it from the effects of harmful enzymes.
   - Below this is a cellular layer with chondrocytes parallel to surface, flat-shaped, high density, many cells 1–3 thick.
   - This layer provides good resistance to shear forces due to tangential arrangement of collagen and provides the greatest tensile strength.
   - Low metabolic activity, hence low healing potential.
   - Thinnest layer with the highest concentration of collagen and water and the lowest concentration of proteoglycan.
   - Water can be squeezed out of the layer to help create lubrication.
   - May function as a barrier to the passage of large molecules from the synovial fluid.

2. **Middle (transitional) zone**: 40–60% of thickness.
   - Collagen fibres arranged obliquely at right angles to each other.
   - Plentiful concentration of proteoglycan.
   - Chondrocytes arranged in random orientation, round shape, progressively lower density and fewer cells.
   - Transitional zone between the shearing forces of the surface layer and resistance to compression in the deep layer.

3. **Deep (radial) zone**: 30% of thickness.
   - Provides resistance to compression.
   - Collagen fibres vertically arranged (perpendicular to articular cartilage) cross the tidemark and are anchored to subchondral bone.
   - Highest concentration of proteoglycans.
   - Chondrocytes spherically arranged in vertical columns.
   - Collagen fibres largest diameter.
   - Lowest water content.

Table 20.3 Constituents of articular cartilage.

Cells (chondrocytes) (5%)			
Extracellular matrix (95%)	Fibres	Collagen (10–20%)	Type II, IX, XI
		Almost exclusively Type II	Type VI, X
		Elastin	
	Ground substance	Water (65–80%)	
		Proteoglycans and glycosaminoglycans (10–15%)	
		Glycoproteins	
		Degradative enzymes (matrix metalloproteinases)	

4. **Calcified zone.**

- This separates the cartilage tissue from the underlying subchondral bone.
- Anchor for the various layers.
- Collagen type X and hydroxyapatite crystals anchor articular cartilage to subchondral bone.
- Forms a barrier to blood vessels supplying subchondral bone.
- Matrix mineralization in the calcified zone allows gradual transition of mechanical properties between cartilage and bone.

Tidemark

- The junction between the deep and calcified zone is called the tidemark.

COMMENT: As a candidate is describing the histological structure of articular cartilage an examiner may start to probe/interrupt/take over[14] and ask esoteric[15] questions.

EXAMINER: What is the tidemark? What attaches to the tidemark?

CANDIDATE: The tidemark provides resistance to shear. It is the boundary between the calcified and uncalcified cartilage. It is cell-free and represents a calcification front. The collagen fibres in the deep zone penetrate through the tidemark into the calcified cartilage to provide structural stability for articular cartilage on the subchondral bone.

It is a smooth, basophilic undulating line that is critical for the transmission of load from cartilage to bone.

EXAMINER: What is the composition of articular cartilage (Table 20.3)?

CANDIDATE: The wet weight proportions of articular cartilage are water (65–80%), collagen (10–20%), proteoglycans (10–15%), chondrocytes (5%) and other matrix components such as adhesives and lipids.

COMMENT: This isn't a wrong answer, but it's a bit unstructured and cumbersome. A better answer would be to say articular cartilage is composed of cells (chondrocytes) accounting for 5% of the wet weight and extracellular matrix the remaining 95%. The extracellular matrix is made up of fibres and ground substance. The fibres account for 10–20% and are almost exclusively Type II collagen. Water accounts for between 65% and 80% of the extracellular matrix, proteoglycans and glycoaminoglycans 10–15% with small amounts of glycoproteins and degradative enzymes.

Or more simply, articular cartilage is mainly composed of chondrocytes, water, Type II collagen, proteoglycans and a variety of matrix proteins.

COMMENT: Do not mix around the wet and dry weight percentages of articular cartilage components; preferably stick to wet weight. If you have to talk about dry weight mention that collagen accounts for 40–70% of the dry weight and that approximately 90% of the dry mass of articular cartilage is made up of proteoglycan aggrecan, type II collagen and hyaluronan.

EXAMINER: What are the contents of articular cartilage?

COMMENT: There is an overlap between describing the layers and discussing the contents of articular cartilage.

Chondrocytes[16]

- Derived from mesenchymal stem cells, chondrocytes produce and maintain ECM, and are the main cell type of articular cartilage.

- Deeper cartilage zones contain no chondrocytes.
- Low metabolic rate.
- Chondrocytes have no contact with neighbouring cells and are spheroidal.
- There are distinct subpopulations of chondrocytes in the different zones of cartilage whose properties differ in terms of their morphology, metabolism, and their response to cytokines.
- Cell morphology varies according to zone.
  - The superficial zone contains a high density of flat cells with approximately three times as many cells in the region compared to the larger cells of the deeper zone.
  - In the deeper zones, they are arranged in columns, reflecting the articular cartilage role in growth of the epiphysis.

Water

- Up to 80% of the extracellular matrix.
- Permits load-dependent deformation of articular cartilage by its movement both in and out and within cartilage.
- Increased water content leads to increased permeability, decreased strength and decreased elasticity.
- Provides a medium for lubrication.

Collagen

- About 10–20% wet weight, 60% dry weight.
- Gives the articular cartilage its tensile stiffness.
- The main collagen in articular cartilage is type II accounting for 90–95% of the collagen.
- Types II, IX and XI form a mesh that serves to trap proteoglycans, providing for stiffness and strength.
- Type VI helps chondrocytes adhere to the matrix. Increases in early OA.
- Type XI constrains the proteoglycan matrix.
- Type X is only found near the calcified zone.

Proteoglycans

- Proteoglycans are complex macromolecules composed of a protein core to which many glycosaminoglycan side chains are attached.

- Proteoglycans trap and hold water, providing the tissue with its turgid nature that resists compression.
- They are secreted by chondrocytes.
- The most common glycosaminoglycan in articular cartilage is chondroitin-sulphate (two subtypes, chondroitin-4-sulphate and chondroitin-6-sulphate), then keratin sulphate and dermatan sulphate.
- Chondroitin-4-sulphate is the most abundant and decreases over the years; chondroitin-6-sulphate remains constant; and keratin sulphate increases with age.
- Glycosaminoglycan can link to a protein core by sugar bonds to form a proteoglycan aggrecan (see Figure 20.14).
- A proteoglycan aggrecan has three globular domains, G1, G2 and G3. G1 and G2 are near the N terminus and separated by a short interglobular domain. The third globular domain, G3, is near the C terminal of the core protein.
- Aggrecan molecules do not exist in isolation within the extracellular matrix, but as proteoglycan aggregates through the interaction with the polysaccharide, hyaluronan.
- Each aggregate is composed of a central filament of hyaluronic acid with up to 100 aggrecan molecules radiating from it, with each interaction stabilized by the presence of a link protein.
- PG aggregation promotes immobilization of the PGs within the fine collagen meshwork.
- PGs have an average lifespan of 3 months and have a great capacity for retaining water, which gives compressive strength and elasticity to the tissue.

EXAMINER: What is the structure of a proteoglycan molecule?[17,18]

COMMENT: This involves differentiating between a proteoglycan aggregate and proteoglycan aggrecan molecule (Figure 20.14). It is not uncommon for candidates to be asked to draw out the structure of either a proteoglycan aggregate or aggrecan molecule (Figure 20.16) or sometimes both.

Volunteer to draw both out for the examiners. As always, rehearse your drawing with dialogue as many times as needed to obtain a smooth, polished flow.

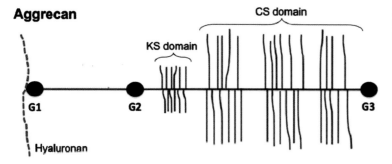

Figure 20.15 Proteoglycan aggrecan. A proteoglycan aggrecan has three globular domains, G1, G2 and G3.

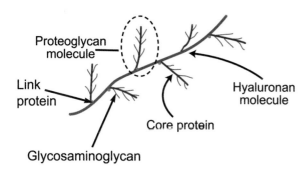

Figure 20.16 Candidate drawing of proteoglycan aggregate.

EXAMINER: How does collagen synthesis take place? (Figure 20.17.)

COMMENT: This question[19] may be asked as part of the main viva theme or as an add-on if a candidate has trail-blazed through previous viva questions and is on for a score 8. The secret is to try and simplify a complex process often poorly described in books. Split the process into intracellular and extracellular events.

CANDIDATE: Procollagen is synthesized by a series of steps within the endoplasmic reticulum of cells such as fibroblasts.

This molecule is then released into the extracellular space by transport through the Golgi apparatus and converted into collagen by procollagen peptidases that cleave the water-soluble, non-helical N- and C-terminal portions of the procollagen molecule to form tropocollagen.

Collagen monomers are then covalently cross-linked with each other after certain residues are oxidized by lysyl oxidase.

Steps that occur INSIDE the cell

- Synthesis of pro-alpha chain.
- Hydroxylation of selected proline and lysine residues.
- Glycosylation of selected hydroxylysine residues.
- Self-assembly of three pro-alpha-chains into triple helix.
- Procollagen triple helix formation.

Then extrusion of procollagen from the endoplasmic reticulum/Golgi compartment into secretory vesicles and then secretion into extracellular matrix.

Steps that occur OUTSIDE the cell

- Cleavage of propeptides. Once secreted, procollagen peptidases remove the N-terminal and C-terminal propeptides.
- Self-assembly into fibril.
- Aggregation of collagen fibrils to form a collagen fibre. Formation of covalent cross-links by the enzyme lysyl oxidase. This enzyme allows hydroxyl groups on lysines and hydroxyl lysines to be converted into aldehyde groups that covalently bond between tropocollagen molecules to form a collagen fibril.

Closely related to synthesis is the structure of collagen and the line of questions may continue on with this subtopic.[20]

EXAMINER: What is the structure of collagen (Figure 20.18)?

CANDIDATE: Collagen is a triple helix of three polypeptide chains.

The amino acids are glycine, proline and lysine.

In articular cartilage collagen is mainly type 2.

EXAMINER: What is the function of matrix glycoproteins?

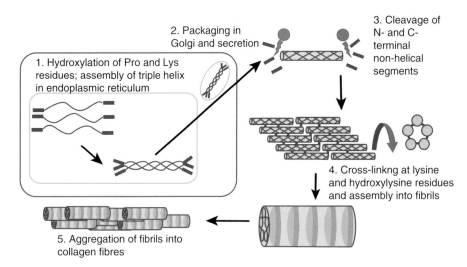

Figure 20.17 Collagen synthesis.

1. Hydroxylation of Pro and Lys residues; assembly of triple helix in endoplasmic reticulum

2. Packaging in Golgi and secretion

3. Cleavage of N- and C-terminal non-helical segments

4. Cross-linkng at lysine and hydroxylysine residues and assembly into fibrils

5. Aggregation of fibrils into collagen fibres

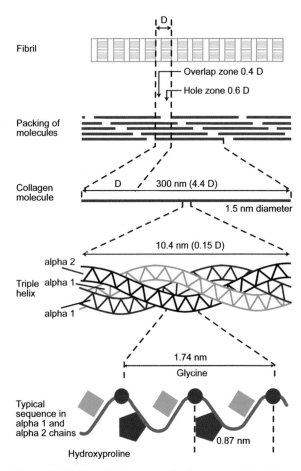

Figure 20.18 Hierarchical structure of collagen ranges from the amino acid sequence, tropocollagen molecules, collagen fibrils to collagen fibres.

CANDIDATE: These interact with collagen fibrils and stabilize the matrix framework.

They help chondrocytes bind to the macromolecules of the matrix.

Matrix glycoproteins are much smaller than aggrecans.

More simply, they act as a tissue glue binding to various matrix components.

EXAMINER: What about matrix metalloproteinases?

CANDIDATE: These degrade collagen and proteoglycan aggregates as part of the normal turnover of the matrix.

EXAMINER: What do we mean by tensegrity architecture?

CANDIDATE:

- Water is attracted and retained in articular cartilage by the ionic pressure created by the high level of negative charges on glycosaminoglycan (GAG) chains on proteoglycan molecules.
- The ionic pressure creates a swelling pressure, which will keep imbibing water until it is resisted by the tension in the fibrous component of cartilage, the collagen fibres.
- As proteogylcans are bound closely, the closeness of the negative charges creates a repulsion force that must be neutralized by positive ions in the surrounding fluid. The amount of water present in cartilage depends on the concentration of proteoglycans and the stiffness and strength of the collagen network. The proteoglycan

aggregates are basically responsible for the turgid nature of the cartilage and in articular cartilage they provide the osmotic properties needed to resist compressive loads. If the collagen network is degraded, as in the case of OA, the amount of water in the cartilage increases because more negative ions are exposed to draw in fluid. The increase in fluid can significantly alter the mechanical behaviour of the cartilage.

COMMENT: Candidates that do not understand this concept particularly well may become trapped quite easily by the examiners (just like water gets trapped by proteoglycans).

EXAMINER: Tell me about matrix metabolism.

CANDIDATE: The production of extracellular matrix, its organization, maintenance and breakdown are controlled by the chondrocyte.

Chondrocyte regulators include hormones, cytokines and growth factors. Turnover of the matrix is needed for remodelling and maintenance. Enzymes include aggracanase and metalloproteinases degrade the matrix. The chondrocytes also make inhibitors of these enzymes called tissue inhibitor of metalloproteinases (TIMP).

EXAMINER: What do we mean by the term matrix region?

CANDIDATE: An alternative zonal classification is by the matrix regions. The matrix is divided into three distinct regions with respect to the distance from the chondrocyte cell membrane.

Matrix regions differ in their collagen content, collagen fibril diameter, collagen fibril orientation and proteoglycan and non-collagenous protein content and organization.

There are three regions.

1. The pericellular matrix is a thin layer adjacent to the cell membrane, completely surrounding the chondrocyte. It contains mainly proteoglycans, as well as glycoproteins and other non-collagenous proteins.

The pericellular matrix region may play a functional role to initiate signal transduction within cartilage with load bearing.

2. The territorial matrix surrounds the pericellular matrix; it is composed mostly of fine collagen fibrils, forming a basket-like network around the cells.

The territorial matrix may protect the cartilage cells against mechanical stresses and may contribute to the resiliency of the articular cartilage structure and its ability to withstand substantial loads.

3. The interterritorial region is the largest of the three matrix regions; it contributes most to the biomechanical properties of articular cartilage.

This region is characterized by randomly oriented bundles of large collagen fibrils and large amounts of proteoglycans.

Structured oral examination question 2

Articular cartilage changes with ageing versus osteoarthritis is more of a section 3 (pathology) topic but there will be a large overlap with section 2 material (structure and function of articular cartilage). Throw in management options for a cartilage defect and this topic is equally at home in an adult and pathology viva.

EXAMINER: Describe the changes in articular cartilage with ageing.

CANDIDATE: Articular cartilage undergoes significant structural, matrix composition and mechanical changes with age. With increasing age there is an age-related decline in the ability of chondrocytes to maintain the tissue. Chondrocytes become less responsive to the proliferative and anabolic effects of growth factors.

There is a marked increase in the formation of advanced glycation end-products (AGEs). This results in increased cross-linking of collagen molecules altering the biomechanical properties of cartilage resulting in increased stiffness and an increased susceptibility to fatigue failure.

COMMENT: Candidates may be asked to directly compare the biomechanical changes of ageing with osteoarthritis in cartilage. This can be rote-learned from various tables, but a more detailed understanding is a safer bet in case follow-up questions focus in on more comprehensive detail.

EXAMINER: Describe the changes in articular cartilage with osteoarthritis.

What pathological processes are involved in the development of osteoarthritis?

CANDIDATE: The process can be divided into three overlapping stages: (1) cartilage matrix damage, (2) chondrocyte response to tissue damage (3) decline of the chondrocyte synthetic response with progressive loss of tissue.

In the early stages of disease, loss of proteoglycan is reversible, whereas at later stages there is irreversible loss. The earliest visible change is loss of collagen integrity resulting in tissue fibrillation and increased water content. Decreased aggrecan concentration and aggregation and decreased glycosaminoglycan chain length all increase the permeability and stiffness of the matrix and make it vulnerable to further mechanical damage. Despite chondrocyte proliferation and increased collagen and proteoglycan synthesis this response fails to halt disease progression. There is progressive loss of articular cartilage and a reduced chondrocyte anabolic and proliferative response. This is related to a downregulation of chondrocyte function.

With osteoarthritis, the cartilage may show areas of softening, fibrillation, fissures or gross erosion. There may be areas of full-thickness cartilage loss with the subchondral bone exposed and often sclerotic.

Microscopic appearances include surface irregularities and erosions, deterioration of the tidemark, fissuring and damage to the cartilage structure. Water content is increased in OA, with a decrease in the proteoglycan content. The proteoglycan chain is shorter, and the chondroitin/keratin sulphate ratio is increased.

Overall, the collagen content is maintained but the presence of collagenase disrupts its organization and orientation.

COMMENT: Have an answer rehearsed.

EXAMINER: What are the management options for osteoarthritis?

CANDIDATE: Conservative measures include targeted physiotherapy, regular oral or topical analgesia/anti-inflammatories, intra-articular injections (corticosteroids or hyaluronic acid) and activity modification.

Surgical management may include joint debridement, osteotomy, arthroplasty and arthrodesis.

EXAMINER: What are the options for treating an articular cartilage defect?

CANDIDATE: There are three main types of cartilage injury: (1) superficial matrix disruption, (2) partial thickness defects and (3) full-thickness defects.

Superficial matrix disruption arises from blunt trauma whereby the ECM is damaged but viable chondrocytes aggregate into clusters and are capable of synthesizing new matrix.

Partial thickness defects disrupt the cartilage surface but do not extend into the subchondral bone. These defects are unable to self-repair.

Full-thickness defects arise from damage that penetrates deep into the subchondral bone. These defects can elicit a repair response due to access to marrow cells; however, they are typically filled with fibrocartilage. This type of repair tissue is much weaker than hyaline cartilage and displays poor long-term performance due to poor compressive strength and durability.

EXAMINER: What are the options for treating a symptomatic focal articular cartilage defect in the medial femoral condyle of the knee of a young active patient?[21]

CANDIDATE: Appropriate management of an articular cartilage defect in a younger patient is often very challenging. Although the natural history of an isolated articular cartilage lesion is not completely understood, these defects may to lead to significant morbidity and progress to diffuse osteoarthritis in time.

Current treatment options fall into three broad categories:

1. Mesenchymal stem cell (MSC) stimulation (microfracture, drilling, abrasion chondroplasty).
2. Substitution options (osteochondral autograft transfer system [OATS], osteochondral allograft).
3. Cell-based, biological replacement options (autologous chondrocyte implantation [ACI], stem cell therapy, tissue engineering).

Marrow stimulation techniques such as abrasion arthroplasty and microfracture penetrate the subchondral bone, causing bleeding within the cartilage defect that leads to fibrin clot formation. Undifferentiated MSCs from the bone marrow migrate into the defect, proliferate and differentiate into fibrochondrocytes. These induce the formation of fibrocartilage repair tissue.

Although excellent short-term clinical outcomes have been reported, the clinical durability of marrow-stimulated repair tissue declines with longer follow-up. The repaired articular cartilage generally fails to replicate the structure, composition and function of normal articular cartilage.

OATS is recommended for smaller lesions, lesions in high-demand athletes, and lesions with associated bone loss.

Microfracture is suited for medium-size defects with little or no bone loss in lower-demand older patients.

COMMENT: Candidates may be asked more specific details about each option such as indications, complications, results, especially if in the adult pathology viva and aiming for score 8.

Structured oral examination question 3

As viva question 1 initially: what are the functions of AC, draw out and describe the layers of AC, etc. and then a focus midway through on the biomechanical properties of articular cartilage.

EXAMINER: What are the biomechanical properties of cartilage?

CANDIDATE: Cartilage is a biphasic, viscoelastic and anisotropic material demonstrating both creep and stress relaxation.

COMMENT: There is a debate whether cartilage is a biphasic (fluid and solid phase) or triphasic material (see below).

EXAMINER: What do you mean by viscoelastic?

CANDIDATE: A viscoelastic material will exhibit a time-dependent behaviour when subjected to a constant load or constant deformation.

EXAMINER: What are the properties of a viscoelastic material?

CANDIDATE: A viscoelastic material demonstrates creep and stress relaxation.

Creep is time-dependent deformation of a material under constant load that is below its yield strength.

Stress relaxation is the decrease in stress required to maintain constant strain over time.

COMMENT: When a constant compressive stress (load/area) is applied to the tissue, its deformation will increase with time; it will creep until an equilibrium value is reached. Creep produces plastic deformation of a material.

When the tissue is deformed and held at a constant strain, the stress will rise to a peak, followed by a slow stress–relaxation process until an equilibrium value is reached.

COMMENT: Viscoelastic materials display four characteristics:

1. Creep.
2. Stress relaxation.
3. Hysteresis.
4. Strain rate-dependent mechanical properties.

Hysteresis occurs when a viscoelastic material is cyclically loaded and unloaded. It is the ability of the material to dissipate energy between loading and unloading cycles. It is due to the fact that materials do not perfectly obey Hooke's law. A viscoelastic material is harder to deform when loading than unloading.

Viscoelastic materials are stiffer, tougher and stronger when loaded at a faster rate (higher strain rate) because there is less time for them to strain. A given load produces less deformation over a shorter period of time than a longer period of time.

EXAMINER: Can you draw out the graphs of creep and stress relaxation (Figures 20.19 and 20.20)?

CANDIDATE: Yes, but my mind has gone blank.

EXAMINER: What about hysteresis and strain-dependent mechanical properties (Figures 20.21 and 20.22)?

CANDIDATE: No, sorry.

COMMENT: These are predictable questions. The viva is heading for a score 4 or at best 5.

EXAMINER: What about articular cartilage permeability with compression?

CANDIDATE: Articular cartilage permeability decreases non-linearly with compression. This serves to regulate the response of cartilage to compression by preventing rapid and excessive fluid exudation from the tissue with compression loading and by promoting interstitial fluid pressurization for load support. It also regulates the ability of cartilage to dissipate energy during cyclic loading.

There are two causes for this nonlinear effect.

As the tissue is compressed:

(1) The water content or porosity is reduced.

(2) The density of the negative charges on the proteoglycans is increased.

There is a direct relationship between permeability and water content and an inverse relationship between permeability and proteoglycan content.

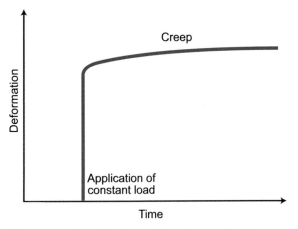

Figure 20.19 Creep. Continuous deformation over time in response to constant load.

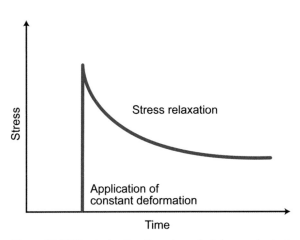

Figure 20.20 Stress relaxation. Time-dependent decrease in stress required to maintain strain.

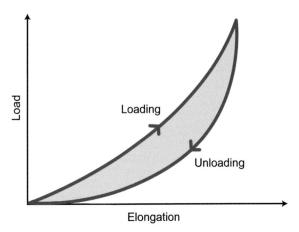

Figure 20.21 Hysteresis. Strain energy loss as heat due to internal friction between loading and unloading.

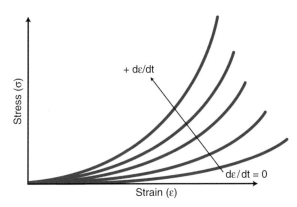

Figure 20.22 Time-dependent strain behaviour. Stress is proportional to strain rate.

COMMENT: This is an esoteric question that tests knowledge of the interaction between proteoglycan and water. This is in the score 8 zone for candidates.

EXAMINER: How does the internal architecture of articular cartilage relate to its biomechanical properties?

CANDIDATE: The presence of water within the tissue allows the support of most of the load through pressurized fluid. This fluid support is not uniform between the different zones of the tissue, with the superficial zone demonstrating the highest support (95%) compared to the deep zone (70% of applied load). Over time there is a decreased interstitial fluid support that causes an increased loading of the solid phase including chondrocytes. As such, articular cartilage can be thought of as a biphasic, porous model.

However, dissolved electrolytes together with fixed charges of the solid matrix bring about mechanoelectrochemical phenomena adding to the load bearing of the tissue and described as a third phase.

The triphasic nature of cartilage explains how fluid is drawn back into the cartilage matrix after being excreted during compression. While the triphasic nature of cartilage is a physically intuitive way to model cartilage, it is also very complex.

COMMENT: The biomechanical properties of articular cartilage can be complicated to understand and tests higher-order thinking relating to structure.

Biphasic creep behaviour of articular cartilage during compression. Rate of creep is governed by the rate at which fluid is forced out from the tissue, which, in turn, is governed by the permeability and stiffness of the porous-permeable, collagen–proteoglycan solid matrix.

Structured oral examination question 4

EXAMINER: What are the properties of articular cartilage?

CANDIDATE: Cartilage is avascular, aneural and alymphatic.

EXAMINER: What are the articular cartilage changes that occur with ageing and osteoarthritis (Table 20.4)?

COMMENT: This is an A-list basic science question. While tables provide a succinct summary they do not give a candidate the opportunity to practise out loud and rehearse their answer. Perhaps best remembered as changes occurring in the composition of articular cartilage, i.e. water, chondrocytes, collagen and proteoglycans.

EXAMINER: What are the changes that occur with osteoarthritis?

CANDIDATE: With osteoarthritis, the cartilage may show areas of softening, fibrillation, fissures or gross erosion. There may be areas of full-thickness cartilage loss with the subchondral bone exposed and often sclerotic.

Microscopic appearances include surface irregularities and erosions, deterioration of the tidemark, fissuring and damage to the cartilage structure. Water content is increased in OA, with a decrease in the proteoglycan content. The proteoglycan chain is shorter, and the chondroitin/keratin sulphate ratio is increased.

Overall, the collagen content is maintained, but the presence of collagenase disrupts its organization and orientation.

COMMENT: The three main areas to consider with OA are (1) macroscopic changes, (2) microscopic changes and (3) synovial joint changes.

Synovial joint changes include changes in periarticular musculature, and in articular and periarticular tendons and ligaments. There is synovial inflammation, joint capsule hypertrophy, meniscal degeneration, thickening of subchondral bone and formation of osteophytes.

EXAMINER: What is the relationship between ageing and osteoarthritis?

CANDIDATE: Ageing does not necessarily cause OA, but age related changes may provide a basis upon which OA can be initiated.

During ageing, an imbalance between the catabolic and anabolic processes occurs. Age-related loss of the ability of chondrocytes and tissues within the ECM to maintain a homeostasis between these pathways leads to a procatabolic state favouring matrix degradation. This loss of homeostasis and inability to adapt to external mechanical stressors can in time become a precursor for the development of OA.

Despite ageing being a significant risk factor for OA, not all aged joints develop the disease.

EXAMINER: What are advanced glycation end products (AGEs)?

Table 20.4 Osteoarthritis versus ageing.

Parameter	Effect of ageing	Effect of osteoarthritis
Water content	Decreased	Increased
Chondrocyte number	Decreased	–
Chondrocyte size	Increased	–
Collagen concentration	Relatively unchanged	Decrease in severe OA
Proteoglycan concentration	Decreased	Initially increased, but with progression becomes decreased
Proteoglycan synthesis	Decreased	Increased
Proteoglycan degradation	Decreased	Increased
Chondroitin-4-sulphate	Decreased	Increased
Keratin sulphate	Increased	Decreased
Modulus of elasticity	Increased	Decreased
Metabolic activity	Unchanged	Increased
Subchondral bone thickness	Normal	Increased

CANDIDATE: Advanced glycation end products (AGEs) are the products of uncontrolled, non-enzymatic glycation, and oxidation reaction between proteins and sugars, and accumulate in the AC as a part of ageing, making the tissue brittle.

Due to its low metabolic activity articular cartilage is particularly susceptible to AGEs accumulation.

The effects of AGEs formation include:

- Modification of type II collagen by cross-linking of collagen molecules:
  - increasing stiffness and brittleness,
  - increasing susceptibility to fatigue failure.

Fragments of collagen and fibronectin are formed because of ageing. These fragments can induce production of inflammatory cytokines and MMPs to continue ECM destruction and also activate innate immune responses or the classic complement pathway. The combination of changes in the mechanical properties of the cartilage tissue, the procatabolic environment, and the innate low capacity for self-repair leads to a tissue that is unable to withstand normal joint loading, which gradually leads to total joint failure.

EXAMINER: What about the use of hyaluronic acid? What is the evidence for its use in osteoarthritis?

CANDIDATE: HA is a macromolecule found naturally within cartilage, with reduced levels found in joints where osteoarthritis is present.

HA injection into degenerative joints has been shown to improve function and to provide good pain relief in knees.

I am not sure about the specifics of the literature, but I believe there has been some recent evidence suggesting beneficial responses in patients with early disease.

EXAMINER: What about PRP. Does this work?

CANDIDATE: PRP can be defined as the volume of the plasma fraction from autologous blood with platelet concentration above baseline.

Platelets contain many important bioactive proteins and growth factors that regulate key processes involved in tissue repair, including cell proliferation, chemotaxis, migration, cellular differentiation, stem cell recruitment, extracellular matrix synthesis and local increased vascularity.

There have been early encouraging clinical results shown in active patients with early knee OA.

NICE guidelines have suggested although there are no concerns regarding safety of PRP in knee osteoarthritis, the evidence for efficacy is weak. It should only be used as a second-line treatment with special arrangements for clinical governance, consent and audit/research.

EXAMINER: What would you say to a colleague who has listed 10 patients with early knee osteoarthritis for PRP injections?

CANDIDATE: This is a delicate situation. I would discreetly suggest PRP injections are quite expensive to perform and can be problematic in blocking up operating list capacity. They perhaps should be used more selectively rather than as a first-line standard treatment for early OA as the evidence for efficacy is fairly weak. If my colleague was still keen to undertake large amounts of PRP injections to patients with early knee OA it could be part of a multicentre RCT with a view to publishing results and giving national guidelines and recommendations for use.

2. Structure and function of cartilage: (b) meniscus

Introduction

This is an A-list topic that candidates should have viva practised beforehand. For a basic 6 the candidate should learn the usual core questions on meniscal structure, function, biomechanics and hoop stresses.

Candidates aiming to score a 7 or 8 will need to put in some detective work to uncover the higher-order thinking and judgement questions that follow on from this. As a general rule the application of basic science in a clinical content is always an excellent starting position.

There are several possible routes into the topic.

Structured oral examination question 1

1. EXAMINER: Here is a picture of the menisci of the knee, which I am sure you recognize. Can you talk me through this picture (Figure 20.23)?

COMMENT: No marks for recognizing the menisci as the examiners have already told you this. Being handed a meniscal diagram is a lucky escape into the topic for those candidates with poor drawing

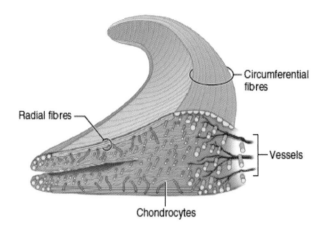

Figure 20.23 A cross-section of the meniscus showing the radial and circumferential collagen fibre orientation. Also shown are blood vessels penetrating the peripheral one-third of the tissue and location of chondrocytes.

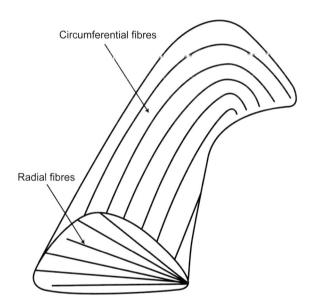

Figure 20.24 Candidate 20-second diagram of meniscal structure.

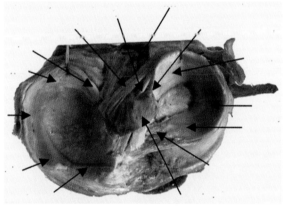

Figure 20.25 Unlabelled axial view of a right tibial plateau showing sections of the meniscus and their relationship to the cruciate ligaments.

skills. The diagram can be tricky to draw and this side-steps the potential for a stumbling start into the topic.[22]

2. *EXAMINER*: Can you draw out a meniscus for me concentrating on the collagen arrangement within the menisci (Figure 20.24)?

COMMENT: Well-prepared candidates would have anticipated this well-known route into the topic and worked out how to draw out and explain the structure within a time period of around 30 seconds.

CANDIDATE: The large collagen fibres within the meniscus are mainly arranged in a circumferential pattern, with a smaller number of fibres in a radial orientation acting as ties.

3. *EXAMINER*: [Bird's eye nest picture of the meniscus shown] Can you identify the unlabelled structures on the diagram (Figure 20.25)?

COMMENT: This diagram could be shown either unlabelled (Figure 20.25) or labelled (Figure 20.26). The unlabelled version is a more precarious way into the topic.

4. *EXAMINER*: [Bird's eye nest picture of the meniscus shown (Figure 20.26)] Describe what you see.

COMMENT: A bird's eye nest picture of the meniscus generally leads to a more focused initial testing of meniscal anatomy.[23] Candidates need to avoid stumbling around

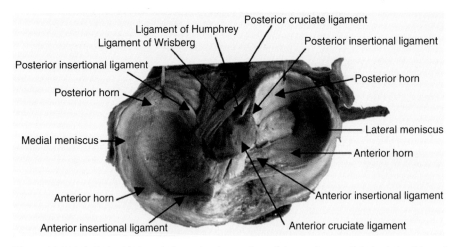

Figure 20.26 Labelled axial view of a knee showing sections of the meniscus and their relationship to the cruciate ligaments.

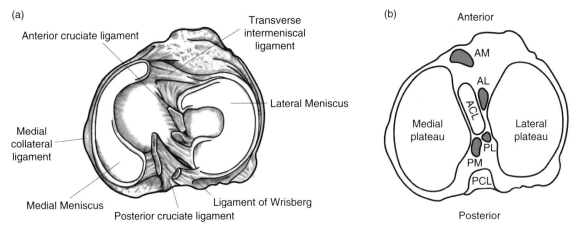

Figure 20.27 (a) Anatomy of the meniscus viewed from above. (b) Axial view of a right tibial plateau showing sections of the meniscus and their relationship to the cruciate ligament. AL, anterior horn lateral meniscus; AM, anterior horn medial meniscus; PCL, posterior cruciate ligament; PL, posterior horn lateral meniscus; PM, posterior horn medial meniscus.

describing the diagram. A well-rehearsed answer would allow a candidate to progress on to the next part of the topic in a timely fashion.

EXAMINER: Describe the anatomy of the medial and lateral meniscus (Figure 20.27).

CANDIDATE: The menisci are specialized intra-articular fibrocartilaginous structures of the knee.

They are triangular in cross-section, with an average thickness of 3–5 mm.

They are divided into three regions: anterior horn, body and posterior horn.

The peripheral, vascular border of each meniscus is thick, convex and attached to the joint capsule. The innermost border tapers to a thin free edge.

The superior surfaces of menisci are concave, enabling effective articulation with their respective convex femoral condyles.

Lateral meniscus

- The lateral meniscus is O-shaped and covers a larger area than the medial meniscus (80–85% of the lateral tibial plateau).
- It is more constant in size between the anterior and posterior horns.

- The anterior horn is attached to the tibia anterior to the intercondylar eminence and posterior to the attachment of the ACL, with which it partially blends.
- The posterior horn is attached posteriorly to the intercondylar eminence of the tibia, anterior to the posterior horn of the medial meniscus.
- No attachment of the lateral meniscus to the LCL, only a loose attachment to the joint capsule that is interrupted posteriorly by the popliteus tendon.
- Occasionally a few fibres of the popliteus are attached to the posterior convexity of the LM.

Medial meniscus

- The medial meniscus is C-shaped and covers 60–65% (~two-thirds) of the medial plateau.
- The posterior horn is significantly wider than the anterior horn.
- It has a larger anterior–posterior dimension than width.
- The anterior attachment is approximately 7 mm anterior to the ACL attachment, in line with the medial tibial tubercle.
- The posterior attachment to the posterior intercondylar fossa of the tibia, anterior to the PCL attachment.
- The MM attaches to the deep part of the MCL and to the capsule around its periphery via the coronary (meniscotibial) ligament. This results in the MM being less mobile than the LM.

EXAMINER: What are the ligaments associated with the meniscus?

CANDIDATE: A number of important ligaments are associated with the menisci.

Both menisci have firm attachments to the tibial surface at their anterior and posterior horns via the insertional ligaments, which are very strong and stiff.

Anteriorly, the transverse meniscal ligament connects the anterior convexity of the lateral meniscus to the anterior horn of the medial meniscus.

Posteriorly, the lateral meniscus may be connected to the lateral side of the medial femoral condyle by one or two meniscofemoral ligaments. The anterior meniscofemoral ligament (ligament of Humphrey) passes in front of the PCL, the posterior meniscofemoral ligament (ligament of Wrisberg) passes behind the PCL.

EXAMINER: What are the functions of the meniscus?

CANDIDATE: The function of the meniscus includes:
- Load transmission (bearing).
- Shock absorption.
- Lubrication.
- Distributes synovial fluid throughout the joint.
- Contributes to joint stability.
- Prevents hyperextension.
- Assists in gliding motion.
- Prevents synovial impingement.
- Proprioception.
- Nutrition.

COMMENT: This is a predictable question and candidates wanting to score higher marks than a basic pass should be able to discuss meniscal function in a more detailed way than the usual bulleted list.

EXAMINER: What are the biomechanical functions of the meniscus?

COMMENT: This is a slightly more probing question than the preceding one and needs a bit more thought. Typical leading-on questions may focus on the development of osteoarthritis.

The meniscus serves several important biomechanical functions. They contribute to load transmission, stability, nutrition, joint lubrication and proprioception. They also function to decrease contact stresses and increase contact area and congruity of the knee.

In most textbooks menisci are described as functioning as shock absorbers in the knee. However, recent evidence has suggested this might not actually be the case.[24]

EXAMINER: What about the load transmission functions of the meniscus?

CANDIDATE: In extension, the posterior menisci bear 50% of the compressive load compared to 85% at 90° flexion. Following meniscectomy, contact areas can be reduced by over 75% resulting in an increase in peak contact pressures as high as 235%.

EXAMINER: How does this lead to the development of osteoarthritis?

CANDIDATE: Medial meniscectomy results in a 50–70% reduction in femoral condyle contact area and a 100% increase in contact stress. Total lateral meniscectomy results in a 40–50% decrease in contact area and increased contact stress in the lateral component to 200–300% of normal.

Increased contact pressures lead to overload of the articular cartilage and the development of osteoarthritis.

EXAMINER: So why is lateral meniscectomy worse than medial meniscectomy?

CANDIDATE: The medial tibial plateau is slightly concave, giving some degree of congruency with the curved femoral condyle. However, with the lateral tibial plateau this is convex, causing a natural tendency to point loading. The lateral meniscus is therefore more important as a load-bearing structure than the medial meniscus and partial or total lateral meniscectomy much more significant than the equivalent medial meniscectomy.

EXAMINER: How are menisci viscoelastic? What do you mean?

CANDIDATE: Viscoelastic materials display properties of both a solid and liquid. The elastic quality or solid phase of the meniscus is due to its collagen–proteoglycan structure, whereas the viscous or fluid phase is due to its permeability and water content.

Under compression, meniscal permeability determines the rate at which fluid is extruded. Meniscal permeability is much lower compared to articular cartilage, giving menisci the ability to maintain their shape during axial loading.

COMMENT: The viscoelastic nature of the meniscus functions to dampen the intermittent shock waves generated by impulse loading of the knee during gait. This shock-absorbing mechanism reduces the risk of osteoarthritic development.

Articular cartilage, tendons and ligaments, intervertebral discs and menisci display viscoelastic properties.

EXAMINER: How does the meniscus assist in lubrication?

CANDIDATE: The menisci serve to increase the congruity between the condyles of the femur and tibia; they contribute significantly to overall joint conformity. This assists in the overall lubrication of the articular surfaces of the knee joint.

COMMENT: Like shock absorption, there is no firm evidence of menisci involvement in knee joint lubrication. Again, similar to shock absorption, it is mentioned as a meniscal function in various textbooks.

EXAMINER: What else?

CANDIDATE: There is fluid exudation across meniscal surfaces. Compression squeezes fluid out into the joint space to allow smoother gliding of the joint surfaces.

EXAMINER: How does the meniscus function in proprioception?

CANDIDATE: The menisci provide a feedback mechanism for joint position sense. Neural elements have been identified within the meniscal tissue. It is thought that mechanoreceptors located in the meniscal horns sense a taut meniscus during extremes of flexion and extension and feed this back to the central nervous system, which contributes to a reflex arc that stimulates protective or postural muscular reflexes.

EXAMINER: What are hoop stresses in the meniscus?

COMMENT: This is very much pass/fail material. Candidates would be expected to know this to score a 6.

The arrangement of collagen fibres in the meniscus convert compressive forces into a radially directed force, which is distributed and resisted as hoop stresses within the meniscus.

The radial fibres act as intrasubstance tie rods to provide structural rigidity and resist against longitudinal splitting of the circumferential collagen bundles.

The development of hoop stresses within the meniscus depends on intact anterior and posterior attachments. Hoop stress also relies on the conversion of axial load into tensile strain through intact longitudinal-orientated collagen fibres.

CANDIDATE: No matter how many times I described hoop stresses in the meniscus, for some reason I never appeared very convinced that I knew what I was talking about. The answer is textbook reading, but something in my delivery either a lack of confidence, poor body language or just not being persuasive enough meant I always failed this question.

Equally frustrating was observing other candidates giving either exactly the same answer or even a slightly incorrect answer but still being passed. Very frustrating!

COMMENT: The candidate has probably rote-learnt the topic rather than fully understood it and the examiners may have sensed this. There may be other complicated reasons that are difficult to analyze in cold print on paper without observing the scenario. Try more to understand basic science principles rather than memorize the subject and sound convincing in your answer, even if you don't feel very confident.

EXAMINER: What is the blood supply of the meniscus?

CANDIDATE: The blood supply to the meniscus is mainly from the medial and lateral genicular arteries (superior and inferior branches). Branches from these vessels give rise to a perimeniscal capillary plexus within the synovial and capsular tissues of the knee joint.

These perimeniscal vessels are orientated predominantly in a circumferential pattern with radial branches directed towards the centre of the joint.

The middle genicular artery also supplies the menisci through the vascular synovial covering of the anterior and posterior horn attachment.

Approximately 10–30% of the periphery of the MM and 10–25% of the LM are relatively well vascularized.

The remaining portion of each meniscus (65–75%) receives nourishment from synovial fluid via diffusion or mechanical pumping (i.e. joint motion).

EXAMINER: What factors influence your decision whether to repair a meniscal tear or resect?

CANDIDATE :

Location of tear

The vascular supply only reaches the peripheral 25–30% of each meniscus. Repair of tears in the well-vascularized red zone (0–5 mm from the periphery) have a good chance of healing. Red–white zonal tears have a reasonable chance of healing, whereas tears in the white zone (3–5 mm from the periphery) are unlikely to heal.

As a general rule, red–red should, white–white won't and red–white might.

Age of tear

Fresh tears are more likely to heal than older tears.

Age of the patient

Meniscal repairs in older patients (> 30 years) have a significantly worse outcome than in younger patients. There is less vascularity in the older tear.

Tear pattern

- Displaced bucket-handle tears should be repaired on an urgent basis whenever possible. Delay of more than a few weeks will lead to scarring and retraction of the bucket-handle fragment. Repetitive compression and abrasion in the displaced position will lead to macerated and damaged tissue and preclude repair.
- Peripheral, vertical, longitudinal tears are ideal for repair in the red–red or red–white zone.
- Complex bucket-handle tears, flap tears, degenerative and radial tears often perform poorly with repair and are more often amenable to excision.
- Horizontal cleavage tears are not repairable, and the unstable leaf should be excised, leaving up to 3 mm of the leaf.

Ligament stability

A meniscal tear should not be repaired in an unstable ACL-deficient knee. Due to the abnormal kinematics of the ACL-deficient knee, the failure rate in the unstable knee is much higher than in a stable or reconstructed knee.

EXAMINER: What percentages of tears are amenable to repair?

CANDIDATE: This depends to a certain extent on the expertise of the surgeon, but a figure around 15% is generally accepted. There is very little guidance in the literature.

If acute and/or a relatively well-preserved joint, consider repair. If the patient is older (> 50 years), degenerative changes are present, or the patient is obese or has inflammatory arthritis, resect.

EXAMINER: How do radial and longitudinal tears differ?

CANDIDATE: A radial tear disrupts the continuity of the circumferential fibres interfering with the distribution of hoop stresses within the meniscus. If the tear reaches the periphery it transects the meniscus and renders the hoop stress distributing capacities of the meniscus ineffective. This is the equivalent of a total meniscectomy. In this situation, consider repair.

In contrast, longitudinal tears do not disrupt the continuity of the circumferentially orientated fibres that bear load. They occur due to fracture of the weak radial tie fibres.

EXAMINER: If radial tears interfere so much biomechanically with hoop stress distribution, why do we not repair more of them?

CANDIDATE: These tears are difficult to repair. There may be a case for attempting repair in a young active person, especially if the lateral meniscus is involved or if the tear extends to the periphery, but success rates can be unpredictable, and the patient needs to be partial weight-bearing for at least 6 weeks following the repair.

EXAMINER: What is a meniscal root tear?

CANDIDATE: A meniscal route tear is where the tear extends to either the anterior or posterior meniscal root attachment to the central tibial plateau. They often tend to be radial tears extending into the root. The tear may lead to meniscal extrusion, secondary osteoarthritis, and subchondral insufficiency fracture.

EXAMINER: Biomechanically?

CANDIDATE: Loss of the root attachment impairs the ability of the meniscus to resist hoop stress when the tibiofemoral joint is loaded. This produces increased joint contact pressure and leads to rapid articular cartilage damage, subchondral bone oedema and sometimes collapse.

EXAMINER: What else?

CANDIDATE: There are two main types of meniscal root tears. The first type is low-energy tear occurring in older patients with pre-existing osteoarthritis. The second type occurs in young athletic patients from a sporting knee injury and are generally repaired. Repair techniques can be difficult but include pull-out (transosseous) techniques, suture anchor repair, and side-to-side suture repair.

EXAMINER: What is the role of meniscal replacement?

CANDIDATE: Meniscal replacement may be indicated in a young patient who develops significant pain and swelling in a compartment specific to a major or total meniscectomy. There should be only early or minimal chondral changes, normal limb alignment and a stable knee. Candidates should be prepared to modify sporting activities after surgery to improve the chances of success.

Cadaveric menisci are matched by size and site and are implanted by various techniques that include a free soft-tissue allograft implantation, separate anterior and posterior bone plugs and bone bridges.

A meniscal allograft may partially replicate the normal meniscus function and significantly reduce pain and improve knee function.

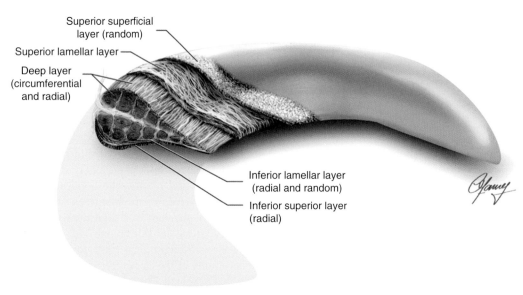

Superior superficial layer (random)
Superior lamellar layer
Deep layer (circumferential and radial)
Inferior lamellar layer (radial and random)
Inferior superior layer (radial)

Figure 20.28 Complex collagen arrangement in meniscus. The outer region is the outer third of the meniscus; the inner region is the inner two-thirds of the meniscus; the superficial region is the surface of the meniscus.

Structured oral examination question 2

Meniscus – draw, structure, function, contents, hoop stresses.

COMMENT: Similar to question 1, but meniscal contents need to be described.

EXAMINER: What are the contents of the meniscus?

CANDIDATE: The meniscus is a dense extracellular matrix (ECM) composed mainly of water (72%) and collagen (22%), interposed with cells. The remaining dry weight is composed of proteoglycans, non-collagenous proteins and glycoproteins (Figure 20.28).

The cells of the meniscus are called fibrochondrocytes because they appear as a mixture of fibroblasts and chondrocytes. Cells in the more superficial layer of the meniscus are more fibroblastic spindle-shaped while those cells located deeper in the meniscus are more chondrocytic ovoid-shaped (Figure 20.29).

The proteoglycans retain water within the meniscus, thus permitting its specific viscoelastic properties.

The outer region of the meniscus is composed of type I collagen while the inner region is 60% type II and 40% type I. As such the outer portion is more fibrous while the inner region displays more hyaline cartilage-like properties.

The collagen fibre arrangement is either circumferential, radial or random. The meniscus is divided into five layers.

- Superior superficial layer: random.
- Superior lamellar: random but with some short radial-orientated fibres at the posterior and anterior horns.
- Deep layer: circumferential fibres interspersed with a few radial fibres.
- Inferior lamellar: radial and random.
- Inferior superficial layer: radial.

Structured oral examination question 3 (Figure 20.30)

Draw me the top of the tibia! Label the structures. How are the menisci attached?

What is the function of menisci – load transfer, shock absorption, hoop stresses, etc.?

How do menisci get injured?

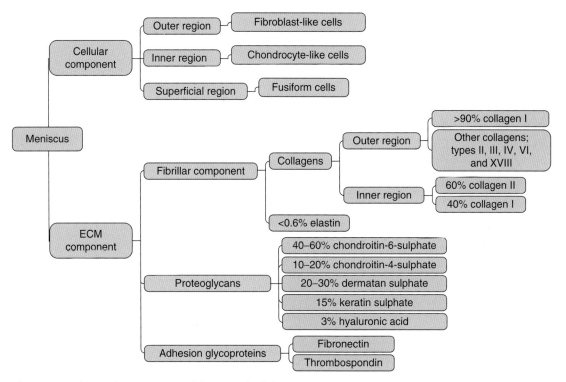

Figure 20.29 The complex composition of the meniscal cellular and meniscal extracellular matrix (ECM) components.

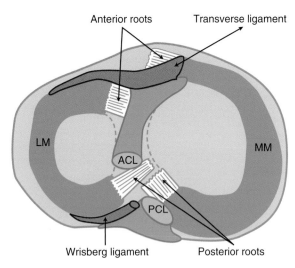

Figure 20.30 Bird's eye picture of the tibia.

CANDIDATE: As a result of circumferential collagen fibres and the insertional features of the anterior and posterior horns, vertical compressive forces are converted into a radially directed force that is taken up as circumferential hoop stresses within the meniscus (Figure 20.31).

EXAMINER: Can you draw this for me?

EXAMINER: Can you explain this free body diagram of forces acting on the meniscus (Figure 20.32)

CANDIDATE: As the femur presses down on the meniscus during normal loading, the meniscus deforms radially but is anchored by its anterior and posterior horns (Fant and Fpost).

During loading, tensile, compressive and shear forces are generated. A tensile hoop stress (Fcir) results from the radial deformation, while vertical and horizontal forces (Fv and Fh) result from the femur pressing on the curved superior surface of the tissue. A radial reaction force (Frad) balances the femoral horizontal force (Fh).

EXAMINER: How do menisci get injured?

CANDIDATE: There are two types of meniscal tears, traumatic and degenerate. Traumatic tears usually occur with rotation as the flexed knee moves towards an extended position. The most common location for injury is the posterior horn and the most common tear pattern is longitudinal.

Degenerative tears occur as the meniscus becomes less compliant and elastic with age.

COMMENT: Bird's eye picture of the meniscus (discussed in earlier questions). Ideally, the anatomical description of each meniscal attachment should be explained while the diagram is being drawn out. Candidates wanting to score well need to get through this opening test material in a timely fashion to set themselves up for the later, more difficult score 7/8 questions.

EXAMINER: What do we mean by hoop stresses?

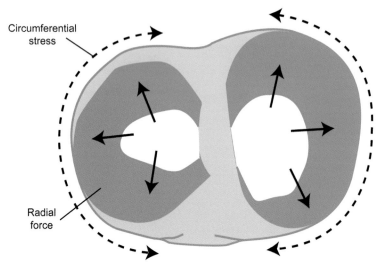

Figure 20.31 Menisci convert a compressive stress into a radial stress that is taken up by a circumferential (hoop) stress within the meniscus.

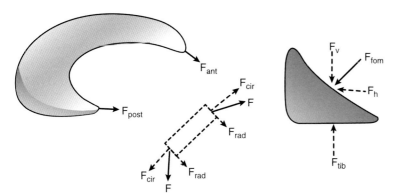

Figure 20.32 Free body diagram of forces acting on the meniscus during loading.

Structured oral examination question 4

Meniscus anatomy and function (see above).

EXAMINER: What is the histology of the meniscus?

CANDIDATE: The meniscus is primarily constituted of interlacing networks of collagen fibres (predominantly type 1 interposed between cells and an extracellular matrix (ECM) of proteoglycans and glycoproteins.

EXAMINER: What about the layers of the meniscus?

CANDIDATE: There are three collagen layers: superficial, lamellar and deep. The surface layer has a random organization of collagen fibres.

There are circumferential collagen fibre bundles and radial 'tie fibres' or tie sheaths. The radial fibres stabilize the meniscus, preventing circumferential splits and also resisting excessive compressive loads. The circumferential fibres function in hoops to accept stress without gross deformation or extrusion from the joint surface. The radial displacement is opposed by posterior and anterior attachments on the tibial plateau.

EXAMINER: When does a meniscus stop growing in a child?

CANDIDATE: The meniscus stops growing in a child when the growth plate closes.

Anatomically, the meniscus is fully vascularized at birth, but the area of vascularity recedes toward the periphery with age, such that, by the age of 10, only the peripheral 10–30% of the meniscus is vascularized, as is seen in the adult meniscus.

COMMENT: The menisci growth closely matches the growth of the femur and tibia.

EXAMINER: What meniscus is usually damaged with ACL injury?

CANDIDATE: Medial meniscus tears are more common in patients with chronic ACL insufficiency, lateral meniscus tears are predominately found in acute ACL injuries.

The lateral meniscus is more mobile than the medial meniscus and can become trapped between the femur and tibia during an acute pivoting episode. Most commonly, the tear occurs in the posterior third of the lateral meniscus, which does not have a strong attachment to the surrounding capsule.

The medial meniscus is a secondary stabilizer of the knee against anterior instability and can be commonly torn in chronic ACL injuries associated with significant knee instability.

3. Invertebral disc structure and function

Introduction

This subject just about makes it as an A-list basic science viva topic. Tipping the balance is that the basic science of degenerative disc disease may additionally find its way into a general adult and pathology viva on PID.

A good starting point is a basic understanding of the anatomy and function of the spine. Although candidates may not be directly asked about spine anatomy, they still need to be familiar with it. If a candidate appears unsure, the examiners may switch focus and start asking them pass/fail questions on spinal anatomy.

Structured oral examination question 1

EXAMINER: Describe the anatomy of the vertebral column

CANDIDATE: The normal adult vertebral column typically consists of 33 vertebrae (seven cervical;

12 thoracic; five lumbar; five fused sacral and four fused coccygeal).

It extends from the occipital condyles of the skull at the atlanto-occipital joint to the apex of the coccyx.

Movement of the vertebral column occurs through the 23 discs in the human spine. Apart from the fused vertebrae of the sacrum and coccyx, the only vertebrae not connected by discs are the atlas and axis, which pivot at the specialized atlanto-axial joint and the articulation between the atlas and the base of the skull at the occipitoatlantal joint.

EXAMINER: What are the individual anatomical features of each vertebral region?

CANDIDATE: In the cervical region there are C1 (atlas) and C2 (axis) which are considered specialized vertebrae. The C3 to C7 section is referred to as the subaxial region. The spinous processes are usually bifid. The vertebral bodies of the subaxial cervical spine have upward projections on the lateral margins called uncinate processes.

In the thoracic region there is a progressive increase in vertebral body mass from T1 to T12, pedicles are small in diameter, laminae are vertical, with a 'roof tile' arrangement, the spinous processes are long, overlapping and projected downwards and the intervertebral foramen is larger with less incidence of nerve compression.

In the lumbar region there is a progressive increase in vertebral body mass, pedicles are long and wider than the thoracic area and oval-shaped, the spinous processes are horizontal, square-shaped, transverse processes smaller than the thoracic region and the intervertebral foramen, although large, has an increased incidence of nerve root compression.

EXAMINER: What are the functions of the spine?

CANDIDATE: Functions of the spine include:
- Protection of the spinal cord.
- Providing for balance and stability of the body.
- It offers attachment points for the ribs and muscles of the back and trunk.
- Allows for flexibility and mobility.
- Supports the structure and weight of the body in various activities.

EXAMINER: What are the functions of the intervertebral disc?

CANDIDATE: The intervertebral disc:

- Allows the spine to twist and bend throughout a wide range of positions.
- Functions to absorb energy and distribute loads applied to the spine.
- Redistributes compressive loads, resists tensile, rotational and shear forces.
- Restricts excessive motion.

COMMENT: If all else fails, reply that the intervertebral disc is a load-bearing structure that gives mobility to the vertebral column. A misconception in the literature is that they act as shock absorbers, but there is no good evidence to support this function.[25] No need to complicate matters for yourself and mention this in the exam lest it alerts the examiners, who may then start asking you difficult questions.

EXAMINER: What is a motion segment?

CANDIDATE: The motion segment is the functional unit of the spine. It consists of the lower half of the upper vertebra, the upper half of the adjacent lower vertebra and the facet joints, intervertebral disc and the ligaments that lie between the adjacent vertebrae.

EXAMINER: What is the structure of the intervertebral disc?

CANDIDATE: There are three main regions to the intervertebral disc each with differing structural compositions: (1) outer annulus fibrosis, (2) inner nucleus pulposus and (3) endplates. Each has different functions.

EXAMINER: What is the structure of the annulus fibrosus?

CANDIDATE: The annulus fibrosis is the outer structure that encases the nucleus pulposus.

It is attached to both the anterior and posterior longitudinal ligaments of the spine and the vertebrae on either side.

It is mainly composed of type I collagen, water and proteoglycans.

It has a high collagen/low proteoglycan ratio.

Fibroblast-like cells are responsible for producing type I collagen and proteoglycans.

Characterized by high tensile strength and its ability to prevent intervertebral distraction.

It remains flexible enough to allow for motion.

Compared to the NP it is a much more fibrous structure with a much higher collagen but lower water content.

The AF can be divided into two regions, the outer third and the inner two-thirds.

The outer annulus fibrosus consists of a number of densely packed layers composed of predominantly type 1 collagen called lamellae. Fibres of each lamella run obliquely between vertebrae at about 30° to the horizon, with adjacent lamella typically running at right angles.

EXAMINER: Why is this?

CANDIDATE: This arrangement allows the disc to resist both torsional, axial and tensile loads (distraction and shear).

COMMENT: This is sometimes referred to as a hands-in-the-pocket configuration or plies in a tyre tread.

CANDIDATE: The lamellae are more abundant and stronger in the anterior and lateral aspects of the disc.

The larger fibrocartilaginous inner annulus fibrosus layer is found more centrally, containing chondrocytes and a less-dense, predominantly type II collagenous matrix lacking lamellar organization.

Therefore, on progressing from the outer to the inner annulus, the type I collagen level declines and that of the type II increases.

EXAMINER: Describe the structure of the nucleus pulposus.

CANDIDATE: The nucleus pulposus is the water-rich, gelatinous central portion of the intervertebral disc that is surrounded by the annulus fibrosis.

It is mainly composed of type II collagen, water and proteoglycans and polysaccharides.

It has a greater water content than the AF.

Chondrocyte-like cells are responsible for producing type II collagen and proteoglycans.

These cells continually maintain the matrix and rely on diffusion of nutrients from the end plates surviving in relatively hypoxic conditions.

The high density of negatively charged sulphate and carboxyl groups on the glycosaminoglycan chains of the major proteoglycan in the disc, aggrecan, are responsible for attracting the high water content.

Aggregates are held together by type II collagen that is cross-linked by type IX collagen. Equilibrium between the aggrecan and type II collagen helps in creating a load-bearing and compression-resisting tissue that gives stability to the disc.

A pressure is generated by swelling from the attraction of water into the IVD from surrounding tissues, resulting in the vertebral bodies being pushed apart. This pressure is resisted by tension in the collagen fibres of the AF.

The balance between expansion of the NP and tension in the AF leads the IVD to resist compression.

COMMENT: The candidate is relating NP structure to function. This should not draw any examiner criticism as to not answering the question,[26] as linking structure to function brings higher-order thinking into the topic.

EXAMINER: What are the functions of the NP?

CANDIDATE: The NP resists compressive loads, dampens mechanical loads and evenly distributes forces onto the end plates.

EXAMINER: What is the function of the matrix?

CANDIDATE: The disc matrix is an elaborate framework of macromolecules that attract and hold water. This viscoelastic matrix distributes forces smoothly to the annulus and the end plates.

The NP contains proteoglycan aggregates entrapped in a collagen fibre network.

The hydration properties of the glycosaminoglycan chains of aggrecan cause the tissue to swell until an equilibrium is reached, in which the swelling potential is balanced by tensile forces in the collagen network.

EXAMINER: What about the end plates? What is the function of the end plates?

CANDIDATE: The end plates are positioned above and below the nucleus and most of the annulus and are thin layers of hyaline cartilage that are considered part of the disc, not part of the vertebral body. The annulus and nucleus are firmly attached to the end plates and separation is difficult. The major function of the end plates is to act as a semipermeable membrane allowing nutrients and metabolites to diffuse into the disc from the capillary blood of the vertebral body and to allow waste products to diffuse out.

EXAMINER: How can oxygen and glucose and other nutrients diffuse through the usually impermeable tough periosteum of the vertebral body?

CANDIDATE: Under normal circumstances, no diffusion would occur; however, the subchondral

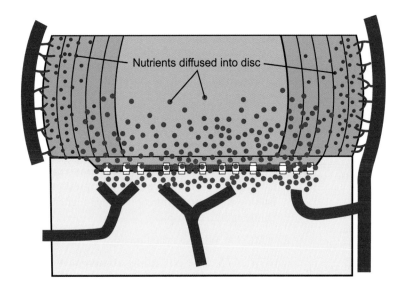

Figure 20.33 Diffusion of nutrients into the intervertebral disc.

Nutrients diffused into disc

bone of the vertebral bodies has special channels called marrow cavities that allow for diffusion to occur (Figure 20.33). Therefore, as long as these channels are open, the cells of the disc can receive oxygen, glucose and other amino acids, as well as have an avenue for waste removal.

EXAMINER: What about the blood supply of the intervertebral disc?

CANDIDATE: Intervertebral discs have no significant vascular supply. They receive their blood supply by diffusion through the vertebral body endplates. A network of vessels located centrally in the end plate allows nutrients to diffuse into the nucleus pulposus and annulus fibrosus (Figure 20.34).

Nutrients are supplied to the disc primarily through diffusion.

Because the disc has a very limited blood supply, invertebral disc cells, particularly those in the centre of the avascular NP, operate in an environment that would be unviable to most other cells. They appear to have adapted to this hypoxic, acidic environment.

EXAMINER: What happens to the disc with ageing?

CANDIDATE: With ageing there is decreased vascularity of the end plates. This reduces the nutrition supply to disc cells resulting in decreased synthesis and concentration of proteoglycans.

This leads to an overall loss of water content within the NP altering the biomechanical

response of the disc to physiological loading stresses. There is an increase in the proportion of type I to type II collagen and an increased ratio of keratin sulphate to chondroitin sulphate. There is conversion to fibrocartilage, which causes a generalized stiffening of the NP, with the net effect being a less biomechanically competent disc.

EXAMINER: What is the nerve supply to the intervertebral disc?

CANDIDATE: The posterior and posterolateral disc are innervated by the sinuvertebral nerve, the lateral disc by the grey ramus communicans (a sympathetic nerve of the autonomic system), and the anterior disc by sympathetic branches from the sympathetic trunk or ganglion that courses anterolaterally over the vertebral bodies (Figure 20.35).

Only the outer third (to a ~3 mm depth) of a healthy annulus is innervated and capable of transmitting pain. The inner two-thirds of the annulus and the entire nucleus are completely avascular (no blood vessels) and aneural (no nerves).

EXAMINER: Describe the natural history of a lumbar disc prolapse.

CANDIDATE: Recurrent torsional strain leads to tears of the outer annulus that lead to herniation of nucleus pulposus.

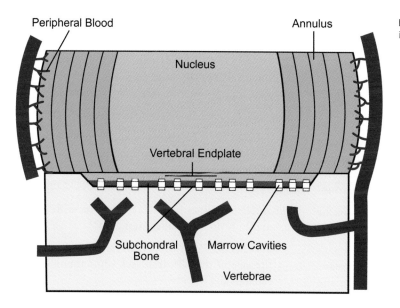

Figure 20.34 Blood supply of the intervertebral disc.

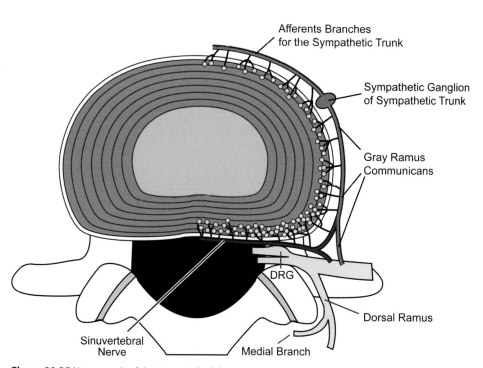

Figure 20.35 Nerve supply of the intervertebral disc.

Size of herniation decreases over time due to reabsorption via macrophage phagocytosis.

Smaller disc fragments are less likely to be resorbed while large sequestered disc herniations show the greatest degree of spontaneous resorption.

Approximately 90% of patients will have improvement in symptoms by 3 months.

EXAMINER: What are the risk factors for developing a disc prolapse?

CANDIDATE: Disc prolapse is related to failure of the annulus fibrosus due to either increased load/pressure or decreased mechanical strength. Pressure within the disc is maximized by forward flexion in a seated position. Torsional movement increases this further. There is also a role of ageing causing degeneration of the annulus, increasing the predisposition to tear. This means the annulus is less well supported and more prone to tearing.

EXAMINER: What are the suggested theories for the mechanism of production of pain in disc disease?

CANDIDATE: There are several possible mechanisms for development of pain in disc disease. The first is due to simple nerve compression and accounts for the radicular pain seen in disc prolapse. There is also a degree of compression in degenerative disc disease due to reduced disc height, causing foraminal stenosis.

The second type of pain is mechanical in nature and is due to the degenerative disc reducing in height and therefore providing a reduced structural role, which causes increased load through the posterior elements (e.g. facet joints) and their subsequent degeneration. The annulus has nociceptors in its outer third and therefore the micro tears due to trauma may be directly painful.

Finally, there is an altered cytokine profile within the degenerative disc with increased IL-1 that may be implicated in discogenic pain.

Structured oral examination question 2

Intervertebral discs, describe parts, contents, effect of ageing, disc function, nutrition, pathophysiology of prolapsed disc, hoop stresses, shock absorption, and what is lumbago vertebra.

EXAMINER: What is this (Figure 20.36)?

CANDIDATE: It is a picture of an intervertebral disc.

EXAMINER: Can you name the various blank labels of the disc?

COMMENT: Be able to name the various structures correctly and if you feel confident and the overall viva table is proceeding well go on to talk about how IVD structure is related to its function.

EXAMINER: Can you describe the various parts and contents of the disc?

COMMENT: Go through the three components of the disc (AF, NP and end plates) and try to link structure to function (see above question 1).[27]

EXAMINER: What are the functions of the disc?

CANDIDATE: The disc essentially functions as a shock absorber to redistribute compressive loads and resist tensile, rotational and shear forces. It allows spinal movement and provides stability.

EXAMINER: What happens to the disc with ageing and how does this affect function?

CANDIDATE: With ageing, the inner AF expands, the size of the NP decreases while the outer AF remains the same.

In the NP the concentration of viable cells decreases, proteoglycan and water concentrations decrease and there is a partial loss of structural integrity.

The NP undergoes a transition from fluid-like to solid-like behaviour, severely limiting the 'shock-absorbing' properties of the disc.

COMMENT: This is a solid score 6, but the answer could be better explained in terms of the changes.

The rate of synthesis of glycosaminoglycans, proteoglycans, link proteins and hyaluronan decreases progressively with age as they undergo continuous proteolytic degradation (MMPs and ADAMs). At the same time, the production of collagen type I increases.

This results in a number of changes.

Aggrecan content in the nucleus pulposus drops significantly, and with it the ability of the ECM to attract, bind and maintain water. The NP becomes progressively more fibrous and opaque, and with increased pigmentation. As the collagen content increases and changes from type II to type I, demarcation between the NP and AF becomes less distinct and separation of adjacent annular laminae occurs. This delamination leads to the development of concentric tears in the annular laminae.

COMMENT: Score 7/8.

EXAMINER: How is ageing different to degeneration?

COMMENT: This is a difficult, controversial topic that is testing higher-order thinking.

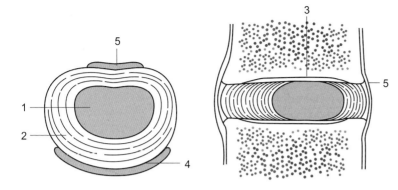

Figure 20.36 The intervertebral disc: 1, nucleus; 2, annulus; 3, cartilaginous end plate; 4, anterior longitudinal ligament; 5, posterior longitudinal ligament.

Although age-related disc changes and disc degeneration are considered separate entities, both share similar biomechanical alterations in the NP with the distinction between the two conditions often blurred.

Intervertebral discs receive the vast majority of their nutrient supply from diffusion across their end plates.

With ageing, the number of vascular channels perforating the osseous vertebral endplates diminishes. This leads to reduced porosity across the vertebral end plates and an accumulation of cell waste products and degraded matrix molecules that impair cell nutrition and function.

This gradual loss of viable cells within the NP further compromises matrix synthesis.

Similar to ageing, the major pathological process associated with disc degeneration is a declining nutritional support reaching the intervertebral disc cells. This leads to a decrease in the number and activity of disc cells.

Factors thought to accelerate disc degeneration include mechanical disc overload, genetic factors, immobilization and obesity.

Additional influences that may compromise disc blood supply leading to disc degeneration include smoking, diabetes and peripheral vascular disease. Each factor mediates its effect by either altering the balance of protein synthesis and degradation and/or the rate of cell death or apoptosis.

EXAMINER: What is the pathophysiology of the prolapsed disc?

CANDIDATE: Degenerative changes in the IVD alter the structural properties of disc components. The NP becomes stiffer with loss of water content and increase in tissue density. There is a more anisotropic stress state with a more non-uniform distribution of stresses. More stress is placed on the collagen fibres of the AF that they are not designed to tolerate. As such, the collagen structure of the AF deteriorates due to impaired formation, increased cross-linking and increased breakdown.

The end plates become thin, sclerotic and prone to microfracture.

This reduces a disc's ability to recover from deformation and predisposes to weakness of the AF, leaving it susceptible to annular fissuring and tearing.

EXAMINER: What are the macroscopic changes that occur?

CANDIDATE: There is narrowing of the disc space, osteophytes at the margins of end plates, increased stress at the facet joints, facet joint degeneration with osteophyte formation, bulging of the annulus and herniation of the NP through an annular fissure.

Osteophytes develop to attempt to stabilize the motion segment, but may encroach on neural structures.

EXAMINER: How do hoop stresses occur in the spine (Figures 20.37 and 20.38)?

CANDIDATE: When loaded from above, the height of the NP is reduced. It attempts to expand out against the annulus and the collagen rings (lamella) of the annulus are stretched. The radial pressure exerted by the NP is quickly balanced by the elastic tension that develops in the lengthening fibres of the annulus.

At the same time, the nucleus is constrained in the up–down sense by the end plates and vertebral bodies.

495

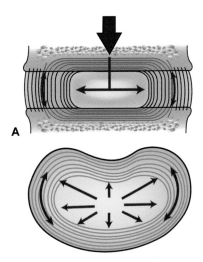

Figure 20.37 Compression force from body weight contraction (straight arrows) raises the pressure in the NP. This, in turn, increases the tension in the AF (curved arrows) and muscle.[29]

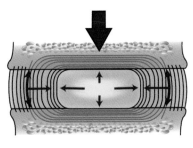

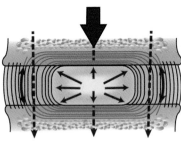

Figure 20.38 The increased tension in the AF inhibits radial expansion of the NP. The rising pressure in the NP is also exerted upward and downward against the vertebral end plates. The weight is partly borne by the AF and NP and is then transmitted across the end plates to neighbouring vertebrae.[30]

In this way, pressure applied to the NP is passed on to both the AF and the end plates. The fibres of the annulus are braced and prevented from buckling.

EXAMINER: How does the disc function as a shock absorber?

CANDIDATE: The conventional view was that a disc works as a shock absorber when the spine experiences a rapidly applied force; the force could be momentarily diverted into the annulus, easing the speed with which it must be transmitted down the chain of vertebrae.

The idea that the intervertebral discs act as a shock absorber has been challenged in recent years, with the view that by far the greatest amount of energy absorbed is from the muscles and tendons surrounding the spine, rather than by the disc.

COMMENT: A controversial and misunderstood concept that perhaps should not have been asked.[28]

The fibre orientation of the AF resists hoop stresses generated by the hydrostatic pressure from the NP (Figure 20.39). The AF provides the ability to absorb significant hoop stresses and maintain stiffness in the presence of tensile forces induced by bending and twisting of the spine. Animal experiments have demonstrated that even a partial thickness laceration in the annulus rapidly produces advanced disc degeneration.

COMMENT: This is probing for a more detailed answer than just concentrating on the gel-like material features of the NP.

Because the nucleus pulposus is gelatinous, the load of axial compression is distributed not only vertically but also radially throughout the nucleus. This radial distribution of the vertical load (tangential loading of the disc) is absorbed by the fibres of the annulus and can be compared with the hoops around a barrel.

EXAMINER: What is lumbago vertebrae?

CANDIDATE: Sorry, I have no idea.

COMMENT: Lumbago is a seldom-used term to mean mild to severe low-back pain. The pain can be acute or chronic and affect old or young patients. Many years ago, lumbago was associated with 'rheumatism', another loosely used term, seemingly brought on by exposure to cold damp winter weather. Low-back pain is a more precise term and should preferably be used instead.

EXAMINER: What is the role of aggrecan and collagen in the ability of discs to resist compression?

CANDIDATE: The NP contains proteoglycan aggregates entrapped in a collagen fibre network.

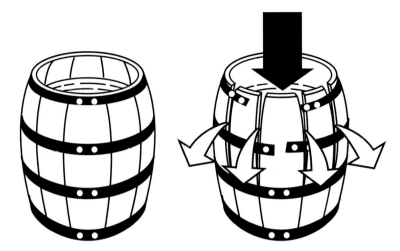

Figure 20.39 Hoop stress. A load of water in a barrel is resisted by the hoops around the barrel. When too great a load is applied, the hoop will break. The annulus functions in a similar manner to that of the hoops around a water barrel.

The hydration properties of the glycosaminoglycan chains of aggrecan cause the tissue to swell until an equilibrium is reached, in which the swelling potential is balanced by tensile forces in the collagen network.

Compressive loading of the spine forces some water from the disc effectively increasing the aggrecan concentration and its swelling potential and resisting further compression.

On removal of the compressive load, disc height is restored as water is drawn back into the tissue to restore the original equilibrium conditions. Any parameter that decreases proteoglycan concentration or weakens the collagen network will be detrimental to disc function.

Structured oral examination question 5

EXAMINER: What is the purpose of the spine?

CANDIDATE: The primary purpose of the spine is to provide protection for the spinal cord and axial support system to allow locomotion and function of limbs. It has three natural curves which provide an S-shape.

[I genuinely didn't know what to say at this stage, which can be seen by the rather pathetic statement above.]

EXAMINER: OK, what is the primary site of movement in the spine?

CANDIDATE: [The penny drops!] Much of the ability to rotate and move within the spinal column is possible due to the intervertebral discs.

EXAMINER: Tell me about the anatomy of the intravertebral disc?

CANDIDATE: Essentially the disc is made up of two parts, the outer annulus fibrosus and the inner nucleus pulposus. In the cervical and lumbar spine, the discs are thicker anteriorly and in the thoracic spine the disc is equal. The largest disc is at the level of L5/S1.

[The largest disc is actually L4/5, but the examiner either didn't know himself or didn't want to push me at this stage.]

The classic paper to quote and read is Coventry et al.[31] There are three parts to this.

EXAMINER: OK, can you tell me about the structure in more detail?

CANDIDATE: The annulus fibrosus makes up the peripheral portion of disk structure and is predominantly made up from fibrocartilage and type I collagen. The fibres run obliquely and are arranged primarily in concentric layers. The orientation of the fibres varies in successive layers and alternates at about 45°. The nucleus pulposus is predominantly type II collagen and has a high water content, which enables it to resist compressive loads. With age, the water content declines, which reduces its resilience.

EXAMINER: What is the nerve supply?

CANDIDATE: The majority of the nerve supply lies in the outer rings of the annulus fibrosus, with supply from the sympathetic chain interiorly.

EXAMINER: And posterior?

CANDIDATE: I can't recall!

[Sinus vertebral nerve dorsally]

EXAMINER: Why is discitis common in children then?

CANDIDATE: Blood vessels occur in the annulus up to late teens, and into the cartilage end plates up to 8 years, which is why discitis occurs in this specific paediatrics group.

A good paper to explain this question is by Rudert *et al.*[32] The vascular pattern of human intervertebral discs and the surrounding tissue at different ages were investigated using histochemical methods.

The occurrence of blood and lymph vessels in growing intervertebral discs helps us to understand childhood discitis without simultaneous affection of the vertebral body.

4. Muscle structure and function

An appreciation of muscle anatomy and physiology is important in the understanding of muscle injury. However, a passive read through of this topic in a standard orthopaedic textbook is quite poor preparation for a viva question. Like most basic science subjects, it takes time and effort to fully appreciate the topic and develop the higher-order thinking needed to master the subject. It is worth knowing this subject well as it is definitely an A-list topic.

Structured oral examination question 1

EXAMINER: What is this picture (Figure 20.40)?

CANDIDATE: This is an electron micrograph picture of skeletal muscle.

EXAMINER: Why do you say this?

CANDIDATE: We can see striations alternating light (I) and dark (A) bands.

EXAMINER: Can you identify sarcomeres, A bands, I bands, Z lines, M lines and H zones (Figure 20.41)?

CANDIDATE: A sarcomere is the basic unit of striated muscle tissue. It is the contractile unit of a muscle cell. It spans from one Z line (disc) to the next.

The Z line represents the attachment of adjacent sarcomeres. This is taken from the German word 'Zwischen', meaning between. Actin fibres are anchored on the Z line.

The I band represents just actin filaments in adjacent sarcomeres where there is no overlap with myosin filaments.

In between the I bands is the A band of the sarcomere. It is darker on the edges where there is a double, overlapping, hexagonal array of thick filaments (mostly myosin) and thin filaments (actin plus the regulating proteins: troponin and tropomyosin). It is anisotropic.

The central H zone of the A band contains only thick myosin filaments. It is a less-dense, lighter region from the German 'Heller' for 'brighter'.

The M-line (or M-band) maintains (anchors) the myosin filaments in a hexagonal lattice and the Z-line (or Z-band) maintains the actin filaments in a tetragonal lattice.

COMMENT: The relationship between the A band and H zone can be confusing.

The A band is a dark overlap of thin and thick filaments that also contains the central H zone composed of thick myosin filaments only (Figure 20.42).

Mentioning the German word 'Zwischen' (between) for some reason seemed to greatly impress the examiners.

CANDIDATE: As the I bands are uniform (iso = same/uniform) in appearance throughout they are called isotropic bands. The dark A bands are not uniform as they have both thick and thin filaments and are therefore called anisotropic.

EXAMINER: What do you mean by isotropic and anisotropic bands?

COMMENT: Candidates need to be careful (especially in the basic science viva) not to use terms they do not fully understand. Better to just stay quiet and not be caught out!

CANDIDATE: Each sarcomere contains an anisotropic (doubly refractive, therefore dark in phase microscopy) band bounded by two isotropic (singly refractive, therefore light) bands. The anisotropic band is called the A band; the isotropic band is called the I band. Actually, each sarcomere contains two half-I bands (one at each end) because a single I band straddles the Z line and therefore is part of two adjacent sarcomeres. In the centre of the A band, there is a lighter region known as the H zone or H band.

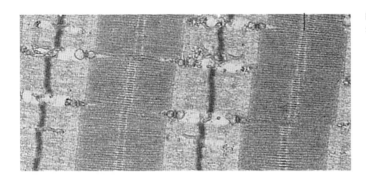

Figure 20.40 Unlabelled electron micrograph picture of skeletal muscle.

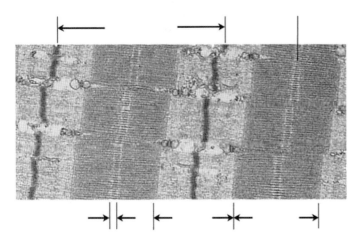

Figure 20.41 Bare labelled electron micrograph picture of skeletal muscle.

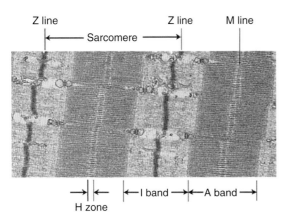

Figure 20.42 Labelled diagram of skeletal muscle.

EXAMINER: What is the structure of actin and myosin?

CANDIDATE: Each myofibril is made of parallel filaments, thick and thin filaments. The thick filaments are made of a protein called myosin. It is shaped like a golf club with two heads.

The thin filament is made of a protein called actin. Actin is a complex globular molecule represented by two chains of beads in a double helix.

Tropomyosin is situated between two actin strands in a double helix configuration. In the resting state, tropomyosin blocks the myosin binding sites on actin.

Troponin is a complex of three separate proteins that is closely associated with tropomyosin. When troponin binds to calcium a conformational change in the troponin complex occurs. This results in a conformational change in tropomyosin, exposing the myosin binding sites on actin.

EXAMINER: What happens to the I and A bands with muscle contracture? Can you identify which sarcomere is contracted in these pictures (Figures 20.43 and 20.44)?

CANDIDATE:

- In a relaxed muscle, actin and myosin myofilaments lie side by side and the H zones and I bands are at maximum width.

499

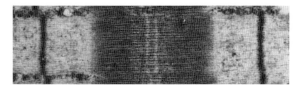

Figure 20.43 Relaxed muscle.

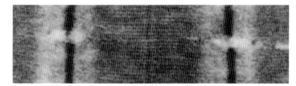

Figure 20.44 Contracted muscle.

- During contracture the actins are pulled towards the centre of each myosin myofilament. As a result, the sarcomeres shorten.
- The Z lines move closer together.
- The I band becomes shorter.
- The A band stays at the same length.
- In a fully contracted muscle, the ends of the actin myofilaments overlap, the H zone disappears and the I band becomes very narrow.

COMMENT: Observations that during muscle contraction, the I and H bands become narrower, while the A band did not, coupled with the observation that thick and thin filaments do not shorten led to the sliding theory model of contracture.

EXAMINER: Can you draw what is happening to the actin and myosin within the muscle sarcomere when the muscle contracts?

CANDIDATE: (Figure 20.45)

COMMENT: This question (we think) tests in equal measure a candidate's drawing ability and muscle sarcomere knowledge.

EXAMINER: How do muscles contract? Explain how skeletal muscles contract.

COMMENT: Having dealt with the microstructure of the sarcomere the second part of the topic deals with how the myosin heads interact with the actin filaments.

An answer would be expected to cover the following points:

- The release of calcium ions from the sarcoplasmic reticulum.

Fully relaxed sarcomere of a muscle fibre

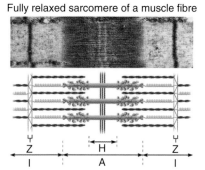

Fully contracted sarcomere of a muscle fibre

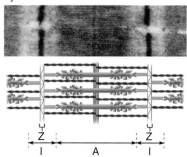

Figure 20.45 Skeletal muscle actin/myosin arrangement with relaxation and contracture.

- The formation of cross-bridges.
- The sliding of actin and myosin filaments.
- The use of ATP to break cross-bridges and reset myosin heads.

When muscles contract, actin slides over the myosin and causes the sarcomere to shorten.

In resting muscle fibres, Ca^{2+} is stored in the sarcoplasmic reticulum. Muscle cells have a unique membrane structure, called the transverse tubule or simply the T-tubule. The T-tubule is an invagination of the muscle membrane that plunges repeatedly into the interior of the fibre.

The T-tubules terminate near the calcium-filled sacs of the sarcoplasmic reticulum. The arrival of the action potential at the ends of the T-tubules triggers the release of Ca^{2+}. The Ca^{2+} diffuses among the thick and thin filaments where it binds to troponin on the thin filaments. This turns on the interaction between actin and myosin and the sarcomere contracts.

Due to the speed of the action potential (milliseconds), the action potential arrives virtually simultaneously at the ends of all the T-tubules, ensuring that all sarcomeres contract in unison. When the process is over, the calcium is pumped

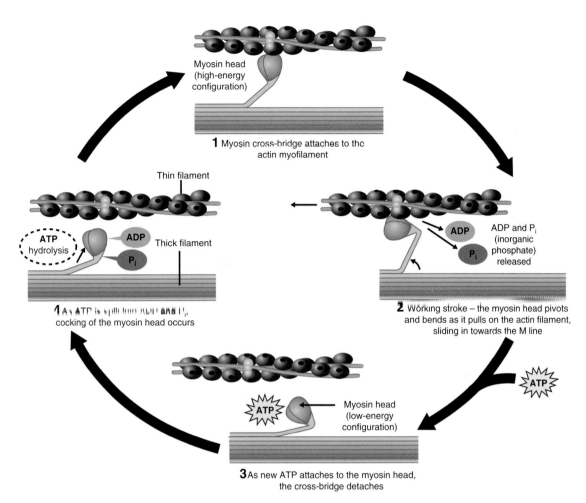

Figure 20.46 Cross-bridge cycle.

back into the sarcoplasmic reticulum using a Ca^{2+} ATPase.

The hydrolysis of ATP causes the myosin heads to change shape and swivel which moves them towards the next actin binding site.

The movement of the myosin heads causes the actin filaments to slide over the myosin filaments, shortening the length of the sarcomere.

Via the repeated hydrolysis of ATP, the skeletal muscle will contract.

EXAMINER: What do we mean by the cross-bridge cycle (Figure 20.46)?

CANDIDATE: The cross-bridge cycle consists of four steps:

1. ATP hydrolysis.

Hydrolysis of ATP reorients and energizes the myosin head.

2. Formation of cross-bridges.

Myosin head attaches to the myosin-binding site on actin.

3. Power stroke.

During the power stroke the cross-bridge rotates, sliding the filaments.

4. Detachment of myosin from actin.

As the next ATP binds to the myosin head, the myosin head detaches from actin. The contraction cycle repeats as long as ATP is available and the Ca^{2+} level is sufficiently high. Continuing cycles applies the force that shortens the sarcomere.

EXAMINER: What is the role of ATP in muscle contracture?

CANDIDATE: ATP is the immediate source of energy for muscle contraction. Although a muscle

501

fibre contains only enough ATP to power a few twitches, its ATP 'pool' is replenished as needed.

EXAMINER: What are the actual events occurring in muscle contraction and relaxation?

CANDIDATE:

Membrane excitation
- Arrival of motor neuron action potential from a nerve cell at the neuromuscular junction.
- Synaptic transmission at the neuromuscular junction with release of acetylcholine into the synaptic cleft and diffusion across to bind to sarcomere receptors.
- Local depolarization occurs with the action potential propagating along the sarcolemma leading to hypopolarization of T-tubules.

Excitation–contraction coupling
- At the end of the T-tubules the depolarization triggers Ca^{2+} release from the sarcoplasmic reticulum.
- Ca^{2+} binds to the troponin C molecule, resulting in a cooperative configurational change in the troponin–tropomyosin complex.
- Release of inhibition of myosin-ATPase.
- Link between thick and thin filaments, swivel of myosin head.
- Tension exerted.
- Shortening by sliding filament.

Muscle recovery
- Ca^{2+} removed from sarcoplasm and transported back into the sarcoplasmic reticulum.
- Mg^{2+} ATP bound by actinomyosin.
- Cross-bridges disconnected.
- Actinomyosin-ATPase inhibited.
- Active tension disappears.

Structured oral examination question 2

Viva question 2 tests similar knowledge to viva question 1, but they are not identical and are probably different diets of the exam rather than a candidate 6 versus a candidate 8 situation.

EXAMINER: How do you classify skeletal muscles?

CANDIDATE: Muscles can be classified according to:
- Shape and fascicular architecture.
- Myoglobin content (red, white).

- Type of contractile activity (isometric, isotonic) (concentric, eccentric and isokinetic).
- The relative magnitude of their stabilizing and rotatory components.
- Orientation of the line of pull to the joint surface (flexors, extensors, abductors and adductors).
- The number of joints over which the muscle crosses.
- Type of muscle action or function (their interaction in joint movement) (agonists, antagonists, synergists and fixators).

EXAMINER: Tell me about the types of muscle contraction that can occur. What do we mean by isometric and isotonic muscle contracture?

CANDIDATE: 1. **Isometric contraction** (iso = equal + metric = length):

Force is generated but the muscle does not shorten (no movement).

Muscle is held at a fixed length. The muscle contraction is activated, but instead of being allowed to lengthen or shorten, it is held at a constant length. Examples include when one pushes against an immoveable object such as a wall or the rotator cuff and its ability to compress the humerus into the glenoid surface.

2. **Isotonic contraction** (iso = equal + tonic = tone or tension):

Constant force with change in muscle length (movement).

a. Concentric contracture.

b. Eccentric contracture.

Concentric contraction (con = towards + centric = centre).

It is a contraction in which the origin and insertion of the contracting muscle are brought closer together due to the action of the muscle. Generation of a force leads to muscle contracture and shortening if the load on the muscle is less than the force the muscle creates.

Eccentric contraction: (Ecc = away from + centric = centre)

It is a contraction in which the origin and insertion of the contracting muscle are moved away from each other by an external force. Despite the muscle contracting the muscle lengthens, as the force generated is less than the external force.

Biceps curls exhibit both concentric and eccentric contraction. During flexion, the bicep is undergoing concentric contraction, and during controlled extension, the biceps is undergoing eccentric contraction.

Isokinetic contraction (iso = equal + kinetics = motion):

This involves keeping the speed (distance per unit time) constant on an actively contracting muscle while the load is changed in order to maintain a constant velocity. Isokinetic exercises require special exercise equipment and are a measure of dynamic strength. The exercises are best used for rehabilitation protocols and are not routinely observed in most muscles during normal activities.

COMMENT: This is the warm-up question!

EXAMINER: What macroscopic types of muscles do you know?

CANDIDATE: Muscles can be broadly classified into either parallel, where the muscle fibres are parallel to the line of pull, or pennate, where the short muscle fibres are oblique to the line of pull (Figure 20.47).

A parallel muscle has an increased range of movement due to increased length of fibres. The total force of contracture is less because there are less numbers of fibres.

Parallel muscles are subdivided into the following subtypes:

1. Strap (sartorius, rectus femoris).
2. Fan-shaped (triangular) (pec major).
3. Fusiform muscles (biceps).

Pennate muscles can be subdivided into:

1. Unipennate.
2. Bipennate.
3. Multipennate.

   1. Unipennate muscles have fibres (fascicles) that insert on only one side of a tendon, thereby

creating a relatively large cross-section and greater strength but smaller change in length.
2. Bipennate muscles insert on two sides of the tendon, increasing relative cross-section, allowing greater strength than a unipennate muscle with smaller changes in length.
3. Multipennate muscles are where a series of bipennate muscles lie side by side in one plane.

The benefit of pennation is that it allows for a greater packing of fibres into a given anatomical cross-sectional area. However, their range of movement is diminished because of the shortness of muscle fibres and oblique direction of pull.

Pennate muscles are located in positions requiring small but powerful movements, parallel muscles are located in positions requiring longer movements with less power.

EXAMINER: What is the role of the horizontal component of a pennate muscle?

CANDIDATE: The force of muscle action is resolved into two component forces – one acts in the line of pull and the other at right angles to it. This muscle force is essentially wasted, but not that much, and while contracting such muscles squeeze themselves, thus becoming more solid and compact.

COMMENT: This is not in the standard orthopaedic textbooks! That's what makes the basic science viva so feared! Trying to work this out from first principles during the viva is tough-going.

EXAMINER: Can you draw me the structure of a muscle?

CANDIDATE:

• Epimysium wraps around an entire muscle.
• Perimysium subdivides each muscle into fascicles, bundles of 10–100 muscle fibres.

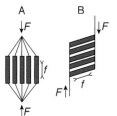

Figure 20.47 The two arrangements of muscle fibres within a muscle. (A) Parallel arrangement. (B) Pennate arrangement. Double-headed arrows (*f*) indicate direction of force exerted by individual muscle fibres.

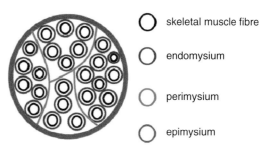

Figure 20.48 Candidate drawing. Cross-section of a skeletal muscle.

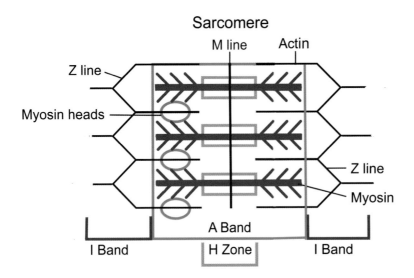

Sarcomere

Figure 20.49 Candidate 20-second exam drawing of skeletal muscle sarcomere. Z line is where the thin filament (actin) creates a zig-zag pattern. One sarcomere is Z-line to Z-line. In between the I bands is the A band (darker on the edges, just myosin present in the H zone).

- Endomysium surrounds individual muscle fibres.

  These connective tissues form a continuous membrane around and within the muscle belly.

COMMENT: The muscle cross-sectional structure/arrangement (Figure 20.48) is universal across all connective tissues (epi, peri and endo) and includes nerves, tendons and ligaments. The sarcomere drawing (Figure 20.49) deals with muscle ultrastructure and is more complicated to draw and explain.

  Actin – thin filaments have actin because if you're active (actin) you will be thin.

  Myosin – o and s short and fat letters.

EXAMINER: What are the different types of skeletal muscles and can you draw them?

CANDIDATE: A. Muscles can be divided into:

1. **Parallel**

Fascicles run parallel to the long axis of the muscle to provide a stronger pull (sartorius, rectus abdominis).

2. **Fusiform**
3. **Pennate**

Fascicles are short.

Attached obliquely to a central tendon that runs the length of the muscle.

Produce more tension (more muscle fibres).

Unipennate (palmer interosseous), bipennate (rectus femoris) and multipennate (deltoid) – to how many sides of the tendon do the fascicles attach?

4. **Convergent (fan-shaped)** Broad at origin converging to a narrower insertion, less pull than parallel muscles (pec major).

5. **Circular** – fascicles arranged in a concentric ring. Act as sphincters, a ring around a body opening (orbicularis oris).

COMMENT: Candidates need to be able to draw out the various types of muscles (unipennate, fusiform, strap) along with examples and be able to discuss the advantages of each type of muscle shape (Figure 20.50).

EXAMINER: What is the hierarchical structure of muscle (Figure 20.51)?

CANDIDATE: Sarcomere > myofibril > muscle fibre (single elongated muscle cell) (endomysium) > muscle fascicle (perimysium) > bundles of muscle fascicles > single muscle (epimysium)

COMMENT: Terminology can be confusing.

  Bundles of muscle fascicles make up a single muscle = muscle bundles (fascicles) make up a single muscle.

  Bundles of 10–100 muscle fibres make up a muscle fascicle.

  A fascicle is the smallest unit of structure visible to the naked eye.

EXAMINER: Draw the structure of striated muscle fibres including the myofibrils with light and dark bands, mitochondria, the sarcoplasmic reticulum, nuclei and the sarcolemma (Figures 20.52 and 20.53).

CANDIDATE: The sarcomere is the smallest contractile unit of skeletal muscle.

  The sarcolemma is the cell membrane that surrounds the muscle fibre and has periodic

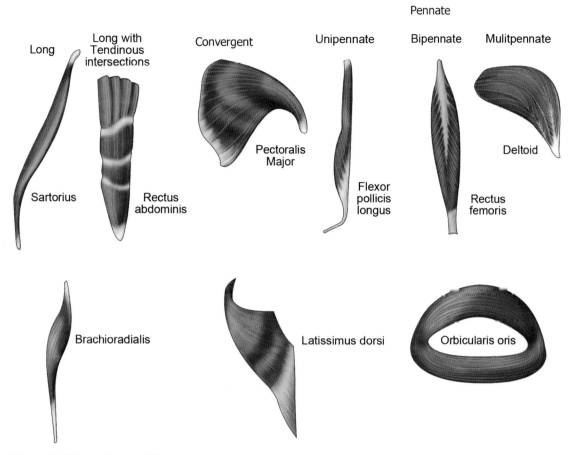

Figure 20.50 Muscle shape and fibre arrangement.

invaginations that descend into the muscle cell forming transverse tubules (T-tubules).

These T-tubules allow the depolarization that occurs during cell contraction to propagate deep into the cell.

The sarcoplasmic reticulum stores calcium (Ca^{2+}) in intracellular membrane-bound channels.

EXAMINER: How does muscle move at a microscopic level, how do troponin, myosin and tropomysin interact?

COMMENT: Similar info to that asked for in oral examination question 2. This is one of the pivotal knowledge areas in the muscle section the Tr & Orth curriculum sets out to test.

CANDIDATE: Sarcomere contraction is regulated by troponin and tropomyosin. Troponin is closely associated with tropomyosin along the actin thin filament and serves as a regulatory protein for contracture. Troponin has three subunits, I, T and C.

Troponin I is inhibitory and is able to block actin–myosin interactions.

Troponin T enables binding of troponin and tropomysin.

Troponin C binds calcium.

When myoplasmic calcium concentrations are low, the troponin–tropomyosin complex is situated on the actin filament in a way that prevents actin–myosin cross-bridge formation (Figure 20.54).

A rise in myoplasmic Ca^{2+} allows Ca^{2+} to bind with troponin C. This binding causes a conformational change in the troponin I molecule complex that removes the troponin–tropomyosin complex from the actin binding sites. This change permits myosin–actin cross-bridge cycling.

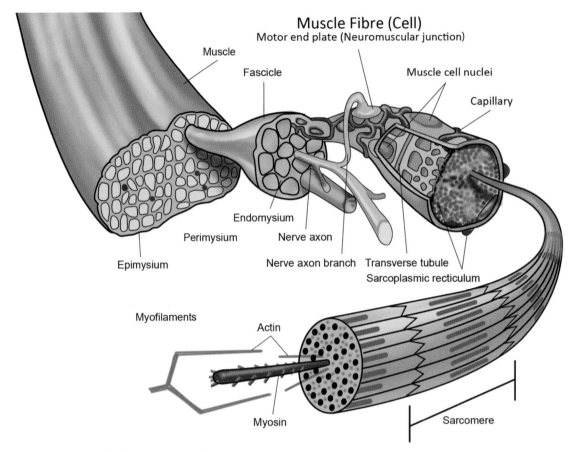

Figure 20.51 Hierarchical structure of muscle.

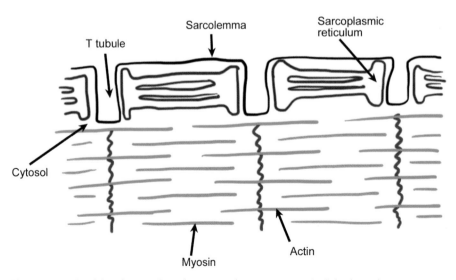

Figure 20.52 Candidate diagram. Sarcoplasmic reticulum arrangement in skeletal muscle.

Myofibril   Sarcolemma   Mitochondrion   T tubule   Sarcoplasmic reticulum

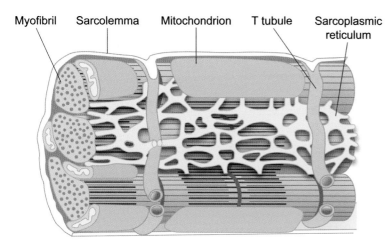

Figure 20.53 Sarcoplasmic reticulum arrangement in skeletal muscle.

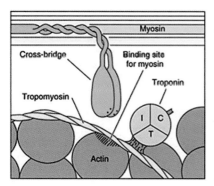 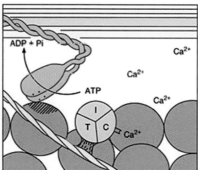

Figure 20.54 Cross-bridge. Troponin T (tropomyosin binding), troponin I (inhibitory protein) and troponin C (calcium binding). Binding of Ca^{2+} to the TnC unit of troponin exposes the myosin binding site on actin.

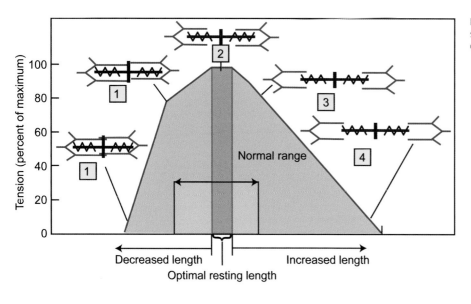

Figure 20.55 Length versus strength of muscle contraction.

Force–Velocity Relationship

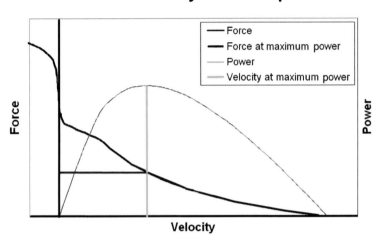

Figure 20.56 Force velocity curve of a skeletal muscle. Right of the vertical axis concentric contractions (the muscle is shortening), left of the axis eccentric contractions (the muscle is lengthened under load); power developed by the muscle in red.

When Ca^{2+} concentrations return to normal resting levels, troponin I reverts to its inhibitory conformation and the actin binding sites are again blocked from forming cross-bridges.

EXAMINER: What about length versus strength of muscle contraction, and the graph, which shows this (Figure 20.54)?

CANDIDATE: Muscles generate the greatest force when at their resting (ideal) length, and the least amount of force when shortened or stretched relative to their resting length.

Skeletal muscle fibre force production is defined in terms of myofilament overlap, i.e. in terms of sarcomere length. At optimal length, where actin–myosin interactions are maximal, muscle generates maximum force (region 2).

As sarcomere length increases (region 3), force decreases owing to the decreasing number of interactions between actin and myosin myofilaments.

At lengths shorter than the optimum (region 1), force decreases owing to double interdigitation of actin filaments with both myosin and actin filaments from opposite sides of the sarcomere.

EXAMINER: What about the force–velocity relationship (Figure 20.56)?

CANDIDATE: The force–velocity relationship in muscle relates the speed at which a muscle changes length with the force of this contraction and the resultant power output (force × velocity = power).

The force generated by a muscle depends on the number of actin and myosin cross-bridges formed; a larger number of cross-bridges results in a larger amount of force. However, cross-bridge formation is not immediate, so if myofilaments slide over each other at a faster rate the ability to form cross-bridges and resultant force are both reduced.

At maximum velocity no cross-bridges can form, so no force is generated, resulting in the production of zero power (right edge of graph). The reverse is true for stretching of muscle.

The amount of force a sarcomere can exert, outside of the relative length at which it functions, is dependent on the speed the sarcomere is contracting.

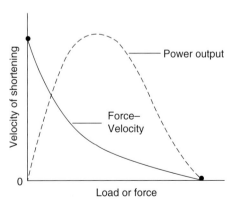

Figure 20.57 Force velocity curve with eccentric contracture. Force and velocity are inversely related such that at zero (0) velocity maximum force is generated, and at maximum velocity zero (0) force is generated.

Making the cross-bridges necessary for contraction takes time. When the filaments are being moved at a higher velocity, fewer myosin heads can bind to the actin filaments at a given time and as a result the total force is lower.

A higher speed during a concentric contraction results in a lower force. At speed 0, or an isometric contraction, the force is greater. When the contraction velocity turns negative and the sarcomere is stretched (eccentric contraction), the force a sarcomere generates increases even further. This can be explained by the force required to stretch passive structures and lengthen the muscle (Figure 20.57).

Although the force of the muscle is increased, there is no velocity of contraction and zero power is generated. Maximum power is generated at approximately one-third of maximum shortening velocity.

5. Structure and function of tendons and ligaments

Introduction

Tendon and ligaments are complex connective tissues often grouped together as they share similar tissue composition and properties.

Candidates should, however, appreciate there are also significant functional and structural differences between these two tissues that the examiners may wish to discuss.

Tendon and ligament disorders are especially common, so it is important to have a clear understanding of their function in both health and disease.

Potential score 7/8 candidates should have something up their sleeve if the examiners probe into new treatment options and evidence for their therapeutic benefit.

Structured oral examination question 1

Tendon structure and function. Leading on to a discussion about tendinopathy versus tendonitis.

EXAMINER: What is the function of tendons?

CANDIDATE: Tendons attach muscle to bone and function to:

- Transmit tensile loads from skeletal muscle contracture to bone resulting in joint movement.

- Enable the muscle belly to be positioned away from the joint so that bulky muscle bodies do not obstruct movement.

EXAMINER: What are ligaments?

CANDIDATE: Ligaments are dense bands of collagenous tissue (fibres) that span a joint and become anchored to bone at either end.

EXAMINER: What is the function of ligaments?

CANDIDATE: Ligaments attach bone to bone and function to:

- Transmit tensile load from bone to bone.
- Provide joint stability by maintaining joint congruency.
- Limit freedom of movement by preventing excessive motion, being a static restraint.
- Contribute to proprioception and position sense.

EXAMINER: What are the differences in structure between ligaments and tendons (Table 20.5)?

COMMENT: If a fairly low-key viva start the generalized details contained in Table 20.5 should be sufficient. However, candidates are often probed in more detail about specific percentage differences in composition between tendons and ligaments (Table 20.6).

- Ligaments have a more random organization with a weaving pattern of collagen orientation compared to a more parallel collagen arrangement seen in tendons. They have a slightly lower collagen content compared to tendons but contain more ground substance.

Table 20.5 Structural differences between tendons and ligaments.

	Ligaments	Tendons
% of collagen	Lower	Higher
% of ground substance	Higher	Lower
Organization	More random	Organized
Strength	Weaker	Stronger
Orientation	Weaving layered pattern	Long axis direction
	Each layer has parallel fibres	
Blood supply	Via paratenon (vascular) Sheathed avascular tendons via single vinculae (mesotendon) and diffusion	Via insertion site, runs longitudinally

Table 20.6 Compositional comparison between tendons and ligaments.

Component	Ligaments	Tendons
Cellular material		
Fibroblasts	20%	20%
Tenocytes	Some present after healing of tendon/ ligament	
Extracellular		
Water	60–80%	60–80%
Solids	20–40%	20–40%
Collagen	70–80%	Slightly higher
Type I	90%	95–99%
Type III	10%	1–5%
Ground substance	20–30%	Slightly less
Elastin	Slightly greater	Less

EXAMINER: What else?

CANDIDATE:

- Ligaments and tendons are composed of cells and extracellular matrix.
- Cells (fibroblasts) occupy around 20% of the total tissue volume, while the extracellular matrix accounts for the remaining 80%.
- The extracellular matrix is composed of water (70%) and solids (30%).
- The solid part of the matrix is mainly composed of collagen, but also ground substance and a small amount of elastin.
- The collagen content is 70–80% in ligaments, slightly higher in tendons. Type I collagen is higher in tendons (95–99%) compared to ligaments (90%) and Type III collagen accounts for 1–5% in tendons and 10% in ligaments.

EXAMINER: What functions does the ground substance perform?

CANDIDATE: The ground substance comprises hyaluronan, proteoglycans (decorin, biglycan, fibromodulin, lumican), structural glycoproteins and a wide variety of other molecules.

The highly viscous and hydrophilic nature of the ground substance acts as a cement-like filling between the long, thin collagen molecules and provides the lubrication and spacing that enables collagen fibres to slide.

It contains proteoglycan aggregates that bind most of the extracellular water of ligaments and tendons, making the matrix a highly structured, gel-like material.

EXAMINER: What about elastin?

CANDIDATE: Elastin isn't usually present in ligaments to any large degree. The ligamentum flava and ligamentum nuchae are the two main exceptions. These ligaments contain large amounts of elastin.

EXAMINER: How is collagen synthesized?

COMMENT: Collagen synthesis again! Candidates need to rehearse an answer based around the cellular collagen synthesis diagram. This can be quite detailed in some textbooks, but it is best to try and keep your answer fairly simply and low key.

CANDIDATE: Collagen synthesis occurs in several stages with both intracellular and extracellular steps.

The first stage in the synthesis of collagen is the formation inside the cell of mRNA for each type of polypeptide alpha-chain.

Messenger RNA translation initiates synthesis of polypeptide chains in the rough endoplasmic reticulum.

Subsequently, the signal peptide is cleaved off, lysine and proline amino acids are hydroxylated and the hydroxylated amino acid residues are glycosylated.

The resultant procollagen is packaged into secretory vesicles in the Golgi apparatus.

On release into the extracellular matrix the ends of the procollagen are cleaved enzymatically by peptides to form tropocollagen fibrils.

Several adjacent collagen molecules pack together (aggregate), overlapping by a quarter staggered array and appear as cross-striations under an electron microscope.

EXAMINER: Describe the structure of a tendon.

CANDIDATE: Tendons are composed of cells and extracellular matrix. The cells are fibroblasts and make up 20% of the total tissue volume. Most of the extracellular matrix is water (70%), but around 30% of the matrix is solid, comprising mainly type I collagen, ground substance and a small amount of elastin.

EXAMINER: What about its hierarchical structure?

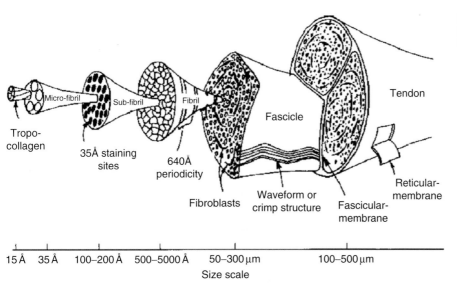

Figure 20.58 Classic tendon hierarchical structure by Kastelic *et al.*

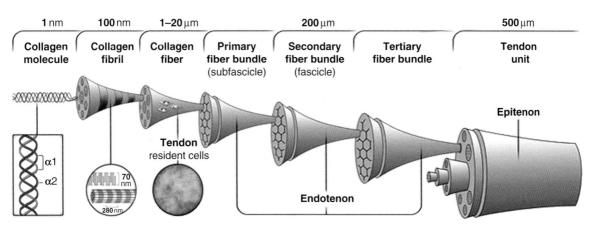

Figure 20.59 Alternative tendon hierarchical structure.

COMMENT: Although there are lots of different ways to draw this diagram there are two main illustrations that regularly appear in textbooks. Although both are quite similar there are also enough differences to cause confusion. We have included both for completeness sake (Figures 20.58 and 20.59). Our own preference is for the classic tendon structure described by Kastelic *et al.* (Figure 20.58).

CANDIDATE:

1. Classic tendon structure and description by Kastelic *et al.*[33]

   Tropocollagen molecules assemble into microfibrils, these microfibrils into subfibrils and several subfibrils give rise to a collagen fibril, with a characteristic 65 nm periodicity visible in scanning electron microscopy.

   Multiple fibrils combine to form a tendon fascicle, and fascicles, separated by the endotenon, join together to form the macroscopic tendon.

2. Alternative hierarchy structure of tendon.

   Collagen molecules assemble into collagen fibrils with a characteristic 65 nm periodicity visible in scanning electron microscopy. Multiple collagen fibrils are packed into larger structures to form collagen fibres. Multiple collagen fibres form primary fiber bundles (subfascicle), groups of which form secondary fibre bundles (fascicle). Multiple secondary fibre bundles form tertiary fibre bundles, groups of which in turn form the tendon unit.

Primary, secondary and tertiary bundles are surrounded by a sheath of connective tissue known as endotenon, which facilitates the gliding of bundles against one another during tendon movement. The endotenon is contiguous with the epitenon, the fine layer of connective tissue that sheaths the tendon unit.

EXAMINER: What is a collagen fibre?

CANDIDATE: A collagen fibre is the smallest tendon unit that can be tested mechanically and is visible under light microscopy.

EXAMINER: Describe the structure of a molecule of collagen.

COMMENT: This question can be asked across a number of section 2 Tr & Orth topics such as bone, articular cartilage or even intervertebral disc.

CANDIDATE: The structural unit of collagen is tropocollagen. Tropocollagen is formed in the fibroblast cell as procollagen that is then secreted and cleaved extracellularly to become collagen. It consists of three polypeptide chains each forming a left-hand helix. The chains are connected by hydrogen bonds and wind together to form a rope-like, right-handed superhelix, which gives the collagen molecule a rod-like shape.

They can be divided into fibrillar and non-fibrillar collagens.

Almost two-thirds of the collagen molecule consists of amino acid triplets (GLY-X-Y), where X is often proline and Y is often hydroxyproline. The structure at the centre of the helix is so spatially restricted that only glycine, the smallest amino acid, can be accommodated.

EXAMINER: What about cross-linking?

CANDIDATE: Tropocollagen molecules are stabilized and held together by cross-linking. Hydroxyproline is involved in hydrogen bonding (intrachain and interchain) between the polypeptide chains.

EXAMINER: Tell me about ligament ultrastructure.

CANDIDATE: The ultrastructure of ligaments is similar to that of tendons, but compared to tendons the tensile strength of ligaments is less, there is a higher percentage of proteoglycans and water and they have a higher elastic content.

Ligaments exhibit non-linear anisotropic mechanical behaviour and under low loading conditions they are relatively compliant, due to recruitment of 'crimped' collagen fibres as well as to viscoelastic behaviours and interactions of collagen and other matrix materials.

EXAMINER: What are the differences in structural collagen arrangement between ligaments and tendons?

CANDIDATE: In tendons, the collagen fibres are arranged completely in parallel, as they need to withstand large tensile loads in one direction only.

In ligaments, collagen fibres are not arranged completely parallel like tendons; fibres are branched and interwoven.

This is because although ligaments need to withstand large loads mainly in one direction, they also need to withstand smaller loads in other directions.

When unloaded the collagen fibres in both tendons and ligaments are 'crimped'. This arrangement allows tendons and ligaments to be initially stretched without too much resistance.

Ligaments exhibit non-linear anisotropic mechanical behaviour and under low loading conditions they are relatively compliant, due to recruitment of 'crimped' collagen fibres as well as to viscoelastic behaviours and interactions of collagen and other matrix materials.

EXAMINER: You have mentioned viscoelastic behaviour; what do we mean by this?

COMMENT: Creep, stress relaxation, hysteresis and rate-dependent deformation. Tendons are less viscoelastic when compared to ligaments.

EXAMINER: How do ligaments fail? What is the reason for midsubstance rupture and bony avulsion?

CANDIDATE: The most common mechanism of ligament failure is rupture of a sequential series of collagen fibre bundles distributed throughout the body of the ligament and not localized to one specific area.

Midsubstance ligament tears are common in adults while avulsion injuries are more common in children.

Bony ligament avulsions usually occur between the unmineralized and mineralized fibrocartilage layers, as this is the weakest link in the ligament/bone complex.

Structured oral examination question 2

EXAMINER: How do tendons and ligaments heal after injury? What factors affect healing?

CANDIDATE: After injury, a large number of growth factors and cytokines are released by the injured tendon and adjacent tissues, including interleukins, vascular endothelial growth factor (VEGF), platelet-derived growth factor (PDGF), fibroblastic growth factor (FGF), transforming growth factor beta (TGF-β), connective tissue growth factor (CTGF), epidermal growth factor (EGF) and insulin-like growth factor 1 (IGF1).

There are three phases of tendon/ligament healing (Table 20.7):

1. Inflammatory.
2. Proliferative.
3. Remodelling.

COMMENT: In strict terms this is section 3 material, but there is almost always some sort of varying overlap between structure and function of connective tissue (section 2) and pathology (section 3).

Phase 1 is characterized by haematoma formation and the initiation of a rapid inflammatory response.

A few days after the injury, phase 2 begins. In this phase, tendon fibroblasts synthesize abundant collagen and other extracellular matrix components such as proteoglycans and deposit them at the wound site.

After about 6 weeks, the remodelling phase starts. This phase is characterized by decreased cellularity and decreased collagen and glycosaminoglycan synthesis. During this period, the repair tissue changes to fibrous tissue, this again changes to scar-like tendon tissue after 10 weeks. During the later remodelling phase, covalent bonding between the collagen fibres increases, resulting in repaired tissue with highest stiffness and tensile strength. Also, both the metabolism of tenocytes and tendon vascularity decline.

EXAMINER: Are there any new methods developed to improve tendon healing?

CANDIDATE: There have been attempts at biological augmentation of tendon healing.

EXAMINER: Such as?

CANDIDATE: These include applying growth factors, singly or in combination, stem cells in native or genetically modified form, and biomaterials, alone or cell-loaded, at the site of tendon damage.

Table 20.7 Cells and matrix changes associated with tendon healing.

	Inflammatory	Reparative (proliferative)	Remodelling (consolidation and maturation)
Cells and matrix changes	Platelets	Cellularity and matrix production	Cellularity and matrix production ⇓
	Neutrophils	Collagen type III ⇑	Collagen type III ⇓
	Monocytes ⇑	Activation of local tendon stem/progenitor cells	Collagen type I ⇑
	Erthyrocytes		
	Circulation-derived mesenchymal stem cells		
Molecular changes	Interleukin-6	bFGF	GDF-5, -6 and -7
	bFGF	GDF-5, -6 and -7	IGF-1
	IGF-1	IGF-1	TGF-β
	PDGF	PDGF	
	TGF-β	TGFβ	
	VEGF	VEGF	

EXAMINER: What is their basis for use?

CANDIDATE:

Growth factors

Tendon injury stimulates the production of a variety of growth factors at multiple stages in the healing process leading to increased cellularity and tissue volume. Increased expression of growth factors is particularly prominent in the early phases of healing.

Growth factors can be applied by local injection, percutaneously or operatively, or by implanting scaffolds or even suture material containing growth factors.

Mesenchymal stem cells

Mesenchymal stem cells can be applied directly to the site of injury or can be delivered on a suitable carrier matrix.

Structured oral examination question 3

EXAMINER: Tell me about ligament ultrastructure.

CANDIDATE: Ligaments are dense bands of collagenous tissue (fibres) that span a joint and become anchored to bone at either end.

The ultrastructure of ligaments is similar to that of tendons, but compared to tendons the tensile strength of ligaments is less, there is a higher percentage of proteoglycans and water and they have a higher elastic content.

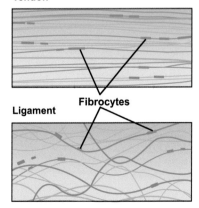

Figure 20.60 Collagen arrangement in tendon and ligament tissue. Tendon: parallel bundles of collagen fibres. Ligaments: irregular wavy bundles of collagen fibres.

EXAMINER: What are the differences in structural arrangement of collagen between ligaments and tendons?

CANDIDATE: In tendons, the collagen fibres are arranged completely in parallel as they need to withstand large loads in one direction only.

In ligaments, collagen fibres are not arranged completely parallel like tendons; fibres are branched and interwoven (Figure 20.60).

EXAMINER: Why?

CANDIDATE: This is because although ligaments need to withstand large loads mainly in one direction, they also need to withstand smaller loads in other directions.

In any single layer the fibres lie parallel to each other, but in subsequent layers they lie in a different direction.

When unloaded the collagen fibres in both tendons and ligaments are arranged in a wavy 'crimped' pattern. This arrangement allows tendons and ligaments to be initially stretched without much resistance, increasing their capacity to absorb energy.

EXAMINER: How do ligaments fail? What is the reason for midsubstance rupture and bony avulsion?

CANDIDATE: The most common mechanism of ligament failure is rupture of a sequential series of collagen fibre bundles distributed throughout the body of the ligament and not localized to one specific area.

Midsubstance ligament tears are common in adults, while avulsion injuries are more common in children.

Avulsion of ligaments usually occurs between the unmineralized and mineralized fibrocartilage layers as this is the weakest link in the ligament bone complex.

EXAMINER: But why is this? What is the reason?

CANDIDIATE: With tendons, ligaments and bones their stiffness increases with increasing strain – they are strain-rate sensitive. Bone is more sensitive to strain rate than tendons or ligaments, so its stiffness increases more proportionally. Therefore, avulsion is more common at slow strain rates and tendon and ligament tearing is more common at higher strain rates. During slow strain rates, avulsion is common, while, as the strain rate increases, the bone becomes stronger than the tendon or ligament and so tearing becomes more common.

EXAMINER: So why do bony avulsions occur in children and midsubstance ligament tears occur in adults?

CANDIDATE: The ligament/bone junction is relatively weak in children resulting in a greater chance of avulsion. In adults the strength of the ligament/bone junction has increased more rapidly than that of ligament tissue so that the strength of the ligament/bone junction exceeds the ligament tissue leading to a greater chance of midsubstance tearing.

Structured oral examination question 5

EXAMINER: Draw the stress–strain curve of a ligament/tendon and describe its various parts as you go along.

COMMENT: There are several minor variations of the stress strain curve for tendons/ligaments seen in textbooks. Although this can become confusing, remember that the principles are more important than absolute specifics. There are, however, specific regions and points on the graph that do need to be understood.

Although the stress–strain curves of tendons and ligaments are broadly similar, there are a few subtle differences. Despite this, they can often be viewed as similar materials sharing comparable features on the stress–strain curve.

Therefore, clarify (if in doubt) whether you have been asked to draw out the stress–strain curve for a ligament, tendon or if the examiners want to focus on a curve demonstrating the composite features of both materials.[34]

Stress–strain curve for ligament

There are four regions that are commonly used to describe the stress-strain curve (Figure 20.61).

1. **Non-linear (toe) region.** Collagen crimped: low stiffness; change in slope as collagen fibres straighten; modulus of elasticity is not constant; the ligament becomes stiffer as more fibres are recruited. The toe region represents 'uncrimping' of the collagen fibrils. Because it is easier to stretch out the crimp of the collagen fibrils, this part of the stress–strain curve shows a relatively low stiffness compared to the linear portion. Toe region ends at about 2% of strain when all crimped fibres straighten.

2. **Elastic linear region.** Slope = stiffness = elastic modulus.
   Elastic modulus stabilizes.
   The ligament deforms in a linear fashion due to the intermolecular sliding of collagen triple helices. If strain is less than 4%, the ligament will return to its original length when unloaded; therefore, this portion is elastic and reversible, and the slope of the curve represents an elastic modulus.

3. **Progressive failure or yield region.** At the end of the linear region there is early sequential failure of a few greatly stretched collagen fibres, causing a

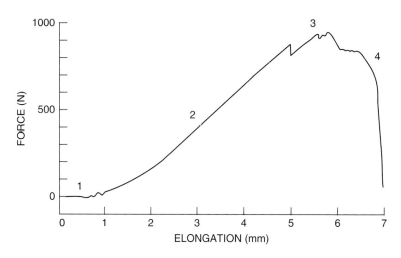

Figure 20.61 Stress–strain curve of ligament (ACL). The stress–strain curve is initially upwardly concave, but the slope becomes nearly linear in the prefigure phase of tensile loading.

series of small force reduction (dips). The load/stress at which this occurs is called the yield point.

As elongation continues, microfibrils begin to tear/rupture and the curve bends towards the strain axis as stiffness is reduced.

The ligament undergoes irreversible plastic deformation. The fibres that fail first will be those that were less crimped, while those that fail last will be those that were initially crimped and so were recruited last.

4. **Complete rupture**. When the ligament is stretched to more than 8% of its original length, macroscopic failure occurs, and the stress–strain curve falls quickly to zero. The ultimate tensile strength is the maximum load/stress that can be achieved before the ligament ruptures. Complete rupture (failure) occurs rapidly after ultimate tensile strength is attained.

EXAMINER: What is the normal operating condition of the ACL within the knee?

CANDIDATE: During everyday activities (such as walking or light jogging) the ACL operates along the 'toe region' of the stress–strain curve. It is thought that ligaments are not generally loaded above a quarter of their ultimate tensile load during these everyday activities.

The early part of the linear region is considered the upper operating range of the ACL during strenuous activities as might be experienced during pivoting while running. Loading of the ACL beyond the linear region which may occur with a bad football tackle or ski accident will result in ligament damage and possible rupture.

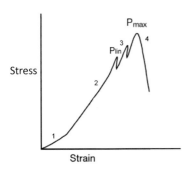

Figure 20.62 Stress–strain curve of tendon tested to failure in tension.

EXAMINER: What about the stress–strain curve of a tendon?

CANDIDATE: The stress–strain curve (Figure 20.62) is very similar to that of ligaments except:

1. Toe region. This is much less prominent than in ligaments because fibres are more aligned. Waxy collagen fibres straighten out with a small increase in load.

2. Elastic (linear) region. Fibres are straightened out and slope represents stiffness which is more or less linear. Elastic recovery at stresses < 4%.

3. End of linear region. The load value at this point is referred to as Plin in certain textbooks. Micro failure takes place after Plin and small force reduction (dips) occur in the curve. Corresponds to strains of 4–8%. Cross-links between collagen fibres fail. Collagen fibres slide past one another, irreversible changes such as tearing or permanent stretching of tendon.

4. Macroscopic failure. The ultimate tensile strength of the material is referred to as maximum load. Pmax in some textbooks. Once maximum load is surpassed complete failure occurs rapidly. Fibres recoil and blossom. Tangled bud at ruptured end.

EXAMINER: Can you draw me the stress–strain curve for the ligamentum flavum?

CANDIDATE: The ligamentum flavum has a high percentage of elastin fibres present so its stress–strain curve is completely different to that of the standard ligament/tendon curve (Figure 20.63).

With tensile testing elongation of up to 50% occurs before the stiffness increases significantly. Beyond this point, the stiffness increases greatly with additional loading and the ligament fails abruptly with little further load.

The elastic fibres allow the ligament to return to its original shape and size after the load has been released.

EXAMINER: What is the difference between force/elongation curves and stress–strain curves?

CANDIDATE: Force/elongation curves are essentially the same as stress–strain curves.

Force/elongation curves involve mounting a specimen in a machine whereas stress–strain curves have been normalized with respect to specimen dimensions.

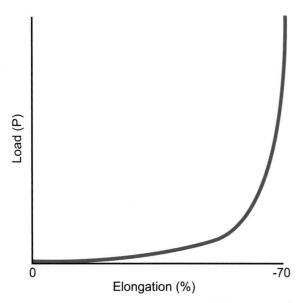

Figure 20.63 Stress strain curve of tendon with large amounts of elastin (ligamentum flavum).

In experiments, you measure load (force) and elongation(displacement). These are properties of the sample under test that change with the size of the sample. For this reason, we often divide load by sample area to get strain and displacement by sample length to get strain. Now any derived quantity is independent of sample size and can be regarded as a true material property.

EXAMINER: How do tendons receive their blood supply?

CANDIDATE: In general, tendons tend to have a sparse but adequate blood supply and low metabolic rate.

Tendons can be divided into vascular or avascular tendons. Vascular tendons are surrounded by loose areolar connective tissue known as paratenon in which the blood supply reaches the tendon. In avascular tendons a true synovial sheath replaces the paratenon.

The vascular supply to a tendon arises from three distinct areas: (1) musculotendinous junction; (2) osseotendinous junction; and (3) vessels from various surrounding connective tissue such as the paratenon, mesotenon and vincula.

Vessels are generally arranged longitudinally within the tendon, passing around the collagen fibre bundles in the endotenon.

The situation is more complicated in sheathed avascular tendons in that the blood supply must enter the mesotenon in vincula that tether the tendon to its sheath in certain locations to supply one tendon segment. Avascular tendon areas receive nutrition via diffusion.

EXAMINER: What is tendinopathy?

CANDIDATE: Tendinopathy is a multifactorial condition often related to a combination of microtrauma, excessive loading and normal ageing. It is characterized by pain, focal tendon tenderness, decreased strength and movement.

EXAMINER: What about pathogenesis of tendinopathy?

CANDIDATE: The pathogenesis is poorly understood. It has been variously defined as a degenerative condition, a failure of the healing process or a region of diminished blood supply just above the tendon insertion.

The role of inflammation in tendinopathy is not clearly established. The exact relationship between tendinopathy and tendon rupture remains unknown. It is thought that tendinopathy could lead to tendon rupture.

EXAMINER: What changes are occurring in the tendon?

CANDIDATE: Tendinopathy can be identified by the following histological characteristics: collagen fibril disorganization, increased proteoglycan and glycosaminoglycan content and increased non-collagenous ECM, hypercellularity and neovascularization.

EXAMINER: How do we treat tendinopathies?

CANDIDATE: First-line treatment involves non-steroidal anti-inflammatory medication for pain relief, physiotherapy with eccentric exercises (involves active lengthening of muscles and tendons) and steroid injections.

EXAMINER: What about PRP injections, how do they work?

CANDIDATE: Platelet-rich plasma (PRP) is a blood derivative containing PRP. It is the plasma fraction of the blood containing concentrated platelets and high levels of growth factors, known to promote tissue healing.

EXAMINER: What is the evidence for their use?

517

CANDIDATE: Current evidence suggests/My understanding of the literature is that PRP is useful for chronic degenerative tendinopathies such as lateral epicondylitis of the elbow or patella tendinopathy.

There is no evidence to support the use of PRP in promoting tendon or ligament-to-bone healing in rotator cuff repair or ACL reconstruction.[35]

The main points are that it should not be considered a first-line treatment but reserved for chronic tendinopathy refractory to standard non-operative management, such as physiotherapy and steroid injections.

EXAMINER: Any other options?

CANDIDATE: Extracorporeal shock-wave therapy has some benefit in calcified tendinitis of the shoulder, and ultrasonography are other treatment options. Stem-cell-based therapy may become available for use in the future.

EXAMINER: What is the difference between tendinitis and tendinosis.

CANDIDATE: Terms can be misleading. Tendinitis suggests inflammation although inflammatory cells are often absent. Patients may experience localized pain, swelling, warmth and redness.

Tendinosis is degeneration of the tendon. This can often be due to repetitive microtrauma.

Tendinopathy is typically used to describe any problem involving a tendon.

EXAMINER: How do tendons and ligaments insert into bone?

CANDIDATE: There is direct and indirect attachment to bone.

Direct insertion into bone is similar for tendon and ligament and consists of four zones.

- Zone 1. Tendon. Parallel collagen fibres at the end of the tendon or ligament.
- Zone 2. Uncalcified fibrocartilage. Collagen fibres intermesh with unmineralized fibrocartilage.
- Zone 3. Calcified fibrocartilage. Fibrocartilage gradually becomes mineralized.
- Zone 4. Bone. Mineralized fibrocartilage merges into cortical bone.

This allows a gradual increase in the stiffness of the tissue, so there is a lesser stress concentration effect at the insertion of a tendon/ligament into bone.

Otherwise, high stress levels will occur at the interface due to the difference in stiffness between the two materials. There is a gradual change in structure, composition and mechanical behaviour between tendon/ligament and bone. The mineralized cartilage tidemark forms deep interdigitations increasing the contact area and reducing the stiffness gradient between mechanically different tissues. This improves the ability of the unit to resist shear and tensile forces.

The continuous change in tissue composition from tendon/ligament to bone aids in the efficient transfer of load between the two materials.

With indirect insertion the deep layer anchors to bone via Sharpey's fibres.

EXAMINER: Can you give me any examples of direct and indirect ligament insertion?

CANDIDATE: ACL direct and indirect superficial.

Structured oral examination question 6

EXAMINER: This is a coronal MRI through the thigh, can you tell me what has happened (Figure 20.64)?

CANDIDATE: [I was not sure exactly what I was looking at initially!] There appears to be a tendon pulled off the bone, along with an associated haematoma.

COMMENT: This is just using your basic understanding of MRI.

EXAMINER: Appears to be, or actually is?

CANDIDATE: There is a definite avulsion of tendon from the bone.

COMMENT: Be confident.

EXAMINER: What's the function of the bone attachment?

CANDIDATE: [I really didn't know where to go, so I gave a very basic answer!] It represents an interface between bone and tendon.

EXAMINER: But what is the function?

CANDIDATE: It allows a load to be transferred from muscle to bone and stores energy. [As you can see, I've not read much on this and gave short answers, so I didn't get into trouble.]

EXAMINER: What type of load?

CANDIDATE: Tensile?

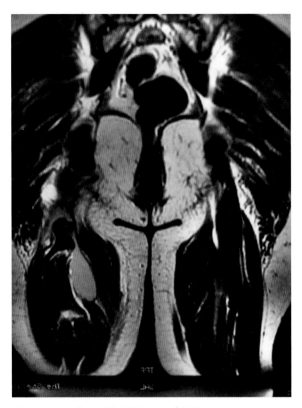

Figure 20.64 Coronal T1 MRI image of thigh.

EXAMINER: What is the difference in general terms between ligaments and tendons?

CANDIDATE: [I started to talk about ligaments attaching bone to bone!]

Mark 4 – poor fail.

EXAMINER: No, I mean structurally!

CANDIDATE: [Finally I can get going now!] Collagen content is higher in tendons and can be up to 80–90% in extremity tendons. [Best answer – up to 99% of dry weight. Remember that tendons and ligaments are made up from 80% ECM and 20% cells.]

EXAMINER: What are the cells found in tendons and ligaments?

CANDIDATE: Fibroblast represents the vast proportion of cells, at about 20% of the total mass.

EXAMINER: You mentioned collagen, which is the common type?

CANDIDATE: Type 1 represents the most common type.

Mark 5 – fail

EXAMINER: That was a little guarded, give me a figure.

CANDIDATE: 70–80 % (actually 90%) [I knew what was coming next!]

EXAMINER: Tell me about type 1 collagen.

CANDIDATE: Type 1 collagen consists of three poly-peptide chains, two alpha and one beta. [This was wrong, it's two (alpha 1) and one (alpha 2). They combine to form a triple helix, which provides the tensile strength.]

If you can't talk at this stage you will fail this section, you must have a broad knowledge base.

Mark 6 – pass

EXAMINER: How does this structure retain its stability?

CANDIDATE: There is cross-linking which is allowed to occur due to hydrogen bonds.

EXAMINER: Can you draw a picture of collagen in a ligament and tendon and explain how they differ?

CANDIDATE: I drew a longitudinal section basically with a well-aligned pattern for a tendon and more haphazard for a ligament. I explained that the less-parallel structure in a ligament means it takes tension in one direction but can also take stresses in other directions. In each layer they are parallel, but in subsequent layers the collagen is at a slightly different angle.

EXAMINER: Can you draw a schematic of this hier-archical structure?

CANDIDATE: [I talked about the layers as I drew, only got to the fibril and he was bored!] (Figure 20.65)

COMMENT: Remember there are lots of different ways to draw this diagram, just use one and learn how to draw it and talk. It is principles not details which are important!

EXAMINER: So, what makes up the extracellular matrix?

CANDIDATE: This essentially is a proteoglycan matrix, with plasma proteins and glycoprotein. These proteoglycans bind water and provide a gel-type matrix. The proteoglycans are glycosaminogly-cans which bind to a protein core, linked to a hyaluronic acid chain which provides a very high molecular weight.

519

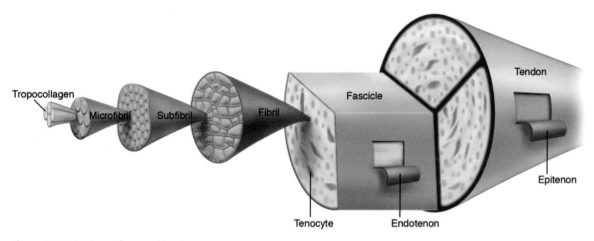

Figure 20.65 Anatomy of a normal tendon.

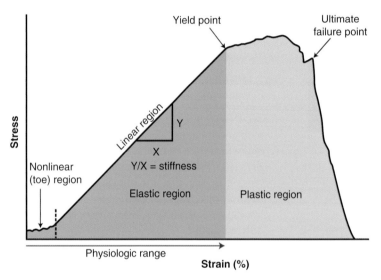

Figure 20.66 Stress–strain curve for tendon and ligament.

Mark 7 – good pass

EXAMINER: Can you draw the stress–strain curve for tendons and ligaments and talk through it (Figure 20.66)?

COMMENT: You can get this from any of the basic science books, just learn it!

CANDIDATE: There are four major regions of the stress strain curve: (1) the toe or toe-in region, (2) the linear region and (3) the yield and (4) failure region. In physiological activity, most ligaments and tendons exist in the toe and somewhat in the linear region. These constitute a non-linear stress–strain curve because the slope of the toe-in region is different from that of the linear region.

In terms of structure–function relationships, the toe-in region represents 'uncrimping' of the crimp in the collagen fibrils. Because it is easier to stretch out the crimp of the collagen fibrils, this part of the stress–strain curve shows a relatively low stiffness. As the collagen fibrils become uncrimped, then we see that the collagen fibril backbone itself is being stretched, which gives rise to a stiffer material. As individual fibrils within the ligament or tendon begin to fail, damage accumulates, stiffness is reduced and the ligament/tendons begin to fail. Thus, a key concept is that the overall behaviour of ligaments and tendons depends on the individual crimp structure and failure of the collagen fibrils.

Mark 8 – excellent Pass

This is an example of a question which is based on one specific topic, which is great if you know it well, but very bad if you don't. This emphasizes the fact you must be able to talk to a basic level on all topics, or you may flounder very early on in the question. This question will be in your basic science viva and last 5 minutes.

6. Structure and function of the nervous system

Introduction

The difficulty with structure/function of the nervous system is that there is considerable overlap with section 3 (nerve injury and regeneration) and section 9 (electrophysiological investigations).

On top of this, the core material is quite dry and complicated but needs to be well understood before candidates would feel confident enough to deal with the viva questions they are likely to be asked.

Structured oral examination question 1

EXAMINER: With reference to nerve conduction studies: what do you see in different types of injury (axonotmesis, neurotmesis, etc.)? The normal reference ranges? Please draw a cross-section of a nerve and label.

COMMENT: This is immediately bang on the money. Candidates need to know straight up their definitions of neuropraxia, axonotmesis and neurotmesis and then they will get hammered with the NCS findings in each specific case. This is a way of grilling candidates about the VERY specifics of NCS while minimizing too much candidate preamble and chit-chat. These are unGoogleable questions.

CANDIDATE: There are three main types of nerve injury:

1. Neuropraxia where the myelin sheath is dysfunctional.
2. Axonotmesis where the axon is damaged but the supporting connective tissues remain intact.
3. Neurotmesis where both the axon and its sheath are damaged.

In clinical reality, nerve trauma usually leads to a mixture of all three to the fascicles within a nerve. However, there will usually be a predominance of one of these, which is important to predicting the prognosis.

Neuropraxia

Myelin is critical to effective signal transmission via saltatory conductance across the Nodes of Ranvier. In neuropraxia, there is focal oedema or breakdown of the myelin sheath which disrupts the nerve's ability to conduct signals and can lead to slowing or 'blocking' of conduction. This type of injury usually arises from a mild stretch or crush injury. As myelin is formed by the Schwann cells, these tend to regenerate quickly, depending on the degree of disruption, from weeks to months. The axon itself is preserved and so there is no Wallerian degeneration and no secondary degeneration of muscle fibres.

There are a number of hallmarks of neuropraxia on nerve conduction studies (NCS) and electromyography (EMG).

NCS will show:

- Conduction slowing or even conduction block across the level of the lesion but should be normal below the level of the lesion.

EMG will show:

- Electrical silence persisting after 3 weeks in a completely stunned state (there won't be any fibrillations as the muscle fibre isn't denervated and there will be no voluntary activity due to the severity of the signal block).
- Single (or limited) motor units at high rates in isolation in a partially stunned state as the brain attempts to generate force via the remaining working fibres.

Axonotmesis

Here there is injury primarily to the axon and its myelin sheath, usually following a more severe crush, or even avulsion. However, the supportive connective tissues remain mostly preserved (endoneurium, perineurium, epineurium) and so the tubes that encapsulate the axons remain preserved.

Wallerian degeneration will occur distal to (and a little proximal to) the site of the lesion and will spread in an anterograde direction, i.e. peripherally over the coming days. Axon degeneration in the distal stump triggers a number of responses in the remaining Schwann cells

521

which are the key to successful regeneration. First, they degrade myelin and signal macrophages to remove debris. Then, they proliferate and form Büngner bands which are bridging tubes as well as signalling molecules to attract the regenerating proximal axon bud into them.

Prognostically, regeneration is likely to occur if the re-innervating fibres follow the pre-existing pathways formed by their original endoneurial tubes. When the distances involved in regeneration are long, then a number of factors may preclude successful re-innervation, particularly if the target muscle fibres have atrophied or fibrosed in the meantime. Occasionally, regenerating axons may follow the wrong endoneurial tube and innervate the wrong fibres. Perhaps the most visible manifestation of this is 'synkinesis' seen in Bell's palsy where a patient may try to smile and ends up blinking.

NCS will show:

- Reduced amplitudes of sensory and motor fibres.
- Relative preservation of conduction velocities (noting that some fast fibre drop out is often expected when there has been severe axonal loss leading to mild slowing).

EMG will show:

- Positive sharp waves and fibrillations following 2 weeks in the upper limbs and 3 weeks in the lower limbs as the denervated muscle fibres upregulate their acetyl choline receptors.
- Reduced interference patterns (i.e. fewer motor units being recruited) for the degree of recruitment (i.e. volitionary effort to generate force) as there are simply fewer working axons to transmit the signal.

Neurotmesis

Here there is complete destruction of the nerve and surrounding supportive tissues, usually caused by serious injuries such as anatomical severance of nerve and/or extensive avulsion or crushing. The axon, Schwann cell and endoneural tube is completely disrupted and the perineurium and epineurium have varying degrees of injury and disruption. Prognosis in these situations is usually poor.

NCS will show:

- Initial preservation of distal responses for the first 3–5 days for motor studies and 6–10 days for sensory studies until Wallerian degeneration reaches distal regions. The earlier impairment of

motor fibres is now thought to relate to neuromuscular junction transmission failure.

- Thereafter there will be absent sensory and motor responses.

EMG will show:

- Where axonal loss is severe, there will be an immediate and complete lack of voluntary activity.
- For the first few weeks there will only be electrical silence and then fibrillations will appear around 2 weeks later in the upper limbs and 3 weeks later in the lower limbs.
- This differentiates this state from severe neuropraxia (see above).
- Fibrillations will be abundant and of large amplitude in the first 6 months, and then diminish as the muscle tissue atrophies and/or fibroses.

EXAMINER: What are nerve conduction studies?

CANDIDATE: Nerve conduction tests are used to evaluate the function of motor and sensory nerves. An NCS may consist of the following:

- Compound motor action potential (CMAP).
- Sensory nerve action potential (SNAP).
- F wave.
- H reflex wave.

Motor nerve conduction studies examine the conduction of a signal along the course of a peripheral motor fibre to its muscle fibres.

- Latency – the time interval between stimulus and the onset of a response.
- Amplitude – the maximal height of the action potential.
- Conduction velocity – speed of the fastest part of the impulse calculated by the time of the recorded impulse between two points of known distance. It is reduced by a reduction in myelin (e.g. external compression or demyelinating conditions).

EXAMINER: Please draw a cross-section of a nerve and label (Figure 20.67).

CANDIDATE: Axons are grouped together in spatially arranged motor or sensory bundles called fascicles. Individual axons are surrounded by a connective tissue layer, the endoneurium, and fascicles are separated by the perineurium. Groups of fascicles are contained within a peripheral nerve surrounded by a connective tissue layer called the epineurium.

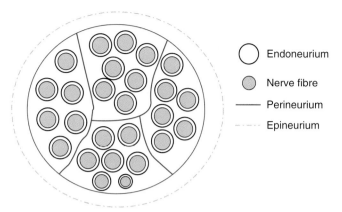

Figure 20.67 Candidate diagram. Cross-section of a nerve fibre.

The epineurium is the outermost layer of dense connective tissue surrounding a peripheral nerve.

The perineurium is the layer that covers individual fascicles and provides tensile strength.

The endoneurium is the inner layer, which is mostly collagenous, that surrounds axons within fascicles and it nourishes and protects the axons.

Structured oral examination question 2

Nerve action potential: explain the graph with relationship of membrane potential to sodium and potassium concentrations, exchange pump, channels.

Neurons exhibit a lipoprotein cell membrane with a negative resting cell (around –70 mV), due to the voltage difference resulting from a high concentration of intracellular potassium (K^+) and low concentrations of sodium (Na^+) and chloride (Cl^-) ions within the cells.

The concentration gradient is maintained by:

- A metabolically active Na^+/K^+ exchange pump.
- A lipid membrane that prevents the passage of water-soluble ions.
- Donnan equilibrium. Irregular distribution of permanent ions across an impermeant membrane when a large impermeable organic ion is present on one side.

EXAMINER: What is a resting potential?

CANDIDATE: A resting potential is a term used to describe the electrical potential across the membrane of a cell in its inactive unexcited state.

EXAMINER: What is an action potential?

CANDIDATE: The whole basis of an action potential is based around a change in permeability to

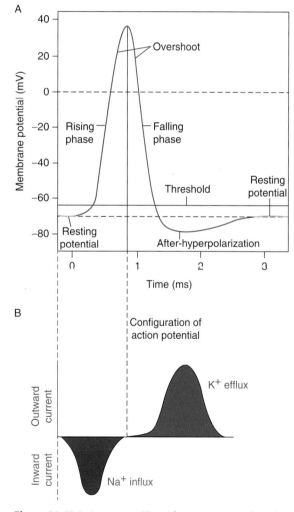

Figure 20.68 Action potential 'hops' from one non-myelinated region (Node of Ranvier) to the next (saltatory conduction). 1, Resting stage. 2, Depolarization stage. 3, Repolarization. 4, Hyperpolarization.

sodium and potassium due to opening/closing of voltage-gated channels in response to a stimulus (Figure 20.68).

When a neuron is stimulated, some of the sodium channels on the membrane open. This allows sodium ions to go into the cell from the outside. As a result, the charge difference between the inside and outside of the cell starts to decrease.

When the membrane potential increases to around –50 mV, most of the voltage-gated sodium channels rapidly open to allow Na$^+$ to enter the cell, and the membrane potential spikes to more than 30 mV.

The inside of the neuron becomes positively charged with respect to the outside.

However, this open channel configuration is unstable and exists for only a fraction of a second before a second conformational change occurs with an inactivation gate to block the sodium channel, thereby stopping the flow of Na$^+$.

For a few ms after closing, they cannot be open again (the refractory period). This limits the number of action potentials a neuron can experience.

The rapid depolarization of the membrane also triggers the more slowly acting voltage-gated potassium channels to open and allows K$^+$ to exit the cell. The flow of K$^+$ from the cell has a longer duration than the flow of Na$^+$ into the cell and the cell begins to repolarize as soon as the sodium channels close.

The electrical potential falls to a level below the original resting potential of –70 mV (repolarization).

The potassium channels eventually close and the sodium–potassium pump will continue to restore the neuron to its original resting potential.

EXAMINER: What do we mean by the threshold stimulus?

CANDIDATE: The threshold stimulus is the minimum stimulus intensity needed to produce an action potential.

A smaller stimulus (subthreshold) will not produce a stimulus. However, summation of a number of subthreshold stimuli is sometimes sufficient to stimulate a response.

Structured oral examination question 3

Nerve picture . . . asked how action potential and muscle contraction produced . . . Cross-bridge theory and

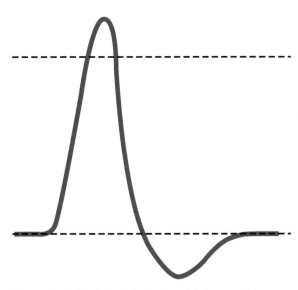

Figure 20.69 Candidate basic drawing of action potential.

power stroke . . . . These are gifts, don't waste them . . . . Wallerian degeneration . . .

EXAMINER: Can you draw out an action potential and tell me what is going on as you go along (Figure 20.69)?

CANDIDATE: Neurons possess a membrane potential of –70 mV due to the voltage difference between the intracellular and extracellular space. This voltage difference is due to the high concentration of potassium ions [K$^+$] and low concentration of sodium ions [Na$^+$] and chloride ions [Cl$^-$].

Action potentials are important for nerve signalling occurring as a result of rapid changes in membrane potential.

The threshold stimulus is the minimum stimulus intensity needed to produce an action potential. An action potential is generated when a neuron is stimulated, resulting in the opening of the Na channels and an in-rush of the Na$^+$ ions into the cell.

EXAMINER: Can you be more specific and point out some features of the diagram (Figure 20.70)?

COMMENT: Point out:

Threshold: Threshold is the membrane potential at which enough voltage-gated sodium channels are open so that the relative permeability of the membrane is higher for sodium ions than it is for potassium ions.

Rising phase/depolarization: When the inside of the membrane has a negative potential, there is a

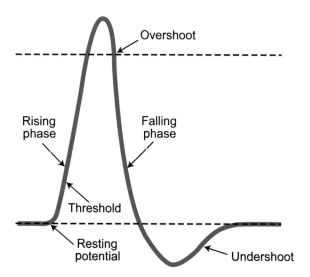

Figure 20.70 Candidate basic drawing of action potential with labels.

large driving force on sodium ions. Therefore, sodium rushes in through the open sodium channels, causing a rapid depolarization of the membrane.

Overshoot: Because of the high permeability to sodium, the membrane potential goes to a value that is close to the equilibrium potential for sodium (~ +55 mV).

Falling phase/repolarization: First, the voltage-gated sodium channels inactivate. Second, the voltage-gated potassium channels open (the delayed-rectifier potassium channels). The driving force pushes potassium out of the cell, causing the membrane potential to become negative again.

Undershoot/hyperpolarization: The open potassium channels add to the normal resting membrane permeability to potassium, and drive the membrane potential close to the equilibrium potential for potassium, thus hyperpolarizing the membrane.

EXAMINER: Tell me about the refractory periods.

CANDIDATE: Refractory periods: the absolute refractory period is due to the inactivation of sodium channels. These channels cannot be opened again until the membrane potential is sufficiently negative to deactivate them.

The relative refractory period is due to the hyperpolarization from the open potassium channels.

This means that more depolarizing current is necessary to initiate another action potential.

EXAMINER: What are the channels dependent on and how does this cause depolarization?

CANDIDATE: The channels are dependent on oxygen and ATP. There is depolarization of the membrane from the initial resting state of −70 mV due to ionic conductance and the polarity across the cell membrane becomes positive.

EXAMINER: What do you mean by ionic conductance?[36]

CANDIDATE: Conductance is the inverse of electrical resistance. If the conductance of the membrane to a particular ion is low, then the resistance to movement of that ion across the membrane is high. High conductance indicates that electrical charge moves easily through a membrane.

The polarity across the cell membrane becomes positive. This also triggers the opening of more Na^+ channels. The Na^+ channels remain open for 1 ms before closing. The refractory period relates to the channels remaining closed for a few milliseconds and not able to reopen, thus limiting the number of stimuli to which a nerve can respond.

Repolarization of the membrane results from the passage of K^+ ions out of the cell through K^+ channels.

EXAMINER: What happens at the motor end plate?

CANDIDATE: The motor end plate includes the terminal portion of the nerve and the muscle membrane. There is a small gap known as the gap junction that separates the nerve from the muscle at the motor end plate.

An action potential is propagated via the axon of the neuron to the nerve terminal.

The presence of an action potential at the nerve terminal triggers the opening of voltage-gated Ca^{2+}.

Ca^{2+} triggers the release of acetylcholine. This is the main neurotransmitter that acts on the motor end plate. It is stored in the presynaptic axon in membrane-encased compartments called vesicles.

Acetylcholine diffuses across the synaptic cleft and binds with specific receptor sites on the motor end plate of the muscle cell membrane.

This binding brings about opening of ion channels with large movements of Na^+ into the muscle cell and smaller movements of K^+ outward. This results in a depolarizing potential called an end plate potential spreading over the surface of the muscle fibre.

This potential triggers the release of calcium (from the sarcoplasmic reticulum), which elicits the movement of actin and myosin filaments, resulting in muscle contraction.

Acetylcholine is destroyed by an enzyme called acetylcholinesterase that inactivates acetylcholine by detaching it from its receptor and hydrolyzing it to acetate and choline.

EXAMINER: What is the postsynaptic membrane?

CANDIDATE: The postsynaptic membrane is the specialized portion of the muscle cell membrane subjacent to the axon terminal, exhibiting a large number of folds that increase the surface area of the muscle cell in contact with the axon terminal.

EXAMINER: Do you know of any diseases affecting the neuromuscular junction?

CANDIDATE: Myasthenia gravis. This is characterized by antibodies that bind to nicotinic acetylcholine receptors with resulting lysis of postsynaptic receptors.

EXAMINER: How is a muscle contraction produced?

CANDIDATE: Depolarization in muscle cell plasma spreads to T-tubules and opens voltage-gated Ca^{2+} channels. This triggers the release of calcium ions (Ca^{2+}) from storage in the sarcoplasmic reticulum (SR). The Ca^{2+} then initiates contraction, which is sustained by ATP. As long as Ca^{2+} ions remain in the sarcoplasm to bind to troponin, which keeps the actin-binding sites 'unshielded', and as long as ATP is available to drive the cross-bridge cycling and the pulling of actin strands by myosin, the muscle fibre will continue to shorten to an anatomical limit.

EXAMINER: What do we mean by the sliding filament mechanism of muscle contraction?

CANDIDATE: In the 1950s Huxley and Hanson discovered that skeletal muscles were composed of hexagonal lattices of actin and myosin filaments and that muscle contraction resulted from relative sliding between the two filaments.

Cross-bridge interaction between actin and myosin brings about muscle contraction. The thin filaments slide inwards over the stationary thick filaments.

EXAMINER: What is a power stroke?

CANDIDATE: The power stroke describes a step in the cross-bridge cycle.

For thin filaments (actin) to slide past thick filaments (myosin) during muscle contraction, myosin heads must pull the actin at the binding sites, detach, re-cock, attach to more binding sites, pull, detach, re-cock, etc. This repeated movement is known as the cross-bridge cycle.

Binding: The active site on actin is exposed as calcium binds to troponin. The myosin head is attracted to actin, and myosin binds actin at its actin-binding site, forming the cross-bridge.

Power stroke: During the power stroke, the phosphate generated in the previous contraction cycle is released. This results in the myosin head pivoting toward the centre of the sarcomere, after which the attached ADP and phosphate group are released.

Detachment: A new molecule of ATP attaches to the myosin head, causing the cross-bridge to detach.

EXAMINER: What do we mean by Wallerian degeneration?

CANDIDATE: When a nerve is cut or crushed Wallerian degeneration occurs. The part of the axon separated from the neuron's cell nucleus degenerates. Distal to the level of injury this involves the whole axon. Proximal to the injury retrograde (primary degeneration) occurs to the next Node of Ranvier.

Macrophages ingest the fragmented myelin to provide a clean endoneural tube for advancement of regenerating axons. Wallerian degeneration is accompanied by marked proliferation of Schwann cells and fibroblasts lining the endoneural tubes.

COMMENT: Viva seems to be jumping around topics.

Structured oral examination question 4

Anatomy of spinal cord and cord syndromes. Candidate is shown an axial CT of C5 (Figure 20.71) with fracture with discussion of why you do not get cord injury at that level commonly.

Central cord syndrome (MUD-E)

Results from bleeding, infarction, or oedema to the central grey matter of the spinal cord.

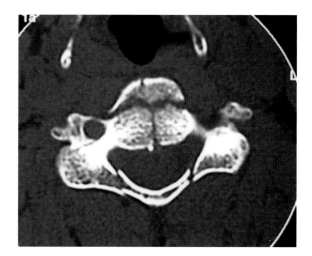

Figure 20.71 Axial CT image of C5 burst fracture.

Blood supply comes from periphery to centre.

Motor loss > Sensory

Motor loss affects **U**pper extremity > Lower extremity

Distal > Proximal

Commonly follows hyper-**E**xtension Injury in an elderly patient with pre-existing spondylosis.

Pain and sensation affected.

Touch and proprioception unaffected.

Dissociative anaesthesia.

Hands and upper extremities are located centrally in corticospinal tract.

Finger and wrist motor function more affected than shoulder and biceps function.

Relatively good prognosis although full recovery rare.

Anterior cord syndrome

Preservation of posterior column-proprioception and vibration sense is intact.

Bilateral loss of motor function, light touch pain and temperature.

Brown–Sequard syndrome

Ipsilateral loss of motor function and proprioception/vibration.

Contralateral loss of pain and temperature (spinothalamic tract crosses over).

EXAMINER: With a C5 fracture, why don't you get cord injury at that level commonly?

CANDIDATE: The spinal cord is situated within the spine. The spine consists of a series of vertebral segments. The spinal cord itself has 'neurological' segmental levels which are defined by the spinal roots that enter and exit the spinal column between each of the vertebral segments. Spinal cord segmental levels do not necessarily correspond to the bony segments.

A patient with a burst fracture of the C5 vertebral body. The burst fracture will typically injure the C6 spinal cord situated at the C5 vertebra and also the C4 spinal roots that exit the spinal column between the C4 and C5 vertebrae. Such an injury should cause a loss of sensations in the C4 dermatome and weak deltoids (C4) due to injury to the C4 roots. Due to oedema (swelling of the spinal cord), the biceps (C5) may be initially weak but should recover.

The spinal vertebral and cord segmental levels become increasingly discrepant further down the spinal column. For example, a T8 vertebral injury will result in a T12 spinal cord or neurological level. A T11 vertebral injury usually results in a L5 lumbar spinal cord level.

Structured oral examination question 5

Photograph of cut section of median nerve shown at wrist all prepared for surgical repair.

EXAMINER: What is this picture (Figure 20.72).

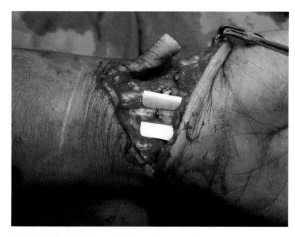

Figure 20.72 Median nerve laceration at wrist.

CANDIDATE: This is picture of a cut nerve at the wrist. The position of the nerve on the radial side of the hand is suggestive of median nerve transection.

EXAMINER: What factors adversely affect recovery of a nerve after repair?

COMMENT: Much better to have a structured answer than a random generation of facts.

List factors in terms of (1) patient, (2) injury, (3) surgical.

Patient

1. Older age.
2. Systemic factors. Diabetes, alcoholism, smoking, rheumatoid arthritis, neuropathies, etc.

Injury

3. High energy of initial injury.
4. Associated vascular or bony injury.
5. Crush or traction injury.
6. More proximal injury (increased time to reach target organ).
7. Nerves that supply multiple sites with sensory and motor components.
8. Large gap.

Surgical

9. Delay in repair (increased time for end-plate degeneration).
10. Repaired under tension. Excessive tension can cause breakdown at the area of repair.
11. Infection.
12. Need for nerve graft. If excessive tension present, use interposition autologous nerve grafts.
13. Quality of repair. It is important to try to suture only the epineurium and not pass the needle and suture through the fascicles, as this can create more damage and scarring, yielding a poorer result. Preservation of blood supply and accurate apposition of the fascicle.

EXAMINER: What happens to a nerve when it is cut? How does it regenerate?

CANDIDATE: During the first few hours chromatolysis and swelling takes place in the cell body and nucleus. Oedema and swelling then continue in the axonal stump for the first few days. Within 2–3 days Wallerian degeneration commences, which involves axonal and myelin disintegration both in an antegrade and retrograde direction. Antegrade Wallerian degeneration then continues with Schwann cells and macrophage infiltration to remove cell debris, leaving only the basement membrane for about 3–6 weeks. Schwann cells then start to proliferate and organize guiding the axonal sprouts between the basement membranes of the two nerve ends. Nerve regeneration then begins on the columns of Schwann cells called Bunger bands. The proximal intact axon then sprouts a growth cone. The lamellipodia and filopodia cytoplasmic extensions allow the axon to explore the new environment and help in guiding the repair. Actin found in the axon allows elongation, within the tube. Growth continues at the restricted rate of 1–3 mm/day, but simultaneously scar tissue interferes with growth.

EXAMINER: Any new developments in nerve regeneration?

CANDIDATE: Sorry, no idea.

Structured oral examination question 6

EXAMINER: Can you draw out a neuron for me?

COMMENT: Have an easy to draw out drawing already rehearsed from your exam preparation (Figure 20.73).

COMMENT: Candidates should be able to describe (talk through) the elements of the neuron as it is drawn.

Neuron

- The functional unit of the nerve.
- Made up of a cell body and an axon.

Cell body

- Gives rise to the axon and dendrites.
- Contains most of the neuron's organelles.

Dendrites

- Thin branching extensions of a neuron that receive messages from other cell bodies and conduct impulses towards the cell body.
- Sensory.

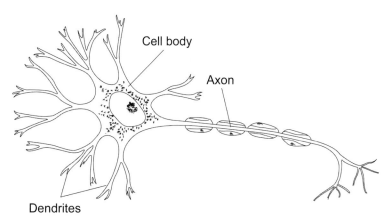

Figure 20.73 Candidate drawing of a neuron.

Axon hillock

- Cone-shaped region of an axon where it joins the cell body, the region where the signals travel down the axon are generated.

Axon

- The extension of a neuron.
- The primary route of conduction to tissues.
- Size of axon is between 0.2 and 20 μm.
- Longest part of the nerve.

Glial cells

- Anchor neurons and form myelin sheath.
- In CNS, glial cells are:
  - Oligodendrocytes (make myelin), astrocytes and microglia.
- In PNS glial cells are:
  - Schwann cells.
- Size of the nerve axon determines whether it will be myelinated.

Myelinated larger axons

- Invaginated by one Schwann cell per axon internode.

Unmyelinated axons

- Bundled together surrounded by one Schwann cell – no myelin.
- Remak bundle.

Myelin

- Lipid- and protein-rich multilaminar substance.
- Laid down in the PNS to form a neurilemma.
- No neurilemma is present around CNS myelinated axons.

Nodes of Ranvier

- Gaps between Schwann cells along an axon.

Structured oral examination question 7

EXAMINER: Draw a cross-section of a nerve and nerve fibre.

CANDIDATE: [I talked about the three layers and the only four components of a nerve fibre I knew] (Figure 20.74).

EXAMINER: How are nerve injuries classified?

COMMENT: For a score 6 pass all you need to know is Seddon[37] and Sunderland.[38]

CANDIDATE: Seddon classified the injury originally into three types and Sunderland defined these into six. Seddon defined neuropraxis as ionic block with possible segmental demyelinization (Sunderland 1), axonotmesis with axon severed but endoneurial tube intact (Sunderland 2), endoneurial tube torn (Sunderland 3) or only epineurium intact (Sunderland 4). Finally, neurotmesis with loss of continuity (Sunderland 5) or a combination of above (Sunderland 6).

529

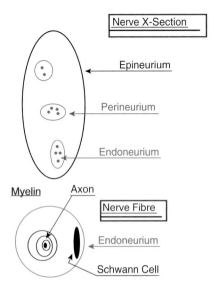

Figure 20.74 Diagram of cross-section of a nerve and nerve fibre.

COMMENT: At this point I could not remember exactly what the implications of all the Sunderland classifications were, so I did not offer them.

Basically, Sunderland 1 and 2 are full recovery, 3 are incomplete, 4 is neuroma, 5 are none and 6 is unpredictable. I think the easiest way to get this down is to draw a box diagram and get used to filling it in.

EXAMINER: If you cut the median nerve during surgery, what factors affect long-term results?

CANDIDATE: The age of the patient is the single most critical factor in sensory recovery after nerve repair and a good result is adversely affected by associated injuries to muscle, arteries, tendons and bone. In children, I believe you get good results in 50% and 40% in adults.

COMMENT: The good results in children are actually 75% and 50% in adults, although this drops on a yearly basis year on year. The examiner either didn't know himself or decided to leave this point. Just be a bit careful of using percentages, as they may ask where this information originates, which you may well not know.

EXAMINER: What will you do if there is a 2-cm graft?

CANDIDATE: If there is going to be tension on the graft, I would either use a nerve graft or a conduit.

[I don't offer any further information at the point as my knowledge is limited! Unfortunately, this strategy does not work very well.]

EXAMINER: What nerve grafts are available for use?

CANDIDATE: Sural nerve, which has up to 20 cm, medial or lateral antebrachial cutaneous nerve.

EXAMINER: What about nerve conduits?

CANDIDATE: I have never seen a nerve conduit, but they may allow up to 2 cm of nerve growth.

[I had never seen a conduit graft, and knew virtually nothing about them, so I justified my answer. The examiner was happy with this and admitted it would be unfair to ask anything further as I had not seen the procedure. Lucky escape.]

COMMENT: A nerve conduit involves reconstruction of a gap defect by the placement of proximal and distal nerve stumps into a tubular repair construct.

A nerve conduit provides a means to approximate nerve stumps within a biologically enhanced microenvironment, which minimizes fibrosis and the potential for ingrowth of external scar tissues. These products can provide directional growth cues and prevent dissipation of pro-regenerative trophic and tropic factors away from the repair site. As a result, these constructs may reduce axonal escape or misdirection, improve regeneration into the distal nerve and enhance functional recovery. Tubular conduits also offer the possibility of avoiding nerve autograft harvest, and thereby avoid the potential morbidity of that procedure.

References

1. Better still, don't mention it.

2. Elliott DS, Newman KJ, Forward DP, *et al*. A unified theory of bone healing and nonunion. *Bone Joint J*. 2016;98(7):884–891.

3. Tactical miscalculation from too long a coffee break and non-focused chitchat.

4. Urist MR. Bone: formation by autoinduction. *Science*. 1965;150(3698):893–899.

5. Wall A, Board T. Bone: Formation by Autoinduction. In P Banaszkiewicz, D Kader (Eds.), *Classic Papers in Orthopaedics*. London: Springer; 2014.

6. This can use up a lot of precious time.

7. Much simpler for candidates to not mention them and just stick with the two above.

8. These contradictions make basic science unnecessarily complicated.

9. You could be given a diagram of articular cartilage or be asked to draw it. A score 8 candidate would be able to continually talk away describing each layer (and fast as well) doing all the work with the examiners (usually) keeping silent, not interrupting and (hopefully) pleased the content is being covered. An excellent candidate with an excellent answer.

    A score 6 candidate would discuss enough detail of each layer for a safe pass, but will need a little prompting from time to time. A score 4 or 5 candidate would struggle with naming the layers, structure and function and require a lot of prompting, giving the impression they hadn't really learnt the subject.

10. If you are proactive you should be able to draw and talk at the same time, so practise this beforehand. If you are given a laminated diagram you have to get on the money straightaway and keep talking.

11. You are only going to be able to do this if you have already practised to perfection drawing out articular cartilage in 30 seconds flat.

12. The candidate was hesitant and needed to be prompted.

13. Dense collagen skin.

14. Depending on your interpretation.

15. The word 'esoteric' perfectly describes the basic science viva questioning.

16. All chondrocytes are not the same. If you grow cartilage in the laboratory and place the surface, deep and middle zone cells in the wrong place, they quickly move to the correct site.

17. You may be asked to draw out a proteoglycan.

18. Looks like a test-tube brush.

19. This is really a subtopic discussion rather than an isolated question.

20. Collagen synthesis and structure can easily take up 5 minutes of a viva, especially if a candidate's answers are sluggish.

21. Testing clinical application of basic science.

22. If a candidate is poor at drawing diagrams they may need to compensate for this by more detailed diagram practice beforehand. In the big scheme of things, poor artistic ability shouldn't make a massive input into a candidate's performance and/or mark. If a candidate has identified this weakness, practised drawing out the relevant diagram and perhaps more

importantly is confident when delivering their discourse, this should be enough.

23. The viva usually develops in a slightly different direction than the previous two viva questions.

24. Andrews S, Shrive N, Ronsky J. The shocking truth about meniscus. *J Biomech*. 2011;44: 2737e40.

25. Smeathers J. Shocking news about discs. *Curr Orthop*. 1994;8(1):45–48.

26. Providing a convoluted answer.

27. If the examiners let you.

28. The question should not have been asked in its present form if at all. It should have been picked up with standard setting on the questions the night before the exam begins and discarded.

29. Neumann DA. *Kinesiology of the Musculoskeletal System, Foundations for Rehabilitation*, 2nd edition. Maryland Heights, MI: Mosby Elsevier; 2010.

30. Neumann DA. *Kinesiology of the Musculoskeletal System, Foundations for Rehabilitation*, 2nd edition. Maryland Heights, MI: Mosby Elsevier; 2010.

31. Coventry MB, Ghormley RK, Kernohan JW. The intervertebral disc: its microscopic anatomy and pathology: Part III. Pathological changes in the intervertebral disc. *J Bone Joint Surg*. 1945;27(3):460–474.

32. Rudert M, Tillmann B. Lymph and blood supply of the human intervertebral disc: cadaver study of correlations to discitis. *Acta Orthop Scand*. 1993;64(1):37–40.

33. Kastelic J, Galeski A, Baer E. The multicomposite structure of tendon. *Conn Tiss Res*. 1978;6(1):11–12.

34. Essentially the four regions of the curve (toe, linear, plastic and failure).

35. Fralinger DJ, Kaplan DJ, Weinberg ME, Strauss EJ, Jazrawi LM. Biological treatments for tendon and ligament abnormalities. A critical analysis review. *J Bone Joint Surg Rev*. 2016;4(6):e5.

36. This info is not contained in your average basic science orthopaedic textbook and requires a deeper level of knowledge to answer. This is why the viva can be difficult. As a candidate, you can't really prepare for this type of question.

37. Seddon HJ. Three types of nerve injury. *Brain*. 1943;66(4):237–288.

38. Sunderland S. Advances in diagnosis and treatment of root and peripheral nerve injury. *Adv Neurol*. 1978;22:271–305.

Design of implants and factors associated with implant failure (wear, loosening)
Tribology of natural and artificial joints

Kiran Singisetti and Paul A. Banaszkiewicz

Introduction

A recent shift in emphasis with basic science from the ICB is to try and link a topic into a clinical problem to make the subject more clinically relevant and less dry. A classic example is the clinical photograph of an explanted worn PE cup leading on to a discussion of wear.

A good understanding of tribological properties helps the orthopaedic surgeon to choose the most suitable bearing solution for each individual patient.

Wear is an A-list topic with similar competency questions in the first part of a viva but unexpected or esoteric higher-order thinking questions in the second part. This is a method to keep the topic fresh with each diet of exams.

Structured oral examination question 1

Clinical photograph of explanted poly cup with wear and cement

EXAMINER: What do you see? Why has this happened?

CANDIDATE: This is a clinical picture of an explanted PE cup demonstrating acetabular wear (Figure 21.1). It may have been explanted because of associated aseptic loosening.

Other causes for revision may include infection or due to recurrent dislocation.

EXAMINER: There is quite obvious wear seen on the inside of the acetabular cup, so what do you think has been the most likely cause for revision?

CANDIDATE: Aseptic loosening.

EXAMINER: What do you mean by aseptic loosening?

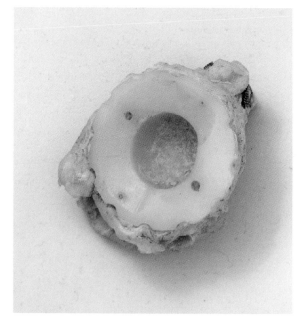

Figure 21.1 Clinical photograph of explanted polyethylene cup demonstrating worn surface.

CANDIDATE: Aseptic (i.e. not caused by infection) loosening refers to the failure of fixation at the bone/implant interface, with resultant micro- or macromotion of the implant relative to the adjacent bone.

EXAMINER: What is the difference between aseptic loosening and osteolysis.

CANDIDATE: [Silence.] They are quite similar processes [more silence].

COMMENT: Although the terms osteolysis and aseptic loosening are often used interchangeably, these processes are different.

Aseptic loosening is an umbrella term that is used to describe total joint arthroplasty failure resulting from inadequate initial fixation, mechanical loss of fixation over time, or biological loss of fixation caused by particle-induced osteolysis around the implant.

Osteolysis refers to the host immunological response that results in implant loosening.

EXAMINER: What do we mean by wear?

CANDIDATE: Wear is the removal of material from two surfaces under load, due to a sliding motion between them.

Wear is the progressive loss of a bearing substance caused by mechanical or chemical (corrosion) action.

COMMENT: There are several definitions of wear. Learn one that you are happy with and stick to it.

EXAMINER: What are the different types of wear that can occur?

CANDIDATE: There are two broad categories of wear, (1) mechanical and (2) chemical.

Mechanical involves:

- Abrasive.
- Adhesive.
- Fatigue.
- Erosive.

Chemical is independent of load and sliding distance:

- Corrosion.

EXAMINER: What are the various types of mechanical wear?

CANDIDATE: Two-body abrasive wear occurs with a hard (cobalt chrome) on soft (UHMWPE) bearing couple.

Asperities on the hard bearing **carve ridges** (plough/cheese grater effect[1]) into the softer bearing.

This generates new particles (wear debris), which become third bodies.

An example is between a metal femoral head and a polyethylene liner.

EXAMINER: What do you mean by adhesive wear?

CANDIDATE: Adhesive wear occurs when opposing asperities of two surfaces bond with each other to form a **junction**.[2] This junction is held by intermolecular bonds and generates friction.

If these bonds are stronger than the **cohesive strength** of the weaker material, then fragments of the weaker material are sheared off.

EXAMINER: What is fatigue wear?

CANDIDATE: With fatigue wear cyclical loading of one surface, at loads greater than the fatigue strength, leads to small cracks forming under the surface.

Cracks propagate, joining together, and the loose material comes away from the surface.

An example is delamination of the polyethylene in TKAs.

EXAMINER: What is erosive wear?

CANDIDATE: Erosive wear occurs when hard particles travelling in fluid interposed between two surfaces remove some of the surface as they collide into it.

An example would be 'third-body' wear from polyethylene wear particles/loose cement travelling in synovial fluid.

EXAMINER: Corrosive wear?

CANDIDATE: Corrosive wear occurs with surface damage due to chemical reactions with the environment.

COMMENT: Do not give a number when mentioning wear mechanisms, i.e. do not say 'wear can occur through five mechanisms (adhesive, abrasive, third body, fatigue, corrosion)'. This is inviting trouble.[3]

Concentrate on the three big wear mechanisms (abrasive, adhesive and fatigue wear) as these are what the examiners are most familiar with.

Although erosive and corrosive wear are less well covered in the textbooks, it is reasonable to briefly mention them and the examiners will decide if they want to further probe you for extra details.[4]

Third-body wear can be either classified as a subtype of abrasive wear or as a separate, distinct type of wear mechanism.

Erosive wear is classified as either a major or minor cause of mechanical wear depending on which textbook is read. It is unlikely that candidates will spend a large amount of viva time discussing this wear mechanism.

EXAMINER: Can you draw out the different types of wear (Figure 21.2a–21.2c)?

COMMENT: In the exam it is difficult to draw if you are caught cold and need to work it out for the first time. To be slick, the drawings need to be practised beforehand. Just as important is a succinct

533

Adhesive wear

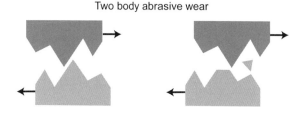

Figure 21.2a Wear mechanisms. Adhesive wear: opposing asperities bond to each other and shear off as one surface slides over the other.

Abrasive wear

Two body abrasive wear

Three body abrasive wear

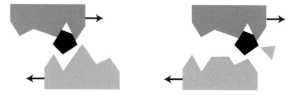

Figure 21.2b Wear mechanisms. Abrasive wear: asperities on the harder material cut into the asperities of the softer material. The new particles become third bodies.

Fatigue wear

Fretting fatigue wear

Tangential cycling load

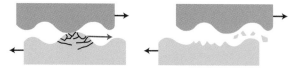

Figure 21.2c Wear mechanisms. Fatigue wear: cyclical loading causes accumulation of micro-damage that breaks off as wear particles.

EXAMINER: How is this wear mechanism in the hip different to that of the knee?

CANDIDATE: Adhesive and abrasive wear is more pronounced for THA while fatigue wear (pitting and delamination) is more problematic for TKA.

EXAMINER: What is the RANKL pathway?

COMMENT: Candidates should be familiar with the RANKL pathway from the Part 1 SBI/EMI paper, but there is a world of difference in answering this topic in a viva exam. Osteolysis is a complicated subject with material sources sometimes lacking focused exam summaries. It is therefore important to go through a dry-run practice viva to refine your answer.

The main biological system that leads to osteolysis-induced resorption of bone is the receptor activator of nuclear factor-κB (RANK)/RANK ligand (RANKL) axis. Activation of this system results in enhanced osteoclast recruitment and activity adjacent to bone implant surfaces, leading to osteolysis. Osteoprotegerin (OPG) is a decoy molecule that blocks RANKL and prevents bone resorption.

The osteolytic response includes various cell types, such as osteoclasts, macrophages and osteoblasts/stromal cells. This is supported by the wide range of factors that are secreted by various cells, including cytokines, growth factors, metalloproteinases, prostanoids and lysosomal enzymes etc. (Figure 21.3).

Once macrophages are activated by particulate debris, they secrete various kinds of mediators to incite a complex cascade of events culminating in recruitment and maturation of osteoclasts, the bone-resorbing cells directly responsible for the pathogenic bone loss in osteolysis.

Other cell types involved in the production of cytokines and inflammatory mediators include

but clear explanation of each wear mechanism while you are drawing.

EXAMINER: What type of wear has occurred on the PE cup surface?

CANDIDATE: The majority of the wear pattern would be abrasive. Third-body abrasive wear is also a possibility. This is like having sand in one's shoes.[5] It is a form of abrasive wear that occurs when a hard particle becomes embedded in a soft surface. The particle acts very similarly to the asperity of a harder material in abrasive wear, removing material in its path. Hard third-body particles such as bone cement can produce damage to both the polyethylene articulating surface and the metal femoral head.

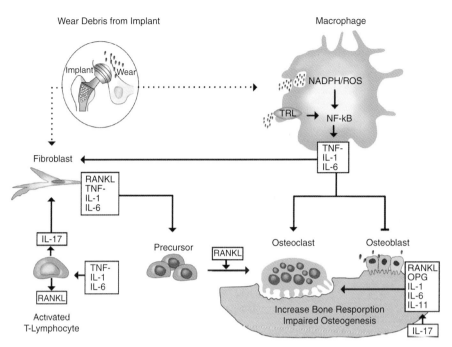

Figure 21.3 Model of interplay between macrophages, fibroblasts, lymphocyte, osteoclasts and osteoblasts in periprosthetic osteolysis. Particles may stimulate macrophages, fibroblasts and osteoblasts directly to induce RANKL and pro-inflammatory cytokines that can induce RANKL. It is thought that T cells stimulated by the pro-inflammatory microenvironment may also promote osteoclast formation, synergized with TNF-α, by secreting IL-17. Thus, RANKL, TNF-α, IL-1, IL-6, IL-17 and M-CSF may mediate the differentiation of myeloid precursor cells into multinucleated osteoclasts.[6] TRL = toll like receptors. Experimentally, polymethylmethacrylate (PMMA) and polyethylene (PE) particles have been shown to activate macrophages via the TRL pathway.

osteoblasts and fibroblasts. Matrix-degradative enzymes and chemokines are also released from several types of cells.

Osteoblasts can also phagocytose small particles, causing adverse effects on viability, proliferation and function of osteoblasts as well as on osteoclasts. Research suggests that UHMWPE increases the release of RANKL from osteoblasts, while OPG is significantly inhibited.

Although wear debris may consist of polyethylene, PMMA cement, or metal, by far the great majority of wear particles derives from polyethylene.

EXAMINER: What factors affect the degree of osteolysis from wear particles?

CANDIDATE: Factors affecting osteolysis severity include:

1. Size of particles:

- Large particles escape active phagocytosis, being recognized as non-digestible foreign bodies. They fail to stimulate macrophages to produce high levels of pro-inflammatory and osteolytic cytokines.

- Particles within the broad size range of 0.1–10.0 μm are phagocytosed by macrophages, leading to cellular activation. Those in the size range 0.1–1.0 μm are the most active.

- Very small submicron particles can escape phagocytosis and fail to stimulate macrophages to produce high levels of pro-inflammatory and osteolytic cytokines.

2. Shape of particles (elongated particles are more active compared to round or spherical particles).

3. Volume of particles (the critical volume is 140 mm^3/year).

4. Total number of particles.

5. Surface area.

6. Immune response to particles.

EXAMINER: What are Gruen zones?

CANDIDATE: This is a widely used system in which the femoral component interface is considered in seven zones (Figure 21.4). These allow the location of cement fractures and of lucent lines either at the cement–bone or the cement–prosthesis interface.

535

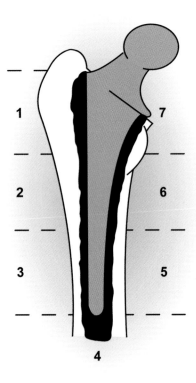

Figure 21.4 Gruen zones. Remember 1–7 starting at GT and ending at calcar.

It is the progressive changes seen in serial radiographs that are important in diagnosing osteolysis and femoral stem loosening.

Structured oral examination question 2

Wear and osteolysis

A clinical picture of a worn polyethylene cup is shown (Figure 21.5).

- Mechanisms of wear.
- Osteolysis.
- Effective joint space.

EXAMINER: What are the mechanisms of wear?

CANDIDATE: The main mechanisms of wear include abrasive, adhesive and fatigue wear (see previous answer).

EXAMINER: What do we mean by the term 'osteolysis'?

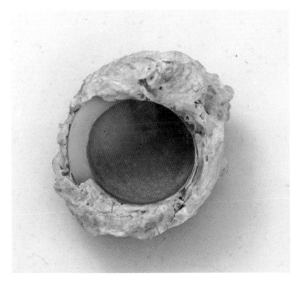

Figure 21.5 Clinical picture demonstrating worn surface of retrieved PE cup.

CANDIDATE: Osteolysis is a cell-mediated biological process that results in the loss of bone as a direct response to stimulation of macrophages by biologically active particles.

The core of the biological response that leads to osteolysis involves the receptor activator of NF-κB ligand [RANKL]–RANK axis for osteoclast precursors, resulting in their differentiation and maturation (see previous answer).

EXAMINER: What about the importance of macrophages in the pathogenesis of osteolysis?

CANDIDATE: The cellular response that occurs in osteolysis is dominated by macrophages. Particles ranging from 0.1 to 10 μm in diameter undergo phagocytosis by macrophages.

Once activated by particulate debris, macrophages secrete various kinds of mediators to incite a complex cascade of events culminating in osteoclast maturation.

Pro-inflammatory mediators such as PGE_2, TNF-α and IL-6 are generated in abundance by particle-challenged macrophages.

The precise nature of stimulation of macrophages by particles remains unknown. However, it is thought that direct interactions between particle and cell surface are sufficient to activate osteoclastogenic signalling pathways. These interactions may include non-specific physical induction of transmembrane proteins or recognition of cell surface molecules by particles. Recently, this phenomenon was explained with the role of toll-like receptor.

EXAMINER: What do we mean by effective joint space[7]?

CANDIDATE:
1. Schmalzried *et al.*[8] coined the term 'effective joint space' to describe all periprosthetic regions that are accessible to joint fluid and thus particulate debris by the pumping action of the joint.
2. All periprosthetic regions that are accessible to joint fluid and its particulate debris.
3. The effective joint space is a concept that describes the entire volumetric area within a hip joint construct that can be infiltrated by PE wear particles and macrophages. Bone breakdown can occur anywhere within the effective joint space.

COMMENT: There are three definitions. Learn one and stick with it.

The presence of particulate matter in joint fluid will initiate a localized macrophage-induced phagocytosis and result in bone resorption. As fluid pressure propels joint fluid and thus particulate debris through the effective joint space, it will result in progressive bone loss.

As bone is resorbed, a bigger sink is produced, encouraging even more flow (preferential flow) into that area, delivering more particles and causing more bone resorption. When sufficient bone has been resorbed, an osteolytic area can be seen on radiographs. If joint fluid is distributed more evenly in an interface, there will be slower resorption of bone, accompanied by a fibroblastic response resulting in the radiographic appearance of linear (diffuse) bone loss.

EXAMINER: How can you reduce effective joint space?

CANDIDATE: Reduction in the effective joint space may reduce the amount of osteolysis that can occur.

The use of bone screws for fixation of acetabular shells is thought to create new voids in the acetabular bone that increase the effective joint space. Implanting acetabular shells without any screw holes in theory reduces the effective joint space.

Cementing seals off the effective joint space.

Using an Exeter stem that subsides into a centralizer blocks off any potential implant/cement space.

The use of circumferential proximal porous coated uncemented stem designs seals off the diaphyseal component of the femoral canal from the effective joint space and may reduce the amount of osteolysis occurring.

EXAMINER: What new designs of hip replacements have been introduced to retard osteolysis by limiting the generation and spread of particulate debris?

CANDIDATE: Improved liner locking mechanisms reduce the amount of motion between shell and PE liner. It has been suggested wear debris can be produced at the interface between the metal acetabular shell and PE liner.

NJR data with a ceramic on a highly cross-linked PE bearing couple compared to a more traditional metal-on-UHMWPE articulation. There have been improvements in the bearing articulation materials, particularly the development of first- and second-generation highly cross-linked PE. UHMWPE has much improved wear characteristics with reduced adhesive and abrasive wear in comparison to the older generation of PE.

Improved results are being reported from traditional metal on UHMWPE articulation.

COMMENT: Candidates could be moved easily towards discussing improvements in PE manufacture, sterilization, shelf packaging, annealing versus heating, amorphous versus crystalline phase, etc. as part of an evolving viva on wear (advanced questions).

EXAMINER: What are the risk factors for osteolysis?

CANDIDATE: Risk factors can be broken down into patient-, surgical- and prosthesis-related factors.

Patient factors include age at surgery and male gender.

The evidence for association between increased body mass index and activity level is contradictory.

Implant factors include prosthetic design, bearing couple, PE (manufacturing process, post-manufacturing sterilization, thickness of PE insert (knee) and liner (hip)).

Surgical factors include cementing technique, correct prosthetic alignment (anteversion, inclination), prosthesis stability.

Structured oral examination question 3

Wear in THA

Picture of aseptic loosening, what is wear, measures to reduce wear, particle size.

A radiograph of aseptic loosening hip is shown to the candidate (Figure 21.6).

EXAMINER: What is wear?

CANDIDATE: Mechanical wear is the removal of material from two surfaces under load, due to the sliding motion between them.

EXAMINER: What are the modes of wear of artificial joints?

CANDIDATE: The four modes of wear are:

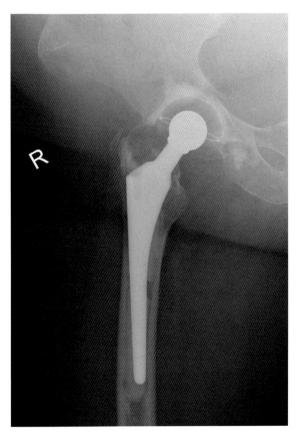

Figure 21.6 Anteroposterior (AP) radiograph, pelvis, demonstrating loose right THA. Cement fracture and femoral stem and cup migration. Gruen mode 1a failure.

Mode 1. Generation of wear material that occurs with motion between the two primary bearing surfaces, as intended by the designers.

Mode 2. A primary surface rubbing against a secondary surface not intended as an articulating surface.

Mode 3. Two primary bearing surfaces with interposed third-body particles.

Mode 4. Two non-bearing surfaces rubbing together.

COMMENT: McKellop's classification. Do not confuse with the four Gruen modes of failure of cemented femoral stems or vice versa.[9]

The fundamental mechanisms of wear include adhesive, abrasive and fatigue wear.

EXAMINER: What measures can be taken to reduce wear?

COMMENT: This is a vague, non-specific question. It is easier to answer if you can turn the question around slightly and discuss factors that affect wear.

One potential answer is to focus on PE. There is more than enough material to discuss that would use up the full 5 minutes of viva discussion if you are allowed to keep on talking (unlikely, but worth trying).

So, a candidate's lead in phrasing to discuss PE wear could be 'The main type of wear particle implicated in osteolysis and loosening of total joint replacements is polyethylene. Methods to improve the wear characteristics of PE include':

- Manufacturing techniques.
- Sterilization techniques.
- Shelf life.
- Using first-/second-generation highly cross-linked PE.

This may not work if the examiners have set questions they are required to ask candidates for the viva topic and PE wear isn't big on this list.

Another possible option is to discuss:

Surgeon (technique) factors:

- Implant selection, avoidance of implant malalignment, avoid impingement (increases wear), accurate restoration of mechanical axis joint, avoidance of debris contamination which will cause third body wear.

Patient factors:

- Weight (weight reduction).

- Activity level (avoidance of excessive activities, e.g. water skiing, treadmill running, etc.).
- Implant design.[10] Decide on whether to discuss hips or knees or both.
- Hips.
  - Offset. Decreasing offset increases joint reaction forces.
  - Choice of bearing couple (MoP, CoP, MoM).
  - Head size.
- Knees.
  - Conformity.
  - Thickness of PE (minimum 8 mm). Thin PE predisposes to accelerated wear by delamination because of concentrated subsurface stress and fatigue wear.
  - Femoral roll back.

Structured oral examination question 4

Wear in TKA

Polyethylene wear in TKA: discuss all factors.[11]

EXAMINER: What does the picture show (Figure 21.7)?

CANDIDATE 1: A worn tibial tray.

CANDIDATE 2: A worn PE tibial insert. It looks like it is a CR-retaining ploy. There is evidence of severe delamination with uneven wear more pronounced medially. Discoloration is as a dark yellow tint representative of polyethylene oxidation.

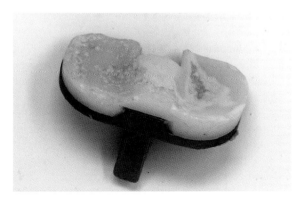

Figure 21.7 Worn PE tibial tray. Delamination is seen as thin sheets of polyethylene separated from the surface.

EXAMINER: Discuss the factors associated with PE wear in TKA.

CANDIDATE: Ultra-high molecular polyethylene wear debris triggering osteolysis is one of the major causes of failure of TKA.

Varus alignment of implants leads to accelerated medial PE wear and the risk of early failure. Varus placement of the tibial component > 3° leads to almost double the PE volumetric penetration rate.

Backside wear between the plastic and metal tray occurs due to micromotions occurring at that interface. Snap-in capture mechanisms combined with manufacturing tolerances may lead to considerable motion under shear and torque. This is compounded by the roughness of the metal tibial tray, resulting in increased PE particle generation leading to osteolysis. This can be particularly severe in tibial trays with holes for fixation screws around which osteolytic lesions can develop.

Additional component features that increase wear include thinner polyethylene inserts, some non-cemented tibial baseplates supplemented with tibial screws, and metal-backed patellar components.

The manufacturing process of PE is important. Direct compression-moulded tibial components have better wear characteristics than components machined from either ram bar extrusion or sheet compression moulding.

The change from sterilization of PE by gamma radiation in air to an inert gas has resulted in much lower rates of osteolysis at 10 years post surgery.

Sterilization of PE by gamma radiation in air creates free radicals that can react with oxygen when stored for an extended period of time in an oxygen-rich environment. This results in a subsurface band of highly oxidized polyethylene that results in decreased mechanical strength and a tendency to premature wear.

Although the benefit of highly cross-linked PE in reducing wear rates in THA have been confirmed, there are concerns with its use in TKA.

These include reduced strength, fatigue resistance and fracture toughness due to additional irradiation and thermal treatment.

THA articulation occurs mostly as a sliding motion in a ball-and-socket joint, while TKA articulation can occur as rolling, sliding and rotating.

The mechanism of wear between these two joints is different. THA wear is mostly due to micro-adhesion and abrasion, while TKA wear can be due to fatigue failure with delamination and pitting.

Most supporting evidence for HXPLE in knee arthroplasty is derived from in-vitro wear simulator studies that show a reduction of wear of up to 60%.

The literature is confusing as three recent mid-term, randomized clinical trials (mean follow-up: 2–5.9 years) comparing HXLPE and conventional UHMWPE bearings have all found no significant difference in clinical or radiological outcomes between the two bearings.[12,13,14]

However, NJR data from Australia have shown higher revision rates with non-XLPE. HXLPE had a lower cumulative percentage revision than conventional polyethylene at 5 years (4.0% vs 2.6%) and 10 years (5.8% vs 3.6%).

It is recognized that failed TKA have larger flake-shaped debris, which elicits a tissue response characterized by fewer macrophages. This is different from failed THA. This larger particle debris may be associated with delamination, pitting and fatigue wear.

COMMENT: A clinical picture of a tibial insert demonstrating a white subsurface oxidized band of PE is another classic lead-in prop to discuss PE wear in TKA. See also the cutting tool effect of machining of PE (Figure 21.8).

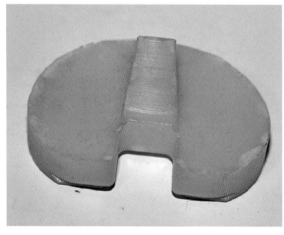

Figure 21.8 Retrieval PE insert demonstrating classic white band defect of oxidation located 1–2 mm below the machined surface of PE.

EXAMINER: What are the wear mechanisms in TKA?

CANDIDATE: Three main wear mechanisms can be seen in TKA.[15] These are adhesive, abrasive and surface fatigue. Tribo-chemical is sometimes mentioned as a fourth mechanism.

Adhesive wear: the bonds formed between different materials are stronger than the specific material properties of either surface and therefore pull out fragments from one surface to another.

Abrasive wear: a harder rougher material ploughs through a softer material.

Surface fatigue: this is a process in which the material near to the surface is weakened by cyclic shear stresses or strains that exceed the fatigue strength of the material.

Tribo-chemical wear: this is a process with a chemical basis that occurs at the interface between the articulating components and the environment. This friction mechanism initiates and propagates cracks at both the surface and subsurface.

EXAMINER: What wear damage occurs at the tibial PE surfaces of a TKA?

CANDIDATE: Hood et al.[16] described seven types of wear mechanism damage at the articulating surfaces of TKA:

- Burnishing (polishing).
- Scratching.
- Abrasion.
- Pitting.
- Delamination.
- Third-body wear (embedded debris).
- Creep (surface deformation).

Burnishing: contact areas are polished due to a combination of abrasive and adhesive wear. This is a less-severe sign of wear, although submicrometre particle size generation can lead to macrophage activation and osteolysis.

Scratching: this is caused by abrasive wear. Differences in roughness and hardness between articulating surfaces lead to ploughing of the softer material.

Abrasion: characterized as a shredding of the polyethylene surface and classified as a mode of abrasive wear.

Pitting: a mode of fatigue wear that is characterized by the formation of millimetre-sized craters (Figure 21.9). It is caused by cracks formed by repetitive tensile and compressive stresses at the

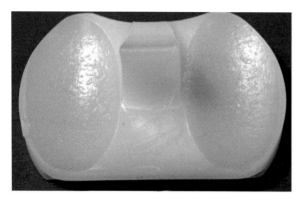

Figure 21.9 Pitting small crater-like surface defects.

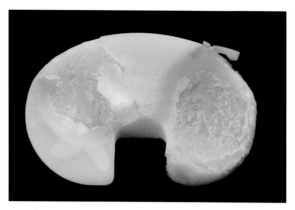

Figure 21.10 Delamination of PE.

surface as the contact areas slide over the surface. It is considered to be a more benign wear mechanism that does not provoke an osteolytic response.

Third-body wear: wear debris can act as third-body particles, initiating wear by rubbing at the bearing surfaces.

Delamination (Figure 21.10): this is a severe form of fatigue wear, involving the removal of sheets of polyethylene, and can result in catastrophic wear.

There is gross disruption of the material to a depth of 0.5 mm or more due to the formation and propagation of subsurface cracks. These cracks are thought to be due to the subsurface shear stresses that fluctuate in direction and magnitude.

Creep (cold flow): the material deforms plastically without release of metal debris. More severe plastic deformation of the tibial insert may be an indication of malalignment or a mismatch of component sizes.

PE wear in knee arthroplasty occurs from a combination of rolling, sliding and rotation motions between the bearing surfaces which in due course leads to fatigue failure of the softer component (PE tibial insert), resulting in pitting and delamination.

Strategies to reduce polyethylene wear include the following.

- Improving implant design.

  . Increased articular conformity increases the articular surface contact area, thereby reducing the subsurface PE contact stress per unit area. Congruent bearing designs lower the amount of cross-shear stresses.

  – 'Double-dished' geometry minimizes contact stresses and edge loading. The sagittal plane should be concave or dished and the individual medial and lateral tibial plateaus should also be dished in the coronal plane.

  . Improved locking mechanisms of modular tibial components to reduce potential backside wear.

  . Highly polished tibial base plate.

  . Mobile bearings rotating platform. A rotating yet flat PE bearing is matched against a highly polished cobalt chromium surface.

  . Monobloc tibial components. The PE bearing surface is direct compression-moulded to the tibial base plate. This design is thought to eliminate backside wear, which may improve long term survivorship in patients receiving TKA.

  . All polyethylene tibial components have been used in an attempt to decrease or eliminate the problems associated with backside wear.

- **Improvements in the quality of ultrahigh-molecular-weight PE.**

  . Improved sterilization techniques (gamma irradiation inert atmosphere).

  . Development of newer, highly cross-linked PE with the introduction of vitamin E and sequential annealing.

- **Refining surgical techniques.**

  . Computer navigation.

  . Fellowship-trained surgeons.

541

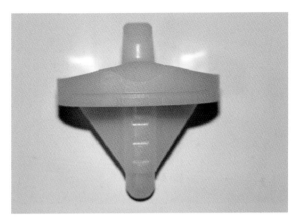

Figure 21.11 All-polyethylene tibial component (APT), posterior stabilized design.

EXAMINER: Is there any evidence that all-polyethylene tibial components reduce wear (Figure 21.11)?

CANDIDATE: The theoretical benefits of using metal-backed tibial components include a more even distribution of weight-bearing stresses to the underlying fixation interface and cancellous bone and a reduction in the potential polyethylene deformity caused by creep. A number of studies have failed to show any difference in survivorship between metal-backed and all-polyethylene tibial components. My understanding is that the newer types of one-piece polyethylene tibial components are best suited for elderly, low-demand patients where survival rates approach those of a metal-backed tibial component.

COMMENT: With all-polyethylene tibial (APT; Figure 21.11) the same amount of tibial resection allows for a thicker PE to be used, potentially increasing the lifetime of the prosthesis if wear rates are equivalent, as less tibial resection will be required to achieve the same poly thickness as a design with a metal tray, resulting in a larger metaphyseal surface area and the ability to use larger tibial component sizes, reducing the magnitude of contact stresses transmitted across the joint while also preserving metaphyseal bone stock.[17]

EXAMINER: What do we mean by conformity?

CANDIDATE: Contact stresses experienced at the PE surface are inversely proportional to the degree of conformity between the femoral condyle and the tibial PE insert.

The greater the conformity at the articulating counter surfaces, the greater the contact area between these surfaces. This reduces detrimental subsurface contact stresses experienced by the PE.

EXAMINER: So why don't we just go with highly conforming knee designs?

CANDIDATE: Highly conforming TKA designs significantly increase the stresses transmitted to the fixation interface and increase the risk of early aseptic loosening. Roll-back is sacrificed, resulting in reduced range of knee movement.

Conversely, reduction of contact area with low-conformity designs leads to accelerated PE wear and early TKA failure.

EXAMINER: What about mobile bearings?

CANDIDATE: In-vitro wear studies have shown that mobile bearing produces less wear compared to fixed designs. This benefit, however, has failed to translate into improved clinical outcomes or survivorship.

EXAMINER: What about surgeon factors?

CANDIDATE: Surgeon-controlled strategies recommended for reduction of PE wear include meticulous attention to ligament balancing, reproduction of anatomic extremity alignment, restoration of the proper joint-line level, and balanced symmetrical flexion/extension gaps.

EXAMINER: What else?

CANDIDATE: Ideally, a fellowship-trained arthroplasty surgeon.

EXAMINER: What else?

CANDIDATE: GIRFT (getting it right first time).

Regular appraisal/assessment including PROMS scores, scrutiny of NJR data including numbers and reasons for any revision knee surgery performed.

Computer navigation.

EXAMINER: Is there any evidence that computer navigation improves the accuracy of implant positioning?

CANDIDATE: There is some evidence that computer navigation reduces the number of TKAs that have a coronal malalignment of more than 3°. Significant outliers are avoided.

EXAMINER: Which paper?

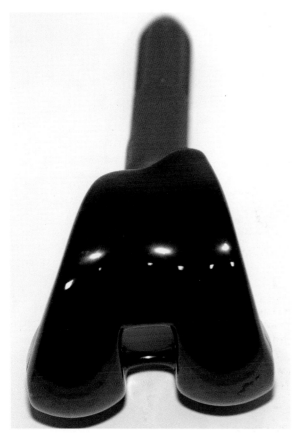

Figure 21.12 Oxium-coated femoral knee implant. During manufacture, OXINIUM implants undergo a process that transforms the implant's surface into a hard, ceramicized metal.

CANDIDATE: I am not familiar with the specific papers, but the general literature suggests better alignment with navigation.

COMMENT: This is a reasonable default statement if you don't know the specifics of a paper. Try not to use it too often as this will irritate the examiners.

Reference

Bauwens K, Matthes G, Wich M, *et al.* Navigated total knee replacement. A meta-analysis. *J Bone Joint Surg [Am]*. 2007;89A:261–269.

CANDIDATE: Although coronal malalignment is reduced, mean alignment and mechanical axis did not differ between navigated and conventional TKRA groups.

COMMENT: The candidate trying to wrangle out of specifics!

EXAMINER: Is there any evidence that computer navigation improves the survival of a knee prosthesis?

CANDIDATE: It is very difficult to prove that computer navigation definitely reduces the need for revision surgery. I am not familiar with the specific papers, but some NJR data from Australia demonstrate a lower revision rate in young patients at around the 10-year mark.

COMMENT: Most studies at mid-term follow-up have failed to show any substantial benefits in terms of functional outcomes, revision rates, patient satisfaction, or patient-perceived quality of life.

Recent Australian Registry data suggest there may be a small advantage, particularly in younger patients, as there is a small reduction in the rate of revision for loosening in this group.

EXAMINER: What about the use of alternative bearings?

CANDIDATE: Some surgeons have begun using oxidized zirconium femoral components as a means of reducing polyethylene wear. This technology incorporates a zirconium oxide ceramic coating on a zirconium metal alloy femoral component. The surface is more scratch-resistant than cobalt chromium, lessening wear debris production.

Another advantage of an oxidized Zr femoral component is that it is safe to use in patients with a nickel sensitivity because there is no traceable nickel in this material.

EXAMINER: Any long-term results reported?

CANDIDATE: Ten-year results were reported by Pinczewski *et al.* from Australia.[18] They showed comparable rates of survival with other implants and excellent functional outcomes 10 years postoperatively.

They did not show any reduction in revisions for PE wear and osteolysis. The main thrust of the paper appeared to be the high level of patient satisfaction with TKA using this bearing surface (WOMAC, KOOS).

EXAMINER: Any concerns with the paper?

CANDIDATE: Single-surgeon series in a tertiary specialized referral centre that may not reflect the average standard knee arthroplasty surgeon practice.

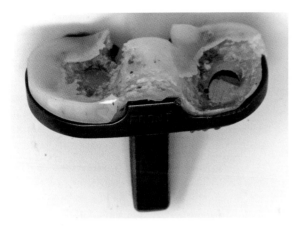

Figure 21.13 Catastrophic failure of PE tibial insert.

Structured oral examination question 5

The candidate is shown a clinical picture of catastrophic PE failure in TKA (Figure 21.13).

COMMENT: Remember to structure your answer (1) PE thickness, (2) articular surface design, (3) knee kinematics, (4) PE manufacture, (5) PE sterilization and (6) surgical technique.

CANDIDATE: This is a clinical photograph of an explanted tibial knee replacement component demonstrating catastrophic PE failure. Causes for this could include low conformity of implant design, inadequate PE thickness, use of low-quality PE . . .

COMMENT: The candidate started well, confidently going straight to the diagnosis of catastrophic PE failure and then was able to talk about possible causes.

The candidate has put their cards on the table and the examiner can then decide where the viva goes next.

Structured oral examination question 6

Charnley THA

Polyethylene cup: what is polyethylene, manufacturing advances, wear, what is the stem made from, stress–strain of the stem

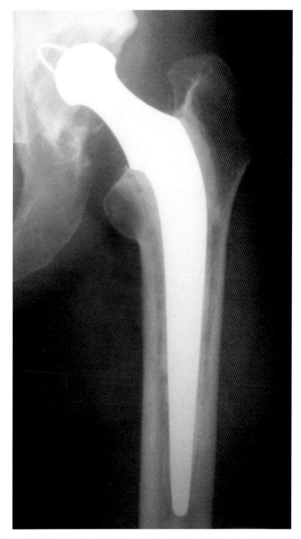

Figure 21.14 Radiograph of Charnley total hip arthroplasty.

EXAMINER: What is polyethylene?

CANDIDATE: UHMWPE is a member of the polyethylene family of polymers with the repeat unit $[C_2H_4]_n$, with n denoting the degree of polymerization.

It is a linear (non-branching), semi-crystalline polymer which can be described as a two-phase composite of crystalline and amorphous phases.

The manufacture of polyethylene is by the Ziegler process, which involves ethylene molecules being polymerized into a high molecular weight by compression-moulding and ram extrusion.

EXAMINER: How is PE manufactured?

CANDIDATE:

Manufacturing processes

- Ram bar extrusion with secondary machining.
  - Polyethylene resin is simultaneously heated and pressurized within an evacuated chamber. As the solid polyethylene forms, it is extruded through an open extrusion port within the chamber. A primitive method of polyethylene manufacture, but cheap.
  - Because the extrusion process is non-continuous, inconsistencies can be found within the solid polyethylene bar stock.
  - Calcium stearate was initially used as a lubricant and release agent in the moulding process. This is no longer added to polyethylene. Calcium stearate crystals could be found between the particles of polyethylene, resulting in fusion defects that became the point of crack initiation and propagation.

- Sheet compression moulding.
  - This is a form of compression moulding used to manufacture large sheets of PE. The resin is poured onto a plate and these plates are brought together and heat is applied.
  - After a specific heating cycle has been completed, the pressure is increased to a desired set point and the material is allowed to cool under pressure.

- Compression moulding into bars with secondary machining.
  - This process produces rods rather than sheets of PE.

- Direct compression moulding.
  - The most advanced form of PE manufacture involves direct compression moulding from PE powder. The resin is directly moulded into the finished implant.
  - There is no secondary machining of the bearing surface. Best wear profile.
  - Direct compression moulding has a lower susceptibility to fatigue crack formation and propagation.

- Hot isostatic pressing (HIPing) into bars.
  - Multistep conversion process of resin powder into stock material.

EXAMINER: What do we mean by the cutting tool effect of polyethylene?

CANDIDATE: In a machined polyethylene insert, machine marks from the lathe create numerous micron-size grooves and shreds on the bearing surface. As the high-speed cutting lathe removes PE, the remaining nearby PE is stretched. The microscopically stretched PE chains are more susceptible to radiation, resulting in greater oxidation in this area. Stretching occurs in the amorphous areas of PE and is most pronounced in the PE 1–2 mm below the surface of the cut PE.

One of the major advantages of direct compression moulding is that the surface of the moulded polyethylene insert is smooth, lacking machine marks or grooves.

EXAMINER: What manufacturing advances have occurred with PE?

CANDIDATE: The advent of highly cross-linked PE (HXLPE) has been shown to improve wear rates in hip arthroplasty.

Compared to standard PE, HXLPE has:
- Better wear resistance.
- The PE particles tend to be smaller in size and produce less osteolytic reaction.
- There is generally a decreased number of particles generated.

Disadvantages include:
- Decreased tensile strength – the pulling force to break.
- Decreased fatigue strength – the maximum cyclic stress the material can withstand.
- Decreased fracture toughness – the force to propagate a crack.
- Decreased ductility – elongation without fracture.

COMMENT: To score a 7 a candidate may need to discuss supportive literature of improved implant survivorship with HXLPE in THA.

To score an 8, a candidate may need to discuss the controversies of HXLPE use in TKA.

EXAMINER: What do we mean by cross-linking?

CANDIDATE: Cross-linking is a process that changes the mechanical and tribological properties of a polymer. By removing atoms or side groups from adjacent chains, covalent bonds can form that link chains together, inhibit relative

545

molecular movement and as such modify the physical properties of the materials.

EXAMINER: What methods are used for PE sterilization?

CANDIDATE: Sterilization methods can be divided into (1) non-energetic (no radiation) and (2) energetic (using radiation) methods.

Ethylene oxide gas may leave residues harmful to tissues.

Both ethylene oxide and gas plasma sterilization avoid free radical production but do not allow cross-linking of PE. As such, they have a higher wear rate compared to cross-linked PE.

Gamma sterilization in air: this makes PE susceptible to oxygenation. Irradiation in the presence of oxygen leads to chain scission of the polyethylene long chain and free radical generation at the crystal surfaces.

Gamma sterilization in an inert atmosphere: irradiation of PE ruptures PE bonds and creates free radicals. In the absence of oxygen, the free radicals will bond with an adjacent chain, resulting in cross-linking of PE. Cross-linked PE has improved resistance to adhesive and abrasive wear.

Shelf ageing: even with gamma sterilization in an inert atmosphere, some free radicals remain in the PE. These free radicals are susceptible to oxidation.

Avoidance of shelf ageing with improved packaging to stop oxygen from diffusing back into the PE through the packaging and causing oxidation.

Highly cross-linked PE:

First generation: high doses of gamma or electron beam radiation are used to promote an elevated cross-link density (i.e. covalent bonds) into UHMWPE. This results in an increase in wear resistance.

Two different approaches are adopted to achieve oxidation resistance.

1. Annealing: this involves a single thermal treatment below the melting temperature of UHMWPE so that crystallinity and mechanical properties are preserved. However, the UHMWPE still contains residual free radicals with the potential to oxidize in vivo.

2. Remelting: post-irradiation remelting of the polymer above the crystalline transition. This strategy allows for elimination of free radicals up to undetectable levels, but at the expense of

crystallinity changes and diminished mechanical properties.

Second generation: use of alternative stabilization strategies, such as natural antioxidants (vitamin E), or sequential irradiation and annealing processes.

EXAMINER: What is the Charnley femoral stem made of?

CANDIDATE: The original stem was a monoblock, flat-backed design with a polished surface manufactured out of EN58J stainless steel (Figure 21.14). The material was changed to 316 low-carbon vacuum-melted stainless steel in 1971 to improve corrosion resistance and fatigue properties.

Score 7

Rates of stem fractures led to change in stem surface in 1969 to a matt finish using the vaquasheen process, which deliberately surface-hardened the metal to resist fracture. This was followed in 1974 by the introduction of the round-backed stem, which significantly increased the cross-sectional area of the stem over the flat-backed stem to increase stem rigidity and further resist fracturing.

In 1975, anteroposterior Cobra flanges were added to the stem to prevent the escape of cement at the level of the neck resection and also pressurize the cement in the femoral canal. This was designed to prevent subsidence of the stems in the femoral canal, as this was reported to be a significant problem related to stem failure.

These changes resulted in a shift in the behaviour of the stem to a composite beam where its predecessor had obeyed the taper-slip principle.

In 1982, the material was again changed to Ortron 90, a cold-worked stainless steel with high fatigue strength.

Gold medal

COMMENT: When Charnley changed his stem from the flatback to the Cobra design, the biomechanical characteristics were changed from a tapered polished (force-closed) to a shape-closed or composite beam biomechanical design.

The biomechanical difference between the loading mechanisms of these two opposing philosophies was not appreciated at the time.

A candidate may get asked about the different stem design philosophies of Charnley (composite beam) and Exeter (taper slip). If you are feeling

- High BMI.
- Higher activity levels.
- Relatively young age.
- Male.
- Varus stem positioning.
- Relatively undersized stem relative to patient's anatomy.

EXAMINER: What is the incidence of Charnley stem fracture?

CANDIDATE: The first generation of Charnley stainless steel femoral stems fractured in approximately 4.1% of patients with fatigue failure attributed to insufficient stem cross-sectional area and inadequate cement support.

Improvements in stem design and metallurgy have markedly reduced the incidence of femoral stem fracture.

COMMENT: This is the basic science viva, so candidates are less likely to be asked how they would revise a broken femoral Charnley stem. This is material for the adult and pathology viva.

Structured oral examination question 7

TKA loose implant

Same discussion of wear, mechanics of loosening and biology of osteolysis as in previous questions.

Discussion about cement – what is it, materials, properties, etc.

Wedges for reconstruction of tibial defect, how wedges work, why wedges and not cement for build up etc.

EXAMINER: What types of tibial bone loss can occur with primary THA?

CANDIDATE: Large posteromedial asymmetrical osseous defects are often seen in the proximal tibia while performing a primary total knee arthroplasty (TKA) in severe varus knees. The majority of these are peripheral uncontained defects. Depending upon the size of the defect, these can be treated with cementoplasty, structural bone grafts or metallic wedges.

Augmented prostheses with a built-up metal wedge are mechanically superior to cement alone in terms of resisting movement when loaded.

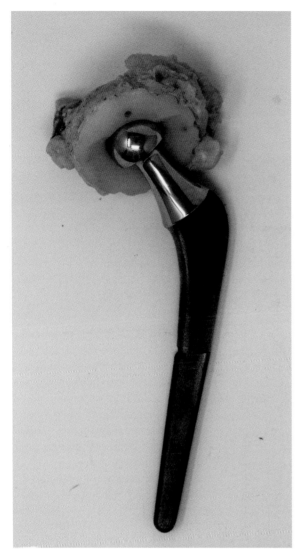

Figure 21.15 Explanted picture of broken Charnley femoral stem.

very confident you can discuss the change in stem behaviour with change in Charnley stem.

EXAMINER: What about the stress–strain curve of the stem?

CANDIDATE: The slope of the stress–strain curve of the stem would be the elastic modulus of stainless steel.

EXAMINER: What are the risk factors for femoral stem fracture (Figure 21.15)?

CANDIDATE: Multiple risk factors for prosthetic stem fracture include:

547

I would prefer to use bone grafting if possible as it is biological, cost-effective and preserves bone stock for future revisions.

EXAMINER: What about cement?

CANDIDATE: Cement is cost-effective, but it cannot be used to address large bony defects. It is reasonable for use for small, shallow, limited defects in elderly patients. It is difficult to pressurize it with large and/or uncontained bone loss. Results are mediocre as its resistance to shear stress and compression is low. Thermal necrosis of bone can occur as well as shrinkage when used in large quantities.

EXAMINER: How do augments work for build-up of bone defects?

CANDIDATE: Metal augments allow rapid filling of bone defects that have been geometrically shaped with instruments. They provide stable support and transfer loading forces to the bone. Results are satisfactory. Using thick augments (30 mm) may result in a painful subcutaneous bulge in the tibia or in the distal femur. Thick augments can prevent bone–intercondylar spacer contact and thus limit stable rotation.

When there is significant bone loss it is often difficult to achieve stable rotational control of the tibial or femoral implant using just a diaphyseal stem with augments. Therefore, to achieve stable fixation a press-fit metaphyseal femoral sleeve can be used to enhance the rotational stability of the femoral component.

EXAMINER: Anything else that can be used to deal with bone loss?

CANDIDATE: Extensive bone loss can be seen with revision TKA.
Management options include:
Metaphyseal sleeves (Figure 21.16). These are indicated in elderly patients where there is metaphyseal deficiency. A broach technique is used to prepare the bone for the press-fit implant.
Metaphyseal filling titanium cones (Figure 21.17a and 21.17b). A high variability of sizes and shapes allows a good adaptability of these modules to the metaphyseal bone deficiency, primarily for those types of cavities in which a reliable cortical shell in the face of a metaphyseal endosteal bone defect is present.

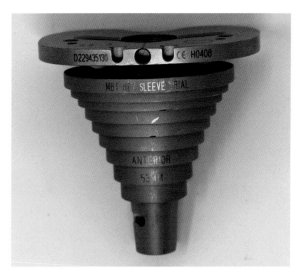

Figure 21.16 Metaphyseal sleeve. The broad tibial sleeve contacts the remaining proximal tibial cortex impacting stability.

My preferred option, if possible, is to use bone grafting, as it is biological, cost-effective and preserves bone stock for future revisions. Its use is especially applicable in young patients in whom a further revision operation is anticipated. I would use impacted morsellized bone graft when there is a contained bone loss larger than 10 mm. I would avoid its use if there was significant cortical bone loss or uncontained defects.

Megaprostheses: high complication rate but the surgical procedure and rehabilitation are rapid. High rate of infection (~5%) that can often be followed by amputation. Best suited for elderly patients with very large bone loss or complex periprosthetic fractures.

Structured oral examination question 8

Cementing technique THA

Picture of broken cement mantle (Figure 21.18) – reasons for this, mantle thickness, asked what would you inform your juniors about too little or too much cement?

EXAMINER: What are the reasons for a broken cement mantle?

CANDIDATE: Initiating events that result in cement failure are due to stresses experienced at the

(a)

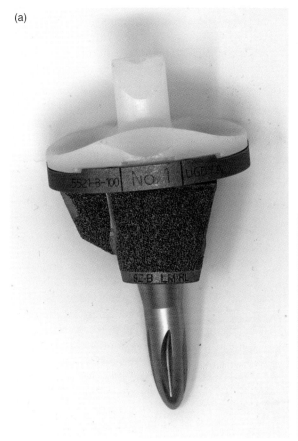

(b)

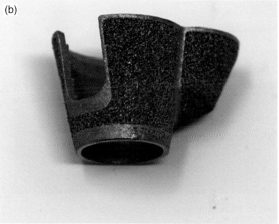

Figure 21.17a and 21.17b Metaphyseal filling titanium cones used to reconstruct metaphyseal bone loss in the tibia or femur.

cement mantle that exceed the fatigue endurance limit of both the stem–cement interface and the cement material itself.

The early development of stem–cement interface debonding (separation) and subsequent cement fracture are thought to be the initiating events of aseptic loosening.

Cement mantle fractures are not benign; they are usually progressive, increasing in number and extent with time.

It is important to reduce cement stresses so as to minimize the risk of cement debonding and fracture.

EXAMINER: So how can high cement stresses be avoided?

CANDIDATE: By the creation of an optimally thick, symmetric and homogeneous cement mantle.

EXAMINER: So how do we achieve this?

CANDIDATE: Stresses experienced in the cement mantle have been shown to be highest at the stem tip and secondarily at the proximal–medial cement mantle.

Stem malalignment produces non-uniform cement mantle thickness in key areas.

Defects or voids in the cement mantle reduce bulk cement thickness and have a substantial effect on cement stresses.

Variations in implant geometry (e.g. diameter and contour) and material have also been shown to affect stresses experienced in the cement mantle.

EXAMINER: Can you be more specific[19]?

CANDIDATE: A varus femoral stem is associated with higher incidence of aseptic loosening. This results in a thin or non-existent cement mantle in the proximal medial and distal lateral zones.

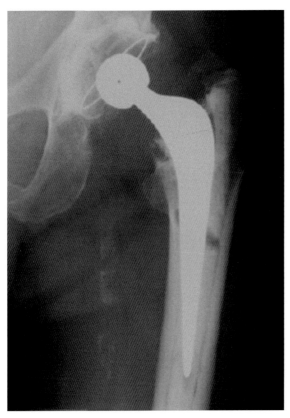

Figure 21.18 Anteroposterior radiograph showing the Exeter total hip replacement with radiolucent lines around the femoral component and fracture of the cement mantle.

Large voids up to 5 mm in diameter are detrimental. The location of voids is important. Small voids in areas of the cement mantle known to experience high strains may result in premature fixation failure.

A proximal–medial cement mantle greater than 10 mm or less than 2 mm in thickness is associated with a significant increase in cement fracture, radiolucent lines at the prosthesis–cement interface and progressive component loosening when compared to proximal–medial cement mantles that measure 2–5 mm in thickness.[20]

An asymmetrical distal cement mantle significantly increases the risk of implant failure.

Inadequate centralization of the stem or malrotation will result in excessively thinned areas of distal cement, increased cement strains and prosthesis bone contact.

Preserving < 2 mm of proximal–medial cancellous bone for 30 mm distal to the femoral neck cut increases cement mantle thickness and reduces proximal–medial cement strain, the incidence of cement fractures, and progressive implant loosening when compared to those cases in which > 2–5 mm of proximal–medial cancellous bone is retained.

COMMENT: Best results for femoral components allow for 2–5 mm proximal–medial thickness of cement mantle, less than 2 mm of proximal–medial cancellous bone thickness, a stem that fills more than half the distal part of the medullary canal and a stem in neutral orientation.

Worst results for femoral components occur with a cement mantle thickness > 10 mm, a femur with more than 2 mm proximal–medial cancellous bone, a stem that fills half or less of the medullary canal and those in varus orientation.

Charnley believed that cancellous bone was weak and incapable of significant load bearing capacity. He believed that removel of weak proximal cancellous bone would improve the long-term fixation of a cemented stem.

Cement mantle stresses are mostly affected by stem design, stiffness and geometry. A stiffer stem reduces cement stress and therefore cobalt chromium is the generally preferred material for cemented THA.

A thin layer of cement will occur if there is lack of removal of proximal–medial cancellous bone.

EXAMINER: What would you inform your juniors about too little or too much cement?

CANDIDATE: The femoral stems of hips that have a 2–5 mm thick cement mantle in the proximal medial region have a better outcome than stems implanted with a thicker(> 10 mm) or thinner (< 2 mm) cement mantle.

EXAMINER: What about the cement, how can this be improved?

CANDIDATE: Improvements in the inherent properties of the cement (increased strength, reduced brittleness, improved interface adherence) to increase strain resistance and thus retard early debonding and microfractures should lead to improved long-term results from cement fixation.

EXAMINER: What measures can be taken intraoperatively to improve the quality of the cement mantle?

CANDIDATE:

1. Canal preparation

Use of correctly sized broaches that allow a mantle of adequate thickness, pulsatile lavage, and brushing and drying of the prepared canal before and during insertion.

Packing of the femoral canal with adrenaline-soaked swabs, hypotensive analgesia to reduce bleeding, suction catheter and avoidance of blood/cement occlusions.

2. Cement preparation

Centrifugation or vacuum-mixing to minimize pore formation and timing of cement injection to achieve optimal viscosity during insertion improves the cement mantle quality. Occlusion of the canal using a distal plug, retrograde filling of the canal and cement gun pressurization of the cement column with a tight proximal seal are essential in achieving an interdigitating, uniform and homogeneous cement mantle.

EXAMINER: How can the cement mantle be optimized. How can we obtain a high-quality cement mantle?

CANDIDATE: Methods for cement fixation optimization include:
- Cement gun pressurization (enhances interdigitation) of the cement column with a tight proximal seal (femoral pressurizer).
- Pulsed lavage (clean dry bone).
- Occlusion of the canal using a distal plug.
- Porosity reduction (vacuum-mixing) which leads to reduced stress points in cement.
- Cement mantle thickness > 2 mm.
- Stem centralizer (reduces risk of stem malpositioning to decrease stress on the cement mantle).
- Absence of cement mantle defects.
- Stiffer stem (results in less bending stress on cement mantle). Increase in stem modulus of elasticity results in elevated cement mantle stresses.
- Improvements in the mechanical properties of cement.

COMMENT: This question approximates to the previous question, but needs a slightly different answer.

EXAMINER: Have you heard of boneloc bone cement?

CANDIDATE: This is a bone cement that was withdrawn quite soon after introduction because of unacceptable revision rates with its use.

Mean fracture toughness and mean tensile strengths were significantly lower than other conventional bone cements.

EXAMINER: What is the ideal cement mantle thickness?

CANDIDATE: I would aim for a cement mantle thickness greater than 2 mm as any less than this increases the risk of cement mantle fracture.

Score 8 candidates

EXAMINER: Have you heard of the French paradox?

CANDIDATE: No, I am sorry I haven't.

COMMENT: The ideal cement mantle thickness is still uncertain. Two philosophies about cement mantle thickness exist. In the UK and USA, the first technique aims to produce a complete cement mantle of at least 2 mm in thickness and without 'windows'. It is believed that 'windows' may allow debris to reach the interface and that thin cement mantles will be highly stressed and may fracture.

The second technique, used in France, is the use of a thinner cement mantle in which the possibility of windows is accepted. This has been called the French paradox in which implantation of a canal-filling femoral component in a line-to-line manner is associated with a thin cement mantle.[21] The reason for good results is thought to be the fact that a thin cement mantle in conjunction with a canal-filling stem was supported mainly by cortical bone and subjected to low stresses.

COMMENT: The discussion could move on to any number of topics related to cement use in arthroplasty surgery depending on how the viva is progressing.
- Barracks grading of cement.[22,23]
- Generations of cementing technique.
- Categories of loosening of cemented stems (Harris).
- Exeter vs Charnley stem design.

Structured oral examination question 9

Wear in TKA

EXAMINER: What types of wear occur in TKA?

CANDIDATE: There are two main types of tibial component wear in TKA, (1) adhesive and abrasive wear and (2) fatigue damage (pitting and delamination).

Fatigue wear occurs during cyclic loading if the yield stress of polyethylene is exceeded (Figure 21.19).

Pitting and delamination are accelerated by the presence of free radicals which cause oxidation.

EXAMINER: Fatigue wear in tibial poly – what, why, where?

CANDIDATE: The appearance of fatigue wear damage is primarily associated with cyclic compressive-tensile loading at the bearing surface, which generates subsurface tensile stresses that initiate and propagate cracks to form delamination and pitting damage.

Instances of fatigue wear and fracture have repeatedly occurred over the history of UHMWPE use in TJR due to changes in molecular weight, fusion defects, crystallinity or cross-linking that can reduce the polymer's resistance to crack initiation and growth.

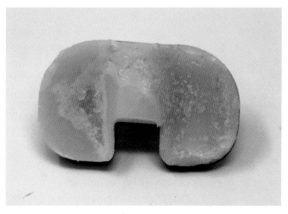

Figure 21.19 Tibial PE insert demonstrating fatigue failure. Fatigue failure is the formation of subsurface cracks in the polyethylene caused by cycles of loading and unloading of the joint, which then propagate and create particles that are shed into the joint space.

Fusion defects (manufacturing processes): the high melt viscosity of UHMWPE can prevent total consolidation of the powders and lead to fusion defects. Fusion defects can exist along particle boundaries, acting as crack nucleation sites for fatigue wear (delamination or pitting) under cyclic sliding contact.

Direct compression moulding results in better consolidation of PE, which likely results in the reduction of defects at particle boundaries when compared to ram bar extrusion.

Degree of cross-linking of PE: cross-linked PE has improved resistance to abrasive and adhesive wear mechanisms.

By limiting the molecular mobility of chains in the amorphous region, cross-linking decreases the creep (cold flow) behaviour of UHMWPE and increases its resistance to wear debris liberation at the contact surface.

However, this also leads to a reduction in plastic deformation processes of UHMWPE that manifests as a reduced resistance to fatigue crack propagation. This renders tibial PE inserts more susceptible to fatigue fracture or delamination wear in the presence of high cyclic contact stresses or at sites of stress concentration, especially in a non-conforming bearing surface.

Sterilization technique: delamination and pitting are common fatigue wear mechanisms after gamma irradiation in air.

Crystallinity of PE: increasing the overall percentage of crystallinity in UHMWPE improves its resistance to fatigue crack growth.

With melting of HCLPE there is lowered crystallinity with improved wear characteristics but reduced mechanical properties. As such, edge loading or excessive PE post loading may result in macroscopic cracks.

Annealing avoids the reduction in the crystalline structure, but there is incomplete elimination of free radicals. Crystalline areas do not cross-link, resulting in an oxidation risk.

COMMENT: The *JBJS* review article 'Osteolysis complicating total knee arthroplasty'[24] provides a good framework for this viva topic. The starting framework for an ICB viva topic may involve basing the viva topic around a well-written credible review article.

Structured oral examination question 10

Osteolysis

The candidate is shown a picture of a THA with femoral osteolysis (Figure 21.20).

COMMENT: This is essentially a question on osteolysis and wear.

CANDIDATE: The principle cell involved in osteolysis is the macrophage. Wear debris from prosthetic materials or bone cement is phagocytosed by macrophages causing release of various mediators.

There is also evidence to suggest a minor role in phagocytosis for fibroblasts and osteoblast cells.

EXAMINER: What size of PE material?

CANDIDATE: Studies have demonstrated that wear particles phagocytosed by macrophages elicited different responses depending on particle size. Particles measuring < 5 μm in size generated a strong mononuclear macrophage response, whereas larger particles resulted in more multinucleated giant cells.

There are many types of wear particles such as polyethylene, PMMA cement, alumina or metal. All have bioactivity and could therefore be involved in the events leading to osteolysis. Evidence suggests that PE wear particles are the most important factor in periprosthetic bone loss around articulations with PE linings.

The debris generated from prosthetic wear triggers a cascade of macrophage cytokines, such as interleukin-1-beta (IL-1β) and tumour necrosis factor-alpha (TNF-α), among others, resulting in osteoclastic bone resorption and eventually leading to osteolysis.

Size: macrophages are most responsive to particles in the size range 0.2–7.0 μm, with larger particles of 90 μm evoking little response.

Shape: the morphology of particles also appears to contribute to cellular responses, with UHMWPE debris with a roughened surface and a fibular shape provoking a greater response in terms of inflammatory cytokine production than particles with a smooth surface and a globular shape.

Material properties (HXLPE vs UHMWPE): higher percentages of small wear particles (0.1–1 μm range) are produced during laboratory wear of HXLPE than conventional PE. Smaller numbers of HXLPE particles compared to conventional PE are required to stimulate cytokine production from macrophages, possibly because of the higher percentage of smaller particles of HXLPE and the increased ability of cells to phagocytose smaller particles.

HXLPE particles may interact with macrophages differently, producing more inflammation and osteolysis compared to conventional PE.

The cellular mechanism of particle-induced osteolysis is that macrophages in the periprosthetic tissues phagocytose wear particles and become activated, releasing an array of cytokines, leading to increased osteoclastic resorption of the adjacent bone and the production of the granulomatous tissue that fills the resorbed space.

The majority of bone resorption occurs from osteoclasts recruited to sites of osteolysis and activated by the osteoclastogenic molecules. To a limited degree, wear particle-activated macrophages present in granulomatous tissue participate directly in bone degradation in periprosthetic osteolysis.

The major pathway of osteoclastogenesis is the production of RANKL by osteoblastic stromal cells and binding of RANKL to its cognate receptor, RANK, on the surface of osteoclast precursors, stimulating these cells to differentiate into mature, active osteoclasts capable of resorbing bone. The natural antagonist of RANKL is

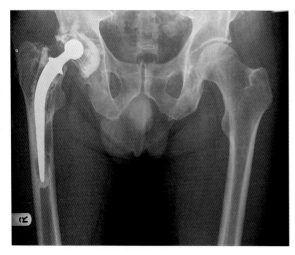

Figure 21.20 Anteroposterior (AP) radiograph, pelvis, demonstrating femoral osteolysis.

553

osteoprotegerin (OPG), whose role is to negatively regulate the activity of RANKL, and therefore bone resorption.

Other cell types, including fibroblasts, osteocytes and activated T cells, also produce RANKL and are capable of stimulating osteoclastogenesis.

There is evidence of direct effects of PE particles on osteoblasts. Exposure of osteoblast-like cells to PE has been shown to induce changes in the rate of cell proliferation, to decrease alkaline phosphatase activity, and to increase the production of osteoclastogenic mediators, such as PGE2, IL-6, GM-CSF, RANKL and nitric oxide.

EXAMINER: Types of wear and modes of wear?

COMMENT: See previous viva questions.

Structured oral examination question 11

Implant materials

COMMENT: Total knee arthroplasty components and the materials used.

Discussions about the advantages of cobalt chrome versus stainless steel and then polyethylene manufacture and sterilization. All standard stuff covered.

The implant biomaterials used in total knee arthroplasty include:

- Stainless steel.
- Cobalt chromium.
- Polyethylene.
- Uncemented implants.
  - Titanium.
  - Tantalum.
  - Oxidized zirconium.

Stainless steel

The advantages of stainless steel include strength, relatively ductile, easy availability, easy to process, easy to fabricate, acceptable biocompatibility and relatively cheap. We know its properties and these are consistent throughout.

Traditionally, its corrosion resistance was poor, being susceptible to pitting, crevice, fatigue, fretting, stress and galvanic corrosion.

Its use in TKA was restricted because other metallic alloys such as Ti-based and Co–Cr-based alloys exhibited superior mechanical (yield strength) and corrosion properties.

Newer implant stainless steel contains a high chromium, molybdenum and nitrogen content, making it stronger and resistant to local corrosion.

The presence of large amounts of nickel within stainless steel is a concern due to worries about Ni sensitivity. In recent years there have been attempts at replacing the nickel content of stainless steel with nitrogen to diminish the possibility of a nickel allergy developing. There are several methods that can be used to modify Young's elastic modulus of stainless steel.

EXAMINER: What does the 316L stand for in stainless steel?

CANDIDATE: The 3 stands for molybdenum (3%), 16 for nickel (16%) and L for low carbon (any stainless steel with less than 0.03% carbon).

EXMAINER: Why low carbon?

CANDIDATE: It is more resistant to corrosion in the body.

Cobalt chromium

The advantages of cobalt chromium are very good wear characteristics, fatigue strength (very strong), toughness and excellent corrosion resistance. Used as a bearing surface as it is very smooth and scratch resistant. It has a high Young's modulus of elasticity and therefore risk of stress shielding. There is a worry it can provoke hypersensitivity reactions.

Titanium

Young's modulus of elasticity is closer to bone; therefore, it is more ductile, with good corrosion resistance, ability to integrate with bone, inert, biocompatible and extremely strong. MRI-compatible. Self passivation. Poor wear characteristics, notch-sensitive and therefore not used as an articulation surface. Expensive.

EXAMINER: Can you give me an example of a titanium alloy used?

CANDIDATE: Titanium alloy 6AL4V (titanium 89%, aluminium 6%, vanadium 4%, others 1%). Vanadium does have potential ion reaction issues, especially if titanium is scratched.

Tantalum: has a high resistance to corrosion, excellent biocompatibility and allows excellent osseointegration with host bone.

Porous tantalum tibial cones or metaphyseal sleeves have been used as a management option for severe tibial bone loss in revision knee surgery.

Oxidized zirconium (OxZr): developed as an alternative bearing material for TJA. This can be used for femoral TKA components and shows significantly less PE wear than chromium. Low friction and high wear resistance.

Higher-order thinking (HOT): putting this all together, cobalt–chromium alloys remain the predominant material (gold standard) used for TKA. There is a worry of increased PE tibial backside wear if titanium is used in place of cobalt–chromium.

All poly tibia inserts were introduced to reduce wear and cost, but had poorer clinical results than conventional metal tibia base plates.

COMMENT: For higher-order thinking, do not just reel off a list of biomaterial properties for each material, but try to match material properties to the function of TKA.

Structured oral examination question 12

Wear and osteolysis

Acetabular cup. Explanted and worn.

What side is up? Divots on the other side may be from neck impingement.

How can you prevent wear? Implant factors/surgical factors.

Implant material, poly manufacturing process and direct compression moulding. Highly cross-linked with gamma irradiation in air vs. vitamin E. Shelf oxidation.

What about the head – we could use ceramics as less rough and better scratch profile.

Tell me about problems with wear – go through the whole RANK/RANKL discussion.

EXAMINER: What side is up?

CANDIDATE: There is eccentric PE wear in the cup superiorly (Figure 21.21).

EXAMINER: What is the difference between PE creep and wear (Figure 21.22)?

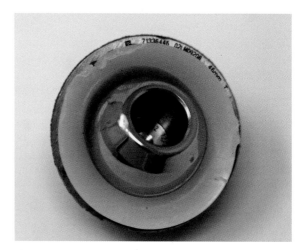

Figure 21.21 PE cup demonstrating superior eccentric wear.

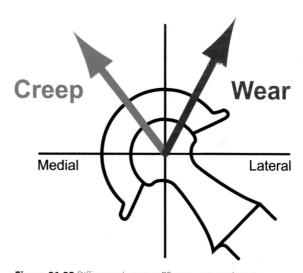

Figure 21.22 Difference between PE cup creep and wear.

CANDIDATE: Creep is normal loading of the polyethylene cup and is superomedial. It is normal to see slight thinning in the area of the weight bearing as the plastic moulds itself. Abnormal loading leads to pressure more laterally, resulting in polyethylene wear on the superolateral side.

EXAMINER: This worn bit here.

CANDIDATE: I pointed out divots on the outer side of the PE cup and said this could be due to neck impingement.

EXAMINER: How do you prevent impingement?

CANDIDATE: Impingement in THA is both implant- and surgeon-dependent.

The implant design factors are those that influence the femoral head–neck ratio as well as features of acetabular design.

The surgeon controls cup position with respect to inclination and anteversion and its depth in the osseous acetabulum. The surgeon also controls the level of the osseous femoral neck cut and the placement of the femoral component for the correct biomechanical restoration of the leg length and hip offset.

EXAMINER: What factors affect the head–neck ratio?

CANDIDATE: The head–neck ratio is affected by femoral head size, femoral neck geometry, and the use of a shirt on the femoral head.

Cam-type impingement can occur with use of a small head on a large circular taper or the use of a skirted femoral head.

A trapezoidal-shaped neck is designed to create a better head–neck ratio, particularly with small heads.

EXAMINER: What features increase acetabular impingement?

CANDIDATE: Features that increase acetabular impingement include the chamfer geometry of the rim of the polyethylene and the presence of an extended-rim (hooded) liner, particularly if the hood is incorrectly positioned in the hip.

Surgeon factors include lateralizing the cup, especially if the cup is also placed in an excessive horizontal position, or failing to remove acetabular osteophytes that can impinge against the metal prosthetic neck or bony femur.

EXAMINER: What do you mean by chamfer geometry?

CANDIDATE: The chamfer geometry is where the liner rim is sloped.

EXAMINER: How do you reduce the chances of impingement occurring?

CANDIDATE: Correct restoration of femoral offset and leg length.

EXAMINER: How do you ensure correct leg length and restoration of femoral offset?

CANDIDATE: It is essential to template the hip pre-operatively and use a calliper-type pin device intraoperatively to check leg length.

EXAMINER: How can you prevent wear?

COMMENT: This is best discussed in terms of patient-related factors, implant-related factors and surgical factors (see above).

Implant material – the poly manufacturing process that has the best wear profile is direct compression moulding into the shape of the desired product. No secondary machining of polyethylene.

CANDIDATE: HXPE with gamma irradiation in an inert atmosphere and vitamin E.

COMMENT: Conventional PE used in hip arthroplasty was sterilized by gamma radiation in air, which offered the benefit of cross-linking but at the same time, this process produced free radicals that oxidized in air, leading to increased wear.

High-dose gamma irradiation of polyethylene is not a sterilization process but a procedure to produce highly cross-linked PE.

First-generation HXPE involves the addition of thermal processing (e.g. annealing or remelting) and gas sterilization (e.g. ethylene oxide or gas plasma) or gamma sterilization in an oxygen barrier packaging with an inert gas (e.g. nitrogen or argon).

Second-generation HXPE involves separate sequential gamma irradiation and annealing steps. The principle behind sequential steps is that smaller doses of radiation in summation can achieve the same levels of cross-linking without generating the number of free radicals created by a single large dose. Vitamin E can also be added as a free radical scavenger.

EXAMINER: Tell me about shelf oxidation.

CANDIDATE: Oxidative embrittlement (characteristically identified as a subsurface white band) is attributed to gamma sterilization in air, and subsequent long-term shelf storage in air has been recognized as a factor contributing to clinical failure (e.g. rim cracking and delamination).

EXAMINER: How does femoral head size affect wear?

CANDIDATE: With conventional UHMWPE the larger the femoral head the greater the volumetric wear. The smaller the head size the greater the amount of linear wear.

Frictional torque increases with head diameter, i.e. the moment arm of the rotating object. The wear of surfaces in rotational relative motion is directly related to frictional torque.

Frictional torque [Nm] = Friction [N] × distance from centre of rotation [m]

Wear of the bearing surface is directly related to frictional torque; therefore, a larger diameter femoral head produces more wear.

Volumetric wear is proportional to the frictional torque of the THA. Therefore, an increase in femoral head size increases frictional torque and related volumetric wear.

COMMENT: This is the basis of Charnley's LFA.

EXAMINER: How can wear of a THA be measured?

CANDIDATE: Wear of the bearing surface of THA can be measured in two ways.

1. Linear wear: the thickness of the acetabular cup decreases as it wears with use. Linear wear is the change in the thickness of the acetabular cup with time.

Linear wear [mm] = original thickness of acetabular cup [mm] – new shortest thickness of acetabular cup [mm]

2. Volumetric wear: this is the actual volume of wear of the acetabular component. Volumetric wear is related to linear wear by the equation

Volumetric wear $[mm^3]$ = π × (radius of femoral head $[mm])^2$ × linear wear [mm]

As such, a larger diameter femoral head produces more volumetric wear for the same linear wear.

EXAMINER: Can you tell me about the scratch profile of ceramic compared to metal (Figure 21.23)?

COMMENT: Best to draw this out if allowed (Figure 21.24).

CANDIDATE: Scratches of the femoral head can lead to an increased rate of PE wear.

Ceramics are harder and more resistant to scratching and damage by third-body wear particles than cobalt–chrome. Ceramic heads have superior surface characteristics. The surface is more wettable and better able to maintain surface lubrication than that of a metal head. Additionally, ceramic has a more rounded surface profile with fewer sharp ridges than a metal surface, thus making it better suited for a bearing surface.

Ceramic is chemically inert. In the aqueous environment of the body, passive oxide films form on the surface of metal femoral heads. This passive film is constantly sheared off and recreated during articulation, a process that increases the surface roughness over time, and also releases potentially damaging third-body particles into the joint space. These consequences are avoided with ceramic heads.

EXAMINER: What factors affect wear of a hard-on-soft bearing surface?

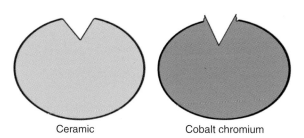

Ceramic   Cobalt chromium

Figure 21.23 Scratch profile of metal and ceramic heads.

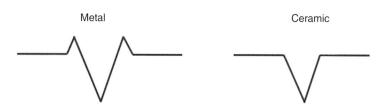

Metal   Ceramic

A pile up of material (ridges) on either side
of the scratch leads to increased rates of wear

Ceramics are harder and
scratching does not cause ridges

Figure 21.24 Candidate drawing of scratch profile.

CANDIDATE: For the head (hard-bearing surface):

- Surface roughness.
- Sphericity of head.
    - Areas out of round are high stress points. These areas increase PE wear.
- Toughness (abrasive wear).
- Hardness (scratch resistance, adhesive wear).

For PE (softer material):

- Manufacturing process.
- Sterilization process.
- Its modification by irradiation.
- PE shelf life.

References

1. Buzz word.

2. Buzz word again.

3. This applies in general to most of your answers. Candidates usually end up forgetting at least one item from a big numbered list and then appear a bit on the backfoot trying to remember it. Unnecessary.

4. If you decide to mention corrosion be careful, as it is chemical rather than mechanical. Although the examiners are more interested in the different types of mechanical wear, we would still mention it.

5. Analogies are helpful for the purpose of explanation or clarification. We don't think there are any major issues using them when appropriate for a principle or idea.

6. Lee S-S, Purdue PE, Nam J-S. Inflammatory periprosthetic bone loss. In *Inflammatory Diseases – Immunopathology, Clinical and Pharmacological Bases*. IntechOpen; 2012. DOI: 10.5772/25558. Available from: www.intechopen.com/books/inflammatory-diseases-immunopathology-clinical-and-pharmacological-bases/biology-of-inflammatory-periprosthetic-bone-loss

7. Banaszkiewicz PA. *Periprosthetic Bone Loss in Total Hip Arthroplasty: Polyethylene Wear Debris and the Concept of the Effective Joint Space*, in *Classic Papers in Orthopaedics*. 2014, Springer. p. 85–87

8. Schmalzried T, Jasty M, and Harris WH. Periprosthetic bone loss in total hip arthroplasty. Polyethylene wear debris and the concept of the effective joint space. *JBJS*. 1992;74 (6):849–863.

9. Quite common in practice vivas in underprepared candidates a few weeks away from sitting the actual part 2 exam.

10. This may be the main thrust of the topic.

11. This is a gift.

12. Kim Y-H, Park JW, Kim JS, Lee JH. Highly crosslinked-remelted versus less-crosslinked polyethylene in posterior cruciate-retaining TKAs in the same patients. *Clin Orthop Rel Res*. 2015;473(11):3588–3594.

13. Kindsfater KA, Pomeroy D, Clark CR, Gruen TA, Murphy J, Himden S. In vivo performance of moderately crosslinked, thermally treated polyethylene in a prospective randomized controlled primary total knee arthroplasty trial. *J Arthropl*. 2015;30(8):1333–1338.

14. Lachiewicz PF, Soileau ES. Is there a benefit to highly crosslinked polyethylene in posterior-stabilized total knee arthroplasty? A randomized trial. *Clin Orthop Rel Res*. 2016;474(1):88–95.

15. Rules need to be broken if needs be.

16. Hood RW, Wright TM, Burstein AH. Retrieval analysis of total knee prostheses: a method and its application to 48 total condylar prostheses. *J Biomed Mat Res Part A*. 1983;17(5):829–842.

17. Doran J, Yu S, Smith D, Iorio R. The role of all-polyethylene tibial components in modern TKA. *J Knee Surg*. 2015;28 (05):382–389.

18. Ahmed I, Salmon LJ, Waller A, Watanabe H, Roe JP, Pinczewski LA. Total knee arthroplasty with an oxidised zirconium femoral component. *Bone Joint J*. 2016;98 (1):58–64.

19. Dennis DA, Lynch CB. Optimizing the femoral component cement mantle in total hip arthroplasty. *Orthopedics*. 2005;28(8):S867–871.

20. Ebramzadeh E, Sarmiento A, McKellop HA, *et al*. The cement mantle in total hip arthroplasty: analysis of long-term radiographic results. *J Bone Joint Surg Am*. 1994;76:77–87.

21. El Masri F, Kerboull M, Kerboull L, Courpied JP, Hamadouche M. Is the so-called 'French paradox' a reality? *Bone Joint J*. 2010;92(3):342–348.

22. Barrack RL, Mulroy R, Harris WH. Improved cementing techniques and femoral component loosening in young patients with hip arthroplasty. A 12-year radiographic review. *Bone Joint J*. 1992;74(3):385–389.

23. Banaszkiewicz PA. Improved cementing techniques and femoral component loosening in young patients with hip arthroplasty: A 12-year radiographic review. In *Classic Papers in Orthopaedics*. 2014, Springer. p. 31–34.

24. Gilbert TJ, Anoushiravani AA, Sayeed Z, Chambers MC, El-Othmani MM, Saleh KJ. Osteolysis complicating total knee arthroplasty. *JBJS Rev*. 2016;4(7): pii: 01874474-201607000-00001. doi: 10.2106/JBJS.RVW.15.00081.

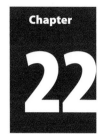

22

Orthotics and prosthetics

Firas Arnaout

Introduction

Orthotics and prosthetics is a subject often neglected during revision, but is an important topic because various aspects may be incorporated into other topics, such as gait, hand injuries or amputations.

This chapter attempts to cover the concepts that have been tested previously in the FRCS (Tr & Orth) exam. The questions and answers provide a high-order thinking framework to build on your answer in the exam oral tables.

Candidates are likely to be shown a clinical photograph, followed by a starting question. You are not normally marked on the starting question – it serves to melt the ice and give you confidence to get going. This will be followed by a competency question, which is a pass–fail benchmark. Once achieved, the examiners will then move on to advanced questions to give you higher scores.

Remember that examiners are looking for a logical and confident approach, testing your higher-order thinking in the application and evaluation of clinical knowledge.

Learn to draw as you talk, this will assist the examiners to understand what you are drawing, especially if your artistic skills are not the best! It will look and feel very awkward to draw silently while examiners are looking at you! Talking while drawing will also save you time and make you look more confident about the topic.

The topics discussed within this chapter are interchangeable, and answers can be mixed according to the scenarios given. Therefore, agility and the ability to adapt your answer to the specific question asked is an essential skill for the FRCS exam, and this is best mastered through repeated practice with other exam candidates and consultants.

Candidates can also be asked about orthotics and prosthetics in both the MCQ and clinical components of the exam. This chapter also helps to cover the knowledge and skills required for these parts of the exam.

Orthotics

EXAMINER: [Hands the candidate a picture of an orthosis] What is an orthosis?

CANDIDATE: The definition that is endorsed by the International Society for Prosthetics and Orthotics is a device that is externally attached to the body to improve function.

It supports weak muscles and corrects or compensates for skeletal deformity.

EXAMINER: What are the ideal characteristics of an orthosis?

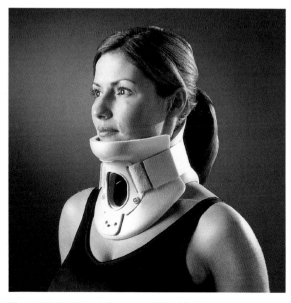

Figure 22.1a Orthosis (courtesy of Blatchford).

CANDIDATE: The ideal orthotic should be effective, lightweight, cosmetically acceptable, easy to put on and take off, and comfortable.

EXAMINER: What are the different types of orthotics that you know of? Can you give me examples of each?

CANDIDATE: Orthoses can be classified according to function into corrective and accommodative.

The corrective ones tend to be hard. They limit joint motion and stabilize flexible deformities. An example is the rocker sole that can lessen the bending forces on an arthritic or stiff midfoot during the midstance as the foot changes from accepting the weight-bearing load to pushing off. It is also useful in treating metatarsalgia and hallux rigidus.

The accommodative ones tend to be soft to allow them to shock-absorb and to accommodate fixed deformities, such as various pressure-relieving insoles that are used to dissipate local pressures over bony prominences to treat diabetic foot.

Sometimes the same orthotic can be used for support and/or correction. An example is the TLSO, which can be supportive in the case of fractures or corrective in the case of idiopathic scoliosis. Another example is the AFO, which can be supportive for weak muscle in polio or corrective in cerebral palsy.

EXAMINER: What different materials are used to make orthotics?

CANDIDATE: Orthotic materials need to be light, strong and sufficiently hard-wearing to survive for the duration of their intended use.

Various materials can be used, such as metal, plaster of Paris, carbon fibre, silicone, leather and plastic.

EXAMINER: [Shows a photo] Can you tell me what this orthosis is made of and the different types of this material that can be used to make an orthosis (Figure 22.1b)?

CANDIDATE: This is made of plastic. Plastic can be thermosetting or thermoforming.

Thermosetting plastics are pliable above a certain temperature and return to solid upon cooling. They are hard and difficult to fabricate as they require high temperature to be moulded. However, they are durable, which makes them good for making prostheses and orthoses that are to be put under great stress.

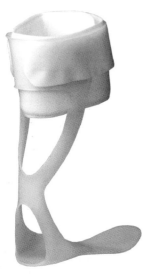

Figure 22.1b Plastic foot drop splint (courtesy Blanchford).

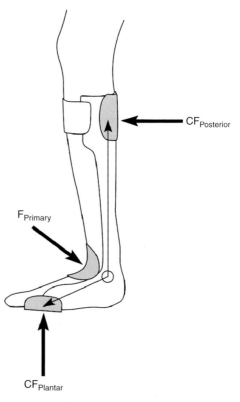

Figure 22.1c Three-point pressure principle for an orthotic.

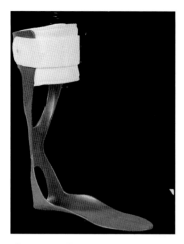

Figure 22.1d Lightweight carbon fibre AFO (courtesy of Steering Group).

Thermoforming plastics have the advantage of allowing to be reshaped by reheating. They can be moulded at high temperatures, such as those used to make AFO (e.g. polyethylene), or a medium temperature, which can be moulded directly on the patients as they have low heat conductivity (e.g. Plastozote). Or moulded at low temperature for making hand therapy splints in clinic; these can be modified if required by gentle heating in water or by a hair dryer (e.g. orthoplast).

EXAMINER: How does an orthotic work?

CANDIDATE: They work according to the three-point pressure principle to control the forces on the body part. This is the same principle that was proposed by Sir Charnley for fracture immobilization.

To control joint movements, one force should be over the joint and the other two act in the opposite direction to the first one.

COMMENT: It would be preferable here to ask for a piece of paper and 'draw as you talk'.

EXAMINER: [Shows the candidate a picture of an orthosis (Figure 22.1d)] Can you describe this orthosis for me?

COMMENT: This can be anything! It could be something you have never seen. It doesn't really matter. Chances are that the examiner also didn't know before the start of the exam. Stick to the below principles and you will impress any examiner.

Start describing the part of the body it supports such as AFO, KAFO, etc.

In the 1960s the American Academy of Orthopaedic surgeons suggested standard reproducible terminology of orthoses. Described by the joint or region of the body it encompasses.

Hence:

Upper limb:	S = shoulder	E = elbow	W = wrist	H = hand
Spine:	C = cervical	T = thoracic	L = lumbar	S = sacroiliac
Lower limb:	H = hip	K = knee	A = ankle	F = foot

Then describe whether it is corrective or accommodative.

Then describe whether it is static or dynamic.

Then describe the materials it is made from.

EXAMINER: [Shows a photo] What can you see and can you explain how it works?

CANDIDATE: This is a GRAFO (ground reaction ankle and foot orthosis).

Ground reaction force (GRF) is a force that is exerted by the ground on the body. It is equal in magnitude but opposite in direction to the force exerted on the ground by the body.

This is based on Newton's third law; for every action, there is an equal and opposite reaction. Therefore, by controlling distal joints one can alter the GRF and affect more proximal joints. The concept of affecting one joint by the position of another is called coupling.

GRAFO is formed from a toe plate and rigid ankle in neutral position, and a rigid anterior tibial shell. It provides knee supports for patients with weak quadriceps and gastrocsoleus by accentuating knee flexion and preventing knee hyperextension in midstance. By fixing the angle of the ankle the

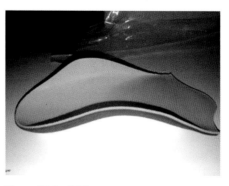

Figure 22.1e UCBL.

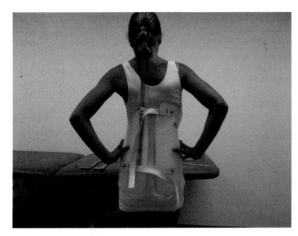

Figure 22.1f Boston brace.

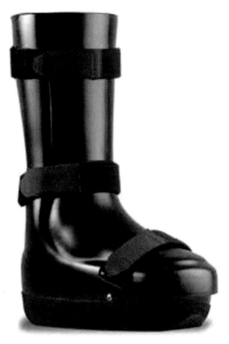

Figure 22.1g Charcot restraint orthotic walker (CROW).

GRF can be positioned anterior or posterior to the knee joint to encourage either flexion or extension.

EXAMINER: What is functional bracing?

CANDIDATE: This was advocated by Sarmiento from the USA. In a review paper he published in the *BJJ* in 2006, he described how his technique has evolved. He believes that rigid immobilization of fractures of long bones is unphysiological, and that movements at the site of fracture during functional activities encourage osteogenesis.

The principle is to stabilize the fracture while allowing weight-bearing and joint movements. Motion at the fracture site is prevented through circumferential compression of the soft tissues.

EXAMINER: [Shows a photo] Tell me about these orthoses.

CANDIDATE: The first one is UCBL (University of California Biomechanics Laboratory) (Figure 22.1e). It is a rigid plastic insert that is fabricated over a cast of the foot with rigid and high posterior, medial and lateral walls to provide a deep cup. It is used to control severe hind foot valgus and midfoot pronation.

The second one is a Boston brace (Figure 22.1f), this is used to treat paediatric scoliosis. It is custom-made and works on the principles of three-point fixation. The bottom part is fixed around the pelvis, and the top part has raised sides for improved sideways support to avoid lateral shift of the spine. Extra padding can also

be used in certain areas to help improve the corrective forces.

The third one is a Charcot restraint orthotic walker (CROW) (Figure 22.1g), which is used in the end-stage foot disease of diabetes.

EXAMINER: How can we prevent complications of orthotics?

CANDIDATE: The principles to minimize orthotic–limb interface pressures are:
1 – Maximize lever arm.
2 – Maximize surface contact area.
3 – Maximize conformity.
4 – Protect bony prominences.
5 – Moist absorbent lining.

Prosthetics

EXAMINER: [Shows a picture of a below-knee prosthesis (Figure 22.2a)] What is a prosthesis?

CANDIDATE: The definition which is endorsed by the International Society for Prosthetics and Orthotics is that a prosthesis is an artificial device that is externally applied to replace the function or appearance of part of the body.

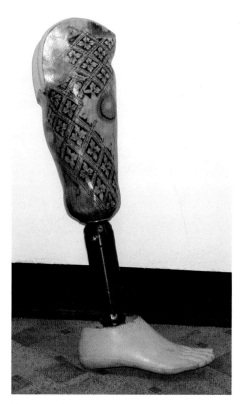

Figure 22.2a Prosthesis.

EXAMINER: How can you classify prostheses?

CANDIDATE: Prostheses can be classified according to structure into exoskeletal or endoskeletal.

Exoskeletal ones have the strength in the rigid external structure, whereas endoskeletal ones are linked by internal struts and covered with external cosmetic.

EXAMINER: Can you describe this prosthesis?

COMMENT: As a candidate describes each component, the examiner may then ask for further details to check the candidate's in-depth understanding and give her/him a higher score. The good candidate who scores 7 and 8 is the one who volunteers relevant information without being asked, hence sending the examiner into a semi-snooze state.

CANDIDATE:

1 – The suspension system that attaches the prosthesis to the residual limb. This can be a belt, straps, or a suction device that has a one-way valve which expels air when the socket is donned.

Some systems use the bulbous shape of the stump for suspension.

2 – The socket which is the connection between the stump and the prosthesis, and is custom-made to the stump shape. Silicon is commonly used here as it provides an airtight seal between the prosthesis and amputated stump due to the pressure differential between the socket and atmosphere. Weight-bearing areas for the socket include the heel pad, transtibial, patellar tendon, lateral tibial flare, medial tibial flare, transfemoral and ischial tuberosity.

3 – The shank, which is a link between the socket and the terminal device, and also serves to restore length. May be made of metal or carbon fibre. This link can be described as articulating or non-articulating based on the presence of a joint mechanism.

4 – The terminal device. This can be a hand or a foot, and is described as static, which is more cosmetic, or dynamic, which is more functional.

The foot terminal device can be described as energy-storing or non-energy-storing.

5 – Cosmetic cover.

EXAMINER: How is the load transferred from the prosthesis to the limb?

CANDIDATE: There are two types of load transfer; direct and indirect.

Direct load transfer or end-weight bearing is accomplished with knee disarticulation or ankle disarticulation (Syme's). Intimacy of the prosthetic socket is necessary only for suspension.

Indirect load transfer is when amputation is performed through a long bone (BKA or AKA) and the end of the stump does not take all the weight and the load is transferred indirectly by the total contact method. This process requires an intimate prosthetic socket fit.

EXAMINER: What are the different types of knee joint mechanism?

CANDIDATE: This can be single-axis, which has the advantage of being lightweight, or polycentric with four bars linkage and a moving centre of rotation that provides controlled flexion during the gait cycle – this is good for longer residual limbs. There is also the hydraulic knee, which allows variable cadence via a piston mechanism and is suitable for shorter residual limbs in patients with higher activity levels. Or simply a manual locking knee, which consists of a constant friction knee hinge with a positive lock-in extension that can be unlocked to allow function – this is used primarily in weak, unstable patients and those just learning to use prosthetics and for blind amputees. The new design development includes a microprocessor-controlled knee plus a motor. Battery life, weight and cost are significant limiting factors.

EXAMINER: [Shows a picture of a foot prosthesis] Can you describe these two prostheses to me and explain the difference?

CANDIDATE: The first photo is of a solid ankle cushioned heel, so-called SACH prosthesis (Figure 22.2b). This is a non-energy-storing device used for patients with low activity levels as it is light in weight, cost-effective and requires little maintenance. It can lead to overload on the non-amputated limb and therefore has been replaced by a single-axis foot, which is based on an ankle hinge that provides dorsiflexion and plantar flexion.

The second photo is of an energy-storing non-articulating foot prosthesis (Figure 22.2c). It is made of carbon fibre. The components are compressible, which provides some energy return.

The third photo is of an energy-storing and articulating hydraulic prosthesis. It allows inversion, eversion and rotation of the foot and is useful for walking on uneven floors.

There is also a motor-powered ankle that has rechargeable batteries and is controlled by a microprocessor. These reduce the energy requirements of walking, but are heavy and costly.

EXAMINER: [Shows a photo of a below-knee prosthesis] What are the most common complications of this prosthesis? And how do you prevent them?

CANDIDATE: One of the most common complications is pistoning, which can occur during the swing phase due to ineffective suspension or during the stance phase due to poor socket fit or stump volume changes. The shear forces from pistoning can cause skin damage and can make the prosthesis feel heavier.

Another common complication is skin damage, blisters and ulcers. To avoid these, a plaster of

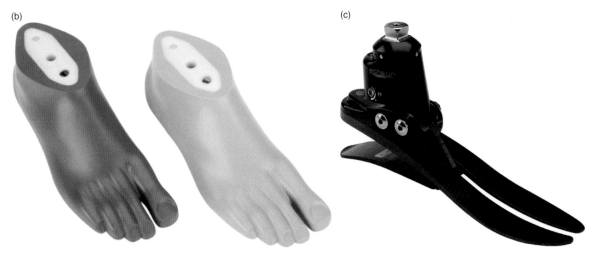

(b)

(c)

Figure 22.2b and 22.c Solid ankle cushioned heel and energy-storing non-articulating foot prosthesis.

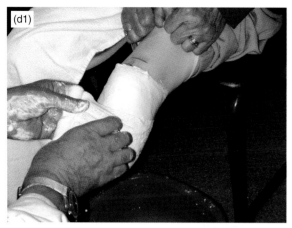

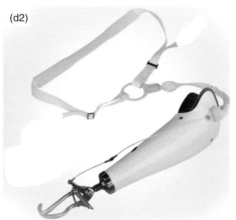

Figure 22.2d Plaster of Paris mould.

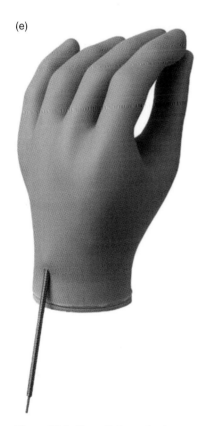

Figure 22.2e Upper limb prosthesis.

Paris mould is made by the prosthetist to mark the pressure-sensitive and pressure-relieving areas which are to be taken into account when the

prosthetic is being fashioned, trying to minimize the pressure through unprotected bony prominences (Figure 22.2d). More recently, computer-assisted technology is used to map the stump.

It is important to try to maximize the surface area through which the forces are applied from the orthotic to the skin and to maximize the conformity between the orthotic and the underlying limb.

The material at the interface should also be moisture-absorbent to avoid maceration of the skin.

EXAMINER: [Shows a photo of an upper limb prosthesis] What do you see (Figure 22.e)?

CANDIDATE: This is an upper limb prosthesis, it looks to be a functional one and is body-powered as it has a figure-of-eight harness.

EXAMINER: What different types of upper limb prostheses do you know of (Figure 22.2f)?

CANDIDATE: Upper limb prostheses can be cosmetic, functional or myoelectric.

The cosmetic ones are passive with no moving parts, but can have some function such as turning a light on. They also improve gait symmetry.

Functional prostheses can be body-powered, activated by shoulder movements via a harness and cables; these tend to have poor cosmesis. They also can be myeoelectric, which are powered by muscles sending signals via attached electrodes to the prosthesis. These signals are magnified and

565

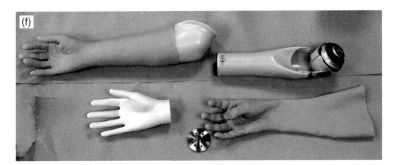

Figure 22.2f Upper limb prostheses.

passed to a microprocessor to operate the terminal device. These prostheses are heavy and therefore best-suited for transradial amputations. They also require maintenance and training, but provide better cosmetic appearance and tend to be more functional with better movements.

The terminal device can be a split hook body-powered device.

Chapter 23

Pain, analgesia and anaesthesia

Christopher Watkins and Bodil Robertson

Introduction

Pain may be asked as part of a viva topic or candidates may be lucky or unlucky enough to have a full 5-minute viva devoted to the topic. It is an important part of orthopaedic practice which is often neglected, but more important now with the push towards day-case surgery and even day-case arthroplasty. Pain is well known to appear as questions in the Part I MCQ/SBA exam.

This viva can be awkward, as bits and pieces such as pain assessment can appear fluffy to orthopods and in real life is best left to the anaesthetists.

Like genetics, ask examiners about pain and one will get a puzzled look back. Suffice to say, it is not an A-list topic and is most likely a C-list category. Again, similar to genetics, the idea is to score a basic 6 for any question asked. Anything else is a bonus.

One word of caution with C list category topics. With the advent of computer generated curriculum sampling C-list topics are quickly becoming the new A list ones.

Section 5 of the Trs+Orth basic science syllabus can be loosely regarded as the pain section. Four topics about which candidates should demonstrate competency are outlined by the JSCFE.

1. Anaesthesia – principles and practice of local and regional anaesthesia and principles of general anaesthesia.
2. Pain management programmes and management of complex regional pain.
3. Pain and pain relief.
4. Behavioural dysfunction and somatization.

If all else fails, try to produce a list of potential pain questions previously asked and work through these in a study group. There is a reasonable chance these questions will be repeated in future diets of exams.

Structured oral examination question 1

Pain

EXAMINER: What is pain?

CANDIDATE: An unpleasant sensory and emotional experience associated with actual or potential tissue damage. (International Association of the Study of Pain (IASP)).

COMMENT: The viva could start off awkwardly with a definition that may catch the unsuspecting candidate off-guard. Go for an uncomplicated, straightforward definition that allows you to build on this foundation if you are able to do so.

EXAMINER: Your patients have pain. You see many patients with pain. How do you assess pain?

CANDIDATE: Pain must be assessed using a multidimensional approach, with determination of the following:

- Chronicity.
- Severity.
- Quality.
- Contributing/associated factors.
- Location/distribution.
- Aetiology of pain, if identifiable.
- Mechanism of injury, if applicable.
- Barriers to pain assessment.

COMMENT: SOCRATES pain mnemonic:

- Site – where is the pain?
- Onset – when did it start? How long ago?
- Character – description: aching, stabbing, burning?
- Radiation – where does it go?
- Associations – impact on QOL: social, emotional, family, financial.

- Time course – does the pain follow a pattern?
- Exacerbating/relieving factors.
- Severity score – how bad is the pain?

Score 7/8 candidate

Pain scales can be useful.

1. Single dimensional scale

Measures a single dimension of pain, usually pain intensity. Useful in acute pain where the aetiology is clear.

2. Multidimensional scale

These measure the intensity, nature and location of pain, and in some cases, the impact that pain is having on a patient's activity or mood. Useful in complex or persistent acute or chronic pain.

Visual analogue pain scales are easy for patients to use. Can be either continuous or discrete.

EXAMINER: What is the difference between acute and chronic pain?

CANDIDATE: With acute pain there is pain of recent onset and probably limited duration. It usually has an identifiable temporal and causal relationship to injury or disease.

Chronic pain persists beyond the time of healing of an injury and frequently there may not be any clear identifiable cause.

EXAMINER: Anything newly introduced for acute postoperative pain relief in orthopaedics?

CANDIDATE: I am not sure what you mean.

EXAMINER: For lower limb arthroplasty surgery?

CANDIDATE: Adductor canal block.

COMMENT: For many years a femoral nerve block (FNB) was used as the main peripheral nerve block for postop analgesia following TKA. One major issue with FNB is quadriceps weakness, which can significantly affect early physiotherapy input and thus interfere with rapid recovery programmes following TKA.

Adductor canal block is a pure sensory nerve block for postop analgesia. The saphenous nerve (sensory nerve) and part of the obturator nerve travelling through the adductor canal of thigh are targeted with local anaesthetics injected into the canal to provide adequate analgesia by blocking these nerves. The block is performed under ultrasound guidance.

This block seems to work well without causing quadriceps weakness.

The candidate should have expanded on their answer if able to do so.

EXAMINER: That's for knee replacements. Anything else?

CANDIDATE: Stop before you block.

EXAMINER: OK, tell me about this.

CANDIDATE: This is a national patient safety initiative aimed at reducing the incidence of inadvertent wrong-sided nerve block during regional anaesthesia. It reduces the chance of a never event occurring.

EXAMINER: What is a never event?

CANDIDATE: The National Patient Safety Agency (NPSA) describes a 'never event' as a serious, largely preventable patient safety incident that should not occur if the available preventative measures have been implemented.

EXAMINER: Have you heard of the sufentanil sublingual tablet system?

CANDIDATE: No.

COMMENT: The sufentanil sublingual tablet system is pre-programmed to dispense a single tablet, when the unique radiofrequency adhesive tag wrapped around the patient's thumb is activated. It provides an alternative option to IV morphine PCA for some people with moderate to severe acute postoperative pain.

Its use is restricted to acute moderate to severe postoperative pain, in the hospital setting and for a maximum duration of 72 hours. It is a user-friendly device that is especially useful in patients for whom improved mobility is an advantage.

EXAMINER: What about day-case lower limb joint replacement?

CANDIDATE 1: In my hospital we don't have the set up for this.

COMMENT: This is a gift question if you have done a bit of homework.

CANDIDATE 2: Enhanced recovery is multidisciplinary standardized perioperative care aimed at early mobility, discharge and return to normal life with both reduced morbidity and potentially mortality.

The strategy has four strands:

1. Improving preoperative care.
2. Reducing the physical stress of the operation.
3. Decreasing postoperative discomfort.
4. Improving postoperative mobility.

There is no single protocol for all hospitals and each centre must develop its own ERAS (enhanced recovery after surgery) programme based on its own strengths and limitations.

Patient selection is important. Ideally, patients should be fully optimized with well-controlled systemic disease and be well motivated to complete the programme.

Preoperative anaesthetic preparation includes correction of anaemia, optimization of hypertension and diabetic control.

Anaesthetic technique is tailored to facilitate enhanced and early mobility.

The use of a widespread local anaesthetic cocktail infiltration may significantly reduce postop pain. In my hospital we use ropivacaine, ketorolac (NSAID) 30 mg and morphine 5 mg. Ketorolac is sometimes omitted if a patient has chronic renal disease and the latest evidence has questioned the effectiveness of morphine. Despite initial concerns over toxicity, this technique has been shown to be safe and aid postoperative recovery. Adrenaline may be added to prolong the duration of action.

EXAMINER: You have mentioned ERAS, but what about day-case surgery?

CANDIDATE 2: This would involve preoperative patient education and motivation for the programme. Anaesthesia should be standardized and would typically involve a low-dose spinal and sedation or light GA, local anaesthetic infiltration, IV paracetamol and use of tranexamic acid.

Perioperative measures would include adequate postop analgesia, physiotherapy, a blood transfusion protocol, standardized discharge medications and arrangements for a nurse specialist to check on the patient to make sure they are safe when discharged.

EXAMINER: Anything else?

CANDIDATE: Sorry.

COMMENT: The patient should be young with no significant comorbidities and live within an acceptable distance from the hospital. Discharge hurdles would include physiotherapy (mobility, stairs, hip precautions), radiographs and dry wound.

Structured oral examination question 2

Managing neuropathic pain

EXAMINER: What do we mean by neuropathic pain?

CANDIDATE: Neuropathic pain arises from damage, or pathological change, in the peripheral or central nervous system.

Neuropathic pain is defined by the IASP as 'pain initiated or caused by a primary lesion or dysfunction in the nervous system'.

EXAMINER: How is neuropathic pain different to nociceptive pain?

CANDIDATE: Nociceptive pain is caused by actual tissue damage, whereas neuropathic pain is produced either by damage to or pathological change in the peripheral or central nervous system, the system that normally signals pain.

EXAMINER: And?

CANDIDATE: The mechanisms of neuropathic pain differ significantly from nociceptive pain.

For example, there is:

- A lower threshold for activation of injured primary afferents causing ectopic discharges from the injured nerve or the dorsal root ganglion.
- There is downregulation of dorsal horn opioid receptors and reduced opioid sensitivity.
- Wind up occurs, that is increased activity of glutamate in the dorsal horn which increases the response to C fibre stimulation.

EXAMINER: Can you give examples of neuropathic pain?

CANDIDATE: Common neuropathic conditions affecting the peripheral nervous system include peripheral diabetic neuropathic pain (PDNP), postherpetic neuralgia (PHN), AIDS polyneuropathy, cervical or lumbar radiculopathy, mechanical compression such as entrapment syndromes (e.g. carpal tunnel syndrome), phantom limb pain after amputation, trigeminal neuralgia and traumatic nerve injury.

Central causes for neuropathic pain include spinal cord injury (SCI), multiple sclerosis (MS) and stroke leading to central post stroke pain (CPSP).

EXAMINER: How does neuropathic pain present?

CANDIDATE: Patients usually complain of dysaesthesias (unpleasant and strange sensations in the skin (tingling, pins and needles)), deep-seated gnawing pain, and abnormal thermal sensations (burning, on fire).

Less commonly, paroxysmal pains such as shooting, stabbing, or electric shocks.

Patients may also complain that the painful area is abnormally sensitive to any innocuous mechanical or thermal stimulus; such as clothes brushing against the area being intensely painful.

EXAMINER: How do we treat nerve pain?

CANDIDATE: Nerve pain can be difficult to treat, as standard treatment with conventional analgesics does not typically provide effective relief of pain. I would use a step-wise ladder:

1. Non-opioid analgesic/basic analgesia paracetamol 1 g QDS. Unlike most other types of pain, neuropathic pain doesn't always respond well to these common painkillers. Higher doses may be better at managing the pain, but are also more likely to cause side effects.
2. Tricyclic antidepressant (TCA). Amitriptyline. TCAs block the reuptake of noradrenaline and serotonin. The pain-relieving effect of TCAs is independent of their antidepressant effect. The most common adverse events include sedation, anticholinergic side effects (namely dry mouth, constipation and urinary retention) and orthostatic hypotension. TCAs can cause or exacerbate cognitive impairment and gait disturbances in elderly patients and may predispose them to falls. They are associated with cardiac toxicity and must be avoided in the elderly and in those with cardiac pathology. They offer moderate relief of neuropathic pain.
3. Anticonvulsant gabapentin. If TCA is contraindicated or there is lancinating pain (electric shock or stabbing).

Proposed mechanism of action is the interaction with the voltage-gated calcium channel alpha-2-delta subunit.

4. Tramadol. Can be used to treat resistant neuropathic pain. Side effects include nausea and vomiting, dizziness and constipation.
5. Secondary pain care referral. Indicated if pain persists or remains uncontrolled.

I would also need to assess a patient's perception of pain, coping strategies, mood changes, disturbed sleep and anxiety.

Treating any associated anxiety or depression may reduce the need for analgesics.

Pain is a subjective, internal experience, and reliable assessment of pain relies heavily on the patient's self-report. Psychosocial factors play critical roles in the development of persistent pain and associated experiences of functional disability and emotional distress.

Structured oral examination question 3

WHO pain ladder

EXAMINER: Your clinic patient has osteoarthritis of the knee. Referred in for a knee replacement, but symptoms aren't severe enough yet for surgery. How would you control his knee pain?

CANDIDATE: I would prescribe him morphine.

EXAMINER: Are you sure?

CANDIDATE: Yes. Morphine is a good choice for pain control.

EXAMINER: What is the WHO pain ladder?

CANDIDATE 1: I have heard of it, but I am not sure.

CANDIDATE 2: The WHO pain ladder was originally introduced as a framework for treating cancer pain in 1986 with modifications in 1997.

Treatment of pain should begin with a non-opioid medication. If the pain is not properly controlled, one should then introduce a weak opioid. If the use of this medication is insufficient to treat the pain, one can begin a more powerful opioid. One should never use two products belonging to the same category simultaneously. The analgesic ladder also includes the possibility of adding adjuvant treatments for neuropathic pain or for symptoms associated with cancer.

The WHO guidelines can be used for all patients with either acute or chronic pain who require analgesia.

Although there has been a number of criticisms due in part to omissions, developments of new techniques and medications, the WHO treatment guidelines are still considered a valid tool to use.

EXAMINER: What are the five recommendations of the WHO ladder?

CANDIDATE 2:

1. Analgesics should be administered orally, wherever possible.

2. Analgesics should be given at regular definite intervals.

3. Analgesics should be prescribed according to pain intensity.

4. The dosing of medication should be adapted to the individual. The correct dosage is one that will allow adequate pain relief.

5. The patient should be given all the necessary information about when and how to administer the medication.

Structured oral examination question 4

Complex regional pain syndrome

EXAMINER: You meet a patient in clinic complaining of severe pain in a wrist preventing them from using it normally after a fracture. It is unrelenting pain, keeping them awake at night, associated with swelling, temperature and skin changes, and light touch provokes severe pain. What are your thoughts?

COMMENT: This is a giveaway diagnosis of CRPS.

CANDIDATE: These features are very suggestive of complex regional pain syndrome. I would like to take a fuller history and examine the patient to confirm my initial provisional diagnosis.

EXAMINER: The patient is a female, 43 years old, right-hand dominant secretary who sustained a straightforward undisplaced fractured radius 10 weeks ago after a fall. Managed conservatively in a Colles' cast.

CANDIDATE: Examination wise I would examine to see if the wrist was red or swollen. I would assess if they hold their limb protectively and if wrist movements were severely restricted and painful.

I would order AP and lateral radiographs of the wrist and look to see if diffuse patchy osteopenia was present.

EXAMINER: What is complex regional pain syndrome?

CANDIDATE: Complex regional pain syndrome is a syndrome associated with severe pain in a distal limb with associated peripheral sensory, vasomotor, sudomotor/oedema and motor/trophic changes.

EXAMINER: How is it diagnosed?

CANDIDATE 1: Diagnosis is based on clinical history and examinations. Investigations can be used as adjuncts.

COMMENT: This is a score 5/6.

CANDIDATE 2: Diagnosis is based on clinical history and examinations. Investigations can be used as adjuncts. However, it is very much a diagnosis of exclusion. It is important to exclude other causes of pain such as fracture malunion or non-union, post-traumatic arthritis, infection, peripheral vascular disease in any patient who develops a red, hot and swollen or cold and poorly perfused limb after a fracture or surgery.

EXAMINER: Any other differentials you need to consider?

CANDIDATE: Diabetic polyneuropathy may also present with pain, skin colour changes and motor deficit.

EXAMINER: Do you know any criteria?

CANDIDATE: No, sorry.

COMMENT: The Budapest Criteria (specificity 0.69) allow a clinical diagnosis to be made on the basis of a combination of symptoms and signs seen in four clinical categories.

- The patient has continuing pain that is disproportionate to any inciting event.
- The patient has at least one sign in two or more categories below.
- The patient reports at least one symptom in three or more categories below.
- No other diagnosis can better explain the signs or symptoms.

571

Category	Symptoms
Sensory	Reports of allodynia and/or hyperalgesia
Vasomotor	Reports of temperature asymmetry and/or skin colour changes and/or asymmetry
Sudomotor/ oedema	Reports of oedema and/or sweating changes and/or sweating asymmetry
Motor/trophic	Reports of decreased ROM and/or motor dysfunction (weakness, tremor, dystonia) and/or trophic changes (hair, nail, skin)

To fulfil diagnostic criteria patients must report at least one symptom in three of the four categories

Signs

Sensory	Evidence of hyperalgesia (to pinprick) and/ or allodynia (to light touch and/or temperature sensation and/or deep somatic pressure and/or joint movement)
Vasomotor	Evidence of temperature asymmetry and/or skin colour changes and/or asymmetry
Sudomotor/ oedema	Evidence of oedema and/or sweating changes and/or sweating asymmetry
Motor/ trophic	Evidence of decreased range of motion and/ or dysfunction (weakness, tremor, dystonia) and/or trophic changes (hair, nails, skin)

Must display ≤ 1 sign at time of evaluation in ≥ 2 of the categories.

EXAMINER: What is the natural history of CRPS?

CANDIDATE: After a year, around half of patients affected will fully recover while the other half may complain of some residual stiffness and pain. A very small number of patients will continue to have significant disabling symptoms which can become chronic in nature.

EXAMINER: What is the pathophysiology of CRPS?

CANDIDATE: It is thought that CRPS develops when persistent noxious stimuli from an injured body region leads to peripheral and central sensitization, whereby primary afferent nociceptive mechanisms demonstrate abnormally heightened sensation, including spontaneous pain and hyperalgesia.

EXAMINER: What do you mean by a noxious stimulus?

CANDIDATE: This is a stimulus that is damaging to normal tissues.

EXAMINER: What is a nociceptor?

CANDIDATE: This is a receptor preferentially sensitive to a noxious stimulus or to a stimulus which would become noxious if prolonged.

EXAMINER: How are nociceptors activated?

CANDIDATE: Peripheral activation of nociceptors is modulated by a number of chemical substances, which are produced and released when there is cellular damage (e.g. potassium, serotonin, bradykinin, histamine, prostaglandins, leukotrienes and substance P).

These substances influence the degree of nerve activity and intensity of the pain sensation.

EXAMINER: What are the current approaches to management?

CANDIDATE 1: A recent paper demonstrating level I evidence looked at the use of antioxidant vitamin C. A dose of 500 mg a day for 50 days was shown to reduce symptoms of CRPS.

COMMENT: Jumping straight in and quoting a paper isn't the best viva tactic approach to use.

CANDIDATE 2: There are several management options which would include:
- Physiotherapy.
- Pharmacological management.
- Nerve stimulation.
- Regional nerve blocks.
- Chemical sympathectomy.
- Surgical sympathectomy.

EXAMINER: What pharmacological management?

CANDIDATE 2: Drugs used include calcitonin, bisphosphonates, steroids and gabapentin. Oral and intravenous biphosphonates, but not calcitonin, have been shown to decrease pain and swelling and increase range of motion in patients with CRPS. A short course of oral steroids may be beneficial but limited evidence exists for the use of gabapentin.

EXAMINER: What about physiotherapy?

CANDIDATE 2: Although we generally refer patients with CRPS to physiotherapy the evidence for its effectiveness is unclear. It may improve ROM of the affected limb but does not affect pain.

EXAMINER: What about regional nerve blocks?

CANDIDATE 2: IV regional sympathetic block typically using guanethidine may help with pain control, but the evidence for improved final outcome is poor.

EXAMINER: How do we minimize the risk of CRPS occurring?

CANDIDATE: Patient risk factors would include complex pain issues pre-surgery, such as if the patient was on lots of pain medication such as gabapentin, codeine or morphine-based tablets before surgery. Surgical factors that would concern me would be if the patient required complex elbow or hand surgery that would need prolonged tourniquet use. Both patient and surgical risk factors for CRPS would mean being proactive preoperatively, perhaps starting them on vitamin C prophylactically and thinking about regional or epidural anaesthesia rather than a general anaesthetic. I would avoid tight casts, painful manipulations of fractures and unphysiological manipulated wrist positions in cast. Mirror physiotherapy postop seems to be a promising new development and TENS may have a role. I would make sure the patient had good pain control postoperatively.

Structured oral examination question 5

Intravenous regional anaesthesia (Bier's block)

EXAMINER: What are the indications for use of a Bier's block?

CANDIDATE: Mainly for manipulation of wrist fractures in A&E. Other indications might include suturing of multiple forearm lacerations, foreign body removal from forearm wounds, excision of wrist ganglia and palmar fasciotomy.

EXAMINER: What are the contraindications to Bier's block?

CANDIDATE: This mainly relates to tourniquet use. Absolute contraindications include:
- Allergy to local anaesthetic.
- Methaemoglobinaemia.
- Severe hypertension (SBP > 200 mmHg).
- Compartment syndrome.
- Uncooperative or confused patient.
- No IV access on affected hand and other limb.

Relative contraindications include:
- Coagulopathy.
- Cardiac conduction abnormalities.
- Peripheral vascular disease.
- Sickle cell disease or trait.

- Epilepsy.
- Local inflammation/infection.
- Children (< 10 years).
- Pregnancy.
- Lymphoedema.

EXAMINER: Anything else?

CANDIDATE: I can't think of anything.

COMMENT: Morbid obesity (as the cuff is unreliable on obese arms), scleroderma and Raynaud's phenomenon.

Paget's disease (local anaesthetic may spread to the systemic circulation via venous channels in bone).

EXAMINER: What local anaesthetic is used?

CANDIDATE: Recommended agents are either prilocaine or lignocaine.
0.5% Prilocaine.
Dose is 3 mg/kg.
A 70 kg patient gets 210 mg (42 ml) 0.5% prilocaine.

EXAMINER: What about cuff deflation?

CANDIDATE: With single cuff use the cuff should not be let down until at least 30 minutes have elapsed. Deflate the cuff briefly (for 5–10 s) then reinflate. If there are no signs of toxicity after 45 s, then deflate again (for 5–10 s). This is repeated once more prior to being permanently removed. This allows some of the local anaesthetic into the systemic circulation at short intervals to avoid local anaesthetic toxicity from large amounts of local anaesthetic being released all at once.

EXAMINER: Why all this protocol?

CANDIDATE: This is because systemic toxic doses of local anaesthetic may be released. After 20 minutes, 30% of the injected drug is fixed within the tissues and is unavailable for immediate release into the systemic circulation.

EXAMINER: What are the dangers of a Bier's block?

CANDIDATE: Major complications include nerve injuries, anaphylaxis, methaemaglobinaemia seizures, arrhythmias, cardiac arrest and death.

Compartment syndrome, but it is difficult to separate out the influence of the distal radius fracture itself as the causative factor.

Tourniquet pain, rash and thrombophlebitis.

EXAMINER: How do you recognize prilocaine toxicity?

CANDIDATE: Symptoms include dizziness, restlessness, anxiety, perioral tingling, metallic taste, altered mental status, muscle twitching and seizures.

EXAMINER: What is a double tourniquet?

CANDIDATE: The double tourniquet is used to increase safety and to reduce tourniquet pain in the awake patient.

EXAMINER: Yes, but what do we mean by the double tourniquet method?

CANDIDATE: This allows better analgesia of the area under the tourniquet.

Step 1: Exsanguinate limb.
Step 2: INFLATE proximal/top cuff of tourniquet to 100 mmHg above the patient's systolic blood pressure.
Step 3: After 10 min INFLATE bottom cuff of the tourniquet. Then ONLY AFTER THE BOTTOM CUFF IS FULLY INFLATED, DEFLATE THE TOP CUFF. The result is that the BOTTOM tourniquet is over a now anaesthetized area of arm.
Step 4: After 30 min from injection deflate the bottom/distal cuff of the tourniquet.

It is important that there is always at least one tourniquet cuff inflated for the full 30 min from injection of prilocaine.

EXAMINER: There has been a prolonged period of icy weather at your local hospital and the trauma list is overloaded with cases. The orthopaedics service manager has called you into their office and asked if you would agree to the temporary introduction of Bier's block use in casualty for distal radius fractures. This is to free up more trauma list time. What are your thoughts?

CANDIDATE: Most wrist fractures managed on a trauma list usually require either ORIF or K-wire fixation rather than just manipulation. I would worry about the risk of fracture re-displacement with just simple manipulation and application of a moulded cast.

If there is a regular list of Bier's block cases taking place in casualty and working well then it may simply be a case of reviewing practice and auditing procedures to ensure optimal patient selection, patient care and clinical governance.

My own hospital does not have a Bier's block list for Colles' fractures. This type of arrangement has generally fallen out of favour, so reintroducing this technique into casualty would need careful planning. I would need to know more about the business plan submitted. My initial thoughts are those of concern about safety.

There is a move by anaesthetists to do a brachial plexus block (axillary approach) instead of a Bier's block for procedures in the forearm. Thus, doing Bier's block may fail with non-anaesthetists such as A&E staff.

COMMENT: This is a soft viva question. If you go in the wrong direction with this type of question you will struggle to score points. Unfortunately, there is a bit of guesswork required as to what to say. Consent, ethics and duty of candour are all creeping into the vivas.

The candidate's answer has sat on the fence a little.

EXAMINER: What do you want to know?

CANDIDATE: We would need to decide if the service was A&E-led, orthopaedic-led or if a combined approach was taken.

We would have to ensure staff had the necessary training. Protocols and procedures would need to be put in place. We would need to have guidelines in place and a business case set out.

The procedure should only be used for fairly straightforward extra-articular distal radius fractures and certainly not in young patients with high-energy displaced intra-articular fractures.

There would need to be an agreed protocol in place for timely patient follow-up, as these fractures may re-displace and require ORIF. Cases that clearly need ORIF should be identified and we should avoid Bier's block use.

It seems like a lot of extra work for a temporary fix of lack of trauma theatre time. My own preference would be to free up some theatre time from elsewhere. An additional trauma list or perhaps cancelling some elective cases would be much better all round.

Again, I must say I do not think it is a good idea. Tourniquets can fail and release toxic doses of local anaesthetic into the systemic circulation, there is a risk of methaemoglobinaemia occurring and there are better methods to anaesthetize a limb.

COMMENT: The candidate has decided not to support the introduction of a Bier's block list. It can

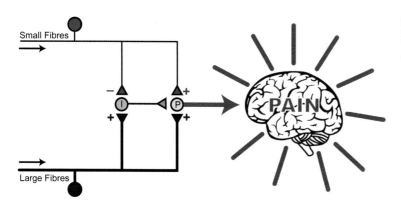

Figure 23.1 Gate theory of pain. I, 'Inhibitory Interneuron' (substantia gelatinosa); P, 'Projection Neuron'; −, inhibition (blocking); +, excitation (activation).

be difficult to decide which way to go with these types of questions, especially if you are not very familiar with the procedure.

EXAMINER: No free theatre time is available.

CANDIDATE: I can only say this would not be a quick-fix solution and needs careful planning and thought and I would be worried this wasn't the correct approach.

COMMENT: This is a soft question dealing with the way the NHS is set up. It is perhaps more suited for a consultant interview, as this type of question is difficult for examiners to differentiate between the different scoring marks.

Structured oral examination question 6

Pain

COMMENT: Three mechanisms need to be mentioned:
1. Segmental inhibition system (gate theory).
2. Opioid system.
3. Descending inhibitory system.

EXAMINER: What is the gate theory of pain (segmental inhibition system)?

COMMENT: This is made unnecessarily complicated in many textbooks. The theory is easier to explain by drawing a diagram (Figure 23.1).

CANDIDATE: Pain sensation is regulated in the spinal cord.
- Synapses between nociceptor fibres (Aδ/Type C) and dorsal root ganglia can be diminished or blocked by an inhibitory neuron (substantia gelatinosa) within the spinal cord.
- The inhibitory neuron is activated by Aβ/Type A fibres (light touch, large diameter).
- Therefore, stimulation of light-touch fibres can block the pain transmission at the nociceptor–dorsal root ganglia synapse.
- Without any stimulation, both large and small nerve fibres are quiet and the inhibitory interneuron (I) (substantia gelatinosa) blocks the signal in the projection neuron (P) that connects to the brain. The 'gate is closed' and therefore there is no pain.
- With non-painful stimulation, large nerve fibres are activated primarily. This activates the projection neuron (P), but it also activates the inhibitory interneuron (I), which then blocks the signal in the projection neuron (P) that connects to the brain. The 'gate is closed' and therefore there is no pain.
- With pain stimulation, small nerve fibres become active. They activate the projection neurons (P) and block the inhibitory interneuron (I). Because activity of the inhibitory interneuron is blocked, it cannot block the output of the projection neuron that connects with the brain. The 'gate is open', therefore, there is pain!

EXAMINER: How does this explain the action of transcutaneous electrical nerve stimulation (TENS) on pain?

CANDIDATE: The development of TENS was the result of stimulating large A fibres that stimulated the inhibitory interneuron (substantia gelatinosa) that blocked the central pain stimulators and thus closed the gate.

Table 23.1 Primary nerve fibre afferents.

Primary nerve fibre afferents	Diameter μm	Myelination	Speed (m/s)	Receptor activation thresholds	Sensation
Aβ	Large (5–12 μm)	Highly	Very fast (35–75 m/s)	Low	Light touch, pressure
Aδ	Large (2–5 μm)	Thinly	Fast (5–30 m/s)	High and low	Rapid sharp pain (epicritic)
C	Smallest (< 2 μm)	Unmyelinated	Slow (< 2 m/s)	High	Slow, diffuse, dull pain (protophytic)

	Destination	Posterior central gyrus
↑	3rd order neuron	Ventral posterolateral nucleus of thalamus
	Pathway	Lateral spinothalamic
	2nd order neuron	Substantia gelatinosa
	1st order neuron	Posterior root ganglia
	Receptor	Free nerve endings

Figure 23.2 Lateral spinothalamic pathway.

EXAMINER: Any other mechanisms of pain?

CANDIDATE: The opioid system.

EXAMINER: OK, what is this?

CANDIDATE: Opioid derivatives are powerful analgesics (morphine, diamorphine, codeine).
- Opioid receptors are present in the spinal cord, periaqueductal grey matter and the ventral medulla. There are three types: μ (mu), δ (delta), κ (kappa).
- Enkephalins, endorphins and dynorphin are naturally occurring peptide ligands that bind to opioid receptors.
- The peptides modulate nociceptive input in two ways:
  1. Block neurotransmitter release by inhibiting calcium influx in the presynaptic terminal.
  2. Open potassium channels, which hyperpolarize neurons inhibiting excitatory action potentials.
- Systemically administered opioid analgesics can bind to the opioid receptors and modulate pain transmission.

EXAMINER: Anything else?

CANDIDATE: Descending inhibitory system (adrenergic and serotoninergic):
- From the periaqueductal grey matter and the rostral medulla descending nerve fibres can modulate the ascent of nociceptor information at the dorsal root ganglia.
- Noradrenaline and serotonin are the main neurotransmitters in this pathway.

Structured oral examination question 7

Pain pathways

EXAMINER: What about primary afferent fibres?

CANDIDATE: There are three main types of afferent fibre (Table 23.1).
- Sensory (Aβ) fibres are highly myelinated and of large diameter, therefore allowing rapid signal conduction. They have a low activation threshold and usually respond to light touch. Under pathological conditions they may become hyperexcitable, leading to stimuli that would usually elicit sensations of tactile touch causing pain.
- Alpha delta fibres (Aδ) are lightly myelinated and smaller diameter, and hence conduct more slowly than Aβ fibres. They respond to mechanical and thermal stimuli. They carry rapid, sharp, shallow pain that is specific to one area. These fast pain pathways composed of Aδ fibres are also responsible for the initial reflex withdrawal response to acute pain. High activation threshold.

- Group C nerve fibres are unmyelinated and are also the smallest type of primary afferent fibre. Hence, they demonstrate the slowest conduction. C fibres are polymodal because they can respond to various stimuli (chemical, mechanical and thermal). C-fibre activation leads to slow, burning pain spread out over an unspecific area (second pain). High activation threshold.

EXAMINER: What about pain afferent fibres?

CANDIDATE: There are two main types of nociceptive nerve fibres: Aδ and C fibres. Aδ fibres transmit rapid, sharp, localized pain. C fibres transmit slow, diffuse, dull pain.

The difference in speeds at which the two types of pain fibres (Aδ and C) conduct nerve impulses explains why, when you are injured, you first feel a sharp, acute, specific pain, which gives way a few seconds later to a more diffuse, dull pain.

EXAMINER: What about the lateral spinothalamic pathway (Figure 23.2)?

CANDIDATE: The lateral spinothalamic tract conveys pain, temperature and crude touch to the somatosensory region of the thalamus.

GABA, glycine, serotonin, norepinephrine, dopamine and acetylcholine have an inhibitory effect on spinothalamic tract neurons, whereas glutamate has an excitatory role.

Destination	Posterior central gyrus
Third-order neuron	Ventral posterolateral nucleus of thalamus
Pathway	Lateral spinothalamic
Second-order neuron	Substantia gelatinosa
First-order neuron	Posterior root ganglia
Receptor	Free nerve endings

The first-order neuron delivers sensations to the CNS: the cell body is in the dorsal root ganglion.

The second-order neuron: an interneuron with the cell body in the spinal cord or brain.

The third-order neuron: transmits information from the thalamus to the cerebral cortex (Figures 23.3 and 23.4).

First-order neuron

Aδ and C primary afferent nerve fibres have cell bodies in the dorsal root ganglia and terminate in the dorsal horn of the spinal cord. Once they have

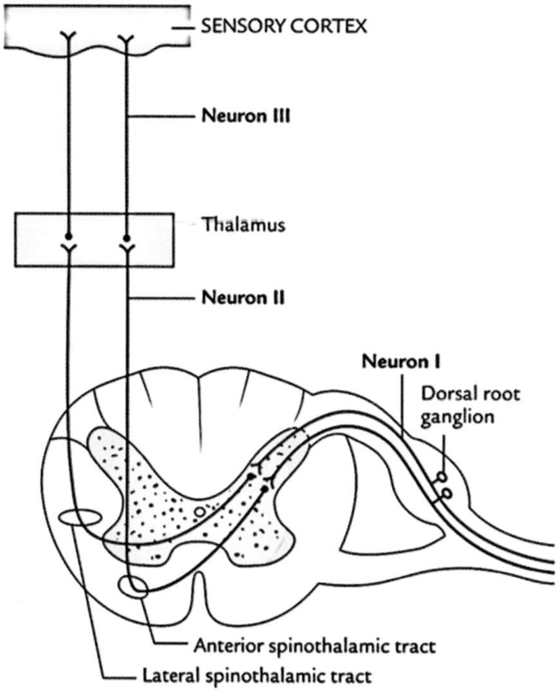

Figure 23.3 Spinothalamic tract.

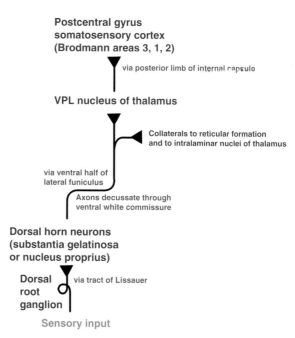

Figure 23.4 Spinothalamic tract. Candidate drawing.

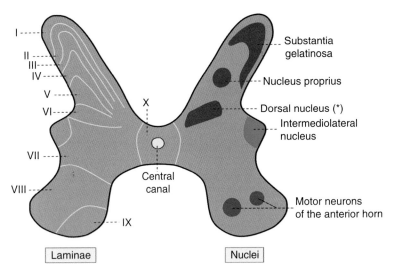

Figure 23.5 Rexed laminae.

Substantia gelatinosa

Nucleus proprius

Dorsal nucleus (*)

Intermediolateral nucleus

Central canal

Motor neurons of the anterior horn

| Laminae | | Nuclei |

*Posterior thoracic nucleus or Column of Clarke

entered the spinal cord the nerve roots may bifurcate into ascending and descending branches, which can enter the dorsal horn one or two segments higher or lower than the segment of origin.

The dorsal horn of the spinal cord is the site where the primary afferent fibres synapse with second-order neurons. It is also where complex interactions occur between excitatory and inhibitory interneurons and where descending inhibitory tracts from higher centres exert their effect.

The dorsal horn is divided into six laminae (called Rexed laminae) responsible for processing sensory information and has an important role in the modulation of pain signals (Figure 23.5).

Lamina II is known as the substantia gelatinosa and this extends from the trigeminal nucleus in the medulla to the filum terminale at the caudal end of the spinal cord. It contains inhibitory and excitatory interneurons.

C fibres terminate in lamina II and Aδ fibres terminate in laminae I and V.

Aβ fibres (light touch and vibration) enter the cord medial to the dorsal horn and pass without synapse to the dorsal columns. They give off collateral branches to the dorsal horn which terminate in several laminae (III–V). They also synapse directly with terminals of unmyelinated C fibres in lamina II.

Laminae II and V are important areas for the modulation and localization of pain.

Second-order neurons

Second-order neurons ascend to higher centres via the contralateral spinothalamic and spinoreticular tracts, which are located in the anterolateral white matter of the spinal cord. Some of these neurons branch out to the periaqueductal gray or the reticular formation.

Third-order neurons

The tertiary neurons in the ventral posterolateral nucleus of the thalamus.

Axons from these thalamic neurons follow the thalamic radiations to terminate in the primary somatosensory cortex (Brodmann's areas 3, 1, 2 of the postcentral gyrus).

EXAMINER: What do you mean by nociceptors?

CANDIDATE:
- Nociceptors are sensory receptors for pain.
- Nociceptive fibres do not have specialized structures (such as Pacinian or Messner corpuscles) at their endings. Instead, they have what are known as free (naked) nerve endings that form dense networks with multiple branches.
- The peripheral activation of nociceptors is modulated by a number of chemical substances, which are produced and released when there is cellular damage (e.g. potassium, serotonin, bradykinin, histamine, prostaglandins, leukotrienes and substance P).

- These substances influence the degree of nerve activity and intensity of the pain sensation.

Structured oral examination question 8

Local anaesthetic

EXAMINER: Local anaesthetics are important in orthopaedics. What do you know about them?

COMMENT: A general start up question that is a gift.
- All local anaesthetics produce their effects by blocking the transmembrane pore of sodium-gated voltage channels. This prevents depolarization of the nerve cell and propagation of the action potential down the nerve (Figure 23.6).
- The duration of action of the drug is dependent on protein binding and its clearance from the injection site.
- Protein binding for the longer-acting agents, i.e. bupivacaine and ropivicaine, is 95%; this is compared to 65% for lidocaine, a shorter-acting drug. The clearance from the injection site is dependent on local blood flow. Short-acting agents, i.e. lignocaine, cause vasodilation, thus potentiating clearance. Vasopressors, i.e. adrenaline, can be added in order to prolong the duration of action. Interestingly, local blood flow has little influence on the longer-acting agents due to their high percentage of protein binding; therefore, the addition of vasopressors does not prolong their duration of action.
- Local anaesthetics block conduction in the following order: small myelinated axons, unmyelinated axons and large myelinated axons. As such, nociceptive transmission in Aδ and C fibres is blocked first and large-diameter myelinated motor fibres last.

EXAMINER: Tell me more about how they work.

CANDIDATE: Local anaesthetics act by inhibiting sodium through sodium-specific ion channels in the neuronal cell. Entry of Na+ is essential for the generation of an action potential. They interact with a receptor within the voltage-sensitive Na+ channel and raise the threshold of opening the channel (Figure 23.7).

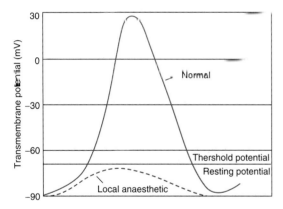

Figure 23.6 Local anaesthetics slow the rate of depolarization of the nerve action potential such that the threshold potential is not reached. As a result, an action potential cannot be propagated in the presence of local anaesthetic, and conduction blockade results.

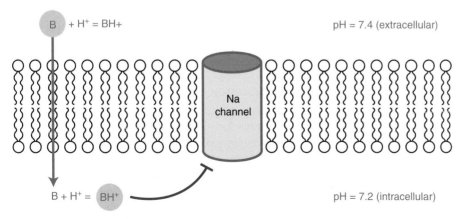

Figure 23.7 Mode of action of local anaesthetics: Na-channel blocker.

Table 23.2 Most commonly used local anaesthetics with their maximum doses and duration of onset and action. A 2% solution of lignocaine contains 20mg in 1ml.

Local anaesthetic agents	Concentration (%)	Onset (min)	Duration (min)	Max. dose (mg/kg)	Max. dose with adrenaline (mg/kg)	pKa
Lidocaine	0.5–2	5–15	40–120	3	7	7.7
Bupivacaine	0.25–0.5	15–30	150–360	2.0	3	8.1
Levo-bupivacaine (Chirocaine)	0.25–0.5	15–30	150–360	2.0	3	8.1
Ropivacaine	0.2–1	5–10	150–300	3.0	Not used	8.1

The rate and rise of an action potential and the maximum depolarization decreases leading to a slowing of conduction. Finally, local depolarization fails to reach threshold potential, resulting in a conduction block.

Local anaesthetic binds more readily to sodium channels in an activated state and slows its reversion to the resting state. The refractory period is increased.

COMMENT: This could easily be asked in the basic science nerve section on action potentials as a score 7/8 question.

EXAMINER: What are the commonly used local anaesthetics and their classes (Table 23.2)?

CANDIDATE: Local anaesthetics can be split depending on their chemical composition into two classes.
1. Amides. Longer-acting. Metabolized by liver enzymes and excreted in urine.
2. Esters. Short-acting, metabolized in the plasma and tissue fluids by a cholinesterase enzyme and excreted in urine.

Amides are more commonly used, i.e. lidocaine, prilocaine, bupivacaine, levo-bupivacaine, ropivacaine.

Esters, e.g. cocaine, chlorprocaine and benzocaine, are now rarely used.

All the amides have an 'I' before the 'caine'.

EXAMINER: What determines the onset and potency of different local anaesthetics?

CANDIDATE: The activity of local anaesthetics is strongly pH-dependent. All local anaesthetics are weak bases which exist in two forms: ionized (BH+) and unionized (B). It is the unionized form that crosses the nerve lipid and once through the ionized form affects sodium depolarization.

The amount that is ionized is determined by the equation

$$pKa - pH = \log [BH+]/[B].$$

EXAMINER: How may the pKa of a local anaesthetic influence its speed of onset?

CANDIDATE: Onset is determined by the pKa. The pKa of a local anaesthetic determines the amount which exists in an ionized form at any given pH. At physiological pH (7.4) all local anaesthetics are more ionized than unionized (as all the pKa values are greater than 7.4). However, the proportions vary between the drugs: lignocaine has a pKa of 7.9 and is approximately 25% unionized at pH 7.4. Bupivacaine has a pKa of 8.1 and hence less of the drug is unionized at pH 7.4 (about 15%).

As the drug must enter the cell in order to have its effect, it must pass through the lipid cell membrane. Unionized drug will do this more readily than ionized drug. Therefore, the drug which is more unionized at physiological pH will reach its target site more quickly than the drug which is less so. This explains why lignocaine has a faster onset of action than bupivacaine.

EXAMINER: What about potency?

CANDIDATE: The aromatic ring structure and hydrocarbon chain length of a particular local anaesthetic determine the lipid-solubility of the drug and hence its potency. A more lipid-soluble drug penetrates the cell membrane more easily to exert its effect. The more potent the drug, the smaller the amount required to produce a given effect. Thus bupivacaine – which is highly lipid-soluble – is approximately four times more potent than lignocaine.

Potency ∝ effect/dose

COMMENT: Potency increases with increased lipid-solubility, which is related to hydrocarbon chain length.

EXAMINER: What about duration of action?

CANDIDATE: Duration of action increases with increased protein binding, which is determined by the length of the intermediate chain which joins onto the aromatic and amine group.

Lignocaine: 65% protein-bound.

Bupivacaine: 95% protein-bound.

As such, bupivacaine will have a longer duration of action than lignocaine.

Lipid-solubility is the second leading determining factor, greater percentage protein-bound and increased lipid solubility = longer duration of action.

EXAMINER: Why do we avoid local anaesthetics use with abscess surgery?

CANDIDATE: There are two reasons.
1. Infection in a tissue decreases its pH, which increases the pKa–pH difference, which leads to more ionized form which does not cross the lipid nerve membrane.
2. Infection is often associated with localized increased blood supply and hence more anaesthetic may be removed from the area before it can affect the neuron.

EXAMINER: You have infiltrated the skin and local tissues for a carpal tunnel release and used the maximum amount of local anaesthetic permitted, but the local anaesthetic doesn't seem to be working. What are your thoughts?

CANDIDATE: Pathological reasons may include infection, previous trauma or surgery or inflammation. Psychological reasons include fear and anxiety. Poor technique with the local anaesthetic injected away from the proposed site of surgery.

I wouldn't inject more than the recommended dose of local and would consider using a GA instead assuming the patient was fully fasted and there was an anaesthetist available to do this in a safe and timely manner.

EXAMINER: Why may levobupivacaine or bupivacaine be preferred for use as a local anaesthetic compared to lignocaine?

CANDIDATE: They are associated with less vasodilation and have a longer duration of action, which is good to cover the operation duration and for postoperative analgesia.

EXAMINER: What are the complications from local anaesthetics?

CANDIDATE: Complications are frequently associated with errors of dose or intravenous administration. Complications are related to membrane destabilization of cells.
- Neurological – perioral and glossitic paraesthesia, dizziness, drowsiness, tinnitus, seizures.
- Cardiovascular – bradycardia, hypotension, cardiac arrhythmias, i.e. ventricular fibrillation and asystole.
- Hypersensitivity and allergy – these are rare and can vary from a mild skin irritation or rash to anaphylactic shock. The main signs and symptoms of anaphylactic shock are chest discomfort, urticaria, stomach pain and dyspnoea. An anaphylactic reaction can rapidly lead to a life-threatening condition due to airway passage obstruction in association with laryngeal oedema and needs immediate treatment.
- Pain at injection – many factors. Low pH and cold solution may irritate the tissue. Fast and high injection pressure may cause rapid swelling of tissues and pain. This can be avoided by a slower injection. Avoid aggressive, rough insertion of a needle.
- Neurological effects are usually witnessed first followed by cardiovascular collapse. Management is supportive. A definitive airway should be established, ensuring adequate oxygenation and ventilation. Benzodiazepines and phenytoin can be used to control seizures. Cardiac monitoring is mandatory, as arrhythmias require urgent treatment.
- The addition of adrenaline to local anaesthetics should not be used on tissues with end arteries, i.e. digit and penis, as the induced vasoconstriction may result in tissue ischaemia. Caution should be used when infiltrating around skin flaps for the same reason. Ear lobes and nose should also be avoided

Structured oral examination question 9

General anaesthesia

Anaesthesia gas machine laminated photo is shown to the candidate (Figure 23.8).

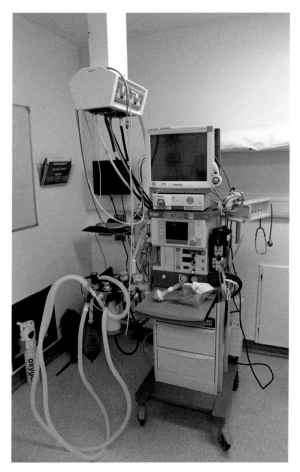

Figure 23.8 Anaesthesia gas machine.

EXAMINER: What are the principles of general anaesthesia?

CANDIDATE: General anaesthesia encompasses the triad of analgesia, amnesia and muscle relaxation. Rather than using a large dose of a single drug to establish the clinical triad, a combination of drugs is used in smaller doses, thus avoiding dose-related adverse effects, and is termed 'balance anaesthesia'.

EXAMINER: What else?

CANDIDATE: General anaesthetic agents act in the CNS to bring about a reversible loss of consciousness, amnesia (memory loss), analgesia, loss of motor reflexes and skeletal muscle relaxation.

EXAMINER: What drugs are used?

CANDIDATE: The three main classes of drugs used for GAs are intravenous induction agents, inhalation induction agents and muscle relaxants. Drugs used as intravenous agents include thiopentone, propofol and ketamine (Table 23.3).

EXAMINER: Do you know which intravenous agents are most useful in certain situations (Table 23.4)?

CANDIDATE: Propofol is mainly used in day case anaesthesia. It would be difficult to do day-case surgery without propofol. Thiopentone has fallen out of favour because it can cause significant bronchospasm and severe extravasation injuries. It has a longer postoperative recovery than propofol. Ketamine is the most cardiovascular-stable induction agent. It is therefore good to use in the trauma situation if there has been a large amount of haemorrhage occurring.

Etomidate is a short-acting intravenous anaesthetic agent historically used for short procedures, such as reduction of dislocated joints.

EXAMINER: You mentioned halothane as an inhalation agent, but what is the problem with using it?

CANDIDATE: It can cause hepatitis and as such is rarely used these days. Around 1 in 50,000 can develop a severe life-threatening hepatitis.

EXAMINER: Why do we use muscle relaxants as part of a GA?

COMMENT: Neuromuscular blocking agents is another way to refer to muscle relaxants.

CANDIDATE: Muscle relaxants are used to facilitate tracheal intubation and provide optimal operating conditions. Muscle relaxants target the neuromuscular junction (NMJ).

EXAMINER: How do muscle relaxants work (Table 23.5)?

CANDIDATE: There are two types of muscle relaxants.
1. Non-depolarizing.
2. Depolarizing.

Non-depolarizing agents competitively block the binding of acetylcholine (ACh) to nicotinic receptors at the post-synaptic membrane. This leaves fewer receptors available for ACH to bind to and initiate channel opening. No end plate potential is generated with paralysis of the affected skeletal muscles.

Depolarizing agents act by depolarizing the post-synaptic plasma membrane of the muscle fibre similar to Ach, but as these agents are

Table 23.3 Intravenous induction agents.

Drug	Mechanism of action	Effects
Thiopentone (barbiturate)	Increases the conductance of chloride ions in nerve cells, mediated by GABA channels causing hyper polarization and neuronal inhibition	Short acting 5–10 minutes Dose-dependent respiratory depression Reduction in CO and SVR leading to hypotension
Propofol	Several mechanisms of action suggested, including reducing the opening time of sodium channels inhibiting depolarization (sodium channel blocker) and potentiation of GABA receptor activity	Obtunds upper airway reflexes (useful for LMAs) Hypotension and decrease in SVR Respiratory depression and apnoea
Etomidate	Activates the GABA receptor	Short-acting and recovery is rapid. Cardiovascular stable with no effect on SVR, myocardial contractility and heart rate. Can cause adrenal suppression
Ketamine	Antagonist effect of the excitatory neurotransmitter glutamate via the NMDA receptor	Potent analgesic Stimulates sympathetic nervous system therefore increases HR, BP and CO

BP, blood pressure; CO, cardiac output; HR, heart rate; LMA, laryngeal mask airway; NMDA, *N*-methyl-D-aspartate receptor; SVR, systemic vascular resistance.

Table 23.4 Inhalation agents.

Agent	Benefits	Limitations/ side effects
Nitrous oxide	Analgesic Used as a carrier for the other volatiles	Not potent enough to be used as sole anaesthetic agent
Halothane	Non-irritant to upper airways Used in paediatrics	Hepatitis and cardiac arrhythmias
Sevoflurane	Non-irritant to upper airways Non-arrhythmogenic	Renal toxicity QT prolongation
Isoflurane	Cheaper	Upper airway irritant
Desoflurane	Rapid recovery	Upper airway irritant

more resistant to breakdown they persistently depolarize the muscle fibre. As such there are two phases to action, the first being an initial depolarization phase where the agent causes muscle fasciculations while the muscle fibres are depolarizing. The second phase involves a desensitizing phase in which the muscle is no longer responsive to neuromuscular transmitter released by the motor neurons.

EXAMINER: How are muscle relaxants reversed?

CANDIDATE: At the end of the procedure muscle relaxants can be rapidly 'reversed' with the use of neostigmine, which has a plasma half-life of 60 minutes, longer than all the commonly used muscle relaxants. Neostigmine is an antagonist to acetylcholine esterase (AChe) (the enzyme that breaks down ACh) resulting in a flux of ACh at the NMJ. Neostigmine is rarely used on its own to reverse as it can cause significant bradycardia, being often given with glycopyrrolate (with a similar but milder action to atropine).

COMMENT: Adjuncts to anaesthesia include antiemetics, which aim to reduce the incidence of postoperative nausea and vomiting. Local anaesthetic and peripheral blocks used in conjunction with general anaesthesia have led to improved postoperative pain relief and aided postoperative physiotherapy.

Analgesia

Anaesthetists use analgesics which are different to those used in non-anaesthetized patients. These often have a very quick onset of action – alfentanil, fentanyl and remifentanil.

Remifentanil has a very short half-life, which is the same even after many hours of receiving the infusion.

In the doses anaesthetists give, these can have a potent respiratory depressant effect (as do most other anaesthetic agents).

EXAMINER: Have you heard of total intravenous anaesthesia (TIVA)?

CANDIDATE: No, sorry.

COMMENT: TIVA has been used for many years as an alternative to inhalational anaesthesia. Some anaesthetists choose to use this as their standard. Others use it for the following reasons:

- Reduced postoperative nausea and vomiting.

Table 23.5 Inhalation agents.

Drug	Mode of action	Benefits	Side effects
Suxamethonium	Mimics ACh, persistent depolarization of NMJ causes muscle relaxation	Rapid-onset and short-acting	Myalgia and hyperkalaemia, anaphylaxis and suxamethonium apnoea
Atracurium	Competitive inhibitor of ACh Non-depolarizing	Intermediate-acting, spontaneously breaks down (Hofmann elimination), useful in hepatic and renal impairment	Histamine release can cause bronchospasm and vasodilation
Rocuronium	Competitive inhibitor of ACh Non-depolarizing	Intermediate-acting, rapid-onset useful in patients at risk of aspiration	

ACh, acetylcholine; NMJ, neuromuscular junction.

Table 23.6 Types of regional anaesthetic used in orthopaedic surgery.

Regional anaesthetic	Surgical procedures
Central neuraxial block (CNB)	
Spinal	Lower limb arthroplasty, pelvic surgery, foot and ankle surgery
Epidural	Postoperative pain relief in lower limb and pelvic surgery (now not common practice with the emphasis on fast-track discharge and enhanced recovery programmes)
Upper limb	
Interscalene block (ISB) level C5/C6	Shoulder surgery
Supraclavicular block (SCB) Axillary brachial plexus block (ABPB) C5–T1	Elbow, forearm and hand
Lower limb	
Femoral nerve block (FNB) L2–L4	Generally used as an adjunct to GA in knee arthroplasty and soft-tissue knee procedures
Sciatic nerve block (SNB)	Foot and ankle surgery and in combination with FNB for complete knee analgesia
Popliteal block	Ankle surgery, foot surgery. Can be unreliable
Adductor canal block	Adjunct to GA for knee arthroplasty and soft-tissue knee surgery. Preserves motor function more than the more proximal femoral nerve block
Ankle block – terminal nerve branches to the foot	Hind, mid and forefoot surgery

- Rapid recovery from anaesthesia.
- Some evidence that it may be better to reduce cancer recurrence (disputed).
- When inhalational agents are absolutely contraindicated – malignant hyperthermia.
- When you wish to avoid muscle relaxant drugs due to certain neurological diseases.
- When you wish to avoid muscle relaxants for endotracheal intubation.

It is possible to intubate without using neuromuscular blocking agents. This can be done with infusions of propofol and remifentanil, or with boluses of propofol and alfentanil/fentanyl.

EXAMINER: What do you understand by the term regional anaesthesia?

CANDIDATE 1: With regional anaesthesia you are rendering a specific area of the body, e.g. foot, arm, insensate to the stimulus of surgery or other instrumentation.

EXAMINER: What types of regional anaesthesia do you know?

CANDIDATE 1: Radial nerve block, brachial plexus block, epidural and spinal anaesthesia.

COMMENT: Scoring 5/6.

CANDIDATE 2: Regional anaesthesia involves infiltration of local anaesthetic to block sensory and motor nerves. Regional anaesthesia makes the operative site insensate and provides peri- and postoperative pain relief. The duration of motor and sensory blockade depends on the type and concentration of local anaesthetic agents and whether any additive agents are used.

EXAMINER: What types of regional anaesthetic are used in orthopaedic surgery (Table 23.6)?

CANDIDATE: A peripheral nerve block involves injecting local anaesthetic near the course of a named nerve. The advantages are that a relatively small dose of local anaesthetic can cover a large area with rapid onset of action. Disadvantages include that it is technically challenging.

To increase the accuracy and safety, nerves or plexuses are located using ultrasound guidance and peripheral nerve stimulation.

A plexus block involves injection of local anaesthetic adjacent to a plexus. The advantages are a large area of anaesthesia can be produced, but the procedure is technically complex with the potential for damage of the plexus.

A spinal anaesthetic involves an injection of local anaesthetic into the CSF and provides profound anaesthesia of the lower abdomen and extremities. It is technically easy (LP technique)

with a high success rate and rapid onset of action. Disadvantages include a 'high spinal', hypotension due to sympathetic block and postdural headache.

An epidural involves injection of a local anaesthetic into the epidural space at any level of the spinal cord. It is used for anaesthesia/analgesia of the thorax, abdomen and lower extremities. Advantages include controlled onset of blockade, long duration of action with catheter use and postoperative analgesia. Disadvantages include postdural puncture headache if the epidural needle is accidentally advanced through the dura, toxicity of doses intended for the epidural space injected into the subarachnoid space as well as higher failure rates than for performing spinal anaesthesia.

Complications of any regional anaesthetic include bleeding, infection, nerve damage and local anaesthetic systemic toxicity (LAST).

COMMENT: Good score 6, possibly 7. Knows the general principles of regional anaesthesia, able to discuss uses and aware of advantages/disadvantages.

Chapter 24

Musculoskeletal oncology

Tomas B. Beckingsale and Kanishka Milton Ghosh

Definitions

As in all other areas of the viva examinations, knowing basic definitions gives you an easy starting point when answering questions and gives the impression to the examiners that you have both a logical and clear thought process, and are in command of the subject matter.

Neoplasm/tumour: A growth or swelling, which enlarges by cellular proliferation more rapidly than surrounding normal tissue and continues to enlarge after the initiating stimuli cease. Usually lacks structural organization and functional coordination with normal tissues and serves no useful purpose to the host.

Malignant tumour: Malignant tumours have a predisposition to invasive and destructive local growth, and to distant metastasis usually via the vascular or lymphatic systems.

Benign tumour: Benign tumours do not metastasize but can still exhibit locally aggressive behaviour.

Sarcoma: A diverse and rare group of malignant tumours of mesenchymal/connective tissue origin. Tumours of peripheral nerves are often included in this group.

Generic structured oral examination question 1

Biopsy

EXAMINER: So how would you obtain a tissue diagnosis?

CANDIDATE: A tissue sample can be obtained by biopsy. In general terms this can be performed by excisional, incisional or percutaneous means, but I would not perform a biopsy without first having discussed the case with a bone and soft tissue tumour MDT.

EXAMINER: Good. Let's suppose you are the bone tumour surgeon now. When might you perform an excision biopsy?

CANDIDATE: The indications for an excision biopsy are narrow. The entire lesion is removed, and the margins are often marginal. Hence, this type of biopsy is really only applicable to benign lesions where the imaging has been diagnostic, for example lipomas, or where the lesion is small and superficial such that excision biopsy would not compromise later re-excision. However, if there is any doubt about the diagnosis I would perform a percutaneous or incisional biopsy first.

EXAMINER: OK, tell me how you would perform an incisional biopsy.

CANDIDATE: First, I would ensure I had appropriate imaging, ideally an MRI scan. I would perform the procedure through a short longitudinal incision. I would plan the incision using the imaging and position it such that the entire biopsy tract could be excised *en bloc* during the definitive resection, and such that it does not contaminate more than one compartment or key neurovascular structures. I would pay close attention to haemostasis and use minimal tissue dissection in order to minimize local tissue seeding.

EXAMINER: We perform most of our biopsies percutaneously now. Do you know any advantages or disadvantages to doing it this way?

CANDIDATE: I've seen biopsy performed by Tru-Cut needle. The procedure can be performed easily in clinic under local anaesthetic, which removes delay and the requirement for theatre time. Welker *et al.* have shown that it is safe, has a low complication rate and reliably provides enough tissue for diagnosis and treatment planning [1]. Other advantages are that it can be combined with imaging modalities, for example ultrasound for soft-tissue lesions and CT for bony lesions. The disadvantage is that necrosis and mitotic rate are less reliable on core needle, but this rarely affects management, and an incisional biopsy can always be performed subsequently if more information is required.

EXAMINER: What do you understand by a marginal margin?

CANDIDATE: A marginal margin, as described by Enneking, is when the resection line passes through the reactive zone of the tumour being excised [2].

EXAMINER: Explain to me what you mean by the reactive zone.

CANDIDATE: Tumours grow in a centifugal fashion and this leads to compression and subsequent atrophy of the surrounding tissue forming a pseudocapsule. Outside the pseudocapsule is an area of oedema where inflammatory cells and micronodules of tumour are present. This is the reactive zone. Hence, if a resection line passes through this reactive zone, as in a marginal margin, then micronodules of tumour are likely to be left behind, increasing the risk of a local recurrence.

EXAMINER: So, what other margins did Enneking describe and what do you understand by them?

CANDIDATE: Enneking described three other possible margins. He described intralesional margins, where the resection line passes through the tumour leaving macroscopic deposits of tumour in the surgical wound. He described wide margins, where the resection line passes outside the reactive zone and the tumour is excised with a surrounding cuff of normal tissue. In wide margins it is still possible that tumour will remain in the form of skip lesions. Finally, he described the radical margin, where the entire compartment in which the tumour resides is excised *en bloc*, in theory removing the entire tumour [2].

Generic structured oral examination question 2

Staging

EXAMINER: So what stage is this tumour?

CANDIDATE: I would stage this tumour using the Musculoskeletal Tumour Society staging system

as described by Enneking [3]. We've discussed that it's a high-grade osteosarcoma, which makes it at least Stage II. It's an intramedullary tumour that's invaded the surrounding soft tissues making it extracompartmental and upstaging it to IIB. We've not discussed whether there is any evidence of metastasis yet, but, if there is, that would immediately make it a Stage III, regardless of the other features we've talked about.

COMMENT: This question will usually follow a discussion about a malignant tumour, for example osteosarcoma as in this example. The Enneking system is the easiest to remember and can be applied equally to bony and soft-tissue sarcomas. The other commonly used system is the American Joint Committee on Cancer (AJCC) system, which is more complicated. The AJCC also has separate systems for bony and soft-tissue tumours.

Structured oral examination question 1

Osteochondroma

EXAMINER: This young lad has been referred to you urgently by his GP after his mum brought him in with a firm lump on the front of his left thigh. Tell me about his X-ray (Figure 24.1).

CANDIDATE: This is a lateral radiograph of his left femur including the knee joint but not the hip joint. There is a bony growth on the anterior aspect of the femur, which looks like a large osteochondroma.

EXAMINER: What makes you think it's an osteochondroma?

Table 24.1 Enneking/MSTS staging system [4].

Stage	Description	Grade	Site	Metastases
IA	Low-grade, intracompartmental	G_1	T_1	M_0
IB	Low-grade, extracompartmental	G_1	T_2	M_0
IIA	High-grade, intracompartmental	G_2	T_1	M_0
IIB	High-grade, extracompartmental	G_2	T_2	M_0
III	Any grade, metastatic	G_{1-2}	T_{1-2}	M_1

587

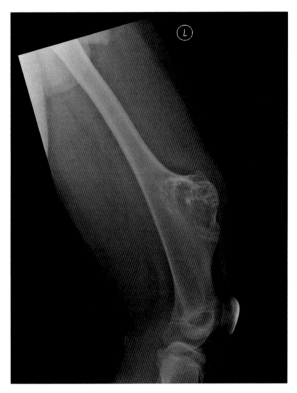

Figure 24.1 Osteochondroma.

CANDIDATE: Well, the cortices are in continuity with the bone as is the medullary cavity, and the lesion is extending out from the metaphyseal region of the distal femur, which is the most common site for these (25%). This is a sessile lesion rather than the pedunculated variety and appears to be a solitary lesion, although I'd want to examine the child to look for other lumps. It is quite a large lesion and there is some slightly atypical sclerosis within it, so I would definitely get an MRI scan.

EXAMINER: OK, so you get an MRI, which shows a nice thin cartilage cap and no worrying features. How are you going to treat it?

CANDIDATE: First I'd take a history and examine the child. I'd want to know if it is tender or symptomatic before I decide what to do.

EXAMINER: It's not tender and it only bothers him occasionally if he knocks it, but his mother is adamant she wants it removed.

CANDIDATE: I would suggest a period of watchful waiting to see if it continues to grow or becomes more symptomatic. Removing it would carry risks

of recurrence and neurovascular damage. There is also a chance of fracture during the operation and afterwards as it's a large sessile lesion and removing it will weaken the anterior cortex of the femur considerably.

EXAMINER: His mum still wants it removed and she's worried that it's going to become cancer.

CANDIDATE: If this is a solitary lesion then malignant change is very rare indeed (< 1%). If the child has multiple hereditary exostoses the risk is a bit higher. The textbooks often quote figures of 10% but it is probably more like 1–5%.

General advice: Examiners may show an example of a solitary osteochondroma in an area that is difficult to access for the purposes of excision, but then insist that the patient wants it removed, e.g. posterior, proximal tibia. The resultant discussion is then used to assess knowledge of anatomy and approaches, e.g. posterior approach to the knee. If the MRI has shown no sinister features, and the lesion is asymptomatic, then you can have a reasoned discussion with the examiner about watchful waiting versus removal, i.e. both answers are perfectly acceptable.

Other points

Continued growth after physeal closure raises the suspicion of malignant transformation.

- A major consideration in determining the malignant potential of an osteochondroma is the thickness of its cartilage cap with thicknesses greater than 1 cm considered worrisome.
- *EXT* gene mutation is the genetic abnormality in multiple hereditary exostoses. It is an autosomal dominant condition.

Structured oral examination question 2

Enchondroma

EXAMINER: Tell me about these radiographs of this chap's right foot (Figure 24.2).

CANDIDATE: Well they're AP and oblique views and they show an expansile, lytic lesion in the proximal phalanx of his second toe.

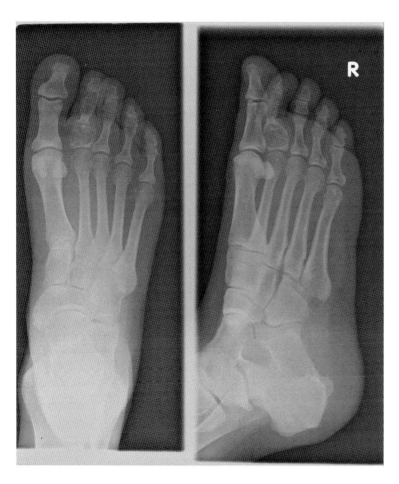

Figure 24.2 Enchondroma.

EXAMINER: What do you think it is?

CANDIDATE: The radiographs show features consistent with an enchondroma. It has a short zone of transition and appears quite well defined. There's also some stippled calcification within the substance of the lesion, which suggests a chondroid matrix.

EXAMINER: How would you treat this lesion?

CANDIDATE: Well I would want to get more information, so I would take a full history and examination. I would also want to get more imaging of the lesion with an MRI or CT and discuss the pictures with a bone tumour MDT. If there's any doubt about the diagnosis they may want to do a biopsy, but in general the surgical treatment of an enchondroma is with curettage, with or without grafting.

COMMENT: Even if the diagnosis appears obvious and is of a benign lesion, don't be rushed into offering surgical treatment. Always work through history, examination and imaging. You will never be criticized for discussing the diagnosis with a bone tumour MDT, but you will end up in a very tricky discussion with the examiners and fail if you have made the wrong diagnosis, it turns out to be malignant, and you've not discussed it with an MDT first.

Other points

- 50% of solitary enchondromas arise in the hands.
- Malignant transformation is very rare, but when it does occur it is usually in large lesions of long bones.
- Enchondromatosis = Ollier's disease (risk of bone malignancy is 10%, but if visceral and brain malignancies are included then the overall risk is 25%).
- Enchondromatosis + haemangiomas = Maffucci's syndrome (risk of malignancy reported anywhere from 25% to 100%).

Structured oral examination question 3

Non-ossifying fibroma

EXAMINER: Tell me about this radiograph (Figure 24.3).

CANDIDATE: This is an AP radiograph of a left lower leg of a child, which includes both the ankle joint and the knee joint. There is a lucent lesion, eccentrically placed in the metaphyseal region of the tibia. The lesion is well-demarcated, and its margin is slightly sclerotic. These features are typical of a non-ossifying fibroma.

EXAMINER: Good. What else can you tell me about this lesion?

CANDIDATE: Non-ossifying fibromas are developmental or hamartomatous lesions. They are actually very common, and some have suggested an incidence of up to 35% in normal children. They are usually asymptomatic and are often discovered as an incidental finding. Occasionally they can present after a pathological fracture, after which they tend to heal up.

EXAMINER: How would you treat this lesion?

CANDIDATE: I can't see any evidence of fracture. I would take a history and examine the patient to ascertain whether the lesion is painful or symptomatic and I would discuss the images with our local tumour MDT to make sure that they were in agreement with the diagnosis. That being the case, this can be treated with observation only as these lesions normally resolve by adulthood. I would plan to keep the patient under review with surveillance radiography.

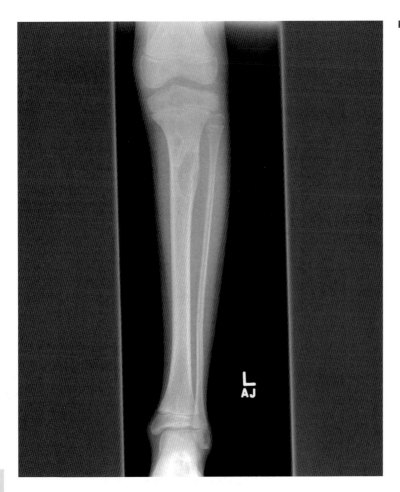

Figure 24.3 Non-ossifying fibroma.

COMMENT: Again, you will not be criticized if you say that would take advice from the bone tumour MDT. You will, however, be in a very difficult situation if you have not stated that you would take their advice and your diagnosis is wrong.

Structured oral examination question 4

Chondrosarcoma

EXAMINER: This 60-year-old lady presented with pain and swelling around her lower back. What can you see on this CT scan (Figure 24.4)?

CANDIDATE: This is an axial section showing the sacrum and iliac wings. There is an expansile lesion in the left iliac wing, which has extended into the soft tissues. The lesion has both lytic and sclerotic elements to it.

EXAMINER: What do you think the diagnosis might be?

CANDIDATE: The expansile nature, as well as the permeative margin and local invasion suggest a malignant process. Malignant tumours of bone can then be broken down into primary, metastatic, or immunohaematopoietic lesions. Metastatic and immunohaematopoietic tumours tend to produce lytic lesions within bones, whereas this lesion has areas of sclerosis and is much more expansile. Primary bone tumours can be classified according to their matrix as either bone-producing, cartilage-

producing, fibrous tissue-producing, or non-matrix-producing. The patchy sclerosis within this lesion is in keeping with either a bone- or cartilage-producing primary tumour, although I would not rule out other diagnoses without further investigations [5].

EXAMINER: You're right to suggest a primary lesion in this case. You've suggested bone- or cartilage-producing as the likely matrix. Which do you think is more likely here?

CANDIDATE: It is most likely to be a chondrosarcoma. The incidence of chondrosarcoma increases with age. This lady is 60 and although there is a second peak in the incidence of osteosarcoma in elderly patients, the majority of cases occur in adolescents around the growth spurt. The site of the tumour also makes chondrosarcoma the more likely diagnosis. Only around 5% of osteosarcomas occur in the pelvis, whereas up to 30% of chondrosarcomas are pelvic in origin. Finally, there is the appearance on the CT. It's not the clearest image, but I'm trying to convince myself that there's stippled calcification, which would indicate a chondroid lesion.

EXAMINER: Very good. What treatment options are there for an aggressive-looking chondrosarcoma like this is?

CANDIDATE: Chondrosarcomas are poorly chemo- and radiosensitive, so the only treatment option is wide local excision plus or minus reconstruction. However, despite surgical excision, longer-term survival is dependent on the presence or absence of metastases.

EXAMINER: So, what do you think the prognosis is for this high-grade lesion?

CANDIDATE: The key is the presence or absence of metastasis and the patient needs staging investigations. In general, low-grade, or grade I, lesions are rarely metastatic and have a better than 90% 5-year survival. High grade III lesions, as you've intimated this one is, are metastatic in over 70% of cases and have only a 30% 5-year survival.

Structured oral examination question 3

Chondrosarcoma

EXAMINER: This is a very fit and well 50-year-old chap, who has come into Accident & Emergency after falling down the stairs at home, sustaining

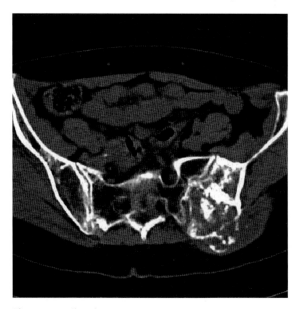

Figure 24.4 Chondrosarcoma.

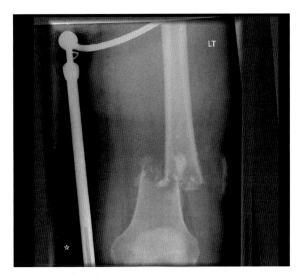

Figure 24.5 Chondrosarcoma 2.

this injury to his left leg. Tell me how you are going to manage this (Figure 24.5).

CANDIDATE: I would manage this patient initially using the principles of ATLS.

EXAMINER: Fine. No issues with ABC and the patient is alert and orientated.

CANDIDATE: Moving on, I want to assess whether the patient has any other injuries, and regarding this injury I want to know whether it is open or closed and whether the limb is neurovascularly intact.

EXAMINER: OK. This is his only injury. It's an open fracture with a 1-cm wound on the lateral thigh. The limb is neurovascularly intact. How are you going to manage this?

CANDIDATE: If it's an open injury then I would take a picture of the wound and cover it with a sterile-soaked swab. The patient needs IV antibiotics and coverage for tetanus, depending on their vaccination history. Some form of immobilization is also important for patient comfort and nursing care. In this case I can see that a Thomas splint has been applied.

EXAMINER: OK. So, shall I book this patient for theatre with a plan to perform a debridement of the wound and nailing of the fracture?

CANDIDATE: Well I know it's an open fracture, but I have some concerns about the X-ray. There's some odd calcification within the medullary cavity, so I'm worried that this is a pathological fracture through a bony lesion.

EXAMINER: Why does that make a difference?

CANDIDATE: It's a rare situation, but if this is a pathological fracture through a bone tumour, and we open up the fracture site and nail it, we would spread tumour the length of the femur and might convert a resectable tumour into one that is unresectable.

EXAMINER: But doesn't the open fracture need washing out?

CANDIDATE: It's a small puncture wound, and I've put the patient on IV antibiotics, so I think the infection risk is low. In this case I would arrange some urgent investigations, get more information and discuss the case immediately with the bone tumour MDT before rushing the patient to theatre.

COMMENT: Always look at the available evidence carefully and look out for any atypical features. If in doubt, say so! You will never be criticized for taking advice, but you will fail if you have blazed on with treatment and taken this patient to theatre for washout and nailing. If there is no threat to life or limb, then there is always time for further investigations, and to seek further opinions.

Always take time to look carefully before answering, especially if a question on a fracture comes up in the adult and pathology viva station!

Other points

- Chondrosarcomas are the second most frequent primary malignant tumour of bone.
- Chondrosarcomas are chemo- and radioresistant because of the presence of hyaline dense extracellular matrix, low mitotic activity and poor vascularity. As such, surgery remains the mainstay of treatment.
- Low-grade (Gd1) tumours can be managed with extensive intralesional curettage with adjuvant therapy such as cryotherapy phenolization or argon beam laser followed by a void-filling procedure.
- High-grade lesions invariably require en-bloc resection.
- Currently a plethora of targeted therapies are under clinical evaluation in patients with chondrosarcoma (e.g. Phase II study using Imatinib).

Structured oral examination question 6

Osteosarcoma [6]

EXAMINER: This young lad presented with a painful knee and a lump after a football injury. What do you think of the X-ray (Figure 24.6)?

CANDIDATE: When I was shown the X-ray I immediately thought that the diagnosis was an osteosarcoma and described the X-ray changes that supported my initial reaction. There is an intramedullary sclerotic lesion with a wide zone of transition and there is extension through the cortices and into the soft tissues. There is sunray spiculation, but at this resolution I can't see an obvious Codman's triangle.

EXAMINER: What's a Codman's triangle?

CANDIDATE: I knew what a Codman's triangle was, but I did not have a clear definition at my fingertips (a triangle of reactive bone at the edge of the tumour where the periosteum is elevated). I struggled for a few seconds but managed to explain that it is indicative of a periosteal reaction.

EXAMINER: So, what do you think the diagnosis is?

CANDIDATE: I think the diagnosis is an osteosarcoma. The imaging shows an osteogenic tumour in an adolescent male. It is also in a classical position in the metaphyseal region of the distal femur, where about 35% of these tumours occur.

EXAMINER: So how would you investigate it further?

CANDIDATE: I would take a history and examine the patient. I would refer the child on to a bone tumour MDT immediately rather than delay the process by organizing more investigations locally.

EXAMINER: OK, so you're working for the bone tumour MDT, what further investigations would you request?

CANDIDATE: I would request investigations to further delineate the tumour itself and I would arrange tests to assess for metastatic disease.

An MRI scan is the best modality for investigating the tumour itself and will delineate the local extent of the tumour, its relationship to key neurovascular structures, and the presence or absence of skip lesions. A CT scan can also be helpful as these lesions are osteogenic and therefore show up well on CT. These investigations can also be used to plan a biopsy.

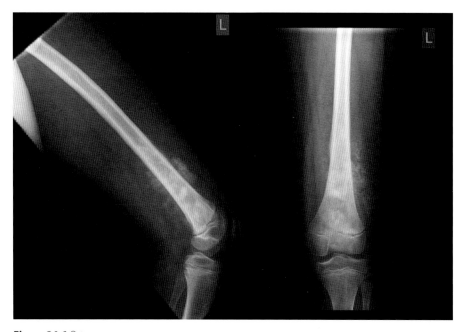

Figure 24.6 Osteosarcoma.

To stage the tumour one might initially get a chest X-ray, but CT scan of the chest is mandatory to look for metastases and these are sadly found in about 30% at diagnosis.

Other investigations you might use are blood tests, for example alkaline phosphatase and lactate dehydrogenase, which, if elevated, are associated with a poorer prognosis.

EXAMINER: Tell me about the general principles of treatment in cases like this.

CANDIDATE: Before commencing treatment, a confirmatory tissue diagnosis is made by biopsy and staging investigations are completed. Treatment for osteosarcoma then follows four distinct phases: neoadjuvant chemotherapy, surgical excision and reconstruction, adjuvant chemotherapy, and follow-up with clinical examination and imaging to look for recurrent disease or distant metastases.

EXAMINER: Why does the treatment start with neoadjuvant chemotherapy? Why don't we start by excising the tumour and then start chemotherapy?

CANDIDATE: There are three main reasons for beginning treatment with neoadjuvant chemotherapy rather than primary surgery. First, to treat occult micrometastases, which are likely to be present in a much greater proportion of patients than the 30% who present with radiologically detectable metastases at diagnosis; second, to reduce the inflammation around the primary tumour, aiding later surgical resection; and finally, to allow assessment of response to the neoadjuvant chemotherapy, determine prognosis, and direct adjuvant chemotherapy.

EXAMINER: You mentioned assessment of response to neoadjuvant chemotherapy. Why is this important?

CANDIDATE: Response of the tumour to chemotherapy treatment is measured as a percentage necrosis on histology of the resected specimen. A greater than 90% necrosis is considered a good response, and this carries a better prognosis than poor or non-responders. The reason for this is that if the tumour has a good response to chemotherapy then occult, but clinically undetectable, micrometastases are more likely to be eliminated by treatment, reducing the risk of then enduring

and developing into detectable metastases, and ultimately fatal disease.

EXAMINER: Do you know of any novel treatments?

CANDIDATE: I have read about muramyl tripeptide (MTP). It is not directly tumoricidal but works by stimulating the immune system, causing macrophages to exhibit cytotoxic antitumour activity. In a randomized trial, Meyers *et al.* showed that, when MTP was added to the standard chemotherapy regime of cisplatin, doxorubicin, and methotrexate, 6-year overall survival improved from 70% to 78% [7]. At the current time, NICE have not permitted its use for osteosarcoma, but this decision is under further discussion and appraisal.

Other points

- Recently, it has been suggested that a more reliable way of predicting the likelihood of local recurrence in high-grade osteosarcoma would be to combine both the measured surgical margin (in millimetres) as well as the tumour necrosis rate [9].

Structured oral examination question 7

Aneurysmal bone cyst

EXAMINER: This is a 20-year-old lad who presents with pain in his proximal left tibia. What do you make of his MRI scan (Figure 24.7)?

CANDIDATE: This is an axial T2 image, which shows a lesion in the posterolateral tibia. It appears well circumscribed with a sclerotic margin, is eccentrically placed, and there are multiple septations and loculations with fluid levels. These appearances would be in keeping with an aneurysmal bone cyst.

EXAMINER: That's right. What's the normal management for these?

CANDIDATE: First, it's important to confirm the diagnosis and I would always discuss bony lesions of this type with a bone tumour MDT. Aneurysmal bone cysts, or ABCs, can often form as a reactive change to another benign lesion, for example an osteoblastoma or giant cell tumour,

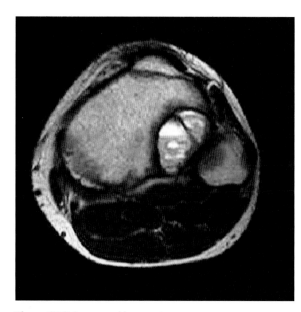

Figure 24.7 Aneurysmal bone cyst.

which needs to be ruled out. The differential diagnosis of an aneurysmal bone cyst also includes a telangiectatic osteosarcoma, which would require very different management. In general, treatment of ABCs is with curettage and grafting, but the recurrence rate can be as high as 50%. I am aware of newer therapies with promising results reported with the use of Denosumab, a RANKL inhibitor; however, its use in ABCs is currently off-label.

Other points

- ABCs and GCTs may have similar appearances on plain X-rays and may only be reliably differentiated radiologically with MRI.
- Traditionally, surgery was the mainstay of treatment.
- 'Denosumab' is a human monoclonal antibody that directly inhibits receptor activator of nuclear kappa B ligand (RANKL) signalling.

  RANKL expression is seen in a variety of benign and malignant bone neoplasms and has higher than normal levels of expression in GCT and ABCs [10].

- Among other things, 'Denosumab' is currently licensed for use in the treatment of skeletally mature adolescents and adults with GCT of bone [11].

- There is growing evidence for its use in ABCs (off-label), with studies showing tumour regression, improved pain and – in the case of spinal lesions – improvement in neurological symptoms [12].

Structured oral examination question 8

Ewing's sarcoma [5]

EXAMINER: This is a histology slide taken from a biopsy of a tumour in the femoral diaphysis of a 16-year-old boy. What does this slide show (Figure 24.8)?

CANDIDATE: This picture shows a magnified view of a stained histology slide. I'm no expert at histology, but I would describe the cells' appearance as small, round and blue, and given the brief history you provided I suspect this may represent a Ewing's sarcoma.

EXAMINER: Excellent. What other features might this patient have presented with?

CANDIDATE: Patients usually present with pain and swelling related to the tumour. They usually present around the knee, with 25% occurring in the distal femur. Frequently, erythema, systemic pyrexia, a leukocytosis and a raised ESR are also presenting features, which can incorrectly lead the unwary to a diagnosis of infection. Hence, it is mandatory to obtain radiographs when patients

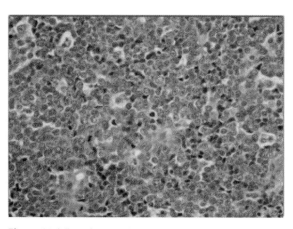

Figure 24.8 Ewing's sarcoma.

present with any unexplained pain or swelling. Patients can occasionally also present with pathological fracture through the lesion or with symptoms related to metastatic disease, such as bone pain in other sites or respiratory symptoms.

EXAMINER: And what would be the characteristic features you'd look for on an X-ray?

CANDIDATE: Ewing's sarcoma leads to a lytic, moth-eaten appearance to the bone. The classic finding, described as onion peel, is seen as a laminated periosteal reaction and probably reflects phases of tumour growth.

EXAMINER: How would you investigate this further?

CANDIDATE: I would start with a full history and examination. MRI scan is essential to delineate the local extent of the tumour and any involvement of key neurovascular structures. It can also be used to plan the biopsy. Other investigations aim to root out any evidence of metastatic disease. A CT chest is required to look for lung metastases, but, in Ewing's sarcoma, a bone scan and bone marrow biopsy are also required to look for widespread bony metastases. Distant bone marrow involvement carries a significantly poorer prognosis.

EXAMINER: In general terms, what is the management for Ewing's sarcoma?

CANDIDATE: There is a national videoconference MDT for all cases of Ewing's sarcoma, which recommends on management. In broad terms, Ewing's sarcomas are both chemo- and radiosensitive and hence these modalities form part of the management protocol. Neoadjuvant chemotherapy is the first-line treatment and usually precedes surgery, which involves wide excision and bony reconstruction where required. Occasionally lesions are treated solely with chemo- and radiotherapy, usually in surgically inaccessible lesions around the pelvis. The response to chemotherapy, like in osteosarcoma, is key to prognosis. Five-year survival is 75% with a good response, but only 20% with a poor prognosis.

Structured oral examination question 9

Lipoma

EXAMINER: This is an MRI of a patient who has presented with a painless mass on the lateral aspect

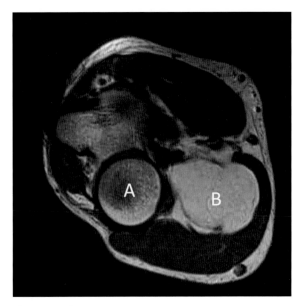

Figure 24.9 Lipoma.

of his right elbow. To orientate you the round structure (labelled A) is the radial head. Tell me about the lesion adjacent to it, which is labelled B (Figure 24.9).

CANDIDATE: There is an intramuscular mass in the extensor compartment adjacent, and lateral, to the radial head. The mass itself appears bland and is of the same intensity as the subcutaneous fat, suggesting a diagnosis of an intramuscular lipoma.

EXAMINER: What is a lipoma?

CANDIDATE: A lipoma is a benign tumour of mature adipocytes, identical to the surrounding adipose tissue, and showing little variation of cell size or shape.

EXAMINER: And how would you treat this lesion?

CANDIDATE: I would want to start by taking a history and examination, in particular looking for any abnormal features like pain or distal neural compromise, which might suggest a more aggressive lesion than a simple lipoma and alter my management. Also, this is only a single image of the lesion and I would want to see the rest of the scan and discuss it with the sarcoma MDT. Bland, innocent-looking lesions are usually treated with excision biopsy with a marginal margin. If there is any doubt, then a biopsy should be taken prior to excision. Histology of lesions below the fascia, like this one, often come back labelled as atypical lipomas by the histologist, despite very bland appearance on MRI.

EXAMINER: What do you mean by an atypical lipoma?

CANDIDATE: The term is quite controversial, and the literature often refers to them as lipoma-like liposarcomas. In essence, an atypical lipoma is a lipoma with some slightly atypical features but no evidence of malignancy. The histology of such lesions shows variation of adipocyte size, in contrast to the bland adipocytes of a simple lipoma, and nuclear atypia, as well as the presence of lipoblasts. These lesions are benign and management is still with marginal excision, but they do have a low rate of local recurrence [8].

Other points

- Atypical lipomas (ALT) and well-differentiated liposarcomas (WDL) are equivalent terms, describing lesions that are identical histologically.
- Site-specific variations in behaviour relate only to surgical resectability.
- In tumours located in the periphery, complete resection is curative. They have no risk of metastasis – for these tumours the designation of ALT is preferred, as they do not behave like sarcomas.
- In tumours that are large, deep-seated (e.g. retroperitoneum, pelvis, etc.), the chance of achieving negative margins is significantly diminished and the risk of local recurrence, dedifferentiation and death are increased.
- These lesions are best regarded as true sarcomas and the terminology of WDL is more appropriate.
- MDM2 amplification using fluorescent in-situ hybridization (FISH) is now a well-recognized method of differentiating WDL and ALT histologically.

Bibliography/Further reading

1. Welker JA, Henshaw RM, Jelinek J, Shmookler BM, Malawer MM. The percutaneous needle biopsy is safe and recommended in the diagnosis of musculoskeletal masses. *Cancer.* 2000;89(12):2677–2686.

2. Enneking WF, Spanier SS, Malawer MM. The effect of the anatomic setting on the results of surgical procedures for soft parts sarcoma of the thigh. *Cancer.* 1981;47(5):1005–1022.

3. Enneking WF, Spanier SS, Goodman MA. Current concepts review. The surgical staging of musculoskeletal sarcoma. *J Bone Joint Surg Am.* 1980;62(6):1027–1030.

4. NCCN. *National Comprehensive Cancer Network Clinical Practice Guidelines in Oncology: Soft Tissue Sarcoma. V.2.2008.* National Comprehensive Cancer Network. 2008.

5. Bullough PG. *Orthopaedic Pathology. Fourth Edition.* Edinburgh: Mosby; 2007.

6. Beckingsale TB, Gerrand CH. Osteosarcoma. *Orthop Trauma.* 2010;24(5):321–331.

7. Meyers PA, Schwartz CL, Krailo MD, *et al* Osteosarcoma: the addition of muramyl tripeptide to chemotherapy improves overall survival – a report from the Children's Oncology Group. *J Clin Oncol.* 2008;26:633–638.

8. Beckingsale TB, Gerrand CH. The management of soft-tissue sarcomas. *Orthop Trauma.* 2009;23 (4):240–247.

9. Jeys LM, Thorne CJ, Parry M, Gaston CL, Sumanthi VP, Grimer JR. A novel system for the surgical staging of primary high-grade osteosarcoma: the Birmingham classification. *Clin Orthop Relat Res.* 2017;475(3):842–850.

10. Yamagishi T, Kawashima H, Ogose A, *et al.* Receptor activator of nuclear kappa b ligand expression as a new therapeutic target in primary bone tumors. *PLoS ONE.* 2016;11(5):e0154680.

11. Van der Hejden L, Dijkstra PDS, Blay JY, Gelderblom H. Giant cell tumour of bone in the denosumab era. *Eur J Cancer.* 2017;77:75–73.

12. Dubory A, Missenard G, Domont J, Court C. Interest of denosumab for the treatment of giant cell tumours and aneurysmal bone cysts of the spine. About nine cases. *Spine (Phila Pa 1976).* 2016;41(11): E654–660.

Tribology and biomaterials

Iain McNamara and Majeed Shakokani

Structured oral examination question 1

Picture of THA with osteolysis shown.

EXAMINER: This is an X-ray of a THA in an elderly patient complaining of pain. What do you see (Figure 25.1)?

CANDIDATE: Plain radiographs of a reverse hybrid THA with a significant area of osteolysis in the greater trochanter.

EXAMINER: What do you think caused this?

CANDIDATE: Potential causes are infection, poly wear . . .

EXAMINER: Tell me about wear.

CANDIDATE: Wear is a progressive loss of material from the surface of a body owing to relative motion at that surface generating debris.

EXAMINER: What types and modes of wear do you know?

CANDIDATE: Well there are four modes of wear and various types of wear (I couldn't remember how many).

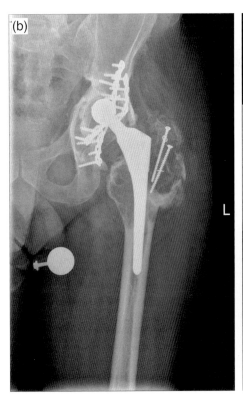
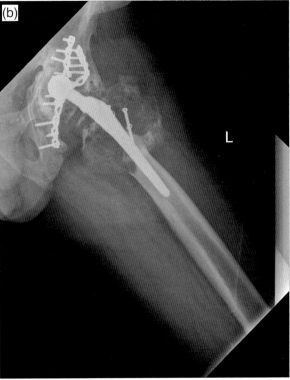

Figure 25.1a and 25.1b Anteroposterior (AP) and lateral radiographs of hybrid THA with areas of osteolysis around greater trochanter.

Mode 1: Wear from two articulating surfaces that are intended to rub together, such as the femoral head and the poly.

Mode 2: Wear from an articulating surface and a non-articulating surface, such as the femoral head and the shell.

Mode 3: Third-body wear, which is particles coming between bearings.

Mode 4: Wear between non-articulating surfaces such as the neck and the edge of the shell.

EXAMINER: OK, how about types of wear?

CANDIDATE: There are mechanical and chemical. Mechanical includes abrasive, adhesive, fatigue, third-body and fretting. Chemical includes corrosive and corrosive fretting.

EXAMINER: Do you know how we can measure wear?

CANDIDATE: There are linear and volumetric wear which are two methods of measuring wear. Volumetric wear measures the volume of material lost in cubic millimetres per year or per million cycles. Linear wear measures the penetration of the component into the other and is measured on X-rays. For example, the bigger the femoral head the greater the volumetric wear and the smaller . . .

EXAMINER: Are you sure? Poly has changed over the last 50 years. So, tell me then, what's the ideal size of a femoral head?

CANDIDATE: [I was waiting for him to ask me this question, I had some papers in mind and drawings.]

McKee and Farrar [1] used large heads and had minimal dislocation but significant wear, Charnley [2,3] initially used size 41.5-mm diameter femoral heads but had massive wear and early failure. He then used 22.25-mm femoral heads and reduced his wear, but bearing in mind that polyethylene quality wasn't like the ones we have these days, highly cross-linked poly. There are various factors that increase wear in a THR, they include thickness < 6 mm, malalignment of components, young patients, men and activity levels.

EXAMINER: OK, let's move on, how does osteolysis happen?

CANDIDATE: It's a histiocytic response to wear debris.

EXAMINER: OK, what does that mean?

CANDIDATE: It's a cascade of events that ends with osteoclast activation. It starts when the macrophages are activated by the debris. They release osteolytic factors like TNF-alpha, osteoclast-activating factor and interleukins. This activates osteoclasts and cause osteolysis. Osteolysis causes micromotion of the prosthesis which then causes further debris. Also, as the patient walks they release the debris into the effective joint space causing further inflammatory response and lysis [4].

References

1. McKee GK, Watson-Farrar J. Replacement of arthritic hips by the McKee–Farrar prosthesis. *J Bone Joint Surg Br.* 1966;48:245–259.

2. Charnley J. Surgery of the hip-joint: present and future developments. *Br Med J.* 1960;1:821–826.

3. Charnley J. Arthroplasty of the hip. A new operation. *Lancet.* 1961;1:1129–1132.

4. Ingham E, Fisher J. The role of macrophages in osteolysis of total joint replacement. *Biomaterials.* 2005;26(11):1271–1286.

Structured oral examination question 2

EXAMINER: Tell me about synovial fluid.

CANDIDATE: Synovial fluid is produced by the synovial membrane in the joint. It is a dialysate of blood plasma without the clotting factors, haemoglobin or RBC. It contains hyaluronic acid, lubricin, proteinase, collagenases and prostaglandins. The main function is to lubricate articular cartilage and nourish it through diffusion. It exhibits non-Newtonian flow characteristics.

EXAMINER: Tell me about lubrication.

CANDIDATE: Lubrication is when a film of lower shear strength is present between two bearing surfaces, reducing friction. There are two main hypotheses surrounding joint lubrication in synovial joints.

EXAMINER: What is friction?

CANDIDATE: The resistance of two surfaces to slide against each other.

EXAMINER: Tell me about the two hypotheses surrounding joint lubrication in synovial joints.

CANDIDATE: The first is fluid-film lubrication, in this hypothesis the joint surfaces are separated by a fluid film which fully supports the applied load, preventing contact between the surfaces. The minimum thickness of the fluid film must exceed the surface roughness of the bearing surfaces in order to prevent asperity contact.

The second is boundary lubrication. In this situation, the bearing surfaces are in contact but separated by a boundary lubricant of molecular thickness, which prevents excessive bearing friction and wear. In boundary lubrication the load is carried by the surface asperities rather than by the lubricant.

It is thought that fluid-film lubrication dominates in synovial joints. However, realistically, both fluid-film and boundary lubrication occur in synovial joints, depending on the specific joint in question and the particular type of loading applied.

EXAMINER: Do you know the lambda ratio?

CANDIDATE: This is the ratio of fluid film thickness to surface roughness, in fluid film it's 3 and in boundary it's less than 1.

EXAMINER: Can you tell me about the different types of fluid-film lubrication?

CANDIDATE: There are various types of lubrication, they include hydrodynamic lubrication (HD), elastohydrodynamic (EHD), micro-elastohydrodynamic (MEHD), squeeze film, weeping and boosted lubrication.

In hydrodynamic lubrication there is no contact between the joint surfaces. The surfaces are separated by a thin fluid film which supports the applied load. In simplistic terms, the movement of the joint surfaces in parallel with one another creates a thin, wedge-shaped fluid film between the surfaces which prevents them from contacting one another.

A model that is more likely in synovial joints is elastohydrodynamic (EHD) lubrication. In this model, the cartilage is not considered to be rigid, as it is in the previous model; rather it is elastic and deformable. In EHD lubrication, elastic deformation of the bearing surface enlarges the area of the surface and traps pressurized fluid. This in turn increases the capacity of the fluid film to carry load and decrease stress within the cartilage.

A modification of the elastohydrodynamic model of lubrication is micro-elastohydrodynamic lubrication (MEHD). The micro-elastohydrodynamic lubrication model assumes that the asperities of articular cartilage are deformed under high loads. This smoothes out the bearing surface and allows a fluid film to be created which is sufficient for fluid-film lubrication.

EXAMINER: Tell me about weeping lubrication.

CANDIDATE: Weeping lubrication happens when cartilage is compressed – tears of lubricant fluid are generated from it. Contrary to boosted lubrication where the water is compressed into the cartilage leaving behind a concentrated fluid pooled with hyaluronic acid in the joint.

EXAMINER: What are asperities?

CANDIDATE: These are the projections from the articular surface; the taller they are, the rougher the surface, also increasing friction.

EXAMINER: OK, what types of lubrication happen in prosthetic joints?

CANDIDATE: Well, it is believed that boundary lubrication predominates but mixed conditions do occur. Lubrication occurs through a pseudosynovial fluid that is created over the surfaces.

Different surfaces have different affinity to the lubricant, this is called wettability and can be measured by the angle of contact at the edge of the drop of the lubricant applied to that surface. For example, ceramics are more hydrophilic than metals, thus they have improved lubrication and lower friction (Figure 25.2).

EXAMINER: OK, so what else decreases friction in the joint?

CANDIDATE: The cartilage.

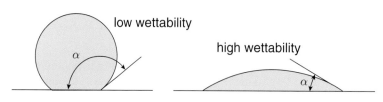

Figure 25.2 Lubrication [I drew this picture at the same time].

EXAMINER: So, tell me about cartilage.

CANDIDATE: Cartilage is a highly differentiated connective tissue made of cells, extracellular matrix (ECM) and water. The cells are chondrocytes and ECM includes fibres, collagen (mainly Type II), elastin, proteoglycans, cartilage oligomeric proteins (COMP) and cartilage matrix protein (CMP).

COMMENT: If you have answered all questions and they have time they might ask you a question to fill the 5-minute time. Cartilage is a very common question and you need to know it by heart. I used the above definition (cells, matrix and water) to answer questions on bone, cartilage, meniscus, ligaments and tendon and just changed the cell component and the ECM (i.e. it is made of water, cells and matrix).

This definition helped me to relax and start building up for that station.

Structured oral examination question 3

Bone

EXAMINER: What makes up bone?

CANDIDATE: Bone is a highly differentiated connective tissue made up of cells (10%) and extracellular matrix 90% (ECM). The cells are: osteoblasts, osteoclasts, osteocytes, bone lining cells. The ECM contains inorganic and organic matrix, the inorganic matrix includes calcium hydroxyapatite and osteocalcium phosphate. The organic matrix includes collagen Type I, proteoglycans, non-collagen matrix proteins (osteocalcin, osteonectin, osteopontin), growth factors and cytokines.

Bone is the primary reservoir of calcium, and also contains the haematopoietic marrow and plays a mechanical role in supporting the body's tissues. It can be divided into woven bone which is immature bone with randomly organized collagen fibres and no lamellae making it weak but flexible. It's found in growing bone and pathological bone.

Lamellar bone is mature bone with organized layers and its structure is arranged according to the stress on the bone. It is found at the periosteal surfaces.

Cortical (compact) bone forms the cortex of long bones. Also in flat bones it comprises 80% of the adult bone.

EXAMINER: Can you draw cortical bone for me (Figure 25.3a)?

EXAMINER: Which cell forms the majority of the bone cells?

CANDIDATE: The osteocyte forms approximately 90% of bone cells, it forms from osteoblasts. It controls the calcium and phosphorus metabolism responding to chemical, mechanical and electrical stimuli.

EXAMINER: Tell me about the osteoclasts.

Figure 25.3a Drawing of cortical bone.

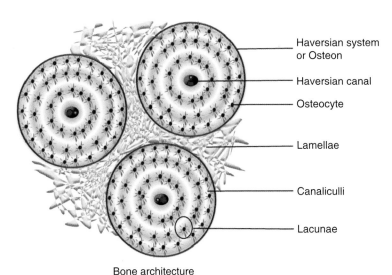

Haversian system or Osteon

Haversian canal

Osteocyte

Lamellae

Canaliculli

Lacunae

Bone architecture

CANDIDATE: Osteoclasts are large multinucleated giant cells; they differentiate from haematopoietic precursors. They resorb bone within pits or depressions known as Howship's lacunae. When laying on bone they have a contact area called ruffled borders which increase their surface area. Bisphosphonates work on the ruffled borders.

COMMENT: I was drawing something like this as I talked (Figure 25.3b).

EXAMINER: How does the blood reach it?

CANDIDATE: Bone receives 5–10% of cardiac output. There are various systems that supply it: nutrient artery system (high-pressure), metaphyseal–epiphyseal system and periosteal system (low-pressure). The nutrient artery enters mid diaphysis and divides into ascending and descending branches supplying the inner two-thirds of the cortex. All three systems are interconnected, and the direction of flow is centrifugal (inside to out).

EXAMINER: How is bone metabolized?

CANDIDATE: A complex interplay and interaction of various hormones, growth factors and cytokines regulate plasma calcium and phosphate levels. They include vitamin D, PTH and calcitonin.

EXAMINER: How does vitamin D regulate calcium?

CANDIDATE: Vitamin D is either taken through diet or activated in the skin by ultraviolet light. Vitamin D enhances the absorption of calcium and phosphorus from the small intestine and enhances osteoclast resorption from bone. In the kidneys it causes increased calcium retention and phosphate excretion (Figure 25.3c).

Structured oral examination question 4

Bone grafts

EXAMINER: So, you have a patient with a tibial plateau fracture on your operating table and you find a big bony defect that needs filling. How do you approach that?

CANDIDATE: Bearing in mind this is a basic science station I went straight for the kill and mentioned bone graft.

EXAMINER: What types of bone grafts do you know?

CANDIDATE: There are autografts, allografts and zenografts. Also, there is demineralized bone matrix (DBM), synthetic, bone morphogenetic protein (BMP) and stem cells.

Autograft utilizes bone obtained from the same patient receiving it. It can be harvested locally or from a distant site like the iliac crest. It has all the good properties of a graft, it is osteoconductive, osteoinductive and osteogenic. It can be cancellous, cortical or vascularized. Cortical provides structural support whereas cancellous is used for its osteogenic properties.

Allografts are obtained from a different patient than the one receiving it. They are taken from cadavers or living donors such as femoral heads. They are available in different methods depending on their processing and preservation, deep frozen –70°C, freeze dried –169°C and fresh. They are not as good as autograft as they have osteoconductive properties only and some osteoinductive properties.

EXAMINER: What would you use for your case?

CANDIDATE: Well it depends on the individual case, but I would prefer to use autograft as it has no immunogenicity, no risks of disease transmission and is cheap, but it has donor site morbidity whereas allografts have no donor site morbidity, but are slow to incorporate . . .

EXAMINER: Ahhh, what's graft incorporation?

CANDIDATE: It is the process by which invasion of the graft by the host cells and the graft is then replaced either partially or completely by host bone or rejected. This happens in stages:

1. Inflammation, stimulated by the necrotic debris.
2. Osteoblast differentiation from precursor cells.
3. Osteoinduction where osteoclasts and blasts are stimulated.
4. Osteoconduction: new bone starts to form.
5. Remodelling, which continues for years.

EXAMINER: So, we know how an autograft is taken, do you know the process of allograft donation and bone banking?

CANDIDATE: Yes, living donors are consented and in case of cadavers as long as there is lack of

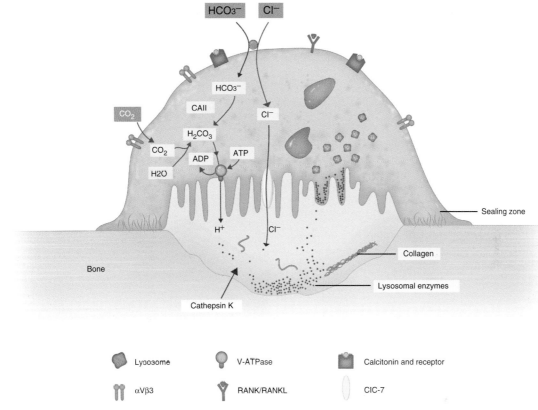

Figure 25.3b Osteoclast.

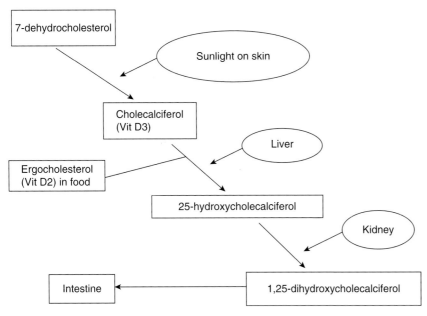

Figure 25.3c Vitamin D metabolism.

objection from next of kin then it can be harvested.

The donors get screened for comorbidities and bloods are taken. They are screened for history of intravenous drug abuse, malignancy TB, steroids. Bloods for hepatitis B & C, HIV, syphilis and Rhesus status.

The graft goes through processing of cleaning then preservation. The graft gets debrided from unwanted tissue, treated with ethanol/antibiotic soaks/irradiation and then preserved either fresh, fresh frozen or freeze-dried.

EXAMINER: OK, quickly tell me about the synthetics and what you are going to use for this tibia?

CANDIDATE: (I realized I have told him all about bone graft but not told him what I will use).

Synthetics are commercially available products. The main constituents are either calcium sulphate, calcium carbonate, calcium triphosphate or hydroxyapatite. I will use calcium phosphate derivative because Russell *et al.* (JBJS Am 2008) performed an RCT of autograft vs. calcium phosphate cement in tibial plateau fractures and showed significantly reduced rates of subsidence, also Buckley published similar results in 2009 in calcaneal fractures.

References

1. Russell TA, Leighton RK. Comparison of autogenous bone graft and endothermic calcium phosphate cement for defect augmentation in tibial plateau fractures. A multicentre, prospective, randomized study. *J Bone Joint Surg Am.* 2008;90(10):2057–2061.

2. Johal HS, Buckley RE, Le IL, Leighton RK. A prospective randomized controlled trial of a bioresorbable calcium phosphate paste (alpha-BSM) in treatment of displaced intra-articular calcaneal fractures. *J Trauma.* 2009;67(4):875–882.

Structured oral examination question 5

THA stem design

EXAMINER: What are these (Figure 25.4a)?

CANDIDATE: The hip replacement on the left is an Exeter hip replacement and the one on the right looks like a Charnley hip replacement.

EXAMINER: OK. What are the differences between the two?

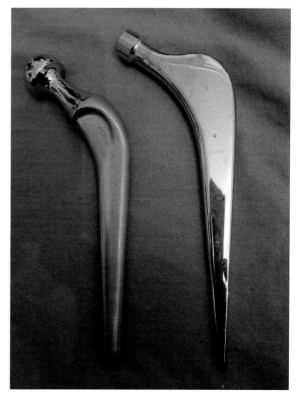

Figure 25.4a Exeter and Charnley femoral stem.

CANDIDATE: The Exeter hip replacement is a collarless, polished double-taper cemented hip replacement. By contrast, the Charnley has a collar to prevent subsidence and is not as smooth.

EXAMINER: By what biomechanical principles are they supposed to work?

CANDIDATE: The Exeter femoral stem works by utilizing a taper slip design and controlled subsidence. It is implanted within a cement mantle and the highly polished nature and the taper allow controlled subsidence of the stem within the cement mantle. The stem will subside on average 1.3 mm in the first 2 years, followed by a period of stability. This subsidence seals off the cement stem interphase, preventing fluid flow leading to loosening. The viscoelastic properties of cement allow for creep to occur. As the stem is loaded the taper engages into the cement, producing radial hoops stress which is distributed to the bone interface minimizing stress shielding. The theory is that it loads all the bone.

By contrast, the Charnley stem works in a composite beam principle, relying on achieving mechanical interlock at the bone–cement interface and sufficient adhesion to achieve force transfer. The load on the femoral head is transmitted through the stem to its tip and then to the cement and bone below it [1].

EXAMINER: What material are they made of?

CANDIDATE: The Exeter stem is made of stainless steel alloy (Orthinox), it has high strength with ductility plus it is resistant to corrosion. The Charnley stem is made of stainless steel alloy as well (Ortron).

EXAMINER: Which one will you use in your practice and why?

CANDIDATE: I will use the Exeter stem based on the theories I mentioned before; also it has excellent survivorship in the NJR and a recent publication by the Exeter team showed the survivorship at 22 years was 99.0% and excellent preservation of bone stock at 20–25 years [2].

EXAMINER: What is cement?

CANDIDATE: Cement is a synthetic polymer of methylmethacrylate (PMMA). PMMA is viscoelastic and the mechanical properties change as a product of time. The important factors that affect cement over time are creep, stress relaxation and fatigue. It is made from mixing a liquid and a powder.

The liquid contains: the monomer, methyl-methacrylate; binding agent, butylmethacrylate; activator, dimethyl-paratoluidine; and a stabilizer, hydroquinone.

The powder contains: the polymer, polymethyl-methacrylate; an initiator, benzyl peroxide; contrast agent and antibiotics.

Cement in a hip replacement acts as a grout. It functions to fill the defect in between the stem and the bone, act for load transfer, allows modulus matching between implant and bone, and in the case of the taper slip stems, allows controlled subsidence of the stem. It is strong in compression and weaker under tension and has a low elastic (Young's) modulus compared to metal and bone.

EXAMINER: Can you draw the relative moduli on a graph and compare it with other materials used in Orthopaedics (Figure 25.4b)? What is 3, what is 2, what is 11?

COMMENT: Figure 25.4b is important as it tests a candidate's ability to appreciate where Young's modulus of bone exists when compared to other implanted materials or connective tissue.

EXAMINER: What are the design principles behind the use of uncemented joint replacements?

CANDIDATE: The uncemented joint replacement can be put in in two ways. The first is a press-fit design, the second is a line-to-line fixation. In the

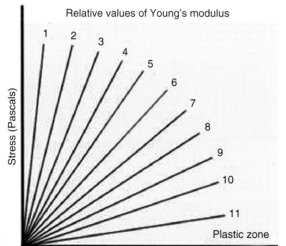

Relative values of Young's modulus

Stress (Pascals)

Strain

Plastic zone

1) Ceramic
2) Cobalt chrome
3) Stainless steel
4) Titanium
5) Cortical bone
6) Polymers
7) PMMA
8) Polyethylene
9) Cancellous bone
10) Tendon/ligament
11) Cartilage

Figure 25.4b Diagram stress/strain curve and Young's modulus.

press fit, the femoral canal is prepared to match the orientation of the eventual stem, but the broach is slightly smaller than the stem. When the stem is inserted it is therefore a tight fit. As it is inserted, the viscoelasticity of the bone allows the slightly larger stem to be inserted and then the stem is gripped by the bone. Theoretically, no additional fixation is required.

In line-to-line fixation, the bone is prepared to be the same size as the eventual implant, e.g. an uncemented cup. A cup the same size as the prepared acetabulum is inserted but, in this case, additional fixation, such as screws, is frequently required.

EXAMINER: What can you tell me about the surface finish of the implant?

CANDIDATE: The surface finish allows either bony ingrowth or ongrowth. Ingrowth surfaces include sintered beads, fibre mesh and porous metals. Ongrowth surfaces are created by grit blasting or plasma spraying. Ingrowth requires a pore size between 50 and 400 μm, and the percentage of voids within the coating should be between 30% and 40% to maintain mechanical strength. Most modern cementless implants rely on bone ongrowth of a plasma-sprayed surface or are a hybrid of ingrowth and ongrowth.

EXAMINER: Do you know anything about the design of the pores?

CANDIDATE: The porosity of the stem should not be greater than 50% otherwise there is the possibility of the pores shearing off.

EXAMINER: How do stems fail?

CANDIDATE: The cemented stems fail in four modes:

1a. Pistoning: stem in cement.
1b. Pistoning: stem in bone.
2. Medial stem pivot.
3. Calcar pivot.
4. Cantilever bending.

EXAMINER: Do you know any name associated with this classification?

CANDIDATE: Sorry.

COMMENT: Gruen's mode of cemented femoral stem failure.

Reference

Gruen TA, McNeice GM, Amstutz HC. 'Modes of failure' of cemented stem-type femoral components: a radiographic analysis of loosening. *Clin Orthop.* 1979;141:17–27.

EXAMINER: And the uncemented stems?

CANDIDATE: Delamination of the HA coating, there is also a mechanism known as flag-staffing. If a relatively small stem is inserted in a patient with strong cortical bone which is stiffer than the implant, then a microenvironment is created allowing for excess stress through the implant, resulting in loosening.

References

1. Shen G. Femoral stem fixation. An engineering interpretation of the long-term outcome of Charnley and Exeter stems. *J Bone Joint Surg Br.* 1998;80(5):754–756.

2. Petheram TG, Whitehouse SL, Kazi HA, *et al.* The Exeter Universal cemented femoral stem at 20 to 25 years: a report of 382 hips. *Bone Joint J.* 2016;98B(11):1441–1449.

Structured oral examination question 6

Articular cartilage

EXAMINER: What do you see (Figure 25.5)?

CANDIDATE: This is a picture of a knee arthroscopy showing a grade IV cartilage defect.

EXAMINER: What is cartilage?

CANDIDATE: Cartilage is a highly differentiated connective tissue made of cells, extracellular matrix (ECM) and water. The cells are chondrocytes, and the ECM includes fibres, collagen (mainly Type II), elastin, proteoglycans, cartilage oligomeric proteins (COMP) and cartilage matrix protein (CMP).

There are three types of cartilage: hyaline cartilage, fibrocartilage and elastic cartilage.

EXAMINER: Draw a cross-section of cartilage.

CANDIDATE: I drew all layers, superficial, middle and deep, arcades of Benninghoff, the tidemark and calcific zone. The examiner was waiting for me to draw the tidemark.

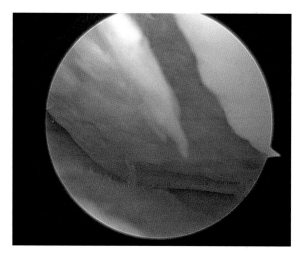

Figure 25.5 Knee arthroscopy picture focal area of cartilage loss.

COMMENT: This is the standard cartilage picture present in the usual textbooks.

EXAMINER: What is the importance of the tidemark?

CANDIDATE: The tidemark is the boundary between the calcified and uncalcified cartilage made visible by histological staining. Clinical importance is that above the tidemark it's avascular and nutrition depends on diffusion, and below it it's vascular.

EXAMINER: What is the importance of water in cartilage?

CANDIDATE: 70% of articular cartilage is water; 30% of it exists between the collagen fibres and this is determined by the negative charge of the proteoglycans (PG) which lie within the collagen matrix. Because the PG are bound closely the closeness of the negative charges creates a repulsion force that must be neutralized by positive ions (hydrogen ions in water) in the surrounding fluid. The amount of water present depends on the amount of PG and the stiffness and strength of the collagen network. The PG aggregates are basically responsible for the turgid nature of the cartilage and in articular cartilage they provide osmotic properties needed to resist compressive loads.

EXAMINER: What happens in osteoarthritis?

CANDIDATE: The collagen network is disrupted either by trauma or an increase in degradation enzymes concentration – this allows the

Table 25.1 Differences between changes in articular cartilage with osteoarthritis and ageing.

	Ageing	Osteoarthritis
Water content	Decreases	Increases then decreases
Synthetic activity	Decreases	Increases
Collagen	Unchanged	Breakdown of cartilage collagen network
PG content	Decreases	Decreases
PG synthesis	Decreases	Increases
PG degradation	Decreases	Increases
Keratan sulphate	Increases	Decreases
Chondrotin sulphate	Decreases	Increases
Hydroxyapatite	Increases	Decreases
Chondrocyte size	Increases	
Chondrocyte number	Decreases	
Modulus of elasticity	Increases	Decreases

proteoglycans to attract more water and softens the articular cartilage, thus reducing its Young's modulus of elasticity and its ability to bear load.

COMMENT: At this stage you will have to draw the table showing the difference between ageing and OA (Table 25.1).

EXAMINER: OK, so how will you treat this defect? [Going back to the arthroscopy picture.]

CANDIDATE: This is grade IV on the Outerbridge Arthroscopic Grading System. Using the hook as a reference, it measures 1.5 cm × 1 cm; as it is below 4 cm^2 then I will treat this with microfracture.

EXAMINER: How would you do that?

CANDIDATE: The goal is to allow access of marrow elements into the defect to stimulate the formation of fibrocartilage.

I would prepare the defect until I achieved stable vertical walls and the calcified cartilage layer was removed. Then using a bone awl, I would make multiple perforations through the subchondral bone 3–4 mm apart, looking for the fat droplets to confirm that I have penetrated far enough. Postoperatively patients are allowed protected weight-bearing with full range of movement of the knee.

607

If that defect was larger than 4 cm^2 then I may consider osteochondral autograft or mosaicplasty; however, I will refer this patient to a knee surgeon expert in this field. I'm also aware of other methods such as autologous chondrocyte implantation (ACI) and matrix-associated autologous chondrocyte implantation (MACI).

EXAMINER: Would you do an ACI?

CANDIDATE: Well, NICE does recommend it, but it has strict criteria and it has to be done at a tertiary centre expert in this field so no I wouldn't, I will refer it on.
www.nice.org.uk/guidance/ta477/chapter/3-Committee-discussion#conclusion

Structured oral examination question 7

Fracture fixation

EXAMINER: Tell me about your approach to the fixation of this fracture (Figure 25.6a).

CANDIDATE: First, I would assess the patient, the soft tissue and then consider the fracture. I would start with ATLS ...

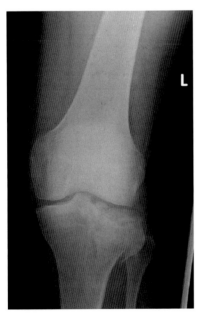

Figure 25.6a Anteroposterior (AP) radiograph of the left knee demonstrating tibial plateau fracture.

EXAMINER: Yes, yes, there are no tricks in this question, everything is fine with the patient, this is a question about the biomechanics of fracture fixation.

CANDIDATE: Right, OK, this is a plain radiograph of a comminuted displaced, intra-articular fracture of the tibial plateau. The principles regarding the fixation of this fracture are anatomical reduction and absolute stability of the articular block and then the restoration of length, axis and rotation of the lower limb by attaching the articular block onto the shaft of the tibia by utilizing a bridging plate and relative stability.

EXAMINER: Tell me about how you would achieve a stable fixation of the articular surface.

CANDIDATE: I would open the joint and reduce the articular fragments under direct vision. I would apply a periarticular clamp to hold the fragments reduced and to compress the fragments. If necessary, I would use K-wires as a temporary fixation device. I would then use 6.5-mm partially threaded cancellous screws to act as both a subchondral raft and also to compress the fracture fragments and achieve absolute stability and primary bone healing.

EXAMINER: Why do you want to achieve absolute stability?

CANDIDATE: As it is an intra-articular fracture, the healing of the bone should be by primary bone healing without the formation of callus. In order for this to happen there has to be no movement at the fracture site. The lack of movement means that the osteoclasts involved in the remodelling of bone will essentially ignore the fracture site and proceed directly across the fracture site using cutting cones, therefore healing by primary bone healing without the formation of callus.

EXAMINER: How does a screw work?

CANDIDATE: A screw converts rotational movement into longitudinal advancement. With a lag screw, the screw is partially threaded therefore as the distal threads bite in the fracture fragment, the proximal smooth barrel can slide over the proximal fragment and so as it is tightened the distal fragment is pulled towards the proximal and compression of the distal piece against the proximal cortex occurs.

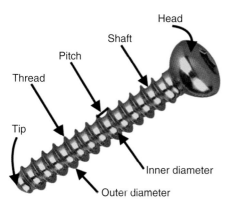

Figure 25.6b Design features of orthopaedic screw.

EXAMINER: What are the parts of the screw?

COMMENT: It is easy to draw and illustrate (Figure 25.6b).

EXAMINER: You said you will use a cancellous screw. What is the main difference between a cancellous and a cortical screw?

CANDIDATE: Pitch, core to outer diameter and tip.
Pitch: closely spaced threads in cortical screws with smaller pitch compared with deeply cut and widely spaced threads in cancellous screws.
Core to outer diameter: cancellous screws have deeper threads, making them better at pull-out strength.
Tip: cortical screws are blunt.

EXAMINER: You mentioned you will use your plate in bridging mode, what other modes do you know?

CANDIDATE: Buttress, bridging, compression, tension band, neutralization.

EXAMINER: So why would you use this one in bridging mode?

CANDIDATE: There is a large amount of comminution in the metaphysis; therefore, it is impossible to compress the fracture fragments. If the other features of length, axis and rotation are correct then the fracture would be expected to heal by secondary bone healing with callus formation.

EXAMINER: What do you understand by Perren's strain theory?

CANDIDATE: Strain is defined as change in length over original length. The theory suggests that the mechanical environment (strain) governs the type of tissue that is laid down between the fracture fragments. Granulation tissue can tolerate 100% strain, fibrous tissue is formed when there is up to 17% strain, fibrocartilage 2–10% and lamellar bone at 2%. As the strain decreased at the fracture site a stiffer tissue is produced.

EXAMINER: Describe the stages of fracture healing.

CANDIDATE: The stages are haematoma and inflammation, soft callus (1 week to months), hard callus (1–4 months) and then remodelling (years). In the first stage, haematoma forms and provides key cells such as macrophages, key inflammatory cytokines (IL1, IL6, TGF-β) are secreted and eventually haematoma is replaced with granulation tissue.
Next phase: soft callus starts to form, providing a bridging role and depending on the mechanical environment, as we mentioned before, osteoblastic differentiation or chondroblastic differentiation happens. Soft callus is converted to woven bone (hard callus) via the process of endochondral ossification. With progression of this process collagen will change from II to I.
Once the fracture has united the final phase of remodelling happens where hard callus is remodelled from woven bone to hard, dense, lamellar bone by the process of osteoclastic resorption followed by osteoblastic bone formation.

EXAMINER: What factors influence fracture healing?

CANDIDATE: Two key factors are involved, mechanical environment and biology. I explained the mechanical environment earlier. The biology is affected by systemic and local factors. Systemic such as smoking, diabetes, age and nutrition. Local factors such as open or closed injury, high mechanism, bone loss, site and type of bone.

Structured oral examination question 8

Osteoporosis

EXAMINER: Could you define osteoporosis for me please?

CANDIDATE: In 1993 WHO defined osteoporosis as a systemic skeletal disease characterized by low bone mass and deterioration in the microarchitecture,

609

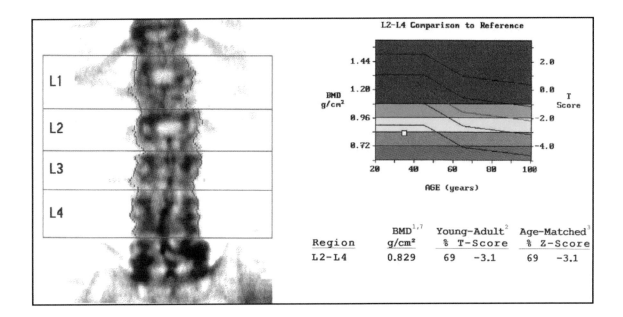

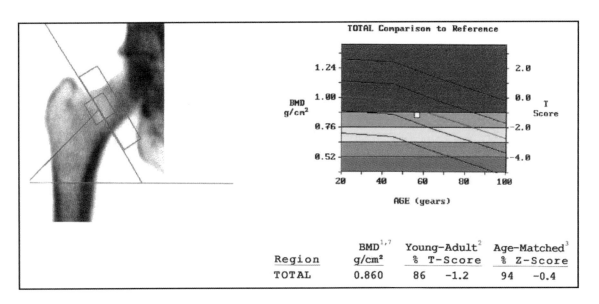

Figure 25.7 DEXA scan report for proximal femur and lumbar spine.

leading to enhanced bone fragility and a consequent increase in fracture risk.

In practice, it is defined on the bases of bone density assessed by a DEXA scan T score. It is considered normal when the bone mineral density is within 1 standard deviation of the mean peak bone mass of a healthy 25-year-old. Osteopenia when it is 1–2.5 below the mean and osteoporosis when it is > 2.5 below the mean.

Osteoporosis can be classified into primary type 1, primary type 2 or secondary.

Type 1 is most common in women after menopause.

Type 2 is senile osteoporosis and occurs after the age of 75 and is seen in both sexes.

Secondary may arise at any age; it's equal in women and men and is a result of a chronic predisposing medical problem or disease, like prolonged steroid use.

EXAMINER: How does a DEXA scan work?

CANDIDATE: DEXA scan is dual-energy X-ray absorptiometry used to assess bone mineral density (BMD). It involves the use of two X-ray beams of different energies passed through the neck of femur or lumbar spine (L2–L4). It provides a value in g/cm^2.

The femoral neck is the preferred site because of its higher predictive value for fracture risk: Kanis and Gluer 2000 [1], Kanis et al. 2008, level 1a Evidence [2].

The result is then compared to a sex- and race-matched BMD of a healthy young adult population (25–30) producing a T score. The Z score refers to the BMD in relation to an age-matched population.

EXAMINER: This is a DEXA scan report (Figure 25.7), how would you interpret it?

COMMENT: You are expected to know how to interpret a DEXA scan report. So, you need to familiarize yourself with one. It will be either of a hip or lumber spine or both. Simplifying it, I just concentrated on the T score and explained that the risk of fracture approximately doubles for each standard deviation decrease in T score. It depends on what the score is, you then can define it as normal/osteopenia or osteoporosis. In my station it was a patient with osteoporosis.

CANDIDATE: Four important numbers to look at in the report:

1. The percentage of normal bone density for the patient's age.
2. The percentage of bone density compared with normal young adults.
3. Z score.
4. T score.

EXAMINER: How would you manage this patient?

CANDIDATE: Prior to obtaining the DEXA scan I would have performed an initial work up which includes detailed history, examination and bloods. In the history I will be looking for risk factors including age, sex, hormonal problems, chronic illness, family history of hip fractures, medication, lifestyle risk such as smoking, alcohol and diet.

I would also use the FRAX tool which computes the 10-year probability of hip fracture or a major osteoporotic fracture.

Treatment will be according to the NOGG [3] and NICE guidelines [4], dividing it into lifestyle changes and pharmacological treatment.

If the patient is at risk or has confirmed OP, then I would provide them with information regarding lifestyle changes. Lifestyle measures to improve bone health include increasing the level of physical activity, stopping smoking, reducing alcohol intake to ≤ 2 units/day, reducing the risk of falls and ensuring adequate dietary calcium intake and vitamin D status.

(www.shef.ac.uk/FRAX)

EXAMINER: How much calcium and Vit D do you give them?

CANDIDATE: In postmenopausal women and older men (> 50 years) at increased risk of fracture a daily dose of 800 IU cholecalciferol should be advised.

In postmenopausal women and older men receiving bone-protective therapy for osteoporosis, calcium supplementation should be given if the dietary intake is below 700 mg/day, and vitamin D supplementation considered in those at risk of or with evidence of vitamin D insufficiency.

EXAMINER: Which pharmacological treatment would you choose?

CANDIDATE: Alendronate 70 mg once-weekly or Risedronate are first-line treatments in the majority of cases. Treatment review should be performed after 3 years of zoledronic acid therapy and 5 years of oral bisphosphonate treatment.

EXAMINER: How do bisphosphonates work?

CANDIDATE: They can be divided into nitrogen-containing (Alendronate) and nitrogen-lacking (Etidronate). They all share the common P-C-P backbone which makes them resistant to metabolism. The nitrogen group inhibits protein prenylation with an end result of loss of guanosine triphosphatase (GTPase) formation, this is needed for ruffled border formation and cell survival. The nitrogen-lacking bisphosphonates are metabolized into a non-functional adenosine triphosphate (ATP) analogue, which induces cell apoptosis.

611

References

1. Kanis JA, Gluer CC. An update on the diagnosis and assessment of osteoporosis with densitometry. Committee of Scientific Advisors, International Osteoporosis Foundation. *Osteoporos Int.* 2000;11:192–202.

2. Kanis JA, McCloskey EV, Johansson H, Oden A, Melton LJ, 3rd, Khaltaev N. A reference standard for the description of osteoporosis. *Bone.* 2008;42:467–447.

3. National Osteoporosis Guideline Group (NOGG). 2017.

4. NICE guidelines:

Compston J, Cooper A, Cooper C, *et al.* Guidelines for the diagnosis and management of osteoporosis in postmenopausal women and men from the age of 50 years in the UK. *Maturitas.* 2009;62:105–108.

Compston J, Bowring C, Cooper A, *et al.* Diagnosis and management of osteoporosis in postmenopausal women and older men in the UK: National Osteoporosis Guideline Group (NOGG) update 2013. *Maturitas.* 2013;75:392–396.

Structured oral examination question 9

Antibiotic prophylaxis

EXAMINER: Which antibiotic do you use for infection prophylaxis in arthroplasty?

CANDIDATE: Our hospital policy recommends cefuroxime 1.5 g at induction provided that the patient is not allergic to penicillin. Alternatively, teicoplanin and gentamycin.

EXAMINER: How does cefuroxime work?

CANDIDATE: Cefuroxime is a beta lactam antibiotic; it inhibits the cross-linking of polysaccharides in the cell wall by blocking the transpeptidase enzyme. Penicillins also work in a similar action.

EXAMINER: Could you tell me about other antibiotics you know and their mechanism of action?

CANDIDATE: In general, I divide the antibiotics by their mechanism of action to antibiotics working on cell wall synthesis, protein synthesis (50S subunit and 30S subunit), nucleic acid synthesis (Figure 25.8).

EXAMINER: How do the bacteria develop resistance?

CANDIDATE: Bacteria can develop resistance either by intrinsic resistance or by acquired resistance to antibiotics. Bacteria can develop the ability to hydrolyze the antibiotic using beta lactamase, or through genetic mutations, like MRSA. Other bacteria can alter the cell wall permeability or create a biofilm barrier.

EXAMINER: How does MRSA develop resistance?

CANDIDATE: MRSA develops resistance through a gene called *mecA*, it produces the enzyme penicillin-binding protein 2a (PBP2a). This enzyme prevents the normal enzymatic acylation of antibiotics.

EAMINER: What is your local trust policy regarding screening and eradication of MRSA?

CANDIDATE: We have a routine preoperative screening involving nasal, groin and axilla swabs for *Staphylococcus aureus*; 20% of patients are staph carriers and 5% are MRSA carriers. Patients must have three negative samples before considering joint arthroplasty.

Carriers are treated with nasal mucopirocin and 4% chlorhexedine bath for 5 days, re-swabbed and repeat if still positive.

EXAMINER: How do you prevent infections in your department?

CANDIDATE: There are various steps performed to prevent infection in our department, I divide them into preoperative, perioperative and postoperative measures.

Preoperative: screening for MRSA, ulcers and UTI. Admission on day of surgery to ring-fenced wards. Optimization of comorbidities, especially diabetes.

Perioperative: laminar flow theatres, minimize theatre traffic, prophylactic IV antibiotics within 1 hour of incision, antibiotic-loaded cement, shaving at time of surgery, good hand-washing technique, draping with disposable drapes and ioband, opening of sets within the laminar flow, efficient surgery, good haemostasis and sound wound closure and avoid hypothermia throughout the procedure.

Postoperative: minimize dressing changes, encourage a culture of infection control, for example using alcohol gel and bare below elbows. Minimize unnecessary transfusions, postoperative antibiotics; however, this is debatable depending on departmental policies, early mobilization and physiotherapy, optimal medical management, timely but safe discharge.

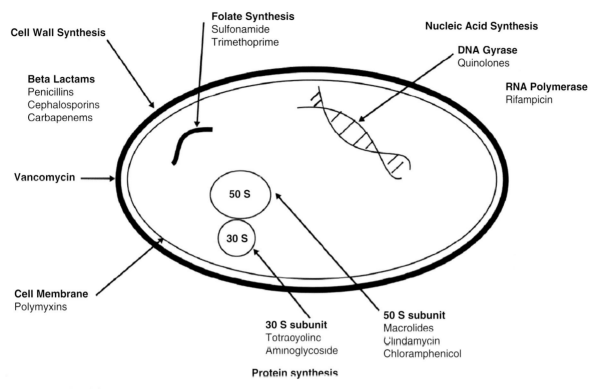

Cell Wall Synthesis

Beta Lactams
Penicillins
Cephalosporins
Carbapenems

Folate Synthesis
Sulfonamide
Trimethoprime

Nucleic Acid Synthesis

DNA Gyrase
Quinolones

RNA Polymerase
Rifampicin

Vancomycin

50 S

30 S

Cell Membrane
Polymyxins

30 S subunit
Totraoyolinc
Aminoglycoside

50 S subunit
Macrolides
Clindamycin
Chloramphenicol

Protein synthesis

Figure 25.8 Simple bacterium (I drew a simple bacterium which is available in most books).

Structured oral examination question 10

Theatre suite

EXAMINER: How would you design a theatre suite?

CANDIDATE: When designing a theatre suite, the first important aspect is theatre location, it needs to be close to related facilities such as ITU, A&E, Surgical wards, and Radiology.

The internal structure is usually thought of in terms of four zones that are intimately linked:

Outer zone: reception (and rest of hospital).

Clean zone: reception to theatre doors.

Aseptic zone: theatre itself.

Disposal zone: sluices (Figure 25.9).

These zones will be connected with corridors that should not cross-contaminate each other.

The design of the theatre itself should be based around the table, with careful attention to lighting, temperature, humidity and ventilation.

Lights should be satellite with 40,000 lux at the wound site.

Temperature and humidity is controlled via thermostats and the ventilation system. Optimum temperature for the patient is 25°C and for the staff is 19°C. We aim to create a microclimate for the patient to prevent hypothermia by using Bair huggers, warmed mattress and fluids . . .

EXAMINER: Which ventilation system is used in your department?

CANDIDATE: We have theatres with a laminar flow ventilation system for elective arthroplasty cases and a plenum type for all other cases.

EXAMINER: What is laminar flow?

CANDIDATE: It is a system that produces an entire body of air flowing in one direction with uniform velocity and along parallel flow lines. Flow rate is 0.3 m/s.

There are three types of air flow: horizontal, vertical and ex-flow.

EXAMINER: Tell me about the ex-flow Howarth system

CANDIDATE: [I had no idea, the only thing I could remember was a trumpet type of air flow.

613

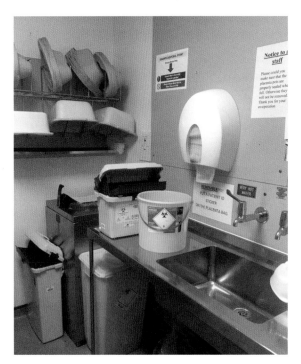

Figure 25.9 Disposal zone. Four zones: outer zone, clean zone, aseptic zone and disposal zone. The purpose of having zones is to have defined boundaries.

I rescued myself by saying I'm more familiar with the vertical laminar flow]

EXAMINER: OK, tell me about the vertical laminar flow.

CANDIDATE: Vertical laminar flow was introduced by Charnley and is the most common type used. It creates a room within a room, with panels from the ceiling to 2 m from the floor. Air flows through a HEPA filter in the ceiling and directed towards the operative field. HEPA stands for high-efficiency particulate air filters. It filters particles of 0.5 μm with 99.9% efficiency.

EXAMINER: Does it filter viruses?

CANDIDATE: Umm, no.

EXAMINER: What are the advantages and disadvantages of horizontal vs. vertical laminar flow?

CANDIDATE: Horizontal is easier to install, but positioning of staff and equipment is restricted because of the sideways flow of air.

Vertical laminar flow does not restrict staff and equipment as long as they are within the marked areas; however, if they stand within the periphery of the laminar flow area they may deflect contaminated air towards the wound.

EXAMINER: What are the sources of infection theatres?

CANDIDATE: Patient, surgeon, instruments and airborne. We shed microorganisms, also when we talk . . .

EXAMINER: How do you measure bacterial contamination in the air?

CANDIDATE: By slit samplers called Casella, it draws in air over 1 minute which passes over culture plates, which are then incubated over 48 hours and colonies formed are counted. It is measured in laminar flow theatre by colony forming units per cubic metre (CFU m^3). Acceptable CFU values for a laminar flow theatre are < 20 CFU in periphery and < 10 in the centre.

EXAMINER: Do you think laminar flow prevents joint infection?

CANDIDATE: I believe it is a combination of multiple factors. Results of the MRC trial in 1982 (Lidwell *et al.*) published in BMJ showed that deep sepsis in arthroplasty was reduced significantly by the use of antibiotic-loaded cement, prophylactic IV antibiotics perioperatively, laminar flow and body exhaust suits [1].

Charnley also showed a reduction in deep infection with the use of vertical laminar flow in combination with other techniques [2]. On the other hand, a review of the New Zealand joint registry questioned the use of laminar flow and space suites as it showed that the rate of revision for early deep infection was not reduced by using laminar flow and space suits [3].

References

1. Lidwell OM, Lowbury EJ, Whyte W, Blowers R, Stanley SJ, Lowe D. Effect of ultra clean air in operating rooms on deep sepsis in the joint after total hip or knee replacement: a randomised study. *Br Med J.* 1982;285:10–14.

2. Charnley J. Postoperative infection after total hip replacement with special reference to air contamination in the operating room. *Clin Orthop Rel Res.* 1972;87:167–187.

3. Hooper GJ, Rothwell AG, Frampton C, Wyatt MC. Does the use of laminar flow and space suits reduce early deep infection after total hip and knee replacement? The ten-year results of the New Zealand Joint Registry. *J Bone Joint Surg Br.* 2011;93(1):85–90.

Structured oral examination question 11

VTE

EXAMINER: How do you set up a VTE protocol in your department?

CANDIDATE: I would set up a protocol to assess all elective and trauma patients. I would have two pathways, one for elective patients and one for trauma.

    The elective patient's pathway starts when listed in clinic identifying correctable risks that can be addressed preoperatively. Risk assessment will be performed using a published tool or guidelines such as the NICE guidelines to balance their risks of VTE against bleeding. They will be stratified into a low-risk group or a high-risk group.

The low-risk group will be offered mechanical prophylaxis only and the high-risk group will be offered both mechanical and pharmacological prophylaxis suitable for them. During their stay they will have a continuous reassessment protocol at senior review or if their clinical condition changes.

EXAMINER: What are the current guidelines for elective hip replacement?

CANDIDATE: The guidelines will be changing in 2018 and aspirin will be considered; however, the current guidelines suggest starting mechanical prophylaxis at admission, either anti-embolism stocking or intermittent pneumatic compression devices. This should continue until the patient no longer has significant reduced mobility or for 4 weeks. Provided there are no contraindications for pharmacological prophylaxis, prophylaxis should start after surgery with either LMWH or Rivaroxiban. Continue prophylaxis for 28–35 days.

EXAMINER: What are the guidelines for total knee replacement and how do they differ from total hip replacements?

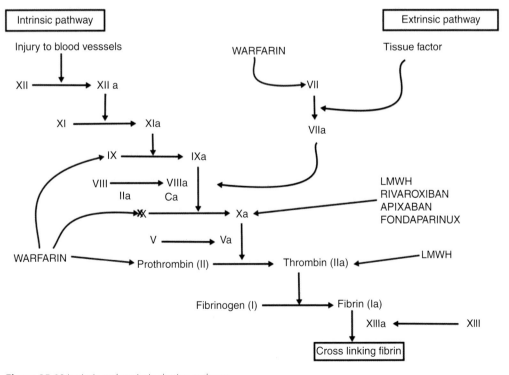

Figure 25.10 Intrinsic and extrinsic clotting pathway.

CANDIDATE: It is the same protocol, but the duration is shorter 10–14 days.

EXAMINER: OK, what is the new guideline that is coming up?

CANDIDATE: For elective hip replacement. In the new guidelines it is recommended to offer VTE prophylaxis to people undergoing elective hip replacement surgery. Choose any one of:
- LMWH (for 10 days) followed by aspirin (for 28 days).
- LMWH (for 28 days) combined with anti-embolism stockings (until discharge).
- Rivaroxaban.

    Consider anti-embolism stockings until discharge from hospital if pharmacological interventions are contraindicated in people undergoing elective hip replacement surgery.

EXAMINER: And for knees?

CANDIDATE: Offer VTE prophylaxis to people undergoing elective knee replacement surgery. Choose any one of:
- Aspirin (for 14 days).
- LMWH (for 14 days) combined with anti-embolism stockings (until discharge).
- Rivaroxaban.

    Consider intermittent pneumatic compression if pharmacological prophylaxis is contraindicated in people undergoing elective knee replacement surgery. Continue until the person is mobile.

EXAMINER: Is there a role for chemical prophylaxis in patient's lower limb immobilization?

CANDIDATE: The new guidelines suggest considering pharmacological VTE prophylaxis for people undergoing foot or ankle surgery, in particular:
- Those requiring immobilization (for example, arthrodesis or arthroplasty).
- When total anaesthesia time is greater than 1 hour.
- When the patient's risk of VTE outweighs their risk of bleeding.

EXAMINER: What is the mechanism of action of LMWH, aspirin and Rivaroxaban?

CANDIDATE: Aspirin is a cyclo-oxygenase (Cox) inhibitor. It inhibits prostaglandin production, preventing platelet aggregation. It also prevents formation of theromboxane A2, which is a prothrombotic agent secreted by platelets.

LMWH: forms a complex with antithrombin 3, but this complex selectively inhibits factor 10a only.

RIVAROXIBAN: direct action on factor 10a.

COMMENT: If you have time, you can draw the intrinsic and extrinsic pathways and explain where each drug works (Figure 25.10).

Chapter 26

Biomechanics

Nick Caplan and Paul A. Banaszkiewicz

Introduction

The stress–strain curve is a triple A-list subject. It always seems to be asked in viva examinations and is a definite top 10 core basic science question. In recent years this topic has been reinvented as it was becoming too predictable. We make no apologies for including the question in all of its various guises.

Structured oral examination question 1

Stress–strain curve

EXAMINER: Can you draw the stress–strain curve for stainless steel?

COMMENT: Drawing is a vital component of the FRCS (Tr & Orth) Exam. A candidate is expected to illustrate to examiners what they are describing to aid discussion and inform techniques. Drawing also helps a candidate deal with the competency-level questions efficiently and accurately, gaining extra time to deal with the higher-order thinking questions, leading to higher scores.

CANDIDATE: The stress–strain curve demonstrates how a material subjected to an increasing tensile load deforms until failure (Figure 26.1).

- Stress is force over area and has units of Newton per square metre.
- Strain is change in length over original length; it has no units. It is usually expressed as a ratio or percentage.

COMMENT: Get this in about strain having no units first. Don't wait to be asked 'what are the units of stress?' by the examiners. Most candidates know it's a fairly blunt question.[1]

EXAMINER: How does force change the cross-sectional dimensions of the area it is acting on?

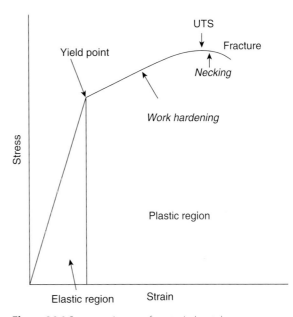

Figure 26.1 Stress–strain curve for a typical metal.

CANDIDATE: An object under stress experiences strain in the transverse direction as well as the horizontal direction.

Transverse strain is usually opposite to longitudinal strain, i.e. as an object gets longer, it gets thinner. As such, force can change the size of the cross-section it is acting upon. However, stress and strain are generally based on the original dimensions of the object.

COMMENT: An initial, slightly off-the-wall question can derail a nervous candidate before they have time to settle and has to be handled with skill. These less-obvious basic science questions are an attempt to move away from conventional book knowledge and force a candidate to apply first principles to problem-solving.

CANDIDATE: The initial section corresponds to elastic deformation. Strain is directly proportional to stress. This is known as Hooke's law.

EXAMINER: What happens to the molecular bonds when in this region of the graph?

CANDIDATE: The molecular bonds are stretched but not broken.

The gradient, i.e. steepness, of the straight line correlates to the material's resistance to deformation. This is called Young's modulus of elasticity.

The higher the Young's modulus of elasticity, the smaller the deformation produced for a given load.

This here is the yield point, which is the maximum stress up to which a material undergoes elastic deformation. The yield point is the point on the stress strain curve that indicates the limit of elastic behaviour and the beginning of plastic deformation.

The non-linear section of the stress–strain curve corresponds to plastic deformation. The deformation is permanent and if the stress is removed, strain is not completely recovered and the material does not return to its original state.

EXAMINER: What happens to the bonds?

CANDIDATE: Molecular bonds are broken, and the molecules move too far apart to return to their original positions.

The ultimate tensile strength is the maximum stress that the material can sustain before fracture.

The fracture point is where the material eventually fails.

Stress at the fracture point can be slightly less than the ultimate tensile strength because the latter can cause the material to neck, which reduces its cross-sectional area and therefore the force required to fracture.

The area under the stress–strain curve represents the energy absorbed per unit volume of the material. It therefore indicates the energy absorbed by the material to failure. This is called toughness. A tough material takes a lot of energy to break it.

Comparing two forces acting on two surfaces can be misleading because this does not take into account the size of the cross-section. Stress indicates the intensity of force acting on a section. As such, it is a fairer comparison of loads acting on different surfaces.

EXAMINER: You seem to be changing around and mixing up stiffness and strength. What exactly do you mean by these terms?

CANDIDATE: Stiffness is stress–strain while strength is the load required to break a material and depends on plastic deformation.

COMMENT: Imprecise answer.

Stiffness and strength are terms often used interchangeably, but they are distinct mechanical properties.

Stiffness is defined as the slope of a force versus displacement graph.

Strength is an imprecise term and represents the degree of resistance to deformation of a material. A material is strong if it has a high ultimate tensile strength.

EXAMINER: Are you sure?

CANDIDATE: The steeper a stress–strain curve, the stiffer the material. The less steep the curve, the more flexible the material.

COMMENT: The slope of the stress–strain curve is the elastic (Young's) modulus of the material.

Mechanical testing measures force on a construct that could consist of bone, ligament and possibly fixation device (plate) and the data obtained relates to properties of the construct as a whole. This is what engineers test in real life. Force and displacement are normalized for an individual material into stress and strain.

Force and displacement data will vary if the specimen dimension changes, even if it is from the same material. That is why we normalize force with its cross-section and displacement with its gauge length to arrive at stress and strain.

Try to understand rather than rote learn your biomechanical definitions otherwise with imprecise terminology you can get drawn into semantics and end up losing marks.

EXAMINER: What is the difference between hardness and toughness?

CANDIDATE: Hardness describes a material's resistance to localized surface plastic deformation, e.g. scratch or dent. Hardness is not a basic mechanical property, but instead derived from a combination of other material properties, e.g. stiffness and strength. Hardness determines the wear resistance of a material. Under the same loading conditions, a harder material has a greater wear resistance than a softer material.

Toughness is a material's ability to absorb energy up to a fracture. Toughness is derived from both strength and ductility of a material.

EXAMINER: So why is hardness important?

CANDIDATE: It has great relevance when considering bearing surfaces and wear with implants.

COMMENT: Basic science applied to clinical relevance.

Structured oral examination question 2

Stress–strain curve

EXAMINER: Stress–strain curve – label all the points, axis and nomenclature and describe what the areas underneath signify.
What is hardness?

CANDIDATE: The x-axis represents strain, which is change in length over original length. It has no units.

The y-axis is stress, which is force per unit area applied and has the units Newton per square metre (N/m^2).

The area under the stress–strain curve up to the elastic limit depicts the modulus of resilience (MR), which signifies the ability of material to store or absorb energy without permanent deformation.

The whole area under the complete stress–strain curve represents the energy absorbed by the material to failure. This is known as the modulus of toughness, which shows the ability of a material to absorb energy up to fracture.

The Young's modulus can be determined from the gradient of the line in the elastic portion of the stress–strain graph.

Hardness is a surface property of a material. It is the ability of a material to resist scratching and indentation on its surface. It has no association with the stress–strain curve.

EXAMINER: How does the Young's modulus differ for isotropic and anisotropic materials?

COMMENT: Differentiating between isotropic and anisotropic materials is factual and rote-learned. The examiner has linked mechanical properties to Young's modulus of elasticity to test whether a candidate is able to demonstrate a more advanced level of understanding.

CANDIDATE: An isotropic material behaves identically, irrespective of the direction of applied force. Examples include most orthopaedic metals, polymers and woven bone. The Young's modulus of elasticity will be constant in all directions the force is applied to the material. With an anisotropic material the Young's modulus varies depending on the direction of loading. Examples include cortical bone, ligaments.

We have the yield point here, which is the start of plastic deformation, and the ultimate stress, which is the maximum stress the material can withstand.

EXAMINER: Hold on; there are lots of different points on the graph that you haven't mentioned (Figure 26.2a).

CANDIDATE: The point separating the elastic region and the plastic region is often difficult to identify in the curve. The usual convention is to define the yield strength, which is the intersection of the curve with a straight line parallel to the elastic deformation of 0.2% on the strain axis.

EXAMINER: There are three points on the graph that in some materials are very close to each other and often difficult to differentiate. These are[2]:

1. Proportionality limit

The stress at which Hooke's law is no longer obeyed.

2. Elastic limit

If the stress slightly exceeds the proportional limit, the stress–strain curve is no longer linear but the material may still respond elastically. The curve tends to bend and flatten out. This continues until the stress reaches the elastic limit.

The elastic limit is the stress at which permanent deformation is seen and beyond this point the deformity will not completely recover if the force is removed.

3. Yield point

The point in the stress–strain curve at which the curve levels off and plastic deformation begins to occur.

EXAMINER: What is the yield point and how does it differ from the elastic limit?

CANDIDATE: Some textbooks describe the yield point as very fractionally later in the curve than the elastic limit. So the elastic limit is the point at which deformation stops being entirely reversible and the yield point is the point at which the material will have an

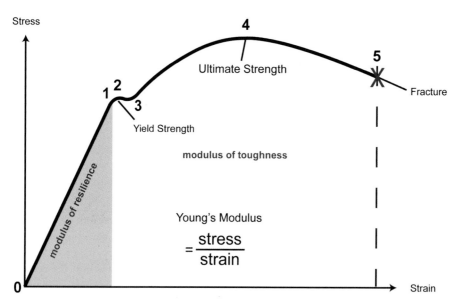

Figure 26.2a Stress–strain curve. Various points on graph include: 1, proportional limit; 2, elastic limit; 3, yield point; 4, ultimate tensile strength and 5, failure.

appreciable elongation or yielding without any increase in load. However, the two values are virtually inseparable for most materials.

EXAMINER: What is the difference between (offset) yield stress and yield point[3]?

CANDIDATE: The yield point is that point at which the material starts to undergo plastic deformation.

As it is often difficult to pinpoint the exact stress at which plastic deformation begins in some materials, the (offset) yield stress is taken to be the stress needed to induce a specified amount of permanent strain, typically 0.2%. To confuse the issue some engineering textbooks define the yield point as the (offset) yield stress.

EXAMINER: What do we mean by the upper and lower yield point (Figure 26.2b)?

CANDIDATE: For certain materials, especially low-carbon steel alloys, the stress–strain curve produces both an upper yield point and a lower yield point. A distinctive ripple pattern following the upper yield point is seen and associated with non-homogeneous deformation.

The upper yield point is the maximum stress at which deformation starts. A fairly dramatic drop is then observed in the stress to the lower yield point, although the strain continues to increase. Eventually the material is strengthened by this deformation and the stress is increased with further straining (strain hardening).

The phenomenon is thought to occur due to dislocations occurring in the material.

Materials lacking this mobility, for instance by having internal microstructures that block dislocation motion, are usually brittle and don't have separate upper and lower yield points.

EXAMINER: What is happening at the yielding, strain hardening and necking stage of plastic deformation?

CANDIDATE: I am not completely sure.

COMMENT: This is not well explained in most revision FRCS (Tr & Orth) textbooks.

For score 8 candidates

The plastic region consists of different parts that are (1) yielding, (2) strain hardening and (3) necking.

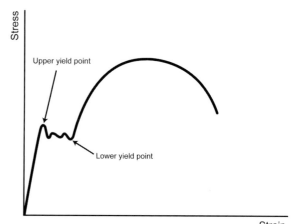

Figure 26.2b Upper and lower yield points on stress–strain curve.

Once the elastic limit (yield point) is passed, the material will undergo considerable elongation (yielding) with little or no increase in stress. This is indicated by the flatness of the stress–strain graph region in the plastic region. When the material is in this state it is often referred to as being perfectly plastic.

Strain hardening is where the plastic deformation increases a material's resistance to further deformation. It occurs due to the material undergoing changes in its atomic and crystalline structure. Lattice defects occurring in the material become too much in number and they restrict each other's movement. Essentially traffic jams have been created that obstruct movement of lattice defects.

An example is cold working of metal alloys. Strain hardening increases the yield point at the expense of lower ductility and toughness. Thus, a material that has received prior deformation will be stronger than an undeformed material.

In the region after the ultimate strength point, stretching occurs with an actual reduction in the stress. This is a result of necking or waisting in the material, whereby the cross sectional area is reduced.

COMMENT: Although the stress the material can withstand is reduced after the ultimate strength point, this is not due to any loss of material strength but due to the reduction in cross-sectional area of the bar. If the cross-sectional area of the narrowest part of the neck is used to calculate the stress, then the true stress-strain curve is obtained.

Structured oral examination question 3

Stress–strain curve

EXAMINER: Draw me the stress–strain curves for materials used in THA (Figure 26.3a).

   What is the stress–strain curve for ceramic, UHMWPE and stainless steel?

COMMENT: Sharp intakes of breath if you haven't read up beforehand, but relatively easy if you have worked through a pre-exam answer.

CANDIDATE: Ceramic is a very brittle material while UHMWPE is plastic. Stainless steel is ductile.

   Ductility is a measure of the ability of a material to be drawn out that is plastically deformed, before failure.

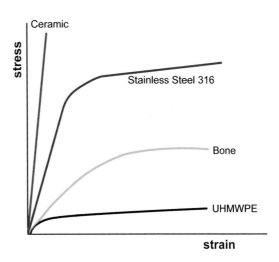

Figure 26.3a Stress–strain curve for materials used in THA.

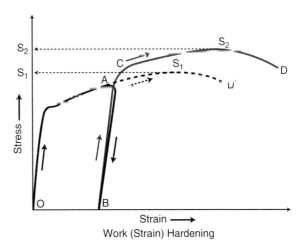

Figure 26.3b Strain hardening of a material

Stainless steel 316 is moderately strong, tough and a highly ductile material (this allows bending before catastrophic failure).

EXAMINER: What is happening with this graph (Figure 26.3b). Can you interpret it for me?

COMMENT: This is demonstrating strain hardening of a material.

- When loaded, the strain increases with stress and the curve reaches the point A in the plastic range.
- If at this stage, the specimen is unloaded, the strain does not recover along the original path AO, but moves along AB.
- If the specimen is reloaded immediately, the strain increases with stress from B to A but via another

path (the slope of stress–strain line is steeper indicating that the material has got stiffer than before) and reaches the point C, after which it will follow the curvature if loading is continued.

- If the specimen would not have been unloaded, after point A, the stress–strain curve would have followed the dotted path AD'.
- Comparison of paths ACD and ACD' shows that due to cold working (plastic deformation), the yield strength and ultimate strength have increased. Ultimate strength increased from S1 to S2. Since the ductility has decreased the work to failure on reloading also decreases. Thus strain hardening reduces toughness.

EXAMINER: What about UHMWPE used in joint arthroplasty. What are its properties?

CANDIDATE: UHMWPE has low friction and high impact strength, excellent toughness and low density, ease of fabrication, biocompatibility and biostability. Its major drawback is wear.

There have been changes in the way PE is manufactured in recent years. Gamma irradiation in air is bad due to generation of free radicals which can become oxidized and . . .

EXAMINER: That's fine, we don't need to go there.

Structured oral examination question 4

Stress–strain curve

EXAMINER: Stress–strain curve of different materials (ceramic, SS, plastic, bone, ligament), how are they different (Figure 26.4)?

COMMENT: Essentially this is describing and interpreting the stress–strain curve for brittle (ceramic), ductile (CoCr) and plastic (elastic) materials. Bone (mostly brittle but with a little plastic deformation before failure) doesn't neatly fit into one of the above categories. Leading on from bone the examiners may choose to throw into the discussion isotropic versus anisotropic material properties. Be careful with bone as the stress–strain curve is different for cortical and cancellous bone.

EXAMINER: Describe how each material behaves when loaded.

COMMENT: Candidates should be able to discuss the elastic and plastic regions of the graph and how they

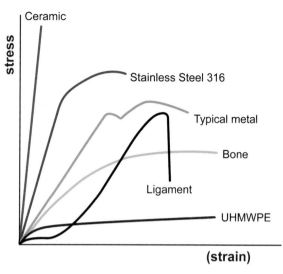

Figure 26.4 Stress–strain curves of different materials.

differ between the various materials. This question is a different way of essentially testing the factual knowledge of the stress–strain curve.[4]

EXAMINER: How is the mode of failure (fracture) different between brittle and ductile materials?

CANDIDATE:

- Materials fracture by a process of crack initiation and propagation.
- All materials are rough and contain defects and cracks at the microscopic level.
- Crack progression in a brittle fracture is associated with little plastic deformation whereas ductile fracture involves significant plastic deformation.
- A brittle material fails suddenly, soon after the yield point.
- The appearance of a brittle fracture is characterized by a clearly defined fracture surface generated across the material.
- With a ductile fracture there is considerable deformation after the yield point that results in a characteristic 'drawn out' appearance.

Structured oral examination question 5

Stress–strain curve

EXAMINER: Can you draw out the stress-strain curve – label all the points, axis and areas of interest (Figure 26.5a)?

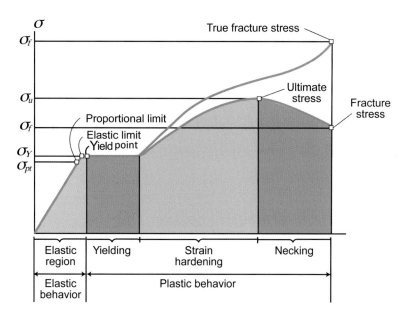

Figure 26.5a Stress–strain curve diagram for ductile material (stainless steel).

What happens at the yielding, strain hardening and necking regions of the graph (see above)?

Stress–strain curve of materials with three different moduli of elasticity. Pick three items from a display in front of me that match those stress–strain curves. Describe their material properties (ceramic/bone/ligament) (Figure 26.5b).

CANDIDATE: A brittle material is one that exhibits a linear stress–strain relationship up to the point of failure. It undergoes elastic deformation only with little to no plastic deformation. Characterized by the fact rupture occurs without any noticeable prior change in the rate of elongation. The classic example to mention is ceramic. Other examples would include PMMA and glass (Figure 26.5c).

Although cortical bone exhibits some plastic deformation it behaves more like a brittle material than a ductile material. It deforms slightly before failure or fracture. Cortical bone displays anisotropic behaviour with its elastic modulus depending on the direction of loading. It is also viscoelastic, with the stress–strain curve varying depending on the rate of loading.

Ligament is also viscoelastic. The toe region of the stress–strain curve is seen predominantly in ligaments and tendons. It denotes a non-linear elastic phase. Initially, a large distance (strain) is travelled under minimal stress as the crimped fibres straighten out. The characteristic shape is produced by the increase in the number of collagen fibrils resisting the strain as the slack fibrils are straightened and stretched, reducing the crimp pattern. Once all the collagen fibrils are straightened and stretched the slope is more or less constant (linear region).

EXAMINER: What about the stress–strain curve of cortical vs cancellous bone (Figure 26.5d)?

CANDIDATE: The compressive stress–strain curve for cancellous bone shows an initially shorter elastic segment (lower yield point) and has a lower stiffness (< 10% that of cortical bone).

Upon reaching the yield point, however, cancellous bone has a very long plastic phase. This phase represents the progressive fracture and collapse of the cancellous trabecula. Once trabecular debris fills the marrow spaces and the cancellous bone compacts, the curve once again turns upward, illustrating the resulting increased stiffness. This prolonged plastic deformation period explains why the total energy absorbed by cancellous bone under compression can exceed that of cortical bone.

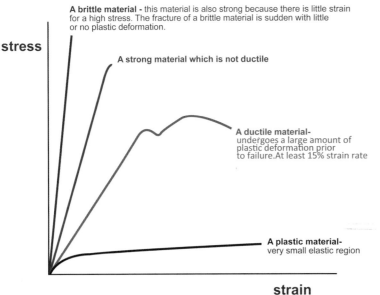

A brittle material - this material is also strong because there is little strain for a high stress. The fracture of a brittle material is sudden with little or no plastic deformation.

A strong material which is not ductile

A ductile material- undergoes a large amount of plastic deformation prior to failure. At least 15% strain rate

A plastic material- very small elastic region

stress

strain

Figure 26.5b Stress–strain curve, different materials.

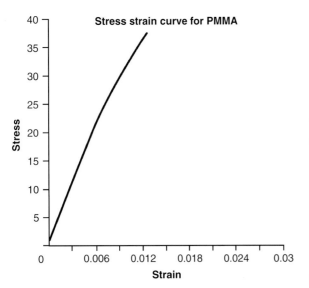

Figure 26.5c Stress–strain curve for PMMA. Essentially brittle with little plastic deformation before failure.

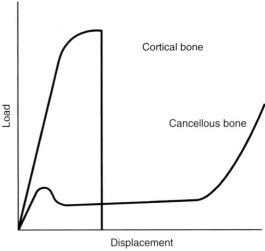

Figure 26.5d Compressive stress–strain curve cortical vs. cancellous bone. There is a prolonged plateau in cancellous loading representing the collapse of trabeculae.

Structured oral examination question 6

S-N curve

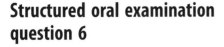

EXAMINER: S-N curve (Figure 26.6a). What is this, what does it mean and label the axis? Relate this to both THA and TKA.

CANDIDATE: Fatigue properties of a material are normally demonstrated on an S-N curve. Stress on the *y*-axis is plotted against number (n) of cycles (millions) on the *x*-axis.

At stresses below the endurance limit, a material can be cycled endlessly without experiencing failure.

The higher the peak stress produced in a given cycle of loading and unloading, the fewer cycles that can be sustained before failure.

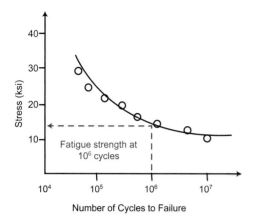

Figure 26.6a S-N curve. Specimens are tested in a series of decreasing stress levels until no failure occurs within a selected maximum number of cycles. The nearly horizontal portion of the curve defines the fatigue or endurance limit. If the applied stress is below the endurance limit of the material, the specimen is said to have an *infinite* life.

Fatigue or endurance limit is normally defined at 10^6 or 10^7 cycles.

Some metals such as aluminium do not have a fatigue limit.

EXAMINER: So, what is the difference between fatigue strength and fatigue limit?

CANDIDATE: For some materials the S-N curve becomes horizontal at higher n values or there is a limiting stress level called the fatigue limit (sometimes called endurance limit) below which fatigue failure will not occur.

For other materials (e.g. aluminium, copper, magnesium) they do not have a fatigue limit, the S-N curve continues its downward trend at increasingly greater n values. As such, fatigue will ultimately occur regardless of the magnitude of the stress. For these materials, the fatigue response is specified as fatigue strength, which is defined as the stress level at which failure will occur for some specific number of cycles (e.g. 10^7, 10^8).

Clinically, THA operate above the endurance limit, while TKA operate at the endurance limit, especially the polyethylene component, predisposing the latter to fatigue failure.

It is important to avoid creating any scratches or dents that can act as stress raisers and so reduce the fatigue properties of an implant.

Fatigue failure in orthopaedic implants is much less common with improved materials and processing.

Mechanical requirements of arthroplasty materials include a high yield point and endurance limit, modulus of elasticity that is similar to bone and wear resistance.

A concern is high and frequent loads on the hip joint. It is estimated around 1 million cycles per year occur at the hip that could potentially lead to fatigue failure.

EXAMINER: What do we mean by notch sensitivity?

CANDIDATE: Notch sensitivity is the extent to which the sensitivity of a material to fracture is increased by the presence of a surface inhomogeneity, e.g. cracks and scratches.

The initial stress concentration associated with a crack is too low to cause a fracture but may be sufficient to cause slow growth of the crack. Eventually the crack becomes sufficiently deep so that the stress concentration exceeds the fracture strength and sudden failure occurs.

In brittle materials a crack grows to a critical size from which it propagates right through the structure in a fast manner, whereas with a ductile material the crack keeps getting bigger until the remaining area cannot support the load and a ductile failure occurs. A notch causes non uniform stress flow lines.

EXAMINER: Stress–strain curve for a viscoelastic compound (Figure 26.6b). What is this? Explain viscoelasticity. Discuss creep/hysteresis/stress relaxation.

CANDIDATE: Most biological tissues are viscoelastic (e.g. tendon, ligament, bone, articular cartilage).[5] A viscoelastic material exhibits stress–strain behaviour that is time and rate dependent i.e. the material deformation depends on the load and its rate and duration of application.

A viscoelastic material is intermediate in properties between an elastic solid (that stores all the energy used to deform it) and a viscous liquid (that dissipates all the energy used to deform it by flow).

Viscoelastic materials demonstrate four properties:

1. Stress relaxation.
2. Creep.
3. Hysteresis.
4. Strain rate sensitivity.

The first three are specific mechanical properties that are present in viscoelastic materials, while the fourth property relates to a material being more rigid when it is rapidly loaded.

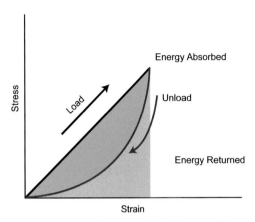

Figure 26.6b Viscoelastic materials exhibit a time delay in returning the material to original shape. Some energy is lost. Loading unloading curves are different.

A viscoelastic material continues to deform when a constant stress is applied to it. This continued deformation is creep. The creep rate decreases with time.

If a viscoelastic material is held at a constant strain, the stress will decrease with time. This is called stress relaxation. Therefore, stress relaxation is the inverse of creep. Stress relaxation time decreases with time.

A viscoelastic tissue does not follow the same path on a stress–strain graph. This is called hysteresis. The area under the initial loading phase represents the energy used to deform the material. The area used for recoil is the area under the unloading curve, and is less than the energy used to deform the material. The area between the two curves is the energy used to change the shape of the material (lost as heat) between loading and unloading. As a result, further energy is required to continue the loading and unloading cycles. This property allows viscoelastic materials to act as shock absorbers.

Viscoelastic materials are usually stiffer, stronger and tougher when loaded at a higher strain rate. This is called strain rate sensitivity and is due to the fact that the material isn't as quick to deform at a higher strain rate.

COMMENT: There are various slightly differently worded definitions of creep/hysteresis/stress relaxation in the textbooks. Just learn one standard definition that you are comfortable with and stick with it.

EXAMINER: Can you give me some everyday examples of creep, stress relaxation?

CANDIDATE: The handle of a heavy shopping bag gets longer and thinner as you walk home. This is creep, a material stretching out over time when subjected to a constant deforming force.

An example of stress relaxation is when a rubber band is wrapped around a newspaper for an extended period of time.

EXAMINER: What about strain rate sensitivity?

CANDIDATE: Sorry, no.

COMMENT: Blu tack.[6]

Structured oral examination question 7

Draw stress–strain curve and mark the events. Draw the curve for a ductile material. Viscoelastic properties, draw the curves for these.

COMMENT: Usual standard question. Remember ductility is the ratio of ultimate strain to yield strain.

EXAMINER: Can you describe the biomaterial behaviour of material A, B and C (Figure 26.7a)?

CANDIDATE: A has high strength, low ductility and low toughness. It is the strongest material.

B has high strength, high ductility and high toughness.

C has low strength, high ductility and low toughness. It extends or stretches the most.

EXAMINER: What do you mean by strength, ductility and toughness?

CANDIDATE: Strength is a somewhat imprecise term, but relates to the degree of resistance to deformation of a material. A material is strong if it has a high ultimate tensile strength.

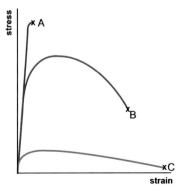

Figure 26.7a Stress–strain curve for various materials.

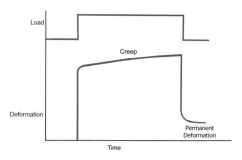
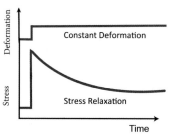
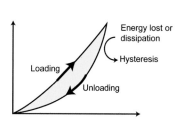

Figure 26.7b, c and d Candidate drawings of creep, stress relaxation and hysteresis.

Toughness is the amount of energy per unit volume that a material can absorb before failure. When comparing brittle and ductile materials with the same ultimate strengths, the brittle material is less tough as it has less area under the stress–strain curve.

Ductility is the amount of plastic deformation that occurs before failure.

EXAMINER. What do we mean by creep, stress relaxation and hysteresis? Can you draw out the relevant graphs (Figure 26.7b–26.7d)?

COMMENT: See previous questions above.

Figure 26.7b, c and d. Candidate drawings of creep, stress relaxation and hysteresis. Talk as you draw making sure your explanation is spot on for accuracy.

EXAMINER: What about elastic materials?

CANDIDATE: Elastic materials do not exhibit energy dissipation or hysteresis as their loading and unloading curve is the same. Indeed, the fact that all energy due to deformation is stored is a characteristic of elastic materials. Furthermore, under fixed stress elastic materials will reach a fixed strain and stay at that level. Under fixed strain, elastic materials will reach a fixed stress and stay at that level with no relaxation.

Structured oral examination question 8

Stress–strain curves for different materials

Materials – what is steel and what is titanium? Stress–strain curves for a variety of different materials. What is HA, why is it on a Ti stem, how is it put on a Ti stem?

EXAMINER: What is stainless steel?

COMMENT: Initial stress–strain curve questions can be a lead in (or prop) to go on and discuss biomaterials.

CANDIDATE: Steel is normally comprised of carbon and iron. If chromium is added it forms an oxide layer on the outer surface that protects it from corrosion – these alloys are stainless steel.

The most common stainless steel in orthopaedics is 316 L. The number 316 refers to 3% molybdenum and 16% nickel added to a normal alloy of iron, carbon and chromium. The letter L indicates a low carbon content < 0.03%.

Molybdenum reduces pitting corrosion.

Carbon content improves corrosion resistance, but too high a level weakens the alloy.

It is usually annealed, cold-worked or cold-forged for increased strength.

It is ductile, stiff and cheap.

Its use in arthroplasty surgery has been limited as Ti and CoCr alloys have better wear and corrosion resistance and lower stiffness. Relatively low biocompatibility and technical difficulties with MRI.

Implant stainless steel contains nickel, which improves corrosion resistance and increases fatigue strength and toughness. However, nickel can cause allergy and there have been recent attempts to reduce its content in SS.

Some newer SS contains a high nitrogen content that makes it stronger and more resistant to localized corrosion.

Titanium is extremely strong, has half the stiffness of cobalt chromium and can osseointegrate with bone. It has excellent biocompatibility.

Undergoes self-passivation to form an adherent oxide layer which decreases corrosion.

High yield strength.

It has poor wear characteristics and a high coefficient of friction, making it unsuitable for use as an articulating bearing surface in THA. Notch-sensitive and rough.

The most commonly used orthopaedic titanium alloy is titanium 64. The numbers refer to alloying elements aluminium (6%) and vanadium (4%).

Calcium hydroxyapatite is the mineral phase of bone.

HA is used as an adjuvant surface coating on prosthetic cup or stem surfaces that are usually made of a titanium alloy (TiAlV).

EXAMINER: Why is this?

CANDIDATE: When compared to cobalt chromium, titanium demonstrates a 33% increase in bond strength.

The modulus of elasticity of titanium is closer to bone, resulting in less stress shielding and bone resorption.

As such, titanium alloy is the preferred metallic substrate of choice.

In addition, although HA can be used on both porous-coated ingrowth and grit-blasted ongrowth femoral implants, for the most part it is mainly used on an ongrowth surface.

COMMENT: The candidate is either very knowledgeable or digging a hole for themselves.

EXAMINER: What is the reason for this?

CANDIDATE: Porous ingrowth surfaces appear to have a greater inherent initial stability which encourages biological fixation. Although HA usage depends somewhat on philosophy, many surgeons believe it has only a limited early role for an ingrowth surface and potential disadvantages outweigh benefit.

The situation is different with grit-blasted implants. Fixation occurs by bony ongrowth on the implant surface, which requires a more extensive area of coating to secure the implant as this is a weaker method of fixation. As such HA is added to improve early stability, reduce micromotion in the immediate postoperative period and accelerate bone ongrowth onto the prosthesis surface.

COMMENT: There is some evidence that HA coating works best on plasma-sprayed ongrowth surfaces rather than grit-blasted ongrowth surfaces.

Odds even with this answer.

EXAMINER: Why do we use grit-blasted stems if ingrowth stems appear to have a better chance of initial stability and obtaining osseointegration?

CANDIDATE: The manufacturing process for porous ingrowth stems can result in diminished fatigue strength properties. This could result in implant failure over time.

EXAMINER: How is HA put on a Ti stem?

CANDIDATE: HA deposition is often achieved through the plasma spray technique, which is performed at high temperature (15,000°C) and under vacuum, by projecting HA particles onto the metallic material at a speed of 300 m/s. The metallic substrate has a rough surface to promote adhesion. The other manufacturing method achieves HA deposition by electrochemical means, although it appears that the plasma spray technique is associated with improved bone ongrowth.

HA is an osteoconductive agent that allows for more rapid closure of gaps. Its surface readily receives osteoblasts and thus provides a bidirectional closure of gaps (i.e. bone to prosthesis and prosthesis to bone), which clinically shortens the time to biological fixation.

The optimal thickness of hydroxyapatite is 50–75 μm. Thicker coatings have been reported to delaminate off the prosthetic interface.

EXAMINER: Is there much difference in the clinical outcome or survivorship between HA-coated stems and uncoated stems.

CANDIDATE: From what I understand of the literature there isn't much evidence to support any difference in outcomes in terms of improved hip function, radiological assessment or survivorship.

EXAMINER: What radiological outcomes are you assessing?

CANDIDATE: Radiological outcomes included the presence of endosteal condensation (spot welds) and the presence of radioactive lines.

Endosteal condensation is considered a sign of endosteal bone ingrowth on the surface of the femoral stem and suggests that femoral stem fixation is optimal. Radioactive lines indicate femoral stem instability and are considered a sign of micromotion and femoral stem loosening.

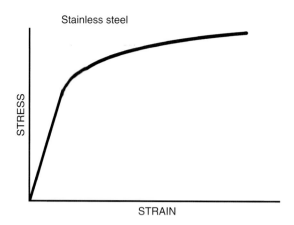

Figure 26.8 Simplified stress–strain curve for steel.

COMMENT: Use of HA-coated femoral stems has several disadvantages. These include high cost and the potential for delamination of the HA coating.

HA particles delaminated from the stem surface may induce osteolysis either by stimulating bone loss or by migration to the joint space producing third-body wear.

EXAMINER: Can you please draw the stress–strain curve for steel?

CANDIDATE: The stress–strain curve for stainless steel is typical of that for a ductile material.

COMMENT: The question may just require a simplified stress–strain diagram to be drawn as for a ductile material (Figure 26.8) or require the full-blown stress–strain diagram to be drawn out with the various regions and points explained (Figure 26.2a).

EXAMINER: The stress–strain curve for ligament vs. tendon?

CANDIDATE: Ligaments and tendons are predominantly made up of collagen. As such their stress–strain relationship is very similar to that of collagen.

There are a few minor differences in the stress–strain curve between ligament and tendon. This is mainly in the toe region of the curve. It takes slightly longer for a ligament to reach the elastic part of the graph as its collagen fibres are more wavy, less unidirectional and less well-structured compared to tendon. The slightly larger content of elastin in ligaments makes them less stiff and slightly weaker than tendons.

The toe-in region represents 'uncrimping' of the crimp in the collagen fibrils. Because it is easier to stretch out the crimp of the collagen fibrils, this part of the stress–strain curve shows a relatively low stiffness. As the collagen fibrils become uncrimped, the collagen fibril is being stretched, which gives rise to a stiffer material. As individual fibrils within the ligament or tendon begin to fail, damage accumulates, stiffness is reduced and the ligament/tendon begins to fail.

Structured oral examination question 9

Free body diagrams: elbow

Quite a large part of biomechanics involves drawing and explaining around free body diagrams (FBD). In the good old days of the past, if the examiners wanted to pass a candidate they would ask them to draw a free body diagram of the elbow. This is probably the easiest joint for a candidate to draw out and explain. Most candidates should breeze through this question with ease.

If examiners were unsure of a candidate they would ask them to draw a FBD of a hip and see how they got on. If a candidate managed to give a reasonably good account of themselves this was great and the candidate was passed with a move on to the next question. If a candidate managed to botch the answer up, the examiners' initial concerns were being realized. The examiners would then begin to unravel the candidate by asking them to draw out another FBD of the hip, but this time with a person holding a stick. This was make or break for the candidate to redeem themselves, but if they messed up again then a couple more FBDs of a person holding a suitcase in one hand, or a suitcase in both hands would usually be enough to sink them.

If the examiners were keen to fail a candidate for whatever reason they would ask them straight up spinal biomechanics. Most candidates will struggle with this and would usually fail miserably. So much for the good old days!

EXAMINER: What do we mean by a free body diagram?

CANDIDATE: This is a method used to illustrate the various forces acting on a structure such as a bone, and to illustrate how far from a joint or other pivot point these forces are acting.

From knowing these forces and distances, the moments of force acting to maintain the structure in static equilibrium can be calculated.

629

COMMENT: FBD show the locations and directions of all forces and moments acting on a body.

They are useful for identifying and evaluating unknown forces and moments acting on individual parts of a system in static equilibrium (i.e. sum of forces and moments is zero).

They can not be used for dynamic equilibrium.

EXAMINER: What are the assumptions made when drawing a free body diagram?

CANDIDATE: The assumptions made are that[7]:

- Bones are rigid bodies.
- Joints are frictionless hinges.
- There is no antagonistic muscle action.
- The weight of the body is concentrated at the exact centre of body mass.
- Internal forces cancel each other out.
- Muscles only act in tension (no compressive forces).
- The line of action of a muscle is along the centre of the cross-sectional area of the muscle mass.
- Joint reaction forces are assumed to be compressive only (no tensile forces).
- The joint acts only as a hinge (other axes of rotation and translation are ignored).

EXAMINER: What do we mean by a joint reaction force?

CANDIDATE: JRF is the force generated within a joint in response to external forces.

It is the vector sum of all forces acting on the joint.

EXAMINER: Can you draw a free body diagram of the elbow joint with an object in the hand (Figures 26.9a and 26.9b)?

COMMENT: Candidates may be straight on asked to draw a free body diagram of a particular joint without the warm up preamble of general free body analysis assumptions (see above). It is reasonable to mention the general assumptions at the beginning of the viva and then go on to joint-specific assumptions afterwards. The examiners will quickly move a candidate on if they don't want them to focus on this.

CANDIDATE: My assumptions when drawing the FBD of the elbow are that:

- The wrist, hand and finger joints are all rigidly fixed.
- Arm is flexed 90°.
- Acting as a class III lever.
- The moment arm of the biceps/brachialis is shorter than the weight of the forearm.
- Brachialis and biceps provide all of the flexion force.
- The force provided by biceps and brachialis is acting vertically upwards.
- Elbow fulcrum for the forearm lever.
- It is a two-dimensional X–Y plane.
- The axis about which an object rotates as the result of a force exerted on the object is called the instantaneous axis of rotation (IAR).
- The entire mass of an object is considered to be concentrated at a point called the centre of mass (COM) and does not depend on gravitational field.
- Centre of gravity (COG) is the point from which a weight is considered to act and depends on gravitational field.

COMMENT: The centre of mass and the centre of gravity of an object are in the same position if the gravitational field in which the object exists is uniform. In most cases this is true to a very good approximation.

It is generally assumed that for most situations COM = COG.

Each joint has specific load interactions because of the particular characteristics of the joint and the muscle actions that cross the joint.

Point O is the IAR of the elbow joint.

Point P attachment of brachialis on the radius.

Point Q is the COG of the forearm.

Point R lies on the vertical line passing through the COG of the weight held in the hand.

Forces acting on the free body include:

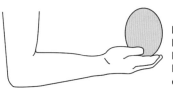

Point O is the IAR of the elbow joint
Point P attachment of brachialis on the radius
Point Q is the COG of the forearm
Point R lies on the vertical line passing through COG of the weight held in the hand

Figure 26.9a Arm flexed at 90° at the elbow, with wrist and fingers rigid, holding a ball in palm of hand.

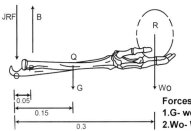

Figure 26.9b Free body diagram showing forearm holding a ball.

Forces acting on the free body include
1.G- weight of the forearm acting vertically downwards 1kg
2.Wo- Weight object 2.5kg
3.B-Force acting through brachialis muscle
4.JRF-Joint reaction force acting between the ulna and humerus

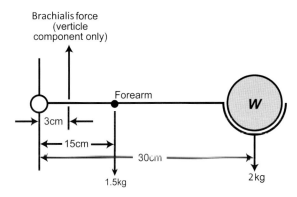

Figure 26.9c Candidate 20-second simplified FBD elbow.

1. G – weight of the forearm acting vertically downwards, 1.5 kg.

2. Wo – weight of object, 2 kg.

3. B – force acting through the brachialis muscle.

4. R – joint reaction force (JFR) acting between the ulna and humerus.

Considering the rotational equilibrium of the forearm about IAR, summation of moments about O will be zero.

Sum of clockwise (extension) = anticlockwise (flexion) moments $\Sigma M = 0$

$$WF \times 0.15 + Wo \times 0.3 = 0.05 \times Biceps$$

$$15N \times 0.15 + 20N \times 0.3 = B \times 0.05$$

$$2.25 + 6 = 0.05B$$

$$165N = B \text{ (Brachialis force)}$$

As the forearm is in translational equilibrium the sum of the forces $\Sigma F = 0$ acting on it is zero.

There is no JRF in the X-axis.

$$B - G - W - J \text{ (JRF)} = 0$$

$$JRF(J) + 15 + 20 = 165 \text{ N}$$

$$JRF = 165 - 35$$

$$JRF = 130 \text{ N}$$

Different textbooks have different values for the load carried in the forearm and different distances for P, Q and R. Learn a simplified FBD of the elbow that can be quickly drawn (Figure 26.9c). Some diagrams have only biceps labelled others only the brachilis muscle. With the elbow flexed to 90° by the side of the body, brachialis is the main muscle that maintains this position.

If you are doing very well or very poorly then the examiners may ask you to calculate JRF on the elbow in extension (Figure 26.9d). Use the same methods as used for elbow flexion.

$\Sigma M = 0$

$(0.1 \times W) - (0.03 \times T) = 0$

If $W = 20N$

$T = (0.1 \times 20N)/0.03$

$T = 67N$

$\Sigma F = 0$

$J - T - W = 0$

$J = T + W$

$J = 67N + 20 \text{ N}$

$J = 87N$

COMMENT: For a brownie point, candidates may be asked what type of lever is occurring in flexion and extension. A class 1 lever with elbow extension whereas a class 3 lever with a flexed elbow.

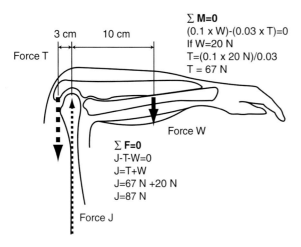

$\Sigma M=0$
$(0.1 \times W)-(0.03 \times T)=0$
If W=20 N
$T=(0.1 \times 20 N)/0.03$
T = 67 N

Force T

3 cm   10 cm

Force W

$\Sigma F=0$
J-T-W=0
J=T+W
J=67 N +20 N
J=87 N

Force J

Figure 26.9d Joint reaction force on the elbow joint during extension using the same method as that for elbow flexion.

The FBD of an extended elbow is approximated to a certain extent in various textbooks in that they show what appears to be a reversed flexed elbow.

The elbow is held in 90° of flexion with the forearm positioned over the head and parallel to the ground. In this position, action of the elbow extensors is required to offset the gravitational force on the forearm. It is assumed that triceps is the major extensor and that the force through the tendon of this muscle acts perpendicular to the longitudinal axis of the forearm.

Structured oral question 10

Hip FBD

The hip joint is somewhere between the elbow and the spine. There are enough scenarios and questions to easily use up 5 minutes of viva time on this topic alone. If a candidate can practise drawing out a standard FBD of a hip in around 20 seconds, then they will create more time to get further on forward with the question chain and score some extra marks.

EXAMINER: Can you draw a free body diagram of a hip joint when a person stands on one leg (Figure 26.10a and 26.10b)?

COMMENT: Mention general assumptions with FBD first and then the specifics for the hip.

CANDIDATE: We are assuming the:

• Body is in a single leg stance.

• Weight of the leg is one-sixth of the total body weight.

• Hip is fixed and the pelvis mobile.

Clockwise moment = Anticlockwise moment

$\Sigma M = 0$ Sum of moments is zero

$F_{AB} \times MF_{AB} = F_W \times M_W$

$\therefore F_{AB} = \dfrac{F_W \times M_W}{MF_{AB}}$

If $MF_{AB} = 0.05$ m

If $M_W = 0.15$ m

If W = 600 N and 5/6 = 500 N

$F_{AB} = \dfrac{0.15 \times 500}{0.05} = 1500$ N

COMMENT: Be careful with the line of action of the abductor muscles. In some textbooks it is assumed they are predominantly acting in a vertical direction while in other textbooks the abductor force is split into My and Mx components.

The abductor force is three times closer to the fulcrum (0.05 m vs. 0.15 m).

A force triangle is then drawn to calculate the JFR. This is estimated by lengths of the limbs (calculate with scale drawings) or by trigonometry (Figure 26.10c).

EXAMINER: What class of lever is this?

CANDIDATE: This is a class I lever between the body weight and abductor force.

EXAMINER: What happens to the joint reaction force in the hip if the patient has osteoarthritis of the hip and is given a walking stick in the opposite hand (Figure 26.10d)? Can you draw this out for me?

• BW = 600 N

• A = 0.05 m

• B = 0.15 m

• C = 0.45 m

• F_{STICK} = 100 N

Sum of moments about the hip is zero

Clockwise = 500 × 0.15

Anticlockwise = FAB × 0.05 + 100 × 0.60

(a)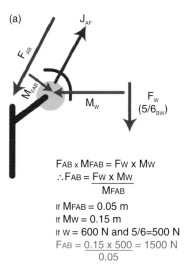

(b)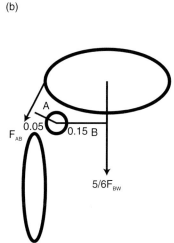

Figure 26.10a and 26.10b Candidate drawing of FBD hip.

$F_{AB} \times M_{FAB} = F_W \times M_W$

$\therefore F_{AB} = \dfrac{F_W \times M_W}{M_{FAB}}$

If $M_{FAB} = 0.05$ m

If $M_W = 0.15$ m

If $W = 600$ N and $5/6 = 500$ N

$F_{AB} = \dfrac{0.15 \times 500}{0.05} = 1500$ N

(c)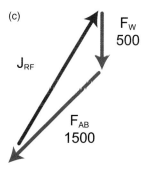

Figure 26.10c A force triangle is drawn to calculate JRF -estimated by lengths of the limbs or by trigonometry $JFR = F_{AB} + F_W$

$0.05 \times F_{AB} = 75 - 60$

$F_{AB} = 15/0.05 = 300$ N (1500 N without stick)

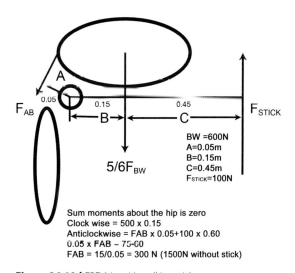

Sum moments about the hip is zero
Clock wise = 500 x 0.15
Anticlockwise = FAB x 0.05+100 x 0.60
0.05 x FAB – 75-60
FAB = 15/0.05 = 300 N (1500N without stick)

Figure 26.10d FBD hip with walking stick.

EXAMINER: What are the properties of a stick?

CANDIDATE: Introducing a stick on the opposite side adds another anticlockwise moment.

The effect is to lower the body weight force and aid the abductors.

As the moment arm on the stick is large there is a significant reduction in JRF.

The joint reaction force is reduced by 80% with using a walking stick in the contralateral hand.

EXAMINER: How do you calculate the optimum length of shaft. How would a person walk if the stick is too short? And too long?

CANDIDATE: A patient should stand upright in shoes they would normally use. The elbow should be slightly flexed and shoulders level. The walking stick should be turned upside down so that the handle is resting on the floor. The distance between the ground and end of the stick should reach to the distal wrist crease (or ulnostyloid joint).

The distance between the ground and distal wrist crease is measured as the optimal length of a stick.

The method of measuring the distance from the greater trochanter to the ground is not accurate or effective.

A number of formulae can be used if a person's height or arm length is known.

If a walking stick is too short, the patient will stoop or lean to one side throwing the patient off balance. If it is too long, using it can cause shoulder pain and be uncomfortable.

EXAMINER: What about carrying a suitcase on the opposite side as the weight-bearing leg. Can you draw this out for me (Figure 26.10e and 26.10f)?

CANDIDATE: Adding a suitcase on the opposite side introduces a clockwise moment which disadvantages/hinders the abductors. This increases the JRF.

BW = 600 N

Weight of suitcase = 250 N

A = 0.05 m

B = 0.15 m

C = 0.45 m

Sum of moments about the hip is zero

Clockwise moment = 500 × 0.15 + 250 × 0.6

Anticlockwise moment = FAB × 0.05

$0.05F_{AB} = 75 + 150$

$F_{AB} = 225/0.05 = 4500$ N

The abductor force that has to be generated is significantly increased by carrying a suitcase in the opposite hand.

Constructing a force triangle to calculate the JRF will show a significantly increased JRF.

EXAMINER: What about carrying a suitcase on the same side as the weight-bearing leg. Can you draw this out for me (Figure 26.10g and 26.10h)?

CANDIDATE: Adding a suitcase on the same side introduces an anticlockwise moment that aids the abductors.

The amount of force needed to be generated by the hip abductors is reduced and JRF is reduced.

BW = 600 N

Weight of suitcase = 250 N

A = 0.05 m

B = 0.15 m

D = 0.20 m

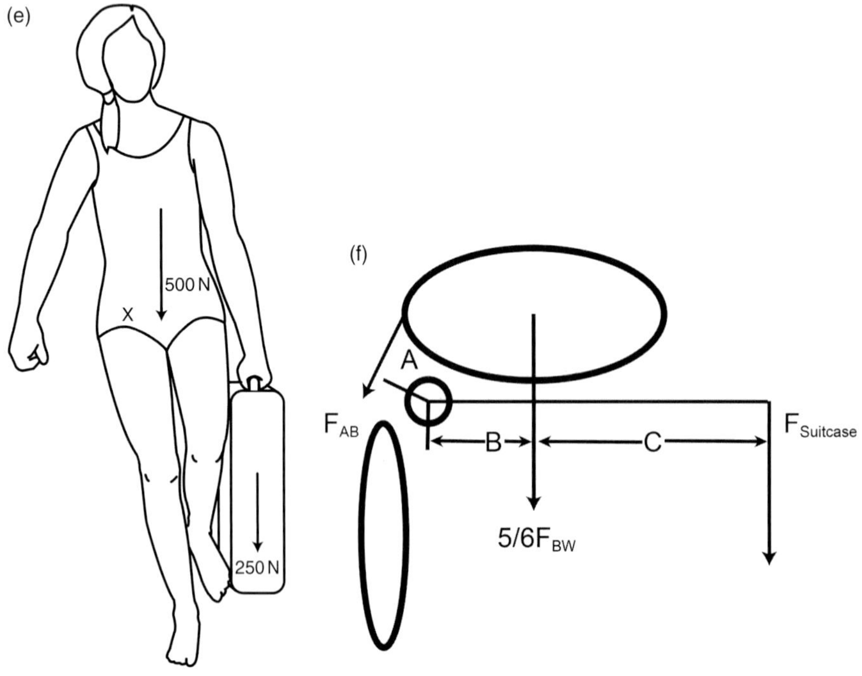

Figure 26.10e and 26.10f
FBD with patient carrying a suitcase opposite side of the weight-bearing limb.

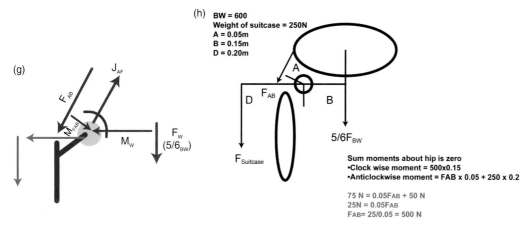

(g)

(h) BW = 600
Weight of suitcase = 250N
A = 0.05m
B = 0.15m
D = 0.20m

5/6F$_{BW}$

Sum moments about hip is zero
•Clock wise moment = 500x0.15
•Anticlockwise moment = FAB x 0.05 + 250 x 0.2

75 N = 0.05F$_{AB}$ + 50 N
25N = 0.05F$_{AB}$
F$_{AB}$= 25/0.05 = 500 N

Figure 26.10g and 26.10h FBD with patient carrying a suitcase on the same side as the weight-bearing limb.

Sum of moments about hip is zero

• Clockwise moment = 500 × 0.15

• Anticlockwise moment – F$_{AB}$ × 0.05 + 250 × 0.2

75 N = 0.05F$_{AB}$ + 50 N

25 N = 0.05F$_{AB}$

F$_{AB}$= 25/0.05 = 500 N

Despite the extra weight carried, the JRF is reduced by carrying a suitcase in the ipsilateral hand.

EXAMINER: What about carrying a suitcase in both hands (Figure 26.10i and 26.10j)?

BW = 600 N

Weight of each suitcase = 250 N

A = 0.05 m

B = 0.15 m

C = 0.45 m

D = 0.20 m

The number of forces acting in this situation is 5

Force from both suitcases 500 N

JRF

Upper body force (5/6 BW) 500 N

Abductor muscle force F$_{AB}$

Sum of moments about hip is zero

• Clockwise moment = 500 × 0.15 + 250 × 0.6

• Anticlockwise moment = F$_{AB}$ × 0.05 + 250 × 0.2

75 N + 150 N = 0.05F$_{AB}$ + 50 N

175 N = 0.05F$_{AB}$

F$_{AB}$= 175/0.05 = 3500 N

There is a large clockwise moment arm when carrying a suitcase in the non-weight-bearing side that is not equally balanced by carrying the second suitcase on the weight-bearing side. As such, the hip abductor force required to be generated is high

COMMENT: In all the above examples, for simplicity's sake we have assumed the centre of mass (COM) is unchanged.

However, if a person carries a suitcase in the left hand during a right leg stance weight the COM usually shifts towards the left of the person. This additionally increases F$_{AB}$ and JRF.

If a person is carrying two suitcases the bodyweight is more balanced, which shifts the COM closer to the femoral head, thus decreasing the moment arm to the COM so the abductor muscles don't have to work as hard (less force) to overcome the moment due to the weights leading to a lower reaction force.

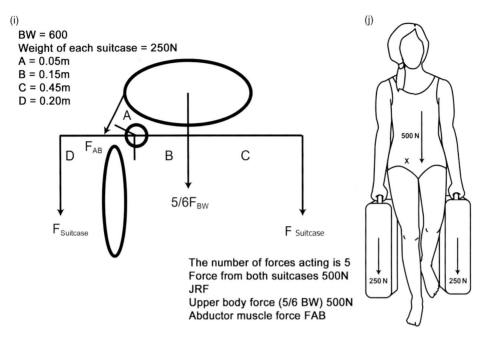

(i)

BW = 600
Weight of each suitcase = 250N
A = 0.05m
B = 0.15m
C = 0.45m
D = 0.20m

F_{AB}

D B C

$5/6F_{BW}$

$F_{Suitcase}$ $F_{Suitcase}$

The number of forces acting is 5
Force from both suitcases 500N
JRF
Upper body force (5/6 BW) 500N
Abductor muscle force FAB

(j)

500 N

x

250 N   250 N

Figure 26.10i and 26.10j FBD with patient carrying a suitcase in both hands.

EXAMINER: What other methods are used to decrease the joint reaction force in the hip joint?

CANDIDATE: Augmenting the abductors or reducing the body weight moment achieves a reduction in the JRF.

Actions that increase the abductor force include:

- Carrying a suitcase on the ipsilateral side.
- Lateralization of GT.
- High offset femoral stem.

Actions that have the effect of reducing body weight moment:

- Losing weight.
- Trendelenberg lurch – shifting body weight nearer to the femoral head, thereby decreasing lever arm.
- Stick on contralateral side.
- Medialization of THA cup (shifts centre of rotation medially thereby decreasing abductor tension).

EXAMINER: What actions increase joint reaction?

CANDIDATE: Valgus neck–shaft angulation – decreases shear across joint.

Structured oral question 8

Spine

The difficulty with a FBD of the spine is that for a candidate to be at their very best in answering this question they need to first understand Pythagoras' theorem.

If a candidate is tight for time the temptation is to go straight to the crux of the question. This can create quite a bit of head scratching for most trainees, as it is many years since they studied A-level maths.

EXAMINER: For the loading conditions shown, calculate the erector spinae muscle force FM and the compressive and shear components of joint reaction force (F_{JC} and F_{JS} at the L5/S1 vertebrae red square) (Figure 26.11a).

CANDIDATE: Assume the person weighs 70 kg and lifts a 20 kg weight.

The spine is flexed approximately 35°.

The three principle forces acting on the lumbar spine at the lumbar sacral level are:

1. Force produced by the weight of the upper body, W.
2. Force produced by the weight of the object, P.
3. Force produced by the contracture of erector spinae muscles, E.

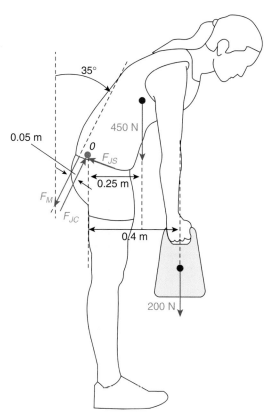

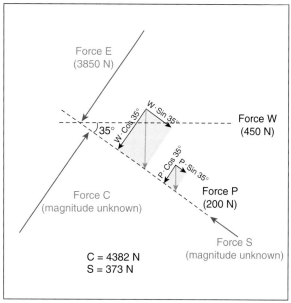

Figure 26.11a FBD of spine.

Because these three forces act at a distance from the centre of motion of the spine, they create moments in the lumbar spine.

Two forward-bending moments and a counterbalancing moment of the erector spinae muscle.

For the body to be in moment equilibrium the sum of the moments acting on the lumbar spine must be zero.

Clockwise and counterclockwise must balance.

$\Sigma M = 0$

$W \times 0.25 \text{ m} + 200 \text{ N} \times 0.4 - FM \times 0.05 = 0$

$450 \text{ N} \times 0.25 \text{ m} + 200 \text{ N} \times 0.4 - E \times 0.05 \text{ m} = 0$

$E \times 0.05 \text{ m} = 112.5 \text{ Nm} + 80 \text{ Nm}$

$E = 3850 \text{ N}$

EXAMINER: Calculate the compressive force exerted on the disc.

CANDIDATE: C is the sum of the compressive forces acting over the disc which is inclined 35° to the transverse plane.

The compressive force produced by the weight of the upper body W which acts on the disc inclined 35°.

$W \times \cos 35°$

The force produced by the weight of the object P which acts on the inclined disc at 35°.

$P \times \cos 35°$

The force produced by the erector spinae muscles, which acts approximately at a right angle to the disc inclination.

The magnitude of C can be found through the equilibrium of forces:

$\Sigma F = 0$

$W \times \cos 35° + P \times \cos 35° + E - C = 0$

$450 \text{ N} \times \cos 35° + 200 \text{ N} \times \cos 35° = 3850 \text{ N} - C$

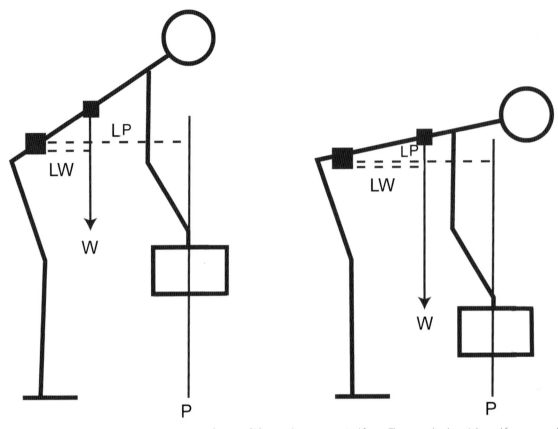

Figure 26.11b Candidate's diagram FBD spine. Influence of lifting technique on spinal forces. The upper body weight and force exerted by the weight act in front of the disc and create forward bending moments. LW:lever arm for body weight, LP-lever arm for weight carried in hand.

C = 368.5 + 163.8 N = 3850 N

C = 4382 N

The shear component for the reaction force on the disc (S) is found in the same way.

450 N × sin 35° + 200 × sin 35° – S

S = 373 N

COMMENT: Practise drawing out a FBD of the spine as it is definitely known to be asked in a viva and trying to draw out for the first time in the exam from first principles is generally going to be doomed to failure (Figure 26.11a). The other viva scenario is the influence of lifting technique on spinal forces. An increase in the distance between the object being lifted and the spine increases the forward bending moment. Reaching too far for an object will induce substantially higher spinal loading (Figure 26.11)

Notes

1. To try and catch a candidate out, to be clever or just because it is something that should be known and tested.

2. In the real exam the test is not about teaching. It is about how much a candidate knows. As such, the examiners will move past a point if a candidate doesn't know it.

3. These terms are often incorrectly interchanged in various internet PPP. Yield strength is often described as the point at which elastic behaviour changes to plastic behaviour.

4. A different route whereby to get to the same destination.

5. As such this viva question can be asked across so many different Section 2 basic science viva topics.

6. Blu Tack is a reusable, putty-like, pressure-sensitive adhesive produced by Bostik, commonly used to attach lightweight objects to walls, doors or other dry surfaces.

7. Practise beforehand being able to trot out these general assumptions while at the same time being able to draw the asked for FBD.

Genetics and cell biology

Stan Jones and Paul A. Banaszkiewicz

Introduction

The average orthopaedic trainee about to sit the FRCS (Tr & Orth) exam requires a basic knowledge of genetics.

This doesn't need to be encyclopaedic, but candidates will need to have a sound grasp of disease inheritance and genetic disorders. Trainees should be able to draw a family pedigree of single gene inheritance and know the gene mutations of the more common orthopaedic conditions.

By comparison, mention genetic viva questions to any examiner and you get a slightly puzzled look back. Safe to say, it is not a major A-list topic for the vivas and probably doesn't even make the B-list. However, the subject does intermittently appear in the vivas and therefore it is definitely worthwhile knowing how the questions will run in order to uncomplicate a potentially complicated topic.

Some genetic material will find its way into Section 1 SBA and EMI papers so common genetic terminology and definitions need to be reasonably well understood.

General information

Nucleic acid structure (Figure 27.1)

There are two main types of nucleic acid, DNA (deoxyribonucleic acid) and RNA (ribonucleic acid), which each consist of a sugar-phosphate backbone with projecting nitrogenous bases. The nitrogenous bases are of two types, purines and pyrimidines.

In DNA, there are two purine bases, adenine (A) and guanine (G), and two pyrimidine bases, thymine (T) and cytosine (C) (Figure 27.2).

RNA also contains adenine (A), guanine (G) and cytosine (C), but contains uracil (U) instead of thymine (T).

In DNA the sugar is deoxyribose, whereas in RNA it is ribose. The nitrogenous bases are attached to the

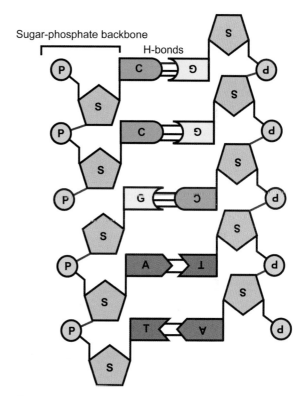

Figure 27.1 Nucleic acid structure.

1′ (one prime) position of each sugar, and the phosphate links 3′ and 5′ hydroxyl groups.

Each unit of purine or pyrimidine base together with the attached sugar and phosphate group(s) is called a nucleotide.

A molecule of DNA is composed of two nucleotide chains that are coiled clockwise around one another to form a double helix with approximately 10 nucleotides per complete turn of DNA (Figure 27.2).

The two chains run in opposite directions (i.e. 5′ to 3′ for one and 3′ to 5′ for the other) and are held together by hydrogen bonds between A in one chain and T in the other or between C and G.

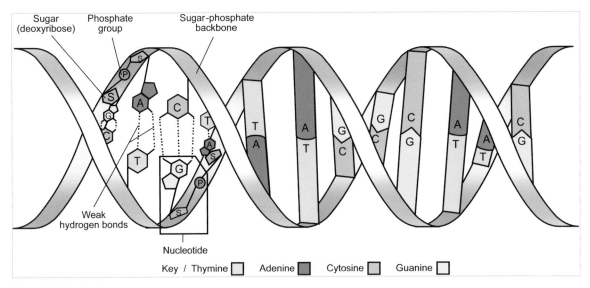

Figure 27.2 DNA structure.

Pedigree charts

Pedigree charts can be complicated to understand if you are unfamiliar with the basics.

A standard set of symbols are used (Figure 27.14). The father is conventionally placed on the left, and all members of the same generation are placed on the same horizontal level. Roman numerals are used for each generation, starting with the earliest, and Arabic numerals are used to indicate each individual within a generation (numbering from the left).

Single gene disorders are due to mutations in one or both copies or alleles of an autosomal gene or to mutations in genes on the X or Y chromosome (sex-linked inheritance). These disorders show characteristic patterns of inheritance in family pedigrees.

Structured oral examination question 1

Autosomal dominant (AD) inheritance

COMMENT: This is much easier to explain if candidates are able to draw out a Punnett square. Just get the pen out and practise (Figure 27.3).

EXAMINER: What pattern of inheritance does the pedigree chart show and why (Figure 27.4)?

CANDIDATE: This is autosomal dominant because:

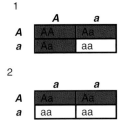

Figure 27.3 Punnett square demonstrating inheritance of an autosomal dominant trait: (1) two heterozygous parents, (2) one heterozygous and one unaffected parent.

- There are people with the disease in each generation.
- Both males and females are affected in approximately equal numbers.
- All forms of transmission are present (male to female, female to male, female to female and, in particular, male to male, which would not be present if the condition were X-linked).
- At conception, each child has a 1 in 2 (50%) chance of inheriting the condition.

COMMENT: Unaffected persons do not transmit the condition if the condition is fully penetrant (e.g. in achondroplasia).

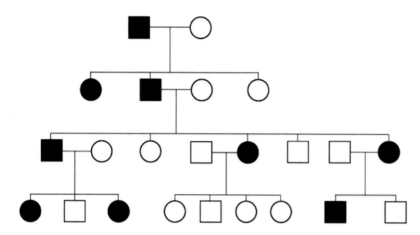

Figure 27.4 Pedigree chart of AD inheritance, one affected heterozygous and one unaffected parent. The disease is passed from father to son – this almost never happens with X-linked traits. The disease occurs in three consecutive generations – this almost never happens with recessive traits.

It is equally likely that a child will receive the mutant or normal allele from the affected parent.

On average there is a 1 in 2 or 50% chance that each child of a heterozygous parent will inherit the gene mutation.

There is usually a variation in time of onset and severity of condition with AD traits. This is likely to be due in part to the effects of other 'modifier' genes and also lifestyle/environmental factors.

EXAMINER: Choose an autosomal dominant condition and discuss the genetics.

COMMENT: A gift if you have done your homework. The three most obvious disorders to choose are (1) achondroplasia, (2) osteogenesis imperfecta or (3) neurofibromatosis. Plenty to talk about with each condition.

It is unwise to choose an obscure disorder that the examiner knows very little about. The conversation will dry up and the examiners will invariably switch back to more difficult basic science questions.[1] Candidates are throwing away easy scoring opportunities.

The other situation is that the clinical condition to discuss has already been decided beforehand.

Achondroplasia

About 80% of people with achondroplasia have the condition as the result of a new mutation; the incidence of the condition increases with increasing paternal age.

Achondroplasia is inherited as an autosomal dominant condition. Each child of someone who has achondroplasia has a 1 in 2 (50%) chance of inheriting the condition.

If both parents have achondroplasia, and a child inherits a copy of the altered gene from both parents, the condition is severe and not compatible with life.

The gene for achondroplasia is on the short arm of human chromosome 4 at locus p16.3.

The condition is the result of a mutation in the gene that codes for fibroblast growth factor receptor 3 (*FGFR3*), which is a key component of cartilage development.

The main defect is abnormal endochondral bone formation in the cartilaginous proliferative zone of the physis.

COMMENT: Clinical features of achondroplasia may be discussed in more detail and these can easily be mugged up in a standard textbook:[2] kyphosis, spinal stenosis, genu varum, trident hand, radial head subluxation, etc.

EXAMINER: What is the genetic mutation responsible for this condition, and what effect does this have?

CANDIDATE: Achondroplasia is caused by a single point mutation in the gene encoding the fibroblast growth factor receptor 3 (*FGFR3*). The *FGFR3* is believed to regulate bone growth by limiting endochondral ossification. Two mutations in the *FGFR3* gene are responsible for 99% of cases of achondroplasia. These mutations both cause substitution of a glycine amino acid by an arginine and lead to prolonged receptor activation after ligand binding and result in excessive growth limitation. Soluble

FGFR3 has successfully been used in mice to act as a decoy for FGF in order to restore normal growth in achondroplasia.

EXAMINER: What is the mode of inheritance of this condition?

CANDIDATE: It is autosomal dominant.

EXAMINER: This child's parents do not have this condition. How is this possible?

CANDIDATE: A large proportion (80%) of cases occur due to a spontaneous (new) mutation.

Osteogenesis imperfecta

There is a qualitative or quantitative defect of type 1 collagen synthesis. Originally classified by Silence[3] into four subgroups, we now know there are many more different subgroups of OI.

The vast majority of cases are autosomal dominant.

Type 1 collagen is the major extracellular protein in bone, skin and tendon.

The structural unit of type 1 collagen is called tropocollagen and is a heterotrimer composed of three polypeptide chains. Two chains are pro-α1(I) and the third chain is pro-α2(I). The three chains form a distinctive unit in which the polypeptide chains wrap around each other for most of their length, forming a tight triple helical braid.

The triple helical structure is not the same as the pro-α helix that is formed by a single polypeptide chain, which is the defining feature of all collagen.

The collagen triple helix forms because both the α1 and α2 chains contain repeat sequences of amino acids (–Gly–X–Y), where Gly is glycine, X is proline and Y is usually hydroxyproline. This arrangement results in a constrained structure that imparts a tight kink in the polypeptide chain with the glycine chain preventing steric hindrance that would otherwise impair wrapping of the helical band.

Only Gly, which has no side chain, can pack into the centre of the triple-helix structure without distortion. A missense mutation[4] leading to the replacement of even one Gly in the repeating (Gly–X–Y)$_n$ sequence by a larger residue may lead to a pathological condition.

The pro-α1(I) chain is encoded from the *COL1A1* gene on chromosome 17 and the pro-α2(I) residue is encoded by the *COL1A2* gene on chromosome 7.

Mutations in the *COL1A1* gene on chromosome 17 or *COL1A2* gene on chromosome 7 are responsible for OI.

In the type 1 condition the *COL1A1* mutant allele results in failure of the production of the pro-α1(I) chain due to a premature codon stop. There is only 50% production of normal pro-α1(I) chain.

In more severe forms of the condition there are mutations of either the *COL1A1* gene or the *COL1A2* gene resulting in a mixture of abnormal and normal collagen chains.

Structured oral examination question 2

Autosomal recessive (AR) inheritance

EXAMINER: Can you please draw a Punnett square demonstrating an autosomal recessive trait (Figure 27.5).

CANDIDATE: Recessive means two copies of the gene are necessary to have the trait/disease. Parents of affected children are both carriers of the condition.

Typically, heterozygotes for the trait/disease are not affected but are gene carriers. Most people do not know they carry a recessive gene for a condition until they have a child with the disease.

If the parents are both carriers the risk of them having an affected child is 25% (1/4) and the risk of them having a child who is a carrier is 50%.

Unaffected adult offspring of carrier parents have a 2/3 risk of carrier status.

COMMENT: Alternatively, candidates may be shown a pedigree chart of autosomal recessive inheritance and asked to identify the pattern of inheritance (Figure 27.6).

1. Males and females are equally affected.
2. On average, the recurrence risk to the unborn sibling of an affected individual is 1/4.
3. The trait is characteristically found in siblings, not parents of affected or the offspring of affected.

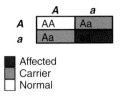

Affected
Carrier
Normal

Figure 27.5 Punnett square demonstrating autosomal recessive inheritance.

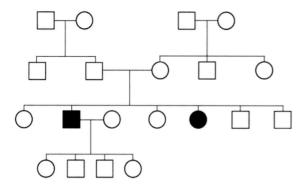

Figure 27.6 Pedigree chart of autosomal recessive inheritance.

4. Parents of affected children may be related (consanguineous). The rarer the trait in the general population, the more likely a consanguineous relationship is involved.
5. The trait may appear as an isolated (sporadic) event in small sibships.
6. Within the completely unaffected siblings of an affected individual the probability of being a carrier is 2/3.

EXAMINER: Can you describe an autosomal recessive disease?

COMMENT: Obvious choices include (1) sickle cell anaemia, (2) mucopolysaccharidoses – all except Type II (Hunter's syndrome, which is X-linked recessive), (3) Gaucher disease and (4) diastrophic dysplasia.

Sickle cell disease

Sickle cell disease describes a group of disorders caused by a mutation in the beta globin gene (*HBB*). The altered haemoglobin produced is HbS. SCA is the commonest of these diseases and is caused by homozygous point mutations in the *HBB* gene on the short arm of chromosome 11. A single nucleotide mutation (base change) from T to A results in glutamic acid changing to valine at the sixth amino acid in the beta haemoglobin chain. This allows polymerization of the HbS but only under conditions of low oxygen concentration.

Heterozygous carriers of *HBB* mutations ('sickle cell trait') have a selective advantage (heterozygote advantage), due to their resistance to malaria. The malarial parasite causes the defective red blood cells to rupture directly, prior to its reproduction. Hence heterozygotes have increased chances of survival in malaria-prevalent areas. Carriers will only have severe symptoms if they are ever deprived of oxygen (e.g. at high altitude) or dehydrate, an important factor in consideration for surgery and when considering using a tourniquet.

Clinical features

SCA is characterized by episodes of pain owing to vaso-occlusive events, chronic haemolytic anaemia and severe infections from early childhood with splenomegaly.

Any organ may be affected but most commonly bones (ON/osteomyelitis), lungs, liver, kidneys, brain and eyes are involved.

Sickle cell crisis presents with severe abdominal pain, chest or bone pain. Management includes analgesia, fluids, oxygen and in severe cases exchange transfusion.

Structured oral examination question 3

X-linked inheritance

EXAMINER: Can you draw the Punnett square for an X-linked dominant condition (Figure 27.7 and 27.8)?

CANDIDATE: [While drawing the Punnett square.] If the father is affected his sons will be unaffected and all his daughters will be affected (Figure 27.7). If the mother is affected (heterozygous) half of her sons will be affected and half of her daughters will be affected. Other sons and daughters will be unaffected (Figure 27.8).

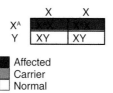

Figure 27.7 Punnett square showing inheritance of an X-linked dominant trait (normal mother and affected father).

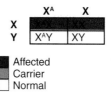

Figure 27.8 Punnett square showing inheritance of an X-linked dominant trait (affected mother and normal father).

643

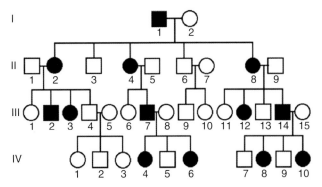

Figure 27.9 X-linked dominant inheritance. The key for determining if a dominant trait is X-linked or autosomal is to look at the offspring of the mating of an affected male and a normal female. If the affected male has an affected son, then the disease is not X-linked. All of his daughters must be affected if the disease is X-linked dominant.

EXAMINER: What is the mode of inheritance here (Figure 27.9)?

CANDIDATE: This is X-linked dominant inheritance. Hallmarks of X-linked dominant inheritance include:

- The trait is never passed from father to son.
- Does not skip a generation. All daughters of an affected male and a normal female are affected. All sons of an affected male and a normal female are normal.
- Matings of affected females and normal males result in 1/2 of the sons being affected and 1/2 of the daughters being affected.
- Males may be more severely affected than females. The trait may even be lethal in males during the embryonic or perinatal periods.
- In the general population, females are more likely to be affected than males, even if the disease is not lethal in males.

EXAMINER: What is the mode of inheritance here (Figure 27.10)?

COMMENT: This is the opposite situation to Figure 27.9 where the male parent is affected.

CANDIDATE: This is still X-linked dominant inheritance. An X-linked dominant trait does not skip generations. Affected sons usually have an affected mother, affected daughters usually have either an affected mother or an affected father.

Affected fathers will pass the trait on to all their daughters.

Affected mothers (if heterozygous) will pass the trait on to half of their sons and half of their daughters.

EXAMINER: Do you know of an example of an X-linked dominant inheritance condition?

CANDIDATE: Hypophosphataemic rickets (vitamin D-resistant rickets).[5]

The condition is caused by mutations in the *PHEX* gene. PHEX protein regulates fibroblast growth factor 23 protein (FGF23). FGF23 inhibits the renal tubular ability to reabsorb phosphate.

In addition, the absence of *PHEX* enzymatic activity may cause accumulation of osteopontin (a mineralization-inhibiting secreted substrate protein found in the extracellular matrix of bone), which contributes to osteomalacia.

Clinical features

Childhood rickets with growth retardation and poor dental development. Short stature and genu varum in males, genu valgum in females.

In middle age, mineralization of spinal ligaments and thickening of neural arches. Loss of mobility of the spine, shoulders, elbows and hips. Treatment with phosphate supplements and large doses of vitamin D.

COMMENT: The condition is caused by mutations in the *PHEX* gene.

The change created in the gene is a loss-of-function mutation, resulting in reduced breakdown and circulatory clearance of FGF23.

FGF23 acts on the kidney to cause increased phosphate excretion and decreased alpha-1 hydroxylase activity.

The gene product is now known to be a zinc-metallopeptidase.

Other X-linked dominant conditions:

- Conradi–Hunermann chondrodysplasia punctata (due to a mutation in the gene encoding EBP).
- Leri–Weill dyschondrosteosis is very unusual. Because of the gene's specific location, it is inherited in a manner that is described as

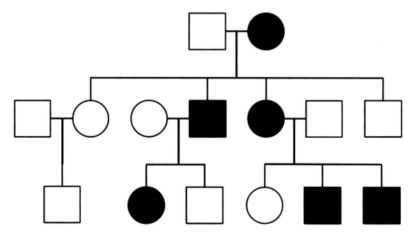

Figure 27.10 X-linked dominant inheritance. Parent female is affected. Affected father does not pass disease on to son.

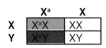

Affected
Carrier
Normal

Figure 27.11 Punnett square showing inheritance of an X-linked dominant trait (affected mother and normal father).

Affected
Carrier
Normal

Figure 27.12 Punnett square showing inheritance of an X-linked dominant trait (normal mother and affected father).

pseudo-autosomal (i.e. similar to autosomal dominant inheritance).

EXAMINER: Can you draw the Punnett square for an X-linked recessive condition?

CANDIDATE: Figure 27.11 and 27.12.

EXAMINER: What is the mode of inheritance here (Figure 27.13)?

CANDIDATE: This is X linked recessive. Hallmarks of X-linked recessive inheritance include:

- As with any X-linked trait, the disease is never passed from father to son.
- Males are much more likely to be affected than females.
- All affected males in a family are related through their mothers.
- The trait or disease may be passed from an affected grandfather, through his carrier daughters, to half of their sons.
- For a carrier female, with each pregnancy there is a one in two (50%) chance her sons will inherit the disease allele and a one in two (50%) chance her daughters will be carriers.

- Affected males transmit the disease allele to all of their daughters who are then carriers, but to none of their sons.
- Females are affected if they have two copies of the disease allele. All of their sons will be affected, and all of their daughters will be unaffected carriers.

Duchenne muscular dystrophy (DMD)

Incidence approximately 1 in 4000 boys.

This is one of the dystrophinopathies caused by a mutation in the dystrophin gene ($Xp21$). The dystrophin protein provides structural stability to the dystroglycan complex of the muscle cell membrane, and its function is lost as a result of the mutation. Females rarely show musculoskeletal signs of the disease, although there is an increased risk of dilated cardiomyopathy in female carriers. There is a relatively high spontaneous new mutation rate.

Clinical features

Age of onset is usually before 6 years. Progressive proximal myopathy of the lower limbs with noticeable calf pseudohypertrophy.

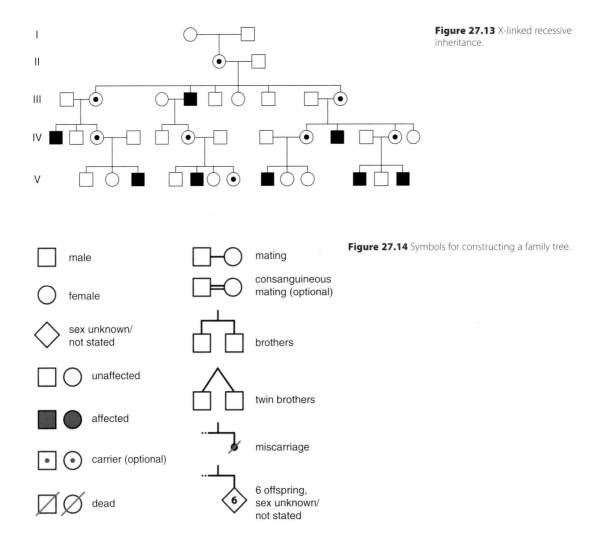

Figure 27.13 X-linked recessive inheritance.

Figure 27.14 Symbols for constructing a family tree.

Compensatory toe walking is an adaptation to knee extensor weakness.

Frequent falls/fatigue.

Speech delay and difficulty with motor skills with learning difficulties in approximately a third of affected boys.

Lumbar lordosis/scoliosis.

Usually wheelchair-bound by 12 years and life expectancy is around 25 years.

Gower's sign positive: the child is unable to jump up quickly from a crossed leg position without bracing their arms against their legs to support the proximally weak muscles.

Other examples of X-linked recessive inheritance:
- Becker muscular dystrophy.
- Mucopolysaccharidosis Type II (Hunter's syndrome).
- Haemophilia A. Genetic defect in factor VIII.
- SED tarda.

EXAMINER: Pick one family pedigree and tell me the mode of inheritance (Figure 27.15).

COMMENT: Be able to justify your answer in terms of pedigree features (see above examples).

Structured oral examination question 4

Stem cells

Potentially an awkward C-list topic, especially if a candidate hasn't read through any structured material beforehand.

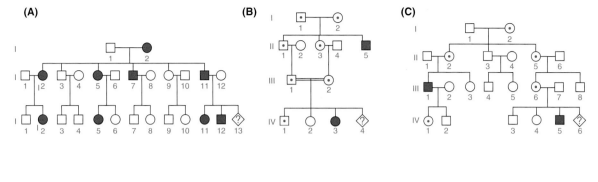

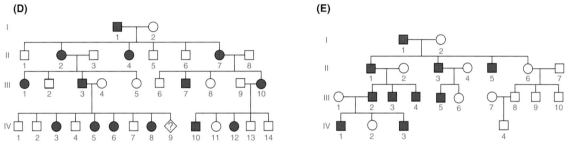

Figure 27.15 Family tree for various modes of inheritance. A, autosomal dominant; B, autosomal recessive; C, X-linked recessive; D, X-linked dominant; E, Y-linked inheritance.

EXAMINER: What are stem cells?

CANDIDATE: Stem cells represent unspecialized cells that have the ability to differentiate into diverse specialized cell types and self-renew to produce more stem cells.

EXAMINER: What two properties must a stem cell demonstrate?[6]

CANDIDATE: The two defining features of a stem cell are:

Self-renewal: the ability to go through numerous cycles of cell division while remaining undifferentiated. If stem cells could not self-renew, tissues would run out of replacement cells for those that had died.

Potency: the capacity to differentiate into specialized cell types. This requires stem cells to be either totipotent or pluripotent – to be able to give rise to any mature cell type.

EXAMINER: What are the different types of stem cells that you know?

CANDIDATE: The two main types of stem cells are:

1. Embryonic stem cells.
2. Adult stem cells.

Other types of stem cell include:

- Foetal stem cells.
- Amniotic stem cells.
- Induced pluripotent stem cells (IPSCs).
- Nuclear transplant stem cells (ovasomes).
- Parthenote stem cells.

EXAMINER: What do you mean by pluripotent?

CANDIDATE:

- Pluripotent cells have the capacity to differentiate into any cell type in the body. They give rise to most, but not all, of the tissues necessary for foetal development.
- Totipotent cells have the capacity to form an entire organism as well as the extraembryonic tissue including the placenta. Embryonic cells within the first couple of cell divisions after fertilization are the only cells that are totipotent.
- Multipotent cells can develop into more than one cell type but are more limited in capacity than pluripotent cells. They can form many types of cell in a given lineage, but not cells of other lineages.

EXAMINER: Can you think of any uses of stem cells in orthopaedics?

CANDIDATE: Stem cells have become a focus of regenerative medicine. Adult stem cells, harvested directly from bone marrow, adipose tissue, muscle or blood have the ability to undergo mitosis as well as multipotent differentiation into a variety of cell lineages.

The goal of stem cell therapy is to replace or replenish diseased tissue through the localized differentiation of transplanted stem cells into cells which advance the healing process or directly restore the tissue physically.

1. Articular cartilage damage/degeneration

    It is hoped that stem cells will create growth of primary hyaline cartilage to restore the normal joint surface. Stem cells assist with growth factor release and alteration of the anatomic microenvironment to facilitate regeneration and repair of the chondral surface. Stem cell application can be combined with microfracture.

    Due to their role in inhibiting the catabolic activity of matrix metalloproteinases (MMP), mesenchymal stem cells (MSCs) have been shown to have a beneficial effect in OA.

2. Bone fractures and nonunions

    Stem cells may stimulate bone growth and promote healing of fractures. Traditionally, bone defects have been treated with solid bone graft material placed at the site of the fracture or non-union. Stem cells and progenitor cells are now placed along with the bone graft to stimulate and speed healing.

3. Ligaments and tendon injury/degeneration

    Mesenchymal stem cells may also develop into cells that are specific for connective tissue. This would allow faster healing of ligament and tendon injuries, such as quadriceps or Achilles tendon ruptures.

4. Rotator cuff tears

    Mixed results reported. Some studies have shown increased rates of healing and repair surface integrity.

5. Spinal cord injury[7]

    There has been recent research into cell-based therapies for spinal cord injury. They may be able to limit cell death, stimulate axonal growth, and replace injured cells.

6. Meniscal injury

    Isolated case reports exist of meniscal regeneration after percutaneous injection of autologous ASCs into an adult human knee.[8] It is not clear whether this is a direct action of the mesenchymal-based cells or is rather mediated by secretion of certain stimulating factors on the existing meniscal tissue.

    Stem cells have also been added to modify the biomechanical environment of avascular zone meniscal tears at the time of suture repair.

7. Intervertebral disc disease

    Various clinical trials have been undertaken using MSCs to biologically repair degenerative disc. Percutaneous stem cell mediated disc regeneration has the potential to establish itself as a possible treatment option in patients with low back pain hoping to avoid invasive spinal surgery.

8. Spinal fusion

    Pseudoarthrosis remains a pressing issue occurring in 13–41.4% of patients undergoing spinal fusion. Risk factors include older age, thoracolumbar kyphosis, smoking, diabetes mellitus, metabolic bone disease and female gender.

    MSCs and adipose tissue derived stem cells (ADSCs) have both demonstrated a significant positive effect on spinal fusion in a number of experimental models. Cellular in-vitro expansion is necessary to increase the number of viable pluripotent cells along with the addition of growth factors and/or bone morphogenic proteins (BMPs).

9. Physeal injury/defects

    Several animal models have investigated the use of stem cells combined with growth factors to promote the regeneration of damaged regions of the growth plate.

10. Osteonecrosis

    Stem cells have angiogenic and osteogenic properties. Core decompression and injection of isolated stem cells have been used in early stages of ON hip.

EXAMINER: What are your concerns with the use of stem cells in orthopaedics?

CANDIDATE:

- MSCs have been reported to promote tumour growth and metastases. There is very limited clinical experience with pluripotent stem cells (embryonal stem cells and IPSC). Based on their features of self-renewal and high proliferation rate, the risks of tumour formation should be considered high.

- Ethical issues and controversies regarding the use of embryonic stem cells and embryos exist.
- Donor site morbidity from stem cell harvesting.
- Processing time (requires separate procedures to harvest and re-implant cells).
- Retroviruses may be used to generate human IPSCs. These viruses are genetically altered to express the genes that are required for transformation into an IPSC. Applying this genetic reprogramming, the used viruses can integrate into the cell genome. Consequently, the cells may contain multiple viral integration sites in their genomes, which could be tumourigenic.
- Cost.
- Microbial contamination during cell amplification.
- Controlling stem cell differentiation into the desired cell lineage.
- Control of their proliferation and differentiation into complex, viable 3D tissues is challenging.
- Lack of adequate vehicles/scaffolds for implantation of stem cells.
- Integration with local tissues.
- Immunological rejection and disease transmission (if allogeneic).

- Potential modulation of host immune system by implanted stem cells.
- Continuous cell amplification of MSCs may lead to chromosomal abnormalities.

Notes

1. This will usually end up making the viva more unnecessarily complicated than would have been the case.

2. Ward J, Gargan A, Smithson S, Atherton G. Orthopaedic manifestations of achondroplasia. *Orthop Trauma*. 2013;27(4):229 232.

3. Sillence D. Osteogenesis imperfecta: an expanding panorama of variants. *Clin Orthop Rel Res*. 1981;159:11–25.

4. A missense mutation is a point mutation in which a single nucleotide change results in a codon that codes for a different amino acid.

5. Best to stick to hypophosphatemic rickets as the rest are just a bit too obscure for your average orthopaedic surgeon.

6. Much better if a candidate volunteers this info rather than being asked.

7. Schroeder GD, Kepler CK, Vaccaro AR. The use of cell transplantation in spinal cord injuries. *J Am Acad Orthop Surg*. 2016;24(4):266–275.

8. Pak J, Lee JH, Lee SH. Regenerative repair of damaged meniscus with autologous adipose tissue-derived stem cells. *BioMed Res Int*. 2014;2014:436029.

Diagnostics

Rajesh Kakwani and Simon Freilich

General radiology viva advice

In the FRCS (Tr & Orth) structured oral exam, most candidates will have anticipated the possibility of being asked a radiology topic and would have (wisely) prepared for this. While candidates will be asked bits and pieces of radiology during a topic discussion the assumption that a stand-alone 5-minute radiology topic is probably too much detailed knowledge for the average candidate (and examiner) to stretch out discussion for is wrong. We know candidates who have had very detailed questioning on the principles of either bone scans or MRI scanners lasting the full 5 minutes of a viva. Bone and MRI scanners would seem to be the most obvious questions that candidates would be asked, although a discussion about X-rays is also fair game. Sometimes, the examiner may put all of them in front of you (X-ray/ultrasound/CT/MRI/ bone scan images) and give you a choice to speak on any one of them. A candidate scoring 6 would start to run out of steam at 3 minutes or struggle if they are seriously probed about the topic in detail. A bit depends on the examiner themselves on how much they really do understand the subject in depth, but you are gambling a bit with this one.

The other aspect of radiology which is extremely important and can certainly set you apart from the average candidate is to be able to describe radiographs, MRI and CT scans well. This is usually at the beginning of an oral question, so it is important to get off to a good start and describe the radiographic or MRI features well. This is not always an easy skill to acquire, so our suggestion would be to arrange one or two tutorials from a local friendly radiologist who will be able to put you on the spot in describing various scans and radiographs. Going on a viva course, closely observing and making mental notes of how other candidates describe various radiographs is another way in which you can refine this technique. If all else fails, then practise out loud describing radiographs and scans from a book.

Structured oral examination question 1

Radiographs

EXAMINER: What are X-rays?

CANDIDATE: X-rays are electromagnetic radiations of wavelength 15–0.01 nm.

EXAMINER: How are X-rays generated?

CANDIDATE: X-rays are released on heating a fine tungsten filament to around 2200°C in a vacuum.[1] Electrons travelling from the filament (cathode) to the target (anode) convert a small percentage (1%) of their kinetic energy into X-ray photons (by the formation of Bremsstrahlung and characteristic radiation).

Bremsstrahlung interactions, the primary source of X-ray photons from an X-ray tube, are produced by the sudden stopping, breaking or slowing of high-speed electrons at the target. When the electrons from the filament strike the tungsten target, X-ray photons are created if they either hit a target nucleus directly (rare) or their path takes them close to the nucleus.

If a high-speed electron hits the nucleus of a target atom, all its kinetic energy is transformed into a single X-ray photon.

Most high-speed electrons have near or wide misses with the nuclei. In these interactions, a negatively charged high-speed electron is attracted toward the positively charged nucleus and loses some of its velocity. This deceleration causes the electron to lose some kinetic energy, which is given off in the form of a photon. The closer the high-speed electron approaches the nuclei, the greater is the electrostatic attraction on the electron, the braking effect, and the greater the energy of the resulting Bremsstrahlung photon.

EXAMINER: How does digital radiography work?

CANDIDATE: Digital radiography uses a phosphor compound detector plate instead of the conventional photographic emulsion film. The detector generates a digital image that can either be printed or sent to PACS (picture archiving and communication system).

EXAMINER: What measures will you take to minimize radiation exposure to staff while using an image intensifier?

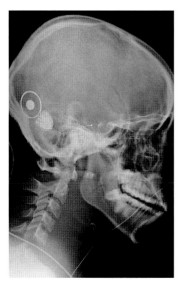

Figure 28.1a X-ray of cervical spine lateral (C5–6 dislocation).

CANDIDATE: The main source of radiation for the surgeon and the team is the scattered radiation from the patient. Measures to minimize the radiation exposure to staff are:

TDS (time/distance/shielding)

(1) *COMMENT*: In the radiation time exposure **A**s **L**ow **as R**easonably **A**chievable (ALARA principle).
(2) Distance: The inverse square law. The amount of scatter radiation is inversely proportional to the square of the distance from the X-ray source. The distance between the X-ray source and the patient should be maximized, i.e. keep the image intensifier as close to the patient as possible. (Staff to stay 1 m away from the X-ray source.)
(3) Shielding: Lead aprons (0.25 mm thick), thyroid shields and protective goggles.

EXAMINER: What is collimation?

CANDIDATE: Reduction in the size of the window through which the X-rays are emitted leads to sharper radiographs as well as reduction in radiation dose.

EXAMINER: What is the maximum safe dose of occupation-related radiation exposure?

CANDIDATE: The whole-body exposure of 20 mSv over a year is the maximum acceptable radiation dose (averaged over 5 years) (UNSCEAR, 2010).

EXAMINER: What does the picture show and what is its use in theatre (Figure 28.1b)?

Figure 28.1b Dosimeter.

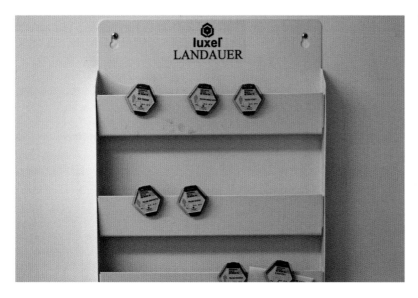

CANDIDATE: This shows a dosimeter. This is a device that measures exposure to ionizing radiation. It is used to estimate the radiation dose deposited in an individual wearing the device.

EXAMINER: Anything else?

CANDIDATE: Ideally all orthopaedic surgeons should wear a personal radiation dosimeter. This should be in a constant position beneath the protective lead gown to record any personal dose.

If dose readings are too high then a review of theatre practice must take place. Dosimeters must be safely stored away from radiation sources and should never be shared.

It is important to also take proper care of the lead apron. Crumpling of the lead apron will break the integrity of the lead fibre shielding. Lead aprons should be properly hung up after use and their integrity checked regularly.

COMMENT: The answer could have been structured into discussion of radiation protection covering five areas: (1) minimization of radiation use, (2) maximizing the distance between the individual and the X-ray source, beam and scatter, (3) use of lead screens, (4) personal protective garments and (5) monitoring personal exposure dose.

Additional notes:
(1) Natural background radiation: 0.01 mSv/day (UK: 2.2 mSv/year).
(2) Cosmic radiation during high-altitude flights: 0.001–0.01 mSv/hour.
(3) X-ray chest: 0.1 mSv.
(4) CT head: 1.5 mSv.
(5) CT abdomen: 9.9 mSv equivalent to 500 chest X-rays.
(6) X-rays were discovered by German scientist Wilhelm Roentgen in 1895.
(7) Lead aprons help in reducing the exposure by a factor of 4 in lateral view and a factor of 16 in posteroanterior view. Thyroid guards decrease the exposure 2.5 times the normal. Eye protection is essential and is the first determinant of workload in all procedures. Lead apron should have at least 0.5 mm equivalent thickness of lead and the goggles should be at least 0.15 mm lead equivalent thick.[2]
(8) Within 2 m of the C-Arm unit, lead protection is a must.

Structured oral examination question 2

Ultrasound

EXAMINER: What is ultrasound?

CANDIDATE: Ultrasound is a form of imaging that utilizes high-frequency sound waves to image interfaces between tissues with different acoustic properties (described as echogenic or hypoechoic). Fluid-filled tissues have low echogenicity while fat is highly echogenic.

EXAMINER: What are the advantages of ultrasound?

CANDIDATE: Ultrasound is cheap, easily available, portable, non-invasive and dynamic. It is safer than CT as it does not emit ionizing radiation and unlike MRI can be used in patients with cardiac pacemakers or metal clips.

EXAMINER: And the disadvantages?

CANDIDATE: Its main disadvantage is that it is operator-dependent.

EXAMINER: What is the physics behind ultrasound imaging?

CANDIDATE: The passage of electric current through a piezoelectric crystal causes deformation of the crystal surface, in turn producing sound waves. When the transducer is then applied to the patient's skin using a lubricating jelly, these waves are then transmitted into the patient's body. The reflected waves when received back by the transducer cause distortion of the crystal surface, producing a voltage, which is then converted to an image. The duration between the sound wave emission and detection reflects the depth of the tissue being studied.[1]

The amount of energy reflected at the interface between tissues depends on the difference in acoustic impedance of those tissues. The acoustic impedance of a tissue is mainly determined by its density. Air has a much lower density than water or soft tissue, which in turn have a much lower density than bone. The larger the difference in acoustic impedance, the more energy will be reflected, and the brighter the resulting image.[3]

However, at the interface between soft tissue and air or bone, nearly all the wave's energy is reflected. No energy is transmitted, and hence no information can be gained about tissues which lie deep to this point. This explains why ultrasound is generally not useful for assessment of bone, bowel or lung. It also explains why a coupling gel is required between the probe and patient's skin to eliminate air.[3]

As a sound wave passes through the body it gradually loses its energy in a process called attenuation. The causes of attenuation are: absorption, reflection, diffraction and refraction.

Refraction causes a transmitted wave to be deflected from its original course. Diffraction is scattering of the wave which occurs particularly when a wave interacts with small structures. Most of attenuation, however, occurs due to absorption. The energy of the sound wave is converted into friction between oscillating tissue particles and is lost in the form of heat. To compensate for this loss of energy, the ultrasound machine uses a process called time gain compensation. This gives greater amplification to those echoes which take longer to return to the transducer, producing an even image.[3]

Frequency 3–50 MHz with a high-frequency probe used for deep tissues and a low-frequency probe for superficial tissues.

EXAMINER: Tell me a few of the practical applications of ultrasound in orthopaedics.

CANDIDATE: A few uses of ultrasound in orthopaedics include:

(1) Hip.
   a. Diagnosis and treatment monitoring in developmental dysplasia of the hip (the viva can drift to Graf's classification of DDH from here).
   b. Detection and guided aspiration of hip effusion (especially in children).
(2) Shoulder: To diagnose impingement and rotator cuff tears.
(3) Tendons: To detect tendon ruptures, swelling/oedema (Achilles/tibialis posterior).
(4) Soft-tissue swelling – size, extent, solid or cystic ± guided biopsy.
(5) Steroid/anaesthetic injections into tender areas (plantar fasciitis), joints (subtalar/sub acromial) and around neuromas (Morton's neuroma) (Figure 28.2).
(6) Regional anaesthesia: Most of the distal limb surgeries are now done under awake-block anaesthesia (administered under ultrasound guidance).

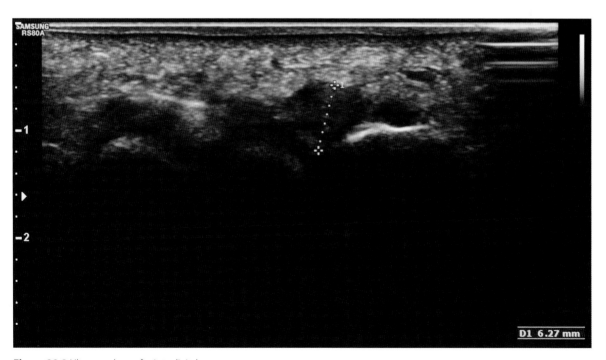

Figure 28.2 Ultrasound scan for interdigital neuroma.

Structured oral examination question 3

CT scanners

EXAMINER: How does a CT scanner work? What are the principles of a CT scanner?

CANDIDATE: The X-rays are liberated from the axially rotating X-ray tube. After passing through the patient, they are received by a circle of stationary detectors. The data collected are processed by the computer and digital images are reconstructed. The scanning gantry rotates helically around the patient, allowing continuous acquisition of data.

With modern multidetector CT transverse (or axial) anatomical sections can be produced with high resolution and reformatted to create reconstructions in any plane. The 3D CT scans allow better visualization of complex intra-articular fracture/spinal problems but at the cost of slight loss of definition (subtle fractures can fade away/be created).

A recent additional feature is the ability to 'ghost out' structures, for example: a ghost outline of the femoral head can be maintained in cases of fractures of the acetabulum to show its relationship to the fracture and at the same time the acetabular fracture can be visualized more clearly.

General information

(1) CT was discovered by Sir Godfrey Hounsfield (Hayes, UK) and the first patient brain scan was done in 1971. Sir Hounsfield was awarded the Joint Nobel prize (with Allan McLeod Cormack of Massachusetts) in 1979.

(2) Hounsfield units are a measure of the attenuation coefficient of the tissue being scanned. (Bone = 1000 HU.) Bone windows are usually centred on 300 HU with a width of 1200 HU.

(3) Limitations.
   a. Radiation dose.
   b. Artefact from orthopaedic metalware reduces image quality.
   c. Soft-tissue detail is limited.

EXAMINER: Give some orthopaedic indications for CT scan.

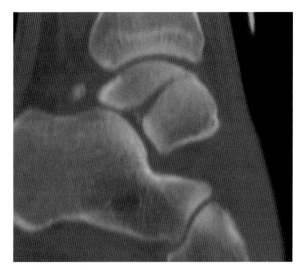

Figure 28.3 Sagittal reformatted image of ankle CT demonstrating talar body fracture.

CANDIDATE:

(1) Complex peri-articular fractures – for example, fractures of the acetabulum, tibial plafond, tibial plateau, proximal humerus, Lisfranc's, talus, calcaneum and vertebrae. CT aids in planning incisions to minimize additional trauma to soft tissues (Figure 28.3).

(2) Polytrauma patients – head, chest and abdominal scanning (in about 30 seconds).

(3) CT arthrography/myelography (if MRI is contraindicated).

(4) Assessment of choice for non-union when radiographs are inconclusive: scaphoid.

(5) Drilling/ablation of osteoid osteoma.

(6) Customized implants: CT scans are increasingly used for patient-specific implants and instrumentation, especially for complex arthroplasty.

Structured oral examination question 4

MRI scanners

EXAMINER: Please describe the findings (Figure 26.4a,b)?

CANDIDATE: This is an MRI scan of the lumbo-sacral spine of . . . Dated . . . Age . . .

EXAMINER: Is it a T1-weighted image or T2?

(a)

(b)

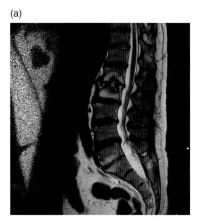 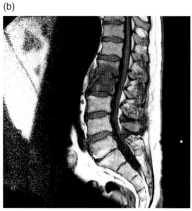

Figure 28.4 Sagittal T2 (a) and sagittal T1 (b) images of the lumbar spine. This demonstrates L1/2-disc space abnormality with adjacent end plate oedema. It could represent either disc space infection or acute inflammatory discovertebral lesion as might be seen in spondylitis.

CANDIDATE: The image to the left is a T1 image as it has a TR (time to repetition) value of (< 1000), whereas the image on the left is a T2 image (TR > 1000).[4]

(Don't rely on fluid/fat signals for judging the type, as they can be confusing in STIR or fat-suppressed images.)

Most imaging protocols will use a combination of different sequences to optimally evaluate the structures and pathologies in question by providing both anatomical and pathological information.

MRI can be utilized in any plane, and this is sometimes crucial in providing additional information.

EXAMINER: What are the differences between T1 and T2 images?

CANDIDATE:

	T1-weighted	T2-weighted
TR	< 1000	> 1000
TE	Short (< 80)	Long (> 80)
Definition	Time constant of exponential growth of magnetism	Time constant of exponential decay of signal following the excitation impulse
	Fat is bright	Water is bright/fat is bright too
	Anatomy	Pathology

EXAMINER: What contrast is generally used with MRI?

CANDIDATE: Chelated gadolinium. It enhances the oedematous tissues on T1 image.

An important but rare complication of gadolinium is nephrogenic systemic fibrosis (a fibrosing dermopathy), which has been reported to occur rarely in patients with Stage 4 renal failure.

Current guidance is that if the eGFR < 30, gadolinium should not be administered.

EXAMINER: What are the contraindications for MRI scan?

CANDIDATE:

(1) Implanted cardiac pacemaker and/or defibrillators.
(2) Internal hearing aids/cochlear implants.
(3) Implanted nerve stimulators/dorsal column stimulators.
(4) Metal objects in orbit of the eye.
(5) Intracranial metal aneurysm clips.
(6) Aortic stent graft.
(7) Mechanical heart valve.

Many coils, filters, coronary stents and grafts are made from non-ferromagnetic materials and MRI can be safely performed. They will require a pre-MRI check regarding their compatibility as some will demonstrate magnetic field interactions and are not safe with MRI use.

MRI is usually used with extreme caution within the first 6 weeks postoperatively when any metallic clip (including skin clips) or implant has been utilized as they will not have become incorporated securely in tissues.

EXAMINER: What else?

CANDIDATE: Certain types of intracranial aneurysm clips are an absolute contraindication to the use of MRI because excessive, magnetically

655

induced forces can displace these clips and cause serious injury or death.

Exposure of internal hearing aids to MRI may damage these components.

In the case of cardiac pacemakers and defibrillators the MR environment can cause movement and heating of pacing leads, temporary or permanent modification of the device, and deactivation of the device.

EXAMINER: What are the advantages of MRI use?

CANDIDATE: MRI provides excellent soft tissue contast. It is particularly good for imaging tumours and occult fractures and does not involve using ionizing radiation.

EXAMINER: What are the disadvantages of MRI use?

CANDIDATE: Patients may be claustrophobic, and it is not as good as CT for cortical bone imaging.

EXAMINER: What are the indications for MR arthrograms?

CANDIDATE:

(1) Shoulder: Suspected capsular/labral tears (Figure 28.4c).
(2) Hip: Labral tears/Impingement.
(3) Knee: Post-meniscectomy for recurrent tear.
(4) Wrist: Scapholunate dissociation, TFCC tear, occult scaphoid fracture.
(5) Ankle: Undisplaced osteochondral lesion of the talus.

EXAMINER: What is the basic principle of an MRI scanner?

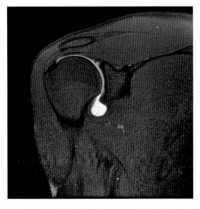

Figure 28.4c MRI arthrogram of shoulder demonstrating dye leakage from rotator cuff tear.

CANDIDATE: The MRI scan involves exploiting the magnetic moment/nuclear spin property of the hydrogen nucleus (in the tissues) when placed in a strong magnetic field. Radiowaves (64 MHz) are then applied using the transmitter coil. Following the cessation of the radiowaves, the individual magnetic moments then precess and the response is recorded in the receiver coil.

The frequency of precession depends on the strength of the external magnetic field.

Larmor equation

Frequency of precession = gyromagnetic ratio (constant) × strength of the external magnetic field

EXAMINER: What do the terms PD, STIR and FATSAT sequences mean?

CANDIDATE: PD = Proton density-weighted image. It is commonly used in knee protocols to image the menisci.

FATSAT and STIR are both sequences used to improve tissue contract by suppressing the response from fat in tissues.

FATSAT: Abbreviation for fat saturation (spectral fat saturation). It can be applied to T1/T2/PD sequences. T1 fat-saturated sequences are commonly used in MR arthrography and after the administration of contrast, and both PD and T2 fat-saturated sequences are commonly utilized to identify pathology.

STIR: Short tau inversion recovery. This is a very robust, commonly used sequence, which is very sensitive to abnormal fluid or oedema and so ordinarily demonstrates pathological processes well.

EXAMINER: What is TE?

CANDIDATE: Time to echo. When a second radiofrequency pulse is applied after the first one is turned off, then the time duration between the first wave and the echo formation is termed TE. TE is used as a controllable factor as timing of application of the second radiofrequency pulse is at the discretion of the user.

EXAMINER: What is extremity MRI?

CANDIDATE: Extremity MRI involves placement of only the involved extremity in the magnetic bore, while the rest of the body remains outside.[5]

Advantages are:

(1) Reduced cost.

(2) Improved patient comfort and reduced claustrophobia.

(3) Facilitated sitting.

(4) Reduced patient risk.

Disadvantage: only the distal two-thirds of the extremity can be scanned.

EXAMINER: What is your option if the patient is claustrophobic in an MRI scanner?

CANDIDATE: Open MRI scanner ± sedation.

Or consider alternative imaging modalities.

Imaging artefacts

1. Chemical shift artefact: fat and water precess at different frequencies in the same external magnetic field. The fat image is slightly shifted with reference to the water image, hence low signal lines can sometimes be seen where these two are shifted away, or high signal lines can be seen where they overlap. These are generally easy to identify as they are generally found at the boundaries between fat and water.

2. Metal artefact: metal distorts the magnetic field, causing major artefacts in its vicinity. T1-weighted images are less susceptible to metal artefacts than T2 images. Hence MARS (metal artefact reduction sequences) are commonly applied to study tissues around hip resurfacing implants.

3. Magic angle artefact: tendons normally yield low signals in all sequences due to low T2 relaxation times. However, if the collagen fibres of the tendon make an angle of 55° to the external magnetic field, the T2 relaxation time increases many fold, causing a high signal on short echo time images. This can be differentiated from tendinopathy by the 55° angle and the absence of a high signal on T2-weighted images.

Structured oral examination question 5

Bone densitometry

EXAMINER: What is bone densitometry?

CANDIDATE: Bone densitometry, also called dual-energy X-ray absorptiometry or DEXA scan, uses simultaneous measurement of the passage through the body of X-rays with two different energies. It uses a low dose of ionizing radiation and is accurate in diagnosing osteoporosis.

The WHO guidelines for interpretation of bone densitometry results (T-score):

Normal	Score not more than one standard deviation below the average value of young adult
Osteopenia	Score more than 1 standard deviation below the young adult average, but not more than 2.5 standard deviations below
Osteoporosis	More than 2.5 standard deviations below the average value for young adult
Severe osteoporosis	Osteoporosis + fragility fracture(s)

EXAMINER: What are its uses?

CANDIDATE: The clinical applications of bone densitometry include:

(1) Assessment of bone status in primary and secondary osteoporosis.

(2) Assessment of the effect of treatment for osteoporosis.

(3) Fracture risk assessment (what is FRAX score?).

(4) Evaluation of preventive measure for bone loss associated with ageing/metabolic disorders.

(5) Measure periprosthetic bone loss (particularly cementless hip arthroplasty).

EXAMINER: OK. You have now started bisphosphonates on this patient for osteoporosis, how will you find out whether your treatment has been effective? Will you repeat the bone density scan? When?

CANDIDATE: Repeated dual-energy X-ray absorptiometry (DXA) has a high within- and between-patient variability. The average annual increase in BMD in patients treated with alendronate is about 0.0085 g/cm^2. This change is smaller than the typical year-to-year (within-person) BMD variation of 0.013 g/cm^2. It would therefore be difficult to differentiate the medication's effect from the random variation inherent in DXA scans.

Response is generally favourable after 3 years of treatment. While there is variation in test results from year to year, longer-term findings are more reliable. After 3 years of treatment, 97.5% of patients taking alendronate had an increase in hip BMD of at least 0.019 g/cm², with a strong correlation between hip and spine measurements.

Hence, if needed I would repeat the bone density scan after 3 years, to evaluate efficacy of the treatment monitored in low–medium-risk patients. The treatment of high-risk patients would need to be considered on an individual case basis.[6,7]

EXAMINER: Name some techniques used to measure bone density in the axial skeleton? (The same question can be asked regarding appendicular skeleton.)

CANDIDATE: Techniques that can be used to measure bone density in axial skeleton are:

(1) DEXA. Dual energy X-ray absorptiometry.

(2) Quantitative CT (rarely used).

(3) Quantitative MRI (rarely used).

EXAMINER: Does DEXA measure true bone density or apparent? (A rather pointed question!)

CANDIDATE: DEXA measures apparent density (obviously) as it is a two-dimensional measurement quantified in g/cm². Quantitative CT gives a volumetric (three-dimensional) true representation of bone density in g/cm³. Even quantitative CT can give false low readings as it also measures intravertebral fat.

EXAMINER: Which of the bone density measurement techniques can differentiate between cortical and trabecular bone?

CANDIDATE: Quantitative CT and quantitative MRI.

EXAMINER: What is FRAX score?

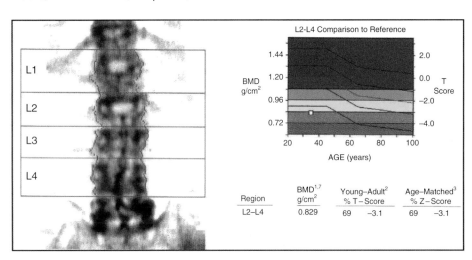

Figure 28.5 DEXA scan.

Region	BMD[1,7] g/cm²	Young–Adult[2] %	T–Score	Age–Matched[3] %	Z–Score
L2–L4	0.829	69	–3.1	69	–3.1

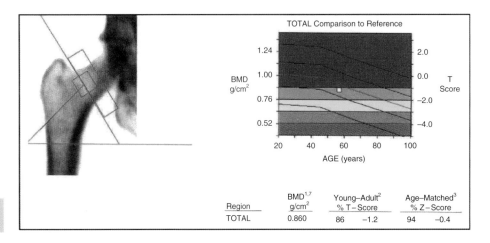

Region	BMD[1,7] g/cm²	Young–Adult[2] %	T–Score	Age–Matched[3] %	Z–Score
TOTAL	0.860	86	–1.2	94	–0.4

CANDIDATE: FRAX (Fracture Risk Assessment Tool) is the tool used to assess 10-year probability of hip/major osteoporotic fracture of patients. It integrates clinical risk factors with bone mineral densitometry for femoral neck. Treatment for osteoporosis is recommended if the FRAX score for hip fracture is more than 3% or that for major osteoporosis-related fracture is more than 20% (National Osteoporosis Foundation 2008).[8,9]

EXAMINER: What is the Singh and Maini index for osteoporosis?[10]

CANDIDATE: The Singh index has been described on the basis of the presence/attenuation of various compressile/tensile trabeculae on a plain anteroposterior(AP) pelvis radiograph. Grade 6 being normal and Grade 1 being severe osteoporosis.

EXAMINER: Any concerns with using the Singh index for measuring osteoporosis?

CANDIDATE: The Singh index traditionally was used in the diagnosis and classification of osteoporosis. Although it is a simple, cheap method for giving a rough measurement of bone mass, it has been shown to be an inaccurate method of estimating the degree of osteoporosis and the technique is not relevant with the current use of DEXA scans. DEXA scan provides a more precise estimate of bone mineral density and is considered the gold standard for diagnosis and quantification of osteoporosis (Figure 28.5).

Structured oral examination question 6

Bone scanning

EXAMINER: What are the principles of bone scanning? How does a bone scan work?

CANDIDATE: Bone scan involves the intravenous injection of 99mT-MDP (technetium methylene diphosphonate compound). The technetium gets adsorbed onto the hydroxyapatite crystals in bone and emits gamma rays, which are then received using a scintillation gamma camera. The gamma camera contains sodium iodide crystals, which absorb 99mT gamma rays. The received signal is amplified using photomultiplier tubes and processed using a computer to produce an image. It reflects blood flow and osteoblastic activity.

COMMENT: Some features of 99mT-MDP that could be asked by the examiners:

(1) Half-life: 6 hours.

(2) Excretion: urine – 70% of the administered dose is excreted within 24 hours.

(3) Dose: 500–600 MBq.

(4) Emits only gamma rays (not alpha or beta).

EXAMINER: What is a SPECT scan and give any uses.

CANDIDATE: Single photon emission tomography involves obtaining tomographic images on a bone scan. The scans are obtained with an arc of 360° around the patient. The images can then be reconstructed in axial, coronal and sagittal planes. The SPECT scan is especially useful to study the posterior spinal elements and to look for areas of decreased uptake in osteonecrosis. Sequential imaging with SPECT and CT with the patient in the same position can provide increased diagnostic accuracy by allowing fusion of the anatomical images.[11]

EXAMINER: What is PET scan and what is it used for?

CANDIDATE: A positron emission scan is mainly used for tumour diagnosis. It involves injection of ^{18}F fluoro-2-deoxy-glucose (FDG), which is a glucose analogue. Half-life: 110 minutes. FDG is transported into cells in a method similar to that of glucose but is not metabolized. Hence it accumulates in areas of high metabolic activity. Successful chemotherapy can cause a decrease in uptake compared to scans before starting chemotherapy.[1]

EXAMINER: What is the duration for which a bone scan can be positive following a fracture?

CANDIDATE: The bone scan usually becomes positive within 24 hours–3 days following a fracture. The dynamic flow component can remain positive for as long as 2–3 weeks following the fracture before returning to normal. The blood pool scan remains positive for approximately 8 weeks. The delayed static scan is usually positive for 6 months–2 years due to continuing bone healing and remodelling. In cases of malunion, it can remain positive indefinitely due to continued bone remodelling.

EXAMINER: What are the phases of a bone scan?

CANDIDATE:

Name	Timing following injection	Significance	Use
Dynamic/blood flow	1–2 minutes	Perfusion	–
Blood pool	3–5 minutes	Extent of bone/soft-tissue hyperaemia	(1) Inflammatory lesions: cellulitis and osteomyelitis (2) Vascular soft-tissue abnormalities such as tumours (3) Dating of traumatic lesions such as fractures or myositis ossificans
Static bone phase	4 hours	Displays sites at which tracer accumulates in skeletal structures when urinary excretion has decreased the amount of the radionuclide in soft tissues	(1) Occult bone or joint pain (2) Metastatic disease (3) Infection: cellulitis, osteomyelitis, multifocal osteomyelitis (4) Trauma: occult, stress fractures (5) Tumour: osteoid osteoma and osteoblastoma, especially spine (6) Primary malignant bone tumours, benign bone tumours (7) Painful joint arthroplasty (8) Avascular necrosis (9) Paget's disease
Delayed	24 hours	–	–

EXAMINER: What is a 'flare phenomenon' in bone scan?

CANDIDATE: The paradoxical increase in uptake and size on bone scan following chemotherapy for metastatic lesions, despite clinical improvement. This can last for up to 6 months following commencement of chemotherapy. This occurs as a result of bone repair following successful chemotherapy.

EXAMINER: Why is a bone scan not the best investigation to study the extent of a bone tumour?

CANDIDATE: The malignant neoplastic lesions may show increased uptake beyond the actual extent of the tumour due to the presence of hyperaemia and bone oedema occurring beyond the actual extent of the tumour.

[NB: Bone scans can be false negative in up to 50% of cases of multiple myeloma.]

EXAMINER: How does [67]gallium localize in sites of infection?

CANDIDATE: No clue.

COMMENT: Answer: Gallium localizes infection due to the following factors:

(1) Gallium is taken up by neutrophils as well as bacteria.
(2) Binding to lactoferrin/plasma transferrin.

(3) Increased vascularity.
(4) Increased capillary permeability.

EXAMINER: What advice will you give the patient after a bone scan?

CANDIDATE:

(1) Drink plenty of fluids for the rest of the day and go to the toilet often. Flush the toilet twice.
(2) Avoid contact with pregnant women.
(3) If travelling abroad in the 7 days following the scan, take a doctor's note along as ports and airports have very sensitive radiation detectors which may pick up tiny amounts of radioactivity remaining after the scan.

EXAMINER: This is a bone scan of a patient with a painful hip arthroplasty. What do you think (Figures 28.6a and b)?

CANDIDATE: The bone scan images are abnormal. They show a large area of intense hypervascularity at the medial aspect of the right proximal femur suggestive of possible infection or gross aseptic loosening.

EXAMINER: Describe the role of a bone scan in the investigations for a painful arthroplasty.

CANDIDATE: In cases of cemented hip and knee replacements, the bone scan can remain positive

(a)

(b)

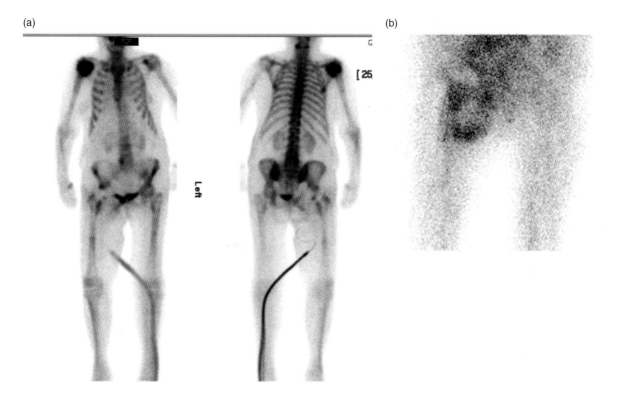

Figure 28.6 The hypervascular abnormality seen on images is suggestive of a soft-tissue abscess with a necrotic centre, possibly related to infection of the right hip prosthesis.

for up to 1 year following the operation. In the case of an uncemented THR, there can be increased uptake around the distal tip of the femoral stem for many years postoperatively. The reactive bone uptake in total knee replacement may persist up to 36 months after surgery.

Painful arthroplasty, more than 1-year postoperative:

- In case of suspected periprosthetic infection with radiographs showing no evidence of loosening, a bone scan generally shows an increased uptake in the delayed static phase as well as hypervascularity in the flow and blood pool phases.
- Mechanical loosening: a bone scan shows increased uptake in the region of loosening in the delayed bone phase due to the increased bone turnover. Blood flow and blood pool phases are normal.

Although a technetium bone scan is sensitive for diagnosing infection, it is not specific. Gallium- and indium-labelled WBC scans are more specific for infection.

Structured oral examination question 7

Nerve conduction studies

EXAMINER: What are nerve conduction studies?

CANDIDATE: Nerve conduction studies examine the electrical function of nerves and muscles. They can detect loss of axons by looking at the amplitude of the responses and loss of myelin by looking at the conduction velocity of the responses.

EXAMINER: How are they performed?

CANDIDATE: Sensory studies are performed by placing recording electrodes over the course of the nerve and stimulating it. The sensory responses are called SNAPs (sensory action potentials) (Figure 28.7). Motor studies are also performed by stimulating the nerve, but the signals are picked up over the muscles. Their

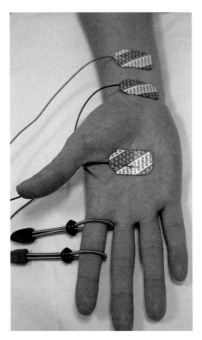

Figure 28.7 Sensory testing (orthodromic stimulation using ring electrodes) of the median innervated digit II.

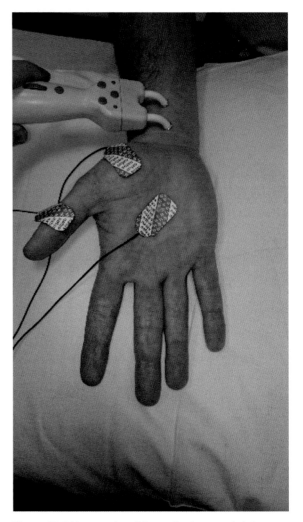

Figure 28.8 Motor testing of the median innervated abductor pollicis brevis (APB) muscle.

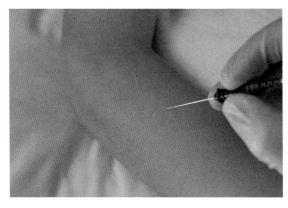

Figure 28.9 EMG studies.

responses are called CMAPs (compound muscle action potentials) (Figure 28.8).

EMG is performed with a fine concentric needle (a needle within a needle to record the potential difference). Here, the extensor digitorum communis (EDC) muscle is being assessed (Figure 28.9).

EXAMINER: Why are the SNAPs so important and draw the anatomy.

CANDIDATE: SNAPs determine whether a nerve lesion is post-ganglionic (i.e. a peripheral

neuropathy) when they are reduced or preganglionic when they are normal (i.e. radiculopathy, polio, motor neuron disease, etc. and some very exceptional neuropathic disorders).

The reason for this is that NCS test the circuitry of nerves up to their cell body. Because the dorsal root ganglion (DRG) is the cell body of the peripheral nerves, and is located outside of the intervertebral foramina, they tend to be spared from radicular compression, even if their dorsal roots are compressed (Figure 28.10). Hence, the SNAPs will be unaffected, even though the patient is experiencing numbness.

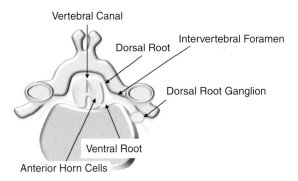

Figure 28.10 Cross-sectional arrangement of dorsal root ganglion.

Structured oral examination question 8

Nerve conduction studies

EXAMINER: Tell me some of the uses of nerve conduction studies? What are the indications for nerve conduction studies?

CANDIDATE: Nerve conduction studies (NCS) are used to assess peripheral nerves. The most common indications are for assessing focal entrapment neuropathies such as carpal tunnel and cubital tunnel lesions. NCS provide an electrical map of large myelinated nerve function and can therefore be used to determine:

(1) The presence and severity of peripheral nerve dysfunction.

(2) Whether it is axonal or demyelinating.

(3) Localization and distribution.

(4) Clues to the underlying aetiology.

(5) Prognosis.

EXAMINER: What is latency, amplitude and conduction velocity?

CANDIDATE: Latency = time between the stimulus discharge and the onset of response in milliseconds.

Amplitude = size of the response. For sensory nerves, this is in microvolts (millionths of a volt) and for motor nerves this is in millivolts (thousandths of a volt). These are usually measured from baseline to negative peak (by convention is displayed upright, see the diagram below).

Conduction velocity (m/s) = is a simple calculation of distance the impulse has travelled divided by the time it has taken to do so.

For sensory nerves where stimulation and recording are directly over the nerve, this is the distance between the stimulation site and the recording site (mm) and divided by the time for signal transmission (ms) (Figure 28.11).

For motor studies, this is a little more complex as while stimulation is over the nerve, the signal is recorded over the corresponding muscle. This will therefore include not only the time taken for the current to pass along the nerve, but also the time taken for neuromuscular transmission and then muscle membrane depolarization and contraction. Distal motor stimulation is therefore recorded and interpreted as a latency. More proximal stimulation points can provide accurate velocity values once the distal latency is removed. Hence the calculation will be the distance (mm) between proximal and distal stimulating sites / (proximal latency (ms) − distal latency (ms)) (Figure 28.12).

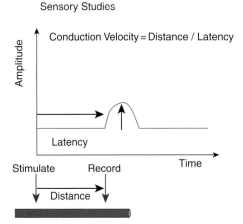

Figure 28.11 Sensory conduction velocity.

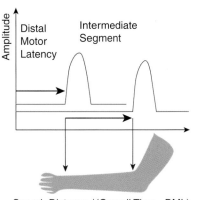

Speed = Distance / (Overall Time - DML)

Figure 28.12 Motor conduction velocity.

EXAMINER: What is the normal conduction velocity?

CANDIDATE: Normal conduction velocities in the upper limb are usually around 50–70 m/s and for the lower limb are around 40–50 m/s. Conduction velocities are sensitive to temperature, as cooling slows the velocities. Performing NCS in the upper limbs above 32°C is therefore a standard of practice to avoid misdiagnosing conditions such as carpal tunnel syndrome. The degree of myelination is less at birth and so conduction values are about 50% of the adult values, increasing to about 75% by 12 months and 100% by 4–5 years.

EXAMINER: What is supramaximal stimulation?

CANDIDATE: When electrically stimulating the nerves, it is important to ensure that all the nerve fibres are fully stimulated to their maximum response. Failure to ensure this will result in inaccurate readings. It is one of the most common reasons for operator error and can lead to reduced amplitudes and prolonged latencies. Stimulus intensity is incrementally increased until a maximal amplitude is reached and then further increased by a further 20–30% to ensure this. Typical intensities are around 30–40 milliamps.

EXAMINER: What are orthodromic and antidromic potentials?

CANDIDATE: Nerve fibres are designed to transmit their signal in one direction only by voltage and time-gating mechanisms. For sensory nerves this is from the peripheries toward the central nervous system (CNS). Motor nerves transmit signals from the CNS to the peripheral nerves and then muscles. However, when nerves are externally stimulated, as in NCS, depolarization is bidirectional.

Orthodromic potentials follow the physiological route, i.e. sensory potentials towards the spinal cord and motor potentials away from the spinal cord.

Antidromic studies (flowing against the physiological direction) can also be performed for sensory potentials.

In the UK, orthodromic responses are preferred in the hands as they provide the most accurate take off latencies which are important for evaluating carpal tunnel. In the feet, antidromic studies are preferred as they provide the most accurate

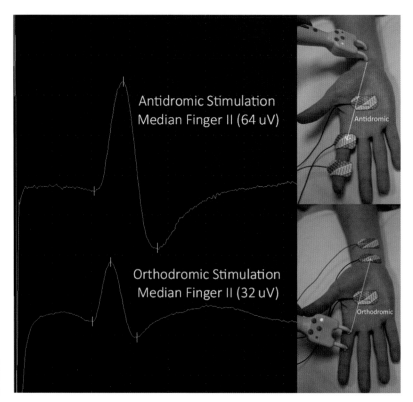

Figure 28.13 Note the difference in amplitude produced by orthodromic and antidromic stimulation.

Table 28.1 SNAP values.

Nerve (Stim, Rec Site)	Amp (uV)	Vel (m/s)	Amp (uV)	Vel (m/s)	Amp (uV)	Vel (m/s)
Age	20		40		80	
Ulnar (Digit 5–wrist)	10	55	5	50	2.5	45
Median (Digit 2–wrist)	20	55	10	50	5	4.5
Superficial Radical (Forearm–snuff box)	30	55	15	50	7.5	45

Nerve (Stim, Rec Site)	Amp (uV)	Vel (m/s)	Amp (uV)	Vel (m/s)	Amp (uV)	Vel (m/s)
Age	20		40		80	
Sural (Posterior lower leg–lat malleolus)	20	45	10	40	5	35
Superficial Peroneal (Anterior lower leg–dorsum ankle)	10	45	5	40	2.5	35

Table 28.2 CMAP values.

Nerve (Stim, Rec Site)	DML (ms)	Intermediate conduction velocity (m/s)	Amplitude (mV)	F-responses (ms)
Ulnar (Wrist–ADM)	3.5	50	10	< 33
Median (Wrist–APB)	4.5	50	5	< 33
Peroneal (Ankle–EDB)	5.5	40	2.5	< 55
Tibial (Ankle–AH)	6.5	40	5	< 55

amplitudes which are important for assessing peripheral neuropathy.

Orthodromic potentials are generally smaller in amplitude but have a cleaner signal definition as only the sensory fibres are stimulated. Antidromic potentials are generally larger amplitude because the sensors are closer to the underlying nerve but are more susceptible to signal artefacts due to co-stimulation of motor fibres (Figure 28.13).

EXAMINER: What are the usual SNAP values you would expect to see in a healthy individual and is there an easy way to remember them?

CANDIDATE: If one takes an average build 40-year-old, the minimal SNAP amplitudes will be 5, 10, 15 microvolts for the ulnar, median and radial responses, respectively, and 5 and 10 microvolts for the superficial peroneal and sural SNAPs.

One can double these for a 20-year-old and halve these for an 80-year-old. The minimal velocities will be roughly 50 m/s at 40, a bit faster at the age of 20 (55 m/s) and a bit slower at the age of 80 (45 m/s) (Table 28.1).

In addition, no side should be less than 50% of the contralateral side.

EXAMINER: What are the typical values of CMAPs?

CANDIDATE: For a typical 40-year-old person, the following values would be expected (Table 28.2). In contrast to the sensory response, there is more variability from overall muscular build, hence a person with a small hand may have a smaller ADM amplitude of around 6–7 mV and a strapping builder would be expected to have a larger ADM amplitude of around 13–15 mV.

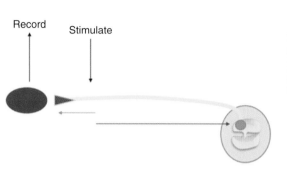

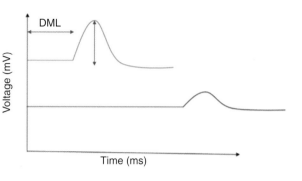

Figure 28.14 F-waves.

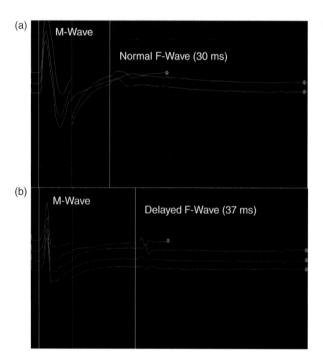

Figure 28.15 Latent responses. (a) F-waves, (b) normal delayed.

A 50% asymmetry in amplitude will also be abnormal.

Further variation will depend on age and height. With increasing age, amplitudes become smaller. Distal motor latencies (DML) and F-waves increase, i.e. prolong, with age and height, and intermediate conduction velocity will reduce with cooling (and therefore age and height as well).

EXAMINER: What are F-waves?

CANDIDATE: Electrical stimulation of a peripheral nerve causes depolarization in both directions (orthodromic and antidromic) (Figure 28.14).

The antidromic passage of current will enter up into the anterior horn cells and irritate a small percentage of them. This causes a secondary orthodromic response to be generated by them down to the muscles. These are small responses which tend to be around 10% of the motor amplitude and are termed F-waves (so-called because they were first described in the feet but are also present in the hands).

They are measured as a latency (ms) and reflect conduction across the entire motor pathway (up and down). They are therefore proportional to limb length and typical values should not exceed

33 ms in the upper limbs and 55 ms in the lower limbs for average height individuals. F-waves are not a reflex as they only travel in the α motor fibres and do not involve any sensory fibres.

Significance:

(1) Evaluation of proximal (nerve root/plexus/proximal segment) lesions of peripheral nerves.

(2) Early loss of these in Guillain–Barré Syndrome where demyelination often commences in the nerve roots.

(3) Radiculopathy (C8/T1 and L5/S1).

Here are two examples of F-waves from the ulnar nerve (Figure 28.15). The first one shows normal latencies of 30 ms (notice how they are much smaller than the direct muscle activation/M-wave). The second shows delayed latencies which were secondary to a cubital tunnel lesion.

EXAMINER: What is the 'H' reflex?

CANDIDATE: Named eponymously after Hoffmann (who worked for Erb). This is a true reflex whereby a selective stimulation of the 1a muscle spindle sensory afferent fibres will activate a monosynaptic spinal cord reflex causing contraction of the corresponding muscle. This requires submaximal stimulation of the mixed nerve. It is the neurophysiological equivalent of an ankle jerk and is only routinely studied in the tibial innervated soleus muscle (Figure 28.16).

The clinical application of H reflex:

(1) In cases of unilateral sciatica, it helps to differentiate S1 (unilateral abnormality of soleus H reflex) from an L5 radiculopathy.

(2) In evaluation of demyelinating neuropathies (early loss in Guillain–Barré Syndrome).

(3) Demonstrating that reflexes are intact when otherwise difficult to obtain clinically, e.g. the elderly.

EXAMINER: How does H-reflex differ from the direct motor or M-wave?

CANDIDATE:

(1) To achieve an H-reflex the sensory fibres need to be selectively stimulated at low intensity. Initially, there are no direct motor responses from direct orthodromic stimulation (M-responses = CMAPs), only via the H-reflex (Figure 28.17a).

(2) As stimulation increases, the direct M-wave will appear. However, there will be collision of

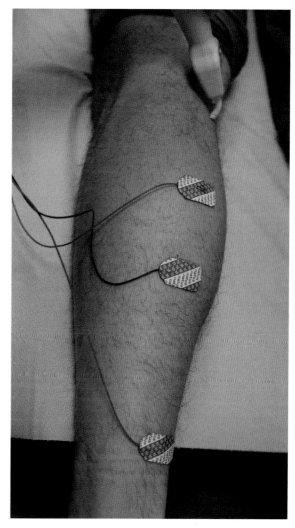

Figure 28.16 Here you can see the tibial nerve being stimulated at the popliteal fossa and the recording electrodes are placed over the soleus and the Achilles tendon (a ground electrode is placed between the stimulation and recording electrodes to reduce artefact).

impulses from the now activated motor fibres (ascending antidromically) which will arrest and diminish the H-reflex (Figure 28.17b). When the motor response becomes maximal, the H-reflex disappears and is replaced by a small late motor response, the F-wave.

(3) Hence, H-reflexes are present at low stimulation and decrease with increasing stimulation and their amplitudes are relatively higher than M-waves for low-intensity stimuli.

(4) H-reflexes are proportional to height and for an average height individual of 170 cm should be less than 33 ms.

(5) After the age of 1 year, the H-reflex tends to persist only in the calf muscle and FCR (flexor carpi radialis).

Structured oral examination question 9

EMG

EXAMINER: Describe 'end plate activity' on EMG.

CANDIDATE: A healthy muscle should be silent at rest. However, if the EMG needle is inserted into the 'end plate' region, i.e. the point where the neuromuscular junctions (NMJs) are located, two types of activity can be detected.

(1) Spontaneous release/leakage of acetyl choline from the NMJs leading to non-propagating contraction of parts of some of the muscle fibres.

(2) Direct irritation of the NMJs leading to some release of acetylcholine.

Because the release of acetylcholine is so small, it is insufficient to depolarize the entire muscle fibre, and these are known as 'muscle end plate potentials'. The neurophysiologist must be able to distinguish these from pathological spontaneous activity such as fibrillations by the following characteristics:

- End plate noise: small, high-frequency, negative, monophasic potentials which sound like seashells.

- End plate spikes: small, biphasic and fire irregularly at high frequency and have a crackling sound. These are believed to be caused by needle irritation of the NMJ.

Both of these usually occur together and the neurophysiologist will usually first be alerted by the patient as these sites of insertion are often quite painful in contrast to other regions of muscle tissue where EMG is usually painless. Adjustment of the needle's position will cease the discomfort and these activities.

EXAMINER: What is 'insertional' activity on EMG?

CANDIDATE: When an EMG needle is inserted into a muscle it causes a brief period of irritation leading to a brief burst of activity lasting up to 300 ms and is called 'insertional' activity.

COMMENT: In Figure 28.18, the needle was just inserted and was followed by sustained elctrical activity with the patient at rest lasting around 700 ms (100 ms is shown here).

Increase: Any cause of muscle membrane irritability – either from a myopathy/myositis or in the very acute stages of a neuropathy.

Decrease: Chronic denervation where muscle fibres have been replaced by fibrosed or fatty tissues.

EXAMINER: Name some of the types of 'spontaneous' activity found in a relaxed muscle.

CANDIDATE: Any activity in a relaxed muscle that lasts longer than physiological insertional activity (i.e. 300 ms) AND is outside of an end plate zone is abnormal and is called 'spontaneous' activity.

Types:

1. Fibrillations:
   a. Action potentials that arise spontaneously from single muscle fibres.
   b. Rhythmic regular firing (their hallmark) which eventually slows and becomes duller over several seconds.
   c. Biphasic or triphasic (initial positive spike).
   d. When abundant, they sound like 'raindrops on a tin roof'.
   e. Present in both myopathic and neuropathic pathologies.
   f. In denervation, they are thought to be caused by secondary upregulation of ACh-receptors, leading to an increased probability of local depolarization.
   g. In myopathies, they are thought to arise from leaky muscle membranes, again leading to increased probability of local depolarization.
   h. In the upper limbs they take at least 14 days to appear and in the lower limbs 21 days, following denervation.
   i. As conditions become chronic, they diminish in amplitude (Figure 28.19).

2. Positive sharp waves (Figure 28.20):
   a. These equate to fibrillations.
   b. Initial positive phase followed by a slow prolonged phase leading to a duller popping sound (see example).

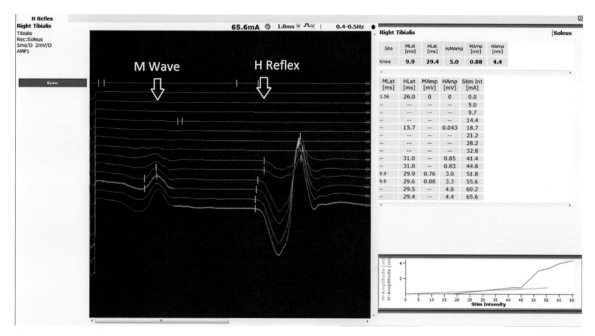

Figure 28.17a H-reflex.

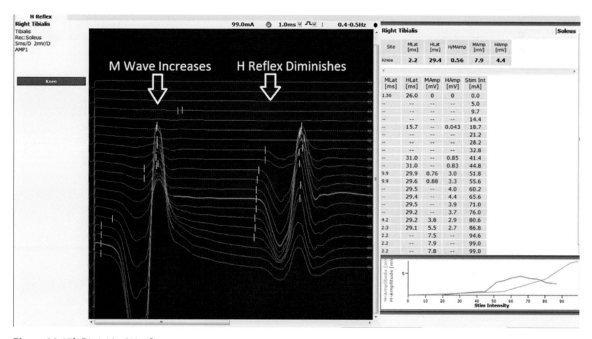

Figure 28.17b Diminished H-reflex.

c. Thought to differ from fibrillations in that the EMG needle may slightly deform the muscle membrane, making it unexcitable and so altering the morphology of the discharge. Movement of the EMG needle can switch the appearances to fibrillations.

d. Sometimes seen prior to fibrillations but usually coexist.

e. Arise from single fibres.

f. Biphasic or triphasic.

3. Fasciculation potentials:

a. Spontaneous single discharges of a group of muscle fibres representing part/whole of

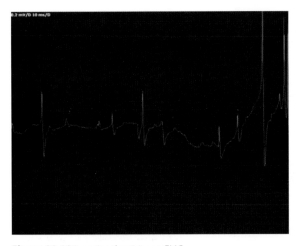

Figure 28.18 Insertional activity on EMG.

a motor unit and the source can be generated anywhere along it. In contrast to fibrillations, they do not arise from muscle pathologies.

b. Characteristic sound similar to 'popcorn' and tend to occur individually. This characteristic differentiates them from voluntary activity which occurs as trains of activity running at a frequency of at least 5 Hz. You can see this in Figure 28.21 with only a single motor unit visible on the screen.

c. Fasciculations are usually visible as twitches. EMG is particularly useful in looking for subtle or subclinical fasciculations.

d. They can occur in benign fasciculation syndrome, but also in any denervating process – and are a characteristic feature of anterior horn cell disease.

4. Myokymic discharges.

a. Group fasciculation potentials resulting from discharge of the same motor unit (Figure 28.22).

b. Characteristic sound of 'marching soldiers'.

c. Most important use is in differentiating radiation-induced plexopathy from tumour infiltration of the plexus, as they are a hallmark of radiation damage.

d. Can be found in any denervating condition.

5. Complex repetitive discharges.

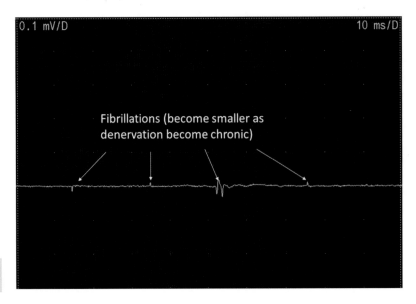

Figure 28.19 Fibrillations diminishing as denervation becomes chronic.

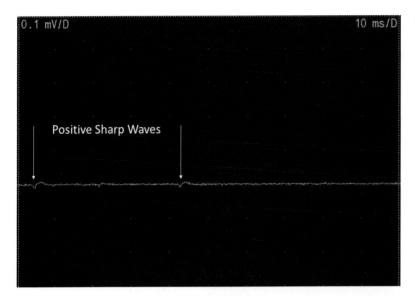

Figure 28.20 Positive sharp waves.

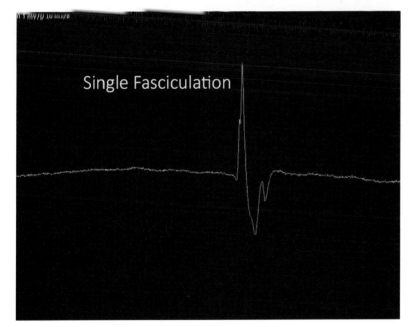

Figure 28.21 Single fasciculations.

a. These result from a circus movement of spontaneous discharges activating adjacent muscle tissues.

b. These often abruptly start and stop and have an 'engine'- or 'motor'-like sound due to their cyclic nature.

c. Because they need adjacent muscles to be in a state of disrepair to allow pathological spread of the currents (either neurogenic or myopathic causes) they tend to be seen in chronic states only, where fibre type grouping of muscle tissues has occurred.

d. In the example in Figure 28.23, you can see just how regular these are firing and some of the preceding discharges are visibly rastered beneath at the same frequency.

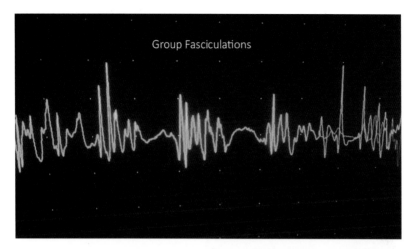

Figure 28.22 Group fasciculations.

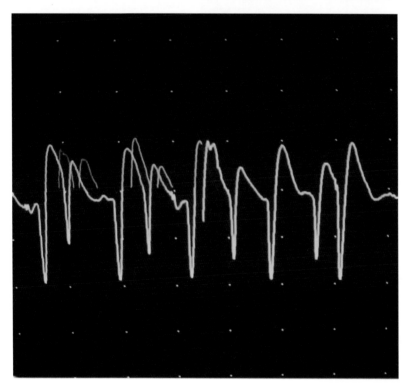

Figure 28.23 Complex repetitive discharges.

Structured oral examination question 10

Motor action potential

EXAMINER: Draw and describe a motor unit action potential.

CANDIDATE: MUAP is the summated electrical activity of the muscle fibres innervated by a single motor neuron. It is generally biphasic or triphasic (see Figure 28.24). In health, they make a sharp and crisp sound.

EXAMINER: Describe and explain the EMG findings in myopathy.

CANDIDATE: The electrical characteristics of MUAPs are proportional to the size of the muscle fibres generating them. In myopathies, the fibres shrink, leading to small-amplitude MUAPs. In

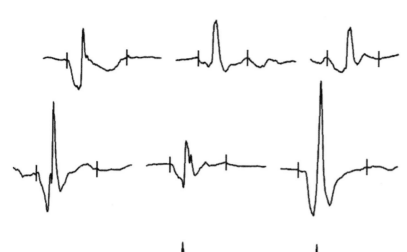

Figure 28.24 Motor unit action potential.

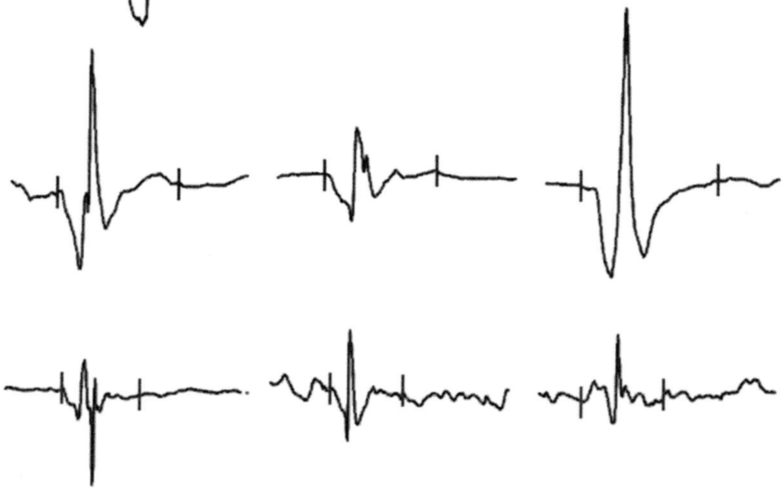

Figure 28.25 Motor unit action potentials in myopathy.

addition, the density of shrunken fibres increases around the needle insertion site in the muscle so the MUAPS appear small and spikey (see Figure 28.25).

Because the brain is trying to generate force, it attempts to force these shrunken fibres to do so by rapidly recruiting them to contract. Hence, early recruitment and full interference patterns of these small spikey units will be present and is the reason why myopathy patients complain of fatigue. Fibrillations/positive sharp waves/complex repetitive discharges may also be present and are a sign of active inflammation, i.e. myositis. In very chronic myopathic conditions, muscle fibre splitting can also cause denervation and so mixed patterns can be seen, e.g. inclusion body myositis.

EXAMINER: Describe and explain the EMG findings in neurogenic conditions.

CANDIDATE: The MUAP configuration will change from the acute to the chronic settings.

(1) Very acute setting (first 2–3 weeks) of complete axonal loss there will be no MUAPS and no fibrillations. Thereafter, fibrillations will appear and there will be no motor units recruited voluntarily as the brain's signals will not reach any of the muscle fibres.

(2) More commonly, axonal loss is partial. Again, fibrillations will not be present for the first 2–3 weeks. However, the remaining axons will be able to recruit their muscle fibres, but in a depleted way. Hence, the number of MUAPs visible on the screen (called the interference pattern) will be reduced.

(3) With time, nerve regeneration will occur. This will be both locally with terminal sprouting (adjacent nerve fibres growing into denervated muscle fibres) and more proximally, at the site of the nerve lesion.

(4) Local recovery will occur first and results in initially leaky and loose connectivity with those adjacent fibres. This will cause the morphology of the remaining MUAPs to widen and become serrated as those additional fibres become incorporated into that motor unit.

(5) As the innervation becomes increasingly stable and established, the additional serrations (= polyphasia) become increasingly incorporated into the main body of the MUAP. The MUAP also enlarges as collectively more muscle tissue is generating electrical activity.

(6) Hence, in chronic denervation, enlarged polyphasic units with reduced interference pattern are present. As regeneration progresses, while they retain their large amplitude, their morphology becomes less complex and their width reduces (Figure 28.26).

Upper motor neuron lesions: will show a reduced recruitment pattern, i.e. a lower firing frequency during maximal contraction as there is less 'drive' to contract the muscles.

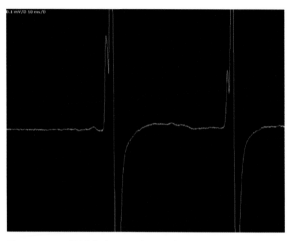

Figure 28.26 EMG findings in chronic degeneration.

Structured oral examination question 11

Nerve conduction studies

EXAMINER: Can you interpret these NCS of a 40-year-old male with tingling in the right radial 3.5 fingers (Table 28.3)?

CANDIDATE: We first analyze the SNAPs to see if this is a pre- or post-ganglionic process. The right F2 is smaller than expected and slower than expected and implies primary demyelination. The right F5 is normal and so there is no evidence of a more widespread neuropathy or brachial plexus lesion. The left F2 is of normal amplitude but is conducting slower than expected. The left F5 is normal. Therefore, we have bilateral focal median nerve lesions, right more than left, which are demyelinating and in keeping with bilateral carpal tunnel lesions.

Next, we check the MCVs (motor conduction velocities). The DML is quite prolonged on the

Table 28.3 NCS results for a 40-year-old male with tingling in the right radial 3.5 fingers.

SAP	Amplitude (uV)	Cond vel (m/s)
Right median (F2–wrist)	6	34
Right ulnar (F5–wrist)	12	57
Left median (F2–wrist)	16	40
Left ulnar (F5–wrist)	11	55

MCV		
Median (SE on APB)	**Right**	**Left**
DML	5.3 ms	3.7 ms
CV (wrist–elbow)	48 m/s	54 m/s
MAP (wrist)	5.4 mV	8.9 mV
MAP (elbow)	4.8 mV	8.6 mV
F latency	32 ms	27 ms
Ulnar (SE on ADM)	**Right**	**Left**
DML	2.3 ms	2.4 ms
CV (wrist–below elbow)	54 m/s	51 m/s
CV (around elbow)	65 m/s	62 m/s
MAP (wrist)	12.3 mV	11.2 mV
MAP (below elbow)	11.5 mV	11.1 mV
MAP (above elbow)	11.6 mV	11.0 mV
F latency	28 m/s	28 m/s

Table 28.4 Carpal tunnel syndrome grading of severity.

Padua scale (Padua 1997)			Canterbury scale (Bland 2000)	
Negative	*Normal findings in all tests	Grade 0	Normal	Normal findings in all tests
Minimal	Standard Negative I, but abnormal comparative or segmental tests	Grade 1	Very mild	Only detected in two sensitive tests
Mild	SNCV F1 < 42 m/s SNCV F3 < 44 m/s DML < 4.0 ms	Grade 2	Mild	SNCV F2 < 40 m/s DML < 4.5 ms
Moderate	Slowing of SNCV Abnormal DML	Grade 3	Moderate	Preserved SNAP 4.5 < DML < 6.5 ms
Severe	Absent SNAP Abnormal DML	Grade 4	Severe	Absent SNAP 4.5 < DML < 6.5 ms
Extreme	Absent SNAP, Absent CMAP	Grade 5	Very severe	Absent SNAP, DML > 6.5 ms
*Normal: SNCV >= 42 m/s, DML < 4 ms		Grade 6	Extremely severe	Absent SNAP, CMAP < 0.2 mV (peak to peak)

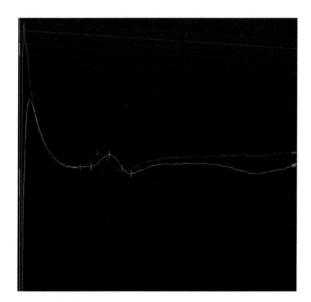

Figure 28.27 Pure sensory fibre conduction slowing.

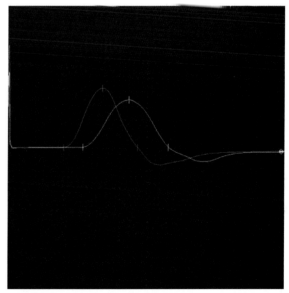

Figure 28.28 Distal motor fibre demyelination.

right and the amplitude is asymmetrically smaller than the left. This implies a focal and distal lesion of this nerve, again in keeping with carpal tunnel lesions. Forearm conduction is preserved. The F-wave is prolonged due to the impulse from the anterior horn cells being delayed through the carpal tunnel lesion. Left-sided median motor nerve studies and both ulnar nerve motor studies were normal.

In summary: there is moderate sensory and motor slowing of median fibres on the right and mild and purely sensory slowing of the median fibres on the left. The grades of the carpal tunnel lesions are therefore moderate on the right and mild on the left.

There are two commonly used neurophysiological grading scales for CTS, by Padua[12] and Bland[13] (Table 28.4). While the precise values of normal and abnormal are different between laboratories, the overall gradings reflect the pattern and degree of fibre involvement. Namely, first the sensory fibres are affected, and this is followed by the motor fibres. For each, the initial loss is of myelin due to the external compression and so the velocities reduce. This is then followed by axonal loss and the amplitudes reduce.

COMMENT: In Figure 28.27 you can see pure sensory fibre conduction slowing (median–digit II) in the green trace compared to the 'normal' side in the grey trace. The waveform has shifted towards the right, i.e. is delayed in time. This is the first stage of a carpal tunnel lesion.

In this second example (Figure 28.28), you can see distal motor fibre demyelination (median–APB) in the green trace, compared with the 'normal' side in the grey trace. The waveform has also shifted towards the right, i.e. is delayed in time. In addition, the amplitude has slightly diminished and the width

of the curve has also increased. This has occurred as more fibres are conducting slowly as they are being compressed. This is a typical finding in a moderate carpal tunnel lesion (Table 28.4).

Structured oral examination question 12

Nerve conduction studies

EXAMINER: Can you interpret these NCS of a 40-year-old male with tingling in the right ulnar 1.5 fingers (Table 28.5)?

CANDIDATE: We first analyze the SNAPs to see if this is a pre or post ganglionic process. The right F2 SNAP is normal. However, the right F5 is smaller than expected and also asymmetrically reduced compared to that on the left. We are therefore dealing with a post-ganglionic lesion, involving right ulnar nerve fibres.

Next, we check the MCVs (motor conduction velocities). These are normal for the right median

Table 28.5 NCS results for a 40-year-old male with tingling in the right ulnar 1.5 fingers.

SAP	Amplitude (uV)	Cond vel (m/s)
Right median (F2–wrist)	14	56
Right ulnar (F5–wrist)	3	48
Left median (F2–wrist)	16	57
Left ulnar (F5–wrist)	11	52

MCV		
Median (SE on APB)	**Right**	**Left**
DML	3.3 ms	3.2 ms
CV (wrist–elbow)	54 m/s	51 m/s
MAP (wrist)	7.4 mV	7.6 mV
MAP (elbow)	7.2 mV	7.4 mV
F latency	31 ms	29 ms
Ulnar (SE on ADM)	**Right**	**Left**
DML	2.3 ms	2.2 ms
CV (wrist–below elbow)	55 m/s	54 m/s
CV (around elbow)	37 m/s	60 m/s
MAP (wrist)	5.8 mV	11.1 mV
MAP (below elbow)	5.4 mV	11.0 mV
MAP(above elbow)	2.4 mV	10.7 mV
F latency	36 m/s	29 m/s

Table 28.6 Padua grading for ulnar nerve compression.

Padua grade	Motor conduction across the elbow
Negative	No motor slowing, i.e. conduction velocity > 50 m/s and above-elbow velocity > below-elbow velocity
Minimal	Motor conduction slowing < 10 m/s across the elbow
Mild	Motor conduction slowing > 10 m/s or absolute velocity < 50 m/s
Moderate	Motor conduction slowing across the elbow AND SNAP < 6 μV
Severe	Motor conduction slowing across the elbow AND absent SNAP

nerve. However, the right ulnar nerve shows conduction slowing across the elbow and some conduction block. This is not present on the left side. The F-wave is also prolonged as the impulses from the anterior horn cells are being delayed through the cubital tunnel.

In summary: there is moderate motor slowing of the ulnar fibres on the right at the level of the elbow together with a reduced sensory amplitude. These are signs of focal demyelination at this level which are in keeping with a moderate cubital tunnel lesion.

The best-described neurophysiological grading scales for cubital tunnel are from Padua[14] (Table 28.6). In contrast to carpal tunnel, the motor fibres tend to be affected first and are followed by the sensory fibres (with rare exceptions and is thought to relate to the orientation of the fibres against the olecranon groove). Initially, the myelin becomes affected and conduction velocity drops due to the external compression. This is then followed by axonal loss with loss of amplitude.

Structured oral examination question 13

Nerve conduction studies

EXAMINER: Can you interpret these NCS of a 20-year-old female with tingling in the right ulnar 1.5 fingers (Table 28.7)?

CANDIDATE: Firstly, analyzing the SNAPs, there is absence of the right ulnar digit V, dorsal cutaneous and medial antebrachial cutaneous responses. These identify a post-ganglionic lesion which is above the level of cubital tunnel, given the involvement of the medial antebrachial cutaneous nerve. MCVs showed a very reduced APB response (median) with sparing of the sensory fibres, so this can't be carpal tunnel-related (notice a little slowing of the DML as a secondary phenomenon to the severe axonal loss). I also see some axonal loss of the ADM muscle, but not as much as the APB or IDIO (first dorsal interosseous). These findings are suggestive of a lower trunk plexopathy. I would wish to see the EMG (Table 28.8)

CANDIDATE: The EMG shows active denervation (fibrillations) with underlying chronic denervation (enlarged, wide, polyphasic units) in the T1–C8 innervated muscles. These are in keeping with the pattern seen in the NCS findings (APB + FDIO smaller CMAP amplitudes than the ADM). Paraspinal EMG was normal and so excludes the possibility of a superimposed C8/T1 radiculopathy.

This combination of sensory and motor axonal denervation is in keeping with a lower trunk brachial plexopathy and at this age, I would consider a thoracic outlet syndrome as the primary differential and arrange for the appropriate imaging. Had this been an 80-year-old patient, I would consider a pancoast tumour as the primary differential.

Structured oral examination question 14

Nerve conduction studies

EXAMINER: Can you interpret these NCS of a 40-year-old with numbness in the left leg and a foot drop (Table 28.9)?

CANDIDATE: All the sensory responses are normal and so this cannot be due to a peripheral neuropathy. Motor responses show significant reduction in the CMAPs on the left side for both the peroneal-EDB and tibial-AH motor studies and prolongation of their F-waves. This suggests a pre-ganglionic lesion. EMG findings corroborate active moderate denervation in the muscles

Table 28.7 NCS results for a 20-year-old female with tingling in the right ulnar 1.5 fingers.

SAP	Amplitude (uV)	Cond vel (m/s)
Right median (F2–wrist)	20	56
Right ulnar (F5–wrist)	Absent	–
Right ulnar (dors cut)	Absent	–
Right med cut (elbow–forearm)	Absent	–
Left median (F2–wrist)	25	57
Left ulnar (F5–wrist)	15	52
Left ulnar (dors cut)	20	58
Left med cut (elbow–forearm)	14	68

MCV		
Median (SE on APB)	**Right**	**Left**
DML	4.1 ms	3.2 ms
CV (wrist–elbow)	49 m/s	51 m/s
MAP (wrist)	0.5 mV	7.6 mV
MAP (elbow)	0.4 mV	7.4 mV
F latency	Absent	29 ms
Ulnar (SE on ADM)	**Right**	**Left**
DML	3.4 ms	2.2 ms
CV (wrist–below elbow)	49 m/s	54 m/s
CV (around elbow)	56 m/s	60 m/s
MAP (wrist)	3.6 mV	11.1 mV
MAP (below elbow)	3.1 mV	11.0 mV
MAP (above elbow)	3.2 mV	10.7 mV
F latency	36 m/s	29 m/s
Ulnar (SE on IDIO)	**Right**	**Left**
DML	3.9 ms	2.3 ms
MAP (wrist)	0.3 mV	8.4 mV

Table 28.8 EMG results.

EMG	
Right biceps	Normal to 2 mV
Right triceps	Normal to 2 mV
Right brachioradialis	Normal to 2 mV
Right ext dig comm	No spontaneous activity. Mild excess of polyphasic units of normal or increased duration. Some rather large units recruiting early to a mildly reduced interference pattern to 4 mV
Right APB	Fibs +. Mild excess of polyphasic units of normal or increased duration. Some rather large units recruiting early to a mildly reduced interference pattern to 5 mV
Right IDIO	Fibs 2+. Moderate excess of polyphasic units of normal or increased duration. Units firing at high rates in relative isolation in a severely reduced interference pattern to 7 mV
Right ADH	Fibs +. Mild–moderate excess of polyphasic units of normal or increased duration. Some rather large units recruiting early to a moderately reduced interference pattern to 5 mV
Right cerv parasp (lower)	Normal
Right thor parasp (upper)	Normal

Table 28.9 NCS results for a 40-year-old with numbness in the left leg and a foot drop.

SAP	Amplitude (uV)	Cond vel (m/s)
Right sural (calf–ankle)	26	49
Right sup peron (calf–ankle)	15	51
Left sural (calf–ankle)	25	52
Left sup peron (calf–ankle)	14	49
MCV		
Common peroneal (SE on EDB)	**Right**	**Left**
DML	4.3 ms	4.9 ms
CV (fib neck–ankle)	49 m/s	47 m/s
CV (pop fossa–neck)	64 m/s	53 m/s
MAP (ankle)	5.6 mV	0.5 mV
MAP (fib neck)	4.3 mV	0.4 mV
MAP (pop fossa)	4.9 mV	0.4 mV
F latency	46 ms	56 ms
Posterior tibial (SE on AH)	**Right**	**Left**
DML	4.5 ms	4.6 ms
MAP (ankle)	15.3 mV	3.6 mV
F latency	47 m/s	57 m/s
EMG		
Left vastus medialis	Normal	
Left tibialis anterior	Fibs +. Moderate excess of polyphasic units of normal or increased duration. Some rather large units recruiting early to a moderately reduced interference pattern to 6 mV	
Left gastroc (medial head)	Fibs+. Individual units of essentially normal configuration. Some rather large units recruiting early to a moderately reduced interference pattern to 6 mV.	

innervated by L5/S1 root levels. The findings are in keeping with an active left L5/S1 radiculopathy.

Structured oral examination question 15

Nerve conduction studies

EXAMINER: Can you interpret these NCS of a 40-year-old with numbness in the left leg and a foot drop (Table 28.10)?

CANDIDATE: The left superficial sensory SNAP is reduced and suggests a post-ganglionic lesion. Motor responses show slowing of motor conduction of the left peroneal nerve across the fibula neck. The F-wave is also prolonged as the signal is passing through the demyelinated zone. EMG confirms moderate active denervation in the tibialis anterior muscle. Absence of denervation in the tibialis posterior muscle excludes a sciatic lesion or L5 radiculopathy. The findings are in keeping with a moderate active left peroneal nerve lesion across the fibular neck.

Notes

1. Ramachandran M. *Basic Orthopedic Sciences*. London: Hodder Arnold; 2007.

2. Theocharopoulos N, Perisinakis K, Damilakis J, Papadokostakis G, Hadjipavlou A, Gourtsoyiannis N. Occupational exposure from common fluoroscopic projections used in orthopaedic surgery. *J Bone Joint Surg Am.* 2003;85:1698–1703.

Table 28.10 NCS results of a 40-year-old with numbness in the left leg and a foot drop.

SAP	Amplitude (uV)	Cond vel (m/s)
Right sural (calf–ankle)	26	49
Right sup peron (calf–ankle)	15	51
Left sural (calf–ankle)	25	52
Left sup peron (calf–ankle)	2.3	45
MCV		
Common peroneal (SE on EDB)	**Right**	**Left**
DML	4.3 ms	4.9 ms
CV (fib neck–ankle)	49 m/s	47 m/s
CV (pop fossa–neck)	64 m/s	33 m/s
MAP (ankle)	5.6 mV	1.2 mV
MAP (fib neck)	4.3 mV	1.2 mV
MAP (pop fossa)	4.9 mV	0.5 mV
F latency	46 ms	56 ms
Posterior tibial (SE on AH)	**Right**	**Left**
DML	4.5 ms	4.6 ms
MAP (ankle)	15.3 mV	14.7 mV
F latency	47 m/s	47 m/s
EMG		
Left vastus medialis	Normal	
Left tibialis anterior	Fibs +. Moderate excess of polyphasic units of normal or increased duration. Some rather large units recruiting early to a moderately reduced interference pattern to 6 mV.	
Left tibialis posterior	Normal	

3. Martin DJ, Wells ITP, Goodwin C, Physics of ultrasound. *Anaesth Intens Care Med.* 2010;16(3):132–135.

4. Miller MD. *Review of Orthopaedics.* 5th Edition. Philadephia, PA: Saunders Elsevier; 2008.

5. Einhorn TA, O'Keefe RJ, Buckwalter JA (Eds.). *Orthopaedic Basic Science: Foundations of Clinical Practice.* 3rd edition. Rosemont, IL: American Academy of Orthopaedic Surgeons; 2007.

6. Burch J, Rice S, Yang H, *et al.* Systematic review of the use of bone turnover markers for monitoring the response to osteoporosis treatment: the secondary prevention of fractures, and primary prevention of fractures in high-risk groups. *Health Technol Assess.* 2014;18(11):1–180.

7. Sharma U, Stevermer JJ. Bisphosphonate therapy: when not to monitor BMD. *J Fam Pract.* 2009;58(11):594–596.

8. Kanis JA. Diagnosis of osteoporosis and assessment of fracture risk. *Lancet.* 2002;359;1929–1936.

9. www.sheffield.ac.uk/FRAX/tool.jsp

10. Singh M, Nagrath AR, Maini PS. Changes in trabecular pattern of the upper end of the femur as an index of osteoporosis. *J Bone Joint Surg [Am].* 1970;52A:457–467.

11. Waller M, Chowdhury F. The basic science of nuclear medicine. *Orthop Trauma.* 2016;30:3,201–222.

12. Padua L, LoMonaco M, Gregori B, Valente EM, Padua R, Tonali P. Neurophysiological classification and sensitivity in 500 carpal tunnel syndrome hands. *Acta Neurol Scand.* 1997;96(4):211–217.

13. Bland JD. A neurophysiological grading scale for carpal tunnel syndrome. *Muscle Nerve.* 2000;23(8):1280–1283.

14. Padua L, Aprile I, Mazza O, *et al.* Neurophysiological classification of ulnar entrapment across the elbow. *Neurol Sci.* 2001;22(1):11–16.

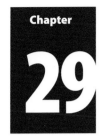

Chapter 29

Clinical environment

Jeevan Chandrasenan and Fazal Ali

Structured oral examination question 1

Sterilization

EXAMINER: What is the difference between sterilization and disinfection?

CANDIDATE: Sterilization is the process that destroys all forms of microbial life and is carried out in healthcare facilities by either chemical or physical methods. Disinfection, however, is a process that eliminates all pathogenic microorganisms, except bacterial spores or viruses.

EXAMINER: What about cleaning?

CANDIDATE: Cleaning is a physical process that removes contamination but does not necessarily destroy microorganisms.

EXAMINER: What forms of sterilization are you familiar with in the orthopaedic setup?

CANDIDATE: High-temperature sterilization of which prevacuum type is most commonly used for sterilization of instruments and linen.

Low-temperature sterilization, of which ethylene oxide and hydrogen peroxide gas plasma sterilization are more commonly used for temperature-sensitive instruments such as arthroscopes and drill and saw systems.

EXAMINER: How are instruments or linen sterilized?

CANDIDATE: Instruments and linen are sterilized in a controlled environment called the central sterile supply department (CSSD) that is divided into areas where the following is carried out:

I. Decontamination: manual or mechanical in water with detergents or enzymatic cleaners. Mechanical cleaners include ultrasonic washers.

II. Packaging: following a visual inspection, instruments are wrapped in a sterilization wrap or kept in rigid containers or instrument trays.

III. Sterilization, either high- or low-temperature depending on the instrument or item.

IV. Instruments or linen are then stored in separate sterile storage rooms.

EXAMINER: Can you think of any factors that can affect the efficacy of the sterilization process?

CANDIDATE: Factors that affect the process are inadequate cleaning beforehand, high residual protein or salt before sterilization, biofilm accumulation, instrument design (e.g. reduced lumen diameter or increased length of arthroscope, sharp bends, screws, hinges).

EXAMINER: How are sterilization processes monitored?

CANDIDATE: Sterilization procedures should be routinely monitored by:

I. Mechanical indicators that record time, pressure and temperature.

II. Chemical indicators that are usually heat- or chemical-sensitive inks that change colour when one or more sterilization parameters are present.

III. Biological indicators are the only process that directly monitors the lethality of a given sterilization process by using commercial preparation of spores. The presence of biological indicators following a sterilization process indicates the inadequacy to kill the microbial contaminates. This is a relatively inexpensive mode of monitoring.

EXAMINER: How are sterile instruments transported from CSSD to theatres?

CANDIDATE: Sterile instruments should be transported in covered or enclosed trolleys with solid-bottom shelves that are cleaned and disinfected after each use.

681

Structured oral examination question 2

Tourniquet use

EXAMINER: What is Figure 29.1 demonstrating?

CANDIDATE: This picture shows a pneumatic tourniquet with an airline to connect to a pneumatic device. Tourniquets are a useful adjunct in maintaining a relatively bloodless operative field.

EXAMINER: Can you tell me how you correctly size a tourniquet and select inflation pressure?

CANDIDATE: A correctly sized tourniquet should be at least one and a half times the circumference of the limb or proportional to the leg or arm diameter. There are no absolute values for inflation pressure and I consider the age of the patient, condition of the skin, and any intercurrent medical conditions such as peripheral vascular disease. In the upper limb, the inflation pressure should be 50 mmHg higher than the systolic pressure while in the lower limb the pressure should be double.

EXAMINER: When would you not use a tourniquet?

CANDIDATE: In patients with severe crush injuries, sickle cell disease, if there is a previous history of tourniquet problems or in severe peripheral vascular disease.

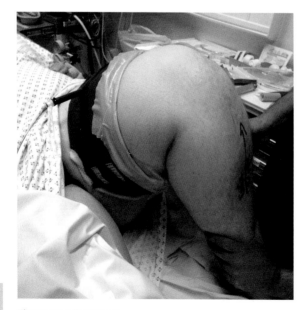

Figure 29.1 Tourniquet.

EXAMINER: What forms of exsanguination are there when using a tourniquet?

CANDIDATE: There is either exsanguination by elevation or expression. In patients with venous thromboembolism, infection or malignancy I would avoid exsanguination by expression as this risks spread by embolism.

EXAMINER: What complications can be encountered when using tourniquets?

CANDIDATE: Local complications can be pain or compression neuropraxia, skin pressure sores, postoperative swelling or compartment syndrome. Systemic complications can be cardiorespiratory decompensation, deep vein thrombosis, cerebral infarction or alterations in acid–base balance.

EXAMINER: What is tourniquet paralysis syndrome?

CANDIDATE: This a flaccid motor paralysis with sensory disturbance usually affecting pain sensation rather than temperature and is caused by cuff pressure and not ischaemia. Usually, colour, skin temperature and peripheral pulses are preserved. Patients with diabetic, alcoholic neuropathy or rheumatoid patients have increased susceptibility.

EXAMINER: How is this different to post-tourniquet syndrome?

CANDIDATE: Post-tourniquet syndrome is a reperfusion injury and is due to ischaemia after release of the tourniquet usually after 2 hours of inflation. Signs include oedema, stiffness, pallor, weakness and subjective numbness.

EXAMINER: What should you do about the tourniquet if you are performing a long operation?

CANDIDATE: Release after 2 hours. The tourniquet should be deflated for at least 20 minutes before re-inflation. After that it can remain inflated for up to 60 minutes.

Structured oral examination question 3

Sutures

EXAMINER: What type of sutures do you use in your practice?

CANDIDATE: I use absorbable sutures like vicryl or non-absorbable such as prolene.

EXAMINER: What are the differences between vicryl and prolene?

CANDIDATE: Vicryl is a form of braided suture and is absorbable while prolene is a monofilament suture and non-absorbable.

EXAMINER: What is the effect of braiding?

CANDIDATE: The effect of braiding is to increase the friction coefficient and hence the ability to fix knots is improved when compared to monofilament sutures.

EXAMINER: Are there any disadvantages of using braided sutures?

CANDIDATE: Braided sutures have an increased risk of promoting infection due to capillarity, as the interstices between fibres can facilitate the spread of pathogens along the fibre and thus to the placement site. In addition, braided sutures have a relatively rough surface which can cause a 'saw effect' when the thread passes through the tissues.

EXAMINER: Can you give me examples of approximate resorption and wound support times for common sutures you use?

CANDIDATE: Monocryl: wound support 20 days
Resorption 90–120 days

Vicryl: wound support 30 days
Resorption 50–70 days

PDS: wound support 60 days
Resorption 6–8 months

Structured oral examination question 4

Electrosurgery

EXAMINER: What does Figure 29.2 demonstrate?

CANDIDATE: This shows monopolar diathermy and a return electrode.

EXAMINER: How does monopolar diathermy work?

CANDIDATE: High-frequency (400 kHz–10 MHz) AC current passes between an active electrode and an indifferent electrode or plate. As the active electrode or instrument has a much smaller surface area than the plate it has a higher current density and creates high temperatures here rather than at the plate.

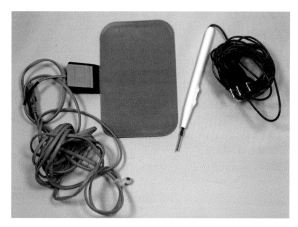

Figure 29.2 Monopolar diathermy.

As a result, it avoids damage through passage of current through surrounding tissue.

EXAMINER: How is this different to bipolar diathermy?

CANDIDATE: In bipolar diathermy the passage of high-frequency AC current is passed from the diathermy machine and then through the patient's tissue that is grasped between a pair of bipolar forceps.

EXAMINER: Are there any contraindications to using diathermy?

CANDIDATE: Although there are no absolute contraindications to using diathermy, care should be exercised when using diathermy in patients with pacemakers (use bipolar diathermy only) and avoidance of application of return electrode plate over internal metal implants such as joint replacements as well as avoiding contact to external metal objects to avoid unintended leakage of current to earth and burns.

EXAMINER: How does diathermy differ to radiofrequency ablation?

CANDIDATE: Radiofrequency ablation is a procedure in which the electrical conduction system of the heart, tumour, or other dysfunctional tissue is ablated using the heat generated from medium frequency alternating current (350–500 kHz). As this does not directly stimulate nerves or heart muscles, it can often be used without the need of general anaesthetic and in the outpatient setting with conscious sedation.

Structured oral examination question 5

Infection control

EXAMINER: What does Figure 29.3 show?

CANDIDATE: This is a slide of Gram-positive cocci demonstrated on Gram staining.

EXAMINER: How is a Gram stain performed?

CANDIDATE: Gram staining initially involves staining with crystal violet solution, then fixing with iodine solution and then finally washing with alcohol. Gram-positive bacteria retain the dye. Gram-negative dye washes out so is restained with safranin-O solution.

EXAMINER: Can you give me some examples of how antibiotics work?

CANDIDATE: Antibiotics can either be bacteriocidal or bacteriostatic or have mixed properties.

- Penicillins, cephalosporins and glycopeptides like vancomycin or teicoplanin inhibit cell wall synthesis.
- Aminoglycosides like gentamycin affect protein synthesis.
- Macrolides like erythromycin inhibit tRNA synthesis.
- Quinolones like ciprofloxacin inhibit DNA gyrase.
- Tetracyclines are bacteriostatic.

EXAMINER: Can you explain to me how resistance to antibiotics develops?

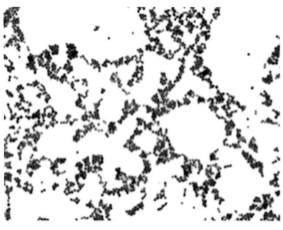

Figure 29.3 Gram-staining Gram-positive cocci.

CANDIDATE: Resistance can be intrinsic, where bacteria have the inherent ability to alter properties such as altering the target site or enzyme. Resistance can also be extrinsic or acquired via plasmids or mutations.

EXAMINER: What is MRSA?

CANDIDATE: It is a Gram-positive bacterium that acquires resistance to methicillin (older antibiotic) through a genetic mutation of the *mecA* gene resulting in penicillin-binding protein PBP2a.

EXAMINER: How do you prevent and treat MRSA in your unit?

CANDIDATE: It is prevented in my unit through an MRSA screening protocol and treated by an MDT approach in line with an infection control team and microbiologists. If screening swabs test positive, then patients are treated with 5 days of nasal mupirocin and 4% chlorhexidine bath and then re-swabbed. Patients undergoing joint arthroplasty should have three negative swabs.

EXAMINER: What would you do if you had four consecutive total hip replacement patients that became acutely infected whilst still inpatients?

CANDIDATE: This is a clinical governance emergency. I would expect a set protocolled action plan in my unit to be activated. I would inform my clinical lead in order to stop all elective operating. The next priority is the appropriate further care of the patients infected. This would involve a multidisciplinary team, barrier nursing and appropriate antibiotics instituted. A committee should be set up in order to investigate the outbreak responsible for reporting at a national level. This should involve the microbiologist and infection control team. Every step of the pathway should be investigated starting from preoperative assessment. All staff should be tested as potential carriers. Theatre suite efficiency and ward cleanliness should be investigated, particularly on whether or not ring-fencing protocols have been adhered to.

EXAMINER: What will you do if you find out you YOURSELF as the surgeon has MRSA?

CANDIDATE: Firstly it is worth noting that it is likely that many clinicians will be carriers. I would take an immediate opinion from my infection control team in the trust in order to inform them and to take their advice. Given that my work as an Orthopaedic surgeon involves working in 'high-risk' clinical areas, the advice that I would expect to receive would be to contact Occupational Health immediately in order to commence eradication therapy and to ensure that this is successful by re-swabbing. I would cease all clinical activity until this is the case. Non-clinical work may sometimes be possible, but this is normally subject to local protocol.

EXAMINER: Would you tell your patients?

CANDIDATE: All clinical work should be cancelled until full eradication therapy success has been confirmed. I will work with my clinical director in order to decide whether to transfer patients to other colleagues in order to balance the waiting list pressures. Patients should be informed of the reasons for their cancellations. In keeping with my duty of candour, I would perform an audit of all surgical cases performed in order to trace any potential MRSA infections contracted post-operatively. Should any cases be identified then these should be discussed as part of a multidisciplinary approach involving microbiology advice.

Structured oral examination question 6

Theatre design

EXAMINER: You are responsible for designing new orthopaedic theatres in your hospital. How would you go about doing this?

CANDIDATE: The theatre suite should be located close to the Emergency Department wards and the Radiology departments. It should be away from the general flow of the public.

There should be separate preparation, aseptic and disposal zones. The zones are there so that there are defined boundaries where specific activities can take place in the theatre environment.

Outer Zone: Rest of the hospital to the theatre reception.

Clean Zone: From theatre reception to the anaesthetic room doors.

Aseptic Zone: Inside the theatre itself.

Disposal Zone: Through the back door to the disposal area.

EXAMINER: What other structural aspects of design are important?

CANDIDATE: Consideration should be given to the walls, floor and doors. Ideally wall and floor coating should allow for easy cleaning. The walls tend to be polyurethane-coated and the floor epoxy resin-coated. The floors are antistatic and the junction between floor and walls are curved to allow more efficient cleaning.

Doors should open outwards as approximately 2 m³ of air is moved when a hinged door is opened. There is a minimal positive pressure gradient of 15 Pascal between the operating room and outside areas which aids the direction of flow of air if the doors open outwards.

Sliding doors cause less disruption and turbulence than hinged doors and are preferred.

EXAMINER: In considering the design of theatres what environmental factors are considered?

CANDIDATE: Lighting, temperature, humidity and ventilation.

- Lighting should cast minimal shadow, should not generate heat and should be at least 40,000 lux. Modern-day LED lights are 120,000 lux.
- The temperature in theatres should be 18–23°C. This is a compromise between what the theatre staff feel comfortable in and the ideal temperature for the patient, which is about 26°C. In order for the patient to achieve this temperature, warming devices are applied to the patient.
  There are two types: forced air warming devices and radiant warming devices. The forced air warming devices have been shown to affect the laminar air flow.
- Humidity should be 30–60%. Excessive humidity causes perspiration, and this will increase the shedding of bacteria.
- Ventilation could be through a plenum system or a laminar flow of ultraclean air.

Structured oral examination question 7

Ventilation

EXAMINER: What forms of air flow in theatre are you familiar with?

685

CANDIDATE: Plenum is air flow down a pressure gradient. This pressure gradient is highest in the preparation area and then air flows into theatres and then into the anaesthetic room and finally the disposal room. This type of airflow is subject to turbulence and eddies. In a plenum system there are 15–25 air changes per hour.

Laminar flow or streamline flow occurs when air flows in parallel layers with no cross-currents, eddies or disruption. Laminar air flow is intended uniform, directional air flow at a constant velocity with no air turbulence. This air flow essentially moves particles floating in the airstream away from the sterile field into the return ducts and filtration systems where they can be disposed of. For airflow to be laminar the velocity of air must be 9 m/s. In a laminar flow system there are about 200 air changes per hour.

EXAMINER: What types of laminar air flow systems are there?

CANDIDATE: Laminar air flow can be horizontal, vertical or newer systems in which the airflow takes the form of an inverted trumpet (exponential flow).

Exponential flow (ex-flow) systems work on the principle of graded velocity, with the flow in the centre being vertical and, in the periphery, radially outwards. Because of efficiency of the ex-flow system they can function at fewer air changes per hour than the traditional laminar flow systems.

EXAMINER: How is ultraclean air achieved in theatres and how is it monitored?

CANDIDATE: Ultraclean air is achieved by high efficiency particulate air (HEPA) filters mounted in the ventilation system. HEPA filters are 99.7% efficient filtering contaminants of 0.5 μm or greater in size. Modern HEPA filters also utilize ultraviolet light in order to increase their efficiency.

Filtration systems are usually monitored regularly where a 1 m^3 sample of air is obtained through a (Casella) slit sampler and introduced over an agar plate. Less than 10 colony forming units/m^3 (CFU/m^3) defines ultra-clean air.

In the plenum system, < 35 CFU/m^3 or < 1 clostridium or staph aureus/m^3 indicates an efficient system. In the laminar system around the theatre table it is < 10 CFU/m^3, but in the periphery of the theatre it should be < 20 CFU/m^3.

EXAMINER: What is the evidence for the use of laminar air flow in theatre?

CANDIDATE: Lidwell et al. (MRC trial) showed a reduction in deep sepsis by 50% with ultraclean air systems (3.4% down to 1.7%). There was a further reduction in deep infection rate by the additional use of systemic antibiotics (0.4%) and body exhaust suits (0.2%).

Recently, there have been some publications which have questioned the effectiveness of laminar air flow. In 2011 the results from the New Zealand joint registry suggested no reduction of early deep infection rate in patients undergoing both total hip and total knee arthroplasty.

An observational study of trauma in England (Pinder et al.) looking at surgical site infection in laminar flow vs. plenum flow theatres showed no difference between the two. In fact, the infection rate was significantly higher in hip hemiarthroplasties when performed in a laminar air flow theatre.

Structured oral examination question 8

Theatre etiquette

EXAMINER: Does the number of people in theatre matter?

CANDIDATE: 95% of theatre-acquired infection comes from air-borne contamination. Most of this is from theatre personnel, from which 90% of skin squames come from below the neck.

Ritter et al. showed that the bacteria count in the operating room air increases 3–4-fold in a theatre with 5 people compared to an empty room.

EXAMINER: So, what is 'entrainment' and how can this be prevented?

CANDIDATE: Entrainment refers to the situation which arises when theatre personnel or equipment disrupt the laminar air flow and the air (and particles) is diverted towards the operative field.

There are two main ways of preventing this. First, the use of a physical barrier (e.g. the 'side screens' that are placed around the tent to a level where they prevent persons or equipment entering the laminar flow field). The second method to prevent entrainment is the use of the ex-flow system via its inverted trumpet effect.

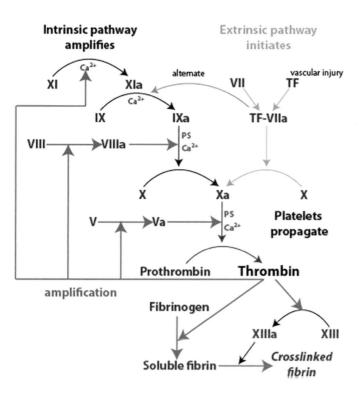

Figure 29.4 Coagulation cascade.

EXAMINER: What are your views on scrubbing?

CANDIDATE: Chlorhexidine decreases the bacterial count by 99% compared to povidone iodine, which is 97%. Chlorhexidine also lasts longer than povidone iodine.

Nicolay *et al.* found that:
- Alcohol rub after scrubbing has been shown to improve the effectiveness of the process.
- Brushes and sponges should not be used.
- Hot water should not be used as it decreases the antimicrobial powers of the antiseptics.

EXAMINER: What should a surgeon wear in theatre to reduce infection?

CANDIDATE: Ideally, protective gear in the form of a cap, mask, eye wear, double gloves, gowns, boots with impervious soles are essential for all surgeries.

Cotton is woven and lets particles less than 80 μm through. Goretex prevents particles greater than 0.2 μm, but is expensive.

Therefore, synthetic, hydrophobic, non-woven, disposable clothing made from spun-laced polyester pulp with mesh size much less than 80 μm is effective and more comfortable and convenient to wear.

Structured oral examination question 9

Perioperative bleeding

EXAMINER: What does Figure 29.4 show, and can you tell me how perioperative bleeding can be influenced by some common medication with reference to this pathway?

CANDIDATE: This demonstrates the coagulation cascade. The common anticoagulants can cause bleeding in the following way:

Aspirin: inactivation of cyclooxygenase (COX) enzyme.

Warfarin: inhibition of hepatic enzymes for vitamin K (factors II, VII, IX, X).

Heparin: antithrombin III inhibitor.

LMWH: indirect factor Xa inhibitor.

Rivaroxaban: direct factor Xa inhibitor.

EXAMINER: What is clopidogrel?

CANDIDATE: Clopidogrel is an irreversible platelet inhibitor with a half-life of 5–7 days. It is used in cardiac conditions and stents. It should be stopped 10 days prior to surgery, giving enough time for healthy platelets to form.

EXAMINER: How does tranexamic acid work? What is its role?

CANDIDATE: Tranexamic acid inhibits fibrinolysis by blocking plasmin effect on fibrin. It does not increase the proclivity for clot formation, but rather prevents the breakdown of a clot.

Tranexamic acid lowers the rate of transfusion without increasing the rate of venous thromboembolism.

Tranexamic acid can be delivered IV, topically or orally. For IV administration the patient requires normal renal clearance and no history of cardiac surgery or venous thromboembolism.

There is little difference in the effectiveness of the different modes.

EXAMINER: What other strategies are available to reduce perioperative blood loss in operations such as TKAs?

CANDIDATE: Although tranexamic acid is the most important, other strategies exist:

- Periarticular injections of analgesia plus adrenalin.
- Fibrin sealants.
- Bipolar sealant – a disposable device that requires its own energy generator but promotes coagulation of periarticular soft tissues.
- Avoidance of tourniquet during the surgery – as this will result in continuous cautery of bleeding during surgery. It is noted that the release of the tourniquet at the end of the procedure may cause a reflex hyperaemia which may increase the blood loss.
- The avoidance of suction drains.

References

Hooper GJ, Rothwell AG, Frampton C, Wyatt MC, et al. Does the use of laminar flow and space suits reduce early deep infection after total hip and knee replacement? The ten-year results of the New Zealand Joint Registry. J Bone Joint Surg (Br). 2011;93:85–90.

Lidwell OM, Elson RA, Lowbury RJ, et al. Ultraclean air and antibiotics for prevention of postoperative infection – a multicentre study of 8,052 joint replacement operations. Acta Orthop Scand. 1987;58:4–13.

McGovern PD, Albrecht M, Belani K, et al. Forced-air warming and ultra-clean ventilation do not mix – an investigation of theatre ventilation, patient warming and joint replacement infection in orthopaedics. J Bone Joint Surg (Br). 2011;93(11):1533–1544.

Nicolay CR. Hand hygiene: an evidence-based review for surgeons. Int J Surg. 2006;4(1):53–65.

Odinsson A, Finsen V. Tourniquet use and its complications in Norway. J Bone Joint Surg (Br). 2006;88B:1090–1092.

Pinder EM, Bottle A, Aylin P, Loeffler MD, et al. Does laminar flow ventilation reduce the rate of infection? An observational study of trauma in England. J Bone Joint Surg (Br). 2016;98:1262–1269.

Ritter MA, Eitzen H, French ML, Hart JB, et al. The operating room environment as affected by people and the surgical face mask. Clin Orthop Relat Res. 1975;111:147–150.

Chapter 30

Statistics and evidence-based practice

Munier Hossain and Sattar Alshryda

Introduction

Many examinees approach medical statistics with a lot of apprehension. This is justified in most circumstances as we do not regularly practise statistics, nor do we study it on a regular basis. Examiners are not different and appreciate this very well. You should remember that when you are asked questions related to medical statistics you are not expected to demonstrate the knowledge of a statistician. The examiners simply wish to satisfy themselves that as an inquisitive orthopaedic surgeon you understand the basic statistical concepts well enough to be able to scrutinize the published orthopaedic evidence. It is very unlikely that you will be asked esoteric questions (unless you do really well). Statistics of direct relevance (for example NJR survival analysis) are very popular with examiners and are frequently asked. Of the six basic science viva questions most of you would probably be asked at least one question related to Medical Statistics.

What kind of statistics question you get asked in the viva would depend on the stage of your viva. If your Basic Science viva commences with a statistics question this would be a 'settling' question designed to get you at ease. Remember when you

answer your question to remain to the point, but whenever you can feel free to use buzzwords designed to show your familiarity and also to tempt the examiner onto your comfort zone.

Below are examples through which we aim to demonstrate what kind of questions you are likely to be asked and how to address them. The answers are deliberately but thoughtfully expanded to better understand the subject around that particular question and to help address potential follow-up questions.

Structured oral examination question 1

EXAMINER: What do these lines represent (Figure 30.1)?

CANDIDATE: These are all bell-shaped curves of a 'Normal' distribution. The x-axis represents a variable (let it be weight, height, Hb level, Na level, hip score, knee score, etc.) and the y-axis represents the frequency of that variable.

EXAMINER: Why do you say this is 'Normal'?

CANDIDATE: A normal distribution of data is one in which the majority of data are relatively similar,

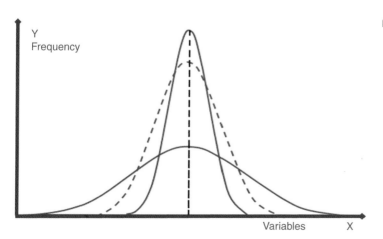

Figure 30.1 Bell-shaped curve normal distribution.

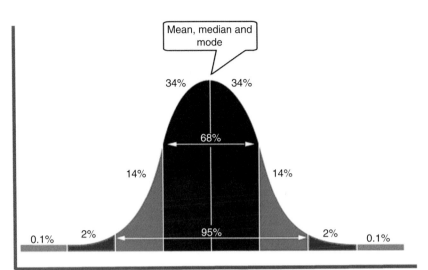

Figure 30.2 Normal distribution curve.

occurring within a small range of values such as height, weight, Hb level, K, Na, etc. Plotting normally distributed data results in a bell-shaped graph as shown here (Figure 30.1).

EXAMINER: What is the significance of this bell-shaped curve?

CANDIDATE: All normal distributions are symmetric and have bell-shaped curves with a single peak. They share important features that make statistical calculation and testing easy and reproducible. Two constant features of normally distributed curve are the mean, where the peak of the density occurs, and the standard deviation, which indicates the spread or girth of the bell curve. Although different variables yield different normal distributions, they all satisfy the 68–95–99.7% rule. Sixty-eight of the observations fall within 1 SD of the mean, 95% of the observations fall within 2 SD of the mean and 99.7% of the observations fall within 3 SD of the mean. Moreover, in normally distributed data, the mean, median and mode are all the same value and coincide with the peak of the curve (Figure 30.2).

EXAMINER: Why is it important to know whether your data are normally distributed or not?

CANDIDATE: So that we can choose the best way to present, analyze and test our findings. For example, I would use mean and SD to present my normally distributed data in contrast to mode, median and range in non-normally distributed data. I would use parametric tests (such as *t*-test, analysis of variance (ANOVA)) in comparing my findings if data were normally distributed, but I would use non-parametric tests (such as Wilcoxon rank test, Mann–Whitney U tests) if I was dealing with non-normally distributed data.

Authors note 1: Describing data

Data are the building stones for any study and it is expected that all candidates are confident in understanding and describing data. In our experience most candidates are; however, there is some confusion about the pros and cons of various methods of presenting data. In this section, we summarize some important aspects.

Data in general are divided into:

1. Categorical data: the objects being studied are grouped into categories based on some qualitative trait; hence, they are also called qualitative data. This is furthered classified into:

   a. Nominal: categories without order, e.g. smoking status, living status, marital status, etc.

   b. Ordinal: categories with order, e.g. social status, ficat grading, and pain score (mild, moderate, severe), etc.

   Either type can be binary (i.e. two categories only e.g. live or dead; married or unmarried; smoker or non-smoker) or not binary.

2. Measurement data: the objects being studied are measured based on some quantitative trait. Hence, they are also called quantitative data. This is further classified into:

Table 30.1 Statistical tests.

Testing	Normal distribution	Non-normal distribution	
		Ordinal, measurement data	Nominal data
Data description – central tendency (spread)	Mean (SD)	Median (range)	Proportion
Intervention in two different groups (such as placebo vs. treatment)	Unpaired *t*-test	Mann–Whitney U test	Chi-square (Fisher's test for sample samples of < 5)
Intervention in the same or matched group (such as Oxford hip or knee scores before and after joint replacement)	Paired *t*-test	Wilcoxon signed rank test	McNemars's test
More than two interventions in different groups (such as pain scores before and after two different non-steroidal anti-inflammatories)	ANOVA	Kruskal–Wallis test	Chi-square test
More than two interventions in the same or matched groups (such as pain scores before and after two different non-steroidal anti-inflammatories)	Repeated-measures ANOVA	Friedman test	Cochrane Q test
Quantifying association between two variables (e.g. recurrent falls and number of fractures)	Pearson correlation	Spearman correlation	Contingency coefficients
Regression analysis † (one variable)	Simple linear or non-linear regression	Non-parametric regression	Simple logistic regression
Regression analysis (several variables)	Multiple linear or non-linear regression		Multiple logistic regression

† Regression analysis involves modelling and analyzing several variables, when the focus is on the relationship between a dependent variable (for example, death) and one or more independent variables (for example, age, weight, comorbidities, haemoglobin level, etc.). It helps to understand how the dependent variable changes when any one of the independent variables is varied, while the other independent variables are held fixed.

a. Discrete: only certain values are possible (there are gaps between the possible values), e.g. number of admissions to an orthopaedic ward, number of spinal metastases, number of patients transfused.

b. Continuous: theoretically, any value within an interval is possible with a fine enough measuring device, e.g. age, height, weight, blood loss.

The type(s) of data collected in a study determine the type of presentation and statistical analysis used. Categorical data are commonly summarized using percentages or proportions and tested using Chi-square or Fisher exact tests. Summarizing measurement data depends on whether the data are normally distributed or not. If they are normally distributed they can be summarized using means and standard deviation and tested by parametric tests. If data are not normally distributed, they can be summarized

using mode, median, range and tested by non-parametric tests (Table 30.1). It is not expected from candidates to know the details of these tests and when to use them. It is acceptable to use a statistician's help to design a study. However, it boosts your answers if you have basic knowledge about the common ones (highlighted in the table).

There are several ways to check data for normality. Plotting normally distributed data produces a symmetrical bell-shaped curve. If the curve is not symmetrical, the data are probably not normally distributed. Alternatively, data can be formally tested using the Kolmogorov–Smirnov test or Shapiro–Wilk's test for normality. The latter tests are too sensitive to sample size and may show data as not normally distributed at the time the violation for normality is not substantive; therefore, graphical methods are generally preferable.

Data can also be presented as risk ratio (RR) or relative risk. These are just ways of expressing

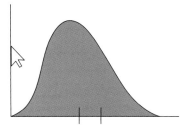 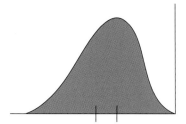

Figure 30.3 Skewed curves.

chance in numbers. For example: 24 people skiing down a slope, 6 fall:

The risk = number of events of interest (falls) / total number of observations = 6/24 = 0.25

The odds = number of events of interest (falls) / number without the event (no falls) = 6/18 = 0.33

- Relative risk or risk ratio (they mean the same thing and are both abbreviated as RR) is simply the risk of the event in one group divided by the risk of the event in the other group. RR value of 1 means no difference between the two groups.
- The risk difference (RD) is the risk difference between two groups. Sometimes this is called the absolute risk reduction and it is equal to risk on treatment – risk on control. RD value of 0 means no difference between the two groups.
- The number needed to treat (NNT) is how many people would need to be treated for one extra patient to be helped and it is the inverse of RD.
- The odds ratio (OR) is simply the odds of the event occurring in one group divided by the odds of the event occurring in the other group. OR value of 1 means no difference between the two groups.

There are pros and cons of using the above ratios. Odds ratios are hard to understand and are often misinterpreted. Risk difference (and derivatives like NNT) is more immediately useful than relative risk and odds ratio. The odds and risk ratio are equally variable whereas the risk difference varies more widely and less consistently. They do not change behaviour when the event of interest is reversed and work well in small samples and for rare events.

EXAMINER: OK, what about these two curves (Figure 30.3), are they also bell-shaped?

CANDIDATE: Not quite, they are skewed curves, they are not symmetric, and the tail is larger on the right for the first image and larger on the left for the second image, respectively called right-skewed and left-skewed data.

EXAMINER: What is the significance of skewed data and where is the mean in these images?

CANDIDATE: They are not symmetrical, therefore the mean is pulled by the outliers, so the mean lies toward the direction of skew (the longer tail) relative to the median. Hence the mean is larger than the median for right-skewed data and smaller than the median in left-skewed data.

EXAMINER: What value would you use to describe this set of data?

CANDIDATE: I would use median and interquartile range.

EXAMINER: OK, what is this chart (shown in Figure 30.4)?

CANDIDATE: It is a box plot. It compares the Oxford hip score changes between distressed and non-distressed groups of patients from pre-operative level to 5 years after surgery. This is another way to present findings graphically. It shows that in both groups of patients, surgery resulted in improvement in Oxford hip score and also that there were more outliers in the non-distressed group compared to the distressed group, postoperative improvement was maintained at 5 years of follow-up and the distressed group appears to have made a comparable if not a slightly larger gain compared to the non-distressed group. This may be a better way to present skewed data graphically.

EXAMINER: What are the different lines?

CANDIDATE: The width of the box shows the interquartile range, the line in the middle is the median value, the whisker shows the lowest and the highest values and the circles are the outliers.

EXAMINER: What is an outlier?

CANDIDATE: A value that is much larger or smaller than the rest of the data.

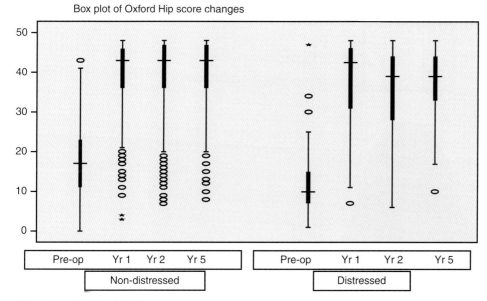

Figure 30.4 Box plot, Oxford hip score.

EXAMINER. Do you know how you can transform non-parametric data to more normal-looking data?

CANDIDATE: No.

EXAMINER: OK, you can do logarithmic transformation or bootstrap technique, thanks.

Authors' note 2

There are several ways to present data numerically and graphically. There is no perfect way and each one has pros and cons. Most candidates are familiar with bell-shaped curves, bar and pie charts. A box plot is another important and common way to present data and has been featured in the exam (Figure 30.5). The middle of the box plots represents the median and the sides (or the bottom and top of the box) are always the first and third quartiles. The ends of the whiskers can represent several possible alternative values, such as the minimum and maximum of all of the data, one standard deviation above and below the mean of the data or the 9th percentile and the 91st percentile. Outliers may be plotted as individual points.

Figure 30.6 compares the box plot to the bell-shaped curve for better understanding.

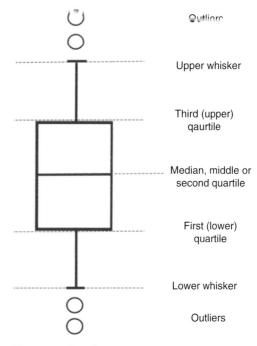

Figure 30.5 Box plot.

Structured oral examination question 2

EXAMINER: Can you tell me how you would design a clinical trial?

Authors' note 3

Frequently, candidates make the mistake of jumping straight onto a randomized controlled trial, the question is designed to see if you have an overall

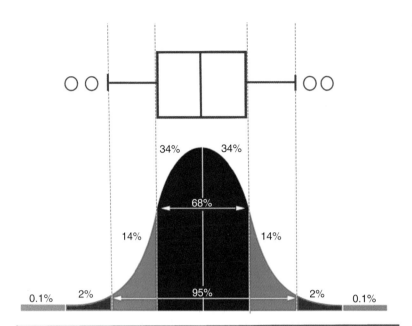

Figure 30.6 Box plot versus bell-shaped curve.

concept of designing a trial and whether you might have any practical experience.

CANDIDATE: Design of a clinical trial would begin with a clinical question that might arise out of a clinical context. In the first instance I would conduct a literature search utilizing the PICO principle [a buzzword that would impress the examiner, PICO stands for Patients, Intervention, Comparison, Outcome]. I would first search for the highest level of evidence in systematic reviews and meta-analyses. If there are none I would search for primary trials and so on [thus demonstrating that you are familiar with level of evidence].

If my search indicates that there is lack of evidence with regard to my clinical question I would proceed to designing a clinical trial. The design of the trial would depend on my underlying clinical question.

EXAMINER: Tell me more about the level of evidence (Table 30.2).

CANDIDATE: Each published (or unpublished) study is considered as an evidence. The importance of this evidence is based on the quality of that particular study. The general principle of the hierarchy is that controlled studies are generally better than uncontrolled ones, prospective are generally better than retrospective, and randomized are generally better than non-randomized studies [1]. Over the last three decades, several systems have emerged to assign a hierarchy for studies based on the aforementioned principles. Examples of these systems are the Oxford Centre for Evidence-Based Medicine (OCEBM) [2], the Scottish Intercollegiate Guidelines Network (SIGN) [3] and the Journal of Bone and Joints Surgery Levels of Evidence [1]. I am familiar with the OCEBM, where the highest level of interventional studies is systematic reviews and meta-analysis of randomized controlled studies with a high homogeneity and the lowest is the expert opinion.

Authors' note 4

Levels of evidence (LOE) are designed to help busy clinicians, researchers, or patients to find the likely best evidence in the shortest possible time. Table 30.1 showed the LOE produced by OCEBM. These levels of hierarchy vary among different systems and over time. They are not absolute. Sometimes 'lower-level' evidence from an observational study with a dramatic effect provides stronger evidence than a 'higher-level' study such as a systematic review of few studies leading to an inconclusive result. There are several examples in orthopaedic practice when a case series (level IV evidence) changed practice significantly. Charnley

Table 30.2 Level of evidence.

Level		Intervention	Prognosis	Diagnosis	Economic and decision analyses
1	a	Systematic review (SR) of randomized controlled trials (RCT) with homogeneous findings	SR (with homogeneity) of inception cohort studies	SR (with homogeneity) of Level 1 diagnostic studies	SR (with homogeneity) of Level 1 economic studies
	b	Individual RCT with narrow confidence interval (CI)	Individual inception cohort study with > 80% follow-up	Validating cohort study with good reference standards	Analysis based on clinically sensible costs of alternatives; systematic review(s) of the evidence; and including multiway sensitivity analyses
	c	All or none studies	All or none case-series	Absolute SpPins and SnNouts	Absolute better-value or worse-value analyses
2	a	SR (with homogeneity) of cohort studies	SR (with homogeneity) of either retrospective cohort studies or untreated control groups in RCTs	SR (with homogeneity) of Level >2 diagnostic studies	SR (with homogeneity) of Level >2 economic studies
	b	Individual cohort study (including low quality RCT; e.g. < 80% follow up)	Retrospective cohort study or follow-up of untreated control patients in an RCT	Exploratory cohort study with good reference standards	Analysis based on clinically sensible costs or alternatives; limited review(s) of the evidence, or single studies; and including multiway sensitivity analyses
	c	'Outcomes' research; ecological studies	Outcomes research		Audit or outcomes research
3	a	SR (with homogeneity) of case-control studies		SR (with homogeneity) of 3b and better studies	SR (with homogeneity) of 3b and better studies
	b	Individual case-control study		Non-consecutive study; or without consistently applied reference standards	Analysis based on limited alternatives or costs, poor-quality estimates of data, but including sensitivity analyses incorporating clinically sensible variations
4		Case series	Case series	Case-control study, poor or non-independent reference standard	Analysis with no sensitivity analysis
5		Expert opinion	Expert opinion	Expert opinion	Expert opinion

1. A complete assessment of the quality of individual studies requires critical appraisal of all aspects of the study design.

2. A combination of results from two or more prior studies.

3. Studies provided consistent results.

4. Study was started before the first patient enrolled.

5. Patients treated one way (e.g. with cemented hip arthroplasty) compared with patients treated another way (e.g. with cementless hip arthroplasty) at the same institution.

6. Study was started after the first patient enrolled.

7. Patients identified for the study on the basis of their outcome (e.g. failed total hip arthroplasty), called 'cases', are compared with those who did not have the outcome (e.g. had a successful total hip arthroplasty), called 'controls'.

8. Patients treated one way with no comparison group of patients treated another way.

This chart was adapted from material published by the Centre for Evidence-Based Medicine, Oxford, UK. For more information, please see www.cebm.net

hip replacement and Ponseti's treatment of clubfoot are classical examples [4].

It is essential to appreciate that LOE are not recommendations for or against certain treatments and several factors must be considered when applying best evidence in practice. These include but are not limited to:

i. Is your patient sufficiently similar to the patients in the studies you have examined?

ii. Does the treatment have a clinically relevant benefit that outweighs the harms (e.g. medicine X reduces blood loss by 50 ml but may be clinically irrelevant)?

iii. Is another treatment better (e.g. a systematic review might suggest that surgery is the best treatment for back pain, but if exercise therapy is useful, this might be more acceptable to the patient than risking surgery as a first option) [5]?

EXAMINER: Suppose that you are trying to test a new treatment? Literature search revealed no useful information.

CANDIDATE: Ideally, I would like to design a randomized controlled trial (RCT) to compare my new treatment to the current (or any another treatment). It is the most rigorous way of determining whether a cause–effect relation exists between treatment and outcome. Good RCT design must ensure [6]:

1. Random allocation to treatment groups.
2. Patients and trialists remain unaware of which treatment was given until the study is completed: this is called 'concealment'.
3. The number of participants is optimum to show a clinically relevant difference.
4. The two groups of treatment are treated identically except for the experimental treatment.

The analysis is focused on estimating the size of the difference in predefined outcomes between intervention groups.

There are two types of RCT; explanatory and pragmatic. It can be debated which one is better in this scenario.

EXAMINER: What is the difference between the two types?

CANDIDATE: Explanatory trials generally measure efficacy – the outcomes of treatments under ideal conditions. For example, if I was testing a new type of cement to help reduce revision rates, I would design my study in such a way that I remove or minimize the effect of any factors that could influence the revision rate. For example, all operations will be done by surgeon X, in centre X using implant X, at room temperature X and using a standardized cementing technique, etc. This design would be likely to show me the real effect of the new cement on revision rate. However, in reality the above design is neither practical nor desirable because we would want to see the tested intervention (the new cement here) work similarly in every centre, for every surgeon and with every implant. Hence the pragmatic trials are more popular. They measure effectiveness – the benefit the treatment produces in routine practice [7].

EXAMINER: How do you randomize?

CANDIDATE: There are many ways of randomization. Ideally this should be performed by a centralized computerized system.

EXAMINER: What is the advantage of randomization?

CANDIDATE: The advantage of randomization is to avoid bias by equally distributing the known and unknown patient variables (that potentially affect the outcomes) so that the difference in treatment effect is most likely to be due to the difference in the intervention.

EXAMINER: What do you mean by bias?

CANDIDATE: Bias is a tendency to deviate from the true value due to an error in the study design and thus over- or underestimate the true value of the treatment effect. Examples of bias include selection bias, allocation bias, assessment bias, performance bias, etc.

EXAMINER: Once you complete your trial how would you know if the new treatment is effective or not?

CANDIDATE: I would perform a statistical test and if the P value is < 0.05 this would suggest that there is less than 5% chance that the observed difference in treatment effect is purely due to chance, therefore I would consider the result to be statistically significant.

EXAMINER: Would you change your practice based on the results of a P value? Can you imagine a situation where the P value is > 0.05 but you might want to reconsider the intervention?

CANDIDATE: Yes, where there is a possibility of a type II error.

EXAMINER: What is a type II error?

CANDIDATE: Where the sample size of the trial might be inadequate and therefore even if there was a significant difference between the intervention and the control group this would not be evident in the statistical test.

EXAMINER: OK, this is known as the power of the study. Time's up. Thank you.

Authors' note 5

Questions about designing RCT are very popular in the FRCS exam. Good understanding increases your marks, even if you do not have personal experience in running a trial. This section summarizes the essential concepts and buzzwords that you need to deliver when you are asked about RCT.

Research is conducted to answer a particular question. Although RCT is the most rigorous way of determining whether a cause–effect relation exists between treatment and outcome, it is not the only way. RCT is conducted to an ethically approved protocol that prospectively sets out its rationale, conduct and plan of analysis. Important design considerations include the following.

1. *A literature search* to establish current knowledge, thus refining the research question and trial methods to take knowledge forward and avoid unnecessary research repetition. Trials are often very expensive and sometimes adequate answers can be found either from the literature or alternative study designs. Information from a previous published work is important to calculate the required sample size.
2. *Sample selection and generalizability*: participants should be representative of the population of interest. Thus, inclusion and exclusion criteria are important trial design features and should be carefully thought about, e.g. excluding pregnant women for safety reasons is often a valid reason for exclusion. However, excluding patients with dementia because consenting is more problematic is not a good reason and may not be ethically acceptable. This would deprive such patients from future evidence-based treatment.
3. *Primary and secondary outcomes*: the primary outcome (or the primary end point) represents the greatest treatment benefit. Some trials have more than one primary outcome if several outcome measures are of equal importance. Secondary outcomes (or secondary end points) may provide information on therapeutic effects of secondary importance, side effects, or tolerability. Both should be clinically relevant, valid, reproducible and sensitive to detect changes. For example, setting a trial to

investigate the value of tranexamic acid in reducing blood loss in joint replacement. Blood transfusion is a good primary outcome. It can be measured easily, accurately and has importance to patient and surgeons. In comparison, drain blood loss, although important, does not tick all the boxes mentioned earlier, hence it is better used as a secondary outcome rather than a primary one (see also the type of data section).

5. *Sample size (power)*. A well-designed study should have the optimal number of participants (adequate sample size) to provide an adequate chance of finding a clinically worthwhile difference between treatments. Over-recruitment is undesirable as it is uneconomic and unethical (exposing more patients to an 'unnecessary' experiment when the answer has been established within reasonable bounds). A smaller number of participants may cause a type II error (not finding a difference between the two treatments although there is a difference).

Sample size is usually calculated for the primary outcome and the following elements are required for calculation:

- Chosen significance level (usually 5%).
- Study power (typically 80% or 90%).
- Chosen clinically important difference in the primary outcome.
- The variability in response (standard deviation in the primary outcome).

There are several pieces of software or websites that provide this calculation.

6. *Bias*: refers to systematic error in trial design, conduct, analysis or reporting. The true effect of the treatment under investigation is systematically under- or overestimated. For example:
   i. *Question bias*: e.g. comparing a new treatment with the most poorly performing alternative will inflate the apparent benefit of the new treatment.
   ii. *Sampling bias*: patients with significant comorbidity are excluded from trial or decline to participate, limiting the generalizability of findings.
   iii. *Selection bias*: patients with underlying prognosis are systematically assigned in larger numbers to one treatment than another.
   iv. *Information bias*: including any of a range of factors that distort the recording of data, e.g. measurement error, recall bias, workup bias, interviewer bias, misconduct.

v. *Windowing bias*: where the investigators' prejudices influence the selection and presentation of findings.

vi. *Publication bias*: studies with negative or no difference are less likely to be submitted, published, quoted or even read.

7. *Randomization*: if adequately conducted, randomization reduces the chance of selection bias because known and unknown prognostic influences are distributed by chance among the different treatment groups.

8. *Blinding (masking or concealment)*: if researchers or patients have a preference for a particular treatment, this can introduce bias. Blinding is an important design feature to manage both explicit and implicit prejudice, although it is not always possible.

9. *Analysis*: this is conducted according to a protocol agreed prospectively before any analysis has begun. Three approaches are described:

i. Intention-to-treat (ITT), meaning that participants are analyzed according to the group allocated regardless of whether they continued with that treatment. ITT is widely considered as the golden standard to analyze RCT because it avoids the bias associated with the non-random loss of the participants.

ii. As-treated analysis: comparing the groups according to the treatment that they received. It does not consider which treatment they were allocated to.

iii. Per protocol analysis includes participants who met all the protocol criteria in the terms of the eligibility, interventions, outcome assessment and follow up.

The cons of the last two analyses are that they potentially overestimate the efficacy of an intervention resulting from the removal of non-compliance and protocol deviations which are likely to occur in actual clinical practice.

10. *Logistics* (ethics approval, local approval, building and training a research team).

Structured oral examination question 3

EXAMINER: If you had the choice of deciding between a highly sensitive test or a highly specific test to diagnose as many of the diseases as possible for a particularly debilitating condition, what kind of test would you go for?

CANDIDATE: I would choose a highly sensitive test.

EXAMINER: Why is that?

CANDIDATE: In a highly sensitive test more of the diseased cases would be positive whereas a highly specific test might miss some disease cases.

EXAMINER: What are the drawbacks of each?

CANDIDATE: A highly sensitive test may pick up more false positive cases and create unnecessary patient anxiety, whereas a highly specific test might have more false negative cases and miss some diseased cases.

EXAMINER: What if you wanted to confirm diagnosis of the disease?

CANDIDATE: I would choose a highly specific test.

EXAMINER: Do you think hip ultrasound is a good screening test for DDH?

CANDIDATE: Yes, ultrasound ticks most of the WHO criteria for a screening test: it is accepted and tolerated by patients and parents, it is safe, it has a high sensitivity to detect the disease before a critical point and has high specificity to reduce false positives.

EXAMINER: Should we screen all newborns for DDH using ultrasound?

CANDIDATE: This is widely debated. Some countries have already started a universal screening programme and showed encouraging results; others opted for a selective screening programme to reach an acceptable cost–effectiveness ratio.

To run a successful screening programme, several criteria should be met. These criteria can be categorized into three groups:

1. Disease criteria.

    i. Disease with significant impact on community.

    ii. Natural history of the disease is known.

    iii. Detection occurs before a critical point (before it is too late).

2. Screening test features.

    i. Accepted and tolerated by patients.

    ii. High sensitivity to detect the disease before the critical point.

    iii. High specificity to reduce false positives.

    iv. Cost-effective.

3. Screened population features.

    i. Disease has high enough prevalence to allow screening.

    ii. Accepted and effective treatment is available.

    iii. Patients are willing to undergo further evaluation and treatment.

DDH as a disease fulfils most (and not all) of these criteria. The condition is 'important' with an accepted treatment and suitable facilities available for that treatment. There is an early stage in which DDH can be picked up, with a sensitive test that is acceptable to the population. However, there is no universal agreement on who should receive treatment and who should not. Furthermore, the cost of the screening programme in comparison to the full costs of delayed detection (including medico-legal costs) has not been established [8].

Authors' note 6: Diagnostic tests

Sensitivity, specificity, positive and negative predictive values of a diagnostic test are commonly featured in the exam. Most candidates are aware of this, yet find it difficult to recall and present their answers succinctly to achieve a high mark to reflect their knowledge. Our advice is to understand the definition rather than memorizing it.

1. Sensitivity (Sn): the probability of identifying a disease (true positive) when the disease is present (true positive + false negative).
Sn = true positive / true positive + false negative.
2. Specificity (Sp): the probability of excluding a disease (true negative) when the disease is not there (true negative + false positive).
Sp = true negative / (true negative + false positive).
3. Accuracy (A): the probability of correct identification of a disease.
A = true positive + true negative / total number.
4. Positive predictive value (PPV): the probability of someone having a disease (true positive) when they have tested positive (all the positives = true positive + false positive).
PPV = true positives / (true positives + false positives).
5. Negative predictive value (NPV): the probability of someone not having a disease (true negative) when they have tested negative (all the negatives = true negative + false negatives).
NPV = true negatives / (true negatives + false negatives).

Unlike sensitivity and specificity, predictive values are properties of the test interacting with the prevalence of disease in the population. A high PPV indicates a strong chance that a person with a positive test has the disease in populations with high prevalence of the condition being examined (true positive is high in such population), whereas a low PPV is usually found in populations with low prevalence of the condition being examined.

6. Likelihood ratio (LR): the ratio of the chances of truly having a disease to not having it, given that a positive test result was obtained.
LR = Sn / (1 − Sp).
We can calculate the LR for every test. The larger the LR, the better the test. Increasing sensitivity and/or specificity would increase the LR (a better test) and vice versa (you can check this by replacing random numbers in the formula).

Plotting Sn against (1 − Sp) produces a characteristic curve called 'receiver operating characteristic' (ROC) curves (see Figures 30.7 and 30.8). An ideal ROC curve rises quickly to the upper left corner of the graph (high Sn and Sp) and stays high, leaving a larger area under the curve. A poor ROC curve rises slowly and has less area under the curve. The overall shape of a test is determined by physical law, biochemical properties, or the financial resources used in the design or manufacturing of the test. Once the overall ROC curve is fixed, the surgeon or experimenter decides how to use the test by choosing a cut-off value. Different cut-off values result in a balanced test, or a test that is optimized for use in screening or confirmation (Figure 30.9).

Structured oral examination question 4

EXAMINER: This is an abstract of an RCT comparing TXA to placebo to reduce blood transfusion in total knee replacement (Figure 30.10). Please, read the result section and tell me your thoughts of the findings.

CANDIDATE: The results of the trial showed that TXA has been effective in reducing blood transfusion rates by 15.4% (from 16.7% to 1.3%). That was statistically significant ($P = 0.0001$). The trial also showed that TXA statistically significantly reduced blood loss. As a surgeon, I consider the first findings are clinically important, but I cannot say the

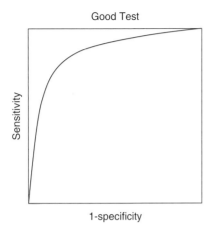

Good Test

Figure 30.7 Good ROC curve.

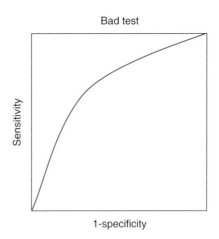

Bad test

Figure 30.8 Bad ROC curve.

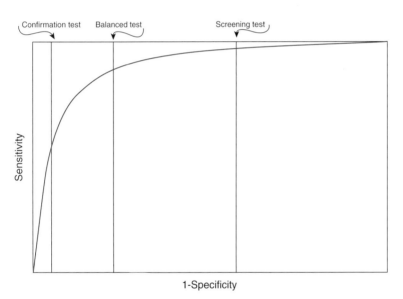

Figure 30.9 Different cut-off values result in a balanced test, or a test that is optimized for use in screening or confirmation.

same about the amount of blood loss. Although it is statistically significant, it is not clinically. The same could be said about the length of stay and cost.

EXAMINER: What do you think about the 95% confidence interval?

CANDIDATE: The 95% CI for the blood transfusion was 7.5–25.4%; a reasonably narrow CI. A confidence interval shows the range within which the treatment effect is likely to lie if the study was repeated again. In other words, if this trial was repeated 100 times, then 95 out of those 100 times, the absolute reduction of blood transfusion would lie within between 7.5% and 25.4%.

EXAMINER: How is CI related to the *P*-value?

CANDIDATE: A *P*-value is calculated to assess whether a treatment effect observed in a study is likely to have occurred simply through chance. Traditionally, researchers accept a *P*-value of less than 0.05. This means that there is a 5% risk that the result I have seen in my study happened by chance and 95% is a true effect of the intervention that I am testing. So, in the above study, there is 1 in 1000 ($P = 0.001$) risk that the 15.4% reduction in

Background: Approximately one-third of patients undergoing total knee replacement require one to three units of blood postoperatively. Tranexamic acid (TXA) is a synthetic antifibrinolytic agent that has been successfully used intravenously to stop bleeding after total knee replacement. A topical application is easy to administer, provides a maximum concentration of tranexamic acid at the bleeding site, and is associated with little or no systemic absorption of the tranexamic acid.

Methods: A double-blind, randomized controlled trial of 157 patients undergoing unilateral primary cemented total knee replacement investigated the effect of topical (intra-articular) application of tranexamic acid on blood loss. The primary outcome was the blood transfusion rate. Secondary outcomes included the drain blood loss, hemoglobin concentration drop, generic quality of life (EuroQol), Oxford Knee Score, length of stay, a cost analysis, and complications as per the protocol definitions.

Results: Tranexamic acid reduced the absolute risk of blood transfusion by 15.4% (95% confidence interval [CI], 7.5% to 25.4%; p = 0.001), from 16.7% to 1.3%, and reduced blood loss by 168 mL (95% CI, 80 to 256 mL; p = 0.0003), the length of stay by 1.2 days (95% CI, 0.05 to 2.43 days; p = 0.041), and the cost per episode by £333 (95% CI, £37 to £630; p = 0.028). (In 2008, £1 = 1.6 U.S. dollars.) Oxford Knee Scores and EuroQol EQ-5D scores were similar at three months.

Conclusions: Topically applied tranexamic acid was effective in reducing the need for blood transfusion following total knee replacement without important additional adverse effects.

Level of Evidence: Therapeutic Level I. See Instructions for Authors for a complete description of levels of evidence.

Figure 30.10 Journal abstract.

the transfusion rate happened by chance and not because of the TXA. For the same reason we should be careful not to discount studies when the *P*-value is close but higher than 0.05. In comparison to CI, the *P*-value does not give any idea about the treatment effect.

EXAMINER: Which one would you prefer?

CANDIDATE: CIs are preferable to *P*-values, as they tell us the range of possible effect sizes. CIs aid interpretation of clinical trial data by putting upper and lower bounds on the likely size of any true effect. A CI that includes no difference between treatments indicates that the treatment under investigation is not significantly different from the control.

EXAMINER: You mentioned that the CI of the above study was narrow. Would you prefer a narrow or a wide CI?

CANDIDATE: I would prefer a narrow CI as this indicates we are more certain about the possible range of treatment effects. A wide CI indicates that we are more uncertain about the range. A suitable example might be of a confident candidate who is 95% confident to have scored between 70% and 80% in his FRCS exam. Contrast this with another candidate who is equally (95%) confident to have scored between 40% and 90%.

In other words, the *P*-value gives you statistical significance, but CI gives you clinical significance.

EXAMINER: Could the above study findings be wrong and TXA does not reduce blood transfusion?

CANDIDATE: Yes, this is called type I error when a study concludes that a supposed effect or relationship exists when in fact it does not. Another example is when a test shows a patient to have a disease when in fact the patient does not have the disease.

EXAMINER: How does it differ from type II error?

CANDIDATE: If this study failed to show that the TXA reduces blood transfusion when really it does, this is type II (Figure 30.11).

EXAMINER: Which one is worse?

CANDIDATE: Both should be considered and minimized. The seriousness of the implication may vary depending on the scenario. A new test that fails to

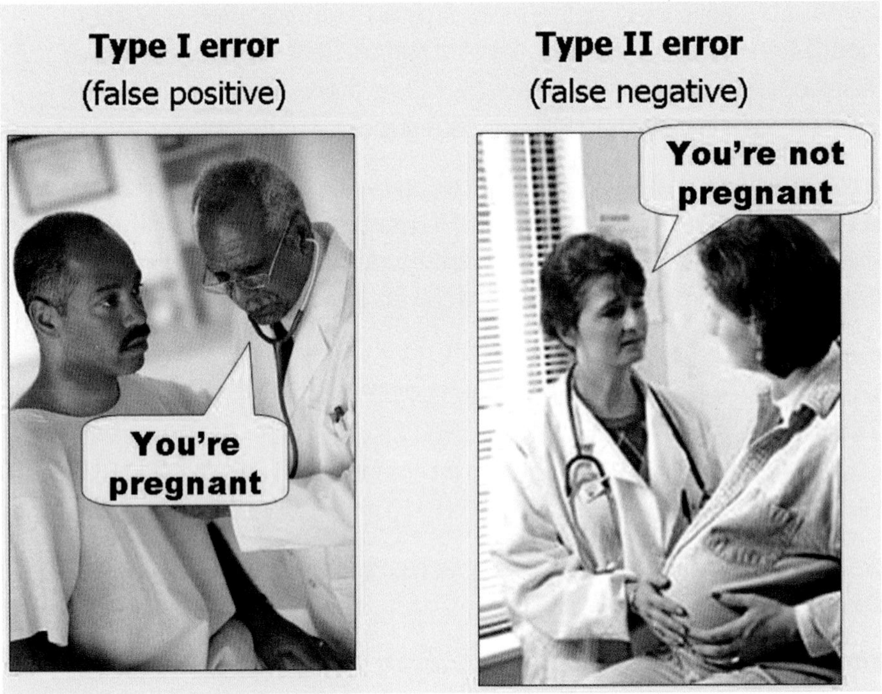

Figure 30.11 Type I and II errors.

detect a cancer when it is there (type II error) is serious. Another test that shows cancer when it is not there (type I error) and the patient then undergoes unnecessary surgery is serious too.

EXAMINER: How do you minimize errors?

CANDIDATE: An integral part of a research study is to formulate and test a hypothesis. Because the test is based on probabilities, there is always a chance of making an incorrect conclusion (type I and type II). In statistical terms, type I error occurs when the null hypothesis is true and gets rejected. The probability of making a type I error is related to the level of significance (*P*-value or α) we set for our hypothesis test. A *P*-value of 0.05 indicates that we are willing to accept a 5% chance that we are wrong when we reject the null hypothesis. To lower this risk, we can lower the *P*-value. The drawback is that we will be less likely to detect a true difference if one really exists.

The probability of making a type II error is related to the size of the study and the power of the test to detect a difference in the primary outcome. We can minimize type II error by increasing the size of the study and/or ensuring our test has enough power (for example, using Hb level drop rather than swab weights to measure blood loss).

EXAMINER: What is the null hypothesis?

CANDIDATE: As I mentioned earlier, an integral part of a research study is to formulate and test hypotheses. The null hypothesis is normally the default position, e.g. that there is no difference between a new and an old treatment. The null hypothesis is paired with a second alternative hypothesis, e.g. there is a difference between treatments. This is because it is easier to prove something exists rather than does not exist. For example, I cannot reject the statement 'all cats are white' by showing you 1000 white cats. However, I could reject it by showing you one black cat!

Structured oral examination question 5

EXAMINER: Have a look at Figure 30.12. Do you know what this plot is?

CANDIDATE: This is called a forest plot (also known as a blobbogram). It numerically and graphically

Study or Subgroup	Control Events	Total	Tranexamic acid Events	Total	Weight	Risk Ratio M-H, Fixed, 95% CI
Alvarez 2008	6	49	1	46	1.3%	5.63 [0.70, 45.01]
Benoni 1996	24	43	8	43	10.3%	3.00 [1.52, 5.92]
Camarasa 2006	23	68	1	35	1.7%	11.84 [1.67, 84.06]
Ellis 2001	7	10	1	10	1.3%	7.00 [1.04, 46.95]
Engel 2001	3	12	0	12	0.6%	7.00 [0.40, 122.44]
Good 2003	14	24	3	27	3.6%	5.25 [1.71, 16.08]
Hiippala 1995	12	13	10	15	12.0%	1.38 [0.94, 2.05]
Hiippala 1997	34	38	17	39	21.6%	2.05 [1.41, 2.98]
Jansen 1999	13	21	2	21	2.6%	6.50 [1.67, 25.33]
Molloy 2007	11	50	5	50	6.4%	2.20 [0.82, 5.87]
Orpen 2006	3	14	1	15	1.2%	3.21 [0.38, 27.40]
Tanaka 2001	26	26	47	73	32.7%	1.53 [1.28, 1.83]
Veien 2002	2	15	0	15	0.6%	5.00 [0.26, 96.13]
Zohar 2004	12	20	3	20	3.9%	4.00 [1.33, 12.05]
Total (95% CI)		403		421	100.0%	2.56 [2.10, 3.11]
Total events	190		99			

Heterogeneity: Chi² = 51.97, df = 13 (P < 0.00001); I² = 75%
Test for overall effect: Z = 9.44 (P < 0.00001)

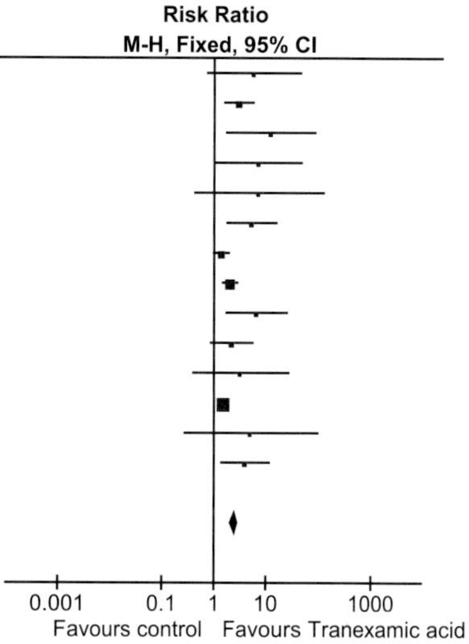

Risk Ratio M-H, Fixed, 95% CI
0.001 0.1 1 10 1000
Favours control   Favours Tranexamic acid

Figure 30.12 Forest plot.

represents a meta-analysis which combines results from a number of studies addressing the same question.

EXAMINER: What is the difference between a review and meta-analysis?

CANDIDATE : A clinical review simply locates and summarizes the findings of several studies. However, a systematic review is a rigorous and prestructured approach to conducting a review. The researchers decide beforehand on their inclusion and exclusion criteria, how they will search the literature, extract data, synthesize and analyze them. The meta-analysis is another stage in conducting systematic reviews when authors combine data from different studies statistically with a view to getting a combined and more precise estimate of the intervention's effectiveness. This is not always possible due to data limitations.

EXAMINER: Why do we need reviews and meta-analyses?

CANDIDATE: For many surgical procedures, there have been a number of clinical studies and it would seem natural to want to combine them to get the most comprehensive overview of the effect of treatment. Properly conducted systematic review and meta-analyses with homogeneity are considered the highest level of evidence in clinical practice.

EXAMINER: What do you mean by homogeneity?

CANDIDATE: In a meta-analysis, investigators combine results from reasonably similar studies. However, findings from these studies are likely to vary due to different methodologies (randomized or not, how allocation is concealed, blinding, etc.); patients (inclusion and exclusion criteria); interventions (type, dose, duration, etc.); outcomes (type, scale, duration of follow up and usage). Such variations can introduce heterogeneity into study findings (variation greater than that expected by chance). Heterogeneity can be formally tested using the χ^2 heterogeneity test (or Q statistic). The significantly high Q test suggests heterogeneity. Homogeneity conversely means that the variations among the study are low and the results of each individual study are compatible with a single underlying treatment effect.

Cochrane software (RevMan) produces I^2, which is the proportion of variation that is due to heterogeneity rather than chance. Roughly, I^2 values of < 50% indicate low, 50–75% indicate moderate, > 75% indicate high heterogeneity.

EXAMINER: Back to Figure 30.12; can you explain the findings?

CANDIDATE: The forest plot represents 14 studies comparing tranexamic acid (TXA) to the control. It is not clear whether the control is a placebo or another medicine. This may be clarified in the methodology section. The forest plot consists of several columns:

1. The first column lists the names of the studies and the date of publication. These can be ordered alphabetically (as in this example) or by the year of publication, the weight of the studies or the treatment effects.
2. The second column represents the events in the TXA group. Again, it is not clear which event the plot represents. It could be blood transfusion, DVT or PE rates. (Examiner: it is blood transfusion rates.)
3. The third column represents the number of participants in the TXA group.
4. The fourth column represents the events in the control group.
5. The fifth column represents the number of participants in the control group.
6. The sixth column is the weight that is given to each study. The weight reflects the precision of the study (size and CI). Tanaka 2001 is the highest weighted study (32.7%).
7. The seventh column represents the treatment effect estimate. In this example it is the risk ratio which is equal to (events/total of the control) divided by (events/total in the TXA group).
   The risk ratio is one of several ways of presenting proportions: others are odds ratios and risk differences.
8. The last column provides a plot of the measure of effect for each study. The area of each square is proportional to the study's weight in the meta-analysis. The higher the weight of the study the larger the square (see Tanaka 2001). On each side of the square there is a horizontal line representing the confidence interval.
   The narrower the CI the more precise the study is. The plots of the weighted effects are scattered on each side of a vertical line representing the no effect line. Here, the no effect line passes through 1 because it represents a risk ratio. It would be 0 if it was a risk difference.

Depending on the outcome of each included study, it can lie on either the left or the right side of the no-effect line. In this example, they all lie to the right of the no-effect line. The further away from the line, the more profound the effect. The overall effect is represented by a diamond. If a study plot touches the no-effect line, it means that its effect does not differ from no-effect for that individual study. The same applies for the diamond (the overall measure of effect): if the points of the diamond overlap the line of no effect the overall result is 'no effect' at the given level of confidence. In this study, the diamond position favours TXA.

EXAMINER: That is very good. What about the word 'fixed' and the letters 'M-H'? What do they signify?

CANDIDATE: The Mantel–Haenszel (M-H) test is used to combine studies in this plot; this is used by the Review Manager (RevMan 5) software that was developed by Cochrane library. The word 'fixed' refers to the fixed-effects model. One of two models used in meta-analysis. The other is called the random-effects model. In the fixed-effects model, it is assumed that the size of the effect is similar in the included studies. In this example, the size of the effect is a participant who had a blood transfusion. It is reasonable to assume the size of the effect is similar and use the fixed-effects model.

EXAMINER: Can you give me an example where a random-effect model should be used?

CANDIDATE: Yes, when the effects are not similar. For example, combining data from two different outcome measures such as Oxford hip score and Harris hip score. Although they measure the hip function, they are not the same.

EXAMINER: How would you interpret the finding in the plot?

CANDIDATE: The plot shows that TXA reduced the risk of transfusion by 2.56 times with 95% CI (2.10–3.11) and P-value 0.00001 (the test for overall effect). This is statistically and clinically significant. However, there is significant heterogeneity as evident by the high I^2 value (75%) and this was statistically significant (P-value < 0.00001). So, my interpretation for the above finding is that there is evidence that TXA does reduce the blood transfusion, but it is difficult to quantify (so the RR of 2.56 shows it is not necessarily true).

EXAMINER: How to deal with heterogeneity?

CANDIDATE: I expect the authors to explore this heterogeneity further. There are several options to do so:

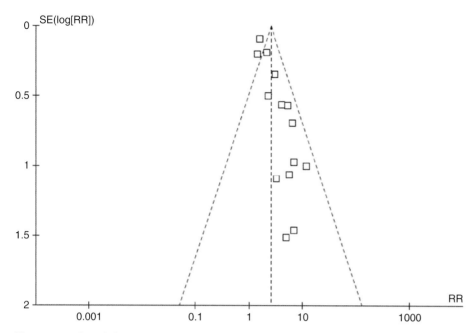

Figure 30.13 Funnel plot.

1. One option is that of not performing a meta-analysis in the first place. They can simply present the findings as a table without pooling them.
2. Subgroups analysis of studies that are more similar. For example, studies with a high dose of TXA, or those receiving TXA earlier rather than later, etc. to see whether this could explain the heterogeneity.
3. In this example, the authors used the fixed-effects model for combining studies. Using the random-effects model may uncover some of the heterogeneity.
4. Investigating heterogeneity using meta-regression. Meta-regression is an extension to subgroup analyses that allows the effects of multiple factors to be investigated simultaneously. It is similar to simple regressions, in which an outcome variable is predicted according to the values of one or more independent variables. In the above example, the outcome variable is the effect estimate (RR). The independent variables are characteristics of studies that might influence the RR such as dose, timing of administration, the use of heparin, the use of transfusion protocol, etc.

EXAMINER: Figure 30.13 is another plot of meta-analysis. In fact, it is from the same meta-analysis in Figure 30.12. Do you know the name of this plot?

EXAMINER: This is called a funnel plot which is a simple scatterplot of the treatment effects (risk ratio – horizontal axis) from individual studies (small squares) against the precision of the studies represented by standard error (SE) (vertical axis). SE is the standard deviation divided by the square root of the sample size. Hence, the larger the study, the lower the SE.

It is expected that larger studies (big sample size) are more precise (low standard errors) and will be scattered very close to each other around the pooled effect at the top of the plot. The smaller studies are scattered widely toward the bottom, giving the classical inverted symmetrical funnel.

The funnel plot shows trials scattered asymmetrically around the pooled RR with small trials having greater effect. There are two explanations for these findings. This may be due to smaller trials of lower quality tending to overestimate the true effect; hence they are on the right side of the pooled effect. It might also reflect publication bias, where small trials that did not show benefit were not published (publication bias).

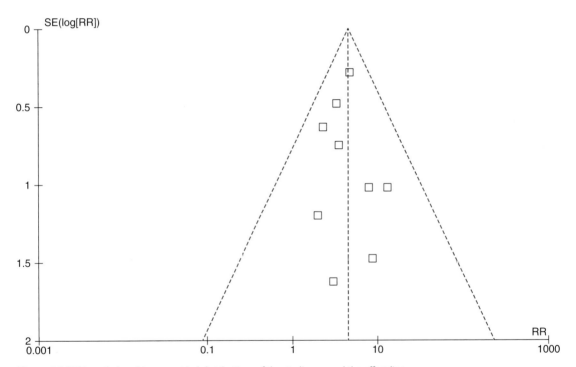

Figure 30.14 Forest plot with homogeneity.

Study or Subgroup	Control Events	Total	Topical TXA Events	Total	Weight	Risk Ratio M.H, Fixed, 95% CI
Canata 2012	2	32	1	32	4.4%	2.00 [0.19, 20.97]
Wong 2010	5	35	4	64	12.4%	2.29 [0.66, 7.97]
Ishida 2011	1	50	0	50	2.2%	3.00 [0.13, 71.92]
Sa-Ngasoongsong 2011	10	45	6	90	17.5%	3.33 [1.29, 8.59]
Roy 2012	7	25	2	25	8.8%	3.50 [0.80, 15.23]
Seo 2012	47	50	10	50	43.8%	4.70 [2.69, 8.22]
Sa-Ngasoongsong 2013	8	24	1	24	44.4%	8.00 [1.08, 59.13]
Georgiadis 2013	4	51	0	50	2.2%	8.83 [0.49, 159.80]
Alshryda 2013 (TRANX-K)	13	78	1	79	4.4%	13.17 [1.76, 98.24]
Total (95% CI)		390		464	100.0%	4.51 [3.02, 6.72]
Total events	97		25			

Heterogeneity, Chi^2 = 3.80, df = 8 (P = 0.87); I^2 = 0%

Test for overall effect Z = 7.38 (P < 0.00001)

Figure 30.15 Funnel plot with symmetrical distributions of the studies around the effect line.

Authors' note 7

See the below figures for comprehension:
Figure 30.14 showed that I^2 is 0% and there is no significant heterogeneity in the included studies. So, the conclusion is that topical TXA reduced blood transfusion significantly by 4.5-fold. The same studies were displayed in a funnel plot (effects against SE) and the plot showed the studies distributed symmetrically around the effect line (4.5 RR), indicating that publication bias is not likely (Figure 30.15).

Structured oral examination question 6

EXAMINER: The following plot (Figure 30.16) is from the Norwegian Joint Registry about the

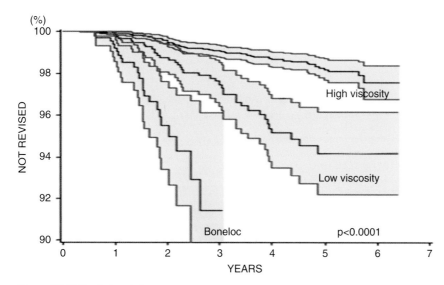

Figure 30.16 Survival analysis curve.

effect of cement on the implant longevity. Can you describe the findings?

CANDIDATE: This is a survival analysis of Charnley femoral prostheses using different types of cements (high-viscosity, low-viscosity and Boneloc). There is a statistically significant difference between the three groups (no overlaps in the confidence interval and *P*-value < 0.0001). The high viscosity cement seems to provide a higher survival rate where about 98% survived to 6 years.

EXAMINER: What is a survival graph, why do you need this, could you not simply measure mean survival with CI?

CANDIDATE: Well, a survival graph measures 'time to event', this graph looks at survival probability and every time the event takes place survival is recalculated.

EXAMINER: What are the different lines in this chart?

CANDIDATE: The midline is the mean value and the upper and lower lines represent the CI.

EXAMINER: Why did the upper and lower lines diverge towards the right?

CANDIDATE: This is because as the study progressed there were fewer patients remaining in the study. With a lower number of patients, the precision of the study and the confidence about the findings become low; therefore, the CI becomes wider.

EXAMINER: Looking at this chart, can you predict the survival probability at 20 years?

CANDIDATE: No, it is not possible to estimate survival probability beyond the maximum follow-up period of the study.

EXAMINER: Can you estimate the mean revision time?

CANDIDATE: No, we cannot as there are differing follow-up times, we can only estimate the cumulative risk of revision.

EXAMINER: What do you understand by 'censored data'?

CANDIDATE: If a patient dies, is lost to follow-up or withdraws from the study then data from that patient are incomplete or censored.

EXAMINER: So, are censored data wasted then?

CANDIDATE: No, they contribute data until the point of censoring.

EXAMINER: Have you noticed any, can you tell me if there is a problem with this chart?

CANDIDATE: Yes, the CI for Boneloc and low-viscosity cement is very wide, and I suspect the population at risk was low, but the numbers are not indicated.

EXAMINER: The below plot is from the National Joint Registry of England and Wales (Figure 30.17). Take a look at this chart and tell me what you understand.

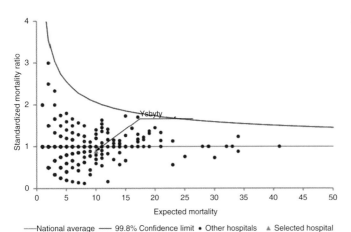

Figure 30.17 **Figure 30.17** National Joint Registry report.

CANDIDATE: This shows the 90-day mortality rate following joint replacement (not specified in this chart whether hip or knee replacement) for a selected hospital (orange triangle). Similar charts are produced for individual surgeons (not shown in this figure). Here the y-axis denotes standardized mortality ratio which is the proportion of deaths compared to the average, the x-axis denotes the expected adjusted mortality for the involved hospitals. The data are 'risk-adjusted' to take account of the fact that different hospitals may operate on higher-risk or lower-risk patients (e.g. because of demographics in the patient population they work with). Although case-mix adjustment is a useful tool, as with any methodological approach it cannot account for all differences including those that may be due to random events. The central green line denotes the average national expected mortality and the red line denotes the 99.8% confidence limit.

Progression along the x-axis means that the hospital has done more cases and/or cases at a higher mortality risk, such as older patients. Progression along the y-axis means the hospital has had more deaths. The y-axis figures are presented as a ratio. This means the values do not represent percentages of patients who have died, but they represent the proportion of deaths compared to the average.

Hospitals on the green (horizontal) line have the average expected mortality taking into account their case mix and number of cases. Hospitals on either side of the green line but below the upper red line have had a level of mortality (when taking into account their case mix and number of cases) that is within the

expected range. Hospitals above the top red line (which represents a '99.8% Confidence Limit line') would have a mortality rate that is higher than expected.

EXAMINER: So, how did this hospital do?

CANDIDATE: The hospital's mortality was well within the expected mortality range.

EXAMINER: Can you tell me anything about the type of patients the hospital operated on?

CANDIDATE: Yes, we can see that the orange triangle is not far along the x-axis denoting that the hospital did not perform surgery on patients with higher expected mortality.

Authors' note 8: Survival analysis

Survival analysis originally studied time from treatment until death, hence the name, but survival analysis is applicable to many other areas as well as mortality. It estimates the time between entry to a study and a subsequent event. Events may include death, injury, revision of an implant, recovery from illness (binary variables) or transition above or below the clinical threshold of a meaningful continuous variable (e.g. CD4 counts in HIV infection). It also compares time-to-event between two or more groups, such as cemented vs. non cemented in total hip replacement. Moreover, it assesses the relationship of co-variables to time-to-event, such as: antibiotic in cement, hinged design, weight of the patients, LMWH, etc.

The following are important definitions.
Time-to-event: the time from entry into a study until a subject has a particular outcome. This is represented by a drop on the survival curve.

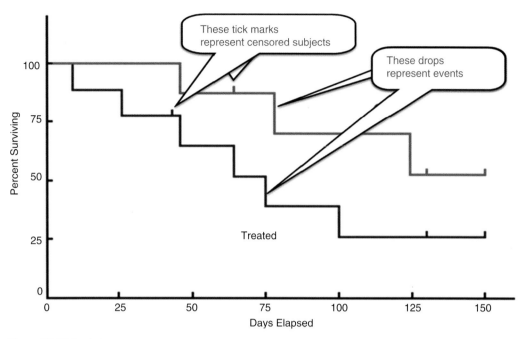

Figure 30.18 Survival curves.

Censoring: subjects are said to be censored if they are: (1) lost to follow-up or (2) drop out of the study, or (3) if the study ends before they die or have an outcome of interest. Censored subjects are represented by a tick mark on the survival curves (Figure 30.18).

The Kaplan–Meier survival curve is a non-parametric estimate of the survival function. Simply put, it is the probability of surviving past certain times in the sample (taking into account censoring). Three assumptions are made in survival analysis:

1. We assume that at any time patients who are censored have the same survival prospects as those who continue to be followed.
2. The survival probabilities are the same for subjects recruited early and late in the study.
3. We assume that the event happens at the time specified.

   The Kaplan–Meier computes the probabilities of occurrence of the event at a certain point of time by multiplying these successive probabilities by any earlier computed probabilities to get the final estimate. For each time interval, survival probability is calculated as the number of patients surviving divided

by the number of patients at risk. Patients who have died, dropped out, or move out are not counted as 'at risk'. These are considered 'censored' and are not counted in the denominator. Total probability of survival until that time interval is calculated by multiplying all the probabilities of survival at all time intervals preceding that time (by applying the law of multiplication of probability to calculate cumulative probability). For example, the probability of a patient surviving 2 days after a kidney transplant can be considered to be the probability of surviving one day multiplied by the probability of surviving the second day given that the patient survived the first day. Although the probability calculated at any given interval is not very accurate because of the small number of events, the overall probability of surviving to each point is more accurate [9].

The survival analysis design is important because:

1. It is not practical to wait until events have happened to all participants (for example, all died) before we conclude a study. Some patients might have left the study early or are lost to follow-up.
2. Although we can compare mean time-to-event between the groups using a *t*-test or linear

regression, this would ignore censoring, i.e. we lose important data.

3. Although we can compare proportion of events between the groups using risk/odds ratios or logistic regression, this would ignore time, which is an important consideration in this design.

Structured oral examination question 7

EXAMINER: What do you understand by PROM?

CANDIDATE: PROMs stand for Patient Reported Outcome Measures. They are short, self-completed questionnaires, which measure the patients' symptoms, functional ability and health-related quality of life from the patient perspective rather than the clinician perspective.

EXAMINER: Can you give me some examples?

CANDIDATE: PROMs can be generic or disease-specific. The European quality of life measure (EuroQol), Short form (SF) 36, SF12 and Nottingham Health Profile (NHP) are examples of generic outcome measures. Disease-specific PROM examples include the Oxford hip score (OHS) for hip arthritis, the Oxford knee score (OKS) for knee arthritis, Disability of the Arm and Shoulder and Hand (DASH) for upper limb, etc.

EXAMINER: What is the advantage of using PROMs?

CANDIDATE: In the past, clinician-based outcome measures were considered objective when the clinician was assessing patient progress using 'hard signs' such as range of motion, strength, swelling, etc. Objectivity was dependent on the reliability or reproducibility of the clinicians' assessments. In contrast, PROMs are subjective and are likely to better measure the outcome of an intervention. Although this is debated, the trend has been the move toward using PROM questionnaires before and after an intervention to provide indication of outcomes or quality of care delivered to patients.

EXAMINER: What do you understand by a 'validated' outcome measure?

CANDIDATE: This means that the outcome measure has been tested and succeeded to show that it measures what it is supposed to measure. There are several rigorous processes in developing and validating an outcome measure. Validation is one aspect. Construct validity: this is the quantitative assessment of validity.

EXAMINER: The following was copied from a paper on treating slipped upper femoral epiphysis. (Figure 30.19). Can you tell me what is meant by the grades (B, C and D) highlighted in yellow?

CANDIDATE: These refer to the grades of recommendation, based on levels of evidence. Several

Recommendation for Treating Slipped Capital Upper Femoral Epiphysis

Although a rare condition, slipped upper femoral epiphysis or slipped capital upper femoral epiphysis (SCUFE) is one of the most common types of paediatric and adolescent hip disorder. SCUFE involves instability of the growth plate at the junction between the head and neck of the thigh bone (femur) resulting in the head of the femur slipping backwards and downwards from the femoral neck. About 30% of patients subsequently developed bilateral SCUFE with the other hip slipping as well [1-3]. With increasing severity, SUFE is associated with increasing pain and disability. Stable SUFE is best treated with single central screw fixation (grade B, C) [4-8]. If a realignment osteotomy is selected for secondary reorientation of a SUFE, the flexion type rather than the Southwick type should be used (grade C) [9-12]. Unstable SUFE treatment is very controversial and our recommendation is urgent gentle repositioning, 1-2 cannulated screw fixation, joint decompression, and protected weight bearing (grades D, C) [13-16].

Figure 30.19 A selected paper with grade of recommendation.

Table 30.3 Grades of recommendation.

Grades	Strength	Descriptions
A	Good	Consistent level I studies for or against recommending intervention
B	Fair	Consistent level II or III studies or extrapolations from level I studies
C	Poor	Level IV studies or extrapolations from level II or III studies not allowing a recommendation for or against intervention
D	Insufficient	Level V evidence or troublingly inconsistent or inconclusive studies of any level

have been described. I follow the one that is recommended by the Oxford Centre for Evidence-based Medicine in which grade A is used for good evidence, grade B for fair evidence, grade C for poor evidence and grade D for insufficient or conflicting evidence [10] (Table 30.3).

Authors' note 9: Outcome measures

Outcome measures have become an essential part of many research projects. In fact, a study is considered weak if outcome measures are not used. Having some core knowledge about how outcome measures are developed is important to understand some of the jargon that you may face in the exam (and clinical practice).

Developing an outcome measure involves several processes. This can be summarized as follows [11].

1. Content: (are the contents of the measure relevant to your population?)
   Content items are generated in several ways. These items are then gradually reduced based on importance and relevance. The following are considered when items are included, excluded or weighed:
   A. Type:
      i. Clinician-based outcome measure (CBOM).
      ii. Patient-based outcome measure (PROM).
   B. Scale: what questions make up the outcome? How are they scored?
   C. Interpretation: do higher scores indicate a better outcome?
2. Methodology: this involves assessing validity, reliability and responsiveness.
   A. Validity: does it measure what it is supposed to measure?

   i. Construct validity: quantitative assessment of validity.
      1. Divergent: two measures do not correlate highly if they measure different things.
      2. Convergent: two measures have a high correlation with each other when they measure the same thing. Outcome measure must show both convergent and divergent validity evidence for construct validity, but neither alone is sufficient for establishing validity.
   ii. Content validity (face validity): are the contents comprehensive and relevant? This is established by content experts: clinicians and/or patients.
   iii. Criterion validity: correlation with golden standard.
      1. Predictive validity: ability to predict the future state of health, e.g. patients with low score will do badly.
      2. Concurrent validity: accurately predict current state of health when compared with other measures.
   B. Reliability: measure the condition the same way every time.

   i. Internal consistency: how consistent are the questions in measuring the same outcome; that is why there are several questions to measure a single dimension.
   ii. Reproducibility: produce the same results when there are no changes.
      1. Intra-observer (test–retest): reproducibility when used on the same patient on two different occasions (provided no changes in patient condition).
      2. Inter-observer: agreement between two or more observers using the same outcome on the same patient at the same time.
   C. Responsiveness: ability of the measure to change as the status of the patient changes.
3. Clinical utility:
   A. Patients' friendliness (acceptability): easy to complete by patients, clear questions, easy to understand, does not take time, etc.
   B. Clinician friendliness (feasibility): easy to use and administer, does it need licensing or special software, does it cost, etc.

References

1. Wright JG. A practical guide to assigning levels of evidence. *J Bone Joint Surg Am.* 2007;89(5):1128–1130.

2. Phillips B, *et al.* Levels of Evidence (March 2009), Oxford Centre for Evidence-Based Medicine 2009 [cited 2012; available from: www.cebm.net].

3. Harbour R, Miller J. A new system for grading recommendations in evidence-based guidelines. *BMJ.* 2001;323(7308):334–336.

4. Alshryda S, Huntley J, Banaszkiewicz P. Chapter 1: Introduction to evidence-based practice. In H Alshryda, JS Huntley, P Banaszkiewicz (Eds.), *Paediatric Orthopaedics: An Evidence-Based Approach to Clinical Questions*, Cham: Springer; 2016: 51–75.

5. Howick J, *et al.* The 2011 Oxford CEBM Evidence Levels of Evidence (Introductory Document). Oxford Centre for Evidence-Based Medicine. www.cebm.net/index.aspx?o=5653. 2011.

6. Sibbald B, Roland M. Understanding controlled trials. Why are randomised controlled trials important? *BMJ.* 1998;316(7126):201.

7. Roland M, Torgerson DJ. What are pragmatic trials? *BMJ.* 1998;316(7127):285.

8. Wright J, Eastwood DM. Clinical surveillance, selective or universal ultrasound screening in DDH. In H Alshryda, JS Huntley, P Banaszkiewicz (Eds.), *Paediatric Orthopaedics: An Evidence-Based Approach to Clinical Questions*, Cham: Springer; 2016.

9. Goel MK, Khanna P, Kishore J. Understanding survival analysis: Kaplan-Meier estimate. *Int J Ayurveda Res.* 2010;1(4):274–278.

10. Grades of Recommendation, Oxford Centre for Evidence-based Medicine. 2009. Available from: www.cebm.net/?o=1025.

11. Suk M, Hanson BP, Norvell DC, Helfet SL (Eds.). *AO Handbook. Musculoskeletal Outcome Measures and Instruments.* Basel: Thieme; 2004.

Chapter

31

Drawings for the FRCS (Tr & Orth)

James Widnall, Catherine McCauley and Lyndon Mason

Drawing has always been an integral part of the FRCS examination, be it as a method to understand a complex process during revision or as a tool for explanation in the viva itself. In order to use drawings in the viva exam the candidate must be able to draw, explain and answer questions simultaneously. Thus, practice and understanding are essential.

In this chapter, we have selected the drawings that we think are most useful, having recently been through the examination or taught on this subject for many years.

By no means are you expected to turn out a quality piece of art, and these drawings are not intended as such. Some of the drawings are deliberately schematic in order to simplify the subject matter and reinforce key points.

We hope, though, that by using these drawings to either act as an aide memoir during revision, or indeed to explain difficult concepts in the viva, the time saved and level of understanding shown will allow you to showcase your knowledge in pursuit of the higher marks.

Good luck.

Tips on drawing

An exam is not just about knowledge but the presentation of that knowledge. Playing the game is important. There is a lot of paper at every station, and sometimes it's useful to draw even if not asked to do so. Remember the old adage 'a picture is worth a 1000 words'. If you are not the first at the viva table, there are often 'paper scars', tales of the last viva! Do not let these distract you.

If using a drawing in the viva, whether as an aid to explain an answer or as the result of being asked to do so, then here are some tips.

1. *Draw big.* Fill the page. Drawing small does not show confidence.
2. *Work from the outside in.* Simplify to the bare image. For example, if drawing a cross-section of a limb, first draw a circle to illustrate the skin then add in the bones, then compartments, then muscles, then NV structures.
3. *Draw schematic.* The examiners will not be assessing you on your artistic skill.
4. *Speak while you draw.* You have limited time to earn marks, so do not lose this time by drawing in silence.

Anatomy

Anatomy is assumed knowledge for surgeons; it is, after all, a subject matter we deal with every day. Thus, an anatomy question in the exam should be dealt with confidently and efficiently, otherwise the examiner may prod more deeply to assess the true level of knowledge. Anatomy will also be the subject that most examiners will revert to if you are struggling with a question.

NB: some of the illustrations below are of cross-sectional anatomy in the limbs. Not only do these convey a knowledge of surrounding structures and relative anatomy of vessels and nerves, but they can be used very succinctly to demonstrate approaches, as seen by the numbered arrows where appropriate. We have given you both anatomically correct and schematic diagrams for these, and it is best to familiarize yourself with one or the other.

Upper limb

Brachial plexus (Figure 31.1)

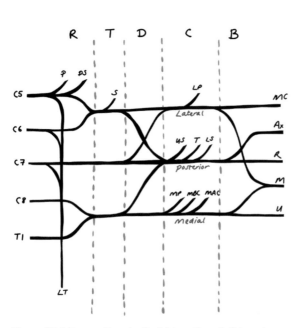

Figure 31.1 R, roots; T, trunks; D, divisions; C, cords; B, branches. P, phrenic nerve (contribution); DS, dorsal scapular; S, suprascapular; LP, lateral pectoral; MC, musculocutaneous; US, upper subscapular; T, thoracodorsal; LS, lower subscapular; AX, axillary; R, radial; MP, medial pectoral; MBC, medial brachial cutaneous (of arm); MAC, medial antebrachial cutaneous (of forearm); U, ulnar; 1st IC: first intercostal; LT, long thoracic nerve (of Bell).

The candidate not only needs to know the anatomy of the brachial plexus but also how to apply it to a clinical picture/examination. Once familiar with the above illustration, the candidate can then picture where the lesion is in accordance to which muscle groups have been affected. There are a number of Youtube videos that teach you how to draw this very quickly.

The candidate can also demonstrate whether the lesion has occurred before (pre-ganglionic) or after (post-ganglionic) the dorsal root ganglion (see Figure 31.2).

Dorsal root ganglion (Figure 31.2)

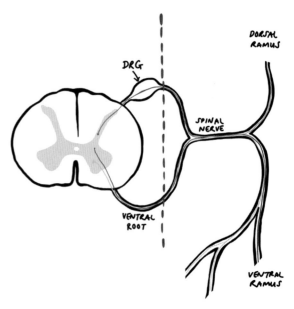

Figure 31.2 DRG, dorsal root ganglion.

Figure 31.2 clearly shows where the division between pre- and post-ganglionic injuries exists. Pre-ganglionic injuries may present with Horner's syndrome, periscapular wasting (rhomboids affected from dorsal scapula nerve) or medial scapula winging (long thoracic nerve). Pre-ganglion injuries carry a poorer prognosis.

Erb's point (Figure 31.3)

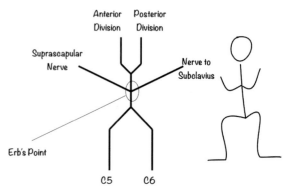

Figure 31.3 Erb's point.

Not to be confused with the cardiology Erb's point (third intercostal space on the left sternal border where S2 heart sound is best auscultated) or the head and neck Erb's point (posterior border of the sternocleidomastoid muscle where four superficial branches of the cervical plexus emerge from). The Erb's point that concerns us is a site at the upper trunk of the brachial plexus located 2–3 cm above the clavicle. It is named for Wilhelm Heinrich Erb, a nineteenth-century German neurologist. Erb's point is formed by the union of the C5 and C6 nerve roots. At the nerve trunk, branches of suprascapular nerve and the nerve to the subclavius also merge. The merged nerve divides into the anterior and posterior division of C5 and C6. Due to this convergence, it is an area that can be torn relatively easily, as its mobility is limited.

Humeral spaces (Figure 31.4)

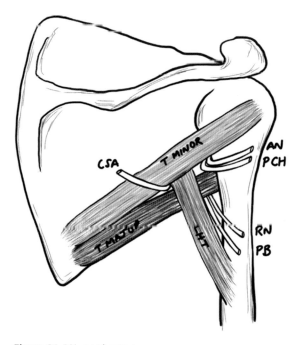

Figure 31.4 Humeral spaces.

A useful aide memoir for this is to place the index and middle fingers of your right hand at right angles to your left hand index and middle fingers to create the same shape. Thus, your left middle finger is teres minor, left index finger teres major. Your right index is long head of triceps and your right middle the humerus.

Clinically, these spaces are important when performing the posterior approach to the shoulder, knowing that finding the interval between infraspinatus and teres minor prevents you from straying too low and thus endangering the axillary nerve and posterior circumflex humeral artery.

Humerus cross-section (Figure 31.5)

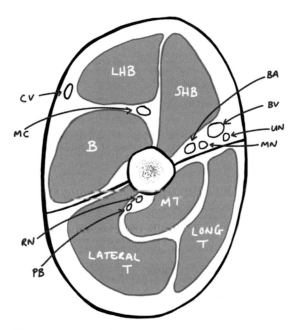

Figure 31.5 CV, cephalic vein; MC, musculocutaneous nerve; BA, brachial artery; BV, basilica vein; UN, ulnar nerve; MN, median nerve; RN, radial nerve; PB, profunda brachii.
LHB, long head biceps; SHB, short head biceps; B, brachialis.
Lateral T, lateral head of triceps; MT, medial head of triceps; Long T, long head of triceps.

The above illustration can be used to succinctly demonstrate the approaches to the humerus.

1. Anterior – retract biceps laterally, identify radial nerve distally, split dually innervated brachialis.
2. Posterior – develop interval between long and lateral heads of triceps, split medial head, protect radial nerve as it sits in the spiral groove.

Schematic drawing (Figure 31.6)

1. First draw a large circle and label the anterior and posterior.
2. Add the humerus centrally and divide the cross-section into anterior and posterior compartments. It initially looks like a Pokemon ball. By drawing

the mid-humeral cross-section you avoid complications of coracobrachialis and deltoid insertions proximally and the forearm musculature distally.

3. In the anterior compartment, divide between the biceps superficially and the brachialis deep. The musculocutaneous nerve lies in the plane between these muscles and supplies the medial half of the muscle.

4. In the posterior compartment the three heads of triceps are drawn easily: medial, long and lateral heads.

5. The radial nerve runs in the spiral groove and supplies the muscles of the posterior compartment. The ulnar nerve, median nerve and medial cutaneous nerve of the forearm run medially with the brachial artery within their own neurovascular compartment.

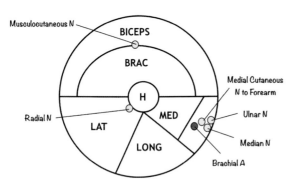

Figure 31.6 Schematic drawing of humerus cross-section.

Mid-forearm cross-section (Figure 31.7)

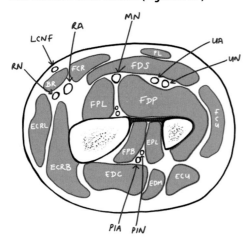

Figure 31.7 RN, radial nerve; LCNF, lateral cutaneous nerve of the forearm; RA, radial artery; MN, median nerve; UA, ulnar artery; UN, ulnar nerve; PIA, posterior interosseous artery; PIN, posterior interosseous nerve.

Schematic drawing (Figure 31.8)

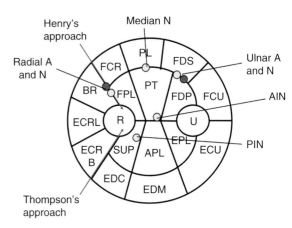

Figure 31.8 Schematic drawing of mid-forearm cross-section.

Drawing the forearm cross-section (Figure 31.8) is a daunting task but can be approached in a similar way to the upper arm.

1. Again, draw a large circle.
2. Draw the radius and ulna and divide the forearm into three compartments – anterior, posterior and the mobile wad.
3. Divide the compartments into superficial and deep and then divide the anterior superficial into four, deep into three; and both in the posterior compartment into three; the mobile wad into three.
4. Fill the mobile wad first – all muscles supplied by the radial nerve. BR lies anterior-most, followed by ECRL and ECRB.
5. Thinking of Henry's approach, FCR can then be added. FCU lies next to FCR on the opposite side. The other superficial muscles are the palmaris longus and FDS.
6. We know the SRN and radial artery lie between FCR and BR.
7. The deep anterior compartment is next, with FDP below FDS. As half of the FDP is supplied by

Caption for Figure 31.7 (cont.)

BR, brachioradialis; FCR, flexor carpi radialis; FDS, flexor digitorum superficialis; PL, palmaris longus; FPL, flexor pollicis longus; FDP, flexor digitorum profundus; FCU, flexor carpi ulnaris.

ECRL, extensor carpi radialis longus; ECRB, extensor carpi radialis brevis; EDC, extensor digitorum communis; EPB, extensor pollicis brevis; EPL, extensor pollicis longus; EDM, extensor digiti minimi; ECU, extensor carpi ulnaris.

the ulnar nerve, this is where the ulnar nerve and artery lie.

8. The remainder of the deep compartment depends on the level, so considering the scotty dog picture in the next section, PT and FPL are drawn here.

9. The median nerve lies deep to palmaris longus and the AIN on the anterior aspect of the interosseous membrane.

10. Posteriorly, start with the superficial compartment. ECU lies adjacent to FCU. On the other side of the superficial compartment lies EDC, which forms the interval for Thompson's posterior approach to the radius.

11. The remaining extensors depend on the level being sectioned. EDM lies centrally.

12. In the deep layer, the supinator lies around the radius; it is likely to only be partially present at this level, but worth drawing for its importance for approaches; EPL and APL fill the other two spaces.

13. The PIN lies within the supinator.

14. Finally, the common approaches to the forearm can be added – Henry's between FCR and BR; Thompson's between ECRB and EDC.

Approaches to the midshaft radius (Figure 31.9)

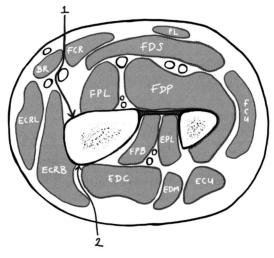

Figure 31.9 Approaches to the midshaft radius.

1. Henry's approach – the true Henry's approach develops the plane between the brachioradialis and the radial artery. The modified Henry's approach (which we use for distal radius fractures) differs by going through the bed of the FCR, creating a plane between the FCR and radial artery.

2. Thompson's approach – develop the interval between ECRB and EDC.

Radius muscle insertions

Radius muscle insertions are often combined with the cross-section of the forearm. This is especially true if Henry's approach is being discussed. The muscles' insertion on the anterior aspect of the radius are simple to understand. There is one supinator (excluding the biceps attachment), two pronators, and two interspersing long flexors to the digits. If you turn the radius on its side the insertions look like a scotty dog. The supinator for the ears, the flexors (FPL and FDS) for the body and the pronators (PQ and PT) for the legs (Figure 31.10).

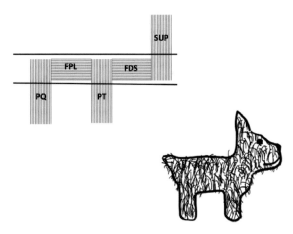

Figure 31.10 Radius muscle insertions.

The deep dissection of Henry's approach to the radius requires the supinator to be incised at its insertion on the radius, when the forearm is in full supination to displace the PIN laterally, away from the operative field. The FDS insertion begins just distal to the bicipital tuberosity and is ulnar to the supinator. Pronator teres in the middle third of the radius is dissected by pronating the arm to better expose its insertion.

Hand and wrist

Carpal tunnel

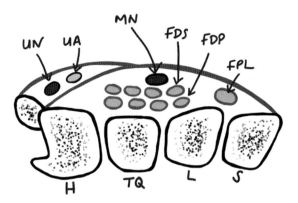

Figure 31.11 UN, ulnar nerve; UA, ulnar artery; MN, median nerve; FDS, flexor digitorum superficialis; FDP, flexor digitorum profundus; FPL, flexor pollicis longus.
  H, hamate; Tq, triquetrum; L, lunate; S, scaphoid.

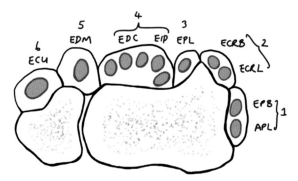

Figure 31.12 Compartment 1: APL, abductor pollicis longus; EPB, extensor pollicis brevis.
  Compartment 2: ECRL, extensor carpi radialis longus; ECRB, extensor carpi radialis brevis.
  Compartment 3: EPL, extensor pollicis longus.
  Compartment 4: EDC, extensor digitorum communis; EIP, extensor indicis proprius.
  Compartment 5: EDM, extensor digiti minimi.
  Compartment 6: ECU, extensor carpi ulnaris.

The contents of the carpal tunnel are easily tested. This diagram (Figure 31.11) can be a quick way to detail the necessary knowledge. The ulnar nerve and artery are clearly shown *not* to be in the carpal tunnel, instead lying separately in Guyon's canal.

The carpal tunnel spans from the scaphoid tubercle and trapezium ridge to the hook of hamate and pisiform. The roof is the transverse carpal ligament with the floor being the proximal carpal row. The contents are the median nerve, FPL tendon, four FDS tendons and four FDP tendons.

As well as the cross-sectional anatomy the candidate should be familiar with the branches of the median nerve, e.g. palmar cutaneous branch and recurrent motor branch and their anatomical variations (recurrent motor branch – extraligamentous 75% of time, subligamentous 13%, transligamentous 12%).

Extensor compartments (Figure 31.12)

Clinically, this illustration can be used to demonstrate approaches to the wrist. It also details the proximity of EPL to Lister's tubercle, which can contribute to attritional rupture of the tendon.

Ulnar canal (Figure 31.13)

The ulnar canal or ulnar tunnel (also known as Guyon's canal or tunnel) is a semi-rigid longitudinal canal in the wrist that allows passage of the ulnar artery and ulnar nerve into the hand. The roof of the canal is made up of the superficial palmar carpal ligament (PCL) and floor by the transverse carpal ligament (TCL).

Anatomy is a possible question especially due to zones of injury.

Zone 1: proximal to bifurcation of nerve (mixed motor and sensory, usually hamate pathology or compression in canal).

Zone 2: Surrounds deep motor branch (motor only, usually hamate pathology).

Zone 3: Surrounds superficial sensory branch (sensory only, usually ulnar artery pathology).

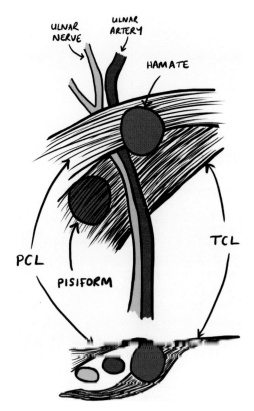

Figure 31.13 Ulnar canal.

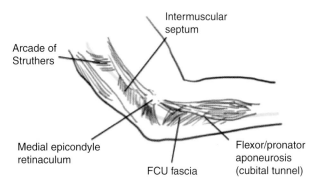

Figure 31.14 Sites of ulnar nerve compression.

Sites of ulnar nerve compression (Figure 31.14)

Management of ulnar nerve compression depends on an accurate diagnosis, yet localizing the site of nerve compression can be challenging. The accepted sites of potential ulnar nerve compression are depicted here: arcade of Struthers, the medial intermuscular septum, the bony retrocondylar groove and the overlying cubital tunnel retinaculum, Osborne's band, the volar antebrachial fascia just proximal to the wrist crease (proximal Guyon's canal), and the leading edge of the hypothenar musculature overlying the deep motor branch of the ulnar nerve (distal Guyon's canal).

Finger cross-sectional anatomy

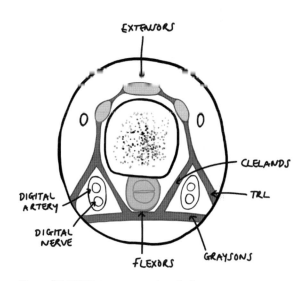

Figure 31.15 TRL, transverse retinacular ligament.

This axial section (Figure 31.15) shows the relationship of the neurovascular bundles to that of the fascial sheets in the finger. This is particularly important in Dupuytren's disease where a diseased Grayson's ligament (remember Cleland's ligament is not involved in Dupuytren's disease) can cause an aberrant path of the neurovascular bundle which the surgeon must be aware of.

Nail anatomy (Figure 31.16)

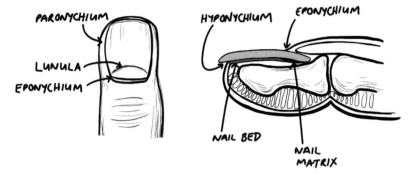

Figure 31.16 Nail anatomy.

Nail tip injuries are commonly seen in orthopaedic practice hence the need for accurate knowledge of the relevant anatomy. With relative ease this viva topic could quickly proceed to high levels talking about potential incisions to extend wounds, nail bed repair or flap coverage.

Lower limb

Blood supply to neck of femur (Figure 31.17)

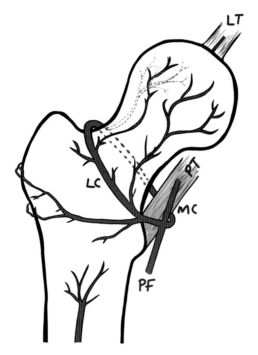

Figure 31.17 LT, ligamentum teres; PT, psoas tendon; PF, profunda femoris; MC, medial circumflex; LC, lateral circumflex.

The blood supply to the femoral head is a large part of what we base our decision-making on when dealing with fractures to the neck of the femur. It is therefore essential knowledge.

The profunda femoris splits into medial and lateral circumflex arteries (so named in their relationship to the psoas tendon as shown). These form an extracapsular ring from which ascending cervical branches travel proximally to supply the femoral head. The posterior superior and posterior inferior branches arise from the medial circumflex. The anterior arises from the lateral circumflex.

A small branch from the obturator artery passes through the ligamentum teres, but the blood supply is negligible in adults.

Femoral triangle (Figure 31.18)

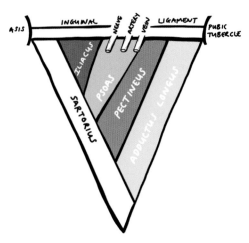

Figure 31.18 ASIS, anterior superior iliac spine.

The femoral triangle (Figure 31.18) is a common testing question given the importance of the structures that lie within.

Boundaries: lateral – medial border of sartorius; medial – medial border of adductor longus; superior – inguinal ligament.

Roof: fascia lata.

Contents: femoral nerve, artery, vein, inguinal lymph nodes.

Floor: iliacus, psoas, pectineus, adductor longus.

Hip cross-section anatomy (Figure 31.19)

Using the retained knowledge from the femoral triangle, we already have the medial aspect of the cross-section of the hip. The only structure not represented is the adductor longus, but this is due to its origin being located below the hip, at the anterior inferior iliac spine. Tensor fascia lata originates next to the sartorius, off the anterior superior iliac spine. The rectus femoris, the gluteal muscles and short rotators can then be added.

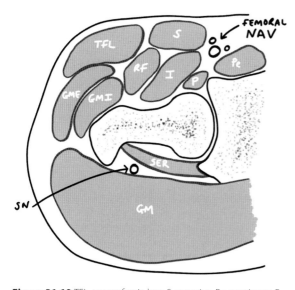

Figure 31.19 TFL, tensor fascia lata; S, sartorius; Pe, pectineus; P, psoas; I, iliacus; RF, rectus femoris; GMI, gluteus minimus; GME, gluteus medius; SER, short external rotators; GM, gluteus maximus; SN, sciatic nerve.

Approaches to the hip (Figure 31.20)

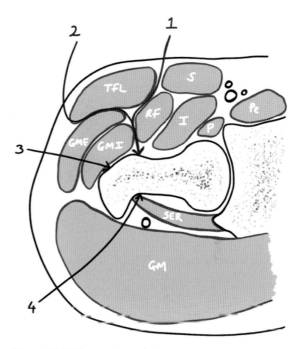

Figure 31.20 Approaches to the hip.

Again, this knowledge of cross-sectional anatomy can be applied to quickly explain the differences between the various approaches to the hip joint.

1. Smith Peterson – superficial plane developed between the sartorius and tensor fascia lata, being mindful of the lateral cutaneous nerve of the thigh and the ascending branch of lateral circumflex. Deeper dissection is between the gluteus medius and rectus femoris.
2. Watson-Jones – develops the plane between the tensor fascia lata anteriorly and the gluteus medius posteriorly.
3. Lateral approach – after incising the fascia lata the abductors (gluteus medius/minimus) are reflected from the greater trochanter to allow access to the anterior capsule.
4. Posterior (southern): split the gluteus maximus to gain access to the short external rotators. The short external rotators can then be elevated from the insertion to gain access to the posterior capsule, protecting the sciatic nerve throughout.

Adductor/Hunter's canal (Figure 31.21)

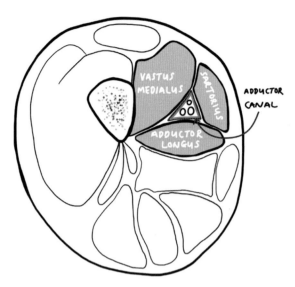

Figure 31.21 Adductor/Hunter's canal.

The adductor canal, or Hunter's (John Hunter, Scottish surgeon, 1728–1793) canal extends from the apex of the femoral triangle to the adductor hiatus. It is located in anterior compartment of the thigh.

Contents: superficial femoral artery, femoral vein, saphenous nerve and nerve to vastus medialis.

Boundaries: medial wall – sartorius; posterior wall – adductor longus (and magnus); lateral wall – vastus medialis.

Mid-thigh cross-section (Figure 31.22)

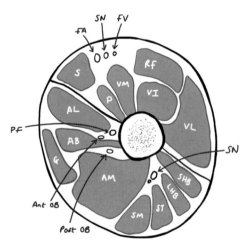

Figure 31.22 FA, femoral artery; SN, saphenous nerve; FV, femoral vein; SN, sciatic nerve; Post OB, posterior branch of obturator; Ant OB, anterior branch of obturator; PF, profunda femoris.

The most common approach to the thigh is that of direct lateral where the surgeon incises the fascia before either lifting or splitting the vastus lateralis to gain access to the femoral shaft. This approach is widely used for DHS fixation.

Schematic (Figure 31.23)

1. Draw a large circle and add the femur centrally.
2. Divide the circle into three compartments: posterior, anterior and adductor. On the peripheries either side of the adductor compartment, add the sartorius and gacillis muscles, which lie in their own muscle fascia.
3. Divide the adductor compartment into two and both the posterior and anterior compartments into four.
4. Add in the muscles, with the adductor compartment containing adductor longus and magnus, the anterior compartment containing the quadriceps (vastus medialis, intermedius, lateralis and rectus femoris) and the posterior compartment the semimembranosus, semitendinosus and two heads of biceps femoris.
5. Add NV structures as shown.

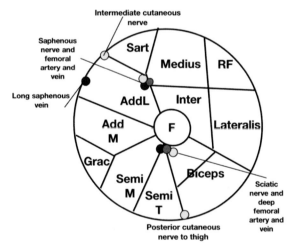

Figure 31.23 Schematic drawing of mid-thigh cross-section.

Caption for Figure 31.22 (cont.)

S, sartorius; P, pectineus; VM, vastus medialis; VI, vastus intermedius; VL, vastus lateralis; RF, rectus femoris.

AL, adductor longus; AB, adductor brevis; AM, adductor magnus; G, gracillis; SM, semimembranosus; ST, semitendinosus; LHB, long head biceps femoris; SHB, short head biceps femoris.

Lower leg cross-section (Figure 31.24)

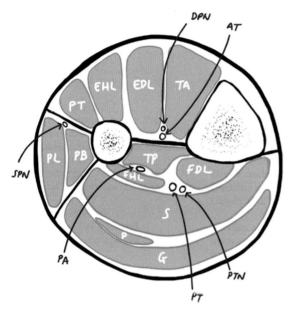

Figure 31.24 Anterior compartment: PT, peroneus tertius; EHL, extensor hallucis longus; EDL, extensor digitorum longus; TA, tibialis anterior; DPN, deep peroneal nerve, AT, anterior tibial artery.
 Posterior compartment (deep): TP, tibialis posterior; FHL, flexor hallucis longus; FDL, flexor digitorum longus; PA, peroneal artery; PT, posterior tibial artery; PTN, posterior tibial nerve.
 Posterior compartment (superficial): S, soleus; P, plantaris; G, gastrocnemius.
 Lateral compartment: PL, peroneus longus; PB, peroneus brevis; SPN, superficial peroneal nerve.

It is important to note that while the peroneal artery runs in the deep posterior compartment, it actually supplies the lateral compartment via perforators. It's called the peroneal artery due to its close relation to the fibula (Greek: *perone*).

The compartments of the lower limb are often asked in the context of the trauma viva as part of wider questioning of compartment syndrome or open fracture management.

Schematic (Figure 31.25)

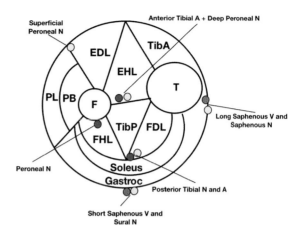

Figure 31.25 Schematic drawing of lower leg cross-section.

1. Draw a circle and add the tibia subcutaneously and fibula.
2. Add the intermuscular septum.
3. Divide and label the four compartments (anterior, peroneal, superficial posterior, deep posterior).
4. Divide the anterior and posterior deep compartment into three, and the posterior superficial and peroneal compartment into two.
5. Add in the muscles; anterior compartment (tibialis anterior, extensor hallucis longus and extensor digitorum longus), deep posterior compartment (tibialis posterior, flexor digitorum longus, flexor hallucis longus). Note the FDL is on the opposite side to the EDL and the same is true for EHL and FHL), peroneal compartment (peroneus longus and peroneus brevis, B close to bone) and posterior superficial (soleus and gastrocnemius).
6. Add in the anterior tibial nerve and artery (anterior to intraosseus membrane), posterior tibial nerve and artery (between the superficial and deep compartments) and peroneal nerve and artery. For extra marks, add in the short and long saphenous veins and the saphenous nerve.

Basic science

Biological materials

Articular cartilage (Figure 31.26)

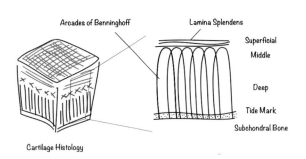

Figure 31.26 Articular cartilage.

Articular cartilage is a common viva question given that it is at the heart of one of the commonest disease processes we treat – osteoarthritis.

The structure can be easily memorized. There is an outer protective layer of the lamina splendens. This covers the superficial layer where the collagen fibres are parallel to the articular surface in order to resist shear forces. This layer has the highest collagen and water but the lowest proteoglycan concentration. The middle layer allows transition from the superficial to the deep layers. In the deep layers the fibres are arranged parallel in order to resist compressive forces. Here, the proteoglycan concentration is the highest, with there being the fewest collagen fibres and water molecules. The tidemark migrates superficially with age, as the cartilage thins. The calcified zone anchors the cartilage to bone via hydroxyapatite crystals. This zone is mostly type X collagen, unlike the other zones which are mainly type II.

Most trainees memorize the histological features with the zones representing columnar areas, cross-hatching and parallel fibres. This truly represents the Arcades of Benninghoff, where the cross-hatching shows the crossings of these arcades.

The candidate needs to know the difference between OA and ageing as well as potential treatment options for varying sizes or cartilage defects.

Differences in ageing and osteoarthritis

This is best remembered if you imagine an elderly individual who is stiff and dry (Figure 31.27). For extra marks, the elderly may have solar keratosis (which will allow you to differentiate with keratin sulphate being high and chondroitin sulphate being low). This is the opposite for OA.

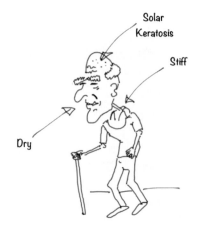

Figure 31.27 Differences in ageing and osteoarthritis.

Proteoglycans (Figure 31.28)

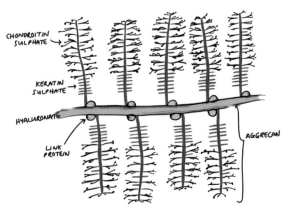

Figure 31.28 Proteoglycans.

Proteoglycans are responsible for around 10% of articular cartilage. They are made of a core of hyaluronate with binding proteins anchoring a feather of keratin sulphate and chondroitin sulphate.

These are hydrophilic (i.e. they attract water). This gives the cartilage volume. Without it the collagen would be flat, like the analogy of oranges in a net bag, with the proteoglycans being the oranges.

Bone (cortical) (Figure 31.29)

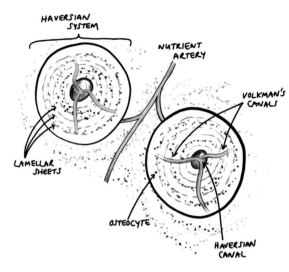

Figure 31.29 Bone (cortical).

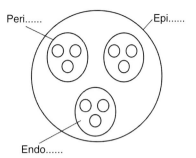

Figure 31.30 Overlying structure of nerve/muscle/tendon.

Nerve

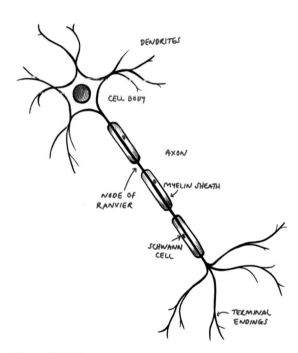

Figure 31.31 Nerve.

Candidates must know about the biological material we treat. It is simply inexcusable not to. One must know the functions, the structure, the composition, the cell types, the blood supply, the regulation mechanisms and the system of remodelling in order to pass a basic science viva on bone.

With regards to cortical bone, one type of lamellar bone (with the other being cancellous), we found the above drawing (Figure 31.29) to be of most use.

It clearly shows the arrangement of haversian systems, which are supplied by a nutrient artery. Within the haversian system there are central Haversian canals surrounded by concentric lamellar sheets, or rings, made of collagen. These haversian canals act as neurovascular channels and the Volkmann canals carry capillaries to and from this central source. Within the lamellae sit osteocytes, which are connected by cannaliculi.

Overlying structure of nerve/muscle/tendon

All these structures can be drawn the same basically as they are all made up of epi-, peri- and endo- (epineural/epitenon/epimysium, etc.). This can be easily drawn as shown (Figure 31.30).

Nerves can open a multitude of avenues of questioning from basic anatomy and physiology to nerve injury and nerve repair. The structure of a standard axon connecting a cell body to terminal endings is a common starting point (Figure 31.31).

Nerve cross-section (Figure 31.32)

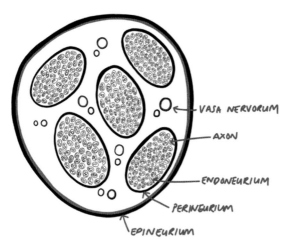

Figure 31.32 Nerve cross-section.

For a nerve this can be more specifically drawn as shown (Figure 31.32). The three covering layers include epineurium as the external layer, perineurium covering nerve fascicles and the endoneurium covering axons. The blood supply is both carried intrinsically within the endoneurium and extrinsically from the vasa nervorum.

Nerve action potential (Figure 31.33)

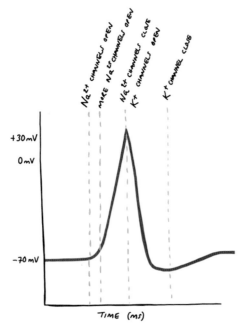

Figure 31.33 Nerve action potential.

The action potential is the mechanism of action of the nerve fibre. It is a rapid depolarization across the membrane which then propagates along the neuron.

The resting potential of the membrane is −70 mV. A threshold stimulus must first be reached (−55 mV) to trigger an action potential. Once triggered, sodium channels open to allow sodium into the cell. This propagates from cell to cell, causing more and more sodium channels to open. The passing of sodium (a positively charged ion) into the cell causes the membrane potential to become positive. As this occurs, the sodium channels close and potassium channels open to allow potassium to leave the cell. This allows the negative resting potential to be restored. For cardiac muscle, the depolarization is halted temporarily by a plateau caused by calcium ions from the sarcoplasmic reticulum.

Nerve injuries (Figure 31.34)

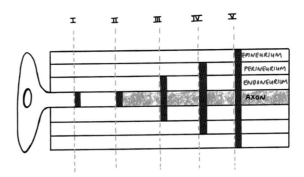

Figure 31.34 Nerve injuries.

Nerve injuries can be classified in accordance with the mechanism of injury (crush, traction, laceration, thermal, etc.), histologically in accordance with Seddon (1943) or anatomically as per Sunderland (1951).

The above illustration details Sunderland's anatomical classification.

1: disruption to myelin/ischaemia to nerve – a block to conduction, *no* Wallerian degeneration.
2: axonal discontinuity – leads to Wallerian degeneration.
3: endoneurium damage (as well as axon) – leads to Wallerian degeneration.
4: perineurium damage (as well as endoneurium and axon) – leads to Wallerian degeneration.
5: total transection of nerve (epi-, peri-, endo- and axon all involved) – leads to Wallerian degeneration. Worst prognosis.

NB: Wallerian degeneration – discovered by Waller in 1850, a process by which damaged axons and myelin are removed via phagocytosis.

Muscle (Figure 31.35)

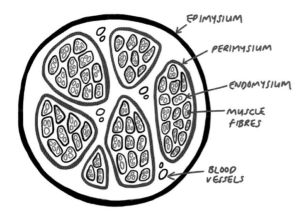

Figure 31.35 Muscle.

As with nerves there are three layers of connective tissue when looking at the macroscopic structure of muscle. The external layer is the epimysium, the perimysium surrounds muscle fascicles (as it surrounds nerve fascicles) and the endomysium surrounds muscle fibres.

Muscle fibres are made from multiple myofibrils, which themselves are made from sarcomeres containing actin and myosin.

Actin and myosin (Figure 31.36)

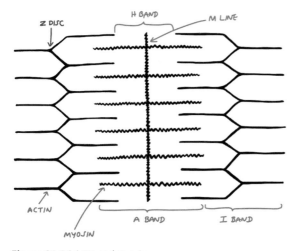

Figure 31.36 Actin and myosin.

Z disc – attachment between adjacent sarcomeres.

H band – only myosin filaments.

M line – connections between adjacent myosin filaments.

A band – both actin and myosin filaments (so-called as it is 'A'nisotropic on electronmicroscopy).

I bands – only actin filaments (so-called as they are 'I'sotropic on electronmicroscopy).

The sarcomere is the motor unit responsible for contraction in the muscle fibre. Each sarcomere consists of actin, myosin, tropomyosin and troponin.

Neuromuscular junction (Figure 31.37)

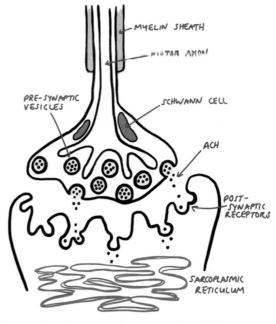

Figure 31.37 ACH, acetylcholine (neurotransmitter).

The candidate needs to know the mechanism of muscle contraction.

When an action potential is delivered to a neuromuscular junction, acetylcholine is released from presynaptic vesicles across the synaptic cleft. Arrival of acetylcholine at postsynaptic receptors triggers calcium release by the sarcoplasmic reticulum. The calcium enters the muscle via T tubules.

In the sarcomeres themselves, tropomyosin blocks binding sites on myosin filaments. The arriving

727

calcium forms with troponin to make troponin C. This troponin C then alters the shape of tropomyosin and thus reveals the myosin binding sites. The myosin filaments then rotate to bind with actin and ATPase activity permits conformational change in the actin which generates the sliding of the two filaments, causing muscle contraction.

Embryology – spinal development (Figure 31.38)

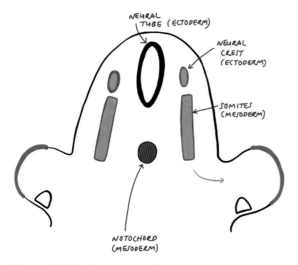

Figure 31.38 Embryology – spinal development.

Embryology is a complex subject, but FRCS candidates only need a basic understanding.

There are three germ layers responsible for embryo growth in the body:

Ectoderm ('outer') – forms the skin and nerves.

Mesoderm ('middle') – forms muscles and cartilage.

Endoderm ('inner') – forms organs.

Figure 31.38 shows a cross-section of an embryo at around day 30. It shows the neural tube and neural crest (both ectoderm) and somites and notochord (both mesoderm).

At day 25, a process called neurulation occurs where the notochord sends messengers to the neural tube (which starts on the outside of the embryo) to fold in on itself, forming a tube, in order to look like it does in Figure 31.38. The neural crest is responsible to ensure that when the neural tube folds in, the skin closes normally above it. If neurulation does not happen correctly, spina bifida occurs.

Following this, spinal development is controlled by the homeobox gene group. The neural tube is

responsible for the spinal cord, the neural crest for the sympathetic chain, basal ganglia and peripheral nervous system. The notochord forms the anterior vertebral bodies and nucleus propulsus and the somites form the rest of the vertebral bodies and annulus fibrosis.

Embryology – limb bud development (Figure 31.39)

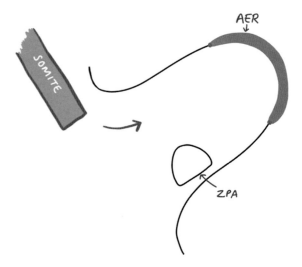

Figure 31.39 AER, apical ectodermal ridge; ZPA, zone of polarizing activity.

Limb development starts at around 4 weeks. At 8 weeks the limb buds rotate, which is why our thumbs are lateral in the anatomical position but our big toes are medial.

There are three axes of growth:

1: Proximal to distal – controlled by the homeobox gene and performed by the AER. If this axis fails then there is transverse limb arrest (i.e. symbrachydactyly).

2: Radial to ulna – controlled by the sonic hedgehog gene and performed by the ZPA. If this axis fails there is longitudinal arrest, e.g. radial longitudinal deficiency.

3: Dorsal to ventral – controlled by the *WnT* gene and performed by the surface ectoderm. This is less important regarding anomalies, but explains the bowing of our long bones as dorsal grows quicker than ventral.

The cartilage and muscle are derived from the mesoderm of the somites which invade the limb bud.

Implant science

Stress–strain curve (Figure 31.40)

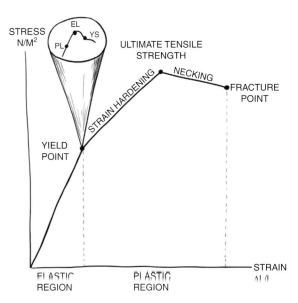

Figure 31.40 Stress–strain curve.

Stress–strain curves are commonplace in the FRCS. Start by drawing and labelling the two axes – stress (N/m^2) and strain (change in length / original length). In the elastic region, the stress–strain relationship is linear in accordance with Hooke's law. The material will undergo recoverable deformation. In this region a specific stress–strain point reveals the material's Young's modulus, a measure of how stiff the material is.

The yield point heralds the change from elastic to plastic region. The yield point is actually made of three points that are very close together:

Proportionality limit – the highest point at which stress is proportional to strain.

Elastic limit – the point at which the forces change from elastic to plastic deformation.

Yield stress – the amount of stress necessary to produce 0.2% deformation.

When looking at metals, strain hardening occurs early in the plastic region. This is where the grains in the metal dislocate and slip, paradoxically increasing the resistance to further strain.

Ultimate tensile strength is the amount of stress that can be applied to the material before fracturing. Necking is where further strain occurs but in a relatively small area of the material, resulting in a decreasing surface area. This occurs until the material breaks, or fractures.

S-N curve (Figure 31.41)

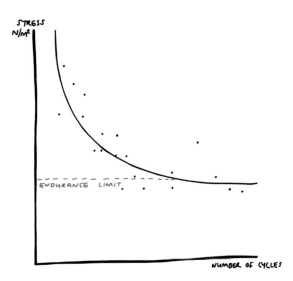

Figure 31.41 S-N curve.

The S-N curve demonstrates the endurance limit of a material and is clinically relevant in fatigue failure of orthopaedic implants. The axes are first drawn with stress (N/m^2) and number of cycles of stress application. The stress is always below that of the ultimate tensile stress, or else the material would break on the first cycle of loading. A point is then made for each level of stress and the amount of times it can be applied before the material reaches fatigue failure and breaks. Unsurprisingly, as you decrease the stress, you can apply the load more times before fracturing the material. A line of best fit is then drawn. Where the line plateaus out corresponds to 10 million cycles of loading for that level of stress without fracturing. This is called the endurance limit. With osteosynthesis it is a race against time between the bone healing and the implant undergoing fatigue failure at that repeated level of stress.

Viscoelastic behaviour (Figure 31.42)

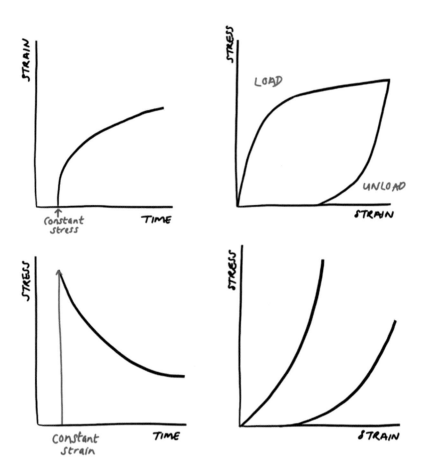

Figure 31.42 Viscoelastic behaviour.

Viscoelastic behaviour demonstrates time-dependent deformation. We encounter four common behaviours in orthopaedics:

Creep – a change in strain over time, under a constant stress. This clinically translates into plaster cast treatment of clubfoot via Ponseti method and the gradual correction of foot shape.

Hysteresis – a different stress–strain relationship is seen between loading and unloading a material. This is often down to energy being lost (often as heat). The more a substance is loaded/unloaded the two curves become more reproducible, hence the cycling of ACL grafts prior to implantation.

Stress relaxation – a change in stress over time, under a constant strain. This can be seen when implanting uncemented femoral stems, with the surgeon waiting between impactions to allow the stress to dissipate through the bone and prevent an intra-operative fracture.

Time-dependent this demonstrates a different
behaviour – stress–strain curve depending
upon how quickly the stress is
applied. Time-dependent behaviour explains why low-energy
injuries result in simpler fracture
patterns and high-energy injuries
result in gross comminution.

Screws (Figure 31.43)

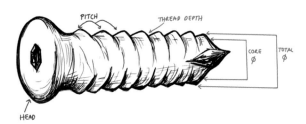

Figure 31.43 Screw.

Tension band (Figure 31.44)

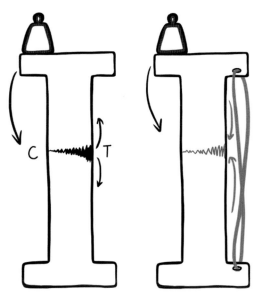

Figure 31.44 Tension band.

Screws are a mechanical device used to convert torque (rotatory load) into linear motion. An FRCS candidate should be able to talk in depth about this common orthopaedic implant. First, the screw itself can be made out of various metals, such as titanium or stainless steel. It can also be cannulated or non-cannulated. The head can be of multiple shapes (hexagonal, star, cross-head, etc.) and on metalwork removal it is imperative to have the correct screwdriver. The neck is often countersunk. The pitch is the frequency of threads and defines the rate of linear motion per 360° turn. The core diameter and the thread depth make up the total diameter. The tip can be blunt, self-tapping or self-drilling. Self-tapping screws are often fluted to remove excess bone chaff. Factors affecting pullout strength (i.e. screw diameter, working length, locking screws, quality of bone) could all be discussed further in a viva scenario.

Candidates could be asked to explain the principle behind a tension band fixation (of an olecranon, for example). We found this easiest when utilizing an illustration such as the one in Figure 31.44. The first picture shows a column (or bone) being loaded eccentrically, creating a compression (C) and tension (T) side. Eccentric loading occurs in curved bones. By applying a tension band (in this case a figure-of-eight wire, similar to that seen in olecranon fracture fixation), the tensile forces from the eccentric load have now been converted to compressive forces. This can be done in a static manner such as in a medial malleolar fixation or in a dynamic fashion such as in patellar fixation. It should be noted that for the fixation to work there *must* be cortical contact on the compression side to prevent bending stresses.

Cement zones (Figure 31.45)

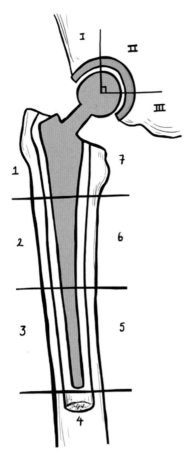

Figure 31.45 Cement zones.

Spinal pathology

Spinal cord anatomy (Figure 31.46)

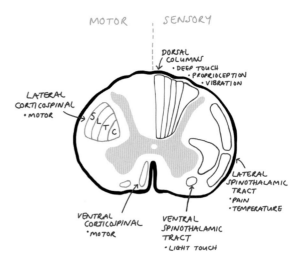

Figure 31.46 Spinal cord anatomy.

Cemented total hips can be assessed radiographically using Gruen's zones in the femur and Charnley's zones in the acetabulum.

Gruen's zones are 1–7. Zones 1 and 7 are at the level of the greater trochanter and lesser trochanter, respectively. Zone 4 is to the tip of the prosthesis but within the cement tail. It should be remembered that zones 8–14 exist in a similar manner on the lateral view.

Charnley's zones are in relation to a line drawn vertically from the centre of the femoral head and a line perpendicular from this. Zone 1 is the superior third, zone 2 is the middle third and zone 3 is the medial third.

Figure 31.46 can be used not only to demonstrate both the anatomy of the spinal tracts but also their clinical implications. On one half the ascending sensory tracts are seen:

Dorsal columns – deep touch, proprioception, vibration. These tracts cross at the level of the medulla.

Lateral spinothalamic tracts – pain and temperature. These tracts cross at the spinal cord, explaining the clinical picture seen in Brown–Sequard syndrome from a cord hemitransection where the ipsilateral side experiences loss of motor, vibration and proprioception functions and the contralateral side demonstrates a loss of pain and temperature modalities.

Ventral spinothalamic tracts – these carry light touch.

On the opposite side the motor tracts are shown:

Lateral corticospinal tracts – carry motor pathways distally. The fibres are arranged with cervical root values carried most centrally, then thoracic root values, then lumbar with sacral fibres being towards the periphery. This explains why in central cord syndrome, the patient will retain more function in their lower limbs than their upper limbs.

Ventral corticospinal tracts – carry motor pathways distally. Both sets of corticospinal tracts cross at the level of the medulla.

Schematic (Figure 31.47)

1. Draw a dumbell shape, and label anterior and posterior.
2. Draw a butterfly within the dumbell shape and label it as 'grey matter' with anterior and posterior horn. Outside the butterfly is 'white matter' because the nerves are myelinated.
3. Divide the spinal cord into halves. On one half, split the posterior part into two, lateral into two and anterior into two.
4. These are then labelled from posterior to anterior with 'G C C S S C'. This is like the GCS or the UK school exam GCSE. This is from the Gracilis, Cuneatus, lateral Corticospinal tract, lateral Spinothalamic tract, anterior Spinothalamic and anterior Corticospinal tract.
5. Topography of corticospinal tracts. This is an important distinction to know as this determines the defects seen in certain spinal cord syndromes. This can be remembered as 'SaLT lake City' if it is located on the right side of the cord (i.e. looking from ground to cephalad) or with some imagination ATLS (if on left side of cord). This is important in the defects it causes in central cord syndrome, where the upper elements are more affected than the lower (i.e. 'man in a barrel') (Figure 31.48).

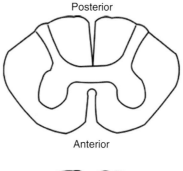

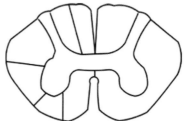

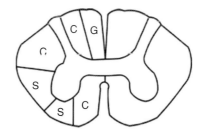

Figure 31.47 Schematic drawing of spinal cord anatomy.

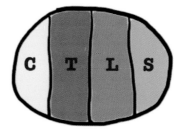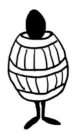

Figure 31.48 Topography of corticospinal tracts.

Vertebral disc (Figure 31.49)

Intervertebral discs consist of an outer fibrous ring, the anulus fibrosus, consisting of several layers (laminae) of fibrocartilage made up of type I collagen, which are obliquely orientated, alternating every layer. This has high tensile strength, like the metal bars on an old wooden barrel.

The inner gel-like centre, the nucleus pulposus, is composed of type II collagen. The nucleus pulposus helps to distribute pressure evenly across the disc. This prevents the development of stress concentrations, which could cause damage to the underlying vertebrae or to their end plates. The nucleus pulposus is a remnant of the notochord.

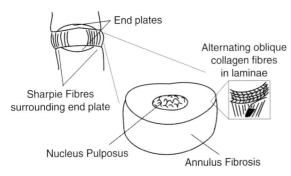

Figure 31.49 Vertebral disc.

Prolapsed intervertebral discs (Figure 31.50)

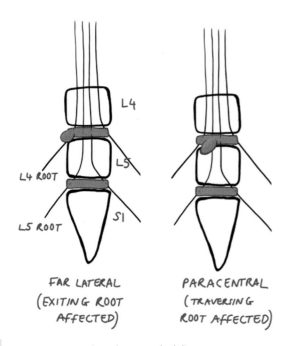

Figure 31.50 Prolapsed intervertebral discs.

Patients with nerve root signs are often seen on the clinical day of the FRCS (Tr & Orth). It is important for the candidate to swiftly determine the level of pathology and be aware of the different potential clinical presentations depending on the location of the disc prolapse, if that is the pathology in question.

At each lumbar level there is an exiting root and a traversing root. For example, at the L4/5 disc, the L4 root is exiting and the L5 root is traversing.

A far lateral disc prolapse will affect the exiting root. Hence a far lateral L4/5 disc will cause L4 root signs. This pathology, if treated surgically, may be best accessed via a Wiltse approach as opposed to the standard posterior approach to the lumbar spine.

A paracentral disc will affect the traversing (in this case, L5) root, leaving the exiting L4 root free from compression.

Paediatrics

Physis (Figure 31.51)

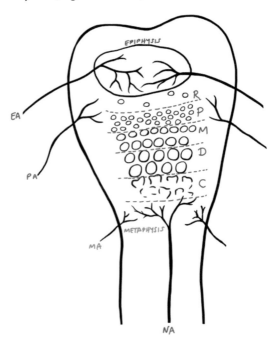

Figure 31.51 EA, epiphyseal artery; PA, perichondrial ring artery; MA, metaphyseal artery; NA, nutrient artery.

R, reserve zone – low oxygen tension, stores glycogen and lipids.

P, proliferative zone – proliferation of chondrocytes.

M, maturation zone – chondrocyte growth.

D, degenerative zone – continued chondrocyte growth (×5 in size), type X collagen produced.

C, calcification zone – chondrocyte death permits calcification.

NB: hypertrophic zone includes maturation, degenerative and calcification zones.

The successful candidate needs to have knowledge both about the physis in health, with regards to structure and blood supply, but also in sickness. One should be aware of the various diseases that can affect each zone of the physis, either from hypo- or hyperactivity, and the clinical manifestations.

Salenius and Vankka graph (Figure 31.52)

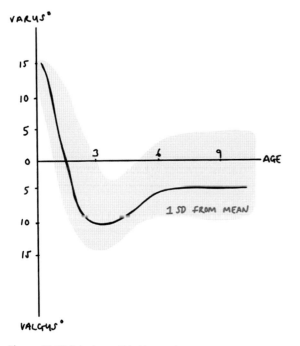

Figure 31.52 Salenius and Vankka graph.

Assessing limb deformities is commonplace in the paediatric clinical cases. Thus an understanding of normality is essential. The causes of genu varum and valgus are multiple, but most are physiological. Following a good history and thorough examination, reproduction of the above graph can be useful to further back your diagnosis of either physiological, or indeed, pathological deformity.

Essentially, newborns exhibit roughly 15° of varus which corrects to neutral by around the age of 2. This progresses to 10° valgus at 3 years and resolves to adult values (5–7°) by 7 years of age. It is important to remember there is wide variability in these milestones, demonstrated by the values covered by one standard deviation.

Index

741